Downey and Darling's
Physiological Basis of Rehabilitation Medicine

Downey and Darling's
Physiological Basis of Rehabilitation Medicine

THIRD EDITION

ERWIN G. GONZALEZ, M.D.
Chief Editor

Clinical Professor Emeritus, Department of Rehabilitation Medicine, Albert Einstein College of Medicine
of Yeshiva University, Bronx, New York; Former Professor of Clinical Rehabilitation Medicine, Columbia University College
of Physicians and Surgeons, New York; Former Professor of Rehabilitation Medicine, Mount Sinai School
of Medicine, City University of New York

STANLEY J. MYERS, M.D.
Co-Chief Editor

A. David Gurewitsch Professor of Clinical Rehabilitation Medicine, Columbia University College
of Physicians and Surgeons, New York; Attending Physician, Department of Rehabilitation Medicine, New York Presbyterian
Hospital, Columbia-Presbyterian Center, New York

JOAN E. EDELSTEIN, M.A., P.T.
Editor

Associate Professor of Clinical Physical Therapy and Director, Program in Physical Therapy, Department
of Rehabilitation Medicine, Columbia University College of Physicians and Surgeons, New York

JAMES S. LIEBERMAN, M.D.
Editor

H. K. Corning Professor and Chairman of Rehabilitation Medicine, Columbia University College of Physicians and Surgeons,
New York; Professor of Rehabilitation Medicine and Division Chief, Weill Medical College of Cornell University, New York;
Physiatrist-in-Chief, Department of Rehabilitation Medicine, New York Presbyterian Hospital

JOHN A. DOWNEY, M.D., D. Phil. (Oxon)
Editor

Simon Baruch Professor of Rehabilitation Medicine, Columbia University College of Physicians and Surgeons, New York;
Attending Physician, Department of Rehabilitation Medicine, Columbia-Presbyterian Center, New York

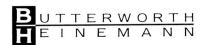

Boston • Oxford • Auckland • Johannesburg • Melbourne • New Delhi

Library of Congress Cataloging-in-Publication Data
Downey and Darling's physiological basis of rehabilitation medicine.—3rd ed./ [edited by] Erwin G. Gonzalez, Stanley J. Myers.
    p. ; cm.
  Includes bibliographical references and index.
  ISBN 0-7506-7179-3
  1. Medical rehabilitation. 2. Human physiology. I. Title: Physiological basis of rehabilitation medicine. II. Gonzalez, Erwin G. III. Myers, Stanley J. IV. Downey, John A., 1930– V. Darling, Robert C., 1908– VI. Physiological basis of rehabilitation medicine.
    [DNLM: 1. Pathology. 2. Physiology. 3. Rehabilitation. QZ 140 D7481 2001]
  RM930 .P48 2001
  612'.0024617—dc21   00-063084

British Library Cataloguing-in-Publication Data
A catalogue record for this book is available from the British Library.

The publisher offers special discounts on bulk orders of this book.
For information, please contact:
Manager of Special Sales
Butterworth–Heinemann
225 Wildwood Avenue
Woburn, MA 01801-2041
Tel: 781-904-2500
Fax: 781-904-2620

For information on all Butterworth–Heinemann publications available, contact our World Wide Web home page at: http://www.bh.com

10 9 8 7 6 5 4 3 2 1

Printed in the United States of America

To Robert C. Darling, M.D., the first Simon Baruch Professor of Rehabilitation Medicine at Columbia University's College of Physicians and Surgeons and founder of its Department of Rehabilitation Medicine.

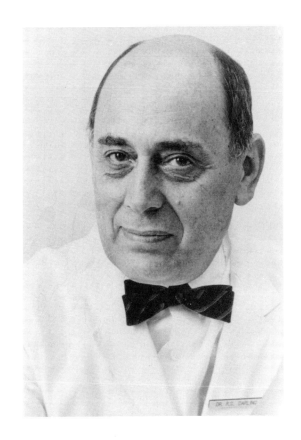

Dr. Darling graduated from Harvard College and Harvard Medical School with high honors. After medical residency at the Presbyterian Hospital in New York, he became a distinguished colleague of Nobel Prize winners Drs. André Cournand and Dickinson Richards, during which time he contributed much to the elucidation of pulmonary and cardiovascular function. He later continued his work in exercise and environmental physiology at the Harvard Fatigue Laboratory, whence came much of the foundation of these fields in modern medicine. He rose to become director of that laboratory before returning to Columbia-Presbyterian Center. He was president of the American Academy of Physical Medicine and Rehabilitation and was a recipient of the Academy's highest honor, the Frank H. Krusen Award. His work in academics, medicine, and science exemplifies the ideal for the future direction of rehabilitation medicine.

Contents

Contributing Authors

Lucinda L. Baker, P.T., Ph.D.
Associate Professor of Biokinesiology and Physical Therapy, University of Southern California, Los Angeles; Consulting Neurophysiologist, Rehabilitation Engineering Program, Rancho Los Amigos National Rehabilitation Center, Downey, California
  31. Functional Electrical Stimulation in Persons with Spinal Cord Injury

Joanne Borg-Stein, M.D.
Assistant Professor of Physical Medicine and Rehabilitation, Tufts University School of Medicine, Boston; Chief, Department of Physical Medicine and Rehabilitation, Newton-Wellesley Hospital, Newton, Massachusetts
  16. Exercise

Julie M. Brody, Psy.D.
Postdoctoral Fellow in Clinical Neuropsychology, Department of Psychiatry, Harvard Medical School, Boston; Clinical Fellow in Neuropsychology, Department of Neuropsychology and Psychology Service, McLean Hospital, Belmont, Massachusetts
  37. Adaptation, Learning, and Motivation

John C. M. Brust, M.D.
Professor of Clinical Neurology, Columbia University College of Physicians and Surgeons, New York; Director, Department of Neurology, Harlem Hospital Center, New York
  30. Aphasia, Apraxia, and Agnosia

Frans L. Bruyninckx, M.D.
Lecturer, Department of Physical Medicine and Rehabilitation, University of Leuven, Leuven, Belgium; Director, E.M.G.-Laboratory, Department of Physical Medicine and Rehabilitation, University Hospital Gasthuisberg, Leuven, Belgium
  14. The Motor Unit and Electromyography

Nancy N. Byl, Ph.D., P.T.
Professor of Physical Therapy and Rehabilitation Science, University of California, San Francisco, School of Medicine
  26. Principles of Neuroplasticity: Implications for Neurorehabilitation and Learning

Mark A. Cabelin, M.D.
Fellow in Neurourology and Urodynamics, Department of Urology, New York Presbyterian Hospital, Columbia-Presbyterian Center; Attending Urologist, Department of Urology, Helen Hayes Hospital, West Haverstraw, New York
  10. Urogenital Physiology

Malcolm B. Carpenter, M.D.*
Former Professor and Chairman Emeritus of Anatomy, Uniformed Services University of the Health Sciences F. Edward Hébert School of Medicine, Bethesda, Maryland
  1. Descending Motor Pathways and the Lower Motor Neuron; 3. Cerebellum and Basal Ganglia

Kenneth J. Ciuffreda, O.D., Ph.D.
Chair and Distinguished Teaching Professor, Department of Vision Sciences, State University of New York, State College of Optometry, New York
  12. Normal Vision Function

W. Crawford Clark, Ph.D.
Professor of Medical Psychology, Department of Psychiatry, Columbia University College of Physicians and Surgeons, New York
  36. Pain and Emotion

*Deceased.

Felicia Cosman, M.D.
Associate Professor of Medicine, Columbia University College of Physicians and Surgeons, New York; Endocrinologist/Osteoporosis Specialist, Department of Medicine, Helen Hayes Hospital, West Haverstraw, New York; Clinical Director, National Osteoporosis Foundation, Washington, D.C.
7. Skeletal Physiology and Osteoporosis

Lucien J. Côté, M.D.
Associate Professor of Neurology, Columbia University College of Physicians and Surgeons, New York; Associate Attending Physician, Department of Neurology, New York Presbyterian Hospital, Columbia-Presbyterian Center, New York
3. Cerebellum and Basal Ganglia

Carol M. Davis, Ed.D., P.T.
Associate Professor of Orthopedics and Rehabilitation, Division of Physical Therapy, University of Miami School of Medicine, Coral Gables; Consultant Physical Therapist, Osteoporosis Clinic, Department of Medicine/Endocrinology, University of Miami Hospital and Clinics
34. Complementary Therapies in Rehabilitation

Ronald E. De Meersman, Ph.D.
Professor of Applied Physiology, Department of Rehabilitation Medicine, Columbia University College of Physicians and Surgeons, New York
4. Autonomic Nervous System

John A. Downey, M.D., D. Phil. (Oxon)
Simon Baruch Professor of Rehabilitation Medicine, Columbia University College of Physicians and Surgeons, New York; Attending Physician, Department of Rehabilitation Medicine, Columbia-Presbyterian Center, New York
21. Thermoregulation and the Effects of Thermomodalities; 22. Peripheral Vascular Function

Robert J. Downey, M.D.
Assistant Professor of Surgery, Memorial Sloan-Kettering Cancer Center, New York
19. Physiological Changes Associated with Bed Rest and Major Body Injury

Joan E. Edelstein, M.A., P.T.
Associate Professor of Clinical Physical Therapy and Director, Program in Physical Therapy, Department of Rehabilitation Medicine, Columbia University College of Physicians and Surgeons, New York
17. Gait; 18. Energy Expenditure during Ambulation; 25. Women's Health Issues

Gerald Felsenthal, M.D.
Clinical Professor of Epidemiology and Preventive Medicine, University of Maryland School of Medicine, Baltimore; Chief, Department of Rehabilitation Medicine, Sinai Hospital, Baltimore
24. Aging of Organ Systems

Tamar S. Ference, M.D.
Attending Physician, Department of Physical Medicine and Rehabilitation, Sinai Hospital, Baltimore
24. Aging of Organ Systems

Walter R. Frontera, M.D., Ph.D.
Earle P. and Ida S. Charlton Associate Professor and Chairman, Department of Physical Medicine and Rehabilitation, Harvard Medical School, Boston; Chief of Service, Department of Physical Medicine and Rehabilitation, Spaulding Rehabilitation Hospital and Massachusetts General Hospital, Boston
16. Exercise

Robert S. Gailey, Jr., Ph.D., P.T.
Assistant Professor of Orthopaedics and Rehabilitation, Division of Physical Therapy, University of Miami School of Medicine, Coral Gables
33. Manual Modalities

Dympna Gallagher, Ed.D.
Assistant Professor of Medicine, Obesity Research, Columbia University College of Physicians and Surgeons, New York; Research Associate, Department of Medicine, St. Luke's-Roosevelt Hospital, New York
20. Obesity and Weight Control

Gary Goldberg, B.A.Sc., M.D.
Associate Professor of Physical Medicine and Rehabilitation, University of Pittsburgh School of Medicine; Director, Brain Injury Rehabilitation, University of Pittsburgh Medical Center–Rehabilitation Hospital
15. Evoked Potentials

Erwin G. Gonzalez, M.D.
Clinical Professor Emeritus, Department of Rehabilitation Medicine, Albert Einstein College of Medicine of Yeshiva University, Bronx, New York; Former Professor of Clinical Rehabilitation Medicine, Columbia University College of Physicians and Surgeons, New York; Former Professor of Rehabilitation Medicine, Mount Sinai School of Medicine, City University of New York
  18. Energy Expenditure during Ambulation

James Gordon, Ed.D., P.T.
Associate Professor and Chair, Department of Biokinesiology and Physical Therapy, University of Southern California, Los Angeles
  6. Receptors in Muscle and Their Role in Motor Control

Daniel J. Hoffman, Ph.D.
Research Fellow, Department of Medicine, Columbia University College of Physicians and Surgeons, New York; Research Fellow, Department of Medicine, St. Luke's-Roosevelt Hospital Center, New York
  20. Obesity and Weight Control

Christopher W. Huston, M.D.
Attending Physiatrist, The Orthopedic Clinic, Scottsdale, Arizona
  35. Diagnostic and Therapeutic Injections

Mary M. Jackowski, Ph.D., O.D.
Research Associate Professor of Ophthalmology and Physical Medicine and Rehabilitation, State University of New York Health Science Center at Syracuse; Coordinator of Low Vision Services, Ophthalmology Service, Veterans Administration Medical Center, Syracuse
  12. Normal Vision Function

Mazher Jaweed, Ph.D.
Director, Clinical Research Education Foundation, Houston
  28. Peripheral Nerve Regeneration

Steven A. Kaplan, M.D.
Given Foundation Professor of Urology, Columbia University College of Physicians and Surgeons, New York; Vice Chairman and Administrator, Department of Urology, New York Presbyterian Hospital
  10. Urogenital Physiology

Neera Kapoor, O.D., M.S.
Assistant Clinical Professor of Clinical Sciences and Director, Head Trauma Vision Rehabilitation Unit, State University of New York, State College of Optometry, New York
  12. Normal Vision Function

Jerie Beth Karkos, M.D.
Associate Professor of Pediatrics, Southern Illinois University School of Medicine, Springfield
  23. Growth and Development

D. Casey Kerrigan, M.D., M.S.
Associate Professor and Director of Research, Department of Physical Medicine and Rehabilitation, Harvard Medical School, Boston; Director, Center for Rehabilitation Science, Spaulding Rehabilitation Hospital, Boston
  17. Gait

David E. Krebs, Ph.D., P.T.
Professor of Physical Therapy and Clinical Investigation, MGH Institute of Health Professions, Boston; Associate in Orthopaedics/Biomotion, Department of Orthopaedics, Harvard Medical School, Massachusetts General Hospital, Boston
  3. Cerebellum and Basal Ganglia

Fredi Kronenberg, Ph.D.
Associate Professor of Clinical Physiology in Rehabilitation Medicine, Columbia University College of Physicians and Surgeons, New York
  25. Women's Health Issues

Phyllis G. Krug, P.T., M.S., C.C.S.
Physical Therapist, Certified Cardiopulmonary Specialist, Teaneck, New Jersey
  9. Cardiopulmonary Physiology

Daniel E. Lemons, Ph.D.
Professor of Biology, City College of New York, City University of New York
  21. Thermoregulation and the Effects of Thermomodalities; 22. Peripheral Vascular Function

James S. Lieberman, M.D.
H. K. Corning Professor and Chairman of Rehabilitation Medicine, Columbia University College of Physicians and Surgeons, New York; Professor of Rehabilitation Medicine and Division Chief, Weill Medical College of Cornell University, New York; Physiatrist-in-Chief, Department of Rehabilitation Medicine, New York Presbyterian Hospital
  5. Skeletal Muscle: Structure, Chemistry, and Function

Robert Lindsay, M.B., Ch.B., Ph.D., F.R.C.P.
Professor of Clinical Medicine, Columbia University College of Physicians and Surgeons, New York; Chief of Internal Medicine, Regional Bone Center, Helen Hayes Hospital, West Haverstraw, New York
7. Skeletal Physiology and Osteoporosis

Brenda S. Mallory, M.D.
Assistant Professor of Clinical Rehabilitation Medicine, Columbia University College of Physicians and Surgeons, New York; Assistant Attending, Department of Rehabilitation Medicine, Columbia-Presbyterian Center, New York
29. Autonomic Function in the Isolated Spinal Cord

John H. Martin, Ph.D.
Associate Professor, Center for Neurobiology and Behavior, Columbia University College of Physicians and Surgeons, New York
1. Descending Motor Pathways and the Lower Motor Neuron

Michael Merzenich, Ph.D.
Professor, Departments of Physiology and Otolaryngology, Keck Center for Integrative Neurosciences, University of California, San Francisco, School of Medicine
26. Principles of Neuroplasticity: Implications for Neurorehabilitation and Learning

J. P. Mohr, M.S., M.D.
Sciarra Professor of Clinical Neurology, Columbia University College of Physicians and Surgeons, New York
2. Anatomy and Physiology of the Vascular Supply to the Brain

Jonathan R. Moldover, M.D.
Associate Professor of Clinical Rehabilitation Medicine, Albert Einstein College of Medicine at Yeshiva University, Bronx, New York; Director, Chronic Back Pain Program, Department of Pain Medicine and Palliative Care, Beth Israel Medical Center, New York
9. Cardiopulmonary Physiology; 16. Exercise

Van C. Mow, Ph.D.
Stanley Dicker Professor of Biomedical Engineering and Orthopaedic Bioengineering and Chair, Department of Biomedical Engineering, Columbia University College of Physicians and Surgeons, New York; Director, Orthopaedic Research Laboratory, Department of Orthopaedic Surgery, New York Presbyterian Hospital
8. Physiology of Synovial Joints and Articular Cartilage

Stanley J. Myers, M.D.
A. David Gurewitsch Professor of Clinical Rehabilitation Medicine, Columbia University College of Physicians and Surgeons, New York; Attending Physician, Department of Rehabilitation Medicine, New York Presbyterian Hospital, Columbia-Presbyterian Center, New York
13. Nerve Conduction and Neuromuscular Transmission; 14. The Motor Unit and Electromyography

Jeri W. Nieves, Ph.D.
Assistant Professor of Clinical Public Health, Department of Epidemiology, Columbia University College of Physicians and Surgeons, New York; Epidemiologist, Clinical Research Center, Helen Hayes Hospital, West Haverstraw, New York
7. Skeletal Physiology and Osteoporosis

Edward M. Phillips, M.D.
Instructor in Physical Medicine and Rehabilitation, Harvard Medical School, Boston; Director, Outpatient Medical Services, Spaulding Rehabilitation Hospital Network, Boston
37. Adaptation, Learning, and Motivation

Janet Hill Prystowsky, M.D., Ph.D.
Associate Clinical Professor of Dermatologic Surgery, Columbia University College of Physicians and Surgeons, New York; Associate Attending, Department of Surgery, New York Presbyterian Hospital
11. Physiology of the Skin

Gale N. Pugliese, M.D.
Assistant Professor of Clinical Rehabilitation Medicine, Columbia University College of Physicians and Surgeons, New York; Assistant Attending, Department of Rehabilitation Medicine, New York Presbyterian Hospital
5. Skeletal Muscle: Structure, Chemistry, and Function

Kristjan T. Ragnarsson, M.D.
Lucy G. Moses Professor and Chairman, Department of Rehabilitation Medicine, Mount Sinai School of Medicine of the City University of New York; Chairman, Department of Rehabilitation Medicine, Mount Sinai Hospital, New York
31. Functional Electrical Stimulation in Persons with Spinal Cord Injury

Michele A. Raya, M.S.P.T., S.C.S., A.T.C.
Instructor, Department of Orthopedics, Division of Physical Therapy, University of Miami School of Medicine, Coral Gables; Senior Physical Therapist, Department of Outpatient Orthopedics, Parkway Regional Medical Center, North Miami Beach
33. Manual Modalities

Georgia Riedel, B.S.
Instructor in Clinical Physical Therapy, Department of Rehabilitation Medicine, Columbia University College of Physicians and Surgeons, New York; Supervisor of Therapy Services, Department of Rehabilitation Medicine, Columbia-Presbyterian East Side, New York
21. Thermoregulation and the Effects of Thermomodalities

Sharon E. Robinson, P.T.
Former Instructor/Distance Site Facilitator, Department of Physical Therapy, Medical College of Georgia School of Medicine at Distance Learning Site, Albany State University; Midwifery student, State University of New York Health Science Center at Brooklyn College of Medicine, State Medical Center, Brooklyn
25. Women's Health Issues

David A. Rohe, M.P.H., P.T.
Former Assistant Professor of Physical Therapy and Coordinator of Distance Education, School of Allied Health Sciences and School of Graduate Studies, Albany State University, Albany, Georgia; Physical Therapy Consultant, Mystic, Connecticut
25. Women's Health Issues

Michael E. Selzer, M.D., Ph.D.
Professor and Associate Dean for Graduate Education, Department of Neurology and Rehabilitation Medicine, University of Pennsylvania School of Medicine, Philadelphia; Attending Physician, Department of Neurology, Hospital of the University of Pennsylvania, Philadelphia
27. Plasticity and Regeneration in the Injured Spinal Cord

Bhagwan T. Shahani, M.D., D. Phil. (Oxon), F.A.C.P., M.B.A.
Professor Emeritus of Rehabilitation Medicine and Restorative Medical Sciences, University of Illinois at Chicago College of Medicine
14. The Motor Unit and Electromyography

Solomon YuChou Shen, M.S., P.T.
Research Assistant, MGH Institute of Health Professions, Massachusetts General Hospital Biomotion Laboratory, Boston
3. Cerebellum and Basal Ganglia

Carl Shin, M.D.
Clinical Associate, Department of Rehabilitation Medicine, Hospital of the University of Pennsylvania, Philadelphia
35. Diagnostic and Therapeutic Injections

Curtis W. Slipman, M.D.
Assistant Professor of Rehabilitation Medicine, University of Pennsylvania Health System, Philadelphia; Director, Penn Spine Center, and Chief, Division of Musculoskeletal Rehabilitation, Hospital of the University of Pennsylvania, Philadelphia
35. Diagnostic and Therapeutic Injections

Jan Weingrad Smith, C.N.M., M.S., M.P.H.
Assistant Professor of Maternal and Child Health Nurse Midwifery Education Program, Boston University School of Public Health
25. Women's Health Issues

Kerstin ML. Sobus, M.D.
Clinical Instructor, University of North Dakota School of Medicine and Health Sciences, Grand Forks; Medical Director, Department of Rehabilitation Medicine, Altru Health Institute, Grand Forks
23. Growth and Development

Neil I. Spielholz, Ph.D., P.T.
Research Professor of Orthopaedics and Rehabilitation, Division of Physical Therapy, University of Miami School of Medicine, Coral Gables
13. Nerve Conduction and Neuromuscular Transmission

Joel Stein, M.D.
Assistant Professor of Physical Medicine and Rehabilitation, Harvard Medical School, Boston; Medical Director, Stroke Rehabilitation Program, Department of Physical Medicine and Rehabilitation, Spaulding Rehabilitation Hospital, Boston
9. Cardiopulmonary Physiology

Nancy E. Strauss, M.D.
Assistant Professor of Clinical Rehabilitation Medicine, Columbia University College of Physicians and Surgeons, New York; Assistant Attending Physician and Director of Residency Program, Department of Rehabilitation Medicine, New York Presbyterian Hospital
   5. *Skeletal Muscle: Structure, Chemistry, and Function*

Irwin B. Suchoff, O.D., D.O.S.
Professor of Clinical Sciences, Head Trauma Vision Rehabilitation Unit, State University of New York, State College of Optometry, New York
   12. *Normal Vision Function*

Matthew T. Sugalski, M.D.
Frank E. Stinchfield Research Fellow, Department of Orthopaedic Surgery, Columbia University College of Physicians and Surgeons, New York; Resident in Orthopaedic Surgery, Department of Orthopaedic Surgery, New York Presbyterian Hospital
   8. *Physiology of Synovial Joints and Articular Cartilage*

Alexis E. Te, M.D.
Assistant Professor of Urology, Columbia University College of Physicians and Surgeons, New York; Director, Incontinence Care Center, Department of Urology, New York Presbyterian Hospital/Maimonides Medical Center, New York
   10. *Urogenital Physiology*

Alan R. Tessler, M.D.
Professor of Neurobiology and Anatomy, MCP Hahnemann University School of Medicine, Philadelphia; Staff Neurologist, Department of Veterans Affairs Medical Center, Philadelphia
   27. *Plasticity and Regeneration in the Injured Spinal Cord*

Stanley F. Wainapel, M.D., M.P.H.
Professor of Clinical Rehabilitation Medicine, Albert Einstein College of Medicine of Yeshiva University, Bronx, New York; Clinical Director of Rehabilitation Medicine, Montefiore Medical Center, Bronx, New York
   12. *Normal Vision Function*

Mary P. Watkins, P.T., M.S.
Clinical Associate Professor, Program in Physical Therapy, MGH Institute of Health Professions, Boston; Research Associate, Department of Rehabilitation, Massachusetts General Hospital, Boston
   16. *Exercise*

Charles Weissman, M.D.
Professor and Chairman, Department of Anesthesiology and Critical Care Medicine, Hebrew University–Hadassah School of Medicine and Hadassah University Hospital, Jerusalem
   19. *Physiological Changes Associated with Bed Rest and Major Body Injury*

Steven L. Wolf, Ph.D., P.T., F.A.P.T.A.
Professor and Director, Research Program, Department of Rehabilitation Medicine, Emory University School of Medicine, Atlanta
   32. *Biofeedback*

Mark Allen Young, M.D., F.A.C.P.
Co-Chair, Department of Physical Medicine and Rehabilitation, The Maryland Rehabilitation Center, Baltimore; Faculty Attending, The Sinai–Johns Hopkins Residency Training Program, Baltimore
   24. *Aging of Organ Systems*

William L. Young, M.D.
Professor of Anesthesia, Neurosurgery, and Neurology, University of California, San Francisco, School of Medicine; Vice Chair, Department of Anesthesia and Perioperative Care and Director, Center for Cerebrovascular Research, San Francisco General Hospital
   2. *Anatomy and Physiology of the Vascular Supply to the Brain*

Adrienne Stevens Zion, Ed.D.
Officer of Research, Department of Rehabilitation Medicine, Columbia University College of Physicians and Surgeons, New York
   4. *Autonomic Nervous System*

Preface

Nearly three decades have passed since Drs. John A. Downey and the late Robert C. Darling published the first edition of this textbook. They shared a common background in basic physiological research, internal medicine, and physical medicine and rehabilitation. Since then, the scope of physical medicine and rehabilitation has greatly expanded, but it continues to be primarily concerned with the management of patients with impairments of function due to disease, trauma, or aging. A distinction should be made between impairments, which are the physical losses themselves, and disabilities, which are the effects of impairments on overall function of the individual. Understanding and application of this distinction require knowledge of normal physiology and the manner in which the human body adapts to and compensates for various forms of stresses. In this way, physiology is the parent basic science in this field of medicine.

This edition has been extensively revised and expanded to reflect the current state of the specialty. This book is a compilation of topics on selected physiological topics most pertinent to adaptation and compensatory adjustments in patients with neurologic, musculoskeletal, and circulatory impairments. In some instances, these physiological topics address reduction of the impairments themselves, but more often they relate to the principles of compensatory adaptations that can reduce the resulting disability. The chapters are not designed to be directly applicable to immediate practice; they are compendia of background knowledge on which practitioners can build as they explore the rationale for a given treatment modality or rehabilitative technique.

We have chosen, when possible, topics on which there is important new evidence and data, but we have tried to avoid areas in which the evidence is so recent that it is likely to be modified or possibly disproved in the near future. In this way, although we may have missed some exciting and useful frontiers of knowledge, we hope our book will have more than fleeting validity.

In this volume, physiology is interpreted broadly. Where structure and functions are closely linked, as in studies of the central nervous system, we have considered neuroanatomy as a physiological topic. Where function is not associated with any local definite structure as in psychology, we have still considered human motivation as a physiological subject as long as it is based on sound observation in a system in which stimulus leads to a predictable response.

Although a number of contributors are former colleagues or residents, a majority of them come from various universities and fields of medicine and the allied health professions and are known for their work in the assigned topics. The contributors were asked to cover their assigned areas thoroughly and not to oversimplify. Yet the result of their efforts, and of the efforts of the editors, is a presentation of material that is easily understandable to physicians and allied health professionals. References listed at the conclusion of each chapter are designed to allow any student or practitioner who so desires to explore the topic in greater depth.

We hope this book also inspires some rehabilitation practitioners to pursue scientific research so as to reduce empiricism, to discard traditions not in accord with scientific fact, and to build up a body of validated knowledge peculiar to this growing field of medicine.

The preceding paragraphs, modified from the first and second editions, set forth the goals shared by the current editors.

Erwin G. Gonzalez, M.D.

Acknowledgments

The editors wish to acknowledge their indebtedness to many former colleagues and students and the following individuals for their contributions to the previous edition: Jose A. Alonso, M.D.; Jerry G. Blaivas, M.D.; Richard Borkow, M.D.; Anne Breuer, M.D.; Elsworth R. Buskirk, Ph.D.; Arminius Cassvan, M.D.; Yasoma Challenor, M.D.; Paul J. Corcoran, M.D.; Leonard C. Harber, M.D.; Martha E. Heath, Ph.D.; E. Ralph Johnson, M.D.; David D. Kilmer, M.D.; Cynthia Lien, M.D.; Robert E. Lovelace, M.D., F.R.C.P. (Lond); N. Venketasubramanian, M.D.; and Jerald R. Zimmerman, M.D. We also honor the memory of the late Malcolm B. Carpenter.

E.G.G. would like to acknowledge all former residents trained by him during the 12 years he directed the Rehabilitation Medicine Residency Program at Columbia-Presbyterian; his mentors, Drs. John Downey, Robert Darling, and Paul J. Corcoran, who became role models for keeping the proper balance between academics, clinical practice, and organizational leadership; and Mark L. Greenley for his support and assistance. S.J.M. wishes to acknowledge the late Dr. A. David Gurewitsch for his example of what a clinician should be. Although not a scientist, he set an example of practicing the "art" and "science" of medicine, which is the end result of this book. J.E.E. is indebted to Elizabeth C. Addoms, P.T., and George Deaver, M.D., for being role models of clinical compassion and scientific curiosity, which are at the core of rehabilitation. She thanks her students and colleagues who have taught her to teach and write. J.S.L. would like to acknowledge his mentors, Professors Gilbert H. Glaser, Sid Gilman, and William M. Fowler, Jr., who were instrumental in developing his interest in and knowledge of the physiology of the nervous system and of muscle. J.A.D. wishes particularly to mention Dr. John B. Armstrong, F.R.C.P.(C), and the late Professors E. C. Eppinger, Sir George Pickering, F.R.S., R. F. Loeb, and R. C. Darling.

The editors also wish to acknowledge Karen Oberheim of Butterworth Heinemann, Sophia E. Battaglia of Silverchair Science + Communications, and Rosemary Bleha of Columbia University for their organizational and administrative assistance.

Erwin G. Gonzalez, M.D.
Stanley J. Myers, M.D.
Joan E. Edelstein, M.S., P.T.
James S. Lieberman, M.D.
John A. Downey, M.D., D. Phil. (Oxon)

Downey and Darling's
Physiological Basis of Rehabilitation Medicine

1

Descending Motor Pathways and the Lower Motor Neuron

JOHN H. MARTIN AND MALCOLM B. CARPENTER

Loss of motor function in parts of the body, caused by a neural lesion, is a distressing and fearful event for anyone. A lesion involving the motor systems often produces debilitating impairments, such as a loss of voluntary movement, muscle weakness, or changes in reflex activity. After a motor systems lesion, movements that were once smooth and effective become awkward and clumsy and can require great effort to produce. During the weeks and months after motor systems damage, the control of some movements improves remarkably, whereas other movements never regain effectiveness. Not surprisingly, the severity of the loss of control after a motor system lesion and the degree to which control recovers depend on the particular structures lesioned and the extent of damage.

In this chapter we examine the organization of the motor pathways that transmit control signals from their origins in the cerebral cortex and brain stem to the spinal cord. These pathways collectively mediate voluntary movements of the limbs and trunk, as well as relatively automatic adjustments in posture and balance. We begin the study of these pathways in the context of the hierarchical organization of the motor systems. We then examine the motor circuits of the spinal cord, which are the targets of action of the motor pathways. Next we focus on the pathways themselves, both those originating in the cerebral cortex as well as those from the brain stem. Finally, we consider the effects of lesion of the motor pathways and their spinal targets.

HIERARCHICAL ORGANIZATION OF MOTOR SYSTEMS

The motor systems of the brain and spinal cord consist of four interrelated (and extensively interconnected) sets of structures (Figure 1-1, gray boxes): (1) the spinal motor circuits, which include motor neurons and interneurons; (2) the supraspinal descending projection systems that originate from the brain stem and primary motor cortex; (3) the basal ganglia and the cerebellum, which are subcortical motor control centers; and (4) diverse regions in the frontal and parietal lobes, which are sometimes termed *higher order motor areas* or *motor association cortex*.

The various components of the motor systems are organized hierarchically. The lowest level of the hierarchy is the lower motor neuron or simply termed the *motor neuron*. The motor neuron is considered the final common path because, on these neurons, all controlling inputs converge. Axon terminations from three principal sources of input converge on motor neurons (see Figure 1-1): (1) the supraspinal motor tracts, (2) spinal neurons (segmental interneurons and intersegmental neurons; see next paragraph), and (3) primary afferent fibers.

Spinal interneurons are the next higher level (see Figure 1-1, lower inset). Whether located in the segments that contain the motor neurons (termed *segmental interneurons*) or at other spinal levels (*intersegmental neurons*), these spinal premotor interneurons also integrate information from primary afferent fibers and descending pathways.

The descending motor pathways make up the next set of hierarchical levels. The neurons that give rise to these motor tracts have been called *upper motor neurons*. The distinction between upper and lower motor neurons derives from differences in the signs produced by their selective lesion, such as after a capsular infarction, for upper motor neurons, or motor axon damage, for lower motor neurons (see the section Effects of Lesions of the

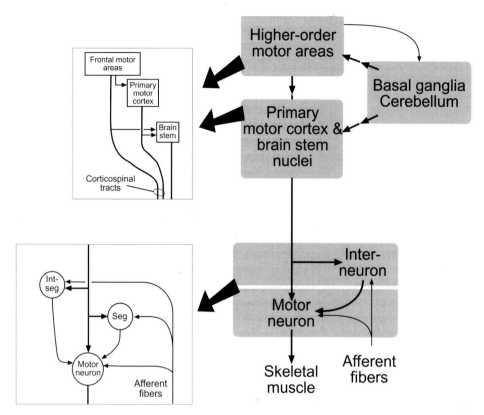

FIGURE 1-1 Hierarchical organization of the motor systems. Gray boxes show the major anatomic components of the motor systems. Upper inset: Organization of projections from higher order and primary motor cortex as well as from the brain stem. Lower inset: Spinal motor circuits. (Int-seg = intersegmental neuron; Seg = segmental interneuron.)

Supraspinal and Spinal Motor Systems). However, the term *upper motor neuron* is misleading. This is because neurons giving rise to the motor tracts have more complex integrative functions than simply specifying muscle contraction. The descending motor pathways, which originate from the brain stem and cerebral cortex, themselves have a hierarchical organization (see upper inset, Figure 1-1). The cortical pathways have extensive connections with brain stem regions that, in turn, give rise to spinal projections.

The highest levels of the motor systems consist of the basal ganglia, cerebellum, and higher order cortical motor areas, all of which provide important inputs to the motor pathways. Although the cerebellum and basal ganglia do not have significant spinal projections, the higher order cortical areas of the frontal lobe do (see Figure 1-1).

ORGANIZATION OF SPINAL GRAY MATTER AND THE LOWER MOTOR NEURON

Organization of the Spinal Gray Matter

The spinal cord has a central cellular region (gray matter) surrounded by a region that contains ascending and descending axons (white matter) (Figure 1-2). Each spinal cord segment contains a pair of nerve roots, the dorsal root, which contains afferent (sensory) axons, and the ventral root, which contains primarily efferent (motor) axons. The dorsal and ventral roots break into rootlets close to the spinal cord surface.

The spinal gray matter has a laminar organization (Figure 1-3A), based on the size, density, and shapes of neurons.[1] The laminae can be grouped into three dorsoventral zones: dorsal horn, intermediate zone, and ventral horn. The dorsal horn, which is the sensory component of the spinal gray matter, consists of laminae I–VI. The dorsal horn receives the densest projections from primary sensory axons and contains neurons whose axons project to supraspinal structures. The intermediate zone contains neurons that receive inputs from the descending pathways and from sensory axon terminals, and in turn, project to motor neurons. Neurons in the intermediate zone mediate spinal reflexes and integrate supraspinal signals with afferent input for movement control. The intermediate zone corresponds approximately to the upper portion of lamina VII. The ventral horn corresponds to the lower portion of lamina VII, as well as laminae VIII and IX. Interneurons and motor neurons are located in the ventral horn, with the

FIGURE 1-2 Schematic drawing of three segments of the spinal cord. (Reprinted with permission from MB Carpenter. Core Text of Neuroanatomy [3rd ed]. Baltimore: Williams & Wilkins, 1985.)

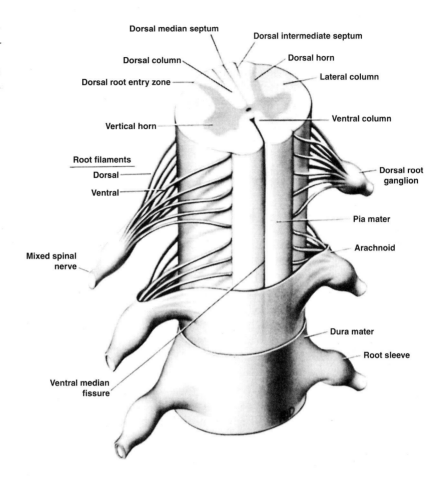

motor neurons localized to the motor nuclear columns in lamina IX (see Figure 1-3).

Neuronal Composition of Spinal Gray Matter

From the perspective of skeletal muscle contraction and movement control, there are three types of spinal cord neurons. (1) *Projection neurons* send an axon to supraspinal structures, such as the cerebellum, or thalamus. These neurons transmit sensory information to motor control structures for the somatic sensory guidance of movement. (2) *Interneurons* have axons that remain within the spinal cord. The axons of segmental interneurons are located within the segment of origin, whereas intersegmental neurons have axons that project to other spinal segments. Spinal interneurons also have axons that project to the opposite side of the spinal cord. (3) *Motor neurons* have an axon that innervates skeletal muscle. Alpha motor neurons give rise to large fibers that innervate extrafusal skeletal muscle, the fiber class that comprises the bulk of the muscle mass and is responsible for generating force. Gamma motor neurons innervate intrafusal fibers in the muscle spindles, which

are muscle stretch receptors (Figure 1-4). The action of intrafusal fibers modulates the response of the muscle spindle stretch receptor. Alpha motor neurons are cholinergic and synapse on skeletal muscle fibers in small, flattened expansions known as motor end-plates, or neuromuscular junction. Hereafter, the term *motor neuron* refers to the alpha motor neuron, unless otherwise specified. Axons of motor neurons emerge through the ventral root and become mixed with dorsal root fibers distal to the dorsal root ganglion. Spinal nerves containing both motor and sensory fibers are referred to as *mixed spinal nerves*. (The fourth major type of spinal cord neuron is the autonomic preganglionic motor neuron, which innervates postganglionic neurons and certain target organs.)

Motor neurons lie in rostrocaudally oriented cell columns in the ventral horn. These cell columns cluster into distinct larger medial and lateral groups. The medial cell column extends throughout the length of the spinal cord and contains motor neurons that innervate the long and short axial muscles. The lateral cell column innervates the remaining body musculature. The lateral column is most prominent in the cervical

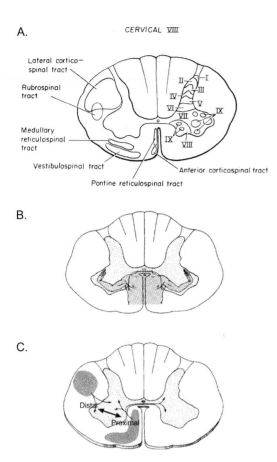

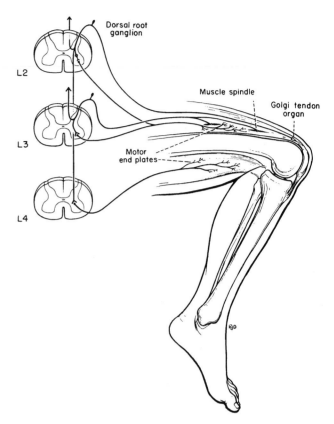

FIGURE 1-3 Segmental organization. **A.** Spinal cord laminar organization and motor path locations. **B.** Somatotopy. **C.** Medial and lateral path terminations. (VST = vestibulospinal tract.) (**B** and **C** reprinted with permission from JH Martin. Neuroanatomy: Text and Atlas. New York: Appleton & Lange, 1996;257 and 264.)

FIGURE 1-4 Schematic diagram of the sensory and motor elements involved in the patellar tendon reflex. Muscle spindle afferents are shown entering only the L-3 spinal segment; Golgi tendon organ afferents are shown entering only the L-2 segment. In this monosynaptic reflex afferent fibers enter L-2, L-3, and L-4 spinal segments and efferent fibers from the motor neurons at these same levels project to the extrafusal muscle fibers of the quadriceps femoris. Efferent fibers from L-4 projecting to the hamstrings represent part of the pathway involved in reciprocal inhibition. (Reprinted with permission from MB Carpenter. Core Text of Neuroanatomy [3rd ed]. Baltimore: Williams & Wilkins, 1985.)

and lumbosacral enlargements, where motor neurons that innervate the muscles of the extremities are located. Cells of the lateral column, located ventrally and laterally, innervate extensor and abductor muscle groups; cells located dorsally and medially to these innervate flexor and adductor muscle groups (see Figure 1-3B). In the thoracic region, the lateral cell column is small and innervates the intercostal and anterolateral trunk musculature.

SPINAL REFLEXES

The myotatic or deep tendon reflex is a monosynaptic reflex dependent on two neurons: one neuron in the dorsal root ganglion that receives afferent impulses from the muscle spindle and the motor neuron that innervates the striated muscle containing the muscle spindles. Sudden, abrupt stretching of a muscle, produced by sharply tapping the tendon of the muscle, causes stretching of the muscle spindle and discharge of the group Ia fibers. (These are the largest diameter primary afferent fibers.) The Ia fibers make synaptic contact with the alpha motor neurons in the ventral horn, and after a brief delay, impulses pass peripherally via the ventral root back to the same muscle and cause it to contract (see Figure 1-4). The myotatic reflex usually involves two or three spinal segments, because most muscles are innervated by fibers arising from several adjacent spinal segments.

Afferent fibers derived from the dorsal root ganglia constitute one of the major sources of input to the motor neuron (see Figure 1-1). In general, input via the dorsal root conveys impulses from a variety of different receptors, both superficial and deep. Golgi tendon organs (see Figure 1-4) are sensitive to the amount of force generated by the muscle; they have no known efferent innervation.[2] These stretch receptors can be caused to discharge by either contracting or stretching the muscle. Impulses from Golgi tendon organs are conveyed by group Ib fibers. Golgi tendon organs have a disynaptic inhibitory influence on alpha motor neurons. The inhibitory influence of the Golgi tendon organ on spinal motor neurons is of clinical importance for understanding the melting away of resistance to passive movement in spasticity.

Activation of nociceptors, which respond selectively to painful stimuli, evokes a flexion reflex that produces withdrawal from the offending stimulus. The flexion reflex is a disynaptic or polysynaptic reflex, with afferents synapsing first on interneurons, which in turn synapse on motor neurons. The flexion reflex, in addition to producing powerful contractions of ipsilateral flexor muscles, also inhibits ipsilateral extensor muscles in a reciprocal fashion, so that an entire limb may be withdrawn. The crossed extensor reflex is part of the flexor reflex.[2] Collateral fibers involved in the flexor reflex cross in the spinal cord and establish reciprocal connections opposite to those that are present ipsilaterally. Contralateral excitation involves extensor muscles; inhibition prevails on flexor motor neurons. In the case of the lower extremity, the crossed extensor response serves to support the body when the ipsilateral lower limb is flexed.

To summarize, segmental input to the lower motor neuron is profuse, direct and indirect, and largely, but not exclusively, ipsilateral. Muscle spindle afferents (group Ia) project directly to the motor neuron, whereas most other receptors, including the Golgi tendon organ (group Ib), influence motor neurons indirectly via interneurons. Group Ia and Ib fibers influence ipsilateral cell groups of the spinal cord, whereas other sensory receptors are distributed by multisynaptic circuits to both sides of the spinal cord. Motor neurons are also under powerful supraspinal control via descending systems. These systems are discussed next.

GENERAL ORGANIZATION OF DESCENDING MOTOR PATHWAYS

The functional organization of the descending pathways parallels the somatotopic organization of the motor nuclei of the ventral horn. As considered previously, motor neurons that innervate limb muscles are located laterally in the ventral horn, whereas those innervating proximal and axial muscle are located medially. The lateral motor nuclei receive projections from pathways that primarily descend in the lateral white matter column (see Figure 1-3C). In contrast, the medial motor nuclei receive projections from pathways that primarily descend in the medial (or ventromedial) portions of the spinal white matter. Although the cortex and brain stem each contribute to the lateral and medial pathways, the lateral paths preferentially arise from the cortex and the medial paths from the brain stem.

There are two important clinical considerations pertaining to this mediolateral organization. First, the lateral systems, which control distal limb movements such as prehension, are predominantly crossed pathways. A unilateral lesion of a lateral pathway produces clear motor deficits that may or may not recover. Second, the medial systems, which control proximal limb and axial movements such as maintaining and adjusting posture, have an overall bilateral organization. A unilateral lesion of a medial pathway does not typically produce clear motor signs because of compensation by the contralateral projection.

We first consider the corticospinal tracts. (A parallel path for cranial muscle control, the corticobulbar tract terminates on cranial nerve motor nuclei in the pons and medulla.) We then consider the brain stem pathways, the rubrospinal, vestibulospinal, and reticulospinal tracts. We also briefly consider the descending autonomic projections.

Corticospinal Tracts

There are separate lateral and ventral corticospinal tracts. The lateral corticospinal tract is the most important limb motor control pathway in humans. It is located in the lateral white matter column in the spinal cord (see Figure 1-3A). The ventral corticospinal tract, which is one of the various medial paths, is located in the ventral white matter column. The term *corticospinal tract* is often used interchangeably with pyramidal tract, which describes the axons in the medullary pyramids. Although the pyramids contain virtually all of the corticospinal axons, they also contain corticobulbar axons. Therefore, it is incorrect to equate the terms *corticospinal tract* and *pyramidal tract*.

Corticospinal tract neurons are located in layer 5 of the cortex. Corticospinal neurons include the largest pyramidal neurons (the Betz cells, which are located in

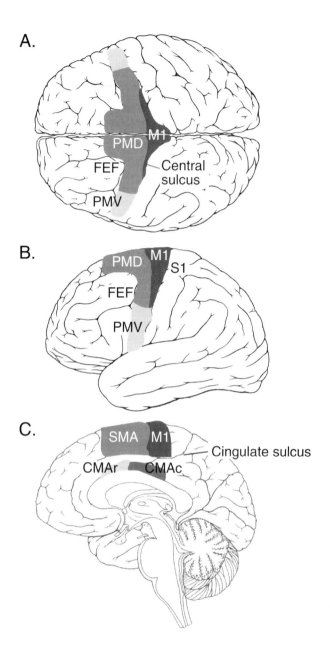

A.

B.

C.

FIGURE 1-5 Organization of the cortical motor areas. **A.** Superior view. **B.** Lateral view. **C.** Medial view. There are four motor areas of the frontal lobe: (1) primary motor cortex (M1); (2) lateral premotor cortex, including dorsal premotor cortex (PMD) and ventral premotor cortex (PMV); (3) supplementary motor area (SMA); and (4) cingulate motor area (CMA), including the rostral (CMAr) and caudal (CMAc) subregions. Some of these areas contain additional subdivisions (see the section Cortical Motor Areas). The location of the frontal eye field (FEF) is also shown. This region participates in the control of saccadic eye movements. (Modified from data summarized by PE Roland, K Zilles. Functions and structures of the motor cortices in humans. Curr Opin Neurobiol 1996;6:773–781.)

the precentral gyrus), as well as smaller pyramidal neurons that are also located in the precentral gyrus as well as rostrally and medially in the frontal lobe.[3,4] Corticospinal neurons are also located in the anterior parietal lobe. The corticospinal projection from the primary motor cortex, located in the precentral gyrus, is thought to be the major projection because it is important in regulating the most basic movement parameters, such as force, movement direction, and the ability to individuate movement. Damage to this area or its projections typically produces incapacitating motor control impairments.

The higher order motor areas that contain corticospinal neurons are located rostral and medial to primary motor cortex (Figure 1-5). In addition to contributing to the corticospinal tracts, the higher order areas also have projections to primary motor cortex. These higher order motor areas are thought to serve important motor planning functions. Indeed, it is a mystery why these areas have direct (and often dense) spinal projections. This mystery has yet to be solved, although functional imaging studies are providing important insights. By mapping changes in cortical neuronal activity during different motor tasks, we hope to identify the distinctive planning and movement control roles of the various cortical motor areas.

The areas that give rise to corticospinal axons, including both primary motor cortex and the higher order motor areas, also contain neurons that project to brain stem regions (e.g., reticular formation) that, in turn, project to the spinal cord (e.g., see Figure 1-1, upper inset). Thus, in addition to contributing to the corticospinal tract, all of these areas contribute to other hierarchically organized descending pathways, such as the corticoreticulospinal tract. For some of these areas, the brain stem projections may be denser than those to the spinal cord.

The corticospinal axons descend through the internal capsule and ventral brain stem en route to the spinal cord (Figure 1-6). Axons that originate from more higher order motor areas (see the section Cortical Motor Areas) descend in the anterior limb of the internal capsule, whereas those from the primary motor cortex and parietal lobe descend in the posterior limb.[5] Corticobulbar axons descend primarily in the genu of the internal capsule.

Corticospinal projections terminate predominantly on the side contralateral to the cell of origin. Most corticospinal axons terminate in the intermediate zone and ventral horn. Corticospinal axons originating from different cortical territories often have different spinal termination patterns, with some axons terminating more dorsally in the gray matter and others terminating more ventrally. These differences in termination patterns forecast different motor control functions. Also, we discuss later how two features of the organization of the corticospinal projections, the distributed cortical origin of corticospinal neurons and the presence of ipsilateral terminations, can contribute to the recovery of motor control function after damage to the spinal projection from primary motor cortex.

Cortical Motor Areas

What constitutes a cortical motor area? Several key criteria have been identified: (1) projections to the spinal cord or cranial motor nuclei, (2) a complete representation of the muscles, joints of the body, or both, and (3) activation during the planning and execution of movements. For any given area, it may not be possible for all of these criteria to be met.[6] Moreover, there may be other, as yet unidentified, important criteria. Although functional imaging studies have expanded our understanding of the human motor systems, anatomic investigation is limited to postmortem tissue.

In humans, there are at least four cortical motor areas located in the frontal lobe (see Figure 1-5)[6]: (1) primary motor cortex, (2) supplementary motor area (SMA), (3) cingulate motor area (CMA), and (4) lateral premotor cortex. Within each of these areas, two or more motor subregions have been identified.[7]

The primary motor cortex (see Figure 1-5, M1) was the first cortical motor area to be identified because this is an area where electrical stimulation in animals produced contraction of contralateral muscles. Primary motor cortex is located on the precentral gyrus, laterally, within the anterior bank of the central sulcus, and medially, on the surface of the gyrus. This corresponds to Brodmann's area 4. It has been shown that the human motor cortex is made up of cytoarchitectonically and histochemically distinct anterior and posterior areas.[8] In animal studies, these two portions of motor cortex have differential anatomic connections and possibly different motor control functions.

Primary motor cortex has a somatotopic organization: Control of the lower extremity is represented medially, the upper extremity is represented on the lateral convexity, and the face, most laterally. Animal studies have shown that the anterior and posterior motor cortex subregions have their own body representations.[9] Within a limb or body part representation, individual muscles and joints are represented at multiple locations.[10] The local organization is thought to be related to interjoint coordination patterns.

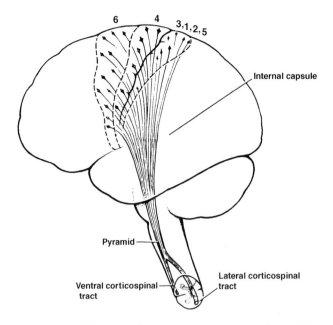

FIGURE 1-6 Schematic drawing of the lateral surface of the brain indicates the origin and course of the corticospinal tract.

The corticospinal tract originating from the primary motor cortex gives rise to dense corticospinal terminations throughout the spinal cord and corticobulbar projections to cranial nerve motor nuclei.[4] Projections from anterior and posterior motor cortex subregions have different laminar termination patterns. The anterior zone projects more ventrally in the intermediate zone and ventral horn, whereas the posterior subregions project more dorsally in the deeper layers of the dorsal horn.[11] The primary motor cortex plays essential roles in regulating force production, steering movement direction, individuation of finger movements, and accurate foot placement during locomotion.[12,13]

The other frontal motor areas are located within the portions of the frontal lobe that make up the higher order motor areas. Anatomic studies show that these higher order motor areas all have projections to the primary motor cortex.[14] The distinction between the higher order and primary area may not be as important as once thought because we now know that the higher order areas also have dense spinal (and cranial motor nuclear) projections. Although the primary motor cortex does not represent extraocular muscles and does not seem to be important in eye movement control, many of the secondary motor areas have demonstrated important roles in eye movement control.[6]

The SMA is located predominantly on medial surface of frontal lobe (see Figure 1-5), in Brodmann's area 6.

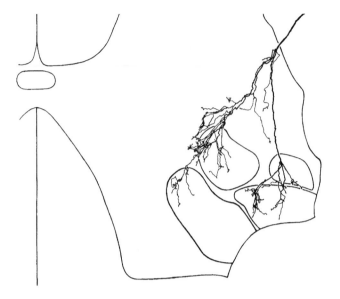

FIGURE 1-7 Partial reconstruction of single corticospinal axon terminals in the spinal cord. (Reprinted with permission from Y Shinoda, J Yokota, T Futami. Divergent projections of individual corticospinal axons to motoneurons of multiple muscles in monkey. Neurosci Lett 1981;34:111–115.)

Research suggests that, in the human, there may be two separate motor representations in the SMA, organized into separate rostral and caudal subregions, and in the monkey, a third area, farther rostrally.[15,16] Corticospinal projections from the SMA have been demonstrated in monkeys, with dense contralateral terminations in the intermediate zone and ventral horn.[3] Imaging studies suggest that the SMA is important in the production of self-generated movements.[16]

The CMA is also located on medial brain surface (see Figure 1-5), in what is traditionally considered limbic association cortex. This corresponds to Brodmann's areas 24 and 25.[15] The CMA appears to have two body representations organized into distinctive rostral and caudal CMAs, and possibly a third area located farther rostrally.[6] The CMA gives rise to dense corticospinal terminations, nearly as dense as those from the primary motor cortex. Although the CMA becomes active during various motor tasks, the distinctive motor control functions of this area are not known.

The lateral premotor area is located in Brodmann's area 6, on the surface of the precentral gyrus and further rostrally into the precentral sulcus (see Figure 1-5).[17] There are at least two distinct motor subregions within lateral area 6, the dorsal and ventral premotor cortical areas. In monkeys, using various anatomic criteria, the dorsal and ventral regions each contain separate rostral

and caudal zones.[18] Parts of the lateral premotor areas contribute to the corticospinal tract.[3] These frontal motor areas are thought to play an important role in initiating and controlling movements that depend on external stimuli, especially vision.[17]

The parietal lobe, clearly important in somatic sensation, also contributes to the corticospinal tracts.[19] Most parietal corticospinal neurons are located within the somatic sensory cortex (areas 1, 2, and 3) and in the posterior parietal cortex (area 5) (see Figure 1-5). Overall, this projection is much smaller than that from the frontal lobes and terminates largely within the dorsal horn. The parietal corticospinal projection is thought to be important for controlling the flow of somatic sensory information to the spinal cord during movements.

Corticomotoneuronal Terminations

A unique feature of the corticospinal system in certain primates is the presence of dense corticomotoneuronal (CM) terminations.[13] These terminations bypass spinal interneurons and provide direct control of motor neuron excitability. Other species may have such connections but they are much less dense. Because corticospinal neurons have extensive terminal branches (Figure 1-7), it is almost certain that neurons giving rise to CM terminations also project to spinal interneurons.[13,20] CM terminations are thought to contribute to the capacity to make individuated finger movements because this motor control function is lost after corticospinal damage in primates (including humans).

Even though CM neurons are the closest to *upper motor neurons* of all descending projection neurons, they do not respond in a manner consistent with their being upper motor neurons. Despite the presence of monosynaptic connections with motor neurons, the discharge of CM cells does not encode muscle activity in a faithful manner. One of the most compelling pieces of evidence is that when monkeys contract particular hand muscles during a fine gripping movement (i.e., precision grip), CM neurons for those muscles become active. However, when the same muscles are contracted while the animal is making a relatively uncontrolled power grip, when the monkey becomes emotionally agitated during task performance, the CM neurons for those muscles do not become active.[21] This finding shows that CM neuronal discharge is contingent on a particular behavioral context, in this example, during motor behavior requiring great skill. Thus, CM neurons do not behave as upper motor neurons, firing like that of the target muscle. Rather, CM neurons, as well as other corticospinal neurons, have a more complex role in directing the contraction of muscles.

Rubrospinal Tract

The red nucleus is located in the midbrain tegmentum (Figure 1-8). It is divided into a large parvocellular region, located rostrally, and a small magnocellular region, located caudally. The parvocellular division gives rise to a projection to the inferior olivary nucleus. By contrast, the magnocellular region gives rise to the rubrospinal tract. Large cells in caudal parts of the nucleus, which give rise to the tract, have axons that cross the midline immediately and descend to spinal levels in the lateral column. These fibers are partially intermingled with those of the corticospinal fibers (see Figure 1-3A). Rubrospinal tract axons terminate on interneurons in the intermediate zone and ventral horn, as well as directly on motor neurons.[22] Like corticospinal tract axons, rubrospinal tract axons have extensive branches. In humans, the rubrospinal tract does not project to the lumbosacral enlargement.[23]

The red nucleus receives input from two major sources, the cerebral cortex and some of the deep cerebellar nuclei. Corticorubral fibers from the motor cortex descend ipsilaterally and are somatotopically organized.[24] Thus, corticorubral and rubrospinal fibers together constitute a somatotopically organized nonpyramidal linkage from the motor cortex to spinal levels that exert effects contralaterally, because the rubrospinal tract is crossed. A second input to the red nucleus arises from the interposed nuclei of the cerebellum; these fibers are crossed and link portions of the opposite cerebellar cortex (i.e., paravermal).[25]

Cerebellar influences on cells of the red nucleus are expressed ipsilaterally because cerebellar efferent fibers and rubrospinal fibers are both crossed. Animal studies have shown that rubromotoneuronal neurons discharge during voluntary limb movements in a manner similar to CM cells.[26] The rubrospinal system is small compared with the corticospinal system, decreasing in size from cats, monkeys, chimpanzees, and humans.[23,27] Its distinctive role in motor control is not known. The rubrospinal system may take on greater functional significance in patients after damage to the corticospinal system, because it is the only brain stem pathway with direct connections to motor neurons innervating distal limb muscles.

Vestibulospinal Tract

The vestibular nuclei constitute a complex in the lateral part of the floor of the fourth ventricle of the pons and medulla (Figure 1-9). The four major nuclei of this complex receive afferents from the vestibular apparatus (semicircular ducts and the otolith organs). These nuclei are concerned with maintenance of equilibrium, posture, and orientation in three-dimensional space. In addition, parts of these nuclei receive input from portions of the cerebellar cortex and the most medial deep cerebellar nucleus (fastigial nucleus). The vestibulospinal tract arises mainly

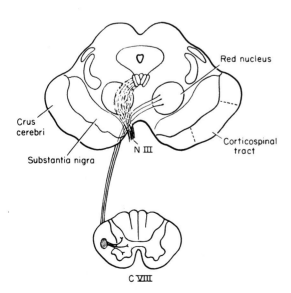

FIGURE 1-8 Schematic diagram of the rubrospinal tract.

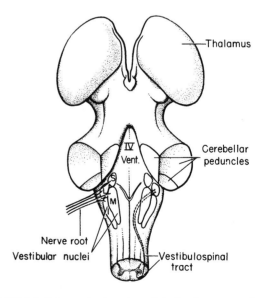

FIGURE 1-9 Schematic drawing of the brain stem and cervical spinal cord shows the locations of the vestibular nuclei in the floor of the fourth ventricle and the course of the vestibulospinal tract. S, L, M, and I indicate the superior, lateral, medial, and inferior vestibular nuclei, respectively.

from the giant cells of the lateral vestibular nucleus and descends in the ventral part of the lateral column of the spinal cord (see Figure 1-9). This tract is somatotopically organized and is present in all spinal segments.[28] Fibers of the tract terminate within the medial parts of Rexed's laminae VII, VIII, and IX.[29-31] Although these vestibulospinal axons terminate ipsilateral to their origin, they synapse on spinal interneurons that have extensive bilateral projections. In this way, the vestibulospinal axons influence axial muscle control bilaterally. Some vestibulospinal tract axon terminals synapse directly on extensor motor neurons. Similar to the other pathways discussed, vestibulospinal tract axons give collaterals to multiple spinal segments.[31,32] Impulses conveyed by the vestibulospinal tract produce increases in ipsilateral extensor muscle tone. Vestibulospinal fibers also originate from the medial vestibular nucleus. These axons descend initially within the medial longitudinal fasciculus and terminate bilaterally within upper cervical spinal segments. Because vestibulospinal neurons in the lateral vestibular nucleus project to all spinal cord levels, they are thought to have a general role in posture and balance. By contrast, vestibulospinal neurons in the medial vestibular nucleus are thought to play a role in neck control because they only project to upper cervical segments.

Vestibular ganglion cells, which innervate the macula of the utricle, appear to project exclusively to the ventral part of the lateral vestibular nucleus.[33] This suggests that stimuli that excite the utricle, such as head tilt, gravity, and linear acceleration, must play an important role in maintaining extensor muscle tone. Direct input to dorsal regions of the lateral vestibular nucleus is derived from Purkinje cells in the anterior lobe vermis of the cerebellum.[34] This pathway exerts inhibitory influences on cells of the lateral vestibular nucleus, mediated by the neurotransmitter gamma-aminobutyric acid.[35] The fastigial nucleus of the cerebellum projects crossed and uncrossed fibers fairly symmetrically to ventral parts of both lateral vestibular nuclei and appears to have excitatory influences mediated by glutamic acid.[36,37] Thus, the excitatory influences of the vestibular end organ can be modulated directly by cerebellar inputs. Lesions of the anterior lobe of the cerebellum in animals produce increases in extensor muscle tone that resemble decerebrate rigidity.

Reticulospinal Tracts

Anatomically, the term *reticular formation* is used to designate the core of the brain stem characterized by aggregations of cells of various sizes enmeshed in a fiber network. The matrix that forms the reticular formation is phylogenetically the oldest part of the brain stem and is surrounded by newer pathways concerned with more specific functions. Development of the reticular formation parallels the process of encephalization. For many years the organization of the reticular formation was considered to be diffuse and nonspecific. In the late 1950s it became apparent that the reticular formation could be divided into regions that possessed a specific cytoarchitecture, distinctive fiber connections, and unique internal features.[38] The reticular formation can be regarded as the principal integrator of motor, sensory, and visceral functions in the brain stem. Basically, the reticular formation can be divided into four major mediolateral subdivisions: (1) the raphe nuclei, (2) a paramedian part related largely to the cerebellum, (3) a medial effector or motor part, and (4) a lateral sensory part.

Spinal projections arise from the medial zone of the pontine and medullary reticular formation. Medullary reticulospinal fibers arise from a large collection of cells dorsal to the inferior olivary complex and project largely uncrossed to all levels of the spinal cord (Figure 1-10). Fibers from this tract descend in the ventral part of the lateral column and terminate largely on interneurons in lamina VII, although some end on processes of cells in lamina IX. Pontine reticulospinal fibers arise from a corresponding larger medial region of the pontine reticular formation. Virtually all fibers of the pontine reticulospinal tracts are uncrossed, descend in the

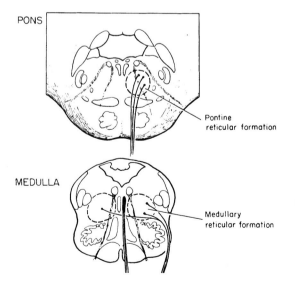

FIGURE 1-10 Schematic diagram of sections of the lower brain stem indicates the origin, course, and regions of termination of the reticulospinal tracts.

ventral column near the midline, and end on interneurons in laminae VII and VIII (see Figure 1-10). Reticulospinal neurons, whether originating in the pons or medulla, can terminate on spinal interneurons with bilateral projections and thereby influence body musculature bilaterally. Unlike the corticospinal, rubrospinal, and vestibulospinal tracts, none of the reticulospinal fibers is somatotopically organized.

One of the characteristic features of the reticular formation is that it receives signals from multiple sources, which include virtually all types of sensory receptors, the cerebellum, and the cerebral cortex. Sensory input to the reticular formation loses its identification with specific stimuli. Functions of the reticular formation are multiple, but some can be related to specific subdivisions. The reticular formation can (1) facilitate or inhibit voluntary motor activity, (2) modify muscle tone and reflex activity, (3) exert a variety of different autonomic responses, and (4) facilitate or inhibit central transmission of sensory signals. Major inhibitory functions appear to be related to the medullary reticular formation. Inhibition produced by reticular formation neurons affects most forms of motor activity, including myotatic and flexor reflexes and muscle tone. Reductions in muscle tone and deep tendon reflexes appear to be mediated by medullary reticulospinal fibers that inhibit gamma motor neurons, which modulate the response of the muscle spindle to stretch and thereby affect alpha motor neuron activity.

A far larger region of the brain stem reticular formation facilitates motor responses, muscle tone, and somatic spinal reflexes. The facilitatory region includes most of the pontine reticular formation and extends into the caudal midbrain. The facilitatory region of the reticular formation includes neurons that do not project directly to spinal cord; thus, effects from these regions must involve polysynaptic pathways. Most of the effects from the facilitatory region appear to involve interneurons at various spinal levels. Not all of the influences of the reticular formation are directed toward modification of spinal neuronal activities. Large regions of both the medullary and pontine reticular formation exert powerful ascending influences that control the electrical excitability of broad regions of the cerebral cortex and affect the state of alertness and behavioral arousal.

Descending Autonomic Pathways

It has been difficult to distinguish supraspinal neurons concerned exclusively with autonomic functions, but axon tracing methods and immunocytochemical techniques have yielded important information. The principal nuclei giving rise to descending autonomic fibers are (1) several regions of the hypothalamus, (2) portions of the parasympathetic nuclei of the oculomotor nuclear complex, (3) the locus ceruleus, (4) parts of the solitary nucleus, and (5) collections of catecholamine neurons in the ventrolateral lower brain stem. In addition, the raphe nuclei, which contain cells rich in serotonin, project bilaterally to spinal levels and modulate pain mechanisms.[39] Large cells in the paraventricular and posterior regions of the hypothalamus project directly to spinal levels, where some of these fibers end on autonomic neurons.[40] Some parasympathetic neurons in the oculomotor nucleus project to spinal levels and end in parts of laminae I and V.[41,42] The locus ceruleus, recognized as a principal source of noradrenergic fibers widely distributed in the neuraxis, projects to parts of the dorsal and ventral horns and the intermediolateral cell column, which gives rise to preganglionic sympathetic fibers.[42] Descending fibers from the solitary nucleus project fibers to neurons of the phrenic nerve nucleus and to ventral horn cells in the thoracic region; these crossed projections are concerned with excitation of inspiratory motor neurons.[43] Ventrolateral noradrenergic neurons located near the facial nucleus project bilaterally to the intermediolateral cell column in thoracic and upper lumbar spinal segments.[44] Lesions in the brain stem and spinal cord often involve the descending autonomic fiber system.

EFFECTS OF LESIONS OF THE SUPRASPINAL AND SPINAL MOTOR SYSTEMS

A lesion involving the motor systems produces such impairments as loss of voluntary movement, muscle weakness, loss of muscle tone, loss or alteration of reflex activity, abnormal postures, and ultimately substitution of inferior motor activity for once effective control. Evaluation of loss or disturbances of motor function should begin by determining the site of the lesion. The location of the lesion frequently provides insights into the specific pathology producing damage. Disturbances of voluntary motor function may involve either the *upper motor neuron*, which involves the origins or axons of the descending pathways, or *lower motor neuron*, the neuron that innervates skeletal muscle for generating joint motion and muscular force. The first step in elucidating the site of damage is to distinguish whether the upper or lower motor neuron is involved. This relatively simple, yet frequently puzzling, distinction is one of the cornerstones of clinical neurology.

Lesions of the Lower Motor Neuron

Lesions selectively involving the lower motor neuron result in weakness or paralysis, loss of muscle tone, loss of reflexes, and muscle atrophy. All of these changes are confined to the affected muscles. Weakness or paralysis has a direct relationship to the extent and severity of the lesion. Because columns of motor neurons that innervate a single muscle extend longitudinally through several spinal segments, and because several such cell columns exist at each level, a lesion confined to one segment causes some weakness, but not complete paralysis, in the several muscles. Complete paralysis of a muscle occurs only when a lesion involves the column of cells in several segments, or ventral root fibers from these cells. Because most appendicular muscles are innervated by fibers arising from three spinal segments, complete paralysis of a muscle resulting from a spinal lesion in the ventral horn indicates involvement of several segments. Neighboring cell columns are likely to be involved at each level, resulting in paralysis of a group of muscles rather than an individual one.

Because the motor neuron consists of the cell bodies in the ventral horn and its axons, which emerge via the ventral root, it is sometimes necessary to distinguish motor deficits that occur as a consequence of lesions in spinal segments from those that involve the ventral root, spinal nerves, or peripheral nerves (Figure 1-11). Lesions of the ventral root usually produce the same motor deficits as destruction of the corresponding motor neurons. These two types of lesions are not the same in thoracolumbar and sacral segments, because in these regions preganglionic autonomic fibers arise from cell groups in the lateral horn but exit via the ventral root. Thus, a lesion involving the ventral root at T-1 produces Horner's syndrome (miosis, pseudoptosis, apparent enophthalmos, and dryness of the skin over the face) in addition to some weakness in the small muscles of the hand.

Section of a single ventral root, for example C-5, would produce weakness in the supraspinatus, infraspinatus, subscapularis, biceps brachii, and brachioradialis muscles, but not complete paralysis of any of these muscles. This pattern of distribution is unique to C-5 ventral root fibers and different from that of any single peripheral nerve. Lesions of mixed spinal nerves produce motor and sensory deficits that correspond to those of combined dorsal and ventral root lesions (see Figure 1-11). The motor deficits correspond almost exactly to those resulting from lesions of the ventral root, but the sensory disturbances follow a dermatomal distribution and tend to be less extensive because of the characteristic overlapping nature of dermatomes. A lesion involving a single dorsal root such as C-5 would not result in detectable sensory loss, because dorsal root fibers from C-4 and C-6 *cover* most of the C-5 area.[45]

These observations are in sharp contrast with the motor and sensory deficits resulting from a peripheral nerve lesion, deficits that correspond to the peripheral distribution of the particular nerve distal to the injury. An ulnar nerve injury near the wrist would produce paralysis of the adductor pollicis, deep head of the flexor pollicis brevis, interossei, inner lumbrical muscles, and muscles of the hypothenar eminence, along with loss of sensation in all of the little finger, the ulnar half of the ring finger, and corresponding portions of the dorsal and palmar surfaces of the hand.

Loss of muscle tone, hypotonia, is a characteristic and constant finding in lower motor neuron lesions. The muscle is flaccid and soft and offers no resistance to passive movement. The reduction in muscle tone results from the withdrawal of streams of efferent impulses that are normally transmitted to the muscle that maintain its tone. Reflexes in the affected muscles are greatly diminished or absent (areflexia) in lower motor neuron lesions because the reflex arc is interrupted. In this type of lesion the effector limb of the reflex arc has been destroyed. Although paralysis, hypotonia, and areflexia occur almost immediately after a lower motor neuron lesion, atrophy, or muscle wasting, does not become evident for

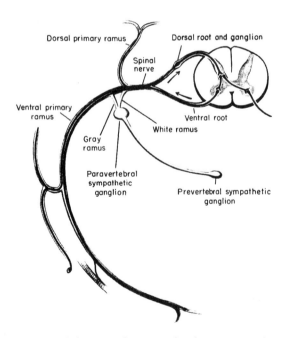

FIGURE 1-11 Schematic diagram of a thoracic spinal nerve shows peripheral branches and central connections. (Reprinted with permission from CR Noback, RJ Demarest. The Human Nervous System [3rd ed]. New York: McGraw-Hill, 1981.)

1 or 2 weeks. Atrophy occurs gradually and in time is obvious on inspection.

In some diseases involving the lower motor neuron the muscles supplied by these neurons exhibit small, localized, spontaneous contractions known as *fasciculations*. These small muscle twitches, visible beneath the skin, represent the discharge of groups of muscle fibers. Fasciculations occur asynchronously in parts of different muscles and are thought to be due to triggering mechanisms within the motor neuron. Fasciculations commonly are seen in amyotrophic lateral sclerosis and sometimes in acute inflammatory lesions of peripheral nerves, but usually they are not seen when motor neurons are rapidly destroyed, as in poliomyelitis.

Lesions of the Descending Pathways and Spinal Cord

Lesions involving the upper motor neuron, both cell bodies and descending axons, at a variety of locations produce paralysis, alterations of muscle tone, and changes in reflex activity. These lesions are rarely selective, are usually incomplete, and frequently involve adjacent structures. The degree of paresis or paralysis is not always directly related to the size of the lesions or the extent of involvement of the corticospinal tract. Such lesions may result from vascular disease, trauma, neoplasms, or infectious and degenerative disease. Unilateral lesions in the cerebral hemisphere or brain stem produce contralateral paralysis, usually hemiplegia. Spinal lesions, most commonly the result of trauma, usually are bilateral and cause paraplegia.

The most common lesion involving the descending pathways is the so-called cerebrovascular accident. Thrombosis of a major cerebral artery, commonly the middle cerebral artery or the main trunk of the internal carotid artery, deprives regions of the brain of blood and oxygen, causing necrosis. Tissues surrounding the infarcted area become edematous. In the majority of patients the onset is sudden. Initial symptoms are both focal and general. Focal symptoms, such as paralysis, sensory loss, and disturbances of speech, usually are related to the site of the lesion. Generalized symptoms include headache, nausea, vomiting, convulsions, and coma. Immediately after the vascular lesion, usually called a stroke, the paralyzed limbs are completely flaccid and the myotatic reflexes are depressed or absent. The plantar response, elicited by stroking the sole of the foot, shows extension of the great toe and fanning of the other toes (i.e., Babinski's response). Although Babinski's response is of great clinical importance, the physiological mechanism is not understood.

Upper motor neuron syndromes caused by lesions of the brain stem are much less common than those involving deep structures of the cerebral hemisphere. Motor disturbances resulting from relatively small lesions are similar, except that cranial nerves and ascending sensory pathways are commonly involved. Large lesions of the brain stem usually are not compatible with survival and often are associated with protracted coma.

Spasticity

Within a variable period of time after cerebral hemisphere lesion, muscle tone gradually returns to the affected limb and ultimately exceeds that of the normal side. This exaggeration of muscle tone is not seen in all muscles. In the lower extremity, the increase in muscle tone develops in the antigravity muscles. In the upper extremity, tone is increased in the adductors and internal rotators of the shoulder, the flexors and pronators of the forearm, and in the flexors of the wrist and digits. In the lower extremity, tone is increased in the adductors of the hip, the extensors of the hip and knee, and the plantar flexors. This increase in antigravity muscle tone is referred to as *spasticity* and is characterized by (1) increased resistance to passive movement, (2) hyperactive deep tendon reflexes (low threshold, large amplitude, and a forceful brisk nature), and (3) the presence of clonus. Clonus represents an extreme exaggeration of the myotatic reflex in which a stretch of the muscle initiates a self-perpetuating stretch reflex in an antagonistic muscle group.

It has been presumed for some time that the upper motor neuron syndrome was due solely to interruption of fibers of the corticospinal tract in their trajectory through the neuraxis. This concept was based on the thesis that this system directly and indirectly conveyed excitatory input to motor neurons and was responsible for voluntary movement. This thesis considered the intact corticospinal system to be associated with voluntary skilled movement and the damaged system to be associated with paralysis, or paresis, and residual spasticity expressed as exaggerated muscle tone in the antigravity muscles. It is difficult to understand how a lesion in this system could produce both paresis and spasticity. The assumption has been that lesions of the corticospinal tract in some way removed inhibitory influences, which resulted in the spasticity. In practice, lesions of the corticospinal system almost invariably involve other neural structures or pathways. The only pure corticospinal lesion is one that destroys the medullary pyramid in the caudal medulla, after all corticobulbar axons have terminated, which is rare. Experimental lesions of the medullary pyramids of monkeys and chimpanzees produce a condition best characterized as *hypotonic paresis.*[46,47] There is no complete paralysis, in the sense that no part of the body is rendered useless, but there is grave and general poverty of movement.

In long-term experiments, a wide range of gross movements shows some recovery, but voluntary movement was stripped of the qualities that endow it with precision and versatility. There is persistent slowness of movement, loss of individual finger movement, and the ability to fractionate movements. In chimpanzees, paresis is more prominent than hypotonia, the deep tendon reflexes are brisk and of large amplitude, and Babinski's sign is evident. If some fibers of the corticospinal tract are preserved, return of motor function, dexterity, and discrete finger movements are more pronounced than with a total lesion.

In addition to raising questions about the mechanisms of spasticity, these studies examined residual motor functions after bilateral section of the medullary pyramids. The results show an important role for subcortical motor systems in initiating and guiding a limited range of motor activities. Thus, nonpyramidal descending systems make important contributions to total motor function, which in normal persons appear to form a basic mechanism on which the functions of the corticospinal system are superimposed. Studies of the nonpyramidal descending systems suggest they are especially concerned with maintenance of erect posture, integration of body and limb movements, and with directing progression movements.[48]

Although these basic studies provide some insights into the contributions made by various components of the descending pathways, they provide little information concerning the mechanism of spasticity. Spasticity is not associated with relatively pure lesions of the corticospinal system or with lesions of the individual descending systems from the brain stem. Although spasticity is a regularly occurring phenomenon with most upper motor neuron lesions, its nature has eluded the most meticulous analysis.

Motor Recovery After Stroke

Motor impairments after stroke tend to become less severe with time. Paralysis that initially involved both upper and lower extremities equally may now appear less severe in one limb. Some voluntary motor function begins to return. The motor functions most affected are those associated with fine, skilled movements. Gross movements that involve the whole limb often show considerable restitution. Many hemiplegics show apprecia-

ble recovery of motor function and become ambulatory. The hemiplegic gait is characteristic: The partially paralyzed leg is circumducted en bloc at the hip and swung forward because of difficulty flexing the knee. The foot is in plantar flexion, and the toe of the shoe is dragged in a circular fashion. The arm on the affected side is flexed at the elbow and wrist, the forearm is pronated, and the digits are flexed.

Techniques for functional imaging and noninvasive activation of cortical motor areas are providing insight into the mechanisms of motor recovery after unilateral hemispheric stroke. Imaging studies have shown that after recovery from infarction of the primary motor cortex, rostrally located cortical motor areas show increased activation compared with healthy subjects.[49] How might this increased cortical activation contribute to recovery? As described previously, anatomic studies show that corticospinal projections arise from multiple regions of the frontal lobes. Although it is believed that normally the various cortical motor areas contributing to the corticospinal tract each serve different motor control functions, after damage to the primary motor cortex (or its descending projection in the posterior limb of the internal capsule) the remaining areas can undergo functional reorganization. The corticospinal projections of the higher order motor areas, which descend through the anterior limb of the internal capsule,[5] could transmit new signals for controlling skeletal muscle.

Another mechanism for functional recovery is thought to involve increased recruitment of ipsilateral corticospinal projections.[50,51] Although the corticospinal tracts are predominantly crossed, there is a small ipsilateral component.[4] This projection is either "double crossed" or strictly unilateral. Increased recruitment of ipsilateral corticospinal projections may be particularly important for recovery of movements produced by midline and proximal muscles.[52]

Spinal Cord Injury

Spinal cord transection immediately produces, below the level of the lesion, (1) loss of all motor function, (2) loss of all somatic sensation, (3) loss of visceral sensation, (4) loss of muscle tone, and (5) loss of all reflex activity. (At the level of the lesion, motor neurons can also be damaged.) Initially there is no evidence of neural activity in the isolated spinal cord caudal to the lesion (i.e., spinal shock). Spinal shock occurs in all animals after transection of the spinal cord and is considered to be caused by the sudden, abrupt interruption of all descending excitatory influences. The duration of spinal shock varies in different animals; in humans it averages approximately 3 weeks. The termination of the period of spinal shock is heralded by the appearance of Babinski's sign.

A fairly orderly sequence of recovery of function follows, with some variations. The phases of recovery of some functions in the isolated portion of the spinal cord have been carefully documented. Recovery phases and their approximate duration are as follows: (1) period of minimal reflex activity (3–6 weeks), (2) period of flexor muscle spasms (6–16 weeks), (3) period of alternate flexor and extensor spasms (after 4 months), and (4) period of extensor muscle spasms (after 6 months). The period of minimal reflex activity is characterized by weak flexor responses to nociceptive stimuli, noted first in distal muscle groups, flaccid muscles, absence of deep tendon reflexes, and Babinski's sign. The phase of flexor muscle spasms is associated with increasing tone in the flexor muscles and stronger responses to painful stimuli. It is during this phase that the triple flexion response is seen, which involves simultaneous flexion at the hip, knee, and ankle in response to a mild nociceptive stimulus. The most exaggerated form of this reflex is the mass reflex provoked by trivial stimuli and resulting in bilateral powerful triple flexion responses. In the mass reflex, afferent impulses spread bilaterally over many spinal cord segments and cause repeated discharge of flexor motor units. This powerful reflex is distressing to the patient, who is unable to prevent it. The mass reflex tends to diminish as extensor muscle tone begins to increase. Extensor muscle tone ultimately predominates, and some patients can momentarily support their weight in a standing position. There is hyperactive deep tendon reflexes, clonus, and bilateral Babinski's signs. Persistent loss of bowel and bladder control presents a major problem.

Acknowledgments

This work was supported by research grants to Malcolm B. Carpenter (C07005 from the Department of Defense, Uniformed Services University of the Health Sciences, and from the NS-26658 from the National Institutes of Health, Bethesda, MD) and John H. Martin (NS36835). The opinions and assertions contained herein are the private ones of the authors and are not to be construed as official or reflecting the views of the Department of Defense or the Uniformed Services University of the Health Sciences. Experiments reported herein were conducted according to the principles set forth in the *Guide for the Care and Use of Laboratory Animals*, Institute of Laboratory Animal Resources, National Research Council, National Institutes of Health Publication No. 80-23.

REFERENCES

1. Rexed B. The cytoarchitectonic organization of the spinal cord in the cat. J Comp Neurol 1954;100:297–379.
2. Gordon J. Spinal Mechanisms of Motor Coordination. In ER Kandel, JH Schwartz, TM Jessell (eds), Principles of Neural Science. New York: Appleton & Lange, 1991;580–595.
3. Dum RP, Strick PL. The origin of corticospinal projections from the premotor areas in the frontal lobe. J Neurosci 1991;11:667–689.
4. Kuypers HGJM. Anatomy of the Descending Pathways. In JM Brookhart, VB Mountcastle (eds), Handbook of Physiology, Neurophysiology. Vol. II. Bethesda, MD: American Physiological Society, 1981;597–666.
5. Fries W, Danek A, Scheidtmann K, et al. Motor recovery following capsular stroke. Role of descending pathways from multiple motor areas. Brain 1993;116(Pt 2):369–382.
6. Roland PE, Zilles K. Functions and structures of the motor cortices in humans. Curr Opin Neurobiol 1996;6:773–781.
7. Zilles K, Schlaug G, Matelli M, et al. Mapping of human and macaque sensorimotor areas by integrating architectonic, transmitter receptor, MRI and PET data. J Anat 1995;187:515–537.
8. Geyer S, Ledberg A, Schleicher A, et al. Two different areas within the primary motor cortex of man. Nature 1996;382:805–807.
9. Strick PL, Preston JB. Two representations of the hand in area 4 of a primate. I. Motor output organization. J Neurophysiol 1982;48:139–149.
10. Sato KC, Tanji J. Digit-muscle responses evoked from multiple intracortical foci in monkey precentral motor cortex. J Neurophysiol 1989;62:959–970.
11. Martin JH. Differential spinal projections from the forelimb areas of the rostral and caudal subregions of primary motor cortex in the cat. Exp Brain Res 1996;108:191–205.
12. Drew T, Jiang W, Kably B, et al. Role of the motor cortex in the control of visually triggered gait modifications. Can J Physiol Pharmacol 1996;74:426–442.
13. Porter R, Lemon R. Corticospinal function and voluntary movement. Oxford: Oxford Science, 1993.
14. Muakkassa KF, Strick PL. Frontal lobe inputs to primate motor cortex: evidence for four somatotopically organized "premotor" areas. Brain Res 1979;177(1):176–182.
15. Picard N, Strick PL. Motor areas of the medial wall: a review of their location and functional activation. Cereb Cortex 1996;6(3):342–353.
16. Tanji J. New concepts of the supplementary motor area. Curr Opin Neurobiol 1996;6:782–787.
17. Jackson SR, Husain M. Visuomotor functions of the lateral pre-motor cortex. Curr Opin Neurobiol 1996;6:788–795.
18. Matelli M, Luppino G, Rizzolatti G. Patterns of cytochrome oxidase activ-

ity in the frontal agranular cortex of the macaque monkey. Behav Brain Res 1985;18:125–136.

19. Coulter JD, Jones EG. Differential distribution of corticospinal projections from individual cytoarchitectonic fields in the monkey. Brain Res 1977;129:335–340.

20. Shinoda Y, Yokota J, Futami T. Divergent projections of individual corticospinal axons to motoneurons of multiple muscles in monkey. Neurosci Lett 1981;34:111–115.

21. Muir RB, Lemon RN. Corticospinal neurons with a special role in precision grip. Brain Res 1983;261:312–316.

22. Cheney PD, Fetz EE, Mewes K. Neural mechanisms underlying coricospinal and rubrospinal control of limb movements. Prog Brain Res 1991;87:213–252.

23. Nathan PW, Smith MC. The rubrospinal and central tegmental tracts in man. Brain 1983;105:223–269.

24. Hartmann-von Monakow K, Akert K, Kunzle H. Projections of precentral and premotor cortex to the red nucleus and other midbrain areas in Macaca fascicularis. Exp Brain Res 1979;34:91–105.

25. Robinson FR, Houk JC, Gibson AR. Limb specific connections of the cat magnocellular red nucleus. J Comp Neurol 1987;257:553–577.

26. Cheney PD, Mewes K, Fetz EE. Encoding of motor parameters by corticomotoneuronal (CM) and rubromotoneuronal (RM) cells producing postspike facilitation of forelimb muscles in behaving animals. Behav Brain Res 1988;28:181–191.

27. Massion J. The mammalian red nucleus. Physiol Rev 1967;47:383–436.

28. Wilson VJ. Vestibulospinal reflexes and the reticular formation. Prog Brain Res 1993;97:211–217.

29. Grillner S, Hongo T, Lund S. The vestibulospinal tract. Effects on alpha-motoneurones in the lumbosacral spinal cord in the cat. Exp Brain Res 1970;10(1):94–120.

30. Shinoda Y, Ohgaki T, Futami T. The morphology of single lateral vestibulospinal tract axons in the lower cervi-

cal spinal cord of the cat. J Comp Neurol 1986;249(2):226–241.

31. Shinoda Y, Ohgaki T, Sugiuchi Y, et al. Morphology of single medial vestibulospinal tract axons in the upper cervical spinal cord of the cat. J Comp Neurol 1992;316:151–172.

32. Abzug C, Maeda M, Peterson BW, et al. Cervical branching of lumbar vestibulospinal axons. J Physiol 1974;243:499–522.

33. Siegborn J, Grant G. Brainstem projections of different branches of the vestibular nerve. An experimental study by transganglionic transport of horseradish peroxidase in the cat. I. The horizontal ampullar and utricular nerves. Arch Ital Biol 1983;121:237–248.

34. Walberg F, Pompeiano O, Brodal A, et al. The fastigiovestibular projection in the cat. An experimental study with silver impregnation methods. J Comp Neurol 1962;118:49–75.

35. Houser CR, Barber RP, Vaughn JE. Immunocytochemical localization of glutamic acid decarboxylase in the dorsal lateral vestibular nucleus: evidence for an intrinsic and extrinsic GABAergic innervation. Neurosci Lett 1984;47:213–220.

36. Carpenter MB, Batton RRI. Connections of the fastigial nuclei in the cat and monkey. Exp Brain Res Suppl 1982;6:250–295.

37. Monaghan PL, Beitz AJ, Larson AA, et al. Immunocytochemical localization of glutamate-, glutaminase- and aspartate aminotransferase-like immunoreactivity in the rat deep cerebellar nuclei. Brain Res 1986;363:364–370.

38. Brodal A. The Reticular Formation of the Brain Stem: Anatomical Aspects and Functional Correlations. Springfield, Il: Charles C Thomas, 1957.

39. Basbaum AI, Ralston DD, Ralston HJD. Bulbospinal projections in the primate: a light and electron microscopic study of a pain modulating system. J Comp Neurol 1986;250:311–323.

40. Saper CB, Loewy AD, Swanson LW, et al. Direct hypothalamo-autonomic connections. Brain Res 1976;117:305–312.

41. Loewy AD, Saper CB. Edinger-Westphal nucleus: projections to brain stem and spinal cord in the cat. Brain Res 1978;150:1–27.

42. Westlund KN, Bowker RM, Ziegler MG, et al. Origins and terminations of descending noradrenergic projections to the spinal cord of monkey. Brain Res 1984;292:1–16.

43. Loewy AD, Burton H. Nuclei of the solitary tract: efferent projections to the lower brain stem and spinal cord of the cat. J Comp Neurol 1978;181:421–449.

44. Loewy AD, McKellar S, Saper CB. Direct projections from the A5 catecholamine cell group to the intermediolateral cell column. Brain Res 1979;174:309–314.

45. Patten J. Neurological Differential Diagnosis. London: Harold Starke Ltd, 1977.

46. Lawrence DG, Kuypers HG. The functional organization of the motor system in the monkey. I. The effects of bilateral pyramidal lesions. Brain 1968;91:1–14.

47. Tower SS. Pyramidal lesions in the monkey. Brain 1940;63:36–90.

48. Lawrence DG, Kuypers HG. The functional organization of the motor system in the monkey. II. The effects of lesions of the descending brain-stem pathways. Brain 1968;91:15–36.

49. Seitz RS, Hoflich P, Binkofski F, et al. Role of the premotor cortex in recovery from cerebral artery in farction. Arch Neurol 1998;55:1081–1088.

50. Benecke R, Meyer BU, Freund HJ. Reorganization of descending motor pathways in patients after hemispherectomy and severe hemispheric lesions demonstrated by magnetic brain stimulation. Exp Brain Res 1991;83:419–426.

51. Carr LJ, Harrison LM, Evans AL, et al. Patterns of central motor reorganization in hemiplegic cerebral palsy. Brain 1993;116:1223–1247.

52. Muellbacher W, Artner C, Mamoli B. The role of the intact hemisphere in recovery of midline muscles after recent monohemispheric stroke. J Neurol 1999;246:250–256.

2

Anatomy and Physiology of the Vascular Supply to the Brain

J. P. MOHR AND WILLIAM L. YOUNG

BRAIN ANATOMY

The brain is divided into two major areas, the large cerebral convexities connected by the white matter pathways known as the *corpus callosum*, and the brain stem, which extends as a narrow stalk from the upper end of the spinal cord through the skull base and links the brain above with the spinal cord below.

Convexities

The surface of the brain is a continuous but highly folded structure that results in a large surface area compacted into the narrow confines of the skull (Figures 2-1 and 2-2). Major and minor clefts, known as *sulci* or *fissures*, separate the two halves of the brain and the major portions (known as *lobes*) from one another. Most of them are readily identifiable.

In each half (hemisphere) of the globule-shaped brain (sphere), these major clefts (sulci, fissures) serve as anatomic landmarks. The most prominent is the fissure of Sylvius (sylvian fissure), which runs from the inferior frontal surface on the side of the brain, broadly separating the upper and anterior (frontal) lobe from the lower, posterior (temporal) lobe. Opening up this large fissure exposes the island (insula) of Reil. Another large fissure or sulcus, the Rolandic fissure, passes up the side of the brain, above the sylvian fissure. This structure is of interest because of its relative constancy of position and because the major motor (forward of the fissure) and sensory (behind the fissure) systems straddle it.

In front of the rolandic fissure, in the frontal lobe of the brain, are fissures that separate other numerous wrinkles (convolutions). The subdivisions of the brain surface resulting from the presence of these major and minor fissures are usually reliably enough present to be described as the *inferior, middle,* and *superior lobules* of the frontal lobe. The frontal lobe is heavily involved in motor activity and it makes up two-thirds of the volume of each cerebral hemisphere. The portion of brain behind the rolandic fissure is known as the *parietal lobe* (Latin for *wall*). Its upper and lower halves, usually slightly divided by the long, curving intraparietal fissure, contain the main sensory functions of the brain. The back portion of the parietal lobe has so many small convolutions that no accepted scheme has been developed for naming all the convolutions. However, some of the commonly found convolutions have names that roughly reflect their shape or position: the angular gyrus, postparietal gyrus, and inferior parietal gyrus, among others. These sites play important roles in mediating reading, writing, and speech and language function in the left (language-dominant) hemisphere. On the lower side of the cerebral hemispheres is the *temporal lobe*, so named because it has long been assumed to govern the temporal sense of time and sleep; its functions also include memory and hearing. This long lobe runs the length of the lower side of the brain, bounded in its anterior half from above by the sylvian fissure and in its posterior half by the parietal lobe. The *temporal lobe* has three barely distinguishable minor sulci, the first, second, and third temporal gyri. The temporal lobe blends at its rear end with the region at the very back of the brain, the occipital lobe. This lobe, much of which is on the under and inner aspects of the brain, is involved with vision. A large mass of fibers, the corpus callosum, binds the two halves of the brain together.

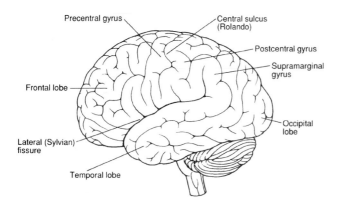

FIGURE 2-1 Lateral view of the brain. Labels show main lobes and gyri.

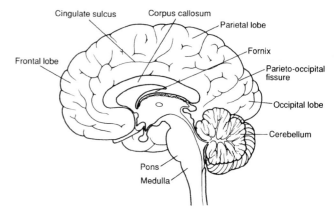

FIGURE 2-2 Medial view of the sagittal section of the brain. Labels show main lobes and gyri.

Depths of the Hemispheres

Each half of the brain contains large collections of cells clustered in formations that could be referred to as *clusters* or *kernels*, but that are given Latin and Greek names as *nuclear groups*, or *ganglia*, respectively. Complex functions are arranged in these masses of nerve cells, among them coordination of the various motor and sensory pathways. A large collection of nuclear groups arranged in the center of the depths of the brain, forming the extreme upper end of the brain stem and supporting much of the brain above, is known as the *thalamus* (Greek for *inner chamber*). Through this structure are routed many of the pathways that connect the brain above with the brain stem and spinal cord below. To either side of the thalamus are the basal ganglia, which process motor movements. The nerve cell bodies are anatomically similar, whether on the crest of a fold (convolution or gyrus) or down in a cleft between folds (fissure or sulcus).

Brain Stem

The brain stem, which is the upward extension of the spinal cord, carries sensory and motor information to and from the brain by means of long bundles of fibers known as *tracts* or *pathways*. Embedded in the brain stem and differentiating it from spinal cord functions are a variety of specialized regions that control breathing, heart rate, blood pressure, and similar functions; movement of the face, mouth, and throat; and sleep and wakefulness.

Cerebellum

Attached to the back of the brain stem is the cerebellum (Latin for *little brain*), a structure that sits astride the brain stem like a small roof. It forms the bulge at the lower back of the head. The cerebellum contains nerve cells important for fine coordination.

VASCULAR ANATOMY AND ISCHEMIC SYNDROMES

Arterial occlusions from thrombosis or embolism produce clusters of findings or syndromes that have distinguishing characteristics for each arterial territory. Many classical syndromes are now recognized, most of them based on long-standing assumptions that occlusive strokes produce predictable effects on the location and size of the brain injury. Modern awareness of the considerable variation in size and location has modified these views, and the classical syndromes should be considered only as models against which the actual clinical picture for a given patient can be compared.[1] The following section reviews the anatomy of each vessel and those syndromes most commonly associated with ischemia in its territory.[2]

Carotid Artery System

Common Carotid Artery

Occlusion of the common carotid artery has the largest variation in clinical syndromes. It may not produce any neurologic effects at all if its flow needs are supplied well enough by collaterals linking it and the vertebrobasilar circulation, either intracranially, extracranially, or both. In some cases the carotid on one side is linked with its opposite side by effective collaterals through the thyroid gland, the tongue, even the vessels across the face. Infrequently, no compensatory replacement (collateral) flow exists and the entire hemisphere depending on the carotid is destroyed, causing total loss of function on the side of the head, trunk, and limb opposite to the occlusion, often with fatal results.

The most frequent sources of collateral develop between the vertebral and the external carotid vessels. The extracranial vertebral artery can form an anastomosis with the occipital branch of the external carotid artery at the skull base, through which retrograde flow reaches the external carotid artery in the front of the neck, fills back to the bifurcation in the common carotid, and through this long route supplies the brain by anterograde flow up the internal carotid artery to the brain. Such patients often surprise their doctors and themselves to learn that an imaging test (see the sections Magnetic Resonance Imaging, Computed Tomography, and Angiography) has discovered an occluded common carotid artery.

Internal Carotid Artery

Arteriosclerosis (also known as *atherosclerosis)* tends to accumulate at the origin of the internal carotid artery at and just above the bifurcation of the common carotid artery. When plaque formation severely limits flow or when the artery (with plaque or previously healthy) is suddenly occluded by a plug of clotted blood carried through the blood stream, or the artery suffers dissection (splitting or fracture) from trauma, the hemisphere on that side has far more limited sources of immediate compensation collateral circulation and symptoms are often produced.[3] The external carotid artery forms anastomoses extracranially with the internal carotid artery via the vessels of the eye and orbit, most often through the ophthalmic artery. Intracranially, collaterals may develop across the circle of Willis, which in many people is capable of linking flow to the endangered carotid territory from the basilar artery below or from the carotid artery from the other side. In some cases the compensatory flow is sufficient to spare the hemisphere any injury. Less commonly, the linkages (border zones) between the major arteries over the surface of the hemispheres may provide some flow to minimize the effects of the reduced flow coming to the brain from the occlusion below. The internal carotid artery supplies the ipsilateral eye (by means of the middle and anterior cerebral artery), the entire frontal lobe, and almost all of the temporal and parietal lobes. Blindness in the eye from occlusion of the ophthalmic artery is rare, owing to the excellent collateral system from the external carotid artery at the level of the eye, collateral not as readily available to the brain above.

The intracranial symptoms of carotid artery occlusion reflect the loss of function of that cerebral hemisphere. When fully developed the syndromes include contralateral hemiparesis with an associated sensory loss. Speech and language disorders (aphasia) occur when the left (language-dominant) hemisphere is infarcted. Disturbance in awareness of the neurologic deficit occurs when the infarct involves the right, or opposite, so-called nondominant hemisphere. An impairment in vision to the opposite side of space (hemianopia), affecting the vision of each eye to the same degree (homonymous hemianopia) is infrequent. The damage to the frontal or parietal lobe often creates an impairment of awareness of objects in the opposite side of space (hemineglect). Coma is rare, because some degree of collateral circulation usually spares the anterior cerebral artery and parts of the middle cerebral artery.

Middle Cerebral Artery

The blood supply to the surface of the cerebrum is composed of some 12–15 individual branches, which are usually grouped into an upper (anterior) division and a lower (posterior) division. The upper division supplies the entire island of Reil (insula, a deep fold of tissue in the sylvian fissure), most of the frontal lobe, and almost all of the convex surface of the anterior half of the parietal lobe. The lower division branches at the posterior end of the sylvian fissure, supplying almost all of the temporal lobe, the posterior half of the parietal lobe, and the adjacent lateral occipital region. At and along a short distance from its origin (this short section is known as the *stem*), the middle cerebral artery gives off the dozen or so small single arteries that penetrate into the depths of the hemisphere to supply the basal ganglia, known as the *lenticulostriate arteries*. These supply the caudate nucleus, anterior limb, genu, and posterior limb of the internal capsule, putamen, external capsule, and claustrum.

The middle cerebral artery and its branches are occluded more frequently by clotted blood particles carried along the blood stream (*embolism*) than is any other intracranial vessel, although the stem is occasionally blocked by atherosclerosis. Occlusion of the main trunk causes infarction of the basal ganglia, internal capsule, and a large portion of the cerebral hemisphere, resulting in contralateral hemiplegia, hemianesthesia, and hemianopia.[4] The speech and language disorder is often quite severe, a syndrome known as *total* or *global aphasia*, and is accompanied by impaired awareness of the opposite side (hemineglect). When the infarct is large, the hemianopia may be caused by involvement of the visual radiations deep in the brain. More often, the hemianopia is part of a syndrome of hemineglect for the opposite side of space and is accompanied by failure to turn toward the side affected by the hemiplegia in response to stimuli from that side.[4]

When the occlusion involves only the upper division of the middle cerebral artery, the sensorimotor syndrome is similar to that of occlusion of the stem. When the hemiparesis involves the face and arm more than the leg, the picture is the opposite of that seen in anterior cerebral artery disease. Isolated weakness of the face, arm, or leg is rare and is seen only with the smallest focal infarcts. Aphasia, when it occurs, is most often of the motor type (Broca's aphasia) because the occlusions usually affect the anterior branches of the upper division. A slightly different syndrome, one featuring speech errors of mispronounced words (known as *literal paraphasias*), occurs if the damage is limited to the posterior (anterior parietal) branches of the upper division. Pure aphasia (grossly deranged comprehension and language errors in spoken and written responses, known as *Wernicke's aphasia*) occurs, typically without any accompanying hemiparesis or hemisensory syndrome when the territory supplied by the lower division in the hemisphere dominant for speech and language suffers infarction, whereas behavioral disturbances featuring hemineglect may appear alone when the same region in the opposite hemisphere is involved. When the involvement is limited to the territory of a small penetrating artery branch of the main stem, a small, deep infarct (lacuna) may occur, affecting the internal capsule, producing a syndrome of pure hemiparesis, without sensory, visual, language, or behavior disturbances.

Anterior Cerebral Artery

The stem of the anterior cerebral artery gives rise to small branches that penetrate into the brain to supply the anterior limb of the internal capsule, the head of the caudate nucleus, and the anterior putamen. The anterior cerebral artery distal to the trunk courses forward, upward, and then backward over the corpus callosum, which it supplies, to reach its major territory, the frontal lobe or pole, upper portion of the anterolateral frontal lobe, and the medial surface of the cerebral hemisphere including the paracentral lobule. The paracentral lobule provides motor and sensory control for the legs and genitalia. Occlusion of the proximal portion of the anterior cerebral artery is rare.

Obstruction of one or more of its surface branches produces paralysis and sensory loss (hemiparesis and hemisensory syndrome) chiefly affecting the leg of the opposite side. Occlusion of the anterior cerebral artery serving the dominant hemisphere may precipitate profound changes in behavior, producing a severe reduction in the rate and complexity of language and speech responses. This syndrome is known as *abulia* (from the Greek, referring to lack of will), or, if severe, as *akinetic mutism*. Involvement of the medial (inner wall) surface of the frontal lobe, and perhaps of the corpus callosum, may lead to ideomotor dyspraxia, which is disruption in the ability of the limbs served by the nondominant hemisphere to respond correctly to verbal commands.

Posterior Cerebral Artery

The area supplied by the posterior cerebral artery includes the inferomedial portions of the temporal and occipital lobes, including the calcarine cortex. This artery usually arises from the basilar artery but is a branch of the internal carotid in 10% of cases. It supplies the midbrain and thalamus via small, deep-penetrating branches arising from the trunk. Thalamic infarction can give rise to delayed development of contralateral, agonizing, burning pain (Déjérine-Roussy syndrome). More often, the infarction involves the cortical territory of the posterior cerebral artery beyond the brain stem. When infarction is confined to the calcarine cortex, contralateral homonymous hemianopia occurs, unaccompanied by other deficits. Commonly, collateral flow from the anterior cerebral artery across the cuneus spares the upper bank of the calcarine cortex; in such cases, the infarct may be confined to the lower bank and may present only as contralateral upper quadrantic homonymous hemianopia. Small infarcts anterior to the calcarine cortex and posterior to the callosum may cause isolated disturbances in spatial orientation. Larger infarcts involving the lingual and fusiform gyri produce disturbances in discrimination and naming of colors and in reading half of words in the contralateral visual field, a syndrome more obvious when the dominant hemisphere is involved. Still larger infarcts affecting the dominant hemisphere may result in total alexia and disturbances in the recall of names for a wide variety of items (amnestic aphasia). The hippocampus is usually affected only by the largest infarcts, but when it is involved as part of a dominant hemisphere infarct, a severe amnestic state occurs, which usually fades over a period of months.

Vertebrobasilar System

Vertebral Arteries

The two vertebral arteries supply muscles of the neck in their extracranial course and form anastomoses with the occipital scalp branches of the external carotid artery. The vertebral arteries also supply branches to the spinal cord via the anterior and posterior spinal arteries. After entering the cranium through the foramen magnum, the vertebral arteries pass across the anterior surface of the medulla oblongata and fuse together at the pontomedullary junction to form the basilar artery.

Occlusion of a vertebral artery at its origin from the subclavian is usually asymptomatic, because collateral flow develops via the ipsilateral occipital branch of the external carotid artery. This form of collateral is the reverse path that may spare the common carotid any effects of occlusion. Intracranial occlusion may result in lateral medullary infarction. If the infarct also affects the cerebellum, owing to involvement of the posterior inferior cerebellar artery (which comes off the vertebral artery near its termination), the edema associated with the cerebellar infarct may produce life-threatening brain stem compression within days, a result that often develops with little warning. Finally, in the few cases in which one vertebral artery provides essentially the entire supply to the basilar artery, its occlusion leads to a full basilar artery syndrome.

Basilar Artery

The basilar artery is formed by the junction of the two vertebral arteries and supplies blood to the pons, midbrain, and cerebellum. It usually forms the two posterior cerebral arteries but may terminate at the level of the superior cerebellar arteries and is connected to the posterior cerebral arteries only by a small trunk. Occlusion of the basilar artery can produce a wide spectrum of syndromes. Which one occurs depends on the site of the occlusion and the efficiency of the collateral circulation.[5] In most instances, the basilar artery is occluded by the process of thrombosis, and the syndrome is usually preceded by transient ischemic attacks. These attacks commonly consist of fragments of the subsequent infarct syndrome. The symptoms most often encountered in vertebrobasilar transient ischemic attacks are dizziness, diplopia, dysarthria, circumoral numbness, ataxia, and hemiparesis or hemisensory disturbances on one or both sides of the body. When thrombosis occludes the basilar artery, collateral flow is often efficient, often limiting the symptoms of basilar occlusion to the region supplied by the small branches at the actual site of the occlusion. Each side of the brain stem can be divided into two areas: the paramedian and the lateral. The paramedian area is nourished by short, perforating arteries that arise from the basilar or vertebral arteries. The lateral area is supplied by surface-conducting arteries that travel some distance from their point of origin before entering the brain stem. Occlusions of paramedian vessels result in paresis of the arm and leg on the contralateral side and involvement of one or more cranial nerves on the same side as the lesion. The usual presentation is ipsilateral ophthalmoplegia from involvement of the third nerve nucleus and pathways; less often it is contralateral hemiparesis from damage to the cerebral peduncle. The majority of symptomatic paramedian branch occlusions involves the pons. Because the bulk of the ventromedial portion of the pons controls motor movements, occlusions result in some form of partial or complete contralateral hemiparesis or ataxia, either alone or as a prominent part of the syndrome.

Depending on how deep the band of infarction penetrates, a number of cranial nerves may be involved ipsilaterally: Infarction of the seventh nerve as it hooks around the sixth nucleus paralyzes the face; infarction of the nucleus of the sixth nerve makes the eye on the side of the lesion deviate inward because of paralysis of the abducting muscles; if the lesion is a little larger, paralysis of conjugate gaze occurs to the side of the lesion, owing to involvement of the medial longitudinal fasciculus and related pathways. Rhythmic contractions of the palate (palatal myoclonus) may occur with damage to the olivodentatorubral connections. The occlusion of paramedian branches supplying the medulla oblongata, a rare event, causes softening of the pyramid, the nucleus of the twelfth nerve, the medial lemniscus, and the medial portion of the olive. The result is paralysis and atrophy of the homolateral half of the tongue, paralysis of the opposite arm and leg, and impairment of the tactile sensation in the trunk and extremities on the paralyzed side.

The circumferential arteries, which arise from the basilar artery, supply the dorsolateral areas of the brain stem and the cerebellum. Occlusion of these vessels disrupts cerebellar projections and the nuclei and tracts in the lateral portion of the brain stem. The important structures in this area of the brain stem are the sensory nuclei of the fifth and eighth cranial nerves, the descending sympathetic pathways, and the ascending spinal lemniscus. The superior cerebellar artery, which arises immediately below the termination of the basilar artery, supplies the lateral area of the midbrain. Its involvement produces a syndrome of cerebellar dysfunction that can be so mild that only slight ataxia is encountered even when the infarct is large; palatal myoclonus is rare, and impairment of pain and temperature of the entire contralateral half of the body occurs only occasionally. The anterior inferior cerebellar artery supplies the lateral area of the pons. Its occlusion produces ipsilateral cerebellar ataxia (brachium conjunctivum), deafness (eighth nerve nucleus), facial paralysis (fifth nerve nucleus), and loss of touch sensibility in the face with contralateral impairment of pain and temperature (lateral spinothalamic tract). Infarction of the lateral area of the medulla usually results from occlusion of the intracranial portion of the vertebral artery, producing Wallenberg's syndrome, manifested by dysphagia and dysarthria; ipsilateral Horner's syndrome of miosis, ptosis, and diminished sweating of the face, neck, and axilla; ipsilateral impairment of pain and temperature on the face; ipsilateral cerebellar ataxia; and contralateral impairment of pain and temperature on the body. Hiccups usually occur, but the lesion site is uncertain. This remarkable syndrome produces little long-term disability itself, but when the cerebellum is infarcted edema may be voluminous enough to produce fatal brain stem compression.

Brain Vascular Physiology

A number of techniques are used to study the blood flow and anatomy of the brain in health and disease: Doppler (named for Christian Doppler, who discovered the compression and expansion effect on sound waves) ultrasonography devices measure blood flow in vessels; angiography, which requires injection of contrast agents directly into the circulation to demonstrate the anatomy of the vessels (Figure 2-3); computed tomography (CT)

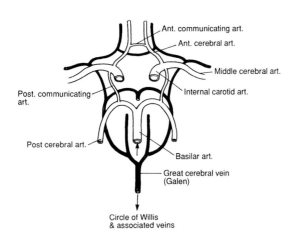

FIGURE 2-3 Schematic representation of the arterial circle of Willis and accompanying veins.

and magnetic resonance imaging (MRI) visualize alterations in tissues directly.

Magnetic Resonance Imaging

MRI (formerly known as *nuclear magnetic resonance* [NMR]) is among the most modern techniques for diagnosing stroke caused by hemorrhage or occlusion. This technique is based on the interaction between magnetically induced radio waves and nuclei of the element hydrogen in the presence of a powerful magnetic field. The strong magnetic field makes the body parts being scanned susceptible to excitation by a radiofrequency pulse. Once excitation occurs, the energy absorbed from the radio transmission is released at a rate that can be measured, and the measurements can be displayed as images. Because bone gives little in the way of an MR signal, MRI offers an imaging advantage over CT for infarcts in the brain stem.

When magnetic field effect is stopped, the tissue being scanned emits the absorbed energy, which is detected by a huge coil surrounding the imaged body parts. In releasing this stored magnetic field energy, the parts imaged undergo complete *relaxation*. During the process of relaxation, the released energy, measured as two tissue-specific relaxation constants known as *T1* and *T2*, is measured and images are reconstructed from the signals obtained. In clinical practice, three types of images are generated: In the favored T2-dependent ones spinal fluid has increased or lighter signal intensity than the brain; in T1-dependent images spinal fluid has decreased or darker signal intensity than the brain, and fat has increased signal intensity; and in *balanced* images the signals from brain and spinal fluid are comparable. Images of brain tissue are obtained in *slices*.

To diagnose and date hemorrhage, pulse sequences known as *T2* and *T1* are necessary, whereas to diagnose small infarcts, a long-interval T2 image is preferred. The changes in tissue water accompanying infarction are easily documented by MRI, making it a useful technique to follow the evolution of cerebral infarction (Figures 2-4 and 2-5).

No signal is obtained from flowing blood, which moves out of a plane of section before it has a chance to give up the stored magnetic energy absorbed earlier, so the vessels appear as nonsignal zones. These signal-empty sites can be inspected to assess the patency of arteries, and current MRI techniques thus allow estimation of the course of vessels, their patency, and even some estimation of narrowing; this imaging is now known as MR angiography (Figure 2-6).

Paramagnetic agents, especially gadolinium, enhance MRI through blood–brain barrier disruption. Constant

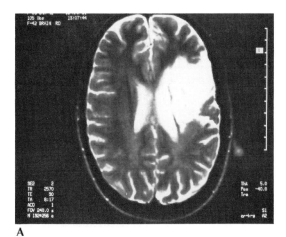

A

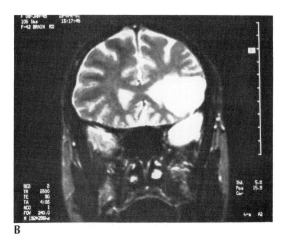

B

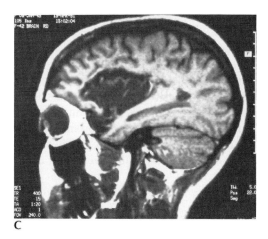

C

FIGURE 2-4 Magnetic resonance imaging shows a large left cerebral infarct: **A.** T2-weighted transverse view. **B.** T2-weighted coronal view. **C.** T1-weighted sagittal view.

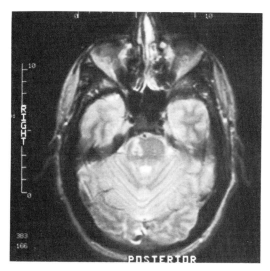

FIGURE 2-5 T2-weighted magnetic resonance image shows a right-sided brain stem infarct.

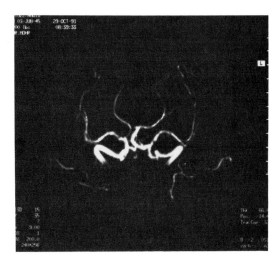

FIGURE 2-6 A normal magnetic resonance angiogram of the distal internal carotid arteries, middle cerebral arteries, and anterior cerebral arteries.

and continued improvements in magnet design and in computer programming are creating images far more detailed than those seen at first. It has even become possible to image ongoing chemical reactions in the brain and assess brain activity through a process known as *MR spectroscopy.*

Computed Tomography

Using computers that measure the tissue absorption of x-rays, it is possible from among the tiny differences in absorption values to magnify and separate x-ray attenu-

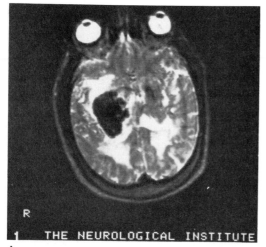

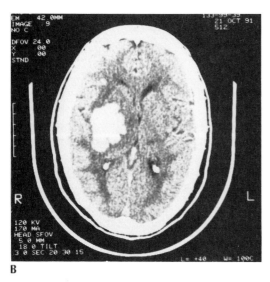

FIGURE 2-7 Magnetic resonance imaging (**A**) and computed tomographic (**B**) images show a large right basal ganglia hemorrhage.

ations of tissues and display the images of air, fluid, brain, and bone as separate shades of gray. The term *attenuation* refers to the degree of loss of the initial x-ray energy through absorption of the x-rays as they are passed through tissues. Air absorbs none, water absorbs little, and bone absorbs a great deal, so signal attenuation is considerable through bone. The actual calculation of the amount of lost energy permits a display of the individual sites inside the head and allows a picture of brain tissue, spinal fluid, skull bone, and an array of attenuations reflecting tissue loss from stroke, compacted blood in an area of hemorrhage, irregular attenuations associated with tumors, and so on. To achieve

this result, a fan beam of x-rays is emitted from a single source, passes through the patient's body, and is received by an array of detectors. The x-ray source rotates around the body, and the attenuated x-ray beams are measured by each of the detectors along various lines through the plane of section, divided into compartments called *pixels*.

Modern CT imaging permits differentiation of white and gray matter, the main divisions of the basal ganglia and the thalamus. Injection of certain chemicals into the blood results in enhanced contrast in a CT scan, increasing the image intensity of the signals from acutely damaged brain tissue, from normal or chronically damaged tissue, and from air, fat, soft tissue, and calcification. Even the major arteries can be imaged. Because of the thick bone and small size of the brain tissue, images from the posterior fossa are still not satisfactory. CT is a reliable means of displaying and measuring the size of intracranial hemorrhages in the first week, when they exhibit their characteristic high density (Figure 2-7). The high signal of fresh blood is lost over days to weeks, owing to chemical changes in the blood. Consequently the CT appearance evolves from initial hyperdensity through an isodense (subacute) phase to hypodensity in the chronic state. During the subacute phase, contrast administration may result in ring enhancement around the hemorrhage. In the chronic state, a hematoma is usually reduced to a slit-like cavity and may disappear entirely. Subarachnoid hemorrhage is even more transient and may not appear on the CT scan at all unless it is particularly dense. With infarction, the CT may be normal for the first 4 days; if the collateral blood supply to the region is large, CT findings are usually positive within 24 hours, showing reduced density of the image because of the fluid accumulation (edema; Figures 2-8 and 2-9) or high-density zones when hemorrhagic transformation has occurred.[6] Infarcts with little collateral supply or edema may remain isodense for days or weeks, later appearing only as focal atrophy. Contrast enhancement of infarction usually occurs within a week and may persist 2 weeks to 2 months. Standard CT techniques do not image the extent of ischemia separate from infarction.

Angiography

Angiography involves the injection of contrast agents directly into the arteries to demonstrate the anatomy of the vessels using either conventional radiographic or digital subtraction techniques. It remains unsurpassed in demonstrating occlusion (Figure 2-10), ulceration and injuries to the large arteries, and stenosis of small arteries. It is relied on for detection of aneurysms and arteri-

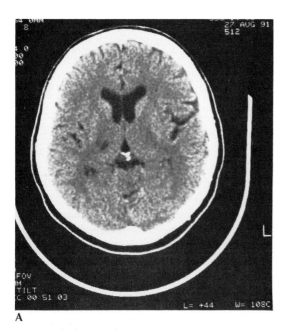

A

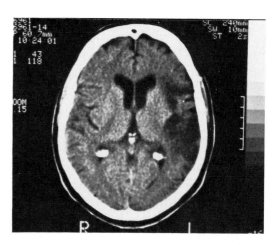

FIGURE 2-9 Computed tomographic image of a large left middle cerebral artery territory infarct.

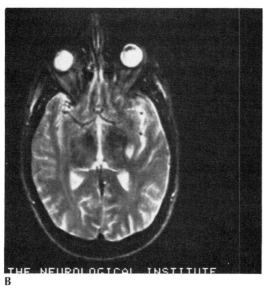

B

FIGURE 2-8 A. Computed tomographic image shows a small, deep infarct in the posterior limb of the right internal capsule. **B.** Magnetic resonance image of a similar infarct in the left internal capsule.

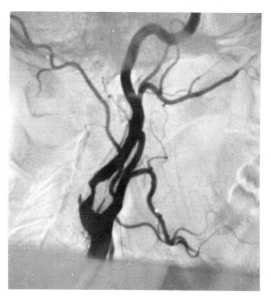

FIGURE 2-10 Digital subtraction angiogram shows tight stenosis at the origin of the right interior carotid arteries.

ovenous malformations. Angiography fails to reliably image vessels smaller than 0.5 mm in diameter and so is not usually helpful in diagnosing the cause of deep infarctions caused by occlusion of tiny vessels. Before direct brain imaging methods were devised, angiography was much relied on to outline intra-axial and extra-axial hematomas, evaluate vasospasm after ruptured aneurysms, and estimate the degree of extracranial arte-

rial stenosis. Many of these conditions are now subject to diagnosis by noninvasive methods.

Angiography is uncomfortable and carries a small risk. At present it is used when alternative noninvasive imaging modalities fail to conclusively diagnose the cause of a stroke. Thus, it requires appropriate fore-thought to maximize the information to be gained. For a diagnosis of embolism, angiography should be under-taken within hours of the ictus, as the embolic particle may fragment early, changing the appearance of the affected vessel from occlusion to one indistinguishable from arterial stenosis or arteritis, and may subsequently appear patent with a normal lumen. In cases in which atheromatous stenosis of large arteries is suspected, pre-angiographic Doppler insonation helps to focus the angiographic study, allowing the angiographer to concentrate on the major territories thought to be diseased.

Doppler Insonation and Imaging

The simplest Doppler ultrasonographic devices pass a high-frequency continuous-wave sound signal over the vessels in the neck, receive the signals reflected from moving blood in the arteries and veins, and feed them through a small acoustic speaker, rather like the police microwave transmitter bounces energy off passing cars to estimate their speed. The examiner detects flow by the changing pitch of the sound waves. Duplex Doppler devices have two crystals, one atop the other (duplex), in a single probe head, one crystal insonating the vessel for evidence of flow, and the other analyzing the reflected sound waves to create an image of the vessel wall (B-mode imaging). Improvements in crystal design are steadily reducing the size of the probe, but its size still makes it difficult to image and insonate the carotid artery high up under the mandible. The crystal in modern Doppler units has an *adjustable range gate* to permit analysis of flow signals from specified depths in the tissues, from a fraction of a millimeter up. This gating eliminates conflicting signals where arteries and veins overlie one another. Some devices have two range gates, allowing an adjustable *volume* or *window* to insonate the moving column of blood in an artery in volumes as small as 0.6 mm, the size of the tightest stenosis. The capacity to interrogate the flow pattern from wall to wall across the lumen makes this technique sensitive for detecting, measuring, and monitoring degrees of vascular stenosis. Because the duplex Doppler unit is sensitive to cross-sectional area and not to wall anatomy, its use before angiography often warns the angiographer to seek stenoses that might not otherwise be noticed. The sonographic images of the vessels are relatively insensitive to most minor ulcerations, which are better seen by conventional angiography. Duplex Doppler methods, although developed to insonate the carotid arteries, can also be used to study the extracranial vertebral artery passing through the intervertebral foramina.

Transcranial Doppler

Using a probe with great tissue penetration properties, it is possible to insonate the major vessels of the circle of Willis, and the vertebral and basilar arteries. Transcranial Doppler devices are range gated but not (yet) duplex, so they document the direction and velocity of

the arterial flow, and spectrum analysis of the signal allows estimation of the degree of stenosis. Extracranial stenosis severe enough to restrict flow (hemodynamically significant) has been shown to damp the waveform in the ipsilateral arteries distal to the stenosis, allowing the effect of the extracranial disease to be measured and followed over time. All these techniques are demanding; patience and skill are required to detect the signal and then to find the best angle for insonation at a given depth. Minor anatomic variations can cause otherwise misleading changes in signal strength; however, as the procedure is fast and safe and uses a probe and microprocessor of tabletop size, the device can be taken to the bedside, even in an intensive care unit. There it can be used to diagnose developing vasospasm, collateral flow above occlusions, recanalization of an embolized artery, and the presence of important basilar or cerebral artery stenoses. When combined with high-field MRI, it is possible to diagnose basilar and middle cerebral artery stem stenoses entirely noninvasively.

Methods of Assessing Cerebral Blood Flow

Regional Cerebral Blood Flow

The techniques of cerebral blood flow (CBF) determination in humans rely on washin or washout of (ideally) freely diffusable and inert indicators (tracers), where the rate of change in brain concentration is proportional to flow. The basic principles of tracer kinetics are generally applicable to newer CBF methodologies such as positron emission tomography (PET) and single photon emission computed tomography. Kety and Schmidt[7] originally described a 10- to 15-minute period of inhalation of 15% nitrous oxide (N_2O). The tracer reaches equilibration between arterial and venous (and therefore tissue) concentrations, and samples are taken intermittently from a peripheral artery and the jugular bulb for determination of tracer concentration. The amount of tracer taken up by the brain over a period of time must equal the amount of tracer delivered to the brain via the arterial blood minus that recovered by the cerebral venous blood in the same amount of time. Assuming that the brain concentration is proportional to venous concentration, CBF can be determined with knowledge of the blood–brain partition coefficient of the tracer used. Ingvar and Lassen[8] offered significant progress in measurement of human cerebral perfusion. The technique involves injecting a radioactive tracer (krypton 85 or xenon 133) as a bolus directly into a carotid artery. After the cerebral washout with external scintillation, counting over the skull allows determination of regional CBF. Modern noninvasive methods were developed primarily by Obrist et al.[9] and later modified by Prohovnik et al.[10] A 1-minute period of inhalation of xenon 133 is followed by a 10-minute period of washout, which is similar to that achieved with intra-arterial concentration. The input of tracer to the brain is not instantaneous, but is smeared, owing to mixing of the tracer in the heart and lungs. The slow compartment (corresponding to white matter flow for the intracarotid method) is contaminated by extracranial clearance, making the noninvasive method suitable principally for assessing gray matter flow. Serial studies are easily done and are limited only by cumulative radiation exposure, which is minimal. CBF may be measured over both hemispheres and in the posterior fossa with a fair degree of spatial (two-dimensional) resolution, because the isotope is delivered to all areas of the brain.

Single Photon Emission Computed Tomography
In one technique of brain imaging, a camera sensitive to radioactivity (gamma camera) is used to count the density of signals emitted from an injected agent minutes after it is given intravenously. The injected agent circulates through the vasculature and is concentrated where the vessels are open and the flow is greatest. In addition to tracers, which are trapped in tissue in proportion to CBF, xenon 133 washout may be used for imaging with single photon emission computed tomography cameras. The emitted signals are assigned to pixels and displayed in slice form, like CT images. The technique is inexpensive, shows regional flow abnormalities from occlusions of individual branches, and is a sensitive test of perfusion disturbances that are larger than the areas of tissue damage.

Positron Emission Tomography
PET also generates axial images using a technique similar to MRI, but the agents that are injected or inhaled are short-lived isotopes. Regional brain metabolic activity is reflected in the emitted metabolic end products of such important substrates as oxygen and glucose. The images obtained are still poorly focused and fuzzy, but PET remains the only currently practical technique for imaging chemical reactions in the living brain.

Cold Xenon Computed Tomography
The cold xenon method uses a standard CT scanner. The patient breathes a relatively high concentration of nonradioactive xenon (30%). The change in x-ray transmission through the brain with washin and washout of the gas can be quantified in a manner analogous to the quantification of radioactive xenon with a gamma camera. This method generates tomographic CBF information similar to that generated by single photon emission computed tomography and PET. Unfortunately, high concentrations of xenon are not physiologically inert and may have mild anesthetic effects.

Magnetic Resonance Imaging of Cerebral Perfusion
Although it is still experimental, progress is being made in developing paramagnetic tracers that will allow washin and washout determinations using standard MRI equipment. This will be a major advance in clinical imaging of cerebral physiological function.

Determinants of Cerebral Blood Flow Autoregulation
Autoregulation entails matching of metabolic demand with the blood supply–bearing substrate. The metabolic demand of the brain is totally dependent on the oxidative metabolism of blood-borne glucose, which fuels all cellular processes. A large part of basal metabolism is devoted to the maintenance of the normal transmembrane ion gradients, the most important being maintenance of intracellular potassium and extracellular sodium. The remainder of basal metabolism is concerned with protein and neurotransmitter synthesis and other basic cellular functions. Two different factors seem to be involved in autoregulation: local metabolic factors and myogenic responses. The exact mechanism by which local metabolic factors are related to CBF is unclear; probably many factors play a role. At one time it was thought that increased hydrogen ion concentration alone controlled vascular resistance, but this is doubtful now. Although extracellular hydrogen ion can increase CBF, it is not required for cerebrovascular dilatation. Extracellular potassium and calcium appear to have minor roles in the control of local CBF. Evidence suggests that endothelium-derived nitric oxide is the predominant metabolic *messenger* between cerebral function and a tightly regulated continuous supply of oxygen, as borne by CBF. Other cellular metabolites that may serve as messengers for regulation of vascular tone include cyclo-oxygenase products of phospholipid membrane metabolism and adenosine. Autonomic nerves do not appear to be necessary for this autoregulatory response, but they may modify it.

Hemodynamic Autoregulation

Vascular autoregulation refers to the intrinsic capacity of the cerebral vasculature to maintain constant blood flow in the face of varying cerebral perfusion pressure. CBF remains constant between mean arterial pressures of 50 and 150 mm Hg in normotensive persons by virtue of active vasomotion at the arteriolar level.[11] Autoregulation may be affected by either disease or concomitant drug therapy. If mean arterial pressure decreases to less than 50 mm Hg, the resistive beds of the cerebral vasculature become maximally dilated. CBF decreases with a further fall in mean arterial pressure. When mean arterial pressure is greater than 150 mm Hg, the cerebral vasculature becomes maximally constricted; CBF increases passively as perfusion pressure further increases. In chronic arterial hypertension, the autoregulatory curve is displaced to the right. Because of this adaptation to higher pressure with vessel wall hypertrophy, marked increases in blood pressure may not result in CBF increases; however, a blood pressure reduction that would be of no consequence in normotensive persons could result in a significant reduction in cerebral perfusion that may be poorly tolerated by the hypertensive patient.[12] There is evidence that with antihypertensive medication and gradual normalization of blood pressure, the autoregulatory curve shifts back toward the left (toward normal) and tolerance of hypotension is improved.

CBF normally is not altered by small changes in central venous pressure, but with severe right-sided heart failure, central venous pressure is greatly increased and cerebral perfusion pressure may be significantly lowered.[13] Arterial oxygen and carbon dioxide concentrations also determine CBF. Oxygen tension exerts its predominant effect at the extremes of oxygen concentration. Moderate changes in arterial oxygen concentration near the physiological range do not influence CBF, although hypoxemia is a most potent stimulus for increasing CBF.

Cerebrovascular resistance is exquisitely sensitive to changes in carbon dioxide tension. The greatest responsiveness to carbon dioxide changes occurs when the PCO_2 is in the physiological range of 20–60 mm Hg. CBF changes by $PaCO_2$ are influenced by the arteriolar tone set by the systemic arterial pressure. Moderate hypotension blunts the ability of the cerebral circulation to respond to changes in $PaCO_2$, and severe hypotension abolishes it altogether.[14] The mechanism by which carbon dioxide exerts its effect on cerebrovascular resistance is not known. Current evidence suggests that cerebrovascular resistance is varied by interstitial pH rather than $PaCO_2$ directly. Carbon dioxide, as a product of oxidation, provides a feedback loop for vasomotor control. With an increase in metabolic rate, carbon dioxide production is increased, causing vasodilatation and increased CBF. The increased blood flow provides a more plentiful supply of nutrients and clearance of lactic and hydrogen ions from the extracellular space, decreasing the amplitude of local pH changes. In the face of continuing hypercapnia or hypocapnia, CBF tends to return toward normal levels. This occurs through a process of pH normalization brought about by varying cerebrospinal fluid bicarbonate concentrations. As a clinical corollary, artificial hyperventilation to reduce intracranial pressure by decreasing CBF is not effective for indefinite periods, and, as these changes in bicarbonate require 24–36 hours to fully evolve, chronic hypocapnia or hypercapnia should not be rapidly corrected.

REFERENCES

1. Mohr JP. Clinical Worsening in Acute Stroke. In N Battistini, et al. (eds), Acute Brain Ischemia: Medical and Surgical Therapy. New York: Raven Press, 1986;173–178.

2. Mohr JP, et al. The Harvard cooperative stroke registry. Neurology 1978; 28:754–762.

3. Castaigne P, Lhermitte F, Gautier JC, et al. Internal carotid artery occlusion: a study of 61 instances in 50 patients with postmortem data. Brain 1970;93:231–258.

4. Caplan LR, et al. Right middle cerebral artery inferior division infarcts: the mirror image of Wernicke's aphasia. Neurology 1986;36:1015–1020.

5. Caplan LR. "Top of the basilar" syndrome. Neurology 1980;30:72–79.

6. Fishman R. Brain edema. N Engl J Med 1975;293:706–711.

7. Kety SS, Schmidt CF. Nitrous oxide method for the quantitative determination of cerebral blood flow in man: theory, procedure and normal values. J Clin Invest 1948;27:475–483.

8. Ingvar DD, Lassen NA. Quantitative determination of regional cerebral blood flow in man. Lancet 61;11:806–807.

9. Obrist WD, Thompson HK, Wang KS, et al. Regional cerebral blood flow estimated by 133-xenon inhalation. Stroke 1975;6:245–256.

10. Prohovnik I, Knudsen E, Risberg J. Accuracy Models and Algorithms for Determination of Fast Compartment Flow by Non-invasive ^{133}Xe Clearance. In P Magistretti (ed), Functional Radionuclide Imaging of the Brain. New York: Raven Press, 1983;87–115.

11. Aatru AA, Merriman HG. Hypocapnia added to hypertension to reverse EEG changes during carotid endarterectomy. Anesthesiology 1989;70:1016–1018.

12. Solomon RA, Fink ME, Lennihan L. Early aneurysm surgery and prophylactic hypervolemic hypertensive therapy for the treatment of aneurysmal subarachnoid hemorrhage. Neurosurgery 1988;23:699–704.

13. Young WL, Prohovnik I, Ornstein E, et al. Monitoring of intraoperative cerebral hemodynamics before and after arteriovenous malformation resection. Anesth Analg 1988;67:1011–1014.

14. Young WL, Solomon RA, Prohovnik I, et al. ^{133}Xe blood flow monitoring during arteriovenous malformation resection: a case of intraoperative hyperperfusion with subsequent brain swelling. Neurosurgery 1988;22:765–769.

3

Cerebellum and Basal Ganglia

DAVID E. KREBS, SOLOMON YUCHOU SHEN, LUCIEN J. CÔTÉ, AND MALCOLM B. CARPENTER

The cerebellum and basal ganglion have separate embryonic origins, but both contribute to motor control. Pathologic changes in the cerebellum or basal ganglion in the adult produce some similar clinical signs such as tremor and hypotonia. Both structures influence brain stem nuclei, but their major effects are exerted on different motor regions of the cerebral cortex via thalamic relays. Differences between cerebellar and basal ganglion motor control functions are presented in this chapter. Despite our understanding of both structures' anatomy, physiology, and neural mechanisms, much of their function remains obscure. Newer findings about cerebellar and basal ganglia motor control give hints of their functional complexity. What is most amazing is that all these functions are compacted within structures no larger than our fists.

CEREBELLUM

The cerebellum is derived from the rhombic lip, a thickening along the superior margins of the fourth ventricle. This region of the embryonic neural tube is regarded as sensory in nature. Although the cerebellum receives sensory inputs from virtually all receptors, it was not until fairly recently that we have been seriously concerned with its involvement with conscious sensory perception.[1] Sensory information transmitted to the cerebellum is used in the automatic coordination and control of somatic motor function. The cerebellum is a prime example of the importance of sensory integration in motor function.

The external appearance of the cerebellum consists of a median portion, the cerebellar vermis, and two lateral lobes, the cerebellar hemispheres. The cerebellum is composed of (1) a superficial gray cellular mantle, the cerebellar cortex, (2) an internal white matter, composed of fibers, and (3) four pairs of intrinsic nuclei deep within the white matter. The cerebellar cortex, unlike the cerebral cortex, is thrown into narrow leaf-like laminae known as *folia*, most of which are oriented in the transverse plane. Three paired cerebellar peduncles connect the cerebellum with the three most caudad segments of the brain stem: the medulla (inferior cerebellar peduncle), the pons (middle cerebellar peduncle), and the midbrain (superior cerebellar peduncle). Three distinctive parts of the cerebellum are recognized based on embryonic and hodologic (Greek: *Hodos*, path; *logos*, science; the study of neurologic pathways) considerations (Figure 3-1). The phylogenetically oldest part, the archicerebellum, consists of the nodulus and paired appendages known as the *flocculi*. This small part of the cerebellum has connections mainly with the vestibular end organ and the vestibular nuclei and is concerned with maintenance of equilibrium and orientation in three-dimensional space. Archicerebellum is also known as the *flocculonodular lobe* in cerebellar literature. All parts of the cerebellum rostral to the primary fissure constitute the paleocerebellum, also known as the *anterior lobe*. This division of the cerebellum receives input from most stretch receptors (muscle spindles and Golgi tendon organs) and from cutaneous receptors. The anterior lobe of the cerebellum plays an important role in automatic regulation of muscle activity.[2] The newest and largest part of the cerebellum, the neocerebellum, forms the posterior lobe. Input to the posterior lobe of the cerebellum arises from broad regions of the contralateral cerebral cortex

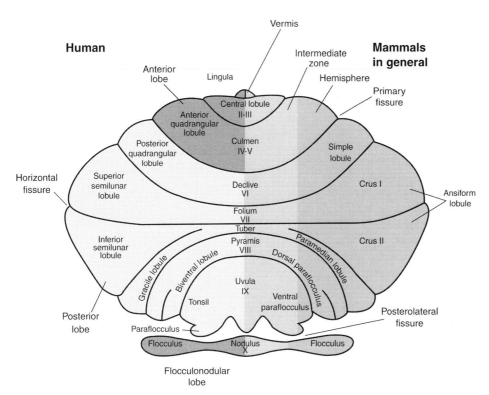

Human

Mammals in general

FIGURE 3-1 Schematic diagram of the fissure, lobules, and functional anatomy of the cerebellum spread out in a single plane. The general division into transversely oriented lobes is indicated on the left side of the diagram, and division into longitudinal zones is on the right. Also on the left side of the diagram are terms classically used for human cerebellum. On the right side are terms from comparative anatomy used more frequently in describing the cerebella of experimental animals. (Reprinted with permission from J Nolte. The Human Brain: An Introduction of Its Functional Anatomy [4th ed]. St. Louis: Mosby-Year Book, 1998;473.)

and is relayed to the cerebellar cortex via the pontine nuclei. The posterior lobe of the cerebellum is concerned with coordination of skilled motor activities initiated at cortical levels. On the other hand, animal studies have led us to view the cerebellum from another perspective. Cerebellums of mammals in general are organized longitudinally instead of horizontally in their anterior and posterior lobes. The spinocerebellum, composed of vermis and the paravermal part of hemisphere, receives multiple somatosensory and special sense outputs. It also controls both proximal and distal motor control and ongoing movement execution. Cerebrocerebellum, the lateral part of the cerebellar hemisphere, receives inputs from the cerebrum. It also involves motor planning, timing, initiation, and motor learning. Studies also suggest cognitive involvement of the cerebellum. Vestibulocerebellum, however, remains consistent with its horizontal structure of flocculonodular lobe.

Cerebellar Cortex

The cerebellar cortex is histologically uniform throughout and consists of three well-defined layers (Figure 3-2). Cells and their processes have specific geometric relationships that are constant and uniform. The three cellular layers of the cerebellar cortex

are (1) a superficial molecular layer, (2) a deep granular layer composed of enormous numbers of small cells, and (3) between these, a ganglionic layer of large flask-shaped Purkinje's cells. The granular layer, closely packed numerous granular cells and little cytoplasm, contains a number of larger inhibitory Golgi cell synaptic complexes known as *cerebellar glomeruli*. Cerebellar glomerulus is a space formed by a bulbus mossy fiber terminal, with multiple granular dendrites and Golgi cell axons. Mossy fibers carry mainly proprioceptive and tactile inputs and indirectly excite the granular cells at the glomerulus. The granular axons send excitatory signals to the molecular layer, which are then carried by parallel fiber to Purkinje's cell dendrites and activate the Purkinje's fiber. The other excitatory input to the cerebellar cortex is climbing fibers, which originate from cerebellum and project into the molecular layer and form numerous synapses. In short, the granular layer receives the principal inputs to the cerebellar cortex and can be regarded as the receptive layer. The Purkinje's cell layer is the discharge layer and gives rise to the only output from the cortex, and it delivers only inhibitory signals. The molecular layer contains a small number of cells and an enormous number of myelinated fibers, a large part of which synapse on Purkinje's cell dendrites. The molecular layer contains axons of granule

FIGURE 3-2 Schematic diagram of the structural elements of the cerebellar cortex. Layers of the cerebellar cortex are indicated on the left. Excitatory inputs to the cerebellar cortex are conveyed by mossy and climbing fibers. Granule cell axons ascend to the molecular layer, bifurcate in a T shape, and form synapses with the dendrites of a number of Purkinje's cells across the width of the cerebellum. Climbing fibers originate from the inferior olivary complex, ascend through all layers, and climb the dendrites of a single Purkinje's cell. Outer stellate, basket, and Golgi cells are all inhibitory. Output from the cerebellar cortex is conveyed by Purkinje's cell axons; these cells inhibit the deep cerebellar nuclei and cells in dorsal regions of the lateral vestibular nucleus. (Reprinted with permission from MB Carpenter. Core Text of Neuroanatomy [3rd ed]. Baltimore: Williams & Wilkins, 1985.)

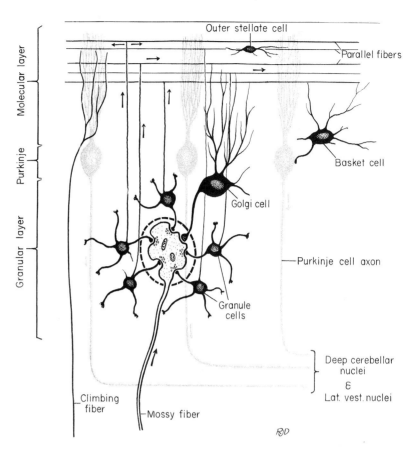

cells, which divide in a T-shaped formation and extend transversely to synapse on the dendrites of a number of Purkinje's cells. Granule cells are excitatory and have glutamate as their neurotransmitter.[3,4] All other neuron types in the cerebellar cortex appear positive for gamma-aminobutyric acid (GABA), an inhibitory neurotransmitter. Golgi cells appear to be the most powerful *GABAergic* neurons in the cerebellar cortex. There is some chemical heterogeneity in Purkinje's cells: Although most contain GABA, some have both GABA and motilin.[5]

All afferent fibers entering the cerebellar cortex lose their myelin sheath and terminate as either mossy fibers or climbing fibers. The most abundant afferents are mossy fibers, which end in the granular layer by breaking up into numerous terminals known as *mossy fiber rosettes*. A single mossy fiber rosette forms the core of a cerebellar glomerulus, a synaptic complex that also contains Golgi cell axons and numerous granule cell dendrites. This synaptic complex controls a major part of the input to the cerebellar cortex because it can inhibit the input to granule cells, which have an excitatory action on Purkinje's cells.[6] Climbing fibers, which originate from the inferior olivary

nuclear complex, are unique because they pass through the white matter, the granular layer, and climb the dendrites of Purkinje's cells (see Figure 3-2). These excitatory fibers, considered to use glutamate as their neurotransmitter, produce all-or-none responses in Purkinje's cells.[7,8] Purkinje's cells are large, GABAergic neurons that serve as the sole output of the cerebellar cortex. Their myelinated axons terminate on neurons of the cerebellar nuclei and certain brain stem nuclei.[9] By sending signals in all-or-none fashion, the nuclei could avoid ambiguity of information. Another example of the importance of Purkinje's cells can be found in research of an individual with complete loss of Purkinje's cells. The individual was unable to consistently produce the same movement direction repeatedly while reaching toward the same target.[10] Without Purkinje's cells, the information collected by the sensory system cannot be integrated, which is the key to the configuration of motor space from sensory input.[11]

Although the cerebellar cortex seems relatively simple and has been regarded in one sense as the *Rosetta stone* of the central nervous system, it has an elaborate structural and functional organization in which multiple

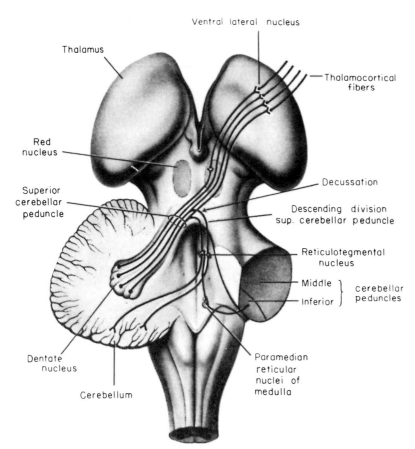

FIGURE 3-3 Diagram of the cerebellum and brain stem shows the cerebellar peduncles and the projections of the superior cerebellar peduncle. Ascending projections from the dentate nucleus project to the rostral third of the opposite red nucleus and to the cell-sparse zone of the thalamus, which includes the ventral posterolateral (pars oralis) and the ventral lateral (pars caudalis) nuclei. (Reprinted with permission from MB Carpenter. Core Text of Neuroanatomy [3rd ed]. Baltimore: Williams & Wilkins, 1985.)

interactions influence conduction of impulses, synaptic articulations, and output, which passes via Purkinje's cell axons to the deep cerebellar nuclei and portions of the lateral vestibular nucleus. The most puzzling feature of the cerebellar cortex is that all excitatory input via mossy and climbing fibers is converted to inhibition[6] (i.e., the entire cerebellar output is inhibitory, so cerebellar pathology results in loss of inhibition or dysmetria and timing difficulties).

Afferent Fibers

Cerebellar afferents are nearly three times more numerous than efferents[12] and, with some exceptions, terminate mainly in the cerebellar cortex. These pathways convey impulses from peripheral receptors and from relay nuclei in the brain stem and spinal cord. Afferents enter the cerebellum largely via the inferior and middle cerebellar peduncles (Figure 3-3).

The inferior cerebellar peduncle conveys input from spinal cord and cerebellar relay nuclei in the medulla. These fibers include the posterior spinocerebellar tract, the cuneocerebellar tract, reticulocerebellar fibers, and olivo-

cerebellar fibers, which numerically form the largest constituent of this bundle. Both the posterior spinocerebellar and the cuneocerebellar tracts convey impulses from stretch receptors (i.e., Ia and Ib fibers) to the anterior lobe of the cerebellum, where they end, topographically.[13]

The middle cerebellar peduncle is the final link in the pathway between the cortex of one cerebral hemisphere and the posterior lobe of the contralateral cerebellum. Corticopontine fibers project to the ipsilateral pontine nuclei, and fibers from pontine nuclei cross in the basilar portion of the pons to enter the cerebellum via the middle cerebellar peduncle. Fibers that form this system are massive and interrelate virtually all regions of the cerebral cortex, including motor, somesthetic, auditory, visual, and associations areas, with parts of the posterior lobe of the cerebellum.

Deep Cerebellar Nuclei

Within the medullary core (white matter) of the cerebellum are four paired nuclear masses, the deep cerebellar nuclei (Figure 3-4). The most lateral and largest is the dentate nucleus, which in section appears as a crumpled bag with the hilus directed medially. This nucleus receives most of its input from Purkinje's cells in the hemisphere. Medial to the dentate nucleus are two smaller nuclei, the emboliform and globose nuclei, which receive inputs from Purkinje's cells in paravermal regions of the cerebellar cortex. Emboliform and globose nuclei are sometimes referred to as *interposed nuclei* in the literature, for most mammals had only one pair of interposed nuclei that carry the functions of emboliform and globose nuclei. The most medial, and second largest of the deep cerebellar nuclei, the fastigial nucleus receives Purkinje's projections from all regions of the cerebellar vermis that converge in a fan-shaped array. The principal efferent fibers from the cerebellum arise from the deep cerebellar nuclei, are excitatory in nature, and are considered to use glutamate as their neurotransmitter.[4] Some direct excitatory influences on the deep cerebellar nuclei arise from extracerebellar sources, such as the red nucleus and the inferior olivary complex. Cortical inhibition of the deep cerebellar nuclei is intermittent and localized.

Efferent Fibers

Two separate cerebellar efferent systems arise from the deep cerebellar nuclei. The largest and most important bundle, the superior cerebellar peduncle, arises from the dentate, emboliform, and globose nuclei, sweeps ventromedially in the caudal midbrain tegmentum, and decussates completely (Figure 3-5; see Figure 3-3). Large numbers of fibers in the emboliform and globose nuclei project fibers and collaterals somatotopically on cells in the caudal two-thirds of the contralateral red nucleus.[14] Fewer fibers from these nuclei project rostrad to terminations in the contralateral thalamic nuclei.[15,16] Fibers from the dentate nucleus contained in the superior cerebellar peduncle project collaterals to the rostral third of the opposite red nucleus and more profusely to terminations in the contralateral thalamus. Projections of these three cerebellar nuclei to the thalamus terminate in parts of the ventral lateral nuclei (pars caudalis) and the ventral posterolateral (pars oralis) nuclei, which have been characterized as the *cell-sparse* zone.[16–18] Fibers from the individual deep cerebellar nuclei terminate in an interdigitating fashion without apparent overlap. Although evidence for a somatotopic representation in the deep cerebellar nuclei is not compelling, the pattern of efferent fiber terminations in the thalamus appears somatotopic: Rostral parts of the body are represented medial in thalamus and anterior body parts (i.e., extremities) ventrally.[16] One of the most important features of the so-called cell-sparse zone of the thalamus is that it

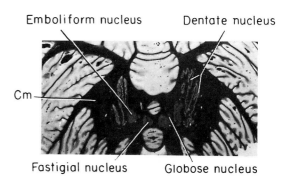

FIGURE 3-4 Section through the cerebellum shows parts of the deep cerebellar nuclei that lie within the white matter of the cerebellum. (Cm = corpus medullare.) (Reprinted with permission from MB Carpenter. Core Text of Neuroanatomy [3rd ed]. Baltimore: Williams & Wilkins, 1985.)

projects directly on the primary motor cortex.[15,19–21] This anatomic circuitry provides a means by which the major output of the deep cerebellar nuclei can influence somatic motor activity.

Fibers and collaterals from the emboliform and globose nuclei projecting somatotopically to the opposite red nucleus can influence ipsilateral flexor muscle activity via the rubrospinal tract (crossed).

Fastigial efferent fibers do not emerge from the cerebellum via the superior cerebellar peduncle. These fibers partially cross within the cerebellum and emerge via the uncinate fasciculus (crossed) and the juxtarestiform body (uncrossed) (Figure 3-6). In the brain stem fastigial efferent fibers are distributed fairly symmetrically in ventral parts of the lateral and inferior vestibular nuclei and in parts of the reticular formation.[22] Smaller numbers of ascending fibers project bilaterally to portions of the cell-sparse zone of the thalamus.[16] Fastigial projections to the lateral vestibular nucleus appear organized to facilitate extensor muscle activity via the vestibulospinal tract (uncrossed). Mori et al. used microtracer mapping stimulus sites of midline cerebellar white matter of the decerebrate cat to demonstrate that the fastigial nucleus is one of the key central sites necessary for the control and integration of posture and locomotor-related neural subsystems within the brain stem and the spinal cord. Cells in the fastigial nucleus are capable of controlling simultaneously the cells of reticulospinal, vestibulospinal, and fastigial pathways origin.[23]

Although most of the cerebellar efferent fibers originate from the deep cerebellar nuclei, regions of the vermal cortex project directly to the lateral vestibular nucleus.[24] Purkinje's cell axons in the vermal cortex project selectively on dorsal regions of the ipsilateral

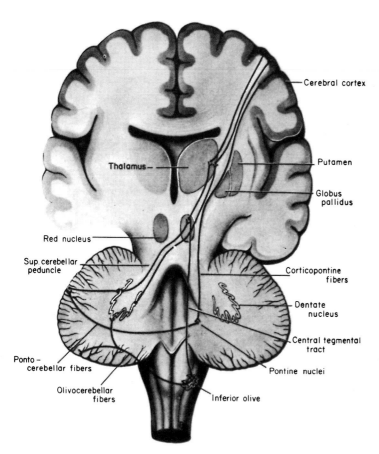

FIGURE 3-5 Schematic diagram of some afferent and efferent cerebellar pathways. Projections from all areas of the cortex pass to the pontine nuclei, which in turn give rise to fibers that pass via the middle cerebellar peduncle to the contralateral half of the cerebellum. Cortical efferents also project to parts of the ipsilateral inferior olivary nucleus, which project crossed climbing fibers to the cerebellar cortex of the opposite side. Purkinje's cell axons project to the deep cerebellar nuclei, which in turn form the superior cerebellar peduncle. Fibers of the superior cerebellar peduncle cross in the midbrain, give collaterals and terminals to the red nucleus, and project to the cell-sparse zone in the ventral lateral thalamus. These thalamocortical fibers are considered to project somatotopically on the primary motor cortex. (Reprinted with permission from MB Carpenter. Core Text of Neuroanatomy [3rd ed]. Baltimore; Williams & Wilkins, 1985.)

lateral vestibular nucleus.[25,26] This connection means that GABAergic Purkinje's cells can directly inhibit extensor muscle activity via their action on cells of the lateral vestibular nucleus.

Cerebellar Functions

Cerebellar function has a major influence on our activities of daily living, which is one of the major concerns for rehabilitation professionals. In fact, children with atrophic cerebellums gave us an insight into cerebellar functions. These children demonstrated muscular hypotonia (deficient muscle activity), delayed development, truncal titubation, and intention tremor. In addition, most of them had fixation nystagmus and esotropia.[27] Important cerebellar functions regarding rehabilitation are equilibrium and balance, coordination, motor learning, speech, and *cognition*. Newer evidence suggests the cerebellum is more than an organ of sensory integration and motor coordination. However, exactly how many functions the cerebellum carries out and a detailed physiological mechanistic analysis of these functions is not yet fully understood.

The cerebellum automatically regulates muscle activity and plays an integral part in virtually all simple and complex motor activities. One of the best ways of demonstrating the important regulatory role of the cerebellum is to describe the disturbances that occur with cerebellar lesions. Several general principles apply to cerebellar lesions: (1) disturbances occur ipsilateral to the lesion, (2) disturbances usually occur as a constellation of related phenomena, (3) disturbances caused by nonprogressive causes undergo attenuation with time, and (4) disturbances are viewed as the physiological expression of the activity of intact structures deprived of the controlling and regulating influences of the cerebellum.

Three distinct cerebellar syndromes are recognized. The most common is the neocerebellar syndrome, associated with lesions of the lateral lobe of the cerebellum involving the dentate nucleus or the superior cerebellar peduncle. This syndrome is characterized by hypotonia and asynergic disturbances. Muscles on the side of the lesion show diminished resistance to movement, are soft, and fatigue easily with minimal activ-

FIGURE 3-6 In a schematic diagram of fastigial efferent fibers, the fastigial nuclei lie in the cerebellar vermis, medial to the other deep cerebellar nuclei. They give rise to fibers that partially cross within the cerebellum (uncinate fasciculus) and ipsilateral fibers that leave the cerebellum via the juxtarestiform body. Crossed and uncrossed fastigial efferent fibers terminate fairly symmetrically in parts of the vestibular nuclei and the reticular formation. Ascending fastigial efferents project bilaterally (not shown), but in smaller numbers, to the cellsparse zone of the thalamus. (FN = fastigial nucleus; MD = mediodorsal thalamic nucleus; RN = red nucleus; [vestibular nuclei: I = inferior; L = lateral; M = medial; S = superior] VL = ventral lateral thalamic nucleus; VPL = ventral posterolateral thalamic nucleus; VPM = ventral posteromedial thalamic nucleus.) (Reprinted with permission from Carpenter MB. Core Text of Neuroanatomy [3rd ed]. Baltimore: Williams & Wilkins, 1985.)

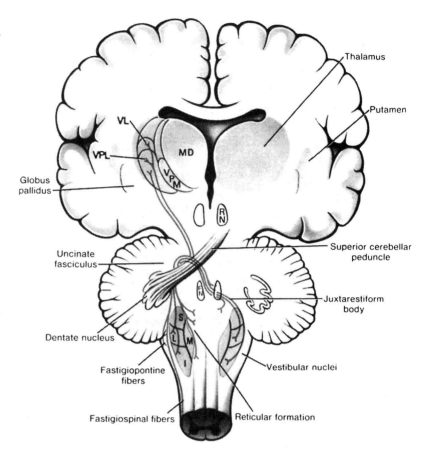

ity. The tendon reflexes often are difficult to obtain and frequently exhibit a pendular quality. Asynergic disturbances are expressed by inappropriate force, direction, and range of muscle contractions. Impairment of ability to gauge distances in the finger-to-nose test is striking. Asynergia underlies the impaired ability to perform rapid successive movements (e.g., alternately pronating and supinating the forearm), the decomposing of complex movements into successive simple movements (e.g., decompensation of movement), and impaired ability to maintain certain positions and postures.[28] The most dramatic asynergic disturbances are tremor and ataxia.[29]

Tremor associated with cerebellar lesions classically occurs during voluntary and associated movement and has a coarse quality, with certain frequencies and irregular amplitude.[30] This tremor is referred to as *intention tremor*, but it is an involuntary motor activity. Cerebellar-induced tremor frequency is predominately 3 Hz.[31-33] On the other hand, tremor amplitude has no clinical value in classification. It can be influenced by a wide range of physiological, psychologi-

cal, and environmental factors. Considerable amplitude variability in pathologic tremor was found even under carefully controlled conditions. In addition to intention tremor, cerebellar patients may also have postural tremor. Various types of postural tremors have been described. The most common consists of oscillations of the arms about the shoulders or of the legs about the hips; it is referred to as *titubation* when it affects the trunk and head. There is also a mild postural tremor that is more rapid (10 Hz) with distal predominance.[31-33] During clinical examination, it is evident on finger-to-nose and heel-to-shin tests. It appears at the initiation and along the course of a movement and has a coarse side-to-side component.[34]

Ataxia is a form of asynergic disturbance that results in bizarre gross and forceful distortions of basic movement patterns. This disturbance involves the large axial muscles and muscles of the shoulder and pelvic girdles that result in wild distortions of gait. The gait is broad based and unsteady, the patient lurches and stumbles, and there is a tendency to overstep and veer to one side. From the preliminary results in our database at the Biomotion Laboratory, Massachusetts General Hospital, we compared the gait profile of cerebellar patients and healthy control subjects. Cerebellar patients spent 20% more time in double-support phase but only 5.8% more time in stance phase as compared with healthy controls. In addition, the swing phases of cerebellar subjects were 7% less than healthy controls. The base of support is 24% larger in cerebellar dysfunction patients than normal control subjects. In other words, cerebellar patients spend more time in a relatively stable double-support phase with a wide base of support. It is a sign of compensated unsteadiness in gait (Figure 3-7). Baloh et al. found patients

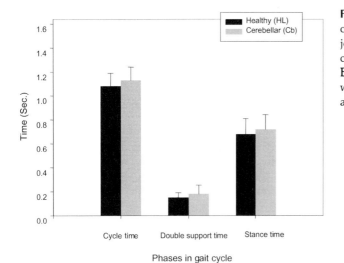

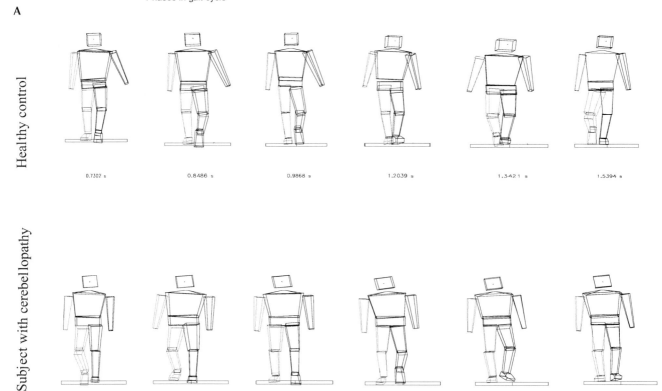

FIGURE 3-7 A. Comparison of different phases within gait cycle of healthy controls and subjects with cerebellopathy. Subjects with cerebellopathy spent more time to complete each gait cycle and spent more time on double support and stance phase. **B.** Androids showing gait cycle of healthy control and subject with cerebellopathy. Subjects with cerebellopathy demonstrated a wider base of support.

with general cerebellar atrophy were unsteady, especially in the anterior-posterior direction in standing, using posturography as a measurement tool. However, posturography did not allow differentiation between cerebellopathy and vestibulopathy patients.[32] From our studies at the Biomotion Laboratory, Massachusetts General Hospital, we were particularly interested in cerebellar ataxic movement under dynamic situations such as moving arms between two horizontal points and negotiating a 7.6-cm step repeatedly. Our studies found lateral postural ataxia actually was exacerbated in dynamic situations (Figure 3-8).[28,35]

In the cerebellum research arena, single or multiple joint arm movements were heavily explored in order to understand the cerebellum's role in coordination. Cerebellar multiple joint movement incoordination was first described in the early twentieth century. Gordon Holmes described cerebellar patients' movements as marionette-like.[2] Individuals with cerebellar dysfunction tend to avoid fast multijoint movements and adopt a slower single-joint movement to improve function and accuracy.[36,37] During upper extremity multiple joint movements, the shoulder and elbow work synergistically in normal subjects,[38] but asynergic shoulder and elbow torques may be present in cerebellar patients.[39,40] Topka et al. further proposed that the asynergy between shoulder and elbow joint was caused by the asynergies of joint antagonists.[41] Although synergy existed between shoulder and elbow, the wrist joint is free from torque synergy. It is, however, sensitive to the velocity and accuracy required for the task.[42,43] Also, subjects with cerebellopathy have more nonplanar movements while pointing ballistically (i.e., cerebellar ataxia). From the database of our laboratory, we found patients with cerebellopathy spent more energy performing upper

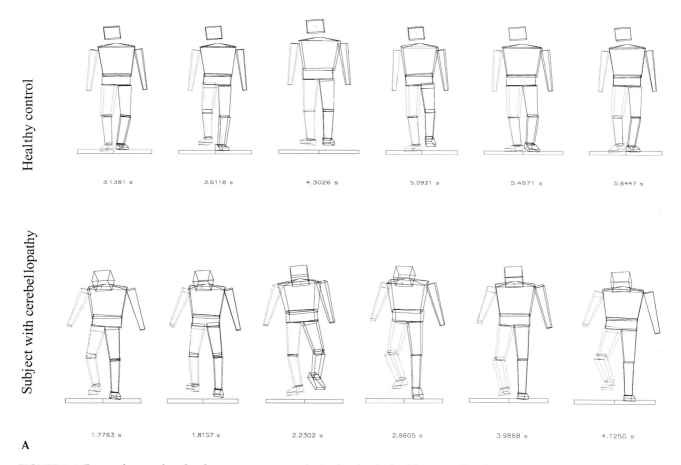

Healthy control

| 3.1381 s | 3.6118 s | 4.3026 s | 5.0921 s | 5.4671 s | 5.6447 s |

Subject with cerebellopathy

| 1.7763 s | 1.8157 s | 2.2302 s | 2.9605 s | 3.9868 s | 4.1250 s |

A

FIGURE 3-8 Postural control under dynamic situations. **A.** Androids of a healthy control and a subject with cerebellopathy while negotiating a 7.6-cm step. Note that the subject with cerebellopathy presented a larger base of support and needed to look down to negotiate the step.

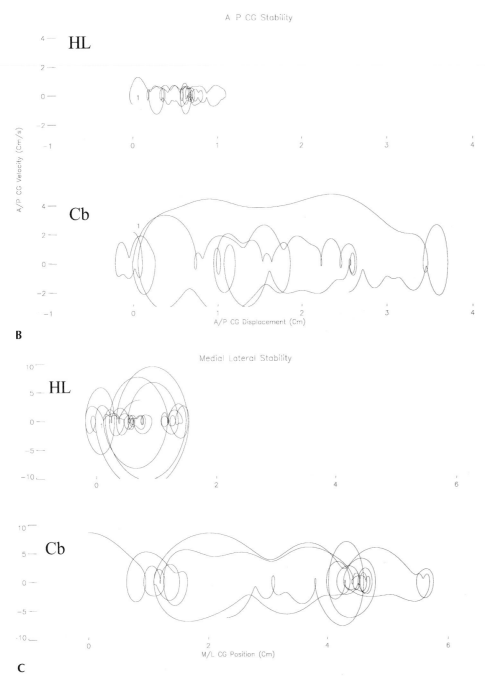

FIGURE 3-8 *(continued)* **B, C.** Anterior-posterior (A/P) and mediolateral (M/L) center of gravity (CG) stability while moving arms between two horizontal points. Subject with cerebellopathy (Cb) has larger CG displacement as well as larger CG velocity in both A/P and M/L directions. This demonstrated the exacerbation of postural stability under dynamic situations. (HL = healthy control.) **D, E.** A/P and M/L CG stability while negotiating a 7.6-cm step. The healthy control subject had a better consistency of CG displacement and velocity.

extremity tasks. The nature of this dexterity problem may not be on individual axial movements and velocities, but on the coordination between multiple axes (i.e., planar movements and velocities) (Figure 3-9).

Patients with cerebellopathy have difficulty with hand dexterity and handwriting. The similarities between handwriting of different amplitude scales in healthy subjects are amazing. Lacquaniti et al. pointed out the existence of two separate but coordinated domains of joint motion: shoulder-elbow complex and wrist. The shoulder and elbow are tightly coupled and work well at large magnitude if wrist motion is limited. On the contrary, wrist movements are dominant when precision was required the most.[44] Animal studies showed damage of anterior interpositus nucleus* and its adjacent dentate impaired preshaping of the hand before grasp and impaired the manipulation of objects, whereas damage to posterior interpositus

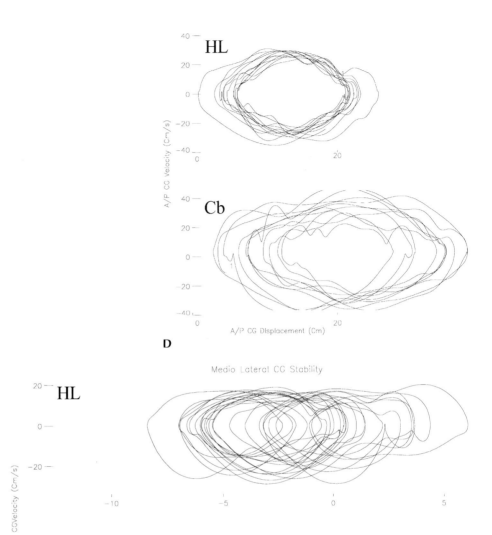

D

Medio Lateral CG Stability

E

nucleus produced deficits in aiming of reach and arm stability.[45]

*Most nonhuman cerebellum has a single nuclear mass called *interposed nucleus*. It is an equivalent to emboliform and globose nucleus combined. Oftentimes *interposed nucleus* is used in the human for the combination of emboliform and globose nuclei.

Common to neocerebellar lesions, cerebellar dysarthria is characterized by slowing down of articulatory movements, increased variability of pitch and loudness, monotonous speech, and articulatory imprecision.[46,47] Over 94% of both learning disabled and the dyslexic samples showed two or more abnormal neurologic test results or electronystagmography (ENG) results, whereas less than 1% had neurologic signs of a cerebral disorder, apparently implying good compen-

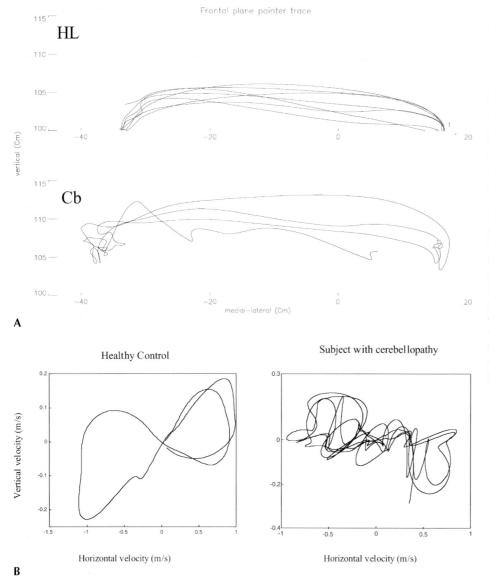

A

B

FIGURE 3-9 A. A comparison of pointing trace between healthy control and subject with cerebellopathy. Subjects were required to move horizontally between two target points in 10 seconds. Healthy control subjects (HL) completed this task not only with a more smooth and flattened trace but also with more repetitions. Subject with cerebellopathy (Cb) is more ataxic at the two ends of the trace, which is one of the contributing factors to why such subjects spent more energy completing upper extremity tasks. **B.** A comparison between healthy control and subject with cerebellopathy on arm coordination. Healthy control subject demonstrates a near perfect figure-of-eight figure when composing the velocities of different axes, whereas subject with cerebellopathy has little control of the velocity. (m/s = meters per second.)

sation for cerebellopathy acquired during youth.[48] A positron emission tomography study also showed lower right cerebellar cortex activity in adults with dyslexia while executing prelearned sequences and during learning new sequences.[49] The underlying neurophysiological mechanism, however, is not yet fully understood.

Lesions involving the posterior vermis (i.e., nodulus and uvula) produce the archicerebellar syndrome. Such lesions particularly affect axial musculature involved in maintenance of equilibrium and in locomotion. This syndrome, seen mainly in children with a midline cerebellar tumor (medulloblastoma), is characterized by unsteadiness in standing, a tendency to fall backward, and ataxic gait. Muscle activity is little affected, and tremor usually is absent.

Nystagmus is common with these lesions and is most pronounced on the lesion side. Most mammals have slight ocular upward drift and torsional skew with prominent downbeat nystagmus following cerebellar lesions. Downbeat nystagmus assumes an inherent vertical asymmetry in the central vestibulo-ocular lesions, as observed in our laboratory (Figure 3-10). Bohmer and Straumann proposed that the vertical asymmetry is caused by the lack of symmetry in the craniocaudal direction. Apparently, each semicircular canal elicits eye movements in the direction roughly of its anatomic plane, and vectorial addition of tonic resting activity of all six canals cancels horizontal and torsional eye movement components, but the vertical (slow phase) upward component remains uncontrolled. This peripheral vestibular bias is normally centrally canceled by archicerebellum (floccular and parafloccular inhibitory pathways), which are related to the smooth pursuit system but disinhibited in the presence of posterior cerebellar lesions.[50]

Although our understanding of human paleocerebellar disease is still limited, some studies indicate that lesions in the anterior lobe of the cerebellum result in severe disturbances of posture and muscle activity.[51,52] Patients with anterior lobe atrophy caused by alcoholism have prevalent anterior-posterior postural sway,[53] wide-based gait, and asynergia of the legs.[2] Positron emission tomography further confirms the involvement of anterior lobe vermis in humans while standing; therefore, the anterior cerebellum aids postural control in humans.[54] However, data from our laboratory suggest that hemispheric and vermal lesions also impair posture, and those anterior lobe lesions impair limb control.[28] In addition, animals with anterior lobe lesions exhibit opisthotonus, hyperactive limb reflexes, increased positive supporting mechanisms, and periodic tonic seizures.[55] Similar tonic seizures occur in humans as a consequence of brain stem compression. Classic studies of Sherrington[56] and Dow and Moruzzi[57] clearly indicate that ablations of the anterior lobe of the cerebellum exacerbate decerebrate rigidity. Exaggerated muscle activity following ablations of the anterior lobe may be caused by the removal of inhibitory influences of Purkinje's cells acting on brain stem nuclei that influence extensor muscle activity.[8,58]

It is indisputable that the cerebellum is a sensory organ, but it may not be exclusively for sensation.[59] The cerebellum receives visual, auditory, and somatosensory information, which is relayed by mossy fibers.[60] The cerebellum contains at least two somatotopic maps of the whole body in the vermal part of the cerebellum, also known as the *projection of spinocerebellum*. Sensory information is carried by mossy fibers to the cerebellum from brain stem or spinal cord, through emboliform and globose nuclei, then projected to cerebellar cortex.[61,62] In animal studies, the projections of sensory input to cerebellar cortex are usually patchily distributed with ill-defined termination and multiple representations of body parts at different locations.[9,61] Moreover, cerebellar representations of different body parts of different sized ani-

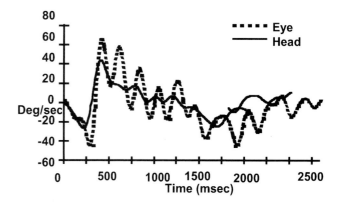

FIGURE 3-10 Patient with impaired vestibulo-ocular pathways eye pitch velocity during chair rise. Note hypermetric eye responses, causing retinal slip.

mals are similarly located, but they differ in size.[63] Considering the evidence and the uniformity of the cerebellar structure, we propose that the cerebellum may be performing approximately similar computations throughout the anterior lobe and cerebellar hemispheres, and this hypothesis seems to fit with the clinical presentation of patients with cerebellar injury.[63] The uncharted territories to cerebellum regarding sensation are the lateral hemispheres. Studies have not been conclusive as to whether the hemispheres have another set of somatosensory maps or are related to any special sense.[64]

It is not fully understood how the cerebellum achieves motor learning. However, from what is known about cerebellar motor learning, the olivocerebellum system is involved. In short, while learning a new task, climbing fibers from inferior olive send signals to Purkinje's cells at glomeruli in cerebellar cortex. An unknown mechanism changes the Purkinje's cell output and sends modified signals to deep cerebellar nuclei. The learning process occurs within this system through repeated movement. With practice, not only is movement improved but the modified signals are also transformed into permanent motor memory. Three major hypotheses have been proposed for cerebellar motor learning: (1) comparator theory, (2) Marr-Albus-Ito theory, and (3) timing and sequencing theory. Comparator theory proposes that the inferior olive is the site controlling information from the central command, transforming it into motor execution. Because the descending and ascending projections to the inferior olive do not converge, it is less likely that the inferior olive nuclei serve as comparators. Marr-Albus-Ito theory proposed that the inferior olive nuclei provide Purkinje's cells with error signals indicating inadequate motor activity, thus serving as a teacher. Timing and sequencing theory proposes that olive nuclei serve as a pacemaker. The pacemaker adjusts its rhythm and sends the rhythm to Purkinje's cells, with resultant changes of motor performance.[62,65] The next question is, Where does the cerebellum store the information once it becomes permanent? Although Marr-Albus-Ito theory indicates it is stored in Purkinje's cells, other researchers suggest such information is probably stored in the deep cerebellar nuclei.[66]

As early as the first half of nineteenth century, clinical neurologists and neuroscientists found that the cerebellum is essential for coordination. Meanwhile, sporadic findings of behavioral problems in cerebellar patients were documented; however, they did not attract enough attention to merit systematic, scientific research.[1] More recently, systematic studies led researchers to other, nonmotor, cerebellar functions. Histoanatomic observation and neuroimaging studies demonstrate that patients with infantile autism actually have a smaller cerebellum, and that the cerebellum is involved with cognitive function.[67,68] Schmahmann and Sherman revealed 11 mental functional category impairments in cerebellar cognitive syndrome patients, which are summarized into four major functions: (1) disturbances of executive func-

tion, (2) impaired spatial cognition, (3) personality change, and (4) linguistic difficulties. These results suggest cerebellar patients not only suffer from incoordination of movement but also have difficulty planning and integrating cognitive response (i.e., disordered and dysmetric thinking). Perhaps all cognitive involvement of the cerebellum is analogous to cerebellar motor control. Although the exact anatomic structures responsible for cerebellar cognitive affective syndrome have not been located, the involvement of the neocerebellum is more impaired than lesions confined to the paleocerebellum.[1,69] However, the extensiveness of cognitive involvement in the cerebellum is not yet fully understood, nor is the underlying physiological mechanism. It is noteworthy that although we discussed cerebellar contribution to cognition, the role of the cerebellum appears to be more of modulation than cognition per se, whereas it is clearly directly involved in motor control.[70]

Clinical Implications

Animal studies from the nineteenth century demonstrated the possibility of cerebellar plasticity. Removal of up to three-fourths of a cat's cerebellum still permits the animal to function.[71] In adult humans with acquired cerebellopathy, there may be some recovery over time. Raymond et al. suggested the histologic uniformity of cerebellar structures implies the uniformity of cerebellar function.[66] They further hypothesized that the whole cerebellum performs the same motor *computations* throughout, but for different parts of the body.[66] Klintsova et al. demonstrated in rats that alcohol-induced pan-cerebellopathy can be rehabilitated through exercise.[72] They concluded that exercise could help surviving Purkinje's neurons retain the capacity for synaptic plasticity.[72] In addition, data from our laboratory demonstrate the benefits of physical therapy to help cerebellopathic patients' dynamic stability during stepping.[73] Thus, there is some evidence that rehabilitation disciplines can help patients with cerebellopathy. Further clinical evidence is needed, however, to support enthusiasm for this notion.

A Case of Acerebellogenesis

We had the opportunity to test a 15-year-old boy with cerebellar agenesis in our laboratory (Figure 3-11). On observation, he was able to walk, turn, and even run, albeit somewhat clumsily. Attention deficit disorder and mild arm and leg incoordination caused his parents to request neurologic consultation at age 11, whereupon

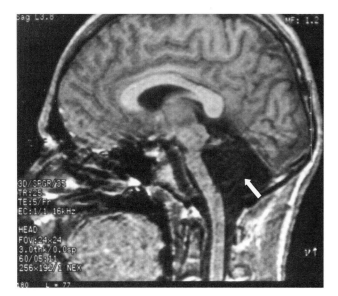

FIGURE 3-11 Magnetic resonance image of a 15-year-old boy with congenital acerebellogenesis. Please note the arrow indicating the empty area where cerebella usually lies.

during magnetic resonance imaging examination the acerebellogenesis was diagnosed. Physical examination demonstrated regular muscle performance, intact sensation, slight muscle hypotonicity, and mild scoliosis. Our laboratory showed he performed gait, chair rise, stair locomotion, and pointing motions similar to healthy control subjects when permitted to attend fully to these tasks. Indeed, upper extremity movements and gait at different speeds revealed only slight timing and accuracy deficits. He required more time to stabilize himself and was hypermetric while responding to standing perturbations.

Mental distracters, however, profoundly impaired his motoric function, especially during activities with an internal or external perturbation, such as chair rise. While singing the national anthem, he interrupted his free-speed, eyes-closed chair rise just after liftoff and literally sat back down. He stated, "I forgot the song!" He showed little difficulty performing chair rise and singing a song separately in prior tests.[74] Having him *sing* silently (to himself) caused a performance decline but no frank interruptions.

We believe this case has at least two interesting features: (1) how highly functional he was and (2) the dramatic change after mental distractions were being added to the motor activities. In the context of the nineteenth century animal experiments we described earlier in this chapter, it is not surprising that our pediatric patient could function well. The cerebellum, although having tremendous influence on sensory, motor, and mental performance in adulthood, always takes a subsidiary role to the cerebrum. Apparently 15 years of life experience required his cerebrum to take over all cerebellar functions. However, the residual deficits were probably the cerebellar functions that are irreplaceable. Given his rather small problems with daily activities, he was well compensated on his sensory, motor, and even cognitive insufficiencies. The problems associated with mental distraction are more substantial and noteworthy. Little evidence was found of cognitive impairment, despite thorough neuropsychiatric testing; there were several clinical reports of cerebellopathy causing difficulty in concentration during complex tasks.[69]

Applying mental distraction is equivalent to performing multiple tasks at the same time. The solutions found in computer science might lead us toward the answer to our question regarding cerebellar function. In the 1980s computer scientists explored the possibility of central processing unit multitasking. Today, most computer models we use are multitasking models, with at least numeric (and usually graphic) copro-

cessors. For example, a PC allows us to play music and surf the Internet at the same time. The technology that made this possible was labeling pieces of information before sending them to the central processing unit so the central processing unit would not be confused about which information belongs to which program. Without the labeling process, the computer would simply crash.[75] To solve the question why our pediatric patient with acerebellogenesis could not perform multiple tasks at the same time may have something to do with this information-labeling process. To date, we are not sure if such a mechanism exists in humans. However, imagine sensory and motor information flowing around the nervous system without labels: It probably only produces confusion. Therefore, individuals with cerebellopathy often need extra attention to function properly and have difficulties performing multiple tasks at the same time. It is still too early to conclude the cerebellum functions as a signal sorter and labeler. Further evidence is needed to tell why patients with cerebellar agenesis have trouble performing multiple tasks.

BASAL GANGLIA

The basal ganglia are five large subcortical structures that are involved in the control of movement. These structures are the caudate, putamen, globus pallidum (GP), subthalamic nucleus (STN), and substantia nigra. Unlike the cerebellum, the basal ganglia do not have direct input or output connections with the spinal cord. The primary input into the basal ganglia is from the entire cerebral cortex to the neostriatum (caudate and putamen), and the output is mainly from the internal segment of the GP and the substantia nigra pars reticulata (SNR) through the thalamus back to the prefrontal, premotor, and motor cortices. Although, the function of the basal ganglia is mediated mainly by the frontal lobes, there are projections from the GPi (internal portion of the globus pallidum) and SNR to the brain stem, including to the pedunculopontine nucleus (PPN) that is involved with locomotion, and the superior colliculi that are involved with eye movements. The basal ganglia are of special interest clinically because pathologic processes in these structures cause abnormal involuntary movements (dyskinesia), changes in posture and muscle tone, and slowness with reduced range of movements (bradykinesia). Although patients with basal ganglia disease often complain of weakness there is little loss of strength as compared with patients with corticospinal tract lesions. Kinnear

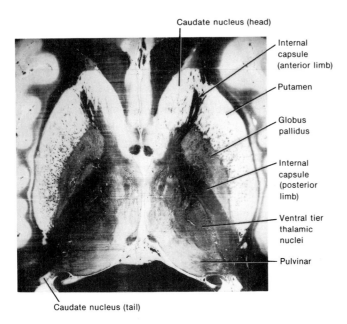

Caudate nucleus (head)

Internal capsule (anterior limb)

Putamen

Globus pallidus

Internal capsule (posterior limb)

Ventral tier thalamic nuclei

Pulvinar

Caudate nucleus (tail)

FIGURE 3-12 Horizontal section through the brain shows the relationships of the corpus striatum (caudate nucleus, putamen, and globus pallidus) to the internal capsule and thalamus.

Wilson, an English neurologist (1877–1937), became interested in studying patients with abnormal involuntary movements, such as tremor, chorea, athetosis, dystonia, and ballism. He observed patients with these abnormal movement disorders and studied their brains at postmortem. He found that many of these patients had lesions in the basal ganglia. He coined the terms *extrapyramidal motor system* for the basal ganglia and *pyramidal motor system* for the corticospinal and corticobulbar tracts. The concept is clinically useful because patients with pyramidal tract lesions present with spasticity and paralysis, whereas those with extrapyramidal tract lesions have involuntary movements, rigidity, and immobility without paralysis. However, these two motor systems are not independent; they are markedly interconnected and cannot be viewed as parallel and separate motor systems. They are highly integrated in the control of movements. In addition, other areas of the brain (i.e., red nucleus, brain stem, and cerebellum) are also involved in movements. Therefore, modern neurophysiologists no longer accept this dichotomy of motor systems. The term *extrapyramidal motor system* is better referred to as the *basal ganglia system*.

Striatum

The caudate nucleus and the putamen together constitute the neostriatum, or striatum, the largest part of the corpus striatum. Both of these nuclear masses are derived from the telencephalon. The putamen lies lateral to the globus pallidus and deep to the insular cortex (Figure 3-12). The caudate nucleus has a C-shaped configuration that follows the curvature of the lateral ventricle (Figure 3-13). Rostrally and ventrally, the caudate nucleus and the putamen are continuous. Cytologically, the caudate nucleus and the putamen appear identical, and both are composed of enormous numbers of primarily small- and medium-sized cells. Two classes of striatal neurons have been identified: those with spiny dendrites and those with smooth dendrites.[76,77] Spiny striatal neurons give rise to seven or eight primary dendrites radiating from the somata and one long axon projecting beyond the striatum (Figure 3-14). Dendrites of these neurons receive all striatal afferents. Axons of these cells provide all efferents. Immunocytochemically, spiny striatal neurons show the presence of GABA, enkephalin (ENK), and substance P (SP).[78-81] Although GABA is the major neurotransmitter, in most cells it coexists with ENK or SP as a neuromodulator.[81]

Three different short-axoned Golgi type II striatal neurons have no dendritic spines (i.e., *aspiny* neurons). These short-axoned cells are intrinsic striatal neurons. The most prevalent type (type I) uses GABA as its neurotransmitter, whereas the giant cells of type II are cholinergic.[82-85]

FIGURE 3-13 Schematic drawing of the isolated neostriatum (caudate nucleus and putamen). The caudate nucleus and putamen are in continuity rostrally and ventrally. The caudate nucleus has a **C** shape that follows the curvature of the lateral ventricle. The tail of the caudate nucleus lies in the roof of the inferior horn of the lateral ventricle and extends rostrally to the amygdaloid nucleus. (Reprinted with permission from MB Carpenter. Core Text of Neuroanatomy [3rd ed]. Baltimore: Williams & Wilkins, 1985.)

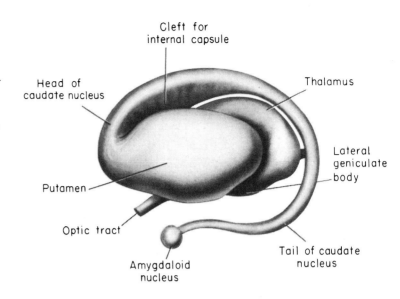

Striatal Afferents

The neostriatum can be regarded as the receptive component of the corpus striatum because it receives massive inputs originating from diverse sources and each input has a different neurotransmitter. All known striatal inputs terminate on dendrites of spiny neurons. Afferents to the striatum originate from (1) broad regions of the cerebral cortex (corticostriate), (2) thalamic nuclei (thalamostriate), (3) the pars compacta of the substantia nigra (SNC; nigrostriatal), (4) the dorsal nucleus of the raphe, (5) portions of the amygdala, and (6) cells of the substantia innominata (Figure 3-15).

Corticostriate Fibers

Corticostriate fibers originate from broad areas of the cerebral cortex and terminate in mosaic patterns.[86-88] The primary motor area projects bilaterally and somatotopically on the putamen in a patchy fashion.[89] Because corticostriate fibers originate from virtually all cortical areas, some of which have no demonstrated motor function, it seems likely that the striatum, or parts of it, may have other functions.[90,91] Corticostriate fibers probably use the excitatory neurotransmitter glutamate.[3,92]

Thalamostriate Fibers

The intralaminar thalamic nuclei have long been identified as a source of input to the striatum.[93] Studies indicate that the centromedian nucleus projects to the putamen and the parafascicular nucleus to the caudate nucleus; few cells in this complex project to both nuclei.[94] The neurotransmitter used by these fibers has not been identified.

Nigrostriatal Fibers

Fluorescence histochemical studies first revealed the extensive nature of the dopaminergic projection system from the pars compacta of the substantia nigra to the striatum.[95-96] Terminal dopamine varicosities form a fine matrix about virtually all striatal neurons; however, clusters of cells within the SNC project to either the putamen or the caudate nucleus, but not to both.[97,98] Pathologic processes that impair the synthesis and transmission of dopamine to the striatum constitute a major feature of Parkinson's disease. Dopamine is regarded as having an inhibitory action on some striated neurons and an excitatory action on others, depending on the receptors (i.e., D_1 and D_2).[99]

Amygdalostriate Fibers

Although the amygdala and the corpus striatum have been considered to have different functions, these structures are in part related by a projection from the amygdala to both the caudate nucleus and the putamen.[100,101] Regions of the striatum that receive afferents from the amygdala are referred to as the *limbic striatum*. In addition, in monkeys approximately 10% of the cells of the substantia innominata (nucleus basalis) project to the caudate nucleus.[102]

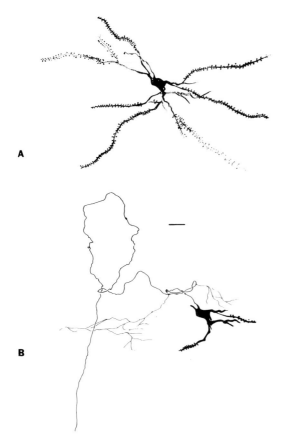

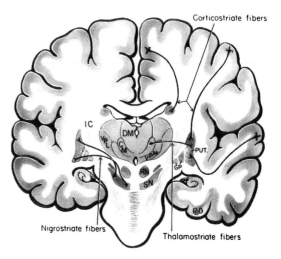

FIGURE 3-15 In a schematic diagram of striatal afferent systems, corticostriate fibers arise from broad areas of the cerebral cortex and terminate in a patchy fashion. Thalamostriate fibers arise from the centromedian (CM) and parafascicular (not shown) nuclei. Nigrostriate fibers convey dopamine to cells in the caudate nucleus and putamen (PUT). Not shown in this schematic are projections from the dorsal nucleus of the raphe, which convey serotonin to ventral parts of the putamen. (DM = dorsomedial nucleus; IC = internal capsule; GP = globus pallidum; SN = substantia nigra; VPM = ventral posteromedial thalamic nucleus; VPL = ventral posterolateral thalamic nucleus.) (Reprinted with permission from MB Carpenter. Core Text of Neuroanatomy [3rd ed]. Baltimore: Williams & Wilkins, 1985.)

FIGURE 3-14 Drawings of a single spiny striatal neuron. All striatal inputs form synapses on dendritic spines of these cells and all axons of these cells project to either the globus pallidus or the substantia nigra. Immunocytochemical studies indicated that these cells have gamma-aminobutyric acid, substance P, and enkephalin as their neurotransmitters; gamma-aminobutyric acid is the dominant neurotransmitter. **A.** Reconstruction of soma and dendrites. **B.** Reconstruction of soma and projecting axon. Calibration in **B** is 20 μm. (Reprinted with permission from MB Carpenter. Core Text of Neuroanatomy [3rd ed]. Baltimore: Williams & Wilkins, 1985.)

Other Striatal Afferents

Other afferents are minor in comparison with those already discussed. They arise from the dorsal nucleus of the raphe, the PPN, the locus ceruleus, and the STN. Serotoninergic neurons in the dorsal nucleus of the raphe project to ventrocaudal regions of the putamen and provide collaterals to the substantia nigra.[103–105] The large cells of PPN are cholinergic and appear to project widely to thalamic nuclei.[106,107] A noncholinergic cell group central to PPN is considered to have projections to the striatum, globus pallidus, substantia nigra, and

STN.[108] The region of PPN is considered to be involved with locomotor functions.[109]

Globus Pallidus

The globus pallidus lies medial to the putamen and consists of two distinct segments separated by thin medullary laminae (Figure 3-16). Unlike the striatum, the globus pallidus is a diencephalic derivative formed from hypothalamic neurons that have migrated lateral to the internal capsule.[110,111] Pallidal neurons are large, ovoid cells with smooth dendrites that ramify in discoid arrays parallel to the medullary laminae.[112,113] Virtually all pallidal neurons appear to use GABA as their neurotransmitter.[3,114,115]

Although the cells in the two segments of the globus pallidus appear morphologically and cytochemically identical, their afferent and efferent connections are different. The medial segment of the globus pallidus (MPS) gives rise to a major part of the output system for the entire corpus; the larger lateral pallidal segment

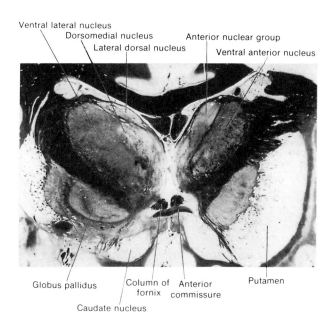

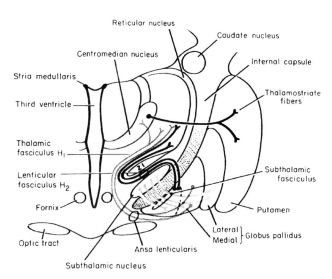

FIGURE 3-16 Asymmetric transverse section through the thalamus, internal capsule, and corpus striatum. On the left, segments of the globus pallidus are well defined by medullary lamina. (Reprinted with permission from MB Carpenter. Core Text of Neuroanatomy [3rd ed]. Baltimore: Williams & Wilkins, 1985.)

FIGURE 3-17 In a schematic diagram of projection fibers from the globus pallidus, pallidal efferent fibers from the medial segment project to rostral ventral tier thalamic nuclei (ventral anterior and ventral lateral) and the centromedian nucleus via the ansa lenticularis and the lenticular fasciculus. These fibers constitute the principal output of the corpus striatum. Fibers from the lateral pallidal segment project mainly to the subthalamic nucleus. The subthalamic nucleus projects mainly to both segments of the globus pallidus but also has a projection to the substantia nigra. (Reprinted with permission from MB Carpenter. Core Text of Neuroanatomy [3rd ed]. Baltimore: Williams & Wilkins, 1985.)

projects mainly to the STN.[116] Surgical attempts to ameliorate dyskinesia due to L-dopa therapy in Parkinson's disease have been directed at interruption of pallidothalamic fibers originating in the MPS.

Pallidal Afferent Systems

Major afferent fibers to the segments of the globus pallidus arise from the striatum and the STN. Unlike the striatum, the globus pallidus does not receive any major inputs from the cerebral cortex, thalamus, or substantia nigra. The most massive inputs arise from spiny striatal neurons and project to both pallidal segments in an organized manner.[117-119]

Striatopallidal fibers traverse the discoid dendritic arbors of pallidal neurons, making multiple synaptic contacts. GABA is the major neurotransmitter of striatopallidal fibers to both pallidal segments,[120] but some of these fibers also contain SP and ENK. ENK fibers terminate selectively in the lateral pallidal segment; fibers containing SP end mainly in the MPS.[121,122]

Subthalamopallidal fibers arise from the STN and project in arrays to both pallidal segments.[123,124] The main neurotransmitter of STN neurons is glutamate.[125]

Pallidal Efferent Systems

Cells in each pallidal segment project to different brain stem nuclei (Figure 3-17). Fibers arising from the MPS project to thalamic nuclei that have access to regions of the motor cortex and in addition have a small descending projection to PPN. Cells in the lateral pallidal segment project almost exclusively to the STN.[124]

Pallidothalamic fibers arising from the MPS must cross through, or go around, the internal capsule to reach the thalamus. These fibers follow both courses. Fibers that loop ventrally around the internal capsule form the ansa lenticularis; those that pass through the internal capsule form the lenticular fasciculus (see Figure 3-17). Both of these fiber bundles merge and project to the rostral ventral tier thalamic nuclei. Pallidothalamic fibers terminate in the ventral lateral (pars oralis) and ventral anterior (pars principalis) nuclei of the thalamus and give off collaterals to the centromedian nucleus.[126,127] Pallidothalamic projections have thalamic terminations distinct and separate from those that originate in the deep cerebellar nuclei.[16,17,20] Thalamic nuclei receiving fibers from the

MPS project to the supplementary motor area (located on the medial aspect of the hemisphere) and to the lateral premotor area.[16,21] Thus, the major influences of the corpus striatum, mediated by striatopallidal, pallidothalamic, and thalamocortical fibers, are on a motor cortical region considered to be concerned with programming of motor activities and known to influence motor function bilaterally.[128] Cells of the MPS have been demonstrated to project collaterals to both the thalamus and the PPN at isthmus levels of the brain stem.[129]

Substantia Nigra

The substantia nigra, the largest single mesencephalic nucleus, lies dorsal to the crus cerebri and extends the length of this brain stem segment (Figure 3-18). The nucleus has two divisions: (1) The pars compacta (SNC), which lies dorsally, contains pigmented (melanin) cells that synthesize dopamine.[95,130] (2) The pars reticulata (SNR), close to the crus cerebri, is composed of less densely packed neurons containing the neurotransmitter GABA.[114] In Golgi preparations of the substantia nigra, cells of the SNC have dendrites oriented dorsoventrally, whereas dendrites of cells in the SNR have a rostrocaudal orientation.[131] Cytologically distinct parts of the substantia nigra have different inputs and outputs. Cells of the SNC consti-

tute the principal source of striatal dopamine, and cells of the SNR form part of the output system from the corpus striatum (i.e., striatonigral and nigrothalamic fibers).

Nigral Afferents

Afferents arise from the striatum, STN, midbrain raphe, and PPN. Each projection has a different neurotransmitter.

Striatonigral fibers form the most massive input to the SNR. Like striatal afferents to the segments of the globus pallidus, these fibers use GABA, SP, and ENK as neurotransmitters. Terminals with different neurotransmitters are segregated in the SNR. GABA is the dominant neurotransmitter.[81]

The neurotransmitter of subthalamonigral fibers projecting to the SNR is as yet unidentified. A single population of STN neurons has been shown to project to both the globus pallidus and the SNR. In rats, virtually all STN neurons project to both sites[132]; in monkeys only approximately 10% of the cells project to both the globus pallidus and the substantia nigra.[133]

Midbrain nigral afferents arise from the dorsal nucleus of the raphe and from the PPN. Cells of the dorsal nucleus of the raphe use serotonin as their neurotransmitter and project to the SNR.[134,135] It is suspected that this projection has an inhibitory influence. Noncholinergic neurons from the midbrain locomotor center near PPN are considered to project to SNR, but their function is unknown.[108]

Nigral Efferent Fibers

Efferent fibers from the two divisions of the substantia nigra project to different nuclei and have different neurotransmitters.

Nigrostriatal fibers arise from the cells of the SNC, have dopamine as their neurotransmitter, and terminate in a fine fiber matrix about all types of striatal neurons. Collections of cells in the SNC project to either the putamen or the caudate nucleus, but not to both.[98] The basic pathologic process in Parkinson's disease involves degeneration of dopaminergic neurons in the SNC, which reduces the synthesis and transmission of dopamine to the striatum. Dramatic improvements result from L-dopa therapy, which raises the level of dopamine in the striatum. L-Dopa, a precursor of dopamine, is given because dopamine does not pass the blood–brain barrier.

Nigrothalamic fibers represent the principal projection from cells of the SNR, which are known to be GABAergic. These fibers project to thalamic nuclei rostral to those that receive fibers from the MPS. In

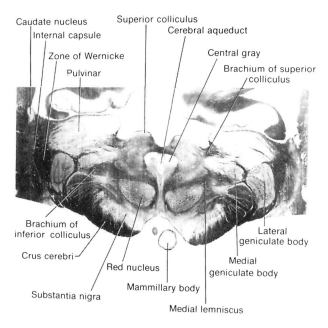

FIGURE 3-18 Transverse section of the midbrain through the substantia nigra. (Reprinted with permission from MB Carpenter. Core Text of Neuroanatomy [3rd ed]. Baltimore: Williams & Wilkins, 1985.)

the thalamus they terminate in the ventral anterior (pars magnocellularis), the ventromedial (pars lateralis), and the paralaminar part of the dorsomedial nuclei.[136,137] These thalamic nuclei are considered to relay signals to the premotor and prefrontal cortex.[138] Fibers that pass to the frontal eye field seem particularly important, as cells in SNR also project large numbers of collaterals to the superior colliculus.[98,139] Although the full significance of the nigrothalamic projection remains unknown, it forms a significant part of the output system of the corpus striatum.

Subthalamic Nucleus

The STN is a small lens-shaped nucleus medial to the fibers of the posterior limb of the internal capsule immediately rostrad to the substantia nigra (Figure 3-19). Like the globus pallidus it is a derivative of the lateral cell column of the hypothalamus. Interest in this nucleus centers around the observation that small lesions in it produce the most violent known form of dyskinesia, hemiballism.[140] Discrete lesions in the STN of monkeys produce a similar form of dyskinesia, the only dyskinesia that can be produced in an animal by a small localized lesion.[141,142]

Neurons of the STN in humans and primates exhibit a wide range of sizes and shapes, have six or seven stem dendrites, and all have long axons. Evolved differences in dendritic development confer on primates the potential for more specific organization.[143,144] Some labeled STN neurons of rats reveal dichotomizing axons with branches that project to both the globus pallidus and the SNR.[145]

Subthalamic Afferents

Projections to the STN arise mainly from the motor cortex and the lateral pallidal segment. Corticosubthalamic fibers project ipsilaterally and somatotopically on lateral parts of the STN[146] and are considered to monosynaptically excite STN neurons.[147] The most massive input to the STN arises from the lateral pallidal segment, to form the pallidosubthalamic projection.[123,124,126,135] It is inhibitory and has GABA as its neurotransmitter.[115,148]

Subthalamic Efferents

Cells of the STN project profusely to both segments of the globus pallidus, and approximately 10% project to both globus pallidus and SNR.[133] The main neurotransmitter of STN neurons is glutamate.[125,149] Claims that it might be GABA[150,151] have not been substantiated by immunocytochemical methods. It has been shown that the STN has excitatory influences on pallidal neu-

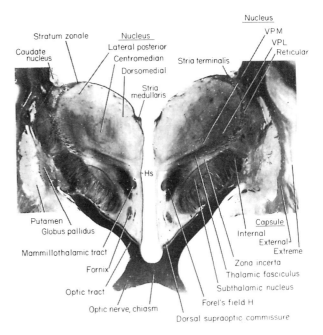

FIGURE 3-19 Transverse section through the diencephalon and corpus striatum shows the subthalamic nucleus on the medial border of the internal capsule. (Hs = hypophysis; VPL = ventral posterolateral thalamic nucleus; VPM = ventral posteromedial thalamic nucleus.) (Reprinted with permission from MB Carpenter. Core Text of Neuroanatomy [3rd ed]. Baltimore: Williams & Wilkins, 1985.)

rons.[152] Although STN neurons have no projection to thalamic nuclei, these cells appear organized to modulate the output systems from the MPS and the SNR that have access to thalamic neurons that can influence activity of cortical neurons.

Functional Considerations

Although considerable progress has been made in understanding the anatomic organization of the corpus striatum and related nuclei, the physiological mechanisms and the neurotransmitters that affect and modulate these activities are just beginning to be understood. The principal thrust of current research is to define anatomic pathways and the respective neurotransmitters. Such information not only provides a key to physiological mechanisms but in some instances leads to specific therapy.

Neostriatum Is Organized into Compartments

The neostriatum (caudate and putamen) is organized into compartments or modules consisting of striosomes (patches) embedded in larger matrices. Histochemically, the striosomes show various neurotransmitters and neuromodulators such as dopamine, ENK, and SP, but are nearly devoid of the cholinergic enzyme acetylcholinesterase. On the other hand, the reverse is seen in matrices. Striosomes receive major inputs from the limbic cortex and project mainly to the SNR, whereas the matrices are more involved with the sensorimotor areas. The relationship of the striosome to the matrix is unclear.[153-155]

Neostriatum Projections to the Globus Pallidum

There are two major projections from the neostriatum to the GP. The direct pathway projects to the GPi and SNR, while the indirect pathway goes first to the external segment of the globus pallidum (GPe), then to the STN, and finally back to both the GPi and GPe, and SNR.[154,156,157]

The direct pathway is GABAergic with SP as the neuromodulator, whereas the indirect pathway is GABAergic with ENK as a neuromodulator. The second set of neurons in the indirect pathway originates in the GPe, is also inhibitory (GABAergic), and acts on the excitatory neurons (glutamatergic) in the STN that go to the GPi and SNR. In Parkinson's disease there is a deficiency of dopamine that leads to an overactivity of the indirect pathway and an underactivity of the direct pathway.

Most of the diseases of the corpus striatum are associated with relatively widespread pathologic processes, but for many syndromes it has been possible to focus on key elements. This has been most successful in Parkinson's disease, which is characterized by tremor at rest (in the absences of voluntary movement), gait and postural reflex impairment, rigidity, bradykinesia (slowness of movement), and certain autonomic disturbances. The tremor is a rhythmic, alternating activity of relative regular frequency and amplitude that commonly involves the digits (pill rolling). Rigidity, which may be progressive, can involve virtually all muscles. Rigidity can easily be demonstrated by passively flexing and extending the limbs or by passively rotating the hand at the wrist in a circular fashion. These movements are interrupted by a series of jerks, referred to as *cog-wheel* phenomena. In addition to these *positive* features, parkinsonism is characterized by what have been called *negative* features. Negative features actually are neural deficits expressed in impairment of locomotion, postural fixation, phonation, or speech. Patients with the parkinsonian syndrome exhibit a masklike face, blink infrequently, and have a stooped posture with characteristic flexion of the neck, trunk, and knees. The gait is slow and shuffling, and the steps are small. There is a loss of

associated movements (swing of the arms when walking), and speech is slow and dysarthric. Many of these patients show amelioration of these disturbances after L-dopa therapy, which supplies the needed striatal dopamine. Although this therapy can bring dramatic improvement initially, it often appears to be less effective over time, probably because the basic progressive pathologic process is not arrested by this drug.

The accidental observation that a clandestinely synthesized meperidine analogue (1-methyl-4-phenyl-1,2,3,6-tetrahydropyridine) produced a severe and chronic form of parkinsonism provided additional evidence implicating the cells of the substantia nigra in this syndrome.[158] With this meperidine analogue it has been possible to produce a Parkinson's-like syndrome in monkeys, associated with degeneration in the substantia nigra.[159] This animal model provides opportunities for studies that cannot be done on humans.

The term *athetosis* is used to describe a form of dyskinesia characterized by slow, writhing, vermicular movements involving the extremities, cervical muscles, and face. Athetosis gives the appearance of a mobile spasm. Dystonia, considered a form of athetosis, involves the axial muscles. Involuntary contractions of the axial muscles result in bizarre distortions and twisting of the trunk. Athetosis and dystonia often occur together.[160] This type of dyskinesia frequently is part of the cerebral palsy syndrome that involves both the cerebral cortex, including the pyramidal tracts, and large parts of the corpus striatum. Paresis and spasticity often are severe. The slow, writhing quality of the dyskinesia appears in part to be related to the paresis and spasticity.

Chorea is the term applied to a variety of dyskinesias characterized by involuntary movements that have a brisk, graceful quality and resemble fragments of purposeful movements. Choreoid activity most commonly is seen in the muscles of the hands, face, and tongue. Moderate degrees of hypotonus occur in this syndrome. Choreoid activity occurs as a consequence of a number of disease processes, but it is most commonly associated with Huntington's disease,[161] a hereditary disorder associated with an autosomal dominant gene localized on the short arm of chromosome 4. Symptoms are progressive and reflect both behavioral and motor disturbances. The cerebral cortex and the corpus striatum bear the brunt of the pathologic process, but changes are not confined to these structures. Brains of patients who died from Huntington's disease demonstrate that striatal neurons have reduced concentrations of GABA and choline acetyltransferase; in these same patients tyrosine hydroxylase and dopamine appeared nearly normal in the striatum.[162] It is well known that large doses of L-dopa given to patients with Parkinson's syndrome may cause choreiform activity to appear. In addition, L-dopa tends to exacerbate choreoid activity in Huntington's disease. It would seem logical to try to increase striatal GABA in this syndrome. Such attempts have met with little success, because GABA does not pass the blood–brain barrier and because GABAergic and cholinergic receptors may be damaged or reduced in number.

Ballism or *hemiballism* is the term used to describe the violent, forceful, flinging movements, primarily of the proximal appendicular musculature. This form of dyskinesia usually appears suddenly in elderly patients with hypertension as a consequence of a small vascular lesion in the STN.[139] The violence of the dyskinesia is exhausting, and without treatment most patients succumb from secondary medical problems. This is the only syndrome of this group that can be produced in monkeys by small, discrete lesions.[140] These animals exhibit marked hypotonus and ballistic activity contralateral to the lesion. Ballistic activity in monkeys shows some attenuation with time but is still recognizable a year after the lesion was produced. This form of dyskinesia can be significantly ameliorated by lesions of the medial pallidal segment or ventral lateral thalamic nuclei that convey signals to the thalamus and the cerebral cortex.[140] Lesions of these types do not produce paresis. The working hypothesis in this unique form of dyskinesia is that destruction of at least 20% of the cells in the STN, which project to the globus pallidus, results in removal of excitatory influences on glutamatergic cells of the medial pallidal segment. The removal of excitatory effect on the inhibitory neurons (GABAergic) in the GPi results in overactivity of the thalamocortical circuitry, causing ballism on the opposite side of the body.

Comparisons of cerebellar and basal ganglia dyskinesia reveal certain common features in their neural mechanisms, even though these structures are widely separate and have different neurotransmitters. Both the cerebellar cortex and the corpus striatum have massive input systems that convey highly varied information. Both output systems have major influences on thalamic nuclei, but each system has descending components that modify activities of brain stem nuclei. Thalamic nuclei, which receive the outputs of the cerebellum and the corpus striatum (from the medial globus pallidus and the pars reticulata of the substantia nigra), are entirely separate and without overlap. These separate thalamic relay nuclei exert their influences on related but different regions of the motor cortex (Figure 3-20). Cerebellar

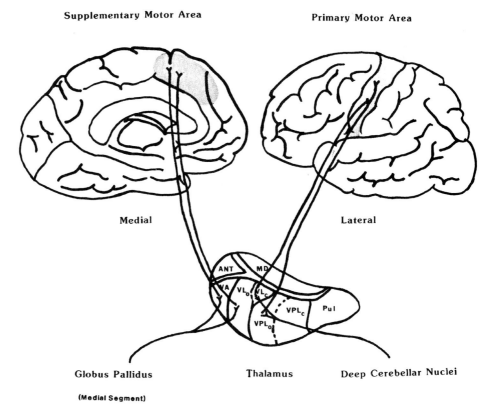

FIGURE 3-20 Schematic diagram compares the thalamic and cortical projections of the globus pallidus and the deep cerebellar nuclei. Fibers from the medial pallidal segment project ipsilaterally to the ventral anterior (VA) and ventral lateral (VL$_o$) thalamic nuclei. These nuclei project on the supplementary motor area located on the medial aspect of the hemisphere. Ascending projections from the deep cerebellar nuclei cross in the midbrain and terminate in the so-called cell-sparse zone of the thalamus (ventral lateral nuclei [VL$_c$] and ventral posterolateral [VPL$_o$]). Cells in the cell-sparse zone of the thalamus project directly to the primary motor cortex. (ANT = anterior nuclei of the thalamus; MD = mediodorsal nucleus; Pul = pulvinar; VPL$_c$ = ventral posterolateral nucleus, pars caudalis.)

Supplementary Motor Area

Primary Motor Area

Medial

Lateral

ANT MD

VA VL$_o$ VL$_c$

VPL$_c$ Pul

VPL$_o$

Globus Pallidus

(Medial Segment)

Thalamus

Deep Cerebellar Nuclei

influences are exerted on the primary motor cortex; influences of the corpus striatum complex act on the supplementary motor area, a region that in part appears to operate through the primary motor area. The primary motor area, associated with skilled, voluntary motor function, acts almost exclusively on contralateral segmental motor neurons. The supplementary motor area is a bilateral system involved in programming motor functions at cortical levels and appears to be involved in most motor activities.

REFERENCES

1. Schmahmann JD, Sherman JC. The cerebellar cognitive affective syndrome [see comments]. Brain 1998;121:561–579.
2. Cohen H, et al. Cerebellum and Motor Control. In H Cohen (ed), Neuroscience for Neuroscience. Philadelphia: JB Lippincott, 1993;196–205.
3. Ottersen OP, Storm-Mathisen J. Glutamate- and GABA-containing neurons in the mouse and rat brain, as demonstrated with a new immunocytochemical technique. J Comp Neurol 1984;229:374–392.
4. Monaghan PL, Beitz AJ, Larson AA, et al. Immunocytochemical localization of glutamate-, glutaminase- and aspartate aminotransferase-like immunoreactivity in the rat deep cerebellar nuclei. Brain Res 1986;363:364–370.
5. Chan-Palay V, Nilaver G, Palay SL, et al. Chemical heterogeneity in cerebellar Purkinje cells: existence and coexistence of glutamic acid decarboxylase-like and motilin-like immunoreactivities. Proc Natl Acad Sci U S A 1981;78:7787–7791.
6. Eccles J, Ito M, Szentagothai J. The Cerebellum as a Neuronal Machine. New York: Springer Verlag, 1967.
7. Hudson D, Valcana T, Bean G. Glutamic acid: a strong candidate as the neurotransmitter of the cerebellar granular cell. Neurochem International 1976;1:73–81.
8. Wiklund L, Toggenburger G, Cuenod M. Selective retrograde labelling of the rat olivocerebellar climbing fiber system with D-[3H]aspartate. Neuroscience 1984;13:441–468.
9. Voogd J, Glickstein M. The anatomy of the cerebellum. Trends Neurosci 1998;21:370–375.
10. Becker WJ, Kunesch E, Freund HJ. Coordination of a multi-joint movement in normal humans and in patients with cerebellar dysfunction. Can J Neurol Sci 1990;17:264–274.
11. Ebner TJ, Fu Q. What features of visually guided arm movements are encoded in the simple spike discharge of cerebellar Purkinje cells? Prog Brain Res 1997;114:431–447.
12. Sinder R. Recent contributions to the anatomy and physiology of the cerebellum. Arch Neurol Psychiatry 1950;64:196–219.
13. Carpenter M. Core Text of Neuroanatomy (3rd ed). Baltimore: Williams & Wilkins, 1985.
14. Courville J. Somatotopical organization of the projection from the nucleus interpositus anterior of the cerebellum to the red nucleus. An experimental study in the cat with silver impregnation methods. Exp Brain Res 1966;2:191–215.
15. Asanuma C, Thach WR, Jones EG. Anatomical evidence for segregated focal groupings of efferent cells and their terminal ramifications in the cerebellothalamic pathway of the monkey. Brain Res 1983;286:267–297.
16. Asanuma C, Thach WT, Jones EG. Distribution of cerebellar terminations and their relation to other afferent terminations in the ventral lateral thalamic region of the monkey. Brain Res 1983;286:237–265.
17. Percheron G. The thalamic territory of cerebellar afferents and the lateral region of the thalamus of the macaque in sterotaxic ventricular coordinates. J Hirnforsch 1977;18:375–400.
18. Thach WT, Jones EG. The cerebellar dentatothalamic connection: terminal field, lamellae, rods and somatotopy. Brain Res 1979;169:168–172.
19. Jones EG, Wise SP, Coulter JD. Differential thalamic relationships of sensory-motor and parietal cortical fields in monkeys. J Comp Neurol 1979;183:833–881.
20. Tracey DJ, Asanuma C, Jones EG, Porter R. Thalamic relay to motor cortex: afferent pathways from brain stem, cerebellum, and spinal cord in monkeys. J Neurophysiol 1980;44:532–554.
21. Schell GR, Strick PL. The origin of thalamic inputs to the arcuate premotor and supplementary motor areas. J Neurosci 1984;4:539–560.
22. Carpenter M, Batton RI. Connections of the fastigial nucleus in the cat and monkey. Exp Brain Res 1982;6:250–295.
23. Mori S, Matsui T, Kuze B, et al. Cerebellar-induced locomotion: reticulospinal control of spinal rhythm generating mechanism in cats. Ann N Y Acad Sci 1998;860:94–105.
24. Carleton SC, Carpenter MB. Afferent and efferent connections of the medial, inferior and lateral vestibular nuclei in the cat and monkey. Brain Res 1983;278:29–51.
25. Walberg F, Jansen J. Cerebellovestibular fibers in the cat. Exp Neurol 1961;3:32–52.
26. Houser CR, Barber RP, Vaughn JE. Immunocytochemical localization of glutamic acid decarboxylase in the dorsal lateral vestibular nucleus: evidence for an intrinsic and extrinsic GABAergic innervation. Neurosci Lett 1984; 47:213–220.
27. Sarnat HB, Alcala H. Human cerebellar hypoplasia: a syndrome of diverse causes. Arch Neurol 1980;37:300–305.
28. Minahan C. Postural Control During Arm Movement in Healthy Subjects and Subjects with Cerebellar Dysfunction [Thesis]. Boston: MGH Institute of Health Professions, 1998.
29. English G. Effects of Vestibular Rehabilitation on Stepping Stability. Post-Professional Physical Therapy Program. Boston: MGH Insitute of Health Professions, 1999.
30. Diener HC, Dichgans J, Bacher M, Guschlbauer B. Characteristic alterations of long-loop "reflexes" in patients with Friedreich's disease and late atrophy of the cerebellar anterior lobe. J Neurol Neurosurg Psychiatry 1984;47:679–685.
31. Vidailhet M, Jedynak CP, Pollak P, Agid Y. Pathology of symptomatic tremors. Mov Disord 1998;13(Suppl 3):49–54.
32. Baloh RW, Jacobson KM, Beykirch K, Honrubia V. Static and dynamic posturography in patients with vestibular

and cerebellar lesions. Arch Neurol 1998;55:649–654.

33. Brown P, Rothwell JC, Stevens JM, et al. Cerebellar axial postural tremor. Mov Disord 1997;12:977–984.

34. Anouti A, Koller WC. Tremor disorders. Diagnosis and management. West J Med 1995;162:510–513.

35. Hudson CC, Krebs DE. Frontal plane dynamic stability and coordination in subjects with cerebellar degeneration. Exp Brain Res 2000;132(1):103–113.

36. Bastian AJ, Martin TA, Keating JG, Thach WT. Cerebellar ataxia: abnormal control of interaction torques across multiple joints. J Neurophysiol 1996;76:492–509.

37. Bastian AJ. Mechanisms of ataxia. Phys Ther 1997;77:672–675.

38. Soechting JF, Lacquaniti F. Invariant characteristics of a pointing movement in man. J Neurosci 1981;1:710–720.

39. Bastian A, Mueller M, Martin T, et al. Control of interaction torques during reaching in normal and cerebellar patients [Abstract]. Taken from Society for Neuroscience 1994;20:408.5.

40. Massaquoi S, Hallett M. Kinematics of initiating a two-joint arm movement in patients with cerebellar ataxia. Can J Neurol Sci 1996;23(1):3–14.

41. Topka H, Konczak J, Dichgans J. Coordination of multi-joint arm movements in cerebellar ataxia: analysis of hand and angular kinematics. Exp Brain Res 1998;119:483–492.

42. Becker WJ, Morrice BL, Clark AW, Lee RG. Multi-joint reaching movements and eye-hand tracking in cerebellar incoordination: investigation of a patient with complete loss of Purkinje cells. Can J Neurol Sci 1991; 18:476–487.

43. Kaminski TR, Gentile AM. A kinematic comparison of single and multi-joint pointing movements. Exp Brain Res 1989;78:547–556.

44. Lacquaniti F, Ferrigno G, Pedotti A, et al. Changes in spatial scale in drawing and handwriting: kinematic contributions by proximal and distal joints. J Neurosci 1987;7:819–828.

45. Mason CR, Miller LE, Baker JF, Houk JC. Organization of reaching and grasping movements in the primate cerebellar nuclei as revealed by focal muscimol inactivations. J Neurophysiol 1998;79:537–554.

46. Ackermann H, Ziegler W. [Cerebellar dysarthria—a review of the literature]. Fortschr Neurol Psychiatr 1992; 60(1):28–40.

47. Ackermann H, Ziegler W. Cerebellar voice tremor: an acoustic analysis. J Neurol Neurosurg Psychiatry 1991;54:74–76.

48. Levinson HN. The cerebellar-vestibular basis of learning disabilities in children, adolescents and adults: hypothesis and study [published erratum appears in Percept Mot Skills 1989 Feb;68(1):preceding 3]. Percept Mot Skills 1988;67:983–1006.

49. Nicolson RI, Fawcett AJ, Berry EL, et al. Association of abnormal cerebellar activation with motor learning difficulties in dyslexic adults. Lancet 1999;353:1662–1667.

50. Bohmer A, Straumann D. Pathomechanism of mammalian downbeat nystagmus due to cerebellar lesion: a simple hypothesis. Neurosci Lett 1998;250:127–130.

51. Ohta S, Mizutani Y, Anno M. [An autopsy case of hereditary cerebellar atrophy (Holmes-type) with mental symptoms and rhythmic skeletal myoclonus]. No To Shinkei 1994; 46(7):663–670.

52. Antoun H, Villeneuve N, Gelot A, et al. Cerebellar atrophy: an important feature of carbohydrate deficient glycoprotein syndrome type 1. Pediatr Radiol 1999;29:194–198.

53. Maki BE, Holliday PJ, Topper AK. A prospective study of postural balance and risk of falling in an ambulatory and independent elderly population. J Gerontol 1994;49:M72–M84.

54. Ouchi Y, Okada H, Yoshikawa E, et al. Brain activation during maintenance of standing postures in humans. Brain 1999;122:329–338.

55. Fulton J. Functional Localization in the Frontal Lobes and Cerebellum. Oxford: Clarendon Press, 1949.

56. Sherrington C. Decerebrate rigidity and reflex coordination of movements. J Physiol 1898;22:319–332.

57. Dow R, Moruzzi G. Albation Experiments. In R Dow, G Moruzzi (eds), The Physiology and Pathology of the Cerebellum. Minneapolis: University of Minnesota Press, 1958;8–102.

58. Huang YP, Tuason MY, Wu T, Plaitakis A. MRI and CT features of cerebellar degeneration. J Formos Med Assoc 1993;92:494–508.

59. Weeks RA, Gerloff C, Honda M, et al. Movement-related cerebellar activation in the absence of sensory input. J Neurophysiol 1999;82:484–488.

60. Glickstein M. Mossy-fibre sensory input to the cerebellum. Prog Brain Res 1997;114:251–259.

61. Ghez C. The Cerebellum. In ER Kandel, JH Schwartz, TM Jessell (eds), Principles of Neural Science (3rd ed). New York: Appleton & Lange 1991;626–646.

62. Guyton AC, Hall JE. The Cerebellum, the Basal Ganglion, and Overall Motor Control. In AC Guyton, JE Hall (eds), Textbook of Medical Physiology (9th ed). Philadelphia: WB Saunders, 1996;715–731.

63. Bower JM. Is the cerebellum sensory for motor's sake, or motor for sensory's sake: the view from the whiskers of a rat? Prog Brain Res 1997;114:463–496.

64. Parsons LM, Bower JM, Gao JH, et al. Lateral cerebellar hemispheres actively support sensory acquisition and discrimination rather than motor control. Learn Mem 1997;4:49–62.

65. De Zeeuw CI, Simpson JI, Hoogenraad CC, et al. Microcircuitry and function of the inferior olive. Trends Neurosci 1998;21:391–400.

66. Raymond JL, Lisberger SG, Mauk MD. The cerebellum: a neuronal learning machine? Science 1996; 272:1126–1131.

67. Courchesne E, Yeung-Courchesne R, Press GA, et al. Hypoplasia of cerebellar vermal lobules VI and VII in autism. N Engl J Med 1988;318:1349–1354.

68. Bauman M, Kemper TL. Histoanatomic observations of the brain in early infantile autism. Neurology 1985; 35:866–874.

69. Schmahmann JD. Dysmetria of thought: clinical consequences of cerebellar dysfunction on cognitive and affect. Trends Cogn Sci 1998;2:362–370.

70. Schmahmann J. From movement to thought: anatomic substrates of the cerebellar contribution to cognitive process. Hum Brain Mapp 1996:174–198.

71. Schmahmann JD. Therapeutic and research implications. Int Rev Neurobiol 1997;41:637–647.

72. Klintsova AY, Matthews JT, Goodlett CR, et al. Therapeutic motor training increases parallel fiber synapse number per Purkinje neuron in cerebellar cortex of rats given postnatal binge alcohol exposure: preliminary report. Alcohol Clin Exp Res 1997;21:1257–1263.

73. Hudson C, Krebs D. Does Rehabilitation Improve Dynamic Stability in Subjects with Cerebellar Pathology? In preparation. 1999.

74. Minahan C, Schmahmann J, Krebs D. Near-normal functional performance

in a subject with cerebellar agenesis. In preparation, 1997.

75. Edstrom J, Eller M. Barbarians Led by Bill Gates. New York: Henry Holt and Company, Inc, 1998.

76. DiFiglia M, Pasik P, Pasik T. A Golgi study of neuronal types in the neostriatum of monkeys. Brain Res 1976;114:245–256.

77. Pasik P, Pasik T, DiFiglia M. The Internal Organization of the Neostriatum in Mammals. In I Divac (ed), The Neostriatum. Oxford: Pergamon Press, 1979;5–36.

78. Jessell TM, Emson PC, Paxinos G, et al. Topographical projections of substance P and GABA pathways in the striato- and pallido-nigral system: a biochemical and immunohistochemical study. Brain Res 1978;152:487–498.

79. Ribak CE. The GABAergic Neurons of the Extrapyramidal System as Revealed by Immunocytochemistry. In G DiChiara, GL Gessa (eds), GABA and the Basal Ganglia. New York: Raven Press, 1981;23–36.

80. DiFiglia M, Aronin N, Martin JB. Light and electron microscopic localization of immunoreactive leu-enkephalin in the monkey basal ganglia. J Neurosci 1982;2:303–320.

81. Penny GR, Afsharpour S, Kitai ST. The glutamic acid decarboxylase-, leucine-, enkephalin-, methionine enkephalin-, and substance P-immunoreactive neurons in the neostriatum of the rat and cat: evidence for partial population overlap. Neuroscience 1986;17:1011–1045.

82. Ribak CE, Vaughn JE, Roberts E. The GABA neurons and their axon terminals in the rat corpus striatum as demonstrated by GAD immunocytochemistry. J Comp Neurol 1979;187:261–284.

83. Kimura H, McGeer RL, Pong JH, et al. The central cholinergic system studied by choline acetyltransferase immunohistochemistry in the cat. J Comp Neurol 1980;200:151–201.

84. Parent A, Csonka C, Etienne P. The occurrence of large acetylcholinesterase-containing neurons in human neostriatum as disclosed in normal and Alzheimer's disease brains. Brain Res 1984;291:54–158.

85. Pasik P, Pasik T, Holstein GR, et al. GABAergic elements in the neuronal circuits of the monkey neostriatum: a light and electron microscopic immunocytochemical study. J Comp Neurol 1988;270:157–170.

86. Goldman PS, Nauta WJH. An intri-cately patterned prefrontocaudate projection in the rhesus monkey. J Comp Neurol 1977;171:369–386.

87. Jones EG, Coulter JD, Burton H, et al. Cells of origin and terminal distribution of efferent cells in the sensory-motor cortex of monkeys. J Comp Neurol 1977;175:391–438.

88. Künzle H. An autoradiographic analysis of the efferent connections from premotor and adjacent prefrontal regions (areas 6 and 9) in Macaca fascicularis. Brain Behav Evol 1978;15:185–234.

89. Künzle H. Bilateral projections from precentral motor cortex to the putamen and other parts of the basal ganglia. Brain Res 1975;88:195–210.

90. Divac I. Neostriatum and functions of prefrontal cortex. Acta Neurobiol Exp 1972;32:461–477.

91. Rolls ET, Williams GV. Neuronal Activity in the Ventral Striatum of Primates. In MB Carpenter, A Jayaraman (eds), Basal Ganglia II Structure and Function—Current Concepts. New York: Plenum Press, 1987;349–356.

92. Fonnum F, Storm-Mathison J, Divac I. Biochemical evidence for glutamate as neurotransmitter in corticostriate and corticothalamic fibres in rat brain. Neuroscience 1981;6:863–873.

93. Powell TPS, Cowan WM. A study of thalamostriate relations in the monkey. Brain 1956;79:364–390.

94. Smith Y, Parent A. Differential connections of caudate nucleus and putamen in the squirrel monkey (Saimiri sciureus). Neuroscience 1986;18:347–371.

95. Dahlström A, Fuxe K. Evidence for the existence of monamine containing neurons in the central nervous system. I. Demonstration of monoamines in the cell bodies of brain stem neurons. Acta Physiol Scand 1964;62:1–55.

96. Andén N-E, Dahlström A, Fuxe K, et al. Ascending monoamine neurons to the telencephalon and diencephalon. Acta Physiol Scand 1966;67:313–326.

97. Parent A, Mackey A, DeBellefeuille L. The subcortical afferents to caudate nucleus and putamen in primate: a fluorescence retrograde double labeling study. Neuroscience 1983;10:1137–1150.

98. Parent A, Mackey A, Smith Y, et al. The output organization of the substantia nigra in primate as revealed by a retrograde double labeling method. Brain Res Bull 1983;10:529–537.

99. Calabresi P, Mercuri N, Stanzione P, et al. Role of D1 and D2 Dopamine Receptors in the Mammalian Striatum: Electrophysiological Studies and Functional Implications. In MB Carpenter, A Jayaraman (eds), The Basal Ganglia II Stucture and Function-Current Concepts. New York: Plenum Press, 1987;145–148.

100. Kelley AE, Domesick VB, Nauta WJH. The amygdalostriatal projection in the rat. An anatomical study by anterograde and retrograde tracing methods. Neuroscience 1982;7:615–630.

101. Russchen FT, Price JL. Amygdalostriatal projections in rat. Topographical organization and fiber morphology shown using lectin PHA-L as an anterograde tracer. Neurosci Lett 1984;47:15–22.

102. Arikuni T, Kubota K. Substantia innominata projection to caudate nucleus in macaque monkeys. Brain Res 1984;302:184–189.

103. Dray A. The physiology and pharmacology of mammalian basal ganglia. Prog Neurol 1980;14:221–335.

104. van der Kooy D, Hattori T. Dorsal raphe cells with collateral projections to the caudate-putamen and substantia nigra: a fluorescent retrograde double labeling study in the rat. Brain Res 1980;186:1–7.

105. Parent A, Descarries L, Beaudet A. Organization of ascending serotonin systems in the adult rat brain. A radioautographic study after intraventricular administration of [³H] 5-hydroxytryptamine. Neuroscience 1981;6:115–138.

106. Sugimoto T, Hattori T. Organization and efferent projections of nucleus tegmenti pedunculopontinus pars compacta with special reference to its cholinergic aspects. Neuroscience 1984;11:931–946.

107. Hallanger AE, Levey AI, Lee HJ, et al. The origins of cholinergic and other subcortical afferents to the thalamus in the rat. J Comp Neurol 1987;262:105–124.

108. Lee HJ, Rye DB, Hallanger AE, et al. Cholinergic versus noncholinergic efferents from the mesopontine tegmentum to the extrapyramidal motor system nuclei. J Comp Neurol 1988;275:469–492.

109. Garcia-Rill E. The basal ganglia and the locomotor regions. Brain Res Rev 1986;11:46–63.

110. Kuhlenbeck H, Haymaker W. The derivatives of the hypothalamus in the human brain; their relation to the extrapyramidal and autonomic systems. Milit Surgeon 1949;105:26–52.

111. Richter E. Die Entwicklung des Globus Pallidus und des Corpus Subthalamicum. Berlin: Springer Verlag, 1965.

112. Francois C, Percheron G, Yelnik J, et al. A Golgi analysis of the primate globus pallidus. I. Inconstant processes of large neurons, other neuronal types and afferent axons. J Comp Neurol 1984;227:182–199.

113. Yelnik J, Percheron G, Francois C. A Golgi analysis of the primate globus pallidus. II. Quantitative morphology and spatial orientation of dendritic arborizations. J Comp Neurol 1984; 227:200–213.

114. Mugnaini E, Oertel WH. An Atlas of the Distribution of GABAergic Neurons and Terminals in the Rat CNS as Revealed by GAD Immunohistochemistry. In A Björklund, T Hökfelt (eds), Handbook of Chemical Neuroanatomy, GABA and Neuropeptides in the CNS. Amsterdam: Elsevier, 1985;436–595.

115. Smith Y, Parent A, Seguela P, et al. Distribution of GABA-immunoreactive neurons in the basal ganglia of the squirrel monkey (Saimiri sciureus). J Comp Neurol 1987;259:50–64.

116. Carpenter MB. Anatomy of the Basal Ganglia. In P Vinken, GW Bruyn, H Klawans (eds), Handbook of Clinical Neurology. Amsterdam: Elsevier, 1987;1–18.

117. Szabo J. Topical distribution of striatal efferents in the monkey. Exp Neurol 1962;5:21–36.

118. Szabo J. The efferent projections of the putamen in the monkey. Exp Neurol 1967;19:463–476.

119. Szabo J. Projections from the body of the caudate nucleus in the rhesus monkey. Exp Neurol 1970;27:1–15.

120. Fonnum F, Gottesfeld Z, Grofova I. Distribution of glutamate decarboxylase, choline acetyltransferase and aromatic amino acid decarboxylase in the basal ganglia of normal and operated rats. Evidence for striatopallidal, striatoentopeduncular and striatonigral GABAergic fibers. Brain Res 1978; 153:370–374.

121. Haber SN, Elde RR. Correlation between metenkephalin and substance P immunoreactivity in the primate globus pallidus. Neuroscience 1981;6: 1291–1297.

122. Haber SN, Elde RR. The distribution of enkephalin immunoreactive fibers and terminals in the monkey central nervous system: an immunohistochemical study. Neuroscience 1982;7:1049–1095.

123. Carpenter MB, Batton RR III, Carleton SC, et al. Interconnections and organization of pallidal and subthalamic nucleus neurons in the monkey. J Comp Neurol 1981;197:579–603.

124. Carpenter MB, Fraser RAR, Shriver J. The organization of the pallidosubthalamic fibers in the monkey. Brain Res 1968;11:522–559.

125. Albin RL, Young AB, Pennly JB. The functional anatomy of basal ganglia disorders. Trends Neurosci 1989; 12(10):366–375.

126. Kuo JS, Carpenter MB. Organization of pallidothalamic projections in the rhesus monkey. J Comp Neurol 1973;151:201–236.

127. Kim R, Nakano K, Jayaraman A, et al. Projections of the globus pallidus and adjacent structures: an autoradiographic study in the monkey. J Comp Neurol 1976;169:263–289.

128. Porter R. Corticomotorneuronal projections: synaptic events related to skilled movement. Proc R Soc Lond 1987;B231:147–168.

129. Parent A, DeBellefeuille L. Organization of efferent projections from the internal segment of the globus pallidus in primate as revealed by fluorescence retrograde labeling method. Brain Res 1982;245:201–213.

130. Hökfelt T, Ungerstedt U. Electron and fluorescence microscopical studies on the nucleus caudatus putamen of the rat after unilateral lesions of ascending nigro-neostriatal dopamine neurons. Acta Physiol Scand 1969;76:415–426.

131. Rinvik E, Grofov I. Observations on the fine structure of the substantia nigra in the cat. Exp Brain Res 1970;11:229–248.

132. van der Kooy D, Hattori T. Single subthalamic nucleus neurons project to both globus pallidus and substantia nigra in rat. J Comp Neurol 1980; 192:751–768.

133. Parent A, Smith Y. Organization of efferent projections of the subthalamic nucleus of the squirrel monkey as revealed by retrograde labeling method. Brain Res 1987;436:296–310.

134. Kanazawa I, Marshall GR, Kelly JS. Afferents to the rat substantia nigra studied with horseradish peroxidase, with special reference to fibres from the subthalamic nucleus. Brain Res 1976; 115:485–491.

135. Carpenter MB, Carleton SC, Keller JT, et al. Connections of the subthalamic nucleus in the monkey. Brain Res 1981;224:1–29.

136. Carpenter MB, Peter P. Nigrostriatal

and nigrothalamic fibers in the rhesus monkey. J Comp Neurol 1972;144:93–116.

137. Carpenter MB, Nakano K, Kim R. Nigrothalamic projections in the monkey demonstrated by autoradiographic technics. J Comp Neurol 1976;144:93–116.

138. Ilinsky IA, Jouandet ML, Goldman-Rakic PS. Organization of the nigrothalamocortical system in the rhesus monkey. J Comp Neurol 1985; 236:315–330.

139. Anderson ME, Yoshida M. Axonal branching patterns and location of nigrothalamic and nigrocollicular neurons in the cat. J Neurophysiol 1980; 43:883–895.

140. Whittier JR. Ballism and the subthalamic nucleus (nucleus hypothalamicus; corpus luysi). Arch Neurol Psychiatry 1947;58:672–692.

141. Carpenter MB, Whittier JR, Mettler FA. Analysis of choreoid hyperkinesia in the rhesus monkey: surgical and pharmacological analysis of hyperkinesia resulting from lesions in the subthalamic nucleus of Luys. J Comp Neurol 1950;92:293–331.

142. Carpenter MB. Brain stem and infratentorial neuraxis in experimental dyskinesia. Arch Neurol 1961;5:504–524.

143. Yelnik J, Percheron G. Subthalamic neurons in primates: a quantitative and comparative analysis. Neuroscience 1979;4:1717–1743.

144. Hammond C, Yelnik J. Intracellular labeling of rat subthalamic neurones with horseradish peroxidase: computer analysis of dendrites and characterization of axon arborization. Neuroscience 1983;8:781–790.

145. Kita H, Chang HT, Kitai ST. The morphology of intracellularly labeled rat subthalamic neurons: a light microscopic analysis. J Comp Neurol 1983;215:245–257.

146. Hartmann-von Monakow K, Akert K, Künzle H. Projections of the precentral motor cortex and other cortical areas of the frontal lobe to the subthalamic nucleus in the monkey. Exp Brain Res 1978;33:395–403.

147. Kitai ST, Deniau JM. Cortical inputs to the subthalamus, intracellular analysis. Brain Res 1981;214:411–415.

148. Tsubokawa T, Sutin J. Pallidal and tegmental inhibition of oscillatory slow waves and unit activity in the subthalamic nucleus. Brain Res 1972;41:101–118.

149. Kita H, Chang HT, Kitai ST. Pallidal inputs to subthalamus: intracellular analysis. Brain Res 1983;264:255–265.

150. Nauta HJW, Cuenod M. Perikaryal cell labeling in the subthalamic nucleus following the injection of [³H]-γ-aminobutyric acid into the pallidal complex: an autoradiographic study in cat. Neuroscience 1982;7:2725–2734.

151. Crossman AR, Sambrook MA, Jackson A. Experimental hemichorea/hemiballismus in the monkey: studies on the intracerebral site of action in a drug induced dyskinesia. Brain 1984; 107:579–596.

152. Kitai ST, Kita H. Anatomy and physiology of the basal ganglia [abstract]. Proc Int Union Physiol Sci 1986; 16:516.

153. Graybiel AM. Neurotransmitters and neuromodulators in the basal ganglia. Trends Neurosci 1990;13(7):244–254.

154. De Long MR. The Basal Ganglia. In ER Kandel, JH Schwartz, TM Jessell (eds), Principles of Neural Science (4th ed). New York: Elsevier Science Publishing Co, Inc, 2000;853–867.

155. Côté LJ, Crutcher MD. The Basal Ganglia. In ER Kandel, JH Schwartz, TM Jessell (eds), Principles of Neural Science (4th ed). New York: Elsevier Science Publishing Co, Inc, 1991; 647–659.

156. Alexander GE, Crutcher MD. Functional architecture of basal ganglia circuits: neural substrates of parallel processing. Trends Neurosci 1990; 13(7):266–271.

157. De Long MR. Primate models of movement disorders of basal ganglia origin. Trends Neurosci 1990;13(7):281–285.

158. Langston JW, Ballard P, Tetrud JW, et al. Chronic parkinsonism in humans due to a product of meperidine synthesis. Science 1983;249:979–980.

159. Kolata G. Monkey model of Parkinson's disease. A contaminant of illicit drugs has caused Parkinson's disease in humans and monkeys. Science 1983;230:705.

160. Carpenter MB. Athetosis and the basal ganglia. Arch Neurol Psychiatry 1950;63:875–901.

161. Gusella JF, Wexler NS, Conneally PM. A polymorphic DNA marker genetically linked to Huntington's disease. Nature 1983;306:234–238.

162. Bird ED, Iversen LL. Huntington's chorea: postmortem measurements of glutamic acid decarboxylase, choline acetyltransferase and dopamine in basal ganglia. Brain 1974;97:457–472.

4

Autonomic Nervous System

RONALD E. DE MEERSMAN AND
ADRIENNE STEVENS ZION

The autonomic nervous system modulates a wide variety of physiological functions without voluntary control. The autonomic nervous system can be functionally and anatomically divided into two branches, the sympathetic and parasympathetic branches. Many of the physiological functions regulated by the autonomic nervous system involve circulatory, hemodynamic, metabolic, and thermoregulatory functions, which are referred to as visceral activities and do not require conscious control. Proper regulation of the previously mentioned functions is generally maintained through a sophisticated synergism of both autonomic branches, rather than through antagonism. Furthermore, the autonomic nervous modulation provides for a fine-tuning of life-sustaining processes within normal homeodynamic ranges. The fibers of the autonomic nervous system are referred to as *visceral efferent fibers.* The autonomic fibers innervate many organ systems, and as such, perturbations in any of these systems appear to translate in autonomic disturbances. Some of these disease models have contributed to furthering our understanding of autonomic regulation. This chapter provides a brief review of the authors' perceptions on how to view the autonomic nervous system. This is followed by a description of the organization and function of the autonomic nervous system. In addition, we describe some of the autonomic adaptations associated with habitual exercise, aging, and spinal cord injury, of which the latter appears to be a model of accelerated aging of the autonomic nervous system. And finally because considerable progress has been made in the assessment of autonomic function, we briefly discuss some noninvasive measurement methods of autonomic modulation.

HOMEODYNAMICS OF THE AUTONOMIC NERVOUS SYSTEM

For many decades the actions of the autonomic nervous system have been viewed as being primarily antagonistic, resulting in the establishment of a homeo*static* state. This view, following the coining of the term *homeostasis* by Walter Cannon, became and still is a major foundation in our view of physiological reasoning.[1] This view of the autonomic nervous system's activities is restrictive and has enhanced the viewing of physiological systems as separate entities.[2]

Because most visceral effectors receive dual innervation by both branches of the autonomic nervous system, these effectors are under constant scrutiny by autonomic modulations.[3] Moreover, the autonomic nervous system is constantly modulating its activities to meet the *homeodynamic* rather than static biological oscillations. Specifically, the parasympathetic branch is primarily concerned with energy-conserving processes, whereas the sympathetic branch is primarily concerned with energy-expending processes.[4] A reciprocal and synergistic relationship appears to exist between the autonomically innervated tissues and organs and the branches of the autonomic nervous system. Clinical evidence of this relationship, as evidenced by a disturbance in the autonomic balance (sympathovagal balance), has been demonstrated in many pathophysiologic conditions.[5] Understanding of these conditions affords us a unique window of physiological study. Some of the following areas of autonomic study described herein will enhance our understanding of the autonomic nervous system and its encompassing physiological function.

ANATOMY OF THE AUTONOMIC NERVOUS SYSTEM

Autonomic visceral efferent pathways consist for the most part of two efferent neuronal pathways. A pathway originates from the central nervous system (CNS) to a ganglion (a group of nerve cell bodies located outside the CNS); the second division originates from the ganglion to its target tissue (organ, gland, and so forth).[6]

The first of the efferent neurons or nerve cells of the autonomic nervous system pathway are known as *preganglionic neurons* and are found within the brain or spinal cord. The myelinated axon originating from this neuron is referred to as a *preganglionic or presynaptic neuron.* The second neuron in this visceral efferent pathway, called *postganglionic or postsynaptic neuron,* travels from the autonomic ganglion, where it synapses with an effector organ. The locations of the autonomic ganglia are part of the differentiation of the divisions of the autonomic nervous system.[7]

Central Autonomic Regulation

Autonomic nervous system regulation is partly achieved via centrally located clusters of neuronal cells. Areas that constitute autonomic integrative centers include the medulla oblongata, pons, diencephalon, and telencephalon. A brief description follows of several of these integrative centers. The *nucleus tractus solitarius* receives information from the gastrointestinal, respiratory, and cardiovascular systems. Projections from the nucleus tractus solitarius migrate down to the brain stem and forebrain that modulate preganglionic sympathetic and parasympathetic functions. The nucleus tractus solitarius is a major area for the regulation of several reflexes involving respiration, blood pressure, and heart rate.[8] The *hypothalamus* is an integrative center that modulates many autonomic responses. Several zones have been identified that are believed to control feeding, fluid regulation, circulatory, and cardiovascular reflexes.[9]

Several areas of the *cerebral cortex* receive information from the hypothalamus that is involved in autonomic regulation. Specifically, the *insular and prefrontal areas* of the cerebral cortex are involved in blood pressure, heart rate, and respiratory regulation.[10] In addition to the few centers mentioned here, there are a vast number of areas involved in autonomic regulation. The main centers modulating the efferent sympathetic activity are located in the brain stem and hypothalamus. Outgrowths of these centers terminate in the *intermediolateral* cell column, which gives rise to the sympathetic preganglionic neurons and represent the final CNS output. Modulation of parasympathetic activity originates primarily from the *nucleus ambiguus* and the *dorsal nucleus of the vagus nerve.* Projections in these nuclei innervate parasympathetic ganglia whose axons terminate in cervical, thoracic, and abdominal viscera.[10]

Autonomic Ganglia

The sympathetic and parasympathetic divisions of the autonomic nervous system share several structural features. Both divisions have myelinated preganglionic neurons within the CNS and unmyelinated postganglionic clusters of neurons (ganglia) that are located outside of the CNS. However, the origins of the preganglionic fibers as well as the location of the ganglia differ for the two divisions.[10]

The autonomic ganglia are divided into three general groups. The sympathetic ganglia are located vertically (opposing, para) along both sides of the vertebral column, starting from the base of the skull down to the coccyx, and are referred to as *paravertebral (lateral) ganglia.* The preganglionic innervation from the sympathetic fibers generally tends to be short in length. An additional group of sympathetic ganglia lies anteriorly to the spinal column and is called the *prevertebral (collateral) ganglion.* These two groups of ganglia receive preganglionic fibers uniquely from the sympathetic division. The third group of autonomic ganglia belongs to the parasympathetic division that is located close to the visceral effectors. These ganglia receive preganglionic fibers belonging to the parasympathetic division. Because the preganglionic fibers of this division travel from the CNS to terminal ganglia or to the innervated organs, these fibers tend to be long.[7]

In postganglionic innervation, sympathetic preganglionic fibers synapse with several (>20) postganglionic fibers at the ganglion; the postganglionic fibers in turn impinge on visceral organs (effectors). Parasympathetic preganglionic neurons generally synapse with few (<5) postsynaptic neurons to a single organ (effector).[10]

Sympathetic Division

The preganglionic sympathetic neurons or fibers that exit from the spinal cord from the first thoracic down to the second lumbar level are also known as the *thoracolumbar division.* The *myelinated preganglionic* fibers originate from the spinal cord via the ventral root. When exiting the *intervertebral foramen,* these preganglionic fibers pass to the sympathetic trunk ganglion. The sympathetic trunks are situated *anterolaterally* to the spinal cord, one on each side. These sympathetic trunk ganglia are named according to their location along the spinal cord (cervical, thoracic, lumbar, and sacral). All of these ganglia receive their preganglionic fibers from the thoracic and lumbar segments (thoracolumbar) of the spinal cord.[11]

The cervical portion of the sympathetic trunk is divided into three ganglionic regions (upper, middle, and lower). The *superior cervical ganglion* is located posteriorly to the internal carotid artery, but anteriorly to the transverse processes of the second cervical vertebra. The *nonmyelinated postganglionic* fibers originating from this ganglion innervate the facial sweat glands, smooth muscle of the eye, blood vessels, and salivary glands. The *middle cervical ganglion* is located near the sixth cervical vertebra, and its postganglionic fibers innervate the heart. The *inferior cervical ganglion*, also called the *stellate ganglion*, is situated at the first rib, anteriorly to the transverse processes of the seventh cervical vertebra. Its postganglionic fibers innervate the heart.[11]

In addition, some preganglionic fibers pass beyond the trunk where they are known as *splanchnic nerves* and where they terminate in the celiac ganglion and the solar plexus, respectively. The *splanchnic postganglionic* fibers innervate the stomach, spleen, liver, kidney, small intestine, and colon. The lower splanchnic fibers innervate the distal colon, rectum, urinary bladder, and genital organs (Figure 4-1). The adrenal medulla of both adrenal glands is only innervated by preganglionic fibers and as such the adrenal medulla is considered a postganglion of the sympathetic nervous system. Because of this configuration, the sympathetic nervous system innervating the adrenal medulla is often referred to as the *sympathoadrenal system*.[10,11]

Parasympathetic Division

The preganglionic fibers of the parasympathetic division, also known as the *craniosacral* division, originate from nuclei in the brain stem, specifically the midbrain and the medulla oblongata, and from the second through fourth sacral segments of the spinal cord. These parasympathetic preganglionic fibers supply the ganglia that are situated within the innervated organs (effectors). Because of this type of innervation, these parasympathetic ganglia are also called *terminal ganglia*. As can be seen from Figure 4-1, unlike sympathetic fibers, most parasympathetic fibers do not travel within the spinal nerves.[10,11] The preganglionic fibers of the *cranial*

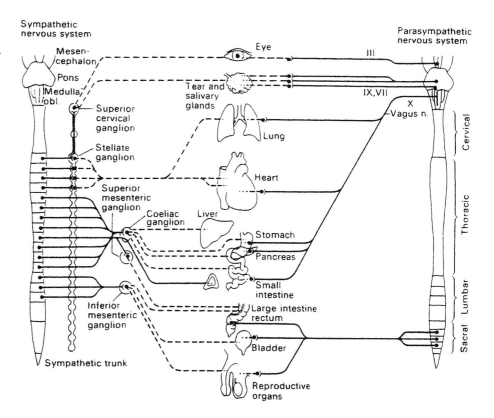

FIGURE 4-1 Schematic illustration of the peripheral autonomic nervous system, including neural pathways and ganglia for specific organs or tissues. Sympathetic innervation of the sweat glands, piloerector muscles, and peripheral vasculature is omitted. (Reprinted with permission from RL Brian. Clinical Neurology [6th ed]. Oxford: Oxford University Press, 1985;124–125.)

outflow portion of the parasympathetic nervous system originate from the brain stem by way of the oculomotor (III), facial (VII), glossopharyngeal (IX), and vagus (X) nerves.

The parasympathetic fibers that originate from the oculomotor nuclei of the cranial outflow synapse in the *ciliary ganglion*, whose postganglionic fibers innervate smooth muscle in the iris of the eye. The preganglionic fibers that originate in the medulla oblongata travel in the facial nerve (VII) to the *pterygopalatine ganglion*. This ganglion is situated lateral to a sphenopalatine foramen and is therefore often referred to as the *sphenopalatine ganglion*. The postganglionic fibers are transmitted to the nasal mucosa, pharynx, palate, and lacrimal glands. Another division of fibers, originating from the facial nerve (VII) innervate the *submandibular ganglion*, which sends postganglionic fibers to the submandibular and sublingual salivary glands. The preganglionic fibers of the glossopharyngeal nerve (IX) synapse in the *otic ganglion* and transmit postganglionic fibers that innervate the parotid salivary gland. Because the terminal ganglia are in close proximity to their visceral effectors, postganglionic parasympathetic fibers are short in comparison with postganglionic sympathetic fibers.[10-13]

Additional nuclei in the medulla oblongata contribute preganglionic fibers to the long and multiple branches of the vagus nerve, which provides approximately up to 80% of the parasympathetic innervation in the body. As the vagus nerve passes through the thorax it forms several plexus (a network of nerves) of which the fibers innervate terminal ganglia supplying the heart or *cardiac plexuses* (superficial and deep cardiac plexus). The vagus nerves that pass through the thorax also contribute postganglionic parasympathetic fibers to the lungs and bronchi. Inferior to the *pulmonary plexuses*, the vagus nerve forms the *esophageal plexuses*. The preganglionic fibers of the vagus synapse with postganglionic neurons that are situated within the innervated organs. These preganglionic fibers from the vagal branch innervate the stomach, pancreas, liver, and upper half of the large intestine. The postganglionic parasympathetic fibers arise from ganglia located inside these organs and innervate the cells. Moreover, the branches of the vagus nerve within the abdomen provide plexus of the abdominal aorta.[10-12]

The sacral portion of the parasympathetic division provides preganglionic fibers from the ventral roots of the second through fourth sacral nerves. Called the *pelvic splanchnic nerves*, these nerves pass into the *hypogastric plexus*. Their parasympathetic postganglionic fibers innervate the colon, ureters, urinary bladder, and reproductive organs.[10-12]

PHYSIOLOGY OF THE AUTONOMIC NERVOUS SYSTEM

The release of the neurotransmitter from the autonomic fibers forms the basis for autonomic fiber classification. Acetylcholine is the neurotransmitter released by all sympathetic and parasympathetic preganglionic axons, all parasympathetic postganglionic axons, and some sympathetic postganglionic axons. Thus, all sympathetic and parasympathetic preganglionic autonomic ganglia as well as the parasympathetic postganglionic fibers are classified as *cholinergic*. The action of acetylcholine is short lived and localized because of the presence of the membrane-bound enzyme acetylcholinesterase.

Norepinephrine or noradrenaline is the neurotransmitter released by most postganglionic sympathetic nerve fibers. Therefore, most postganglionic sympathetic fibers are classified as adrenergic. Because norepinephrine is inactivated more slowly and norepinephrine can enter the blood stream, consequently the action of sympathetic stimulation lasts longer and is more diffuse than parasympathetic stimulation. The adrenal medullae are considered to be postganglionic sympathetic extensions and produce norepinephrine and epinephrine. In addition to norepinephrine and epinephrine, a transmitter is produced within the CNS, called *dopamine*. All three transmitters are collectively referred to as *catecholamines*.[10-12]

Receptor Physiology

Excitatory and inhibitory effects are produced in different tissues and organs by the same neurotransmitters. Clearly the response depends on factors other than the chemical property of the transmitter. The major factor responsible for the specific response relates to the membrane receptor proteins. Two major classifications for these proteins have been identified and are designated as alpha (α) and beta (β) receptors. Additional subtypes of receptors have been identified and designated as α_1 and α_2 and β_1 and β_2.[10-13]

The effects of the *adrenergic* neurotransmitters, norepinephrine and epinephrine, depend on the type of postsynaptic receptors that are being activated. These receptor subtypes in various organs precipitate specific physiological effects of the autonomic neurotransmitters. As a general rule, binding to an α receptor results in an influx of sodium ions followed by a membrane depolarization (excitation). β-Receptor binding generally results in an efflux and influx of potassium and chloride ions, respectively, bringing about hyperpolarization of the postsynaptic membrane (inhibition). Most effector organs contain either α or β receptors; some effector cells contain both receptors.[10-13]

In general, norepinephrine stimulates primarily α receptors, and epinephrine tends to stimulate both α and β receptors. It is important to note that there are many exceptions to these general rules, and as such, this area of study is often confusing and extremely complex.[10-13]

The *cholinergic* neurotransmitter acetylcholine is synthesized and released from the vesicles stored in the axon terminals of the cholinergic fibers. As with the adrenergic neurotransmitter responses, the cholinergic postsynaptic responses are largely determined by the type of cholinergic postsynaptic receptors. Cholinergic receptors consist of two types and are known as *nicotinic* and *muscarinic* receptors. This classification was derived because of a similarity in the receptors' actions when occupied by the two chemicals nicotine and muscarine. Nicotinic receptors are found on sympathetic and parasympathetic postganglionic neurons. Muscarinic receptors are found on all parasympathetic postganglionic effectors and some sympathetic postganglionic effectors. Molecular cloning studies have demonstrated the existence of multiple subtypes for both muscarinic and nicotinic receptors. In addition to acetylcholine, cholinergic neurons contain other transmitter substances: Preganglionic neurons contain enkephalins.[10-13]

EFFECTS OF AEROBIC TRAINING ON AUTONOMIC MODULATION

Endurance exercise elicits a vast number of cardiovascular adaptations, most notably a decrease in heart rate. Several theories have been advanced that include reductions in sympathetic activity and enhancement of both vagal cardiac activity and baroreflex sensitivity. Endurance exercise training has been shown to modify autonomic outflow favorably. A modification of the autonomic nervous system, specifically a reduction in sympathetic activity (sympathetic nervous system), was suggested after evidence was seen of reduced concentrations of catecholamines in the heart of physically trained animals.[14] In addition, human studies using pharmacologic blockade (e.g., atropine) have indicated that trained compared with untrained subjects possess higher vagal tone.[15-16]

Human studies performed in our laboratories have provided additional support for endurance training as a beneficial modulator of cardiac autonomic nervous system activity. Our earliest work compared 72 male New York road runners, aged 15-83 with 72 age-, weight-,

and socioeconomic level–matched sedentary control subjects for their amplitude in heart rate variability.[17] The amplitude of the heart rate variability was used as an index of parasympathetic activity. Fitness level for both groups was determined using on-line, open-circuit spirometry, during an incremental stress test. Overall results in this cross-sectional study showed that the physically active group had significantly higher fitness levels, which were associated with a higher amplitude in heart rate variability when compared with their sedentary counterparts.[17] Because of the cross-sectional nature of the study, these findings provided suggestive evidence for habitual aerobic exercise as a beneficial modulator of heart rate variability in an aged population. To further verify the beneficial effects of aerobic exercise on autonomic modulation, we investigated in a longitudinal study the effects of intense aerobic training on autonomic modulation. Nine middle- and long-distance male track athletes were tested before and following an 8-week high-intensity regime (7 days/week). Aerobic capacity was tested on both occasions using on-line, open-circuit spirometry. Parasympathetic activity was assessed as described previously during carefully controlled breathing. Our findings revealed that a 7.3% increase in aerobic capacity was associated with a 23% augmentation in heart rate variability, a noninvasive marker of parasympathetic activity (peripheral nervous system).[18] These data are suggestive of several important factors, namely that aerobic training of sufficient intensity to elicit significant improvements in aerobic capacity improves parasympathetic modulation, and secondly, that autonomic changes appear to be more sensitive to change than the improvement in aerobic capacity itself.[18]

These findings of enhanced parasympathetic modulation to the heart over a 24-hour period were again documented by our colleagues. Specifically, in a cross-sectional investigation, comparing 24-hour time and frequency domain measures of vagal modulation, they found significantly higher parasympathetic cardiac modulation in the highly trained endurance athletes when compared with sedentary age-matched controls.[19] In addition to the work by our group and colleagues, several other laboratories have demonstrated augmentations in peripheral nervous system activity and a reduction in sympathetic nervous system. Furthermore, in one study in which young and middle-aged trained subjects were compared for parasympathetic nervous system and sympathetic nervous system activity, there were no differences.[20] It would appear that regular physical activity promotes the maintenance of cardiovascular fitness in middle-aged individuals and attenuates the effects of aging. Could this then possibly reduce the risk of cardiovascular disease? The answer to this question remains to be seen. However, the clinical relevance of loss of vagal cardiac activity, augmentation in sympathetic activity, or both has been demonstrated via the association with increased cardiovascular morbidity and mortality. The quantitative relationship between level of activity or fitness and magnitude of cardiovascular benefit may extend across a wide variety of activities. However, physical activity must be performed frequently to maintain these effects. Moderate-intensity activity performed by sedentary individuals or by individuals recovering from illness results in functional capacity improvements.[21] Specifically, in this investigation they found that low-intensity exercise training significantly reduced systolic, diastolic, and mean blood pressure in spontaneously hypertensive rats.[21] These findings have been corroborated in human studies in which exercise training at 55% of $\dot{V}O_2$max reduced high blood pressure in men more when compared with exercise training in excess of 75% of $\dot{V}O_2$max.[22] Therefore, we recommend people increase their regular physical activity level appropriate to their capacities, needs, and interests.

EFFECTS OF AGE ON AUTONOMIC MODULATION

Aging is associated with changes in sympathovagal balance, specifically, an exaggerated shift toward sympathetic activity has been reported. Multiple mechanisms appear to be responsible for this age-related increase in sympathetic modulation, and autonomic as well as nonautonomic influences appear to play a role. One hypothesis that has been suggested to explain these age-dependent alterations in sympathovagal balance is that aging is associated with loss of vascular compliance or increased stiffness of the vessels. Therefore, a prior cross-sectional investigation from our laboratory assessed the relationship between aging, vagal cardiac activity, and arteriolar compliance. The respiratory sinus arrhythmia and pulse wave analyses were used to determine vagal cardiac activity and arteriolar compliance, respectively, on 70 normotensive male subjects (age range, 15–81 years).[23] Both respiratory sinus arrhythmia and arteriolar compliance decreased with age. These findings support the notion that there is an age-related loss of vagal cardiac activity that can be partly explained by the loss of arteriolar compliance in a normotensive population.[23] The majority of heart rate variability studies appears to suggest a gender difference in autonomic modulation.

Specifically, women appeared to have greater parasympathetic activity and lesser sympathetic activity while at rest and during orthostatic stress, respectively.[24] These results could be a major factor in the recognized lower risk of cardiovascular disease in women and deserve further study. A possible explanation could be that estrogen plays a role; however, to date few studies have been carried out comparing autonomic modulation in the elderly of both genders.

ESTROGEN REPLACEMENT AND AUTONOMIC MODULATION

Several studies have demonstrated beneficial associations between postmenopausal estrogen use and cardiovascular mortality, morbidity, and risk factors.[25-30] Estrogen replacement therapy has been associated with decreased overall mortality, decreased cardiovascular mortality, and improved risk factor profiles. Few studies have studied the autonomic modulation associated with estrogen replacement. Studies by our laboratory demonstrated favorable alterations in autonomic modulation following estrogen replacement when compared with placebo.[31] Specifically, we found a reduction in low-frequency modulation with concomitant augmentation in vagal modulation to the heart. To explain these adaptations we studied baroreceptor sensitivity and found a rapid and significant improvement in baroreceptor sensitivity. Furthermore, this significant improvement in baroreceptor sensitivity was significantly correlated with improved vasodilatory capacity of the arterioles. These salutary effects of estrogen on autonomic modulation and vessel distensibility appear to have direct beneficial implications on cardiovascular morbidity and mortality. However, despite the well-established efficacy of estrogens in protecting women against cardiovascular disease, a reluctance to use them still exists, because of their uterotropic effects. A new group of nonuterotropic estrogens does not have these cancer-promoting abilities and has been demonstrated to confer protective effects on bone. No information is currently available on the effects of nonuterotropic or selective estrogen receptor modulators on cardiac autonomic modulation.

CARDIAC AUTONOMIC MODULATION IN SPINAL CORD INJURY

Since 1995 we have investigated autonomic modulation in spinal cord injury patients using power spectral density analyses. The noninvasive nature of these methodologies allows for information to be obtained without undue stress. However, because of uncertainties surrounding the autonomic activity represented by low frequency modulation we will emphasize the high frequency modulation, which is considered to be a valid marker of vagal cardiac activity.[32] This initial work indicated that complete quadriplegia patients experienced a significant down-regulation of vagal cardiac activity.[32] This shift in autonomic modulation would lead to unfavorable long-term cardiovascular outcomes and prompted us to further explore cardiac autonomic physiology in spinal cord injury patients. Subsequently, we studied the autonomic modulation in healthy incomplete quadriplegic, complete quadriplegic, and paraplegic patients in response to provocations and compared these autonomic responses with healthy matched controls.[33] All subjects were studied under resting conditions and during provocative maneuvers (tilt, cold pressor, and isometric contraction). Analyses revealed and confirmed our earlier observation of a loss of vagal modulation in spinal cord injury. The findings in this investigation further support our earlier observations of an attenuation of vagal cardiac modulation at rest and an exaggerated withdrawal during provocative maneuvers. Furthermore, we observed a positive relationship between the magnitude of loss of vagal cardiac modulation and level and completeness of injury.[32] Moreover, cardiac output in paraplegia is greatly reduced because of the loss of the muscle pump. To compensate for this loss, there is an increase in sympathetic modulation with concomitant increases in heart rate. These increases in heart rate attenuate cardiac filling time, which reduces the cardiac output even more. Consequently, a greatly augmented sympathetic modulation feeds this debilitating cycle.

Prior cross-sectional research has demonstrated greater hemodynamic efficiency in paraplegic subjects following aerobic training.[34] To date no longitudinal study has been carried out investigating the effects of habitual aerobic exercise on cardiac output and autonomic modulation in paraplegic patients. However, some preliminary data from our laboratory seem to suggest favorable autonomic alterations and improved stroke volumes in these patients with aerobic training.[35] Further research in this area is warranted because spinal cord injury leads to a sedentary lifestyle. Wheelchair ambulation appears to be an insufficient stimulus to elicit cardiovascular and autonomic improvements in these patients. Perhaps a physically active lifestyle could attenuate these accelerated degenerative processes in these populations and reduce overall cardiovascular morbidity and mortality.

NONINVASIVE ASSESSMENT OF AUTONOMIC ACTIVITY

It has been shown that the measurement of autonomic activity is a powerful predictor of overall cardiovascular morbidity and mortality.[36,37] Therefore, the determination of autonomic activity may be a valuable tool in the overall prognosis of patients at high risk for cardiovascular morbidity and mortality. Today computerized analysis of digitized electrocardiographic signals and readily available software afford us a rapid window on the patient's autonomic activity. We briefly discuss two methods for determining autonomic activity using frequency-domain and time-domain analyses. For the appropriateness of data collection and interpretation we refer the reader to the standards put forth by the European Task Force.[38] However, for an appropriate reflection of the activity of the sympathetic and parasympathetic branches, a minimum of 3 minutes of data collection has been suggested.[38]

Principle of Frequency-Domain Analysis

Most organ systems possess an inherent rhythm (i.e., our mean breathing rate is around 12 breaths per minute, and our mean heart rate tends to be around 70–80 beats per minute, and so forth). These rhythms or frequency modulations are also specific for the branches of the autonomic nervous system, and they happen to differ dependent on the branch or division. Specifically, the sympathetic activity tends to have a rhythm or frequency modulation that occurs at a low frequency. The parasympathetic activity tends to occur at a higher frequency. Therefore, if we are able to delineate or demodulate the frequency of our heart rate variability and blood pressure variability, we then can infer (with some limitations) the magnitude of activity (power) of the two branches of the autonomic nervous system. Briefly, frequency-domain analyses convert data from the time domain into the frequency domain. These frequency domains are delineated in Hertz or cycles per second. Additionally, the area of the derived spectrum represents the energy or power present ($msec^2$ or $mm\ Hg^2$) of the branch of the autonomic nervous system. Pharmacologic studies have revealed frequency bandwidths representative of the two branches of the autonomic nervous system.[38] Clinically relevant frequency bands have been established, in which low-frequency bandwidth (0.06–0.15 Hz) is considered primarily representative of sympathetic activity and some parasympathetic activity. The power centered around 0.15–0.4 Hz is referred to as the *high-frequency band* and is considered to be primarily representative of parasympathetic activity.[38] The ratio of these frequency modulations is the assessment of the so-called sympathovagal balance.[38] There is, however, some controversy regarding this assessment as a measure of sympathovagal balance.[39] One of the reasons for this controversy is the unclear magnitude of contribution of the two branches of the autonomic nervous system to the low-frequency bandwidth. Prior work in our laboratory has demonstrated that low-frequency power of blood pressure (systolic pressure) variability is a more precise marker of sympathetic activity.[40,41] Computation of these specific area measurements (spectra) is greatly facilitated by our microcomputer technology.

The most commonly used transformational techniques (transforming time-domain data to frequency-domain data) are based on autoregressive models and the fast Fourier transforms.

Time-Domain Analyses

Analysis of heart rate variability in the time domain has been shown to provide insight in the prognosis of myocardial infarction.[42] Simple descriptive statistics can be computed from a time series. Of these, the standard deviation has been found to be a key variable in predicting myocardial infarction.[42]

REFERENCES

1. Cannon WB. Organization for physiological homeostasis. Physiol Rev 1929;399–431.
2. Dinner DS (ed). The autonomic nervous system [review articles]. J Clin Neurophysiol 1993;10:1–82.
3. Loewy AD. Anatomy of the Autonomic Nervous System: An Overview. In AD Loewy, KM Spyer (eds), Central Regulation of Autonomic Functions. New York: Oxford University Press, 1990;3–16.
4. Gaskell WH. The Involuntary Nervous System. London: Longmans, Green, 1916.
5. Bannister R, Mathias C. Testing Autonomic Reflexes. In R Bannister (ed), Autonomic Failure. A Text Book of Clinical Disorders of the Autonomic Nervous System. Oxford: Oxford University Press, 1988;289–307.
6. Spyer KM. The Central Nervous Organization of Reflex Circulatory Control. In AD Loewy, KM Spyer (eds), Central Regulation of Autonomic Functions. New York: Oxford University Press, 1990;168–188.
7. Fox SI. Human Physiology. Dubuque, IA: WC Brown, 1996;208–225.
8. Strack AM, Sawyer WG, Hughes JH. A general pattern of CNS innervation of the sympathetic outflow demonstrated by transneuronal pseudorabies viral infections. Brain Res 1989;491:156–162.
9. Dale HH. Nomenclature of fibers in the autonomic system and their effects. J Physiol (Lond) 1933;80:10p–11p.
10. Van de Graaf K, Fox SI. Concepts of Human Anatomy and Physiology (2nd ed). Dubuque, IA: WC Brown, 1989.
11. Tortora GJ, Anagnostakos NP. Principles of Anatomy and Physiology (6th ed). New York: Harper & Row, 1990.
12. Hole JW. Human Anatomy and Physiology (5th ed). Dubuque, IA: WC Brown, 1990.
13. Fox SI. Human Physiology (4th ed). Dubuque, IA: WC Brown, 1993.
14. Tipton C. The influence of atropine on the heart rate responses of nontrained, trained, and detrained animals. Physiologist 1976;12:376.
15. Ekblom B, Kilbom A, Soltysiak J. Physical training bradycardia, and autonomic nervous system. Scand J Clin Lab Invest 1973;32:251–256.
16. Smith ML, Hudson DL, Grazier HM, Raven PB. Exercise training bradycardia: the role of autonomic balance. Med Sci Sports Exerc 1987;21:40–44.
17. De Meersman R. Heart rate variability and aerobic fitness. Am Heart J 1993;125:726–731.
18. De Meersman R. Respiratory sinus arrhythmia alteration following training in endurance athletes. Eur J Appl Physiol 1992;64:434–436.
19. Goldsmith RI, Bigger JT, Steinmann RC, Fleiss JL. Comparison of 24-hour parasympathetic activity in endurance-trained and untrained young men. J Am Coll Cardiol 1992;20:552–558.
20. Boutcher SH, Stein P. Association between heart rate variability and training response in sedentary middle-aged men. Eur J Appl Physiol 1995;70(1):75–80.
21. Krieger EM, Brum PC, Negrao CE. Influence of exercise training on neurogenic control of blood pressure in spontaneously hypertensive rats. Hypertension 1999;34(2):720–723.
22. Esler MD, Lambert G, Jennings G. Regional norepinephrine turnover in human hypertension. Clin Exp Hypertension 1989;11(Suppl 1):75–89.
23. De Meersman R. Aging as a modulator of respiratory sinus arrhythmia. J Gerontol A Biol Sci Med Sci 1993;48:2,B74–B78.
24. Lipsitz, L. Syncope in the elderly. Ann Intern Med 1983;99:92–105.
25. Colditz GA, Willett WC, Stampfer MJ, et al. Menopause and the risk of coronary heart disease in women. N Engl J Med 1987;316:1105–1110.
26. Barrett-Connor E, Bush TL. Estrogen replacement and coronary heart disease. Cardiovasc Clin 1989;19:159–172.
27. Barr DP, Russ EM, Elder HA. Influence of estrogens on lipoproteins in atherosclerosis. Trans Assoc Am Physicians 1952;65:102–113.
28. Ross RK, Paganini-Hill A, Mack TM, Henderson BE. Estrogen Use and Cardiovascular Disease. In DR Mishell (ed), Menopause Physiology and Pharmacology. Chicago: Year Book Medical, 1987;209–223.
29. Henderson BE, Ross RK, Pagannini A, Mack TM. Estrogen use and cardiovascular disease. Am J Obstet Gynecol 1986;54:1181–1186.
30. Henderson BE, Pagannini-Hill A, Ross RK. Decreased mortality in users of estrogen replacement therapy. Arch Intern Med 1988;108:358–363.
31. De Meersman R, Zion AS, Giardina EGV, et al. Estrogen replacement, vascular distensibility, and blood pressures in postmenopausal women. Am J Physiol 1998;274(43):H1539–H1544.
32. Grimm D, De Meersman R, Almenoff P, et al. Sympathovagal balance of the heart in subjects with spinal cord injury. Am J Physiol 1997;272(41):H1427–H1431.
33. Grimm D, Almenoff P, Bauman W, De Meersman R. Baroreceptor sensitivity response to phase IV of the Val-

salva maneuver in spinal cord injury. Clin Aut Res 1998;8:111–118.

34. Huonker M, Schmid A, Sorichter S, et al. Cardiovascular differences between sedentary and wheelchair-trained subjects with paraplegia. Med Sc Sports Exerc 1998;30(4):609–613.

35. Wecht J, De Meersman R, Weir JP, et al. The effects of spinal cord injury and inactivity on venous vascular function. Am J Physiol 2000;278: H515–H520.

36. Kleiger RE, Miller JP, Bigger JT, et al. Decreased heart rate variability and its association with increased mortality after acute myocardial infarction. Am J Cardiol 1987;59:256–262.

37. Bigger JT, Hoover CG, Steinman RC. Frequency domain measures of heart period variability in patients to assess risk after myocardial infarction. J Am Coll Cardiol 1990;66:497–498.

38. Pagani MF, Lombardi S, Guzetti O, et al. Power spectral analysis of heart rate and arterial pressure variabilities as a marker of sympatho-vagal interaction in a conscious dog. Circ Res 1986;59:178–193.

39. Eckberg DL. Sympathovagal balance: a critical appraisal. Circulation 1997;96:3224–3232.

40. Sloan R, De Meersman R, Shapiro P, et al. Cardiac autonomic control is inversely related to blood pressure variability responses to psychological challenge. Am J Physiol 1997; 272(41):H2227–H2232.

41. Sloan R, De Meersman R, Shapiro P, et al. Blood pressure variability responses to tilt are buffered by cardiac autonomic control. Am J Physiol 1997;272(41):H1427–H1431.

42. Bigger JT, Kleiger RE, Fleiss JL, et al. Components of heart rate variability measured after acute myocardial infarction. Am J Cardiol 1988;61(1):208–215.

5

Skeletal Muscle: Structure, Chemistry, and Function

JAMES S. LIEBERMAN, GALE N. PUGLIESE,
AND NANCY E. STRAUSS

A majority of the basic elements of skeletal muscle structure and function and the mechanics of muscle contraction have been known for many years. More definitive understanding of the anatomy, chemistry, and physiology of muscle contraction has come only after the development of modern investigative techniques such as electron microscopy, x-ray diffraction studies, and magnetic resonance spectroscopy.

In this chapter we provide a concise overview of the development, anatomy, chemistry, physiology, and energetics of skeletal muscle and skeletal muscle contraction.

MUSCLE DEVELOPMENT

Prenatal Development

Embryonic development of skeletal muscle is treated in standard textbooks,[1-3] most data being derived from nonhuman mammalian species. Skeletal muscles of the limbs and trunk are derived from mesodermal somites, whereas cervical and craniobulbar muscles originate in the branchial arches. When the somitic cells migrate into the limb bud they become subject to a set of guidance and patterning cues.[4] By the eighth week of gestation, the primordia of many individual muscles are identifiable as groups of primitive myotubes. These multinucleated syncytia contain the first traces of myofibrils in their cytoplasm. The myotubes are formed by fusion of mononucleate stem cells termed *myoblasts*.

Individual skeletal muscles are well formed by the tenth week of gestation, and in the next 6 weeks myotubes proliferate by fusion with specific neighboring cells until the ultimate number of muscle fibers has been formed in a given muscle. Division by mitosis does not occur in striated muscle cells.[5] As myotubes mature, their myofibrils increase in number and size until they are densely packed, and the nuclei migrate to their familiar location beneath the sarcolemma, at which time they are termed *myofibers*. Maturation of the sarcotubular system and initiation of motor innervation occur concurrently. The first fetal movements at around 14–16 weeks' gestation probably reflect functionally active neuromuscular junctions. The second half of fetal life is associated with exponential growth of skeletal muscles, primarily by hypertrophy of individual muscle fibers.[6] Mean fiber diameter increases exponentially.[7]

Histochemical staining properties of fetal muscle are uniform until approximately the fifth month of gestation. At 20 weeks, a few type I fibers can be identified by staining characteristics, but they are sparse until 34 weeks, when they rapidly increase in number in a linear fashion to constitute 40% of total fibers at term.[7] Types IIa and IIb, as well as newly discovered fiber types,[8] gradually differentiate from fetal type II fibers, often called *type IIc fibers*. Maturity of the innervating motor neurons may be the determining factor in fiber type differentiation.[9]

Postnatal Growth

Between birth and puberty, muscle mass increase is the result of both fiber hypertrophy and lengthening. Sarcomeres are added to the ends of the muscle fiber in series adjacent to the musculotendinous junction, resulting in increased fiber length.[10] The amount of muscle stretch seems to affect sarcomere growth. For example, immobilization of growing mouse muscle in a shortened position decreases the addition of sarcomeres, but the ability to fully recover is not affected by the period of immobilization or the stage of development.[11] Most of the increase in myofiber cross-sectional area is caused by the increased number of myofibrils, although the number of nuclei per fiber also increases with age.[10]

MUSCLE STRUCTURE

Muscles are divided into fascicles, each containing many muscle fibers. These vary in length up to 40 cm; diameter varies from 10–100 μm and generally run the entire length of the fascicle without interruption. Owing to the pennate arrangement of most muscles, few fibers are longer than 10 cm and most are shorter than the overall length of the muscle.

Connective Tissue

Muscle fibers are bound by collagenous connective tissue that has three separate components. The epimysium is the tough elastic envelope for the entire muscle merging at its end with the tendon. Connective tissue septa that divide fibers into fascicular bundles are termed the *perimysium*. The final connective tissue component, the endomysium, separates individual muscle fibers from each other.

Each individual muscle fiber is surrounded by a structural framework called the *sarcolemma*, a connective tissue scaffold made up of basal lamina and endomysial reticula. This is differentiated by anatomists from the

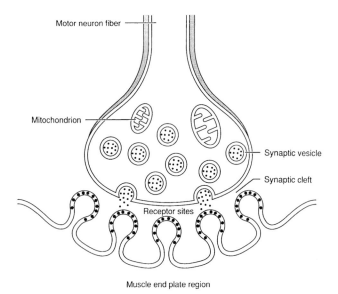

Muscle end plate region

FIGURE 5-1 Structure of the neuromuscular junction shows major structures and release of acetylcholine from synaptic vesicles.

plasmalemma, the cell membrane of each muscle syncytial fiber, but in practice these terms are often used interchangeably.

Vascular Supply

The vascularization of skeletal muscle varies considerably. Generally, five main types of intramuscular arterial vascularization patterns are seen in muscles[12]: (1) Separate nutrient vessels enter the muscle throughout its length, forming an anastomotic chain (soleus and peroneus longus). (2) A single group of arteries forms a longitudinal pattern, but they arise from a common stem and enter one end of the muscle (gastrocnemius). (3) A radiating pattern of collaterals is formed from a single vessel that enters the middle of the muscle (biceps brachii). (4) A series of anastomotic loops is present throughout the muscle length. The loops are formed from a succession of entering vessels (tibialis anterior, extensor hallucis longus, long leg flexors). (5) The final type is an open quadrilateral pattern with sparse anastomotic connections (extensor hallucis longus).

A significant capillary bed is present in muscle. At rest, few capillaries are open. With muscle contraction, however, a great number open.[12] As a general rule, in any particular muscle, blood flow at rest is proportional to the number of slow fibers, whereas during increasing muscle activity it is proportional to the number of fast fibers.[13]

Nerve Supply

The nerve supply to a muscle enters near the end-plate zone and may consist of one or several branches that contain both efferent and afferent fibers. In fact, only 50–60% of large myelinated fibers are typically efferent in a muscle branch[14] in the muscle itself. The major afferent fibers (types Ia and Ib) are from muscle spindles and Golgi tendon organs. Significant branching occurs at nodes of Ranvier, resulting in the presence of many intramuscular nerve bundles.[13] Efferent fibers are myelinated until the terminal portion of the nerve at the neuromuscular junction.[13]

Neuromuscular Junction

As a terminal axon of a muscle nerve nears its muscle fiber, it loses its myelin sheath and develops a slightly bulbous terminal (Figure 5-1).[15] The terminal lies within a groove on the surface of the muscle fiber, and the presynaptic (neural) portion of the neuromuscular junction comes to within 50 nm of the postsynaptic (muscular) portion. This 50-nm gap is the synaptic cleft. One or more

Schwann's cells cover the nerve terminal and form the membrane of the postsynaptic portion of the muscle fiber.

The muscle membrane on the postsynaptic side is constructed with multiple folds that much increase its surface area. Within these junctional folds are acetylcholinesterase receptors and storage sites for acetylcholinesterase. The muscle sarcoplasm underlying the neuromuscular junction contains a large number of muscle nuclei and mitochondria.

On the presynaptic side, the nerve terminal contains a number of mitochondria as well as large numbers of 40- to 50-nm vesicles that contain the neurotransmitter acetylcholine. Although the vesicles are distributed diffusely within the terminal, they cluster at several thicker portions of the presynaptic membrane, the *active sites*.[16]

Two proteins that are important in synaptic formation and vesicle recycling have been described.[17] Syntaxin is associated with synapse formation, whereas dynamin is associated with synaptic vesicle recycling.[17]

Muscle Fiber Histochemistry

With histochemical techniques it is possible to differentiate fiber types based on activity of key enzymes and constituents. This has important functional and metabolic consequences, as each individual muscle has a unique fiber makeup that generally supports its function in the body.

Originally, two major fiber types were identified, based on a difference in reactivity of myofibrillar adenosine triphosphatase (ATPase) at pH 9.4 and verified with histochemical activity of oxidative enzymes and phosphorylase. Type I fibers are characterized by high activity of oxidative enzymes and low relative activity of phosphorylase and myofibrillar ATPase at pH 9.4. They also have greater lipid and myoglobin concentrations as well as capillary density, but less glycogen storage. This suggests that type I fibers have greater capacity for oxidative metabolism.

Type II fibers have a contrasting profile with fibers specialized for anaerobic or glycolytic metabolism (Table 5-1). Type II fibers can be subgrouped into IIa, IIb (Figure 5-2), and IIc[18-19] by using the pH sensitivity of the myofibrillar ATPase reaction and acid preincubation. The IIa fibers seem to represent an intermediate class that has both oxidative and glycolytic characteristics. Type IIc fibers may be intermediate as well, and they are often regarded as an immature fiber type. The more recently described type IID and IIX fibers are also intermediate types.[8]

An important finding is that muscle fibers that belong to a single motor unit are of a single histochemical type.[20,21] These fibers are not grouped together but are interspersed throughout a larger volume of muscle with many fibers from other motor units. Functionally, this

TABLE 5-1

Muscle Fiber Type Classification

	Type I	*Type IIa*	*Type IIb*	*Type IIc*
Color	Red	Red	White	—
Myoglobin content	High	High	Low	—
Glycogen content	Low	High	High	—
Capillary density	High	High	Low	—
Mitochondria	Many	Many	Few	—
Lipid content	High	Intermediate	Low	—
Muscle fiber type: contraction and metabolism	SO	FOG	FG	—
Physiological motor unit type	S	FR	FF	F(int)
Contraction	Slow	Fast	Fast	Fast
Fatigue resistance	High	High	Low	Intermediate
Enzyme activity				
ATPase (pH 9.4)	Low	High	High	High
ATPase (pH 4.6)	High	Low	Moderate	Moderate
ATPase (pH 4.3)	High	Low	Low	Low
Phosphorylase	Low	High	High	—
Oxidative enzymes	High	Intermediate	Low	—

ATP = adenosine triphosphatase; FF = fast twitch, fatiguable; FG = fast twitch, glycolytic; F(int) = fast twitch, resistance to fatigue intermittent between FF and FR; FOG = fast twitch, oxidative-glycolytic; FR = fast twitch, fatigue resistant; S = slow twitch; SO = slow twitch oxidative.

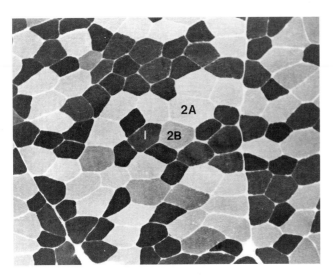

FIGURE 5-2 Photomicrograph of vastus lateralis from a 21-year-old man stained for adenosine triphosphatase at pH 4.6 showing type I, type IIa (2A), and type IIb (2B) fibers (original magnification × 185). (Courtesy of Dr. William Ellis, Department of Pathology, University of California at Davis.)

spreads the contractile force generated by a single unit across a larger area of muscle.

Correlations between histochemical fiber type and physiological properties demonstrate that type I fiber motor units contract slowly and are fatigue resistant.[20] Type IIb motor units tend to have the opposite characteristics (i.e., fast twitch and relative susceptibility to fatigue). As expected, type IIa units are intermediate, having both fast twitch and fatigue-resistant properties. In humans, predominantly tonic postural muscles such as the soleus contain primarily type I fibers, whereas phasic muscles such as the orbicularis oculi contain principally type II fibers.[22] The physiology of the newly described type IID and IIX fibers is not yet worked out.[8]

Although cross-innervation experiments demonstrate the ability to change the histochemical profile of a predominantly slow muscle,[23] until fairly recently it was not considered possible to change fiber type proportions using specific training techniques or electrical stimulation, but there is now evidence to the contrary. Long-term low-frequency stimulation induces transformation of fast muscle fibers into slow ones in both rats and rabbits.[21,24] High-intensity interval training has been shown to increase the proportion of type I fibers in both rats[25] and humans[26] at the expense of type IIb. This suggests that the proportions of fiber types may not be solely under genetic control and may respond to specific environmental influences.

Structural Organization Within the Muscle

A skeletal muscle is composed of a number of discrete bundles of muscle fibers termed *fascicles*, each sheathed in connective tissue. Each muscle fiber, in turn, is composed of a number of myofibrils. The myofibrils are composed of myofilaments arranged in units called *sarcomeres*. There are two types of myofilaments, thin filaments containing actin, troponin, and tropomyosin, and thick filaments containing myosin. The arrangement of myofibrils into sarcomeres is responsible for the striated appearance of skeletal muscle under the light microscope; thus, the derivation of the term *striated muscle*.

Ultrastructure

The sarcomere, the functional unit of the myofibril, can be seen with electron microscopy. One sarcomere is defined as extending from Z line to Z line (Figures 5-3 and 5-4). The dark A band of the sarcomere is composed of thick myosin filaments and overlapping thin actin filaments, whereas the pale I band, transected at its midpoint by the Z line, is made up only of thin actin molecules. The H zone is the central area without filament overlap and is relatively lighter than the A band because it contains only myosin filaments. However, the H zone is darker than the I band, which contains only thin filaments. The dark central M line represents the point at which myosin filaments are bound together with their neighbors, lending stability to the thick filaments during contraction.[27] The Z lines serve as the junction between sarcomeres and are the attachment point for thin filaments; thus, they appear to be the point of tension transmission between sarcomeres during muscle contraction.

Changes in the sarcomere during contraction were described by Huxley and Hanson, who noted that during stretch and contraction the size of the A band remained constant whereas the length of the I band and the H zone changed. From this they derived the sliding filament theory of muscle contraction[28] (i.e., the thin filaments slide toward the center of the sarcomere [M line], whereas thick filaments remain stationary) (Figure 5-5).

INTERNAL NONCONTRACTILE STRUCTURES

Sarcoplasmic Reticulum

The sarcoplasmic reticulum (SR) is a network of tubules and cisternae that surrounds the myofibrils.[29] The SR

FIGURE 5-3 Electron micrograph of muscle shows a typical sarcomere. Major structures are labeled, including Z and M lines and I and A bands (original magnification × 40,000). (Courtesy of Dr. William Ellis, Department of Pathology, University of California at Davis.)

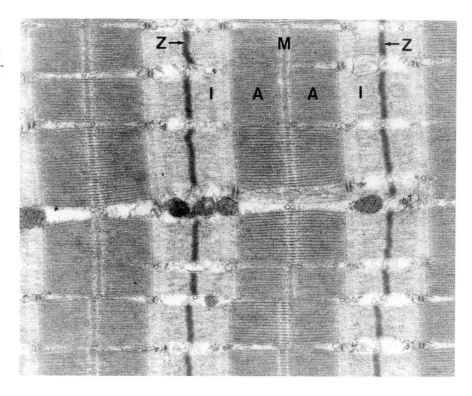

maintains a specific relationship to the transverse tubular system (T system), which is described presently. The SR consists mainly of tubules arranged longitudinally, parallel to the long axis of the myofibrils. At the junction of the A and I bands, where the SR is adjacent to the T system, the SR tubules fuse to two terminal cisternae, one on either side of the T tubule.

The SR is the primary calcium storage and release site in muscle. Portions of the SR function as a calcium pump, and the terminal cisternae have the special ability to convert an electrical impulse from the T system into calcium release. In addition, the SR interior contains large amounts of calsequestrin, a protein that binds calcium. The SR contains a specific calcium channel receptor ryanodine that aids in the release of Ca^{++} that activates contraction.[30,31]

T System

An extension of the plasma membrane, the T system, or tubule, penetrates the muscle fiber in the region of the terminal cisternae of the SR at the junction of the A and I bands.[29] The T system assists in the propagation of electrical impulses from the surface to the interior of the muscle. The T system, with two transverse tubules per sarcomere, occupies approximately 0.1–0.5% of the volume of the muscle fiber[32]; the SR occupies greater than 1.0–9.0% of muscle volume in some animal species.[33,34]

Triads

The combination of two SR terminal cisternae and one transverse tubule, known as a *triad* (Figure 5-6), is where the electrical impulse is converted into calcium release, which initiates muscle contraction.[29]

At the triad there is a gap of 11–14 nm between the SR cisternae and the T tubule. Periodic densities, called *feet*, have been described in this space.[35] It still is not clear whether these feet have a functional role in muscle contraction or only a structural one. Finally, a series of indentations in the terminal cisternae have been

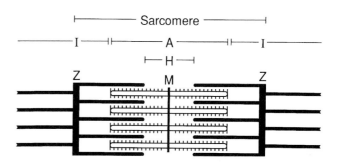

FIGURE 5-4 Diagram of the sarcomere shows thick filaments, thin filaments, cross-bridges, as well as subdivisions of the sarcomere, including Z lines, the M line, H zone, I band, and A band.

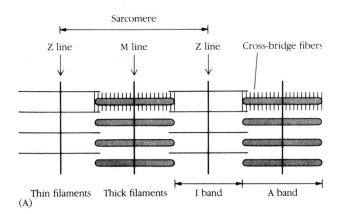

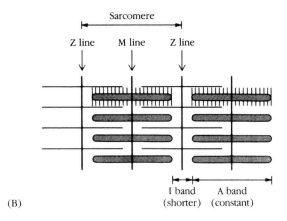

FIGURE 5-5 The sarcomere, showing the relationship between thick and thin filaments at **(A)** rest and **(B)** during contraction, illustrating the sliding filament theory. (Reprinted with permission from GG Matthews. Cellular Physiology of Nerve and Muscle [3rd ed]. Boston: Blackwell Scientific, 1998.)

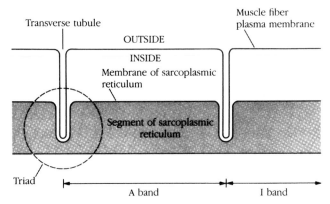

FIGURE 5-6 The transverse tubule and sarcoplasmic reticulum in the region of the triad. (Reprinted with permission from GG Matthews. Cellular Physiology of Nerve and Muscle [3rd ed]. Boston: Blackwell Scientific, 1998.)

described. At least one group of investigators[36] believes that these indentations mark sites of calcium release.

Mitochondria

Muscle mitochondria are seen in two locations, between the myofibrils and beneath the plasmalemma. Most mitochondria between myofibrils are near the Z lines at the I-band level.

Satellite Cells

Mature muscles include certain cells located in a characteristic position between the basal lamina and the plasma membrane of muscle fibers.[37,38] These satellite cells retain their myogenic capabilities. They cannot be distinguished from normal muscle nuclei without special techniques. Their numbers increase and they show significant mitotic activity in growing, injured, or denervated muscle.[39]

SKELETAL MUSCLE PROTEINS

Contractile Proteins

The force of skeletal muscle contraction is generated by thick filament myosin molecule projections (cross-bridges), which cyclically attach to adjacent actin thin filaments during contraction and relaxation.[40] Therefore, a review of muscle protein structure and chemistry is essential for understanding the mechanism of skeletal muscle contraction.

Each muscle fiber is composed of 10^2–10^3 myofibrils enveloped by SR and suspended in sarcoplasm containing potassium, magnesium, phosphate, and protein enzymes. Each myofibril is 1–3 μm in diameter. Mitochondria producing ATP are found between myofibrils.

Each myofibril has 1,500 thick myosin filaments and 3,000 thin actin filaments that interdigitate. The pattern of interdigitation in polarized light produces the sarcomere's typical appearance, with isotropic I light bands, which contain actin filaments, and anisotropic A dark bands, which contain myosin filaments and overlapping actin filaments (see Figure 5-3). Actin filaments are attached to Z discs comprised of several filamentous proteins different from actin and myosin. These act as structural attachments for actin filaments. The length of the fully stretched sarcomere at rest is approximately 2.0 μm.

Thick Filaments

Myosin

The myosin filament is an essential functional component of the sarcomere. Each myosin filament contains some 200–300 myosin molecules of approximately 480

A

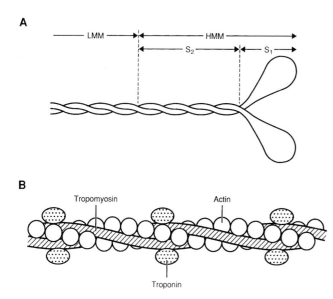

B

FIGURE 5-7 Structure of the contractile proteins. **A.** The myosin molecule. **B.** The thin filament showing actin, tropomyosin, and troponin. (HMM = heavy meromyosin; LMM = light meromyosin.)

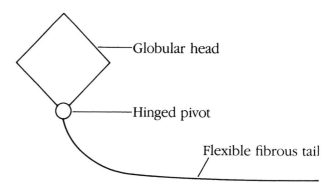

FIGURE 5-8 The myosin molecule, showing the flexible pivot area of the myosin head as well as the flexible portion of the fibrous tail. (Reprinted with permission from GG Matthews. Cellular Physiology of Nerve and Muscle [3rd ed]. Edition Boston: Blackwell Scientific, 1998.)

kD molecular weight, organized as six polypeptide chains, two heavy chains (weight, 200 kD each), and four light chains (weight, 20 kD each).[41,42]

Trypsin splits myosin into two components, light meromyosin (LMM), which forms the tail or rod portion of the molecule, and heavy meromyosin (HMM), primarily a globular protein termination of the molecule called a *head* (Figure 5-7). Papain splits HMM into an S_1 globular protein and a rodlike S_2 protein that is attached to LMM. The two myosin-heavy chains are arranged in a double-stranded α helix of 146 nm called the *tail* or *rod*. Each heavy chain terminates in an unstranded globular head of 17–20 nm. Each head contains two polypeptide light chains. One light chain can be phosphorylated and has a single site for binding bivalent cations, known as the *P light chain*. The second is the alkali or A light chain. Both light chains regulate actomyosin interaction.

The two heads of the myosin molecule are roughly pear shaped, 6–7 nm wide at the tip and 5.4 nm thick, and have a 3.5–4.0 nm, slightly curved neck.[43] Each head is mobile and rotates and angulates at the neck hinge or fulcrum, which is located at the junction of the S_1 and S_2 subfragments. A hinge in the myosin molecule at the junction of the S_2 and LMM provides additional flexibility, allowing a portion of the rod (tail) to act as a trunk or arm to move the head toward the actin filaments (Figure 5-8). The myosin head has ATPase activity, hydrolyzing ATP to release a high-energy phosphate bond.[44] The ATPase activity of myosin is located in the HMM or HMM-S_1 fragments and correlates with the shortening velocity of skeletal muscle contraction. The myosin head and neck form the cross-bridges (Figure 5-9).

Thin Filaments

Actin, Tropomyosin, and Troponin

The second essential component of the skeletal muscle sarcomere is the actin filament approximately 1 μm long and containing a double-stranded helix F-actin, a polymer of 300 G-actin monomers of 42 kD molecular weight. Each G-actin monomer is attached to one molecule of adenosine diphosphate (ADP). Interaction between the actin and the myosin heads occurs at the ADP loci. These active sites are staggered every 2.7 nm. Each actin monomer interacts with three or four other

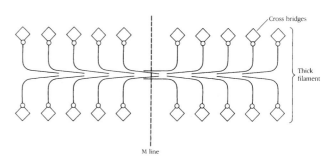

FIGURE 5-9 Structure of the thick filaments shows the formation of the cross-bridges by the myosin heads. (Reprinted with permission from GG Matthews. Cellular Physiology of Nerve and Muscle [3rd ed]. Boston: Blackwell Scientific, 1998.)

actin monomers in the polymer as well as with tropomyosin and troponin.[43]

The thin filament is actually a complex of three proteins: actin, tropomyosin, and the troponin complex in a 7:1:1 ratio. Tropomyosin and the troponin complex are regulatory proteins that assist in the control of the actin-myosin interaction. These two regulatory proteins are a structural component of the thin filament (see Figure 5-7).

Tropomyosin is an elongated polymer of approximately 70 kD molecular weight, 41 nm in length, and 20 μm diameter, consisting of two α helix coiled chains located 180 degrees apart in two F-actin grooves.

Troponin is a complex of three separate proteins. Troponin T (30 kD molecular weight) binds the other two troponins to tropomyosin. Troponin C (18 kD molecular weight) is a calcium receptor lying between troponin T and troponin I. Troponin I (22 kD molecular weight) is involved with inhibition of the actin-myosin interaction during muscle relaxation. This inhibition may be stereotactic. At concentrations of calcium less than 10^{-5} mol/L, troponin I participates in stereotactic blockage of the actin active site, which inhibits the attachment of myosin to actin.[45] One molecule of troponin complex containing one molecule of troponin I regulates the interaction of seven actin monomers with myosin.[46,47]

Noncontractile Proteins

Thick Filaments
C protein is a nonmyosin component of the thick filament, a monomer with a single polypeptide chain of 140 kD molecular weight. C protein binds to LMM and S_2 myosin fragments. Its function is not known. It has no ATPase activity.[48]

Thin Filaments
Alpha actinin is a protein localized to the Z line. Alpha actinin is believed to attach F-actin to the Z line. Beta actinin is located at the free end of the actin filament and is believed to function as a polymerization terminator for actin.

Sarcoplasmic Reticulum

Calsequestrin
Calcium ions released from the SR are essential in initiating the actin-myosin interaction. Normal Ca^{++} concentration in myofibrillar cytosol is 10^{-7} mol/L, too small to initiate the actin-myosin interaction. Maximal muscle contraction requires a calcium concentration of 10^{-5} mol/L. There is an active calcium pump that concentrates Ca^{++} in the SR to 10^{-4} mol/L. Calsequestrin is a SR protein that provides another 40-fold increase in calcium storage. Through these mechanisms the myofibrillar cytosol is essentially depleted of Ca^{++} during muscle relaxation. Excitation of the T tubules in the sarcoplasmic reticular system releases Ca^{++} to the myofibrillar fluid in concentrations as high as 2×10^{-4} mol/L. Ca^{++} release involves structurally complex proteins at loci that are dihydropyridine-sensitive receptors.[49] The receptor peptide has a molecular weight of 212 kD, binds dihydropyridine, is phosphorylated by ATP, and is similar to the large peptides of voltage-sensitive sodium channels.

Parvalbumin
Parvalbumin[50] is an intracellular calcium-binding protein that may play a role in the diffusion of Ca^{++}. Speed of relaxation is correlated with parvalbumin content in mammalian skeletal muscle. Fast skeletal muscle, which is rich in parvalbumin, relaxes much faster than slow fibers, which are almost devoid of it.

Other Proteins

Myoglobin
Myoglobin functions as a store for oxygen and speeds its diffusion from the periphery into the muscle fiber.[51] Type I fibers are richer in myoglobin than type II fibers.

Dystrophin
Dystrophin is a structural protein localized to the sarcolemma of the surface muscle membrane in the triad region. Its normal role is unknown, but it may play a role in signal transduction.[52] It is absent in Duchenne's muscular dystrophy and decreased in Becker's dystrophy.[53] It is believed to be the gene product of the Duchenne's dystrophy gene locus.

Utrophin
Utrophin is an autosomally encoded homologue of dystrophin.[54] It may be expressed in a manner reciprocal to dystrophin. Utrophin is found at the neuromuscular junction, whereas dystrophin is found at the sarcolemma. Because its structure is similar to dystrophin, it may be able to replace dystrophin in dystrophin-deficient muscle.

Titin/Connectin and Nebulin
These are giant proteins that have been described fairly recently.[55] Titin/connectin may be associated with the *cytoskeleton* of muscle. Nebulin is found along the contractile proteins. Titin/connectin is the largest protein known to date.

MUSCLE CONTRACTION

Presynaptic Events

Muscle contraction is initiated by the arrival at the synaptic terminal of a presynaptic nerve action potential. With the arrival of the action potential the synaptic terminal is depolarized, leading to the opening for calcium of voltage-sensitive membrane channels, which are closed when the terminal is in its resting state.

As the calcium concentration in the extracellular fluid is much greater than that inside the nerve terminal, calcium enters the terminal when the channels open. When the calcium concentration within the synaptic terminal reaches the appropriate level, acetylcholine is released from the presynaptic membrane.

The acetylcholine is packaged in the synaptic vesicles in multimolecule units termed *quanta*, each containing approximately 10,000 molecules of acetylcholine. In the resting state in a synaptic terminal, the release of single quanta of acetylcholine occurs regularly and spontaneously. This release can be recognized as the miniature end-plate potential when recording from the neuromuscular region with a microelectrode. Release of single quanta with their resultant miniature end-plate potentials does not lead to propagation of a potential along the muscle fiber, so miniature end-plate potentials do not stimulate muscle contraction.

A nerve action potential, however, leads to simultaneous release of 100–200 quanta of acetylcholine. The release of this amount of acetylcholine generates an end-plate potential in the postsynaptic muscle fiber. The end-plate potential is propagated along the muscle fiber, and muscle contraction follows.

Postsynaptic Events

The acetylcholine released from the nerve terminal enters the synaptic cleft and diffuses across the cleft to the postsynaptic muscle membrane. This membrane contains acetylcholine receptor sites, which act as gates controlling acetylcholine-sensitive sodium and potassium channels (Figure 5-10). These channels open when two acetylcholine molecules bind to them.

After acetylcholine binding has occurred, the channel opens. This ion channel allows both sodium and potassium to cross the membrane in equal amounts. The equal permeability to sodium and potassium results in depolarization of the muscle membrane, as the relative concentrations of these two ions are changed in a direction that leads to depolarization of the muscle membrane. This depolarization is then propagated throughout the muscle, and contraction results. The contact of acetylcholine with the

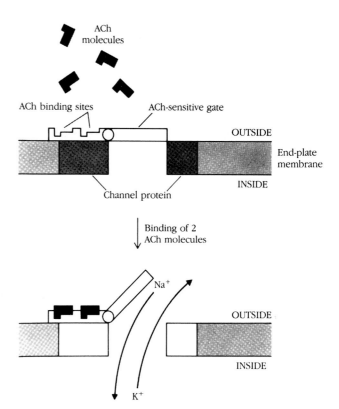

FIGURE 5-10 The acetylcholine (ACh)-sensitive channel in the end-plate membrane. (Reprinted with permission from GG Matthews. Cellular Physiology of Nerve and Muscle [3rd ed]. Boston: Blackwell Scientific, 1998.)

receptor site lasts approximately 1 msec. At this time, acetylcholine is inactivated by acetylcholinesterase and is split into acetate and choline. The choline is taken up again by the nerve terminal and acetylcholine is resynthesized.

The calcium available for release from the SR accumulates because of a calcium pump in the SR membrane. The calcium pump causes the transport of calcium ions into the SR and uses ATP for energy. Following the release of calcium from the SR, actin-myosin interactions are triggered and actual contraction begins. The calcium pump also serves to terminate contraction by pumping calcium back into the SR after it has reacted with the protein troponin on the thin filament.

Excitation-Contraction Coupling

Actual contraction of muscle with shortening of the sarcomere (see Figure 5-5) occurs because of the interaction of the myosin head cross-bridges with myosin-binding sites on the actin filament. The myosin head contains an area that binds ATP, forming myosin ATP. A high-energy phosphate bond is then split off, yielding an

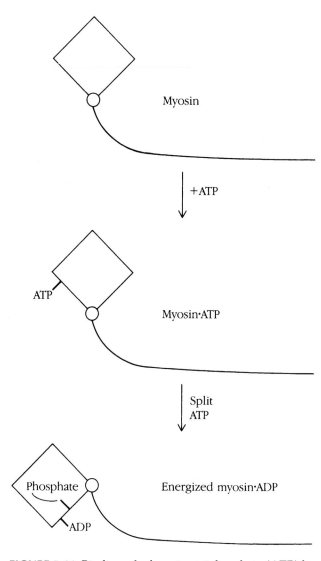

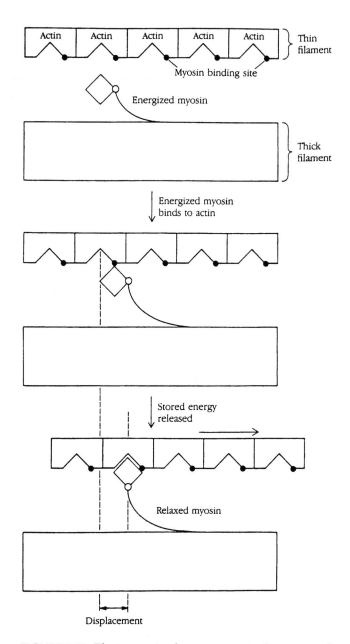

FIGURE 5-11 Binding of adenosine triphosphate (ATP) by the myosin molecule, and the energized state of the myosin head with rotation of the head about the pivot point. (ADP = adenosine 5' diphosphate.) (Reprinted with permission from GG Matthews. Cellular Physiology of Nerve and Muscle [3rd ed]. Boston: Blackwell Scientific, 1998.)

FIGURE 5-12 The interaction between energized myosin and actin according to the sliding filament hypothesis. (Reprinted with permission from GG Matthews. Cellular Physiology of Nerve and Muscle [3rd ed]. Boston: Blackwell Scientific, 1998.)

energized myosin head (Figure 5-11) that is capable of binding to the myosin-binding site on the actin filament (Figure 5-12). After binding, energy is released and thin filament displacement occurs, as shown in the diagram.

The regulation of the actin-myosin interaction depends on the interrelationship between troponin, tropomyosin, and actin in the thin filament. Without regulation, as long as ATP was present every muscle would be constantly contracting because of continual actin-myosin head binding.

During the resting state, the myosin-binding sites on the thin filament are unavailable to the myosin head

because they are blocked by tropomyosin held in position by troponin. The calcium released by the SR interacts with troponin to shift its position. As a result, the position of tropomyosin is also shifted and the myosin-binding sites become available to the myosin heads. These events are summarized in Figure 5-13.

Postsynaptic skeletal muscle plasma membrane depolarization is propagated when the resting membrane

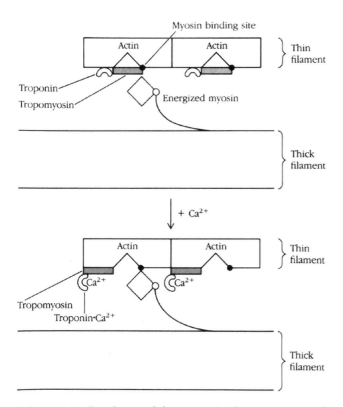

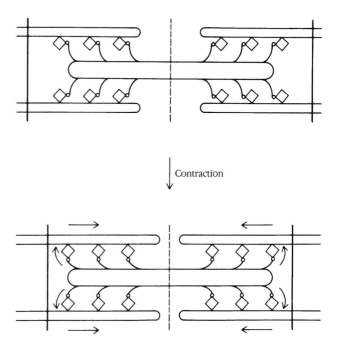

FIGURE 5-13 Regulation of the interaction between actin and myosin by calcium ions, troponin, and tropomyosin. (Reprinted with permission from GG Matthews. Cellular Physiology of Nerve and Muscle [3rd ed]. Boston: Blackwell Scientific, 1998.)

FIGURE 5-14 The mechanism of sarcomere shortening as well as the flip of the myosin heads during contraction. (Reprinted with permission from GG Matthews. Cellular Physiology of Nerve and Muscle [3rd ed]. Boston: Blackwell Scientific, 1998.)

potential is raised from –90 to –50 mV and is conducted at a velocity of 4 m per second.[56] The electromotive force changes during depolarization are rapidly spread to the sarcoplasmic T-tubule system at a radial propagation velocity of 0.064 m per second.[57–59] The wave of depolarization then travels via the T tubule from the surface to the interior of the muscle, where it causes release of calcium by the SR.

The exact molecular mechanism by which the electrical depolarization in the T tubule causes calcium release in the SR is unknown; however, both electrical and chemical mechanisms are possible, including calcium-induced calcium release. In this regard, it is interesting to note that T tubules contain Ca^{++} ATPase capable of concentrating and sequestering Ca^{++} in the tubule lumen.[60] Whatever the mechanism, the radially propagated electromotive force initiates a release of Ca^{++}, raising the cytosol Ca^{++} concentration from 10^{-7}–10^{-5} mol/L.[61] This results in movement of tropomyosin and the uncovering of the myosin-binding site on the thin filament.

Myosin heads are then activated. The binding of a single calcium ion may activate both myosin heads. The hinged myosin rod and hinged myosin neck move to place

the myosin heads at the active site[62] via the high myosin affinity for actin, thus producing an actomyosin complex.

The myosin heads then move or flip to a new position (Figure 5-14), initiating a more acute angle, with the myosin rod producing 5–7 nm of shortening or sliding of the myosin filament on the actin filament, which is stabilized at the Z line. ATP is hydrolyzed by the ATPase activity of myosin in the presence of actin to produce the energy required for contraction.[63,64] Myosin extracted from fast and slow muscle fibers produces the same velocity of contraction.[65]

After the flip stroke of the cross-bridge actin myosin interaction, sustained and continued contraction is produced by sequential attachment and angulation of myosin heads on adjacent actin-active sites. Muscle relaxation is initiated with rapid depletion of Ca^{++} by the pumping mechanism described previously. As the Ca^{++} concentration in the myofibrillar cytosol decreases, the tropomyosin-troponin complex folds to cover the actin-active site and the contractile cycle ends.

ENERGY PRODUCTION

Energy for the various processes in muscle contraction and relaxation is derived from ATP. The ATP content of resting muscle is approximately 5×10^{-6} mol/g. This *stored* energy can sustain maximal muscle contraction for only a few seconds; regeneration of ATP by phosphorylation of ADP is necessary for sustained contraction.

Creatine phosphate provides a substrate for rapid resynthesis of ATP via the transfer of a phosphate bond to ADP in the presence of MM creatine kinase, which is localized exclusively at the M line.[66] The energy bonds of creatine phosphate are present in four to six times the concentration of resting muscle ATP; however, the combined stored energy of ATP and creatine phosphate in muscle is adequate to maintain maximal contraction for only a few seconds more than resting ATP alone. Additional sources of ATP are required for sustained contraction.

Glycolytic breakdown of glucose via the Embden-Meyerhof pathway provides two ATP molecules per molecule of glucose degraded (Pi = inorganic phosphate):

$$Glucose + 2\,ADP + 2\,Pi + 2\,pyruvic\ acid + 2\,ATP$$

Glycolytic degradation of glucose produces new ATP two and one-half times as rapidly as oxidative mechanisms. However, glycolytic end products build rapidly to prevent maximal contraction beyond 1 minute.

Muscle glycogen provides a large source of the energy required for sustained muscle contraction. During 1 hour's heavy exercise muscle glycogen content decreases to approximately zero, after which no further work can be done in the absence of regeneration or glycogen or oxidative mechanisms for ATP regeneration.[67] When glucose is infused to maintain a high serum concentration, glycogen use is reduced only 25%, indicating that glycogen is the primary energy source for muscle contraction, even in the presence of a high serum glucose concentration.

Synthesis of mammalian skeletal muscle glycogen requires a cell permeable to the hexose molecule and an effective intracellular phosphorylating mechanism to produce glucose-6-phosphate. Insulin increases the permeability and transport of several hexoses and pentoses across the cell membrane. The pentose pathway is not used for mammalian muscle energy bond production. Skeletal muscle has high glucose phosphorylating capacity relative to glucose uptake, even at maximal insulin transport effect. Thus, there is no significant free intracellular glucose in resting muscle under normal conditions. Glucose is converted to glycogen by several mechanisms:

1. Phosphorylation of glucose to glucose-6-phosphate requires a high-energy phosphate bond:

$$Glucose + ATP - Glucose\text{-}6\text{-}phosphate + ADP$$

2. Conversion of glucose-6-phosphate to glycogen occurs via several enzymes, including uridine triphosphorylases and glycogen synthase.

Glucose-6-phosphate cannot be reconverted to free glucose in skeletal muscle, as it lacks glucose-6-phosphatase, which is present in liver, kidney, and small intestine.

Glycogen is a highly branched homopolymer of glucose that is stored predominantly in the I-band sarcoplasm near the tubule system.[68] Fast twitch and slow twitch fibers have similar amounts of glycogen at rest. In 80% of both fiber types, glycogen content at rest is between 300 and 750 mmol/kg dry weight. At the end of 2 hours' work, however, fast twitch fibers averaged 150 mmol/kg and slow twitch fibers 70 mmol/kg.[69]

Glycogenolysis of glycogen to glucose-6-phosphate requires several enzymes. Glucose-6-phosphate generated from glycogenolysis or glycolytic degradation of glucose is further metabolized to pyruvic acid, generating ATP via the citric acid–cytochrome oxidase aerobic pathway or lactic acid via the anaerobic pathway. Lactic acid is then converted to pyruvic acid when oxygen is available.

Complete oxidation of glucose to carbon dioxide and water yields 686,000 cal/mol or 38 ATP molecules per molecule of oxidized glucose. As 456,000 calories are available for production of ATP, 66% of the energy is converted to ATP, while the remainder is released as heat. Complete degradation of a molecule of glycogen yields 39 ATP molecules per glucose unit. The one ATP difference occurs in the energy bond required to convert glucose to glucose-6-phosphate. Under anaerobic conditions, glucose degradation stops at lactic acid and yields 56,000 cal/mol, an aerobic-anaerobic ratio of approximately 12:1.

REFERENCES

1. Carpenter S, Karpati G. General Aspects of Skeletal Muscle Biology. In S Carpenter, G Karpati (eds), Pathology of Skeletal Muscle. New York: Churchill Livingstone, 1984;1–38.
2. Kukulas BA, Adams RD. Embryology and Histology of Skeletal Muscle. In BA Kakulas, RD Adams (eds), Diseases of Muscle: Pathologic Foundation of Clinical Myology. Philadelphia: Harper & Row, 1985;3–60.

3. Landon DN. Skeletal Muscle: Normal Morphology, Development and Innervation. In FL Mastaglia, J Walton (eds), Skeletal Muscle Pathology. New York: Churchill Livingstone, 1987;1–87.

4. Blagden CS, Hughes SM. Extrinsic influences on limb muscle organization. Cell Tissue Res 1999;296:141–150.

5. Kelly AM, Zacks SI. The histogenesis of rat intercostal muscle. J Cell Biol 1969;42:135–153.

6. Stickland NC. Muscle development in the human fetus as exemplified by m. sartorius: a quantitative study. J Anat 1981;132:557–579.

7. Schloon H, Schlottmann J, Lenard HG, et al. The development of skeletal muscles in premature infants. Eur J Pediatr 1979;131:49–60.

8. Zhang M, Koishi K, McLennan IS. Skeletal muscle fibre types: detection methods and embryonic determinants. Histol Histopathol 1998;13(1):201–207.

9. Haltia M, Berlin O, Schucht H, et al. Postnatal differentiation and growth of skeletal muscle fibres in normal and undernourished rats. J Neurol Sci 1978;36:25–39.

10. Williams PE, Goldspink G. Longitudinal growth of striated muscle fibres. J Cell Sci 1971;9:751–767.

11. Williams PE, Goldspink G. The effect of immobilization on the longitudinal growth of striated muscle fibres. J Anat 1973;116:45–55.

12. Jerusalem F. The Microcirculation of Muscle. In AG Engel, BQ Banker (eds), Myology. New York: McGraw-Hill, 1986;343–356.

13. Slater CR, Harris JB. The Anatomy and Physiology of the Motor Unit. In J Walton (ed), Disorders of Voluntary Muscle (5th ed). New York: Churchill Livingstone, 1988;1–26.

14. Schmalbruch H. Motorneuron death after sciatic nerve section in newborn rats. J Comp Neurol 1984;224:252–258.

15. Grinnell AD. Dynamics of nerve-muscle interaction in developing and mature neuromuscular junctions. Physiol Rev 1995;75(4):789–834.

16. Hubbard JI. Microphysiology of vertebrate neuromuscular transmission. Physiol Rev 1973;53:674–723.

17. Noakes PG, Chin D, Kim SS, et al. Expression and localization of dynamin and syntaxin during neural development and neuromuscular synapse formation. J Comp Neurol 1999;410(4):531–540.

18. Brooke MH, Kaiser KK. Muscle fiber types: how many and what kind? Arch Neurol 1970;23:369–379.

19. Gauthier F. Skeletal Muscle Fiber Types. In AG Engel, BQ Banker (eds), Myology. New York: McGraw-Hill, 1986;255–283.

20. Burke RE, Levine DN, Zajac FE III. Mammalian motor units: physiological-histochemical correlation in three types in cat gastrocnemius. Science 1971;174:709–712.

21. Kugelberg E, Edstrom L. Differential histochemical effects of muscle contractions on phosphorylase and glycogen in various types of fibres: relation to fatigue. J Neurol Neurosurg Psychiatry 1968;31:415–423.

22. Johnson MA, Polgar J, Weightman D, et al. Data on the distribution of fibre types in thirty-six human muscles: an autopsy study. J Neurol Sci 1973; 18:111–129.

23. Dubowitz V, Newman DL. Change in enzyme pattern after cross-innervation of fast and slow skeletal muscle. Nature 1967;214:840–841.

24. Pette D. Activity-induced fast to slow transitions in mammalian muscle. Med Sci Sports Exerc 1984;16:517–528.

25. Luginbuhl AJ, Dudley GA, Staron RS. Fiber type changes in rat skeletal muscle after intense interval training. Histochemistry 1984;81:55–58.

26. Simoneau JA, Lortie G, Boulay MR, et al. Human skeletal muscle fiber type alteration with high-intensity intermittent training. Eur J Appl Physiol 1985;54:250–253.

27. Craig R. The Structure of the Contractile Filaments. In AG Engel, BQ Banker (eds), Myology. New York: McGraw-Hill, 1986;73–123.

28. Huxley H, Hanson J. Changes in the cross-striations of muscle during contraction and stretch and their structural interpretation. Nature 1954;173:973–976.

29. Cullen MJ, Landon DN. The Ultrastructure of the Motor Unit. In JN Walton (ed), Disorders of Voluntary Muscle (5th ed). New York: Churchill Livingstone, 1988;27–73.

30. Franzini-Armstrong C, Protasi F. Ryanodine receptors of striated muscles: a complex channel capable of multiple interactions. Physiol Rev 1997;77(3):699–729.

31. Sutko JL, Airey JA. Ryanodine receptor Ca^{++} release channels: does diversity in form equal diversity in function. Physiol Rev 1996;76(4):1027–1071.

32. Eisenberg BR. Quantitative Ultrastructure of Mammalian Skeletal Muscle. In LD Peachey, RH Adrian (eds), Handbook of Physiology. Sec 10: Skeletal Muscle. Bethesda, MD: American Physiological Society, 1983;73–112.

33. Schmalbruch H. The membrane systems in different fiber types of the triceps surae muscle of cat. Cell Tissue Res 1979;204:187–200.

34. Davey DF, Wong SYR. Morphometric analysis of rat extensor digitorum longus and soleus muscle. Aust J Exp Biol Med Sci 1980;58:213–230.

35. Franzini-Armstrong C. Structure of sarcoplasmic reticulum. Fed Proc 1980;39:2403–2409.

36. Dulhunty AF, Gage PW, Valoes AA. Indentations in the terminal cisternae of denervated rat extensor digitorum longus and soleus muscles. J Ultrastruct Res 1984;88:30–34.

37. Mauro A. Satellite cells of skeletal muscle fibers. J Biophys Biochem Cytol 1961;9:493–495.

38. Campion DR. The muscle satellite cell: a review. Int Rev Cytol 1984;87:225–251.

39. Klein-Orgus C, Harris JB. Preliminary observations of satellite cells in undamaged fibres of the rat soleus muscle assaulted by a snake-venom toxin. Cell Tissue Res 1983;230:617–676.

40. Huxley A. Prefatory chapter: muscular contraction. Annu Rev Physiol 1988;50:1–16.

41. Huxley HE. Electron microscope studies on the structure of natural and synthetic protein filaments from striated muscle. J Mol Biol 1963;7:281–308.

42. Cooke R. The mechanism of muscle contraction. Crit Rev Biochem Mol Biol 1986;21:53–118.

43. Elliott A, Offer G. Shape and flexibility of the myosin molecule. J Mol Biol 1978;123:505–519.

44. Engelhardt WA, Ljubimowa MN. Myosine and adenosine triphosphatase. Nature 1939;44:668–669.

45. Adelstein RS. Regulation and kinetics of the actin myosin-ATP interaction. Annu Rev Biochem 1980;49:921–956.

46. Perry SV, Cole HA, Head JF, et al. Localization and mode of action of the inhibitory protein component of the troponin complex. Cold Spring Harb Symp Quant Biol 1973;37:251–262.

47. Perry SV. The regulation of contractile activity in muscle. Biochem Soc Trans 1979;7:593–617.

48. Moos C, Mason CM, Besterman JM, et al. The binding of skeletal muscle C protein to F actin and its relation to the interaction of actin with myosin subfragment 1. J Mol Biol 1978;124:571–586.

49. Agnew WS. Proteins that bridge the gap. Nature 1988;334:299–300.

50. Kretsinger RH. Calcium-binding proteins. Annu Rev Biochem 1976;45:239–266.

51. Wittenberg JB. Myoglobin-facilitated oxygen diffusion: role of myoglobin in oxygen entry into muscle. Physiol Rev 1970;50:559–636.

52. Ozawa E, Hagiwara Y, Yoshida M. Creatine kinase, cell membrane and Duchenne muscular dystrophy. Mol Cell Biochem 1999,190:143–151.

53. Hoffman EP, Brown RH, Kunkel LM. Dystrophin: the protein gene product of the Duchenne muscular dystrophy locus. Cell 1987;51:919–928.

54. Blake DJ, Tinsley JM, Davies KE. Utrophin: a structural and functional comparison to dystrophin. Brain Pathol 1996;6(1):37–47.

55. Wang K. Titin/connectin and nebulin: giant protein rulers of muscle structure and function. Adv Biophys 1996;33:123–134.

56. Buchthal F, Guld C, Rosenfalck P. Propagation velocity in electrically activated muscle fibres in man. Acta Physiol Scand 1955;34:75–89.

57. Huxley AF, Taylor RE. Local activation of striated muscle fibers. J Physiol (Lond) 1958;144:426–441.

58. Costantin LL. The role of sodium current in the radial spread of contraction in frog muscles fibers. J Gen Physiol 1970;55:703–715.

59. Nakajima S, Gilai A. Radial propagation of muscle action potential along the tubular system examined by potential-sensitive dyes. J Gen Physiol 1980;76:751–762.

60. Brandt NR, Caswell AH, Brunschwig JP. ATP energized Ca pump in isolated transverse tubules of skeletal muscle. J Biol Chem 1980;255:6290–6298.

61. Endo M. Calcium release from the sarcoplasmic reticulum. Physiol Rev 1977;57:71–108.

62. Lehman W, Kendrick-Jones J, Szent-Gyorgi AG. Myosin-linked regulatory systems: comparative studies. Cold Spring Harb Symp Quant Biol 1973;37:319–330.

63. Goldman YE, Hibberd MG, Trentham DR. Relaxation of rabbit psoas muscle fibres from rigor by photochemical generation of adenosine-5-triphosphate. J Physiol 1984; 354: 577–604.

64. Goldman YE, Hibberd MG, Trentham DR. Initiation of active contraction by photogeneration of adenosine-5-triphosphate in rabbit psoas muscle fibres. J Physiol 1984;354:605–624.

65. Altringham JD, Yancey PH, Johnston IA. Limitations in the use of actomysin threads as model contractile systems. Nature 1980;287:338–340.

66. Walliman T, Turner DC, Eppenberger HM. Localization of creatine kinase isoenzymes in myofibrils. J Cell Biol 1977;75:297–317.

67. Bergstrom J, Hultman E. A study of the glycogen metabolism during exercise in man. Scand J Clin Lab Invest 1967; 19:218–228.

68. Wanson JC, Drochmans P. Rabbit skeletal muscle glycogen. A morphological and biochemical study of glycogen B particles isolated by the precipitation centrifugation method. J Cell Biol 1968;38:130–150.

69. Essen B, Henriksson J. Glycogen content of individual muscle fibres in man. Acta Physiol Scand 1974;90: 645–647.

6

Receptors in Muscle and Their Role in Motor Control

JAMES GORDON

Mammals are richly endowed with an extensive network of sensory neurons that convey information from the body to the nervous system. Although many of these somatosensory neurons have their receptors in the layers of the skin and are thus concerned with the sensations of touch, pain, and temperature, the majority of the somatosensory neurons has receptors in the deep tissues of the body, including the muscles, tendons, joints, and fascia. But, while the functions of cutaneous sensations are self-evident, the functions of the sensations that arise from the deep receptors have not been easy to establish, perhaps because in ordinary experience they are not even recognized as distinct sensations.

Indeed, the very idea that there is a "muscular sense," as Sherrington referred to it, was not definitively established until the end of the nineteenth century.[1] Before that time, the idea was a controversial one; the prevalent view was that our sense of movement derives not from peripheral receptors but rather from our estimate of the effort required to move. In the nineteenth century, however, detailed descriptions by Ruffini and Golgi of the receptors in muscles began to turn the tide.[2,3] The matter was definitively resolved in 1894, when Sherrington demonstrated that when the ventral roots were cut a rich supply of afferent fibers to the muscles remained after the motor fibers degenerated.[4] The largest sensory fibers, which were as large as the motor fibers themselves, innervated two types of receptors, called *muscle spindles* and *Golgi tendon organs*. The muscle spindle, perhaps because of its intriguing combination of sensory and motor elements, became the focus of intensive study throughout the twentieth century.[5] Nevertheless, a full understanding of muscle spindle structure was slow to develop. It was not established until 1945 that its motor innervation is independent of the innervation of the skeletal muscles themselves, and many important details of its ultrastructure are still emerging today.

An explanation of the functional role of muscle receptors in motor control has been even more difficult to achieve. The early recognition that muscle spindles provide the stimulus for stretch reflexes, such as the well-known knee jerk, provided the impetus for intensive studies during the first half of the twentieth century of the properties of these reflexes. The principle that guided these studies was that simple reflexes such as stretch reflexes provide the nervous system with a set of building blocks from which to construct more complex behavioral acts, but the overly simplistic corollary, that voluntary movements can be reduced to simple reflexes chained together, fell gradually into disfavor, especially as evidence emerged that complex movements can be executed in the absence of sensory input. A more recent insight, which emerged along with the science of cybernetics at the end of World War II, was that muscle receptors and stretch reflexes could be profitably analyzed as components of feedback loops, capable of providing automatic compensation for errors in motor output. Nevertheless, although this type of analysis deepened our knowledge of the function of muscle receptors, it has gradually given way to the recognition that nature's round pegs do not so easily fit into the square holes of engineering theory.

The current attitude toward the functional role of muscle receptors has become more eclectic. The contemporary emphasis on motor control has brought with it the recognition that the properties of the musculoskeletal system are complex and change from moment to moment. Thus, to accurately plan motor commands, the brain requires information about the state of the musculoskeletal system, including the current length and tension of the muscles. This information derives in large part from muscle receptors and is undoubtedly used in myriad ways, depending on the external context and overall goal or intent.

This chapter presents a basis for understanding the role of muscle receptors in motor control. No single theory is presented. Rather, the structure and functional properties of muscle receptors are discussed, their central connections are considered, and some of the current views of their role in motor control are reviewed. For more detailed information on these subjects, several excellent reviews are available.[2-4,6-15]

SENSORY RECEPTORS IN MUSCLE

The classic studies of Ruffini, Golgi, and Sherrington showed that skeletal muscles are richly supplied with a variety of receptors. Indeed, afferent axons outnumber efferent axons in most muscles.[2] The afferent fibers arising from muscle are classified according to a system introduced by Lloyd and Chang.[16] Because larger diameter axons conduct impulses faster, these investigators were able indirectly to estimate the sizes of axons in peripheral nerves by measuring their conduction velocity. They found that the axons of myelinated fibers fall into three groups, according to their diameters (Table 6-1). Group I fibers are the largest and fastest-conducting afferent axons in the peripheral nervous system. Group II and group III fibers are smaller and conduct impulses more slowly. Unmyelinated axons are classified as group IV. Among

the different receptors in muscles, two have been studied most thoroughly, the muscle spindles and the Golgi tendon organs. Muscle spindles are innervated by both group I and II axons. Tendon organs are innervated by group I axons. The group I axons from spindles are, on average, slightly larger than those from tendon organs and are referred to as *group Ia axons*, whereas those from tendon organs are referred to as *group Ib axons*.

Muscle Spindles

The muscle spindle is a remarkable sensory receptor whose supporting structure has a complexity that is often compared with that of the eye. Each spindle consists of a set of specialized muscle fibers, called *intrafusal fibers*, embedded within the extrafusal muscle fibers. Each intrafusal fiber is innervated by one or more sensory receptors that are sensitive to stretch of the spindle. In addition, the spindle has motor innervation, which allows the central nervous system (CNS) to control the firing properties of the sensory endings. Thus, just as the brain can move the eyes and change the shape of the lens to focus on objects of interest, it can also control the degree of contraction of the muscle fibers on which the sensory endings terminate to adjust the sensitivity and dynamic range of the sensory output from the spindle.

This simple description of spindle structure and function disregards considerable complexity of both structure and function. Spindle endings transmit information about both dynamic and static aspects of muscle length, and the CNS can selectively control the sensitivity to

TABLE 6-1
Muscle Afferents and Efferents

Afferent axon type	Receptor	Sensitive to:
Group Ia	Primary spindle ending	Muscle length and rate of change of length
Group Ib	Golgi tendon organ	Muscle tension
Group II	Secondary spindle ending	Muscle length (little rate sensitivity)
Group II	Nonspindle endings	Deep pressure
Groups III and IV	Free nerve endings	Pain, chemical stimuli, and temperature (important for physiological response to exercise)
Efferent axon type	**Innervation**	**Function**
Alpha motor neurons (skeletomotor)	Extrafusal muscle fibers	Control tension of muscle
Beta fibers (skeletofusimotor)	Intrafusal muscle fibers (collaterals from alpha motor neurons)	Control sensitivity of spindles (no independent control of spindle sensitivity)
Gamma motor neurons (fusimotor)	Intrafusal muscle fibers	Control sensitivity of spindles (independently of alpha motor neuron activation)

these different aspects of length change. These physiological properties of muscle spindles derive from the fine structure of the muscle spindle and, in particular, from differences in the physiological properties of the different types of intrafusal fibers. Indeed, the most significant advances since the 1970s have been in working out the *internal operation* of the spindle.[11]

Muscle spindles are found in almost all skeletal muscles. In human muscles, counts of spindles have ranged from six in the small stylohyoideus muscle and 35 in the lumbrical muscles up to 500 in the triceps brachii and 1,300 in the quadriceps femoris.[2,8] In general, they are more dense in the small muscles responsible for fine movement or postural control. The greatest density of spindles has been found in the small intervertebral muscles of the neck, whereas in large muscles such as the gluteus maximus, spindles are relatively less dense. There is no evidence for greater density of spindles in either extensor or flexor muscles.[2]

Spindles are encapsulated structures with a fusiform or spindle shape (Figure 6-1). They range in length from a few millimeters to 10 mm and usually lie deep within muscle bellies, close to the intramuscular nerve branches and blood vessels. Each spindle consists of a bundle of intrafusal muscle fibers (usually two to 12) arranged in parallel with each other and with the larger extrafusal fibers of the muscle within which they lie. The connective tissue capsule that surrounds the intrafusal fibers is thickest in the central region, giving the spindle its fusiform shape, and it encloses a gelatinous substance within this region. Presumably this substance facilitates sliding of the intrafusal fibers on each other.

It was recognized as long ago as the nineteenth century that there were two morphologically distinct types of intrafusal fibers and that there were differences in the sensory and motor innervation of the two.[4] One type, referred to as a *nuclear bag fiber*, is distinguished by a concentration of many nuclei in the central region of the fiber, so that in cross-section three or four nuclei may be seen. The other type of fiber, referred to as a *nuclear chain fiber*, is shorter than the bag fiber, and its nuclei are arranged in a row, so that only one is visible at a time in cross-section. It is now understood that there are two distinct types of nuclear bag fibers that differ in structure, physiological properties, and innervation. They are referred to as *dynamic* and *static* nuclear bag fibers. A typical mammalian muscle spindle contains two nuclear bag fibers, one of each type, and a variable number of chain fibers, usually approximately five. The different properties of these three intrafusal fiber types and their roles in how the spindle operates are discussed in the following sections.

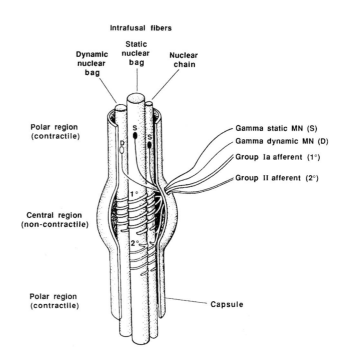

FIGURE 6-1 Simplified illustration of a muscle spindle. Capsule is cut away to show pattern of connections of afferent and efferent axons to different types of intrafusal fibers. Three intrafusal fibers are shown, one of each type; however, there are typically as many as five nuclear chain fibers in a spindle. Sensory endings wrap around the central regions of the intrafusal fibers; these are responsive to stretch of the intrafusal fibers. There are two types of sensory endings, each has different firing properties (see Figure 6-4). A primary (1°) ending consists of the terminations of a group Ia afferent, usually on all three types of intrafusal fibers. A secondary (2°) ending consists of the terminations of a group II afferent, usually only on nuclear chain and static nuclear bag fibers. There are also two types of gamma motor neurons. Gamma dynamic (D) motor neurons (MN) innervate only the dynamic nuclear bag fibers. Gamma static (S) motor neurons innervate both static nuclear bag fibers and nuclear chain fibers. The gamma motor neurons regulate the sensitivity of the muscle spindle by causing contraction of the polar regions of the intrafusal fibers (see Figure 6-5). (Reprinted with permission from M Hulliger. The mammalian muscle spindle and its central control. Rev Physiol Biochem Pharmacol 1984;101:1–110.)

The central region of each intrafusal fiber is noncontractile and is innervated by one or more sensory endings that are sensitive to stretching of the central portion of the intrafusal fiber. In many cases the afferent terminals spiral around the intrafusal fiber in what is referred to as an *annulospiral ending*. The polar regions of the intrafusal fibers connect to the aponeuroses of the whole muscle, so that as the length of extrafusal fibers changes, the length of the intrafusal fibers changes in parallel. When the central region of an intrafusal fiber is lengthened, the rate of firing of the sensory endings accelerates; when it shortens, the rate of firing slows. Thus, the firing of the sensory endings of the muscle spindle encodes information about changes in length of the whole muscle.

There are two types of afferent terminals in muscle spindles, primary and secondary. A *primary ending* consists of multiple branches of a single group Ia axon that terminate on all the intrafusal fibers in the spindle, including dynamic bag, static bag, and chain fibers. There is usually just one primary ending on each spindle. A *secondary ending* consists of the terminations of a single group II afferent on one or more chain fibers or static bag fibers. There may be as many as five secondary endings in a muscle spindle. Both types of endings respond to stretch of the intrafusal fibers; however, the primary and secondary endings have different firing properties.

The polar regions of the intrafusal fibers are contractile and are innervated by small myelinated motor

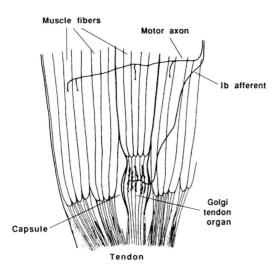

FIGURE 6-2 Illustration of a Golgi tendon organ and its relationship to muscle fibers. A capsule surrounds the collagen fibers that connect a set of muscle fibers to the common tendon. A group Ib afferent axon enters the capsule and splits into many fine, unmyelinated branches that intertwine among the collagen fibers. When the tendon is stretched, especially by a muscle contraction (see Figure 6-3B), these sensory endings are compressed and increase their firing rate. Note that each tendon organ is connected in series to a small number of muscle fibers, but because these are typically from different motor units, the firing rate of the afferent fiber is sensitive to the effects of recruitment. (Reprinted with permission from JC Houk, PE Crago, WZ Rymer. Functional Properties of the Golgi Tendon Organs. In JE Desmedt [ed], Spinal and Supraspinal Mechanisms of Voluntary Motor Control and Locomotion. Basel: Karger, 1980;33–43.)

axons called *gamma motor neurons*. The motor axons that innervate extrafusal fibers are larger and are referred to as *alpha motor neurons*. Because the central region is noncontractile, contraction of the intrafusal fibers elongates the central region by pulling on it from both ends. Depending on the type of intrafusal fiber (see the section Dynamic and Static Gamma Motor Neurons) and the current state of the muscle, intrafusal contraction may either increase the rate of firing of sensory endings or make them more sensitive to changes in length of the muscle. Thus, by controlling the firing rate of gamma motor neurons, the CNS can modulate the sensitivity of the spindle.

Golgi Tendon Organs

Golgi tendon organs are slender encapsulated structures approximately 1 mm long and 0.1 mm in diameter.[7] Like muscle spindles, they are plentiful in almost all skeletal muscles. Although referred to as *tendon organs*, they rarely are found within the tendon itself but more typically are located at the musculotendinous junction, where collagen fibers arising from the tendon attach to the muscle fibers (Figure 6-2). The tendon organs consist of bundles of such collagen fibers, which are in series with approximately 15–20 extrafusal muscle fibers.[8] Within the capsule of the tendon organ these collagen fibers have a braided appearance.

Each tendon organ is innervated by a single group Ib axon, which loses its myelination after it enters the capsule and branches into many fine endings, each of which intertwines among the fine collagen fibers. When the extrafusal muscle fibers contract, they cause the collagen fibers to straighten, compressing and stretching the nerve endings, which causes their firing rate to increase. The braided arrangement of the collagen fibers gives them a significant mechanical advantage in deforming the nerve endings, making these axons sensitive to minute changes in muscle tension.[17] Moreover, because the muscle fibers in series with a given tendon organ are members of many different motor units, the firing rate of the tendon organ's afferent fiber is sensitive to the effects of recruitment.[18]

Other Muscle Receptors

Relatively little is known about afferents that do not arise from spindles and tendon organs, even though they outnumber those that do. Most of these have smaller diameters and are classified as group III or IV. Most have free nerve endings and probably subserve nociceptive and thermoregulatory functions. It is presumed, but not proven, that some of these afferents play an important role in regulating the response of the body to exercise, including changes in blood pressure and breathing.[8] Some nonspindle afferents in the group II range respond to pressure, such as squeezing the muscle belly. There is indirect evidence that these afferents have significant influences on motor neurons and so may play some role in motor control.[19]

FUNCTIONAL PROPERTIES OF SPINDLES AND TENDON ORGANS

Complementary Information from Spindles and Tendon Organs

The functional differences between muscle spindles and Golgi tendon organs were first demonstrated by Matthews in 1933.[20] In the first direct recordings from muscle afferents, Matthews found that when he recorded from the afferent axon of a muscle spindle or a tendon organ and stretched the muscle, the spindle afferent increased its rate of discharge, whereas the tendon organ afferent showed only small and inconsistent increases in discharge rate. On the other hand, if the muscle was made to contract actively while still stretched (e.g., by stimulating the motor neuron that innervates the muscle), the firing rate of the tendon organ increased markedly, but the firing rate of the spindle decreased or ceased altogether.

The main reason for this difference in response lies in the different anatomic relationships of the two types of receptors to extrafusal muscle fibers. The muscle spindles are arranged in parallel with the extrafusal fibers, whereas the Golgi tendon organs are arranged in series (Figure 6-3A). Passive stretching of the muscle elongates and distorts the spindle receptors, leading to an increased firing rate. The tendon organ is relatively less responsive to stretch than the muscle spindle, because the collagen fibers emanating from the tendon are stiffer than muscle fibers. Therefore, most of the stretch is taken up by the more compliant muscle fibers and little direct stretching of the tendon organ takes place. When the muscle contracts, however, the muscle fibers pull directly on the collagen fibers and thus transmit more effective stretch to the tendon organ (Figure 6-3B). As a result, tendon organs always respond more robustly to muscle contraction than to passive stretch of the muscle. The arrangement in series of tendon organs therefore makes them most responsive to the tension of muscles. Spindles, on the other hand, decrease their firing rate when the muscle contracts, because, as the extrafusal fibers shorten with active contraction, the parallel intrafusal fibers also shorten. The resultant unloading of the intrafusal fibers causes them to slacken, often to the point of kinking, leading to a

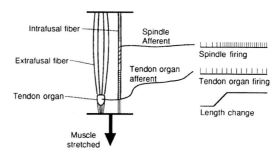

A Muscle stretch

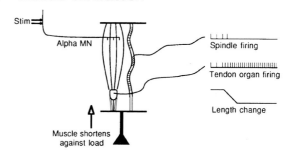

B Muscle contraction

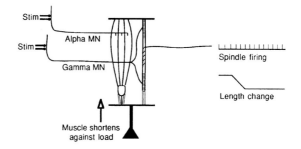

C Alpha-gamma coactivation

FIGURE 6-3 Functional properties of muscle spindles and Golgi tendon organs. The intrafusal muscle fibers of muscle spindles are arranged in parallel with extrafusal muscle fibers. Tendon organs are arranged in series with extrafusal fibers. Because of this difference in anatomic arrangement, the spindles sense changes in length of the muscle, whereas the tendon organs sense changes in tension. **A.** When the muscle is stretched, the spindle is also stretched, and its afferents increase their discharge rate. The tendon organ shows little response, because most of the stretch is taken up by the muscle tissue. **B.** When the muscle contracts, the spindle shortens and its afferents decrease their firing rate and eventually fall silent as the intrafusal fiber becomes slack. The tendon organ is sensitive to contraction because the tendon is pulled directly by the muscle fibers. **C.** The nervous system can prevent the muscle spindle from slackening during muscle contraction by activating the gamma motor neurons (MN). The resulting contraction of the polar regions of the intrafusal fibers maintains the central region taut and allows the spindle to continue to sense small changes in length during muscle shortening.

decrease in or cessation of firing. Thus, the muscle spindles, because of their parallel relationship to extrafusal fibers, are sensitive to changes in length of the muscles. Because the length of a muscle is directly related to the angle of the joint or joints it crosses, muscle spindles indirectly provide the CNS with information about the positions of the limbs in space.

Therefore, although muscle spindles and tendon organs are both sensitive to stretch, because of their different anatomic arrangements within muscles they provide the CNS with complementary information about the state of the muscle. The muscle spindles inform the nervous system about changes in length of the muscle; the tendon organs signal changes in tension exerted by the muscle. The complementary information coming from spindles and tendon organs is thought to be important in allowing the CNS to distinguish between changes in internal state of the muscle (e.g., fatigue) and changes in external loads acting on the muscle.[8]

Primary and Secondary Endings of Muscle Spindles

When a muscle is stretched or released from a stretch we can distinguish two phases of the change in length: a dynamic phase, the period during which length is changing, and a static phase, after a new steady-state length is achieved (Figure 6-4). The primary and secondary endings of muscle spindles respond quite differently during the dynamic phase of a change in length.[21] Although both receptors discharge similarly when the muscle is held at a constant or static length, the primary ending shows a distinct high-frequency burst during the dynamic phase of a stretch, whereas the secondary ending does not.

Thus, the firing rates of both primary and secondary endings always reflect the final static or steady-state length. When a muscle is stretched to a longer length, both endings respond by increasing their firing rates to a higher steady-state level. When a muscle shortens, both endings decrease their firing rates to a lower rate, reflecting the shorter final length. The primary endings of the muscle spindle are additionally sensitive to the rate of change in length, a property sometimes referred to as *velocity sensitivity*. During the dynamic phase of stretch of the muscle the primary ending shows a distinct burst in firing, achieving much higher rates than during the later steady-state phase. The firing rate of the secondary ending increases more gradually, and the firing rate is not much higher during the dynamic phase

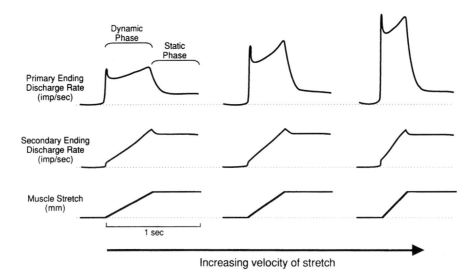

FIGURE 6-4 Differences in the firing properties of primary and secondary endings of muscle spindles. The traces show the time-varying changes in discharge rate of the afferent axons during muscle stretches of different velocities. During the static phase, when the muscle has stabilized at a new, longer length, the firing rate of both types of endings is faster than before the stretch. The firing rate during this phase is roughly proportional to the length of the muscle. During the dynamic phase, when the muscle is stretching, the firing rate of the primary ending increases. The magnitude of this transient increase in discharge rate reflects the velocity of the length change. Thus, the primary ending has the additional capacity for signaling the velocity of length change. Note also the brief increase in firing of the primary ending at the beginning of muscle stretch. This occurs because the primary ending is most sensitive to small changes in length. (imp = impulse.)

than during the steady-state phase. The instantaneous rates of firing in the primary ending that occur during a change in muscle length reflect the rate of length change; higher rates occur during faster stretches. A similar velocity sensitivity is also present for shortening of muscle; the primary ending often shows a pause in firing during a fast shortening before achieving a new steady-state firing rate. Because primary endings are so sensitive to phasic length changes, they typically fire in bursts in response to stimuli such as vibration or quick taps of the muscle. As these stimuli do not change the steady-state length of the muscle, the secondary endings are relatively unaffected by them.

The high degree of rate sensitivity of primary endings implies that the firing rates of spindles can encode both the length of a muscle and the velocity of length change, thus allowing the CNS to compute the speed of movements as well as the static positions of joints. The strength of this interpretation must be tempered, however, by several additional properties of primary endings.[3,8] First, and most important, primary endings are most sensitive to small changes in length (<0.1 mm). For large changes the dynamic sensitivity of the primary endings decreases dramatically. This high degree of sensitivity of primary endings to small stretches is often reflected by a transient increase in firing rate at the beginning of a stretch (see Figure 6-4). Second, the primary ending has the ability to reset its responsiveness to small stretches after it comes to a new length. Consequently, it is able to sense small changes in length at whatever new length it comes to. Third, these first two properties indicate that the actual relationships of muscle length and rate of length change to rate of spindle firing are highly nonlinear (i.e., they depend in complex ways on multiple factors, such as the initial length and the recent history of spindle firing). This has confounded physiologists attempting to *decode* signals from muscle spindles: It means that there are no simple formulas by which the nervous system can compute muscle length and velocity of length change from spindle firing. It thus appears that primary endings are most useful for detecting small movements or unexpected changes in rate of length change, rather than for direct velocity transduction.

Dynamic and Static Gamma Motor Neurons

Although it was known since Ruffini's descriptions of the spindle in the nineteenth century that intrafusal fibers had motor innervation, an understanding of the source and function of this innervation awaited a series of classic studies in the period between 1945 and 1955.

Until this time it was believed that the motor innervation of the spindle derived from the same motor axons that innervated the extrafusal muscle fibers, as had been demonstrated in amphibian muscle spindles. However, in 1945 Leksell used pressure to block conduction in the large alpha motor axons in ventral roots so that stimulation of the ventral roots excited only smaller motor axons, classified as *gamma motor neurons*.[22] He discovered that although such excitation of the gamma fibers produced no significant increase in muscle tension, multiunit recordings of spindle afferents showed a greater discharge rate. These findings were soon refined and confirmed by Hunt and Kuffler, who developed a method for stimulating single gamma efferents and simultaneously recording from single spindle afferents.[23] Their experiments established that the motor innervation of the spindle derived from a separate system of smaller gamma efferents and that excitation of these efferents led to higher rates of discharge of spindle afferents. The separate system of efferents to spindles is often referred to as the *fusimotor* system; the alpha motor neurons that innervate extrafusal muscle fibers are referred to as the *skeletomotor* system.

The gamma efferents do more than simply change afferent discharge, however. The changes in contractile state of intrafusal fibers that result from modulation of gamma discharge alter the sensitivity of spindle endings to changes in length. Moreover, there are two types of gamma motor neurons, *static* and *dynamic*, which selectively alter the dynamic and static responsiveness of spindle afferents (Figure 6-5). This was demonstrated in an experiment carried out by Crowe and Matthews in 1964.[24] They recorded from isolated Ia afferent fibers while stretching the muscle at a controlled rate. The primary ending typically showed a high rate of discharge during the dynamic phase of the stretch and a higher steady state rate during the static phase. They then repeated the procedure many times, while at the same time stimulating different gamma motor neurons. Activation of some gamma motor neurons produced marked enhancement of the steady-state discharge from the primary afferent during the static phase, with little effect on the dynamic responsiveness of the afferent. These efferents are thus classified as gamma *static* motor neurons. Activation of gamma static motor neurons has a similar effect on the output of secondary endings, increasing their firing rate at a given length. Activation of other neurons produced marked enhancement of the high-frequency burst during the dynamic phase with only slight enhancement of the static responsiveness. These efferents are classified as gamma *dynamic* motor neurons.

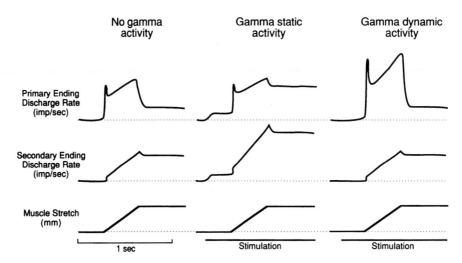

FIGURE 6-5 The effects of activating different types of gamma motor neurons on the firing properties of primary and secondary endings of muscle spindles. Here, as in Figure 6-4, each trace shows the discharge rate of spindle afferents during muscle stretch. In the middle column, the effect of stimulating a gamma static motor neuron is shown. Both types of endings show increases in discharge rate during the static phase. Note that because the firing rate during the static phase increases without any change in the firing rate during the dynamic phase, the primary ending shows relatively less dynamic responsiveness. In the column on the right, the effect of stimulating a gamma static motor neuron is shown. This increases the sensitivity of primary endings during the dynamic phase of length change but has little effect on the secondary ending. Thus, the nervous system can, by selective activation of these two types of gamma motor neurons, adjust the input from the spindles so that it predominantly reflects either steady-state length or rate of length change. (imp = impulse.)

Because activation of gamma static motor neurons increases the static discharge rate of spindle afferents relative to their dynamic response, it diminishes the relative intensity of the dynamic response (the dynamic response is that over and above the final steady-state firing level; see Figure 6-5). Thus, selective activation of gamma static motor neurons has the overall effect of making the ensemble spindle input to the CNS more related to current length of the muscle, whereas selective activation of gamma dynamic motor neurons makes the overall spindle input more phasic (i.e., related to small and quick changes in muscle length).[11] The CNS, therefore, has the capacity to modify the predominant quality of the information it is receiving.

Relationships between Structure and Function

The reason for the different actions of the two types of gamma motor neurons, as well as the different firing properties of primary and secondary afferents, is not that the neurons themselves have intrinsically different properties, but rather that they innervate different types of intrafusal fiber (Table 6-2).[2,8] Primary spindle endings terminate on all the intrafusal fibers within a spindle, including dynamic bag fibers, static bag fibers, and nuclear chain fibers. Therefore, the firing pattern of primary endings derives from the combined influence of all three types of fiber. Secondary endings, on the other hand, innervate principally nuclear chain fibers but also some static bag fibers. Their firing patterns, therefore, reflect only the properties of these intrafusal fibers. Gamma dynamic motor neurons innervate only the dynamic bag fibers. Gamma static motor neurons innervate nuclear chain fibers as well as static bag fibers.

The dynamic sensitivity of primary afferent fibers derives from the mechanical behavior of the dynamic nuclear bag fibers, referred to as *intrafusal creep*.[25] This type of intrafusal fiber has nonuniform characteristics along its length. The central region acts much like a spring, whereas the polar regions exhibit a kind of viscous friction. Thus, when the intrafusal fiber is stretched, the central region lengthens immediately, and the polar regions only gradually stretch out to the new length. As the polar regions slowly stretch, the initially lengthened central region *creeps* back to a slightly shorter length. Because the sensory endings are located in the central region, they respond to the stretch with a burst of firing, which then adapts to a lower level as the central region shortens. Furthermore, the contraction of one of these intrafusal fibers is not propagated throughout its length, as in normal muscle fibers. Activation of

TABLE 6-2
Different Types of Intrafusal Muscle Fibers

Type	Sensory Innervation	Motor Innervation
Dynamic nuclear bag	Primary ending (Ia)	Gamma dynamic
Static nuclear bag	Primary ending (Ia)	Gamma static
	Secondary ending (II)	—
Nuclear chain	Primary ending (Ia)	Gamma static
	Secondary ending (II)	—

these fibers by gamma dynamic motor neurons leads not to shortening of the intrafusal fiber but rather to stiffening of the polar regions, with a concomitant increase in the viscous friction. This has the effect of enhancing the intrafusal creep and, in turn, the dynamic sensitivity of the primary ending, without much effect on the steady-state discharge rate.

Nuclear chain fibers, on the other hand, have properties much more like those of ordinary skeletal muscle. They exhibit a rapid, propagated contraction when stimulated, leading to shortening of the intrafusal fiber. Thus, stimulation of these fibers by gamma static efferents brings about an increase in steady-state discharge rate of both primary and secondary endings. The static nuclear bag fibers seem to have intermediate properties, but at present the view is that they behave more like nuclear chain fibers.

Role of the Gamma System

An important role of gamma motor neurons was first suggested by Hunt and Kuffler in the early 1950s.[23,26] They reasoned that during large muscle contractions the spindle becomes slackened and therefore is unable to signal further changes in muscle length. They suggested that one role of the fusimotor system is to sustain tension in the muscle spindle during and after active contraction, in order to maintain its responsiveness at different lengths. Experiments carried out by Hunt and Kuffler demonstrated the feasibility of this hypothesis.[27] If the discharge rate of spindle afferents is recorded while alpha motor neurons are stimulated, the firing of the afferent shows a characteristic pause during the contraction, because the muscle is shortening, and therefore unloading (slackening) the spindle (see Figure 6-3B). If, however, a gamma motor neuron is activated at the same time as the alpha motor neuron, the pause becomes filled in because contraction of the intrafusal fibers keeps their central regions loaded, or under tension (see Figure 6-3C).

Thus, an essential role of fusimotor innervation is to prevent the spindle from falling silent when the muscle

shortens as a result of active contraction, thus enabling it to signal length changes over the full range of muscle lengths. This mechanism maintains the spindle firing rate within an optimal range for signaling length changes, whatever the actual length of the muscle. If alpha motor neurons were activated more or less in parallel with gamma motor neurons, a pattern referred to as *alpha-gamma coactivation*,[28] automatic maintenance of sensitivity, would result.

It is now known that, in addition to gamma efferents, there are collaterals from alpha motor neurons that innervate intrafusal fibers.[9,11] These are referred to as *skeletofusimotor* or beta efferents. A significant, although still unquantified, amount of skeletofusimotor innervation has been found in both cat and human spindles. These efferents provide the equivalent of alpha-gamma coactivation; when skeletofusimotor neurons are activated, unloading of the spindle by contraction of extrafusal fibers is at least partially compensated by loading caused by intrafusal contraction. Nevertheless, the existence of a skeletofusimotor system, with its forced linkage of extrafusal and intrafusal contraction, serves to highlight the importance of the independent fusimotor system, the gamma motor neurons. Apparently, mammals have evolved a mechanism that allows for uncoupling the control of muscle spindles from the control of their parent muscles. On logical grounds, this would give the organism greater flexibility in controlling the spindle output in different functional contexts; however, the degree to which such independent control is achieved remains a matter of controversy and is taken up again in the section Alpha-Gamma versus Independent Modulation.

Role of Muscle Spindles in Perception of Limb Position and Movement

One of the most venerable controversies in neurophysiology is whether muscle receptors, particularly spindles, are responsible for our conscious perception of limb position and movement. This controversy has raged for at least 100 years, since Helmholtz attributed our ability to perceive limb position and movement to a "sense of effort" (i.e., we know where our limbs are by monitoring the neural output that has gotten them to where they are).[1] Sherrington, on the other hand, proposed that there is a "muscular sense" that accounts for position and movement sense, and he used the term *proprioception* to refer to the general sense of where limbs are in relation to each other. The notion that muscles are insentient and that our sense of position derives purely from monitoring neural effort became less attractive as the rich sensory innervation of muscles was detailed by different investigators. Thus, for a time, Sherrington's view that muscle receptors are the source of proprioception became the accepted account.

More recently, however, the controversy was revived. Many investigators argued that, rather than muscle receptors, receptors in the joints themselves were the chief source of information about the positions of the limbs. These receptors respond to tension in the joint capsule and often show a preferential joint angle at which they fire; usually at the extremes of range. In 1956, Skoglund[29] showed that some slowly adapting joint receptors discharged at intermediate joint angles and argued that these could be used to detect joint position. This idea held sway for approximately a decade, until Burgess and Clark,[30,31] in extremely detailed studies, showed that the overwhelming majority of joint receptors fires at the extremes of range. The few receptors found that fired at intermediate angles could not possibly account for our sense of position. Thus, the notion that joint receptors account for position sense became less tenable.

At the same time, a number of psychophysical experiments lent weight to Sherrington's original idea that it was the muscle spindles that account for position sense. Perhaps the most dramatic of these was first performed by Goodwin and colleagues[32] and later by several other groups.[33-35] They showed that vibration of a muscle, known to be a powerful stimulus to primary endings of spindles, induced large errors in sense of position. If, for example, a vibration was applied to the biceps muscle of a subject, the subject perceived the elbow as being more extended than it actually was. Often these errors could be as great as 40 degrees. Thus, the error in perception was consistent with a stimulus to the spindle, because if the spindle was active, the CNS would interpret this as a stretching of the biceps muscle, leading to a perception that the elbow was extended.

The current consensus, therefore, is that muscle spindles play a primary role in our sense of position and movement.[1] Joint receptors, cutaneous receptors, and sense of effort also play a role in position sense, but the relative importance of their contributions is still being worked out.[36]

REFLEX CONNECTIONS OF SPINDLES AND TENDON ORGANS

Until now, we have been discussing spindles and tendon organs as sensory receptors, transducers of muscle length and tension, but the intrinsic role of these receptors in motor control cannot be fully appreciated without discussing their participation in stretch reflexes. Stretch reflexes are automatic contractions of muscle in response to passive lengthening of the muscle. Although once thought to result from intrinsic properties of muscles themselves, Sherrington's demonstration at the turn of the century that stretch reflexes could be abolished by cutting either the dorsal or the ventral roots established that they require sensory input from the muscle to the spinal cord and a return path to the muscles.[11]

Liddell and Sherrington carried out an extensive series of investigations of the properties of the stretch reflex.[37] They used the decerebrate cat preparation, in which the brain stem is surgically transected at the level of the midbrain, between the superior and inferior colliculi. Decerebrate animals have simplified and usually heightened spinal reflexes, making it is easier to examine the factors controlling their expression. Liddell and Sherrington found that the stretch reflex has two components: a brisk but short-lived phasic component, which is triggered by the change in muscle length, and a weaker but longer-lasting tonic component, which is determined by the static stretching of the muscles at the new longer length. The phasic component can be seen in isolation in intact animals by briskly tapping a muscle or its tendon, which produces a brief contraction of the muscle. Tonic stretch reflexes are more subtle and less obvious in intact animals. Typically, they are not seen unless the muscle is already contracting. A critical finding of Liddell and Sherrington was that stretching one muscle often produced effects in other muscles. Synergist muscles, those with a similar mechanical action, also contracted. Most interestingly, when a muscle was stretched its antagonist muscles tended to relax. Sherrington referred to this as *reciprocal innervation*.

Although Sherrington believed that the receptor responsible for the stretch reflex was the muscle spindle, it remained for other investigators to definitively identify the afferent fibers responsible and to work out the spinal circuitry. Investigators such as Lloyd [16,38,39] and Eccles[40,41] using increasingly refined techniques, have given us a fairly complete picture of the central connections of Ia fibers, and it is now known that these afferents are largely responsible for the phasic component of the stretch reflex.

Spinal Connections of Group Ia Afferents

Ia fibers from muscle spindles enter the spinal cord through the dorsal roots and immediately diverge into numerous collateral fibers (Figure 6-6). Some collaterals pass to the ventral horn of the gray matter, where they make direct (monosynaptic) excitatory connections with alpha motor neurons that innervate the same muscles (homonymous motor neurons). The distribution of Ia fibers to alpha motor neurons supplying homonymous muscles is quite extensive. A single Ia afferent makes monosynaptic connections with virtually all of the motor neurons innervating the same muscle from which the Ia afferent arises. Thus, Ia afferent fibers provide a strong excitatory drive to the muscle in which they originate, a phenomenon referred to as *autogenic excitation*. Other Ia collaterals make monosynaptic excitatory connections with alpha motor neurons innervating synergist muscles. These connections, although widespread, are not quite as strong as the connections to homonymous motor neurons. The strength of these connections varies from muscle to muscle in a complex way, according to the similarity of the mechanical actions of the synergists.

Ia collaterals also make excitatory connections with a special class of inhibitory interneurons that project to alpha motor neurons supplying muscles that are antagonistic to the muscles from which the Ia fibers originate. Thus, Ia afferents inhibit antagonist motor neurons disynaptically (i.e., through an interposed inhibitory neuron). This connection accounts for the reciprocal innervation observed by Sherrington. As motor neurons supplying homonymous and synergist muscles are excited, motor neurons to antagonist muscles are reciprocally inhibited.

Many Ia collaterals make connections with propriospinal and other interneurons, whose targets and functions are not well understood. Besides the monosynaptic stretch reflex, Ia afferents also participate in other, more complex reflex pathways. Finally, some Ia collaterals ascend in the dorsal columns to the brain stem, where they make connections to sensory tracts that ultimately reach the cerebral cortex and other higher centers.

Monosynaptic Stretch Reflex

How does this spinal circuitry account for the stretch reflex? Brisk passive extension of the limb lengthens the

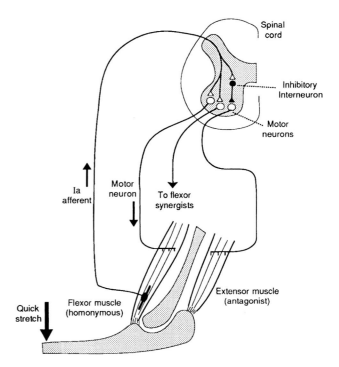

FIGURE 6-6 The spinal connections of Ia afferents from muscle spindles and their role in the stretch reflex. Ia afferents make excitatory connections (*unfilled triangles*) to motor neurons that innervate the same muscle and synergist muscles. They make inhibitory connections (*filled triangle*) through an interneuron to motor neurons that innervate antagonist muscles. The primary endings of muscle spindles respond to a quick stretch with an increase in firing rate of the Ia afferent. This increase in firing rate causes the motor neurons to fire, and the muscle contracts briskly. At the same time, the antagonist muscle is inhibited. The stretch reflex thus enhances the intrinsic stiffness of the muscle because it acts to oppose stretch of the muscle.

flexor muscles (see Figure 6-6), causing an increase in the discharge rate of Ia fibers arising in these muscles. The Ia fiber discharge excites both homonymous and synergist muscles monosynaptically, causing a contraction that tends to oppose the passive lengthening. By virtue of the Ia afferent's connection to inhibitory interneurons, antagonist motor neurons are inhibited, and the antagonist muscles tend to relax, an action that indirectly assists the reflex resistance to the imposed stretch.

Thus, it would appear that the stretch reflex acts to resist changes in joint position. It certainly functions in this way in decerebrate cats, whose standing position is maintained by virtue of tonic stretch reflexes in the extensor muscles. In intact animals tonic stretch reflexes are not nearly strong enough to prevent changes in joint position, and the monosynaptic stretch reflex produced by Ia afferents is primarily phasic. Because Ia afferents terminate in primary endings, which are highly sensitive to the dynamic phase of a length change, it is usually necessary to quickly stretch the muscle to elicit an observable reflex. A sharp tap on a tendon, for example, produces brief but effective stretching of most or all of the spindles in a muscle. The ensuing volley of Ia afferent discharge reaches the homonymous and synergist motor neurons synchronously, and, owing to the widespread divergence and convergence patterns of Ia afferents, the result is both temporal and spatial summation of excitatory potentials in the motor neurons. This leads to a brisk phasic contraction in the stretched muscles, sometimes referred to as a *tendon jerk* or a *deep tendon reflex*. Despite the widespread clinical use of this terminology, it must be emphasized that the receptors responsible are in the muscle and not the tendon. In fact, it is now believed that tapping a tendon with a reflex hammer causes a wave of vibration to pass through the whole muscle, which gives a powerful stimulus to many if not most of the primary endings within the muscle.[42]

Spinal Connections of Group II Spindle Afferents

The central connections of group II afferents from the secondary spindle endings have proven more difficult to trace, primarily because there are other muscle afferent fibers in the group II diameter range that arise from nonspindle receptors and free nerve endings. Group II spindle afferents from the secondary endings do participate in the monosynaptic stretch reflexes, although this connection is thought to be relatively weak.[43,44] Early findings by Eccles and Lundberg[45] suggested that group II afferents were excitatory to motor neurons innervating flexor muscles and inhibitory to those innervating extensor muscles and that these connections were polysynaptic, as the latencies of these effects were relatively long. It is clear now that at least some of the afferents producing these effects arise from free nerve endings and are not directly involved in sensing muscle length.[19] These connections are now seen as part of a widespread system of reflex pathways, referred to as *flexion reflex afferent* pathways. Lundberg et al. more recently suggested that the spinal reflex pathways in which group II afferents participate can be switched on and off by higher centers.[46-48] They further proposed that these pathways are important for organizing whole limb movements, as for locomotion, and that the afferent

input serves to reinforce muscle contraction and modulate its timing.

Spinal Connections of Group Ib Afferents from Tendon Organs

Group Ib afferents from Golgi tendon organs also show widespread divergence in the spinal cord. Stimulation of tendon organ afferents produces disynaptic or trisynaptic inhibition of homonymous motor neurons, called *autogenic inhibition*, and excitation of antagonist motor neurons. Because stimulation of Golgi tendon organs produces an effect that seems opposite to that of stimulating the spindle afferents, this is often referred to as an *inverse myotatic reflex*.

The action of Ib afferents is a good deal more complex than this, however, primarily because the interneurons that mediate these effects receive convergent input from many different types of receptors as well as descending pathways. Moreover, Ib afferents make more diffuse connections than Ia afferents, with significant effects on motor neurons innervating remote muscles. Therefore, the central connections of tendon organ afferents, like those of group II afferents, are thought to be part of spinal reflex networks responsible for regulating whole limb movements.[49]

Golgi tendon organs were originally thought to have a protective function, preventing damage to muscle, because it was assumed that they fired only when high tensions were achieved. In 1966, however, Houk and Henneman[50] demonstrated that they signal minute changes in muscle tension, thus providing the nervous system with precise information about the state of contraction of the muscle. Lundberg et al.[49] have proposed that the convergence of afferent input from tendon organs, cutaneous receptors, and joint receptors onto interneurons that inhibit motor neurons allows for precise spinal control of muscle tension in activities such as active touch. Combined input from these receptors would inhibit muscle contraction when the limb contacts an object.

In addition, it is now clear that stimulation of Ib afferents may, under certain conditions, produce excitation rather than inhibition of homonymous motor neurons, along with a corresponding reciprocal inhibition of antagonist motor neurons. Pearson and colleagues[51-53] have demonstrated that, during locomotor activity, stimulation of group Ib afferents in extensor muscles excites motor neurons that innervate extensor muscles. This excitation serves a functional purpose, because the tendon organs in extensor muscles would be maximally stimulated while the limb was bearing weight. Thus, the input from tendon organs serves to increase extensor muscle activity in order to assist in weight bearing during the stance phase of locomotion.

STRETCH REFLEX IN MOTOR CONTROL

Historically, the analysis of stretch reflexes has served as a useful model system in which to examine the processes by which neurons communicate with each other and by which neural signals are integrated. Indeed, well before modern techniques for intracellular recording were developed, Sherrington and his contemporaries, by careful measurement of muscle responses to stretch and other stimuli, were able to infer the basic rules governing synaptic transmission, including excitation and inhibition, as well as spatial and temporal summation.[28,54] Modern neurobiology continues to exploit simple reflexes as model systems for analyzing the elementary mechanisms of neural processing.

Because of the relative simplicity of the neural circuits responsible for the monosynaptic stretch reflex, testing the strength of phasic stretch reflexes is also an extremely useful tool in clinical diagnosis. Absence or weakness of phasic stretch reflexes often indicates a disruption of one or more of the peripheral components of the reflex arc: peripheral motor or sensory axons, the cell bodies of motor neurons, or the muscle itself. However, because the excitability of motor neurons is dependent on both excitatory and inhibitory descending influences, hypoactive (decreased relative to normal) stretch reflexes can also result from lesions of the CNS. This is especially evident after transection of the spinal cord, which produces a phenomenon referred to as *spinal shock*, in which all spinal reflexes are depressed. The spinal shock is usually transient, lasting several days to weeks, and reflex excitability usually increases gradually, with the result that stretch reflexes ultimately become hyperactive (increased relative to normal). Hyperactive stretch reflexes always result from central lesions that disrupt the normal balance of excitatory and inhibitory influences on the motor neurons. Hyperactive stretch reflexes are often associated with spasticity, a condition in which muscles show abnormally high resistance to passive stretch, especially rapid muscle stretches. The association of hyperactive stretch reflexes with weakness or paralysis and spasticity is often referred to clinically as *upper motor neuron disease*, as it is presumed that, either directly or indirectly, the lesion disrupts the descending motor pathways that converge on the alpha (lower) motor neurons.

Despite the experimental and clinical significance of the stretch reflex, its role in normal motor control has not been easily defined. Nevertheless, the spinal stretch reflex is the only known monosynaptic reflex in the mammalian nervous system, and its afferent and efferent neurons are among the fastest conducting of the nervous system. Thus, it provides a relatively fast system for influencing motor neuron excitability. Furthermore, the sheer magnitude of spindle input to the spinal cord, with widespread convergence and divergence patterns, implies that these reflex pathways play an important role in motor control. Some possible explanations of the functional role of stretch reflexes are therefore considered.

Reflex Generation of Posture and Movement

During the first half of the twentieth century it was generally believed that stretch reflexes were directly responsible for triggering many simple motor acts, especially in relatively automatic behaviors. For example, postural adjustments in standing were thought to result from simple stretch reflexes. Thus, if the body swayed forward, posterior muscles of the legs would be stretched, initiating reflex contractions that would resist the sway. Rhythmic behaviors, such as locomotion, that require alternation between flexion and extension, were believed to be generated by alternating reflex contractions. In this scheme, flexion movements of the legs would trigger stretch reflexes in the extensor muscles that would initiate the next phase of the cycle, and so on.

More recent research, however, indicates that even automatic behaviors such as postural adjustments and locomotion are controlled by central neural circuits that generate relatively complex sequences of muscle contractions. Postural adjustments, for example, typically occur in advance of a disturbance, if that disturbance can be anticipated, and they involve synergic contractions of groups of muscles.[55,56] Furthermore, the alternating patterns of muscle contraction seen in locomotion persist even when all afferent information from the limbs is blocked.[57,58] Nevertheless, even though stretch reflexes may not be directly responsible for generating these motor actions, they still play an important role in modulating and refining the motor output. Under certain conditions stretch reflexes may reinforce certain motor patterns; in other situations they may assist in correcting for unanticipated disturbances.[13]

Stretch Reflex as a Feedback Loop

An important class of functional hypotheses about stretch reflex function depends on the idea that the stretch reflex can function not only as a discrete reflex but also as a closed feedback loop (Figure 6-7). For example, stretch of a muscle produces an increase in spindle discharge,

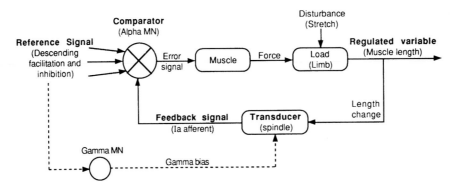

FIGURE 6-7 The stretch reflex as a feedback loop. The spindle acts as a transducer, sensing changes in the regulated variable muscle length. If the actual length is different from the intended or reference length, the motor neuron (MN) either increases or decreases its firing rate, producing the appropriate change in muscle force to bring the muscle back to the intended length. Such a system can in principle act to maintain an intended posture at the joint, but in normal situations the stretch reflex is not strong enough to overcome a large disturbance. It is more probable that it acts to correct for small perturbations. The dotted lines show the hypothetical effect of activating gamma motor neurons. This gamma bias could produce indirect activation of muscles by inducing the spindles to signal a change in length (see text). In effect, the gamma bias would signal the intended length of the muscle. This hypothesis that the stretch reflex acts as a servomechanism for initiating movement has not been validated, but it did stimulate intensive interest in the stretch reflex as a feedback loop.

leading to muscle contraction and consequent shortening of the muscle. But this muscle shortening leads to a decrease in spindle discharge, a reduction of muscle contraction, and a lengthening of the muscle. Thus, the stretch reflex loop, in theory, can act continuously, tending to keep muscle length close to a constant value. This is referred to as *feedback* because the output of the system (a change in muscle length) is *fed back* and becomes the input. The stretch reflex is a *negative* feedback system because it tends to counteract or reduce deviations from a reference value of the regulated variable (i.e., it tends to keep muscle length constant). The reference value is set by descending signals that act on the alpha motor neurons. Because the regulated variable is length, the spindle feedback loop enhances the spring-like properties of muscle, tending to resist changes in length.

How might such a feedback loop function in motor control? In 1952, Merton[59,60] put forward an ingenious hypothesis that, although it was ultimately proven erroneous, drew attention to the possible roles of feedback in motor control. Merton suggested that the higher centers might activate muscles indirectly, by way of gamma motor neurons, rather than directly, through the alpha motor neurons (see Figure 6-7). Activation of gamma motor neurons would cause contraction of the intrafusal fibers, thereby activating Ia afferent neurons. The Ia afferent neurons would then activate alpha motor neurons, causing the muscles to contract. The advantage of indirect activation through this gamma loop would be that the amount of gamma activity

(referred to as *gamma bias*) would in effect signal the intended length of the muscle. The automatic stretch reflex would continue to produce contraction of the muscle until it shortened to the point where the spindle was unloaded, at which point stable equilibrium would be achieved. According to Merton's hypothesis, the stretch reflex serves as a *servomechanism* (i.e., a feedback loop in which the output variable [actual muscle length] automatically follows a reference value [intended muscle length]). This mechanism, therefore, would bring the muscle to the intended length, regardless of the actual load being moved. Thus, the nervous system could produce a movement of a given distance without having to know in advance the actual load or weight to be moved.

Merton's hypothesis was attractive because it postulated a mechanism for simplifying movement control. Unfortunately, such compelling and explicit hypotheses often turn out to be oversimplifications, and such was the case here. A central prediction of Merton's hypothesis was that a voluntary movement is initiated in a specific sequence of events in peripheral axons: (1) activation of gamma motor neurons, (2) activation of Ia afferent neurons, and (3) activation of alpha motor neurons. In the early 1970s, Swedish investigators developed a technique known as *microneurography* for recording from the larger afferent neurons in peripheral nerves, and this method allowed direct testing of Merton's hypothesis. In 1972, Vallbo[61] recorded from Ia afferent neurons while at the same time recording the electromyographic (EMG) activity in muscles (EMG activity is an indirect measure of the activation of alpha motor neurons). Vallbo's experiments demonstrated conclusively that Ia afferent activity always followed EMG activity, so the initial activation of the muscle could not be through the gamma loop.

Nevertheless, the fact that Ia fibers increase their rate of discharge during the movement in Vallbo's recordings indicates that gamma motor neurons must have been activated, not before, but rather in synchrony with the alpha motor neurons. If there were no gamma activation, spindle discharge should decrease or pause during a contraction, because of unloading of the spindle. This finding led Vallbo and others[4,62,63] to suggest a revision of the Merton hypothesis, referred to as *servoassistance*. They argued that the afferent discharge from the spindle is insufficient to bring about large changes in muscle length, especially when significant loads are to be moved. Further, muscle spindles are most sensitive to small changes in length. Therefore, according to this view, alpha and gamma motor neurons are normally coactivated during shortening contractions. The stretch reflex feedback loop then serves to compensate for small disturbances, allowing automatic correction of small errors in the movement trajectory.

Alpha-Gamma Coactivation versus Independent Modulation

Although alpha-gamma coactivation may often be used, especially in the slow, precise movements that Vallbo studied, it is by no means the only possible mode of interaction of the fusimotor and skeletomotor systems. Although it is inherently difficult to record simultaneously from alpha and gamma motor neurons during natural movements, indirect evidence strongly suggests that the nervous system adjusts fusimotor activation in different ways, according to the specific task. For example, Loeb and Hoffer[64] recorded from Ia afferents in hind limb muscles during locomotion in cats and showed that they behaved differently depending on whether the muscle they originated from was lengthening or shortening. During certain phases of locomotion, muscles contract while shortening; during these phases, gamma motor neurons appear to be activated, presumably to maintain sensitivity of the spindle. During other phases, however, some muscles contract while lengthening; during these phases, there appears to be relatively little gamma activation. Loeb points out that gamma activation is not necessary for maintaining sensitivity of the spindle during lengthening contractions, and it might even be counterproductive, because spindle firing would saturate (i.e., reach its highest level and become

unresponsive to further increases in muscle length). Thus, Loeb emphasizes the importance of different patterns of gamma activation for maintaining optimal sensitivity of the spindle as a transducer.[10]

A particularly elegant series of experiments aimed at discovering natural patterns of gamma activation was carried out by Prochazka and colleagues.[12,65-67] These investigators recorded, during natural movements of cats, the activity of Ia afferents and the movements of the associated joints. They then electrically stimulated gamma motor neurons in anesthetized cats while at the same time reproducing the exact joint movements with a computer-controlled motor and recording from Ia afferents with similar characteristics to those they had recorded in awake animals. By using a computer to adjust the fusimotor stimulation until the patterns of Ia discharge exactly matched the records in natural movements, they were able to *reconstruct* the specific type of gamma activation that had been used.

The overall results of these experiments indicate that, rather than a strict linkage of alpha and gamma activation, the amount and type of gamma activation (static or dynamic) are preset at a certain tonic level, depending on the specific task or context. Prochazka and coworkers[66] referred to this as *fusimotor set*. A summary of some of their findings is illustrated in Table 6-3. Gamma static activation predominates when the animal is carrying out slow and predictable movements. On the other hand, high levels of gamma dynamic activation appear to be preset when the animal is moving fast or attempting a difficult or unpredictable task, such as beam walking. Thus, it would appear that the nervous system is capable of tuning the spindles so that they provide information most appropriate for the specific task conditions.

Adaptive Control of Muscle Tone

Stretch reflexes play an important role in the neural regulation of muscle tone (i.e., the force with which a muscle resists being lengthened). One component of muscle tone derives from the intrinsic elasticity, or stiffness, of the muscles themselves. Muscles have both series and parallel elastic elements, which resist lengthening; thus, a muscle behaves like a spring. In addition to this intrinsic stiffness, however, there is a neural contribution to muscle tone; the stretch reflex also acts to resist lengthening of the muscle. Thus, stretch reflexes enhance the spring-like quality of muscles.

Normal muscle tone serves several important functions. First, the tone of muscles helps maintain posture. As we sway back and forth while standing, the muscles resist being stretched, preventing the amount of sway

TABLE 6-3
Relative Activity of Gamma Static and Gamma Dynamic Motor Neurons in Cats during Different Motor Activities

Motor Activity	Gamma Static Firing	Gamma Dynamic Firing
Resting	0	0
Sitting	+	0
Standing	+	0
Slow walking	+ +	0
Fast walking	+ + +	+
Imposed movements	+	+ + +
Paw shaking	+	+ + +
Beam walking	+ + +	+ + +

0 = no firing; + = low firing rate; + + = moderate firing rate; + + + = high firing rate.
Source: Adapted from A Prochazka, M Hulliger, P Trend, et al. Dynamic and Static Fusimotor Set in Various Behavioural Contexts. In P Hrik, T Soukop, R Vejsada, et al. (eds), Mechanoreceptors. New York: Plenum, 1988;417–430.

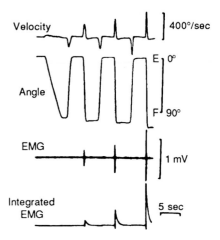

FIGURE 6-8 Electromyographic (EMG) responses in the quadriceps muscle of a spastic patient to stretches of different velocities. The downward changes in knee angle stretch the quadriceps muscle, causing a phasic reflex contraction of the muscle. Each successive stretch is faster, as indicated by the progressively higher velocity peaks in the top trace. A normal subject would show little or no EMG activity under these conditions. Note that there is no EMG activity except during the static phase of the stretches, even when the muscle is fully lengthened. Thus, spasticity is a phasic phenomenon, reflecting an abnormal increase in the velocity-dependent stretch reflex. (Reprinted with permission from D Burke. Spasticity as an Adaptation to Pyramidal Tract Injury. In SG Waxman [ed], Functional Recovery in Neurological Disease. New York: Raven Press, 1988;401–423.)

from becoming too large. Second, muscles, like springs, can store energy and release it later. This is particularly important in walking and running. As weight is accepted on a limb, the muscles stretch and store mechanical energy. When the leg pushes off, some of this energy is released and assists the active contraction of muscles. Thus, the elasticity of muscles makes locomotion more efficient: Less active contraction of muscles is required to propel the body forward. Finally, the spring-like qualities of muscles help to smooth movements. If muscles acted simply like the motors that control a robot's limbs, movements would be jerky, with sudden starts and stops. The elasticity of muscles smoothes out these jerks, because the muscle achieves an equilibrium length more gradually, like a spring.

The neural circuits responsible for stretch reflexes provide the higher centers of the nervous system with a mechanism for adjusting muscle tone under different circumstances. For example, during walking, the strength of monosynaptic stretch reflexes is continuously modulated to provide greater stiffness during the period when weight is being accepted on the limb and reduced stiffness when the limb is swinging.[68] Descending pathways regulate stretch reflex sensitivity, both directly, through synaptic connections with alpha and gamma motor neurons, and indirectly, through interneurons.

Because stretch reflexes are controlled by higher brain centers, disorders of muscle tone are frequently associated with lesions of the motor systems, especially those that interfere with descending motor pathways. These

may involve both abnormal increases (hypertonus) and abnormal decreases (hypotonus) in tone. The most common form of hypertonus is spasticity, which is characterized by hyperactive tendon jerks and an increase in velocity-dependent resistance to muscle stretch.[69] In a patient with spasticity, slowly applied stretch of a muscle may elicit little resistance, but as the speed of the stretch is progressively increased, resistance to the stretch progressively increases in magnitude (Figure 6-8). Thus, spasticity is principally a phasic phenomenon. An active reflex contraction occurs only during a rapid stretch; when the muscle is held in a lengthened position, the reflex contraction subsides. In some patients, however, there is also a tonic component to the hypertonus (i.e., the reflex contraction continues even after the muscle is no longer being lengthened).[69]

The pathophysiology of spasticity is still unclear. It was long thought that the increased gain of stretch reflexes in spasticity resulted from hyperactivity of the gamma motor neurons. More recent experiments, however, have cast doubt on this explanation.[70] Although gamma overactivity may be present in some cases, it is probable that changes in the direct input to alpha motor neurons and interneurons play a more important role. Thus, the presence of spasticity is clear evidence of disordered descending input to motor neurons.

It would logically seem that spasticity in certain muscles should interfere with rapid movements in which the antagonist muscles are spastic. This assumption has led to attempts to reduce spasticity with drugs, biofeedback, nerve blocks, and physical therapy techniques. Often, however, little functional improvement has been associated with reduction in spasticity.[71,72] The inability of spastic patients to make rapid movements is more likely caused by direct impairments of motor unit control than indirect resistance by overactive stretch reflexes,[73,74] although in some patients overactive stretch reflexes may indeed interfere with fast movement.[75] It is, therefore, important to keep in mind Landau's caution that spasticity is a positive symptom and cannot necessarily explain negative symptoms also associated with upper motor neuron syndromes.[76]

Long-Loop Stretch Reflexes

It should be emphasized that the monosynaptic reflexes are not the only means for providing active resistance to stretch. When a muscle that is already contracting is stretched, it typically contracts after a short latency (approximately 20–30 msec in arm muscles), a response that can be attributed to monosynaptic spinal circuits. This contraction is associated with a brief burst in the EMG signal from the muscle. Usually, however, the muscle shows later EMG bursts (approximately 40–60 msec); these are often larger than the short-latency burst and provide greater resistance to stretch than the monosynaptic component. Voluntary responses to stretch (i.e., those that can be consciously controlled and modulated) take at least 100–120 msec to appear in the EMG record. The neural circuits responsible for the medium-latency responses, often referred to as *long-loop* stretch reflexes, have not been definitively identified. Some have argued for a transcortical loop[77]; others contend that polysynaptic spinal circuits can account for these responses.[78] There is now strong evidence that at least some long-loop reflexes involving distal muscles must involve transcortical loops. Patients with abnormal bilateral cortical projections who make mirror movements during voluntary efforts also demonstrate bilateral long-latency stretch reflexes on the side contralateral to a stretch stimulus.[79]

Whatever their mechanism, long-loop stretch reflexes are functionally important. As Hughlings Jackson argued more than a century ago, there is a continuum between reflex and voluntary control.[80] Short-latency stretch reflexes provide the quickest response to stretch, and they help to compensate for intrinsic irregularities in the initial passive response of a muscle tissue to stretch.[81] The long-loop stretch reflexes fall somewhere in the middle of the continuum. They are under greater adaptive control than monosynaptic stretch reflexes. In contrast to monosynaptic stretch reflexes, which are most automatic and stereotyped, long-loop responses can vary considerably, according to prior expectations and intentions of subjects.[82] Voluntary responses to stretch provide the greatest degree of intentional control. Rather than viewing each of these as a discrete entity, we should perhaps view the entire response to stretch, from monosynaptic to voluntary, as providing a smooth stiffness with progressively greater adaptive control over its strength as the response unfolds.[83]

MOTOR CONTROL IN PATIENTS WITH ABSENCE OF PROPRIOCEPTION

One way to assess the role of muscle receptors and spinal reflexes in motor control is to observe the movements of patients or experimental animals whose sensory nerves are damaged or transected. In the early years of the twentieth century, experiments by Sherrington and others, involving transection of dorsal roots in experimental animals, appeared to indicate that intact sensory pathways from the limbs are essential for movement.[84,85] This view held sway until the early 1960s when experiments by Taub and others, demonstrated that such *deafferented animals* are able to initiate movements, although with reduced smoothness and elegance of movement.[86–88]

Then, in 1982, Rothwell and colleagues published a study of the motor control of a man with large-fiber sensory neuropathy.[89] This rare condition causes degeneration of the large-diameter afferent fibers that transmit proprioceptive input from the muscles and joints. Although there is no pathology in the motor axons of these patients, they have severe impairments in both feedback control and programming of movement.[89–95] Moreover, their movements are poorly coordinated, their balance is poor, and, because they must rely on vision to substitute for absent proprioception, they move slowly and awkwardly. Patients with lesions of the somatosensory areas of the cerebral cortex, where proprioceptive information is processed, have similar problems.[96] Thus, there is convincing evidence that sensory input from the limbs, especially from muscle receptors, is essential for both planning movements in advance and monitoring them during their course.

CONCLUSION

Since the end of the nineteenth century, the study of muscle receptors, especially spindles, and their central connections has attracted the attention of succeeding generations of motor physiologists. Although much has been learned, especially about their structure and basic physiology, there is still no clear picture of the roles they play in motor control. Nevertheless, there can be no doubt that proprioceptive input from the limbs is crucial for motor control.

Though the lack of consensus concerning the role of muscle receptors in motor control initially may be discouraging to beginning students, an appreciation for the elegance of their structure and operation, and for their usefulness in clinical diagnosis, should more than compensate. Moreover, we should expect that continuing interest in muscle receptors will soon resolve at least some of the questions about how the brain uses them to control movement.

REFERENCES

1. Matthews PBC. Where does Sherrington's "muscular sense" originate? Muscles, joints, corollary discharges? Ann Rev Neurosci 1982;5:189–218.
2. Boyd IA, Smith RS. The Muscle Spindle. In PJ Dyck, et al. (eds), Peripheral Neuropathy (2nd ed). Philadelphia: WB Saunders, 1989;171–202.
3. Matthews PBC. Muscle Spindles: Their Messages and Their Fusimotor Supply. In VB Brooks (ed), Handbook of Physiology. Sec 1: The Nervous System. Bethesda, MD: American Physiological Society, 1981;189–228.
4. Matthews PBC. Mammalian Muscle Receptors and Their Central Actions. London: Arnold, 1972.
5. Granit R. Comments on History of Motor Control. In VB Brooks (ed), Handbook of Physiology. Sec 1: The Nervous System. Bethesda, MD: American Physiological Society, 1981;1–16.
6. Baldissera F, Hultborn H, Illert M. Integration in Spinal Neuronal Systems. In VB Brooks (ed), Handbook of Physiology. Sec 1: The Nervous System. Bethesda, MD: American Physiological Society, 1981;509–595.
7. Crago PE. Golgi Tendon Organs. In PJ Dyck, et al. (eds), Peripheral Neuropathy (2nd ed). Philadelphia: WB Saunders, 1989;203–209.
8. Hasan Z, Stuart DG. Mammalian Muscle Receptors. In RA Davidoff (ed), Handbook of the Spinal Cord. Vol 2–3: Anatomy and Physiology. New York: Marcel Dekker, 1984;559–607.
9. Hulliger M. The mammalian muscle spindle and its central control. Rev Physiol Biochem Pharmacol 1984;101:1–110.
10. Loeb GE. The control and responses of mammalian muscle spindles during

normally executed motor tasks. Exer Sports Sci Rev 1984;12:157–204.
11. Matthews PBC. Evolving views on the internal operation and functional role of the muscle spindle. J Physiol (Lond) 1981;320:1–30.
12. Prochazka A, Hulliger M. Muscle Afferent Function and Its Significance for Motor Control Mechansims During Voluntary Movements in Cat, Monkey, and Man. In JE Desmedt (ed), Motor Control Mechanisms in Health and Disease. New York: Raven Press, 1983;93–132.
13. Pearson K, Gordon J. Spinal Reflexes. In ER Kandel, JH Schwartz, TJ Jessell (eds), Principles of Neural Science (4th ed). New York: McGraw-Hill, 2000;713–736.
14. Prochazka A. Proprioceptive Feedback and Movement Regulation. In LG Rowell, JT Sheperd (eds), Handbook of Physiology. Sec 12: Exercise: Regulation and Integration of Multiple Systems. New York: Oxford University Press, 1996;89–127.
15. Jami L. Golgi tendon organs in mammalian skeletal muscle: functional properties and central actions. Physiol Rev 1992;72:623–666.
16. Lloyd DPC, Chang H-T. Afferent fibers in muscle nerves. J Neurophysiol 1948;11:199–207.
17. Swett JE, Schoultz TW. Mechanical transduction in the Golgi tendon organ: a hypothesis. Arch Ital Biol 1975;113:374–382.
18. Houk JC, Crago PE, Rymer WZ. Functional Properties of the Golgi Tendon Organs. In JE Desmedt (ed), Spinal and Supraspinal Mechanisms of Voluntary Motor Control and Locomotion. Basel: S Karger, 1980;33–43.
19. Rymer WZ, Houk JC, Crago PE.

Mechanisms of the clasp-knife reflex studied in an animal model. Exp Brain Res 1979;37:93–113.
20. Matthews BHC. Nerve endings in mammalian muscle. J Physiol (Lond) 1933;78:1–53.
21. Cooper S. The responses of primary and secondary endings of muscle spindles with intact motor innervation during applied stretch. Q J Exp Physiol 1961;46:389–398.
22. Leksell L. The action potential and excitatory effects of the small ventral root fibres to skeletal muscle. Acta Physiol Scand Suppl 1945;10:1–84.
23. Hunt CC, Kuffler SW. Stretch receptor discharges during muscle contraction. J Physiol (Lond) 1951;113:298–315.
24. Crowe A, Matthews PBC. The effects of stimulation of static and dynamic fusimotor fibres on the response to stretching of the primary endings of muscle spindles. J Physiol (Lond) 1964;174:109–131.
25. Boyd IA, Ward J. Motor control of nuclear bag and nuclear chain intrafusal fibres in isolated living muscle spindles from the cat. J Physiol (Lond) 1975;244:83–112.
26. Kuffler SW, Hunt CC, Quilliam JP. Function of medullated small-nerve fibers in mammalian ventral roots: efferent muscle spindle innervation. J Neurophysiol 1951;14:29–54.
27. Kuffler SW, Hunt CC. The mammalian small-nerve fibers: a system for efferent nervous regulation of muscle spindle discharge. Res Publ Assoc Res Nerv Ment Dis 1952;30:24–47.
28. Granit R. The Basis of Motor Control. London: Academic Press, 1970.
29. Skoglund S. Anatomical and physiological studies of knee joint innervation in the cat. Acta Physiol Scand 1956;124:1–99.

30. Burgess PR, Clark FJ. Characteristics of knee joint receptors in the cat. J Physiol (Lond) 1969;203:317–335.

31. Clark FJ, Burgess PR. Slowly adapting receptors in cat knee joint: Can they signal joint angle? J Neurophysiol 1975;38:1448–1463.

32. Goodwin GM, McCloskey DI, Matthews PBC. The contribution of muscle afferents to kinaesthesia shown by vibration induced illusions of movement and by the effects of paralysing joint afferents. Brain 1972;95:705–748.

33. Eklund G. Position sense and the state of contraction: the effects of vibration. J Neurol Neurosurg Psychiatry 1972;35:606–611.

34. Roll JP, Vedel JP. Kinaesthetic role of muscle afferents in man, studied by tendon vibration and microneurography. Exp Brain Res 1982;47:177–190.

35. Ferrell WR, Gandevia SC, McCloskey DI. The role of joint receptors in human kinaesthesia when intramuscular receptors cannot contribute. J Physiol (Lond) 1987;386:63–71.

36. Gandevia SC. Kinesthesia: Roles for Afferent Signals and Motor Commands. In LG Rowell, JT Sheperd (eds), Handbook of Physiology. Sec 12: Exercise: Regulation and Integration of Multiple Systems. New York: Oxford University Press, 1996;128–172.

37. Liddell EGT, Sherrington CS. Reflexes in response to stretch (myotatic reflexes). Proc R Soc Lond B Biol Sci 1924;96:212–242.

38. Lloyd DPC. Conduction and synaptic transmission of the reflex response to stretch in spinal cats. J Neurophysiol 1943;6:317–326.

39. Lloyd DPC. Integrative pattern of excitation and inhibition in two-neuron reflex arcs. J Neurophysiol 1946;9:439–444.

40. Eccles JC, Fatt P, Koketsku K. Cholinergic and inhibitory synapses in a pathway from motor-axon collaterals to motoneurones. J Physiol (Lond) 1954;126:524–562.

41. Eccles JC. The Physiology of Synapses. Berlin: Springer-Verlag, 1964.

42. Lance JW, McLeod JG. A Physiological Approach to Clinical Neurology. London: Butterworth, 1981.

43. Matthews PBC. Evidence that the secondary as well as the primary endings of the muscle spindles may be responsible for the tonic stretch reflex of the decerebrate cat. J Physiol (Lond) 1969;204:365–393.

44. Kirkwood PA, Sears TA. Monosynaptic excitation of motoneurones from secondary endings of muscle spindles. Nature 1974;252:243–244.

45. Eccles JC, Lundberg A. Synaptic actions in motoneurones by afferents which may evoke the flexion reflex. Arch Ital Biol 1959;97:199–221.

46. Lundberg A, Malmgren K. Schomburg ED. Reflex pathways from group II muscle afferents. 1. Distribution and linkage of reflex actions to α-motoneurones. Exp Brain Res 1987;65:271–281.

47. Lundberg A, Malmgren K, Schomburg ED. Reflex pathways from group II muscle afferents. 2. Functional characteristics of reflex pathways to α-motoneurones. Exp Brain Res 1987;65:282–293.

48. Lundberg A, Malmgren K, Schomburg ED. Reflex pathways from group II muscle afferents. 3. Secondary spindle afferents and the FRA: a new hypothesis. Exp Brain Res 1987;65:294–306.

49. Lundberg A, Malmgren K, Schomburg ED. Convergence from Ib, cutaneous and joint afferents in reflex pathways to motoneurones. Brain Res 1975;87:81–84.

50. Houk JC, Henneman E. Responses of Golgi tendon organs to active contractions of the soleus muscle of the cat. J Neurophysiol 1967;30:466–481.

51. Pearson KG, Collins DF. Reversal of the influence of group Ib afferents from plantaris on activity in model gastrocnemius activity during locomotor activity. J Neurophysiol 1993;70:1009–1017.

52. Pearson KG, Ramirez JM, Jiang W. Entrainment of the locomotor rhythm by group Ib afferents from ankle extensor muscles in spinal cats. Exp Brain Res 1992;90:557–566.

53. Whelan PJ, Hiebert GW, Pearson KG. Stimulation of the group I extensor afferents prolongs the stance phase in walking cats. Exp Brain Res 1995;103:176–179.

54. Sherrington CS. The Integrative Action of the Nervous System. New Haven, CT: Yale University Press, 1947.

55. Marsden CD, Merton PA, Morton HB. Human postural responses. Brain 1981;104:513–534.

56. Cordo PJ, Nashner LM. Properties of postural adjustments associated with rapid arm movements. J Neurophysiol 1982;47:287–302.

57. Forssberg H. Spinal Locomotor Functions and Descending Control. In B Sjolund, A Bjorklund (eds), Brain Stem Control of Spinal Mechanisms. New York: Elsevier, 1982;253–271.

58. Grillner S, Wallen P. Central pattern generators for movement, with special reference to vertebrates. Ann Rev Neurosci 1985;8:233–261.

59. Merton PA. Speculations on the Servo-Control of Movement. In GEW Wolstenholme (ed), The Spinal Cord. London: Churchill Livingstone, 1953;247–255.

60. Merton PA. How we control the contraction of our muscles. Sci Am 1972;226:30–37.

61. Vallbo ÅB. Discharge patterns in human muscle spindle afferents during isometric voluntary contractions. Acta Physiol Scand 1970;80:552–566.

62. Granit R. The functional role of muscle spindles-facts and hypotheses. Brain 1975;98:531–556.

63. Stein RB. The peripheral control of movement. Physiol Rev 1975;54:215–243.

64. Loeb GE, Hoffer JA. Muscle Spindle Function During Normal and Perturbed Locomotion in Cats. In A Taylor, A Prochazka (eds), Muscle Receptors and Movement. London: Macmillan, 1981;219–228.

65. Prochazka A, Wand P. Independence of Fusimotor and Skeletomotor Systems During Voluntary Movement. In A Taylor, A Prochazka (eds), Muscle Receptors and Movement. London: Macmillan, 1981;229–243.

66. Prochazka A, Hulliger M, Zangger P, et al. "Fusimotor set": new evidence for α-independent control of γ-motoneurones during movement in the awake cat. Brain Res 1985;339:136–140.

67. Prochazka A, Hulliger M, Trend P, et al. Dynamic and Static Fusimotor Set in Various Behavioural Contexts. In P Hnik, T Soukop, R Vejsada, et al. (eds), Mechanoreceptors. New York: Plenum Press, 1988;417–430.

68. Stein RB, Capaday C. The modulation of human reflexes during functional motor tasks. Trends Neurosci 1988;11:328–332.

69. Burke D. Spasticity as an Adaptation to Pyramidal Tract Injury. In SG Waxman (ed), Functional Recovery in Neurological Disease. New York: Raven Press, 1988;401–423.

70. Burke D. A Reassessment of the Muscle Spindle Contribution to Muscle Tone in Normal and Spastic Man. In RG Feldman, RR Young, WP Koella (eds), Spasticity: Disordered Motor Control. Miami, FL: Symposia Specialists, 1980;261–278.

71. McLellan DM. Co-contraction and stretch reflexes in spasticity during treatment with baclofen. J Neurol Neurosurg Psychiatry 1977;50:30–38.

72. Neilson PD, McCaughey J. Self-regulation of spasm and spasticity in cerebral palsy. J Neurol Neurosurg Psychiatry 1982;45:320–330.

73. Sahrmann SA, Norton BJ. The relationship of voluntary movement to spasticity in the upper motor neuron syndrome. Ann Neurol 1977;2:460–465.

74. Tang A, Rymer WZ. Abnormal force-EMG relations in paretic limbs of hemiparetic human subjects. J Neurol Neurosurg Psychiatry 1981;44:690–698.

75. Corcos DM, Gottlieb GL, Penn RD, et al. Movement deficits caused by hyperexcitable stretch reflexes in spastic humans. Brain 1986;109:1043–1058.

76. Landau WM. Spasticity: the fable of a neurological demon and the emperor's new therapy. Arch Neurol 1974;31:217–219.

77. Marsden CD, Merton PA, Morton HB. Stretch reflexes and servo actions in a variety of human muscles. J Physiol (Lond) 1976;259:531–560.

78. Ghez C, Shinoda Y. Spinal mechanisms of the functional stretch reflex. Brain Res 1978;32:55–68.

79. Matthews PBC. The human stretch reflex and the motor cortex. Trends Neurosci 1991;14:87–90.

80. Walshe FMR. Contributions of John Hughlings Jackson to neurology: a brief introduction to his teachings. Arch Neurol 1961;5:119–131.

81. Nichols TR, Houk JC. Improvement in linearity and regulation of stiffness that results from actions of stretch reflex. J Neurophysiol 1976;39:119–142.

82. Houk JC. Participation of Reflex Mechanisms and Reaction-time Processes in the Compensatory Adjustments to Mechanical Disturbances. In JE Desmedt (ed), Cerebral Motor Control in Man: Long Loop Mechanisms. New York: S Karger, 1978;193–215.

83. Brooks VB. The Neural Basis of Motor Control. New York: Oxford University Press, 1986.

84. Mott FW, Sherrington CS. Experiments upon the influence of sensory nerves upon movement and nutrition of the limbs. Proc Royal Soc Lond B Biol Sci 1895;57:481–488.

85. Twitchell TE. Sensory factors of purposive movement. J Neurophysiol 1954;17:239–252.

86. Taub E. Somatosensory Deafferentation Research with Monkeys: Implications for Rehabilitation Medicine. In LP Ince (ed), Behavioral Psychology in Rehabilitation Medicine: Clinical Implications. Baltimore: Williams & Wilkins, 1980;371–401.

87. Polit A, Bizzi E. Characteristics of motor programs underlying arm movements in monkey. J Neurophysiol 1979;42:183–194.

88. Bossom J. Movement without proprioception. Brain Res 1974;71:285–296.

89. Rothwell JL, Traub MM, Day BL, et al. Manual motor performance in a deafferented man. Brain 1982;105:515–542.

90. Sanes JN, Mauritz K-H, Dalakas MC, et al. Motor control in humans with large-fiber sensory neuropathy. Hum Neurobiol 1985;4:101–114.

91. Ghez C, Gordon J, Ghilardi MF, et al. Roles of proprioceptive input in the programming of arm trajectories. Cold Spring Harb Symp Quant Biol 1990;55:837–847.

92. Ghez C, Gordon J, Ghilardi MF, Sainburg R. Contributions of Vision and Proprioception to Accuracy in Limb Movements. In MS Gazzaniga (ed), The Cognitive Neurosciences. Cambridge, MA: MIT Press, 1995;549–564.

93. Gordon J, Ghilardi MF, Ghez C. Impairments of reaching movements in patients without proprioception. I. Spatial errors. J Neurophysiol 1995; 73:347–360.

94. Ghez C, Gordon J, Ghilardi MF. Impairments of reaching movements in patients without proprioception II. Effects of visual information on accuracy. J Neurophysiol 1995;73:361–372.

95. Gordon J, Ghez C. Roles of Proprioceptive Input in Control of Reaching Movements. In H Forssberg, H Hirschfeld (eds), Movement Disorders in Children: International Sven Jerring Symposium, Stockholm, 25–29 August 1991. Medicine and Sport Science: Vol 36. New York: Karger, 1992;124–129.

96. Jeannerod M. The Neural and Behavioral Organization of Goal-Directed Movements. Oxford, UK: Clarendon Press, 1988.

7

Skeletal Physiology and Osteoporosis

JERI W. NIEVES, FELICIA COSMAN, AND ROBERT LINDSAY

PHYSIOLOGY OF BONE METABOLISM

Functions of the Skeletal System

The skeleton has critical mechanical functions, including protecting vital organs, acting as a framework for the body, and anchoring muscles. The skull and vertebral column protect brain and spinal cord, sternum and ribs protect thoracic and upper abdominal viscera, and the pelvis protects genitourinary structures. Additionally, bones surround and protect hematopoietic marrow, creating a physically secure, compartmentalized microenvironment in which blood cells are made and subsequently released into the circulation. In infants, this hematopoietic activity occurs in all bones; in adults it occurs primarily in the flat bones (sternum, ribs, skull, vertebrae, and innominate bones) and in only the proximal ends of long bones such as the humerus and femur. In addition to its protective mechanical functions, the skeleton serves to maintain erect posture, acts as a focus of locomotion, and provides a system of levers to which muscles attach for all movement. Muscles attach through the collagenous fibers of tendons, interweaving through the periosteum, the fibrous outer sheath surrounding bone surfaces.

Bone also acts as the storage site for calcium and phosphate. To serve this function, a readily accessible part of bone is always available for dissolution when the supply of electrolytes diminishes. Likewise, minerals can be redeposited into bone when the ion supply is plentiful. Finally, toxins, again usually minerals such as lead or aluminum, are stored in bone until they can be excreted.

The skeletal system's function in maintaining a normal extracellular calcium level takes precedence over its mechanical functions. In times of calcium deficiency, for example, in order to maintain serum calcium, mineral can be rapidly reabsorbed from the skeleton, causing it to weaken, fracture easily, and lose the ability to protect and to support posture and locomotion.

Gross Structure and Growth of the Skeleton

The skeleton consists of bones that differ markedly in their gross structures, so that no two bones are identical. Microscopically, however, there is much less variability. Generally, long bones are laid down on a cartilaginous anlage, whereas flat bones are ossified in a membranous matrix. Flat bones make up the axial skeleton, whereas tubular bones generally form the appendicular skeleton. Linear growth of bones is a phenomenon that occurs only at the specialized cartilaginous growth plates (epiphyseal plates) that separate bone into shaft (diaphysis) and end (metaphysis). The regulation of bone length involves different genetic, endocrine, and environmental controls than those that regulate bone shape, thickness, or diameter. Although genetic endowment probably defines the basic structure of each bone, environmental influences modify the structure significantly. Genetic endowment also controls (at least in part) environmental factors such as body mass and muscle mass. Figure 7-1 provides a model of how genetic and environmental factors may operate and interact to determine ultimate bone size and structure.[1]

Bone modeling, the sculpting of size (diameter) and gross architecture (macrogeometry), occurs during growth of the skeleton in all known bony vertebrates and continues into adulthood. Modeling of bone shape and thickness should be distinguished from cartilagi-

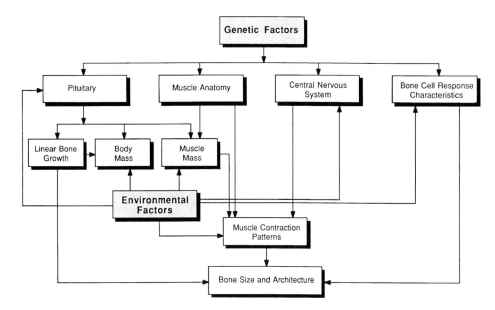

FIGURE 7-1 A schematic representation of the association between genetic and environmental factors as determinants of bone size and structure. (Adapted from HM Frost. Mechanical determinants of bone remodeling. Metab Bone Dis Rel Res 1982;4:217–229.)

nous phenomena such as linear growth. Modeling must also be distinguished from remodeling, which is a preventive maintenance process of coupled resorption and formation that occurs throughout life as old bone is replaced with new to maintain structural integrity. Remodeling does not affect the external shape of bone or move bone through space relative to a defined body axis, as bone modeling does.[2]

Wolff hypothesized more than a century ago that altered mechanical loads could induce appropriate architectural changes in bone. In general, mechanical use increases cortical (compact) bone mass and lack of it has the opposite effect. The difference in bone mass between congenitally paralyzed and normally mobile growing limbs suggests that mechanical use during growth is responsible for 20–50% of the ultimate dimensions of the normal young adult skeleton.[3] Figure 7-2 exemplifies the difference in thickness and structure of an animal bone after a period of disuse.[4]

Frost's flexural strain theory extends Wolff's law. In essence, he states that, in growing mammals (or in adults during fracture repair), under repetitive, uniformly oriented, nontrivial, dynamic flexural strains (causing slight bending or angular deformation of bone), bone growth proceeds in the direction of the concavity, with bone formation on the concave surface and resorption on the convex surface.[1] It is generally well accepted that compression strain stimulates bone growth, and tension strain stimulates bone resorption.[5] The resultant drift or movement of the bone in space ultimately reduces compression stress and strain in the concave cortex and tension stress and strain in the con-

vex cortex. This general principle explains to some extent the final macrogeometry of ribs, clavicles, and vertebrae and predicts the eventual correction of fracture malunions. Figure 7-3 is a schematic representation of the events that normally follow a femoral fracture that healed with angulated malunion and ultimately corrected through the modeling process.[1] Tension forces probably contribute in a different way (nonresorbing stimulus) to a few highly specialized macroscopic cortical thickenings or outpouchings, such as those that occur at the insertions of powerful tendons from the iliopsoas and gastrocnemius muscles.[5]

Exactly how mechanical factors (such as compression strain) translate into the cellular processes of bone modeling is still poorly understood. Mechanisms that may be involved include the strain itself (directly stimulating or inhibiting bone cells, especially osteocytes), release of local matrix factors or cellular growth factors, changes in intrabone pressure, fluid flow, pH, oxygen tension, and streaming electrical potentials.[4] These signals are communicated between bone cells by a complex network of intercellular connections.

Macroscopic Bone Structure

Just as genetic codes specify some aspects of general skeletal size and shape, they encode some differences in the internal structure of bone. One variable is the relative amounts of cancellous (spongy or trabecular) and cortical (compact) bone. Overall, the skeleton contains 80% cortical and 20% trabecular bone by mass.[6] Nearly every bone in the skeleton contains some cancellous and

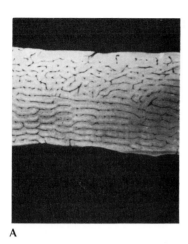

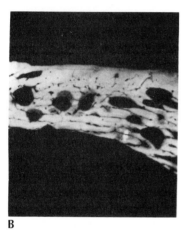

A

B

FIGURE 7-2 A. Microradiograph of a 100-mm thick transverse section from the midshaft of a normal male turkey ulna. **B.** Similar microradiograph from a bone after 8-week loss of functional load bearing. Bone is thinned and porous from endosteal resorption. (Reprinted with permission from LE Lanyon. Functional strain as a determinant of bone remodeling. Calcif Tiss Int 1984;36:556–561.)

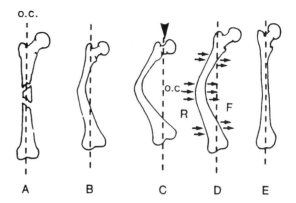

FIGURE 7-3 A. Fractured femur of a young child. (O.C. = original centroid of bone.) **B.** Healing with angulation of the diaphysis. **C.** With each vertical load, angulation increases slightly. **D.** Modeling occurs with bone formation on the side of the concavity (*right*) owing to increased stress and strain components (F). Bone resorption (R) occurs with increased tension in the lateral cortex (*left*). This causes the diaphysis to move back toward the original centroid. **E.** Modeling has resulted in a return of the original configuration of the bone. (Adapted from HM Frost. Mechanical determinants of bone remodeling. Metab Bone Dis Rel Res 1982;4:217–229.)

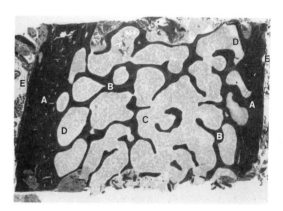

FIGURE 7-4 A full-width iliac crest bone biopsy specimen showing cortices (A), cancellous bone (B), marrow cavity (C), corticoendosteal surfaces (D), and periosteal surfaces (E). (Courtesy of Dr. David Dempster, Helen Hayes Hospital and Columbia University, New York, New York.)

some compact bone, although the proportions of each are highly variable. The calcaneus contains almost solely cancellous bone, whereas the midshaft regions of the femur and radius are almost entirely compact bone. Vertebrae contain 45–80% cancellous bone, and the femoral neck contains 75% cortical bone. Various proportions occur in other parts of the skeleton.[7,8]

Compact and trabecular bone contain all the same elements, although they are organized differently. In cancellous bone, each small bone fragment (trabecula) is surrounded by marrow rather than by other packets of bone. Compact bone contains bone units that are densely packed, and only the few that form the corticoendosteal (inner cortical) surface are contiguous with

bone marrow (Figure 7-4). Cancellous bone, therefore, has a much higher surface-to-bone volume ratio, providing a large diffusion surface or bone-blood vessel interface for mineral exchange from bone to blood.

Cortical bone contains longitudinally oriented, parallel, cylindrically shaped packets called *haversian systems* or *osteons*. Each haversian system consists of a central blood vessel, nerve, and lymphatic channel sur-

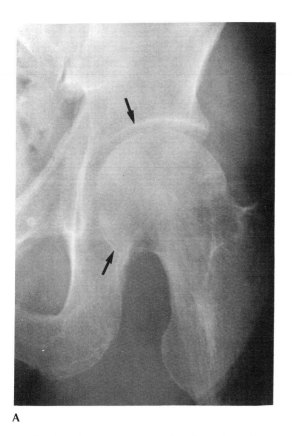

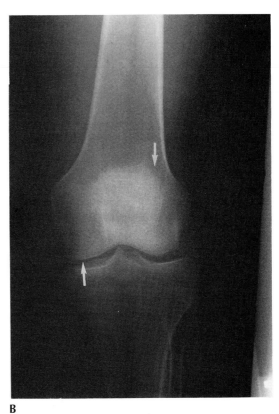

A   B

FIGURE 7-5 A. Note that two major trabecular orientations are seen in the femoral head. The major vertical orientation (*top arrow*) is parallel to the major weight-bearing forces on the bone. The arched, transversely oriented trabeculae (*bottom arrow*) correspond to deformational forces produced by compression against the lower acetabulum. **B.** In the femoral condyles, note that almost all trabeculae are vertically oriented, because almost all compressive forces are exerted vertically and there is little transverse or lateral pressure.

rounded concentrically by rings of osteocytes (mature osteoblasts) embedded in calcified bone matrix. Each osteocyte is interconnected to other osteocytes and to a central blood vessel by filamentous cell processes that course through tiny canals (canaliculi) in the mineralized matrix. The haversian system has an average cross-sectional diameter of 250 μm; thus, no cell is farther than that from a blood vessel.[2] The fluid that bathes the bone cells is a specialized derivative of extracellular fluid maintained by both the capillary endothelial cells and the membranous osteocyte cell processes.

Cancellous bone is composed of a series of interconnected plates, often arranged in parallel. Just as mechanical factors help determine the shape and thickness of cortical bone during modeling, they also influence the structure of trabecular bone during skeletal remodeling. This trajectorial theory of trabecular bone architecture was first put forth by Culmann and von Meyer and expounded by Wolff and Roux.[5] In addition

to affecting the overall trabecular bone mass, mechanical vectors affect the orientation of the trabeculae, the degree of connectedness, the thickness, and the separation between trabeculae. The long axis of trabecular orientation is parallel to the deformational forces of weight bearing and muscle contraction.[9] Figure 7-5 shows the predominant trabeculae and their orientation parallel to the major compressive forces in the femoral head and tibial plateau.[5] The relative stiffness or strength of trabecular bone depends, as does that of cortical bone, on its overall mineral density.[10] Trabecular contiguity, the frequency of perpendicular trabecular interconnections and thus reinforcement of strength (Figure 7-6), however, is also important.[11] Moreover, the age of bone tissue is a critically important factor in determining strength and ability to resist fatigue damage.[2]

Cancellous bone has a greater surface and is more richly vascular; therefore, it contributes much more toward the function of mineral exchange than compact bone, even though it makes up only a small proportion of the overall skeletal mass. The relative stiffness or strength of cancellous bone is an order of magnitude smaller than that of cortical bone,[10-12] and it is lighter than cortical bone. It is, therefore, structurally economical, preventing bone from being unnecessarily heavy while still contributing significantly to compressive strength (e.g., in the vertebrae, where estimates suggest that cancellous bone is responsible for 25–90% of the total compressive strength).[10,12,13] Although cancellous bone is not as stiff as cortical bone, it is more resistant to deformation (strain or bending forces); resistance to fracture is associated with a greater proportionate length change than of cortical bone. Cancellous bone is thus more compliant, allowing better protection of joint surfaces and transmission of forces from joints to bone shafts.[12]

Microscopic Bone Structure

Like all connective tissue, bone is composed of cells, matrix, and organic fibers. Its compressive strength is due principally to hydroxyapatite mineral and its tensile strength to type I collagen fibers. The extracellular matrix of bone is 35% organic by weight (50% organic by volume).

Organic Phase

The organic component of bone matrix is 90% collagen, a triple polypeptide helix that associates into fibrillar networks, giving bone its tensile strength and serving as a framework for the deposition of bone mineral and bone cell attachment.[14] The major noncollagen proteins, at least in terms of quantity, are osteocalcin (bone gla protein [BGP]), osteonectin, and osteopontin. The functions of these proteins are unknown. In addition to collagen and noncollagen proteins, the organic phase of bone contains a small amount of lipid.[15]

BGP, a major noncollagen protein, accounts for 15–20% of noncollagen proteins or 1–2% of total bone protein. This 49-amino acid protein has three glutamic acid (gla) residues, which become γ-carboxylated in a posttranslational modification. The protein is highly conserved among mammals, birds, and fish.[16] It is also highly specific, being found in only dentin and plasma besides bone matrix. BGP is secreted by osteoblasts during bone formation and has an affinity for hydroxyapatite when fully γ-carboxylated, and thus is incorporated into bone matrix. The protein is chemotactic for monocytes and may induce formation of osteoclast precursors and initiate bone resorption.[17] It has also been reported to inhibit the precipitation of hydroxyapatite, and thus prevents excess mineralization. During Coumadin treat-

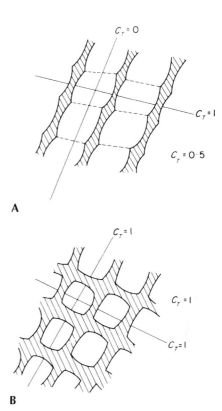

FIGURE 7-6 Idealized trabecular bone structure. **A.** Since trabecular contiguity (C_T) is 0 in vertical direction and 1 in horizontal direction, overall $C_T = 0.5$. **B.** Overall C_T is 1, with much greater strength. (Reprinted with permission from JW Pugh, RM Rose, EL Radin. Elastic and viscoelastic properties of trabecular bone: dependence on structure. J Biomech 1973;6:475–485.)

ment, gla residues cannot be added to BGP. Whether this affects bone formation or not has yet to be determined.[18] Matrix gla protein (MGP), with 79 amino acids and five gla residues, has significant sequence homology with BGP, suggesting common derivation. It is also secreted by some osteoblast-like cells, in addition to cartilaginous cells.[19] MGP is often found in association with bone morphogenetic protein[16] and may reflect an earlier stage in bone formation than BGP.[19]

Osteonectin is as abundant as BGP, is 15% of noncollagen proteins, and is both glycosylated and phosphorylated. It binds both hydroxyapatite and collagen through different regions of the molecule. In vitro, this protein promotes mineral deposition onto collagen. It is possible that in vivo, after binding to collagen, it nucleates hydroxyapatite crystal deposition. Osteonectin, which is immunologically and electrophoretically identical to bone osteonectin, is also found in platelets. During clotting, osteonectin is released into the circulation so that the majority of serum osteonectin is derived from platelets, not bone. Osteonectin may also be made by megakaryocytes.[20] In general, the amount of osteonectin in bone correlates with the amount of lamellar bone. Osteonectin is distinct from both fibronectin and thrombospondin, larger proteins that also bind collagen and probably contribute to cell attachment capability.[21,22]

Mineral Phase

The mineral phase of bone matrix accounts for 50% of its volume and 65% of its weight. The mineral phase contains both well-formed hydroxyapatite (calcium and phosphate) crystals and amorphous calcium phosphates. The amorphous form has a lower calcium-to-phosphate ratio than hydroxyapatite, but the two forms are rapidly interchangeable. Mineral deposition occurs in close relation to collagen fibrils (within spaces between triple helices) and within 2–10 μm from the osteoblast cell surface. Mineralization normally begins within 5–10 days after newly synthesized osteoid is laid down.[15]

Bone Cells

Bone cells account for only 3% of bone volume. They include osteoblasts, osteoclasts, and osteocytes (mature osteoblasts or bone-lining cells) as well as bone cell precursors. Osteoblasts derive from stromal tissue in the bone marrow, which also gives rise to fibroblasts, adipocytes, and reticular cells in addition to preosteoblasts.[23] Osteoblasts are the cells primarily responsible for bone formation, and they have an important role in activating bone resorption. Osteoblasts elaborate a variety of organic matrix components, including collagen, BGP, osteonectin, thrombospondin, osteopontin, and MGP, in addition to various growth factors (including bone morphogenetic protein [BMP]) and osteoclast-stimulating factors including the ligand for osteoprogerin, some of which are prostaglandins that stimulate resorption and activate bone remodeling. BMP was originally described by Urist et al. as an extract of bone that had the ability to induce endochondral bone formation from extraskeletal mesenchymal tissue in rats.[24] More recently, BMP was recognized as a family of proteins belonging to the transforming growth factor-β superfamily, each independently having similar potential bone induction activity. Differences in the ability to secrete these products occur among different osteoblast-like cell lines and at different stages in cell differentiation.[6,21,25] Osteoblasts also secrete alkaline phosphatase, which is expressed on the cell membrane. This enzyme degrades inorganic pyrophosphates

(inhibitors of bone mineralization) and may promote mineralization. Osteoblasts probably also synthesize 1,25-dihydroxyvitamin D from 25-hydroxyvitamin D.[26] When active, osteoblasts are cuboidal and contain intracellular organelles characteristic of cells engaged in active protein synthesis.[6] As synthesis of osteoid by osteoblasts progresses, some osteoblasts become incorporated into the organic phase. These cells become osteocytes, incorporated deeply into bone, with a complex syncytium of canaliculi connecting them to surface osteoblasts. Osteocytes are probably important as initiators of signals to surface osteoblasts. In some fashion these cells can indicate the strain that is being placed on the skeletal structure and activate or depress the resting osteoblasts on the surface. Osteocytes may also report internal microdamage and thereby initiate remodeling.

Osteoblast function is mediated by numerous hormones and local factors, including endocrine factors and growth factors. Parathyroid hormone (PTH) probably signals osteoblasts to activate osteoclasts, which then begin resorption, and exerts a direct trophic effect on osteoblasts.[6] There is also accumulating evidence that PTH may stimulate the formation of some osteoblast products, such as BGP[27] and alkaline phosphatase under certain conditions.

Calcitriol regulates some aspects of osteoblast function, such as increasing production of BGP (in vivo and in vitro), MGP, and alkaline phosphatase and modulating osteoblast proliferation.[17,19,28] Calcitriol probably also stimulates rapid bone resorption through osteoblastic activation of osteoclasts.[28]

Glucocorticoids inhibit osteoblast function with respect to BGP formation both in vivo and in vitro[29,30] and reduce bone formation rates as determined by analysis of bone biopsy specimens, probably through a direct inhibitory effect on osteoblast function.[31] They also diminish the stimulatory effect of calcitriol on BGP formation in vivo.[30] On the other hand, glucocorticoids may serve a permissive role in the differentiation of osteoblasts.[32]

Estrogens may exert at least some of their skeletal effects directly on osteoblasts. Estrogen receptors were identified on osteoblasts and osteoblast-like cells,[33,34] but the responses of these cells in vivo are unknown. In vitro, estradiol stimulates osteoblast proliferation and collagen synthesis,[35] and it has been shown to increase the secretion of various products of osteoblast-like cells, including alkaline phosphatase, other cellular enzymes, and type 1 insulin-like growth factor (IGF-1).[36–38] Estrogen may also affect the skeleton indirectly through reducing monocytic interleukin 1 synthesis.[39] Interleukin 1, a potent bone-resorbing factor, exerts some of its effects directly through the osteoblast.[6]

Insulin probably increases bone formation directly and acts indirectly by modulating levels of IGF-1.[32] Thyroid hormones stimulate osteoblastic function directly and nonspecifically.[40] Certain prostaglandins may stimulate bone resorption indirectly through osteoblasts, whereas others are capable of increasing bone formation.[6] Tumor necrosis factors stimulate bone resorption through osteoblastic regulation.[6]

Osteoclasts derive from mononuclear cells (most likely of the monocyte-macrophage series) in hematopoietic tissue. Precursors undergo first differentiation and then fusion to become multinucleate giant cells with many mitochondria and lysosomes. Once activated (a process that appears to be under osteoblastic control), osteoclasts demonstrate a ruffled, membranous border with numerous projections and a large surface area where bone resorption occurs. The ruffled border is surrounded by a clear zone delineated by relatively smooth plasma membrane in direct apposition to underlying bone. Attachment to bone requires the synthesis of the integrin alpha-v beta-3.[41] The clear or sealing zone has no organelles but contains bundles of actin that attach the osteoclast tightly to the underlying bone surface, separating the bone and cell compartment from the surrounding extracellular space to create and maintain a favorable microenvironment for bone resorption. It is generally well accepted that osteoclasts are responsible for resorption of both the mineral and the organic phase of bone matrix. Osteoclastic carbonic anhydrase and ruffled border proton pump enable osteoclasts to secrete acid into the subosteoclastic resorption zone to dissolve hydroxyapatite and create the acidic environment optimal for the function of lysosomal enzymes, including acid phosphatase and cysteine proteases, which solubilize and remove the organic matrix.[42-44]

Calcitonin is a potent inhibitor of bone resorption, causing rapid obliteration of the active ruffled border and loss of osteoclastic motility.[45,46] Certain prostaglandins may also transiently inhibit osteoclastic function directly. Estrogen receptors have also been found on osteoclasts, although their physiological role is unclear. Osteoclast function may be stimulated by PTH, calcitriol, prostaglandins E_2 and I_2, thyroxine, and many cytokines including interleukin 1, tumor necrosis factors, tissue growth factors, transforming growth factors, and osteoclast-activating factors, all probably acting indirectly through osteoblasts.[6,42] Glucocorticoids stimulate osteoclastic activity, probably indirectly by secondary hyperparathyroidism (possibly by hypersecretion of PTH).[31]

BONE REMODELING

Bone remodeling is a process of cyclic resorption and formation that begins in childhood and continues throughout life, at varying rates. It maintains the strength and integrity of bone, prevents mechanical failure, and repairs microfractures. Remodeling also maintains a dynamic state that allows mineral release into extracellular fluid when needed and subsequent redeposition into bone. Remodeling activity is proportionately much greater in the trabecular part of the skeleton: At any one time, approximately 20% of the trabecular surface is actively undergoing remodeling, but only 5% of the intracortical bone surface. Consequently, 25% of the total trabecular bone mass, but only 5–10% of the cortical bone mass, is renewed each year.[2]

There are several important distinctions between remodeling and modeling of bone. Remodeling is a coupled process of erosion and repair on the same bone surface with long quiescent periods between remodeling cycles. Modeling may involve formation and resorption, each on separate bone surfaces, and these processes may continue long without interruption. Remodeling does not result in grossly perceptible changes in bone shape, whereas the purpose of modeling is to alter the macrostructure of the bone. Finally, the net effect of remodeling in adults is bone loss and the net effect of modeling is bone accrual.[2]

Bone remodeling occurs in anatomically discrete packets of bone in which the bone and cells involved are called *bone remodeling units*. The process involves a characteristic sequence of events: activation, resorption, reversal, formation, and quiescence (Figure 7-7).[43,47] Remodeling occurs on all bone surfaces, including those deep within cortical bone, where the surface is adjacent to a haversian canal. Rates of remodeling vary, not only in different regions of the skeleton but also in different areas of any bone, areas commonly divided into periosteal, intracortical, corticoendosteal, and trabecular bone envelopes (see Figure 7-4). How a systemic hormone such as PTH, probably the most important activator of skeletal remodeling, can activate the remodeling sequence in some quiescent bone regions without affecting others is unknown.

Osteocyte lining cells (the terminal cells of the osteoblast lineage) probably play a role in local remodeling activation. These cells retract their cell processes, removing the nonmineralized lining material and exposing the mineralized bone surface, which is probably chemotactic for osteoclast precursors.[2] Activated multinucleated osteoclasts then resorb bone, creating cavities of a characteristic shape and depth over a 1- to 3-week

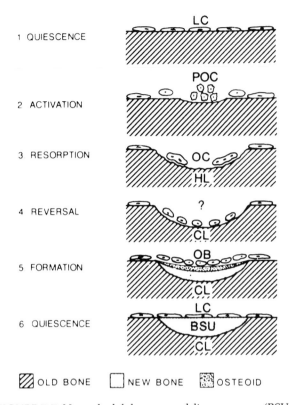

1 QUIESCENCE

2 ACTIVATION

3 RESORPTION

4 REVERSAL

5 FORMATION

6 QUIESCENCE

OLD BONE   NEW BONE   OSTEOID

FIGURE 7-7 Normal adult bone remodeling sequence. (BSU = bone structural unit; CL = cement line; HL = Howship's lacuna; LC = lining cell; OB = osteoblast; OC = osteoclast; POC = preosteoclast [mononuclear cell].) (Reprinted with permission from AM Parfitt. The cellular basis of bone remodeling: the quantum concept reexamined in light of recent advances in the cell biology of bone. Calcif Tiss Int 1984;36:537–545.)

period. Resorption cavities are called *Howship's lacunae* in trabecular bone and *cutting cones* in cortical bone. Although the initial cavity is formed by osteoclasts alone, the final resorption stage, which is much slower, includes mononuclear cells.

The reversal stage, which follows resorption, lasts 1–2 weeks and appears to be responsible for the coupling of formation to resorption, although the precise mechanisms are unknown. Some of the reversal (mononuclear) cells deposit a thin layer of cement substance, smoothing and preparing the surface for bone formation. Osteoblast precursors from connective tissue or marrow stroma are recruited to the resorption cavity and mature into osteoblasts.

Osteoblasts commence formation by secreting the organic components of bone matrix. Mineral deposition begins through basically unknown mechanisms approximately 5–10 days after the first osteoid has been

secreted but generally before the organic phase of formation is completed. As the resorption cavity is filled, osteoblasts make a gradual morphologic and functional transformation from highly active cells to the quiescent bone lining cells, called *osteocytes* at this stage. Maturation and increasing density of bone mineral continue to occur, extending the total formation phase to approximately 3 months and the total remodeling sequence to an average of 4 months (range, 3–24 months).[48]

The duration of the remodeling sequence, extent of resorption cavities, extent of repair with newly formed bone, and rate of remodeling site activation are some of the variable parts of this process that are under complicated regulatory control, including genetic, endocrine, nutritional, mechanical, and age-related factors. In general, although formation is coupled to resorption, the exact balance of these processes is such that at any one surface there may be a net loss or gain of bone. Characteristically, in adulthood, there is a small net gain of bone on the periosteal surface and a net decrease of bone on endosteal and trabecular surfaces. The latter overwhelms the periosteal increases and results in net loss of bone from the skeleton over time. This is a universal age-related phenomenon, although it occurs in varying degrees depending on the factors already mentioned.

MINERAL HOMEOSTASIS

Calcium

Nearly all of the body's calcium (99%) is stored in bone, and only 1% is spread throughout other tissues, extracellular fluid, and blood. Approximately one-half the circulating calcium is bound to protein and one-half is in ionized form with a small amount complexed to bicarbonate, citrate, or phosphate.[49] It is critical to maintain the extracellular calcium within tight limits because small increases or decreases can cause severe neurologic, neuromuscular, or renal disturbances that can lead to death. Calcium intake is highly variable, usually correlating with total calorie, protein, and phosphorous intake. Calcium absorption occurs primarily in the upper intestine through both an active mechanism, dependent on the presence of active vitamin D (1,25[OH]$_2$D), and passive diffusion, purely dependent on dose. We normally absorb only approximately 25% of the calcium we consume. Although the total amount of calcium absorbed increases with increased intake, the proportion of dietary calcium absorbed, particularly the active fraction, declines with increased intake.[50] Excess dietary calcium, together with calcium secreted into the gastrointestinal tract, is eliminated in the feces. Under normal circumstances, the kidney excretes much of the absorbed calcium. Although 98% of the filtered calcium normally is reabsorbed, this can be increased to almost 100% when strict calcium conservation is required. During states of calcium deprivation, increased PTH causes increased renal tubular reabsorption of calcium and increased bone resorption. It also increases the level of 1,25(OH)$_2$D, which in turn increases the efficiency of intestinal calcium absorption. These three mechanisms maintain a normal serum calcium level despite great fluctuations in intake.

Phosphorous

A large proportion of the body's phosphorous is also in the skeleton, both in association with calcium in the hydroxyapatite crystal and in the organic bone matrix with organophosphorous compounds such as phospholipids, phosphoproteins, and nucleic acids. In the blood, only 13% of phosphorous is protein bound, and of the rest approximately equal amounts are present as ions and complexes. We normally absorb approximately 90% of the phosphate that we consume. Absorption is mostly passive and less dependent on vitamin D than is calcium absorption. Dietary phosphorous deficiency and malabsorption are, therefore, rare. The kidney is the major site of phosphorous regulation; renal tubular reabsorption rates depend on the PTH level.[49]

Endocrine Control of Mineral Homeostasis

PTH and calcitriol are the major hormonal controls on mineral metabolism; calcitonin has a less important role. Other regulators such as thyroid hormone, gonadal steroids, glucocorticoids, and catecholamines, among others, may also affect mineral homeostasis, especially when they are frankly low or high.

PTH is synthesized initially as preproparathyroid hormone, which then undergoes two intracellular cleavages, ultimately being secreted as the intact PTH molecule with 84 amino acids. It undergoes rapid peripheral metabolism to amino (N)-terminal fragments, most containing 34 amino acids, and carboxy (C)-terminal fragments. Bioactivity seems to reside in the N-terminal portion of the molecule, as the N-terminal fragments and intact molecule are active while the C-terminal fragments are biologically inert.[49] PTH causes an increase in bone resorption, calcitriol production, and renal reabsorption of calcium. It also decreases the renal threshold for phosphate reabsorption, causing phosphaturia. PTH

secretion is increased by low serum calcium or high serum phosphate. The hormone acts by increasing both cyclic adenosine monophosphate[47] and intracellular calcium in its target tissues, bone and kidney.[51,52]

Intake of vitamin D is variable. It is present primarily in fortified foods and foods that contain small bones such as fish. Despite tremendous dietary variability, vitamin D deficiency is rare in young adults because the body is able to synthesize the vitamin from a precursor in the skin (7-dehydrocholesterol) when the skin is exposed to sunlight. The elderly or people who avoid the sun or who live in areas of the world where penetration of sunlight is limited are still vulnerable to vitamin D deficiency.[53] Absorption of dietary vitamin D, a fat-soluble vitamin, depends on normal hepatobiliary, pancreatic, and probably gastric function to digest fat and on a normal intestinal surface to absorb it. Figure 7-8 gives an overview of this and subsequent steps in vitamin D metabolism.[54]

Once in the blood, choleciferol associates with D-binding protein, an α-globulin, and is transported to the liver, where it is converted to 25(OH)D. This conversion is not strictly regulated and correlates well with dietary intake and cutaneous formation. 25(OH)D is the principal circulating metabolite and occupies the majority of D-binding protein. It is converted to 1,25(OH)$_2$D by the renal 1-α-hydroxylase enzyme. This enzyme is regulated principally by PTH, which increases its activity, and by phosphorous, which decreases its activity.

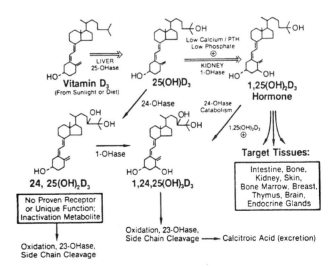

FIGURE 7-8 The vitamin D endocrine system. (Reprinted with permission from P Meunier, P Courpron, C Edouard, et al. Physiological senile involution and pathological rarefaction of bone. Clin Endocrinol Metab 1973;2:239–256.)

Because of tight regulation of this enzyme, calcitriol levels are constant over a large range of 25(OH)D levels. In states of suppressed PTH secretion, as when calcium supply is abundant, 25(OH)D is preferentially converted to 24,25-dihydroxyvitamin D, a metabolite presumed, but not proven, to be essentially inactive.[28] That the most active form of vitamin D is 1,25(OH)$_2$D is relatively indisputable, but possible contributions from other metabolites to the regulation of bone and mineral homeostasis cannot be fully excluded.

1,25(OH)$_2$D increases fractional calcium absorption from the intestine, its major target organ. Through this indirect effect on calcium supply, it exerts its major influence on bone formation. 1,25(OH)$_2$D has been shown to modulate several aspects of osteoblast function directly, but the physiological relevance of these effects is unknown. The better characterized effect on the skeleton is its ability to resorb bone and mobilize calcium. This activity occurs both rapidly (within hours) and slowly (over days). The latter effect is probably mediated by an increased number of osteoclast cells resulting from increased precursor differentiation. Like other steroid hormones, 1,25(OH)$_2$D complexes with an intracellular receptor and enters the target cell nucleus, where it exerts its effects by modulating mRNA production. Some cellular effects are thought to be too rapid to have occurred through this mechanism and consequently other nongenomic pathways of 1,25(OH)$_2$D action have been proposed. The plasma half-life of 1,25(OH)$_2$D is on the order of minutes; its biological half-life is hours. 1,25(OH)$_2$D is excreted mostly in bile and reabsorbed through the enterohepatic circulation.[28]

Calcitonin is a small peptide hormone (32 amino acids) synthesized by parafollicular or C cells in the thyroid gland. The physiological function of this hormone is unknown. In pharmacologic doses, it inhibits osteoclast activity, resulting in decreased bone resorption and increased renal calcium clearance. These two effects can cause a moderate decrease in serum calcium. Unlike deficiencies of PTH and 1,25(OH)$_2$D, which cause well-described diseases, no definite disease state has been described as a result of calcitonin deficiency or excess. It is likely, therefore, that calcitonin plays a less important physiological role in mineral metabolism than PTH or calcitriol.[55,56]

Numerous other hormones and factors affect mineral metabolism, particularly frank excesses or deficiencies, but they only rarely produce changes in serum levels of calcium because of dominant regulation by PTH and calcitriol. For example, deficiency of estrogen is well known to cause increased skeletal turnover, but it does not produce frank hypercalcemia because PTH release may be suppressed. Likewise, excessive adrenal or exogenous glucocorticoid causes osteoblastic dysfunction and calcium malabsorption, resulting in osteoporosis but not hypocalcemia, because excess PTH is secreted. In contrast, thyrotoxicosis (excess thyroid hormone), particularly when severe, may occasionally cause mild hypercalcemia, despite complete suppression of PTH and calcitriol, suggesting that certain disease states can overwhelm the physiological adaptations of the calciotropic hormones.

METABOLIC BONE DISEASE

Metabolic bone disease is generally defined as a disorder of the skeleton secondary to alteration in bone cell function. In most cases these are diffuse diseases that result from abnormalities in the hormones, minerals, or other regulators of function. Although the abnormal cell processes usually occur throughout the skeleton, they may cause more marked changes or symptoms in characteristic localized areas. Generally, although the mechanisms underlying these diseases are different, the common end point is most often loss of skeletal integrity and strength and a predisposition to fracture with minimal trauma or none. The major metabolic bone diseases are osteoporosis, Paget's disease, hyperparathyroidism, osteomalacia, renal osteodystrophy, and congenital diseases such as osteogenesis imperfecta and osteopetrosis.[57-62] As osteoporosis is by far the most common of these disorders for the rehabilitation physician, the remainder of this chapter focuses on that disease.

Osteoporosis

Definition
Osteoporosis is a skeletal disorder characterized by a reduction in bone mass with accompanying microarchitectural damage that increases bone fragility and the risk of fracture.[57,58] The histologic changes include thin and porous cortices and fewer, thinner trabeculae that are less connected than they are in normal bone. Primary osteoporosis refers to this condition when it occurs in the aging population when a secondary predisposing condition cannot be found. Thus, the primary condition includes both postmenopausal osteoporosis and osteoporosis of aging, the most common forms of the disorder, as well as a few rare forms. The clinical hallmark of the disease is fracture, which most characteristically occurs in the

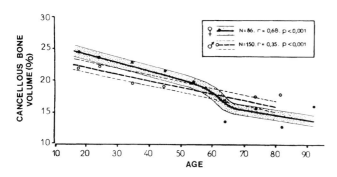

FIGURE 7-9 Changes in iliac trabecular bone volume with age and sex in 236 controls (curves statistically smoothed). (Reprinted with permission from P Meunier, P Courpron, C Edouard, et al. Physiological senile involution and pathological rarefaction of bone. Clin Endocrinol Metab 1973;2:239–256.)

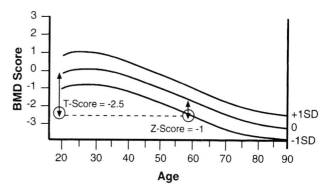

FIGURE 7-10 Relationship between Z and T scores in a woman aged 60 years. (BMD = bone mineral density.)

spine, femoral neck, or distal radius, although it may occur in the pelvis, humerus, or any other bone and is associated with minimal trauma.

Bone loss is universally associated with aging (Figure 7-9)[7,63–65]; therefore, any person who lives long enough will develop osteoporosis. Acceleration of the bone loss process, especially when accompanied by low peak bone mass, increases the likelihood of osteoporotic fracture.

Patients of all ages who present with fractures sustained from minimal trauma that have no evidence of other underlying bone disorders probably have osteoporosis. We also consider patients osteoporotic if their bone mass value is more than 2.5 standard deviations below the average bone mass values for young normal persons (Figure 7-10). This definition includes 50% or more of the population older than 70 years (i.e., even those with average or above average bone mass for that age are considered osteoporotic). This definition makes no distinction between a natural aging process and a more extreme or exaggerated process that probably occurs in only a small percentage of the population and is perhaps more consistent with the usual definition of a disease process. This difficulty in separating natural aging from disease is common to other aging phenomena, such as memory loss, systolic hypertension, glucose intolerance, and aortic atherosclerosis.

The absolute amount of bone, rather than the relationship of bone mass to others of that age, predicts the risk of fracture. Not surprisingly, then, bone mass values of patients who fracturedo overlap bone mass measurements of those who are "normal for age" and who have not had a fracture.[66] However, numerous studies have shown that bone mass values are the best predic-

tors of fracture risk in an individual, and this is demonstrated in Figure 7-11.[67]

Epidemiology

As bone mass declines with menopause and age, fracture frequency also increases with age.[68,69] Osteoporotic fractures are most common in postmenopausal women and in elderly persons of both sexes and typically occur with moderate trauma. Fractures in younger patients are considered unrelated to osteoporosis. The most common fractures are compressions of the vertebrae of which an estimated 500,000 cases occur annually in the United States, approximately 90% in women. The female-to-male ratio is somewhere between 2 and 8 to 1.[70,71] Accurate incidence and prevalence rates of these

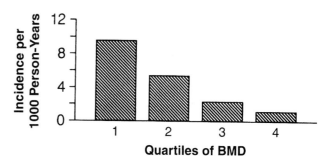

FIGURE 7-11 Relationship between femoral neck bone mass and fracture occurrence from the Study of Osteoporotic Fractures. (BMD = bone mineral density.) (Reprinted with permission from SR Cummings, MC Nevitt, WS Browner, et al. For the Study of Osteoporotic Fractures Research Group. Risk factors for hip fracture in white women. Unadjusted mean percent change in bone mineral density in the hip by treatment assignment and visit: adherent PEPI participants only. N Engl J Med 1995;332:767–773.)

fractures are difficult to obtain, because the fractures are often asymptomatic and are not recorded in epidemiologic data. Approximately 25% of all women older than the age of 65 have evidence of vertebral fractures.[70,71] The prevalence of vertebral fracture increases as vertebral bone mass declines such that women with bone mass in the osteoporotic range have an incidence of vertebral fractures of greater than 40%. Hip fracture is the most serious complication of osteoporosis; approximately 300,000 of these occur each year in the United States. Although the female-to-male ratio is only approximately 2 to 1, 80% of hip fractures occur in women because more women live to an older age.[46,72-74] The number of hip fractures is expected to increase as the percentage of aged persons in the population increases. At the age of 50, the average woman has a lifetime risk of 15% for hip fracture and one in three of the very old have had a hip fracture. The mortality of hip fracture is 12–20% within the first year and a large proportion of hip fractures result in disabilities. Fractures of the distal radius are the third most common form of osteoporotic fracture with 150,000–200,000 Colles's fractures occurring each year in the United States. The other sites of fracture that are most common include the pelvis proximal, humerus, ribs, and tibia.

Pathophysiology

Bone Mass   Bone mass is the major determinant of fracture risk (see Figure 7-11), with bone strength being 80–90% dependent on bone mass. Several additional factors contribute to fracture risk independently of bone mass. These include falling risk, personal history of adult fracture, history of fracture in a first-degree relative, current cigarette smoking, or low body weight. Although bone mass measurements in patients with fractures overlap those without fractures, the prevalence of vertebral fracture and incidence of hip and radius fracture are inversely proportional to bone mass values at the respective sites. Bone mass at any adult age

TABLE 7-1
Factors That Affect Peak Bone Mass

Genetics: race, sex, body build, skin type
Genetic diseases: Turner's syndrome, osteogenesis imperfecta, homocystinuria, Ehlers-Danlos syndrome
Calcium intake
Level of physical activity
Late menarche
Periods of hypogonadism (exercise, anorexia nervosa, hyperprolactinemia, idiopathic)

is determined by peak bone mass and the amount of bone subsequently lost, a product of both rate and duration of loss.

Peak Bone Mass   Peak mass is achieved some time after puberty (between ages 18 and 30) and is primarily determined genetically. Peak bone mass can be maximized through normal endocrine function and adequate exercise and adequate dietary intake (especially calcium).

Factors thought to affect peak bone mass are listed in Table 7-1. The major determinants are probably genetic, including race, gender, and body build. Men have approximately 5–10% higher bone density than women throughout youth and early adulthood, and the difference increases as ovarian failure occurs.[65,66,72] Blacks have bone densities approximately 5–10% higher than whites from an early age.[75,76] Thin, small, pale-skinned women are at greater risk than large, obese, or dark-skinned women.[61,72,75] Studies have shown a high level of concordance of bone mass measurements between monozygotic twins as compared with dizygotic pairs.[77-79] Daughters of osteoporotic mothers have exhibited reduced bone mass in the lumbar spine, and possibly, the femoral neck, in some,[80] but not all, studies.[81] Both male and female children and siblings of osteoporotics have been found to have lower spinal bone mass than control subjects.[82] Certain genetic diseases such as Turner's syndrome and osteogenesis imperfecta are associated with low peak bone mass.[61,83,84]

The total duration of the skeleton's exposure to estrogen levels that are compatible with menstrual function is a major determinant of bone mass, affecting peak mass as well as the rate of bone loss. Thus, those who have late menarche (after age 16) are more likely to have diminished peak bone mass compared with those whose menarche occurred at the average age.[85] Women who experience periods of amenorrhea in youth (induced by exercise, anorexia nervosa, or endocrine diseases) suffer lower peak bone mineral density (BMD).[86-91] Estrogen deficiency is at least one of the causes of low bone mass in Turner's syndrome.[84] Furthermore, all of the factors listed in Table 7-2 that increase bone loss might reduce peak bone mass if they occurred during the period of skeletal accrual.

In addition to genetic influences and gonadal insufficiency in youth, peak bone mass is affected by dietary calcium intake during childhood, adolescence, and young adulthood.[92] A study of two Yugoslavian populations that differed primarily in their lifelong calcium intake showed higher peak bone density to be associated with higher calcium intake.[93] Studies of postmenopausal women showed that those who reported consuming much milk during childhood and adolescence had higher bone density than age-matched women whose milk intake during youth was lower,[94-98] and women with higher lifetime calcium intakes have been associated with lower hip fracture rates.[93] A review of calcium intake in premenopausal women concluded that calcium supplementation led to an average increase in bone density at the spine and forearm of 1.1% per year as compared with placebo.[99]

Several studies in young adults show a correlation between BMD and physical activity level, suggesting that exercise might increase peak bone mass.[100-102] Physical activity level, measured as daily energy expenditure in walking (using a pedometer) and non-walking leisure activity, was found to correlate significantly with vertebral BMD in young premenopausal female subjects.[100] In another study of premenopausal women, activity level measured by a motion sensor correlated with both spinal BMD and total body calcium.[101] In young men, spinal BMD was significantly greater in those who engaged in regular, vigorous exercise than in relatively sedentary persons.[102] Lifelong cross-country runners (longer than 25 years in sport) had greater bone mineral mass in seven sites in their skeletons than sedentary age-matched controls.[103] A study comparing male athletes and nonathletes showed higher femur densities in the athletic group. Of the nonathletes, the exercisers had greater bone density than the nonexercisers.[104] Weight lifters and ballet dancers who began training early in life had higher forearm and leg densities and bone widths than healthy age-matched controls.[105] In general, weight-bearing exercise is associated with increased peak bone mass.[106] The type of exercise that confers the greatest benefit to bone are exercises with high impact forces. All of these studies suggest that the amount of various types of physical activity in youth is an important determinant of peak skeletal mass. Along the same lines, immobilization or reduction in weight-bearing physical activity is well known to reduce bone mass, as demonstrated in paraplegia, poliomyelitis, space flight, and bed rest for unrelated conditions.[107]

Bone Loss

In women, the rate of bone loss accelerates for several years before actual menopause (during partial ovarian failure), and for as long as 10 years after complete cessation of ovarian function.[65,68,108-112] The majority of evidence supports the importance of estrogen deficiency at menopause as the major factor in rapid bone loss and subsequent osteoporotic fractures.[112-115]

TABLE 7-2

Causes of Increased Bone Loss

Premature hypogonadism
Early menopause[80,101]
Oligomenorrheal amenorrhea
Exercise induced[81,82]
Anorexia nervosa[83,84]
Hyperprolactinemia[85-88]
Low testosterone in male subjects
Idiopathic[88,90,91]
Anorexia nervosa[89,124]
Other endocrine disorders
    Cushing's syndrome[31,92]
    Thyrotoxicosis[61,93]
    Insulin-dependent diabetes mellitus[61,94]
    Primary hyperparathyroidism[61,93]
    Addison's disease[95]
Lifestyle
    Smoking[61,91,96,97]
    Alcohol consumption[91,97,98,112]
    Thin body habitus[61,91,96]
    Immobilization/inactivity[93]
    Insufficient dietary calcium
    Too much protein, caffeine, phosphorus, sodium[61,99,100]
Drugs
    Glucocorticoids[31,92]
    Excessive thyroid hormone[102,103]
    Antiepileptics[104]
    Chemotherapy[105,107]
    Heparin[107]
Systemic disease[79,105]
Gastrectomy
Malabsorption
Chronic obstructive pulmonary disease
Some hematopoietic/neoplastic disorders (lymphoma/leukemia)
Radiotherapy (localized)

Estrogen Deficiency

The loss of estrogen at menopause increases the activation rate of more bone remodeling sites. Because resorption slightly exceeds formation in remodeling units (after peak bone mass is achieved), this elevated activation rate causes a net increase in skeletal resorption and hence bone loss, particularly on the endosteal surface of cortical bone and in cancellous bone. In addition, estrogen withdrawal may result in actual eradication of some trabecular units, this being caused by increased size or depth of resorption cavities.[116] This results in decreased trabecular connectivity or contiguity (see Figure 7-6), causing loss of reinforcing strength. These additional architectural changes cause more loss of bone strength than would be expected by the loss of mass alone.[116-120]

The increased skeletal remodeling associated with estrogen withdrawal is consistent with the biochemical and calcium kinetic changes observed across menopause. Levels of calcium and phosphate in the serum and urine increase but remain within the normal range.[112] Increases in biochemical markers of bone turnover in the blood and urine are consistent with increased skeletal turnover.[21,112] In a series of studies, Heaney et al. showed that at menopause there is increased transit of calcium into and out of the skeleton, decreased intestinal calcium absorption, and decreased renal tubular calcium reabsorption.[121-123] These latter effects are probably secondary to the increased skeletal liberation of calcium, which in turn suppresses PTH and calcitriol.

Estrogen receptors, both alpha and beta, have been detected on a variety of cells within marrow and on cells of osteoblast and osteoclast lineage. Estrogen's action depends on a variety of cell-cell interactions and the release of a variety of local cytokines and growth factors.[124] Those that might play a role in estrogen action on the skeleton are interleukins 1, 6, and 11; prostaglandin E_2; tumor necrosis factor-α; transforming growth factor-β; IGF-1; and perhaps IGF-2.[125-137] Estrogen may also have direct effects on bone including control of cell lifespan for osteoblasts, osteoclasts, osteocytes, or all three.[138-140] One alternative hypothesis for bone loss after menopause is that there is a primary renal leak of calcium that is offset by increased skeletal remodeling[141] as well other effects on mineral metabolism.[142]

Age

The mechanism of the slower, continuous bone loss associated with age alone is also ill understood, although a portion of age-related loss may be also attributed to estrogen deficiency. From the fourth decade onward, there is a remodeling imbalance at individual foci such that less bone is formed than is resorbed in most modeling units. This may be caused by impaired regulation of the osteoblast population rather than by intrinsic cellular osteoblast dysfunction.[68] Fasting urine calcium increases with age. Intestinal calcium absorption efficiency decreases with age and is concomitant with decreased $1,25(OH)_2D$ level.[50] PTH usually increases with advancing age, often in association with reduced serum 25(OH)D. The primary defect may be in $1,25(OH)_2D$ production or increased resistance to $1,25(OH)_2D$ at the gastrointestinal tract, associated with a compensatory and secondary increases in PTH to maintain calcium homeostasis,[50,143] which would result

in a net increase in bone resorption. Other age-related factors, such as decreased mechanical stress from decreased activity, muscle mass, or weight loss, may also be involved in bone loss associated with aging.

Other Causes of Bone Loss

Other factors besides age and menopause that are thought to affect the degree of bone loss are listed in Table 7-2.[144] Early age at menopause or any significant periods of hypogonadism in both women and men (from anorexia nervosa, hyperprolactinemia, extreme exercise, or other cause) are likely to result in more bone loss than unaffected persons exhibit.[86-91,117-123] Endocrine diseases such as thyrotoxicosis, Cushing's syndrome, insulin-dependent diabetes mellitus, and primary hyperparathyroidism may accelerate bone loss.[31,72,145-148] Smoking increases bone loss because of its association with a thin body habitus, its ability to induce early menopause, and perhaps through the stimulation of estrogen degradation and metabolism and consequent lowering of serum estrogen levels.[149-152] Excessive alcohol ingestion increases skeletal loss by inducing a defect in bone formation resulting in greater net resorption of bone.[118,119,151,153,154] Immobilization is well known to accelerate bone loss,[107] and increased physical activity may help prevent bone loss. Medicines, including glucocorticoids, excess thyroid hormone, antiepileptics, heparin, and some chemotherapy drugs (methotrexate) all adversely affect the skeleton.[31,136,145,155-159] Underlying systemic diseases such as postgastrectomy states, malabsorption, certain liver diseases, and chronic obstructive lung disease have all been associated with low bone mass.[150,158]

The influence of dietary calcium intake on bone loss and fracture rates in postmenopausal adults remains controversial. In one review, the response of bone to calcium supplementation in 20 trials of postmenopausal women has estimated that the calcium-supplemented group lost approximately 1% less per year than the placebo groups.[160] Calcium intake alone and in combination with vitamin D has been found to reduce the risk of spine, hip, and other nonspine fractures.[161-164] Other dietary factors, including excessive protein, phosphorous, caffeine, or sodium intake, may also increase bone loss to some extent by either decreasing calcium absorption or by increasing calciuria.[165,166]

Qualitative Factors

In addition to bone mass or quantity, several qualitative factors increase the probability of fracture. One is the phenomenon of complete elimination of trabecular plates that occurs during bone loss after ovarian failure.

Highly active remodeling with deep resorption cavities results in trabecular perforation followed by resorption of the remaining free ends of trabeculae (Figure 7-12). The actual eradication of trabecular units causes loss of structural reinforcement, which, as described earlier, is a major determinant of the strength of trabecular bone. This architectural abnormality causes a greater predisposition to fracture than the loss of bone mass alone.[116,119,120] The age of bone is also important in determining its ability to resist fracture. Bone that is not remodeled effectively can accumulate fatigue damage that weakens it and makes it more liable to fracture.[118] Other changes in the chemical composition of bone may occur, such as a reduction in the calcium content per unit volume of bone. Age-related changes such as increased diameter of the medullary canal of bones and increased cortical bone diameter are adaptations that maximize strength in the face of an overall reduction in mass. This is accomplished to some extent through local remodeling imbalances that favor endosteal bone resorption and periosteal bone formation.[167,168]

Falls

Though vertebral fractures may occur spontaneously, almost all other fractures occur only after a traumatic event, usually a fall. Falling is especially common in elderly persons; poor sight, balance problems, postural hypotension, dementia, and drugs such as hypnotics, antidepressants, antipsychotics, antihypertensives, diuretics, and hypoglycemics all probably play a role. Alcohol ingestion, with its effects on vision, coordination, and concentration, is also potentially dangerous and likely to cause falls in elders.[169] Certain acute and chronic diseases, including those that cause nocturia, may precipitate falls. Environmental hazards in the home such as slippery surfaces, especially in the shower and bath, poor room lighting, floor wires, throw rugs, and poorly placed furniture also contribute to the risk of falling. Ill-fitting shoes or excessively long trousers or skirts are additional risks for tripping and falling. Moreover, elders may not tolerate falls as well as younger persons because of their reduced soft tissue padding, weaker muscles, and slowed reflexes with consequent greater force transmission to bones.[170]

Patient Evaluation

Clinical Evaluation of the Patient

All women who reach menopause should be counseled about the risk factors for osteoporosis. All postmenopausal women who have clinical risk factors should have a bone density test. Any women who have not had

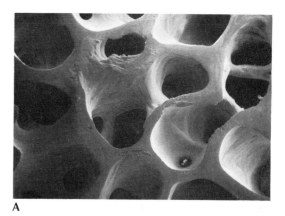

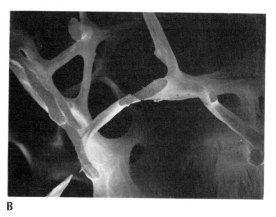

FIGURE 7-12 Low-power electron micrographs of iliac crest biopsies. **A.** Healthy 44-year-old man. **B.** A 47-year-old osteoporotic woman. Notice substantial loss of bone volume with complete eradication of many trabecular plates. (Reprinted with permission from DW Dempster, E Shane, W Holbert, et al. A simple method for correlative light and scanning electron microscopy of human iliac crest biopsies. J Bone Miner Res 1986;1:15–21.)

a bone density test by the age of 65 should have one. Many asymptomatic women come to discuss the results after a bone density test has been done. At this time a careful history and physical examination would complement the bone density results. When there is suspicion of secondary disease, whether identified by medical history or a low Z score based on a dual-energy x-ray absorptiometry (DXA) result (Z < –2.0), further investigation may be needed.

For patients who present with fractures it is important to determine whether the fractures are a result of either trauma or osteoporosis, as determined by a bone density test, and not secondary to underlying malignancy. In some circumstances routine radiography cannot make this distinction, and computed tomography, magnetic resonance imaging, or radionuclide scans may be helpful. It is important to remember that radiography can allow diagnosis of fractures (Figure 7-13), but a bone density test should be used to diagnose the underlying disease of osteoporosis. The presence of height loss exceeding 1.5 inches or significant kyphosis or back pain (particularly with an onset after menopause) is an indication for radiography to rule out asymptomatic vertebral fractures.

Assessment of Bone Mass

The major clinical tools for evaluation of skeletal status are noninvasive techniques that are available for estimating skeletal mass or density. These techniques include radiography and ultrasound. Bone mass measurement devices are also defined based on the site of measurement, either central or peripheral skeleton. The technique of bone mass measurement that is considered the gold standard is DXA. This x-ray–based technique allows measurement of any skeletal site, as well as the complete skeleton. The technique is highly accurate and precise.[171] Attenuation of x-ray through the skeleton

allows estimation of bone mineral for each region of interest within the spine, hip, forearm, or total body. The use of two levels of x-ray energy allow for correction for soft tissue. A measure of the area of mineral is used to provide a result that is in part corrected for the size of the skeleton. Results are reported as bone mineral content or BMD (content in grams divided by area in centimeters squared). Different manufacturers produce DXA equipment, however, and the measured density from each can vary. It has become standard practice to compare the results obtained from any machine with a normal distribution of bone density values. Individual results are compared with those obtained in a reference population of the same race, age, and sex. This comparison results in a score commonly called the *Z score* (see Figure 7-10). In addition, the individual's results are compared with the normal values obtained in a young population (peak bone mass) of the same race and sex; this is known as the *T score* (see Figure 7-10). In each case, if the individual's value falls at the mean of the population value, the score is zero. Scores are obtained using the difference (in standard deviations of the popu-

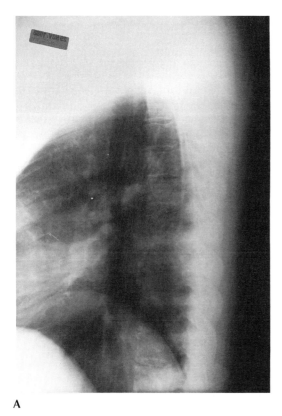

A

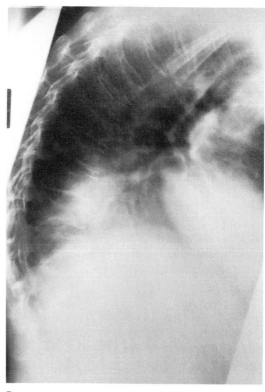

B

FIGURE 7-13 A. Thoracic spine of normal 60-year-old woman with preservation of vertebral height in all vertebrae. **B.** Severely kyphotic thoracic spine with compression fractures of essentially all vertebrae.

lation) between an individual's measurement and the population mean. A working group of the World Health Organization has defined osteoporosis as a T score that is more than 2.5 standard deviations below the mean for bone mass of a young normal population. The T score was developed only for postmenopausal women using central DXA and is accurate in those circumstances. The Z score can be clinically useful in determining those individuals who may have secondary causes of bone loss (Z score below –2.0).

Other methods of bone mass measurement include computed tomography that can be used to measure the spine. Peripheral computed tomography units can be used to measure bone in the forearm or tibia. The results obtained from computed tomography are different from all others currently available because this technique yields a pure sample of trabecular bone. However, there is less information regarding fracture risk using this technology than using DXA. Specialized dual-energy x-ray machines are also available to measure peripheral bone, usually the forearm or the heel. Ultrasound can also be used to measure bone mass. This technique depends on the attenuation of a band of ultrasound as it passes through bone or the speed with which the ultrasound traverses the bone. Each produces somewhat different results, although both are related to the amount of bone that is present.

All of these techniques have been approved by the Food and Drug Administration based on their capacity to predict the risk of fracture, and measurement of BMD is simply that: the estimation of a risk factor for fracture. Hip fracture risk is best predicted by measurements of the hip, which are also good predictors of the risk of other osteoporosis-related fractures. The hip, as measured by DXA, is the preferred site of measurement in most individuals; although the spine is often also measured at the same time. In younger individuals (i.e., closer to menopause) the spine measurement may be a more sensitive indicator of bone loss.

Routine Laboratory Evaluation

When a diagnosis of osteoporosis is made, either because of asymptomatic low bone density or because of a fracture, a general evaluation including complete blood count, serum calcium, and urine calcium may be justified to rule out secondary causes, particularly in women with fractures or low Z scores. When there is clinical suspicion of hyperthyroidism or Cushing's syndrome, a thyroid-stimulating hormone or urinary cortisol test should be performed. Thyroid-stimulating hormone should be routinely checked in patients on replacement therapy. In excessively thin women, in

whom bowel disease or malabsorption is suspected, serum cholesterol and albumin should be checked. Elevated serum calcium suggests hyperparathyroidism or malignancy, whereas reduced serum calcium could indicate malnutrition and osteomalacia. In the presence of hypercalcemia, serum PTH differentiates between hyperparathyroidism and malignancy, and high PTH-related protein levels can help document the presence of humoral hypercalcemia of malignancy. Severe malnutrition can be confirmed by low albumin levels or anemia. Asymptomatic malabsorption might be suspected if there is anemia (macrocytic, B_{12} or folate, microcytic, iron), low serum cholesterol, or low urinary calcium. If there is a suggestion of malabsorption, further evaluation is required. The most common finding is asymptomatic celiac sprue with selective malabsorption, which requires antigliadin and antiendomysial antibody tests and often a small bowel biopsy. A test of a gluten-free diet may also be confirmatory. In some individuals, 24-hour urine calcium can be helpful, especially in male subjects and younger women, or when the Z score falls below –1.5. A low urine calcium (< 50 mg/24 hours) suggests osteomalacia, malnutrition, or malabsorption. A high urine calcium (> 300 mg/24 hours) is indicative of hypercalciuria and must be investigated further. Hypercalciuria could result from a renal leak of calcium or absorptive hypercalciuria or in situations associated with excessive bone turnover including Paget's disease, hyperparathyroidism, and hyperthyroidism. Myeloma can masquerade as generalized osteoporosis, although it more usually presents with bone pain and characteristic punched-out lesions on radiography. Serum and urine electrophoresis and evaluation for light chains in urine are required to exclude this diagnosis. A bone marrow biopsy may be required to rule out myeloma in some patients and can also be used to rule out mastocytosis, leukemia, and other marrow infiltrative disorders, such as Gaucher's disease.

Several biochemical tests are now available that provide an index of the overall rate of bone remodeling. Biochemical markers are usually characterized as those related primarily to bone formation or bone resorption. These tests measure the overall state of bone remodeling at a single point in time. Their clinical use has been limited by high biological and analytic variability within and between individuals. Markers of bone resorption may help predict the risk of fracture, particularly in older individuals, adding to the predictive value of bone densitometry results.[44] In women 65 years of age or older when bone density results are above the treatment cut points noted previously, a high level of bone resorption may indicate a need for treatment nevertheless.

Another use of biochemical markers at present is in monitoring response to treatment. With the introduction of an antiresorptive therapeutic agent, bone remodeling declines rapidly, with the decrease in resorption occurring earlier than the decrease in formation. With all current therapies, bone resorption reaches its nadir within 3–6 months. Thus, a measure of bone resorption before initiating therapy and 4–6 months after starting therapy can provide an earlier estimate of patient response than can bone densitometry. Despite the variability in the results of these biochemical tests, for women being treated with bisphosphonates or hormone replacement therapy, declines in the results of most assays are detectable. This is less clear with either raloxifene or intranasal calcitonin treatment. It may also be possible that the resorption marker could assist in long-term compliance with osteoporosis medications, although supportive evidence is lacking.

The dysfunctional remodeling unit that leads to an increase in the risk of fractures with declining bone mass[46,74,172–177] suggests that biochemical markers should correlate with the risk of fracture. Several studies have now indicated that biochemical markers do predict the risk of fracture in several populations, perhaps independently of bone mass.[178–182]

The use of bone biopsy is rarely clinically required. Bone biopsy after tetracycline labeling of the skeleton allows evaluation for other metabolic bone diseases and determination of the rate of remodeling. Today, the careful use of biochemistry, including serum 25(OH) vitamin D (recommended if serum calcium is low), and biochemical markers of remodeling has largely replaced the biopsy.

Treatment

Management of Fractures

Treatment of the patient with osteoporosis involves management of acute fractures, as well as treatment of the underlying disease. Hip fractures almost always require surgical repair if the patient is to become ambulatory again, with procedures potentially including open reduction and internal fixation with pins and plates, hemiarthroplasties, and total arthroplasties depending on the location and severity of the fracture, condition of the neighboring joint, and general status of the patient. Long bone fractures often require either external or internal fixation. Some fractures such as vertebral, rib, and pelvic fractures require only supportive care, with no specific orthopedic treatment.

Vertebral compression fractures only occasionally present with a sudden onset of back pain. For those fractures that are acutely symptomatic, treatment with analgesics, including nonsteroidal anti-inflammatory agents, acetaminophen, or both, sometimes with the addition of a narcotic agent, is required. Short periods of bed rest may be helpful for pain management, although early mobilization is advantageous to help prevent any further bone loss. In some cases the use of a soft elastic style brace may help the patient become mobile sooner. Muscle spasms, which often occur with acute compression fractures, can be treated with muscle relaxants, moist or dry heat treatments, and physical therapy, including electric stimulation and massage.

Constipation, which may be a secondary symptom of ileus related to acute compression fracture, should be treated with a mild cathartic agent to help prevent exacerbation of back pain. All these recommendations are based on anecdotal experience, rather than clinical trials. A few randomized clinical trials have demonstrated that subcutaneously administered or perhaps intranasal calcitonin might be helpful to reduce the duration of pain related to acute vertebral compression fracture.[183–185] A still experimental technique involves percutaneous injection of artificial cement (polymethylmethacrylate) into the vertebral body and has been reported to offer significant immediate pain relief in the majority of patients.[186]

There are no informative studies indicating the usual course of pain associated with acute vertebral compression. It is highly variable among individuals. Clinical experience suggests that the severe pain usually resolves within 6–10 weeks. Chronic pain, which is probably not bony in origin, but related to abnormal strain on muscles, ligaments, and tendons associated with change in thoracic and abdominal shape, is difficult to treat effectively. The pain may require analgesics, sometimes narcotic analgesics, but sometimes responds to back-strengthening exercises (paraspinal) and frequent intermittent rest in a supine or semireclining position to allow the soft tissues, which are under tension, to relax. Heat treatments can also help relax muscles and reduce the muscular component of discomfort. Various physical modalities, such as ultrasound and transcutaneous nerve stimulation, may be beneficial in people who are particularly troubled by chronic pain. Pain might also occur in the neck region, not as a result of compression fractures (which almost never occur in the cervical spine as a result of osteoporosis), but because of the chronic strain associated with trying to elevate the head in a person with a severe thoracic kyphosis and may be helped with a soft collar. Symptoms such as early satiety, anorexia, and abdominal discomfort associated with multiple compressions and reduced volume of the abdominal cavity, should be treated symptomatically and by eating small meals frequently throughout the day. Constipation should also be avoided to prevent increased abdominal pressure with evacuation that can increase likelihood of further vertebral compression.

Management of the Underlying Disease

The management of the underlying disease, including risk factor reduction, is the next important step in caring for the osteoporotic patient to improve bone mass and reduce falls. Patients should be thoroughly evaluated to reduce the likelihood of concomitant risks associated with bone loss and falls. Medications that might cause bone loss should be reviewed to make sure that the drug is truly indicated and is being given in minimally effective doses. For those on thyroid hormone replacement, thyroid-stimulating hormone testing should be performed to ensure that an adequate, but not excessive, dose is being used, as this treatment can be associated with increased bone loss. In patients who are smokers, efforts should be made toward smoking cessation, and alcohol abuse should be evaluated and treated accordingly. Modifying the risk of falls also includes alcohol abuse treatment as well as a review of the medical regimen for any drugs that might be associated with orthostatic hypotension, sedation, or both, including the hypnotics and anxiolytics. Furthermore, patients should be instructed about environmental safety with regard to eliminating exposed wires, curtain strings, slippery rugs, and mobile tables and about providing good light in paths to bathrooms as well as just outside the home. Avoiding stocking feet on wood floors and checking carpet conditions, particularly on stairs, are good preventive maintenance. Treatment for any underlying visual problem is recommended, particularly problems with depth perception, which are specifically associated with increased risk of falls.

Optimization of Nutritional Status

A huge body of literature indicates that optimal calcium intakes can help reduce bone loss and suppress bone turnover. All patients with postmenopausal osteoporosis should be consuming least 1,200 mg of calcium per day, preferably from food sources, but with dietary supplements as needed. Patients who are taking calcium supplements should be instructed to look at the elemental calcium content of the supplement. The optimal calcium intake should be obtained with a good diet, high in fruits and vegetables, low in fat and salt, and moderate in protein. If a supplement is required, it should be taken in doses less than or equal to 600 mg at a time, as the calcium absorption fraction decreases with content

greater than that. Calcium supplements containing carbonate are best taken with food because they require acid for solubility. Calcium citrate supplements can be taken at any time. The efficacy of taking all calcium supplements at night to prevent a nocturnal increase in bone resorption has not been proven. Some patients may experience constipation, distention, or excess gas as side effects of calcium supplements. Those patients who have had kidney stones should have a 24-hour urine calcium determination before increasing calcium intake because hypercalciuria might be exacerbated at higher intakes. Furthermore, a thiazide-containing diuretic might be indicated in those patients to increase renal tubular calcium reabsorption and reduce urine calcium levels. Another important nutrient, vitamin D, should be taken at doses of approximately 400 IU per day in individuals below the age of 65 and at doses of 600–800 IU per day in those 65 years of age and older. There are no other routine recommendations for use of other nutritional supplements. Magnesium is abundant in foods and magnesium deficiency is quite rare in the absence of serious chronic diseases such as inflammatory bowel disease, celiac sprue, chemotherapy, severe diarrhea, malnutrition, and alcoholism.

Physical Activity and Exercise

High physical activity throughout the lifespan is likely to have a significant effect on bone mass. Postmenopausal women who initiate weight-bearing exercise (done while standing), can help prevent bone loss, but are unlikely to result in substantial bone gain. Specific muscle-strengthening exercises can also help prevent bone loss, and exercise is also recommended for effects on neuromuscular function. Exercise can improve coordination, balance, and strength, and thereby reduce the risk of falling. It is important that exercise is consistent, optimally at least three times a week, but any exercise is better than none. Walking itself is associated with reduced mortality and may be enough particularly for people with other coexisting medical conditions.

The best exercise regimen for the patient population with asymptomatic low bone mass has not been determined. Weight-bearing activity is thought to be critical to skeletal integrity, but the optimal level is unknown. Generally, aerobic exercises such as rapid walking, running, or upright calisthenics or aerobics are recommended. Several studies suggest that these weight-bearing aerobic exercises may increase or maintain BMD. Aloia and colleagues studied postmenopausal women. Those who exercised 3 hours per week for 1 year increased their total body calcium, whereas the calcium level of controls decreased significantly, although forearm BMD did not change significantly in either group.[187] After both 9 and 22 months Dalsky and coworkers found a significant increase in lumbar BMD above baseline and above the values for bone-losing controls in postmenopausal women who exercised 3 hours per week.[188] Chow's group randomized postmenopausal women to participate in aerobic, aerobic plus strengthening, or no exercise three times per week for 1 year and found significantly increased bone mass in the exercising groups, as compared with those who did not exercise.[189] Smith and associates found various indices of bone mass in the forearm to be increased in middle-aged women who performed approximately 3 hours of aerobic exercise per week over a 4-year period.[190] Not all studies are supportive, however. In a 3-year randomized trial of the effects of walking on postmenopausal women, forearm bone density decreased in both groups although in a subset of patients (those with high grip strength), radius cross-sectional area increased in the exercisers but not in the controls.[191] Additionally, another study of brisk walking in postmenopausal women showed equivalent decrements in bone mass of the spine in both walkers and nonwalkers after 1 year.[192]

Whether or not exercising specific muscle groups adds density or prevents loss of mass in the underlying skeletal site has yet to be determined. BMD of the lumbar vertebrae was found to correlate significantly with the strength of back extensor muscles.[193] Spinal extension exercises have been shown to increase spinal muscle strength[194] but have not yet been shown to increase bone mass. It is possible that strengthening back extensors may help protect against vertebral bone loss and subsequent fracture. In tennis players, BMD values are well known to be significantly higher in the dominant arm than in the other one.[195] Clinical trials are required to investigate whether building muscle strength in the spine, hip, wrist, or intercostal region in the postmenopausal age group increases BMD and decreases fracture rates in the respective sites.

Patients who have already sustained a fracture represent a more challenging problem than those with only asymptomatic low bone mass. Appropriate medicine for pain relief (i.e., anti-inflammatory agents, muscle relaxants, if necessary narcotic analgesics) is critical. Physical modalities should be tried, including hydrotherapy, hot packs, ultrasound massage, and transcutaneous nerve stimulation and massage. Although bed rest right after a fracture is usually recommended, patients should be mobilized as soon as pain is tolerable, as more prolonged immobilization could aggravate osteoporosis. Occasionally, a thoracic brace, usually made of soft elastic material, helps patients feel better and become ambulatory faster. Stiff metal and plastic braces are not recommended because they are extremely uncomfortable, they facilitate awkward and potentially imbalanced movements, and they often encourage patients to spend more time in bed than they would otherwise. Proper body mechanics should be taught, including avoidance of unnecessary spinal compression forces like those associated with spinal flexion, twisting, rapid jarring, and forward reaching movements.[196]

When the patient is ready, a program of both weight-bearing aerobic exercise (low impact) and spinal extension exercise should be prescribed. These recommendations are based on a few preliminary studies of the effects of exercise in osteoporotic women. Krolner and coworkers studied middle-aged osteoporotic women (all had had a wrist fracture), half of whom participated in a supervised and varied exercise program 2 hours per week for 8 months. BMD of the lumbar spine increased in exercisers while it decreased significantly in controls, although forearm BMD decreased slightly in both groups.[197] Sinaki and Mikkelsen studied the effects of spinal exercises on postmenopausal osteoporotics. Those who performed regular spine extension exercises had a lower fracture recurrence rate than those who performed flexion exercises or had no exercise regimen.[198] Over 5 months, various dynamic loading exercises of the forearm increased radius BMD in postmenopausal osteoporotics, as compared with decreased BMD in controls.[199] More studies are obviously required to confirm and extend these results so that specific exercise programs can be prescribed for osteoporotic women.

Pharmacologic Therapies

It is currently recommended that all postmenopausal women with a BMD T score of –2 or below begin medical treatment or those with T score of –1.5 or below begin treatment if any of the major osteoporotic risk factors are present.

Estrogens   There are numerous clinical trials indicating that estrogens of various types and routes of administration (conjugated equine estrogens, estradiol, estrone, esterified estrogens, ethynylestradiol, and mestranol) reduce bone turnover, prevent bone loss, and actually increase bone mass of the spine, hip, and total body.[200] This is true in women at both natural and surgical menopause and is also true in late postmenopausal women and in women with established osteoporosis. Combined estrogen and progestin preparations are now available in many countries. One of the largest clinical trials, the Postmenopausal Estrogen/Progestin Intervention Trial (Figure 7-14) indicated that

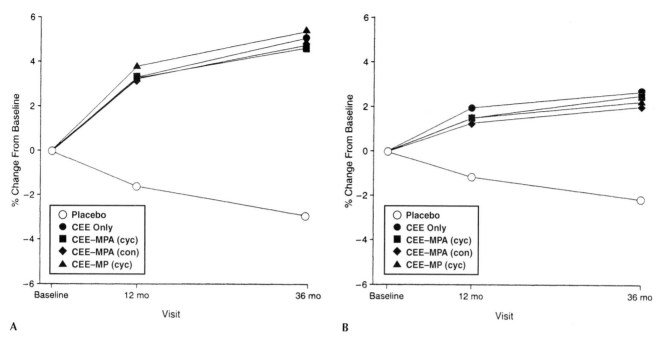

FIGURE 7-14 Results of various hormone replacement therapy regimens on bone mineral density of the spine **(A)** and hip **(B)**. Unadjusted mean percent change in bone mineral density in the hip by treatment assignment and visit: adherent PEPI participants only. Results from the Postmenopausal Estrogen/Progestin Intervention Trial. (CEE = conjugated equine estrogen, 0.625 mg per day; CEE-MPA [cyc] = CEE + medroxy progesterone acetate, 10 mg per day for 12 days per month; CEE-MPA [con] = CEE + medroxy progesterone acetate, 25 mg daily; CEE-MP [cyc] = CEE + micronized progesterone, 200 mg per day for 12 days per month.) (Reprinted with permission from TL Bush, et al. Effects of hormone therapy on bone mineral density. JAMA 1996;276:1389–1396.)

progestins did not augment the effect of conjugated equine estrogen alone on bone mass.[201]

The effects of estrogens on fracture occurrence have been less well studied than the effects on bone mass.[202–205] The majority of data is from large epidemiologic studies (Study of Osteoporotic Fractures, Upsala, Nurse's Health, Framingham, Leisure World, and Rancho-Benardo Studies). These studies indicate overall that estrogen use is associated with an average reduction of 50% in the risk of various osteoporotic fractures, including hip fractures.[206] The fracture prevention diminishes after discontinuation of estrogen. Approximately 10 years after discontinuation, there is no residual effect against fracture occurrence.[206,207] Clinical trial data evaluating the effect of estrogen administration on fractures are sparse. The ongoing Women's Health Initiative, a large-scale randomized trial of the benefits of hormone replacement versus placebo, will help determine if estrogen treatment reduces fracture risk. In addition to the effects on the skeleton, estrogens have effects throughout the body, including the urogenital and cardiovascular systems, breast, and brain.[208–210] Estrogen use is also associated with minor side effects including

breast tenderness and engorgement and vaginal bleeding or spotting. However, with a daily continuous regimen of estrogen and progestin bleeding in most patients usually abates within 6 months.

Selective Estrogens Receptor Modulators Two selective estrogens receptor modulators are currently being used in postmenopausal women. Raloxifene is approved for prevention and treatment of osteoporosis, and tamoxifen is approved for the prevention and treatment of breast cancer. Tamoxifen has been shown to reduce bone turnover and bone loss in postmenopausal women when compared with placebo groups in patients with and without breast cancer.[211,212] Thus, tamoxifen is believed to act as an estrogenic agent in bone. There are two clinical trials that have looked at the effects of tamoxifen on fracture risk. In a group of patients with breast cancer who were followed for an average of 8 years after 1 year of treatment with tamoxifen provided no protection against hip fracture risk. The Breast Cancer Prevention Trial showed a nonsignificant trend toward reduction in risk of hip, clinical spine, and wrist fractures in healthy postmenopausal women over 4 years of use.[213] No spine radiographs were done in this trial to evaluate asymptomatic vertebral compression deformities. Tamoxifen, like estrogen, has effects throughout the body. The major benefit of tamoxifen is on breast cancer occurrence.[213] Tamoxifen does increase the risk of venous thromboembolic disease approximately threefold, similar to the increased risk seen in patients treated with estrogens. Tamoxifen also increases occurrence of both benign and malignant uterine disease, but there is no evidence that it increases the risk of ovarian cancer.

Raloxifene has estrogenic effects on bone turnover and bone mass that are similar to those of tamoxifen. The efficacy of raloxifene as well as tamoxifen, on improving bone density (1.4–2.8% versus placebo in the spine, hip, and total body) is of somewhat smaller magnitude than that of standard-dose estrogens.[214] In a large treatment study, over 7,700 women with osteoporosis were randomly assigned to receive one of two different doses of raloxifene versus placebo in addition to 500 mg of calcium and 400–600 units of vitamin D per day provided to all groups.[215] The major outcome in this study was vertebral fracture occurrence, and raloxifene reduced the occurrence of vertebral fracture by 30–50%, depending on the subpopulation (Figure 7-15). In this trial there was no suggestion of reduced risk of any other osteoporotic fracture other than that of the ankle. However, the study was not designed nor did it have adequate power to evaluate risk of other fractures. Raloxifene, like tamoxifen and estrogen, has

effects throughout other organ systems. The most positive of these effects appears to be a reduction in invasive breast cancer occurrence of approximately 70% in women taking raloxifene compared with placebo, primarily in estrogen receptor–positive disease (90% reduction).[216] In addition, raloxifene in multiple studies is not associated with an increase in the risk of uterine cancer or any benign uterine disease. Raloxifene, like tamoxifen, however, increases the risk of thromboembolic disease and may increase the occurrence of hot flashes.

Bisphosphonates   The bisphosphonate class of drugs is approved for treatment and prevention of osteoporosis as well as Paget's disease and hypercalcemia of malignancy. Two agents, alendronate and risedronate, are currently approved for osteoporosis therapy. Alendronate decreased turnover and increased bone mass up to 8% versus placebo in the spine and 6% versus placebo in the hip over 3 years in patients with osteoporosis.[217] In addition, reduction in the occurrence of vertebral fracture and reduced height loss were found in the alendronate treated women. The Fracture Intervention Trial has subsequently provided evidence in over 2,000 women with prevalent vertebral fractures that daily alendronate treatment (5 mg/day for 2 years and 10 mg/day for 9 months afterward) reduces the risk of vertebral fractures by approximately 50%, multiple vertebral fractures by up to 90%, and hip fractures by up to 50% (Figure 7-16). In this trial of over 4,000 women with low bone mass, a reduction in vertebral

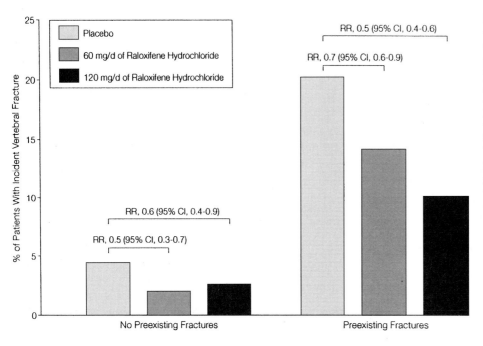

FIGURE 7-15 Incidence of new vertebral fractures in 6,828 women who completed the MORE Study. (CI = confidence interval; RR = relative risk.) (Reprinted with permission from B Ettinger, DM Black, BH Mitlak, et al. Reduction of vertebral fracture risk in postmenopausal women with osteoporosis treated with raloxifene. Results from a 3-year randomized clinical trial. JAMA 1999;282:637–645.)

fractures was shown over 4 years.[218] The reduced risk of hip fracture, however, was limited to those patients who had osteoporosis by bone mass criteria alone. In a subsequent fracture study of over 1,900 women with low bone mass who were treated with alendronate (10 mg/day versus placebo), the treatment group had a 47% reduction in incidence of all nonvertebral fractures after just 1 year.[219]

Alendronate must be given on an empty stomach, because all bisphosphonates are poorly absorbed. It is contraindicated in patients who have stricture or inadequate emptying of the esophagus because of the potential for esophageal irritation. Patients are recommended to remain upright after taking the medication for at least 30 minutes to avoid this possible esophageal irritation. Although cases of esophagitis, esophageal ulcer, and esophageal stricture have been described, the true incidence of gastrointestinal toxicity from this agent is probably quite low. In clinical trials there was no increased risk from alendronate in overall gastrointestinal symptomatology. Postmarketing experience suggesting that gastrointestinal effects are common may be related to the underlying high risk of these symptoms in the elderly. Flexible dosing for alendronate (higher dose less frequently) may avoid some of the apparent gastrointestinal toxicity.

Risedronate is another potent bisphosphonate that is currently available for Paget's disease, treatment of osteoporosis, and treatment and prevention of glucocorticoid-induced osteoporosis. This agent also produces dramatic effects on bone mass and bone turnover and has been shown to reduce the risk of vertebral fractures by more than 40% over 3 years (Table 7-3).[220,221] These studies report a reduction of approximately 33% in all nonspine fracture in risedronate-treated patients, but no significant reduction in hip fracture. Preliminary reports from studies designed specifically to look at hip fracture suggest that risedronate is also associated with a reduction in hip fracture of approximately 40% in patients with osteoporosis.[222] Risedronate must be given in a similar fashion to alendronate to avoid upper gastrointestinal toxicity. Flexible dosing for risedronate may help avoid any possible gastrointestinal toxicity.

Etidronate was the first bisphosphonate to be approved for use in Paget's disease and hypercalcemia, and this agent has also been used in osteoporosis trials; however, these trials were smaller than those performed for alendronate and risedronate. This agent probably has some efficacy against vertebral fracture when given as an intermittent cyclical regimen (2 weeks on, 2.5 months off). There are no data indicating protection against any nonspine fracture.

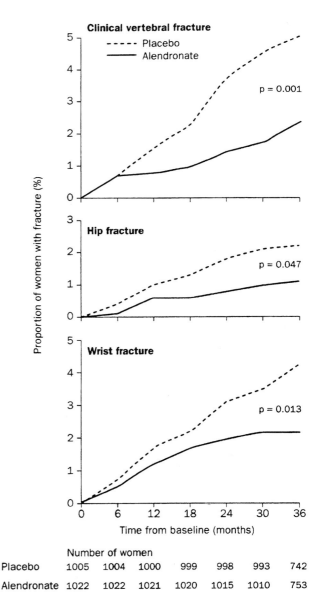

FIGURE 7-16 Cumulative proportions of women with osteoporosis who suffered clinical vertebral hip or wrist fracture during 3 years of treatment with alendronate or placebo. (Reprinted with permission from DM Black, S Cummings, D Karpf, et al. Randomized trial of effect of alendronate on risk of fracture in women with existing vertebral fractures. Lancet 1996;348:1535–1541.)

Another agent, ibandronate, can be administered intravenously once every 3 months and is currently under investigation. It may provide an effective alternative to an oral regimen of bisphosphonates, particularly in people who have upper gastrointestinal disease.

Calcitonin Calcitonin is a polypeptide hormone normally produced by the thyroid gland. It can be either

TABLE 7-3
Cumulative Incidence of Fractures

Treatment Group by Time	No.[a]	Subjects with Incident Fracture, No. (%)[b]	Relative Risk (95% Confidence Interval)[c]	P Value[d]
New vertebral fractures				
Year 0–1				
Placebo	660	42 (6.4)	—	—
Risedronate, 2.5 mg	618	23 (3.8)	0.54 (0.32–0.91)	.02
Risedronate, 5 mg	669	16 (2.4)	0.35 (0.19–0.62)	< .001
Years 0–3				
Placebo	678	93 (16.3)	—	—
Risedronate, 5 mg	696	61 (11.3)	0.59 (0.43–0.82)	.003
Nonvertebral fractures				
Years 0–3				
Placebo	815	52 (8.4)	—	—
Risedronate, 5 mg	812	33 (5.2)	0.6 (0.39–0.94)	.02

[a]For the vertebral fracture assessments, the number of subjects is those with evaluable radiographs both at baseline and after treatment.
[b]Proportion is based on Kaplan-Meier estimate of the survival function.
[c]Based on Cox regression model.
[d]Based on log-ranked test.

injected or administered intranasally. Its physiological role is unclear, as no skeletal disease has been described in association with calcitonin deficiency or calcitonin excess. Calcitonins are approved by the U.S. Food and Drug Administration for Paget's disease, hypercalcemia, and osteoporosis in postmenopausal women who are more than 5 years from menopause.

Injectable calcitonin produces small increments in bone mass of the lumbar spine. However, difficulty of administration and frequent reactions including nausea, often with vomiting, and flushing of the face limit general use. A nasal spray containing calcitonin (200 IU/day) was approved in 1995 for treatment of osteoporosis in late postmenopausal women. Several studies have indicated that nasal calcitonin can produce small increments in bone mass.[223-225] Furthermore, the risk of new vertebral fractures was reduced in calcitonin-treated patients versus those on calcium alone.[224] Calcitonin did not produce lumbar spine bone mass increments in recently postmenopausal women, but in women more than 5 years postmenopausal, lumbar BMD did increase compared with placebo by approximately 3%.[225] The largest study of nasal calcitonin was a 5-year multicenter study of three different doses of calcitonin (100, 200, and 400 units) versus placebo in patients with low bone mass and prevalent vertebral fractures at entry. Of the original 1,255 patients, whose mean age was 68 years, almost 70% dropped out of the study, thereby rendering conclusions of this study difficult to interpret. All participants received 1,000 mg of elemental calcium

and 400 units of vitamin D daily. Overall, using intent-to-treat analysis, vertebral fracture reduction was significant at 36% in the 200-unit dose of calcitonin only, with no statistically significant effect on nonspine fractures.[226] Calcitonin is not indicated for prevention of osteoporosis and is not sufficiently potent to prevent bone loss in early postmenopausal women. In the subcutaneous and possibly the nasal form, calcitonin may have an analgesic effect on bone pain.

Experimental Agents Endogenous PTH is an 84-amino acid peptide, which is largely responsible for calcium homeostasis. Observational studies in the past indicated that mild elevations in PTH could be associated with maintenance of cancellous bone mass, although elevated levels might be detrimental to cortical bone mass. On the basis of these observations, preclinical and early clinical studies were performed that indicated that exogenous PTH (1-34 PTH) could produce dramatic increments in bone mass. The first randomized controlled trial in postmenopausal women showed that PTH, when added to ongoing estrogen therapy, could increase bone mass by approximately 13% over a 3-year period compared with estrogen alone.[227] This increment in bone mass was also associated with a reduction in risk of vertebral compression deformity (Figure 7-17). In premenopausal women rendered amenorrheic by gonadotropin-releasing hormone therapy for endometriosis, PTH treatment prevented bone loss and actually resulted in bone gain compared with placebo.[228] The PTH and estrogen study was repeated by other investigators who

FIGURE 7-17 Number of incident vertebral deformities (15% and 20% reductions) in women with osteoporosis on hormone replacement therapy (HRT), compared with hormone replacement therapy + parathyroid hormone (PTH) over 3 years. (Reprinted with permission from R Lindsay, DM Hart, C Forrest, C Baird. Prevention of spinal osteoporosis in oophorectomised women. Lancet 1980;2:1151–1154.)

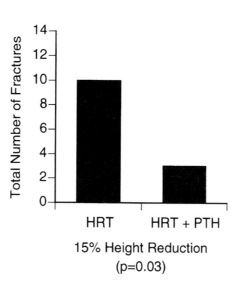

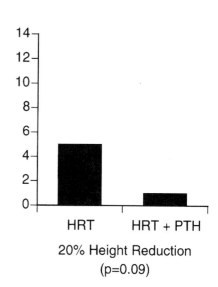

found even more dramatic effects on bone mass.[229] Use of PTH plus estrogen in patients on corticosteroid therapy has also been shown to produce substantial increments in bone mass. PTH might also be effective on bone mass when used in high doses for 1 month of every 3.[230] Data confirming the antifracture efficacy of PTH in postmenopausal women have recently been presented.[231] PTH use may be limited by mode of administration, which currently must be subcutaneous injection, although alternative modes of delivery are being investigated.

Fluoride has been available for many years and has been used in multiple osteoporosis studies with conflicting results. A substantial effect of sodium fluoride against vertebral fracture was not seen, but there was a possible trend toward increased risk of nonvertebral fracture, particularly of the hip. Side effects were substantial including lower extremity pain syndrome and gastrointestinal side effects, including hemorrhagic ulceration. There was a dramatic improvement in both spinal and hip bone mass that was clearly not reflected in improvement in bone strength and resistance to fracture. A subsequent trial involving slow-release sodium fluoride (50 mg/day) showed improvement in bone density that was associated with a substantial reduction (70%) in the risk of new vertebral compression deformities.[232] This study has yet to be confirmed by other work. At this time sodium fluoride is still a promising compound. However, it is purely experimental, limited by side effects and by concerns that bone quality may be compromised by incorporation of the fluoride into bone crystal, thereby reducing the competency of the crystalline component or resulting in immature mineralization of the bone.

Several small studies of growth hormone alone or in combination with other agents have not shown consistent or substantial positive effects on skeletal mass. The effects of growth hormone and the IGFs are still under investigation. Anabolic steroids, mostly derivatives of testosterone, act primarily as antiresorptive agents to reduce bone turnover, but may stimulate osteoblast proliferation and differentiation in vitro. Effects on bone mass remain unclear, but in general are weak and have been associated with frequent masculinizing side effects. Investigations of strontium's possible antiresorptive and bone-stimulating effects are ongoing.

Nonpharmacologic Approaches

Protective pads worn around the outer thigh, which cover the trochanteric region of the hip, were found to prevent hip fractures in elderly nursing home residents. In this study, no patient who fell while wearing a hip protector had a hip fracture. This was a dramatic improvement over those patients who fell without protective pads, where the fracture frequency was substantial. The use of hip protectors is limited largely by compliance and comfort, but new devices are being developed that may resolve these problems, so that these agents might serve as adjunctive treatments to those pharmacologies mentioned previously for prevention of hip fractures.

CONCLUSION

We now have effective, inexpensive, noninvasive, no-risk ways of diagnosing osteoporosis in its asymptomatic stage. We know reducing risk factors associated with bone loss and optimizing nutrition and exercise can help influence the course of the disease. We also have multiple agents, some multisystemic and some bone-specific, that can reduce fracture occurrence by approximately 50% overall. Ultimately these agents help reduce disability and death from this disease. Various nonpharmacologic approaches including reducing falling risk and supplying hip protectors can also be helpful.

REFERENCES

1. Frost HM. Mechanical determinants of bone modeling [Review article]. Metab Bone Dis Rel Res 1982;4:217–229.
2. Parfitt AM. Bone Remodeling: Relationship to the Amount and Structure of Bone, and the Pathogenesis and Prevention of Fractures. In BL Riggs, LJ Melton III (eds), Osteporosis: Etiology, Diagnosis and Management. New York: Raven Press, 1988;45–93.
3. Frost HM. Vital biomechanics: proposed general concepts for skeletal adaptations to mechanical usage. Calcif Tissue Int 1988;42:145–156.
4. Lanyon LE. Functional strain as a determinant for bone remodeling. Calcif Tissue Int 1984;36:S56–S61.
5. Trueta J. Mechanical Forces and Bone Shape. In J Trueta (ed), Studies of the Development and Decay of the Human Frame. Philadelphia: WB Saunders, 1968;37–41.
6. Martin TJ, Ng KW, Nicholson GC. Cell Biology of Bone. In TJ Martin (ed), Bailliere's Clinical Endocrinology and Metabolism. Vol 2: Metabolic Bone Disease. London: Bailliere Tindall, 1988;1–29.
7. Riggs BL, Wahner HW, Seeman E, et al. Changes in bone mineral density of the proximal femur and spine with aging. J Clin Invest 1982;70:716–723.
8. Wasnich RD, Ross PD, Vogel JM. Letter to the editor. N EngI J Med 1985; 313:325–326.
9. Cowin SC. Wolff's law of trabecular architecture at remodeling equilibrium. J Biomech Eng 1986;108:83–88.
10. Hayes WC, Gerhart TN. Biomechanics of Bone: Applications for Assessment of Bone Strength. In WA Peck (ed), Bone and Mineral Research. Vol 3. Amsterdam: Elsevier, 1985;259–294.
11. Pugh JW, Rose RM, Radin EL. Elastic and viscoelastic properties of trabecular bone: dependence on structure. J Biomech 1973;6:475–485.
12. Melton LJ III, Chao EYS, Lane J. Biomechanical Aspects of Fractures. In BL Riggs, LJ Melton III (eds), Osteporosis: Etiology, Diagnosis, and Management. New York: Raven Press, 1988;111–131.

13. Rockoff SD, Sweet E, Bleustein J. The relative contribution of trabecular and cortical bone to the strength of human lumbar vertebrae. Calcif Tissue Res 1969;3:163–175.
14. Kleinman HK, Klebe RJ, Martin GR. Role of collagenous matrices in the adhesion and growth of cells. J Cell Biol 1981;88:473–485.
15. Robey PG, Fisher LW, Young MF, et al. The Biochemistry of Bone. In BL Riggs, LJ Melton III (eds), Osteporosis: Etiology, Diagnosis, and Management. New York: Raven Press,1988; 95–109.
16. Price P. Osteocalcin. In WA Peck (ed), Bone and Mineral Research. Vol 1. Amsterdam: Excerpta Medica, 1983; 157–190.
17. Lian JB, Gundberg CM. Basic science and pathology. Osteocalcin biochemical considerations and clinical applications. Clin Orthop 1988;226:267–291.
18. Menon RK, Gill DS, Thomas M, et al. Impaired carboxylation of osteocain in Warfarin-treated patients. J Clin Endocrinol Metab 1987;64:59–61.
19. Fraser JD, Otawara Y, Price PA. 1,25-Dihydroxy vitamin D_3 stimulates the synthesis of matrix gamma-carboxyglutamic acid protein by osteosarcoma cells. Mutually exclusive expression of vitamin K-dependent bone proteins by clonal osteoblastic cell lines. J Biol Chem 1988;263:911–916.
20. Tracy RP, Shull S, Riggs BL, et al. The osteonectin family of proteins [Review]. Int J Biochem 1988;20:653–660.
21. Robey PG, Young MF, Fisher LW, et al. Thrombospondin is an osteoblast-derived component of mineralized extracellular matrix. J Cell Biol 1989;108:719–727.
22. Yamada KM, Olden K. Fibronectins-adhesive glycoproteins of cell surface and blood [Review article]. Nature 1978;275:179–184.
23. Owen M. Lineage of Osteogenic Cells and Their Relationship to the Stromal System. In WA Peck (ed), Bone and Mineral Research. Vol 3. Amsterdam: Elsevier, 1985;1–25.

24. Urist MR, Nillsson OS, Hudak R, et al. Immunologic evidence of a bone morphogenetic protein in the milieu interieur. Ann Biol Clin 1985;43:755–766.
25. Noda M, Rodan GA. Transcriptional regulation of osteopontin production in rat osteoblast-like cells by parathyroid hormone. J Cell Biol 1989;108: 713–718.
26. Turner RT, Howard GA, Puzas JE, et al. Calvarial cells synthesize 1,25-dihydroxyvitamin D_3 from 25-hydroxyvitamin D3. Biochemistry 1983;22:1073–1076.
27. Noda M, Yoon K, Rodan GA. Parathyroid hormone (PTH) enhances osteocalcin mRNA expression in rat osteosarcoma cells [Abstract]. J Bone Miner Res 1988;3(Suppl 1):sl44.
28. Reichel H, Koeffler HP, Norman AW. The role of the vitamin D endocrine system in health and disease. N Engl J Med 1989;320:980–991.
29. Ekenstam E, Stalenheim G, Hallgren R. The acute effect of high dose corticosteroid treatment on serum osteocalcin. Metabolism 1988;37:141–144.
30. Beresford JN, Gallagher JA, Poser JW, et al. Production of osteocalcin by human bone cells in vitro: effects of 1,25(OH)₂D₃, 24,25(OH)₂D₃, parathyroid hormone and glucocorticoids. Metab Bone Dis Rel Res 1984;5:229–234.
31. Dempster DW. Perspectives. Bone histomorphometry in glucocorticoid-induced osteoporosis. J Bone Miner Res 1989;4:137–141.
32. Raisz LG, Kream BE. Regulation of bone formation [Part 2]. N Engl J Med 1983;309:83–89.
33. Komm BS, Terpening CM, Benz DJ, et al. Estrogen binding, receptor mRNA, and biologic response in osteoblast-like osteosarcoma cells. Science 1988; 241:81–84.
34. Eriksen EF, Colvard DS, Berg NJ, et al. Evidence of estrogen receptors in normal human osteoblast like cells. Science 1988;241:84–86.
35. Ernst M, Schmid C, Froesch ER. Enhanced osteoblast proliferation and collagen gene expression by estradiol. Proc Natl Acad Sci U S A 1988;85: 2307–2310.

36. Gray TK, Flynn TC, Gray KM, et al. 17-Beta-estradiol acts directly on the clonal osteoblastic cell line UMR106. Proc Natl Acad Sci U S A 1987;84: 6267–6271.

37. Bankson DD, Rifai N, Williams ME, et al. Biochemical effects of 17-beta-estradiol on UMR106 cells. Bone Miner 1989;6(1):55–63.

38. Gray TK, Mohan S, Linkhart TA, et al. Estradiol stimulates in vitro the secretion of insulin-like growth factors by the clonal osteoblastic cell line, UMR106. Biochem Biophys Res Commun 1989;158:407–412.

39. Pacifici R, Rifas L, McCracken R, et al. Ovarian steroid treatment blocks a postmenopausal increase in blood monocyte interleukin-1 release. Proc Natl Acad Sci U S A 1989;86:2398–2402.

40. Rizzoli R, Poser J, Burgi U. Nuclear thyroid hormone receptors in cultured bone cells. Metabolism 1986;35:71–74.

41. Aubin JE, Bonnelye E. Osteoprotegerin and its ligand: a new paradigm for regulation of osteoclastogenesis and bone resorption. Osteoporos Int 2000. In press.

42. Vaes G. Cellular biology and biochemical mechanism of bone resorption. A review of recent developments on the formation, activation, and mode of action of osteoclasts. Clin Orthop 1988;231:239–271.

43. Arnett TR, Dempster DW. Effect of pH on bone resorption by rat osteoclasts in vitro. Endocrinology 1986;119:119–124.

44. Miller PD, Baran DT, Bilezikian JP, et al. Practical clinical application of biochemical markers of bone turnover. J Clin Densitometry 1999;2(3):323–342.

45. Murrills RJ, Shane E, Lindsay R, et al. Bone resorption by isolated human osteoclasts in vitro: effects of calcitonin. J Bone Miner Res 1989;4:259–268.

46. Melton LJ III, O'Fallon WM, Riggs BL. Secular trends in the incidence of hip fractures. Calcif Tissue Int 1987;41:57–64.

47. Parfitt AM. The cellular basis of bone remodeling: the quantum concept reexamined in light of recent advances in the cell biology of bone. Calcif Tissue Int 1984;36:S37–S45.

48. Recker RR, Kimmel DB, Parfitt AM, et al. Static and tetracycline-based bone histomorphometric data from 34 normal postmenopausal females. J Bone Miner Res 1988;3:133–144.

49. Auerbach GD, Marx SJ, Spiegel AM. Parathyroid Hormone, Calcitonin, and the Calciferols. In JD Wilson, DW Foster (eds), Williams' Textbook of Endocrinology (7th ed). Philadelphia: WB Saunders, 1985;1137–1217.

50. Heaney RP, Gallagher JC, Johnston CC, et al. Calcium nutrition and bone health in the elderly. Am J Clin Nutr 1982;36:986–1013.

51. Reid IR, Civitelli R, Halstead LR, et al. Parathyroid hormone acutely elevates intracellular calcium in osteoblastlike cells. Am J Physiol 1987;252:E45–E51.

52. Hruska KA, Goligorsky M, Scoble J, et al. Effects of parathyroid hormone on cytosolic calcium in renal proximal tubular primary cultures. Am J Physiol 1986;251:F188–F198.

53. Audran M, Kumar R. The physiology and pathophysiology of vitamin D. Mayo Clin Proc 1985;60:851–866.

54. Haussler MR, Mangelsdorf DJ, Komm BS, et al. Molecular biology of the vitamin D hormone. Recent Prog Horm Res 1988;44:263–305.

55. Talmage RV, Cooper CW, Toverud SU. The Physiological Significance of Calcitonin. In WA Peck (ed), Bone and Mineral Research. Vol 1. Amsterdam: Excerpta Medica, 1983;74–143.

56. Hurley DL, Tiegs RD, Walmer HW, et al. Axial and appendicular bone mineral density in patients with long-term deficiency or excess of calcitonin. N Engl J Med 1987;317:537–541.

57. Bijvojet OLM, Vellenga CJLR, Harinck HIJ. Paget's Disease of Bones: Assessment, Therapy, and Secondary Prevention. In M Kleerekoper, SM Krane (eds), Clinical Disorders of Bone and Mineral Metabolism. New York: Mary Ann Liebert, 1989;525–542.

58. Bilezikian JP. Clinical Disorders of the Parathyroid Glands. In LG Raisz, TJ Martin (eds), Clinical Endocrinology of Calcium Metabolism. New York: Marcel Dekker, 1987;53–97.

59. Labat M, Milhaud G. Osteopetrosis and the Immune Deficiency Syndrome. In WA Peck (ed), Bone and Mineral Research. Vol 4. Amsterdam: Elsevier, 1986;131–212.

60. Ritz E, Drueke T, Merke J, et al. Genesis of Bone Disease in Uremia. In WA Peck (ed), Bone and Mineral Research. Vol 5. Amsterdam: Elsevier, 1987;309–374.

61. Sillence D. Osteogenesis imperfecta: an expanding panorama of variants. Clin Orthop 1981;159:11–25.

62. Marel GM, McKenna MJ, Frame B. Osteomalacia. In WA Peck (ed), Bone and Mineral Research. Vol 4. Amsterdam: Elsevier, 1986;335–412.

63. Consensus development conference: prophylaxis and treatment of osteoporosis. Osteoporos Int 1991; 1:114–117.

64. Consensus development conference: diagnosis, prophylaxis, and treatment of osteoporosis. Am J Med 1993; 94(6):646–650.

65. Mazess RB. On aging bone loss. Clin Orthop 1982;165:239–252.

66. Riggs BL, Walmer HW, Dunn WL, et al. Differential changes in bone mineral density of the appendicular and axial skeleton with aging. Relationship to spinal osteoporosis. J Clin Invest 1981;67:328–335.

67. Cummings SR, Nevitt MC, Browner WS, et al., for the Study of Osteoporotic Fractures Research Group. Risk factors for hip fracture in white women. N Engl J Med 1995;332:767–773.

68. Riggs BL, Melton LJ III. Involutional osteoporosis. N Engl J Med 1986;314:1676–1686.

69. Hui SL, Slemenda CW, Johnston CC Jr. Age and bone mass as predictors of fracture in a prospective study. J Clin Invest 1988;81:1804–1809.

70. Cooper C, Melton LJ. Epidemiology of osteoporosis. Trends Endocrinol Metab 1992;3:224.

71. Kanis JA, McCloskey EV. Epidemiology of vertebral osteoporosis. Bone 1992;13(Suppl 2):S1–S10.

72. Cummings SR, Kelsey JL, Nevitt MC, et al. Epidemiology of osteoporosis and osteoporotic fractures. Epidemiol Rev 1985;7:178–208.

73. Melton LJ III. Epidemiology of Fractures. In BL Riggs, LJ Melton III (eds), Osteoporosis: Etiology, Diagnosis and Management. New York: Raven Press 1988;133–154.

74. Lindsay R, Dempster DW, Clemens T, et al. Incidence, Cost, and Risk Factors of Fracture of the Proximal Femur in the USA. In C Christiansen, CD Arnaud, et al. (eds), Osteoporosis I, Copenhagen International Symposium, Aalborg Srifts bogtrykkeri Copenhagen, Denmark, 1984;311–315.

75. Liel Y, Edwards J, Shary J, et al. The effects of race and body habitus on bone mineral density of the radius, hip, and spine in premenopausal women. J Clin Endocrinol Metab 1988;66:1247–1250.

76. Weinstein RS, Bell NH. Diminished rates of bone formation in normal black adults. N Engl J Med 1988;319:1698–1701.

77. Moller M, Horsman A, Harvald B, et al. Metacarpal morphometry in monozy-

gotic and dizygotic elderly twins. Calcif Tissue Res 1978;25:197–201.

78. Pocock NA, Eisman JA, Hopper JL, et al. Genetic determinants of bone mass in adults. A twin study. J Clin Invest 1987;80:706–710.

79. Dequeker J, Nijs J, Verstracten A, et al. Genetic determinants of bone mineral content at the spine and radius: a twin study. Bone 1987;8:207–209.

80. Seeman E, Hopper JL, Bach LA, et al. Reduced bone mass in daughters of women with osteoporosis. N Engl J Med 1989;320:554–558.

81. Gardsell P, Lindberg H, Obrant KJ. Osteoporosis and heredity. Clin Orthop 1989;240:164–167.

82. Evans RA, Marel GM, Lancaster EK, et al. Bone mass is low in relatives of osteoporotic patients. Ann Intern Med 1988;109:870–873.

83. Beals RK. Orthopedic aspects of the XO (Turner's) syndrome. Clin Orthop 1973;97:19–39.

84. Stepan JJ, Musilova J, Pacovsky V. Bone demineralization, biochemical indices of bone remodeling, and estrogen replacement therapy in adults with Turner's syndrome. J Bone Miner Res 1989;4:193–198.

85. Johnell O, Nilsson BE. Lifestyle and bone mineral mass in perimenopausal women. Calcif Tissue Int 1984;36:354–356.

86. Drinkwater BL, Nilson K, Chesnut CH, et al. Bone mineral content of amenorrheic and eumenorrhic athletes. N Engl J Med 1984;311:277–281.

87. Marcus R, Cann C, Madvig P, et al. Menstrual function and bone mass in elite women distance runners. Ann Intern Med 1985;102:158–163.

88. Rigotti NA, Nussbaum SR, Herzog DB, et al. Osteoporosis in women with anorexia nervosa. N Engl J Med 1984;311:1601–1606.

89. Biller BMK, Saxe V, Herzog DB, et al. Mechanisms of osteoporosis in adult and adolescent women with anorexia nervosa. J Clin Endocrinol Metab 1989;68:548–554.

90. Klibanski A, Greenspan SL. Increase in bone mass after treatment of hyperprolactinemic amenorrhea. N Engl J Med 1986;315:542–546.

91. Schlechte J, El-khoury G, Kathol M, et al. Forearm and vertebral bone mineral in treated and untreated hyperprolactinemic amenorrhea. J Clin Endocrinol Metab 1987;64:1021–1026.

92. Kleerekoper M, Tolia K, Parfitt AM. Nutritional, endocrine, and demographic aspects of osteoporosis. Orthop Clin North Am 1981;12:547–559.

93. Matkovic V, Kostial K, Simonovic I, et al. Bone status and fracture rates in two regions of Yugoslavia. Am J Clin Nutr 1979;32:540–549.

94. Cauley JA, Gutai JP, Kuller LH, et al. Endogenous estrogen levels and calcium intakes in postmenopausal women. Relationships with cortical bone measures. JAMA 1988;260:3150–3155.

95. Halioua L, Anderson JJB. Lifetime calcium intake and physical activity habits: independent and combined effects on the radial bone of healthy premenopausal Caucasian women. Am J Clin Nutr 1989;49:534–541.

96. Murphy S, Khaw KT, May H, Compston JE. Milk consumption and bone mineral density in middle aged and elderly women. BMJ 1994;308:939–941.

97. Sandler RB, Slemenda C, LaPorte RE, et al. Postmenopausal bone density and milk consumption in childhood and adolescence. Am J Clin Nutr 1985;42:270–274.

98. Soroko S, Holbrook TL, Edelstein S, Barrett-Connor E. Lifetime milk consumption and bone mineral density in older women. Am J Public Health 1994;84:1319–1322.

99. Welton DC, Kemper HCG, Post GB, Van Staveren WA. A meta-analysis of the effect of calcium intake on bone mass in young and middle aged females and males. J Nutr 1995;125:2802.

100. Kanders B, Dempster DW, Lindsay R. Interaction of calcium nutrition and physical activity on bone mass in young women. J Bone Miner Res 1988;3:145–149.

101. Aloia JF, Vaswani AN, Yeh JK, et al. Premenopausal bone mass is related to physical activity. Arch Intern Med 1988;148:121–123.

102. Block JE, Genant HK, Black D. Greater vertebral bone mineral mass in exercising young men. West J Med 1986;145:39–42.

103. Dalen N, Olsson KE. Bone mineral content and physical activity. Acta Orthop Scand 1974;45:170–174.

104. Nilsson BE, Westlin NE. Bone density in athletes. Clin Orthop 1971;77:179–182.

105. Nilsson BE, Andersson SM, Havdrup T, et al. Ballet dancing and weight lifting effects on BMC [Abstract]. AJR 1978;131:541–542.

106. Snow-Harter C, Marcus R. Exercise, bone mineral density, and osteoporosis. Exercise Sport Sci Rev 1991;19:351–388.

107. Steinberg FU. The Effects of Immobilization on Bone. In FU Steinberg (ed), The Immobilized Patient: Functional Pathology and Management. New York: Plenum, 1980;33–64.

108. Krolner B, Nielsen SP. Bone mineral content of the lumbar spine in normal and osteoporotic women: cross-sectional and longitudinal studies. Clin Sci 1982;62:329–336.

109. Meunier P, Courpron P, Edouard C, et al. Physiological senile involution and pathological rare-faction of bone. Quantitative and comparative histological data. Clin Endocrinol Metab 1973;2:239–256.

110. Genant HK, Cann CE, Ettinger B, et al. Quantitative computed tomography of vertebral spongiosa: a sensitive method for detecting early bone loss after oophorectomy. Ann Intern Med 1982;97:699–705.

111. Johnston CC, Hui SL, Witt RM, et al. Early menopausal changes in bone mass and sex steroids. J Clin Endocrinol Metab 1985;61:905–911.

112. Lindsay R. Sex steroids in the pathogenesis and prevention of osteoporosis. In BL Riggs, LJ Melton III (eds), Osteoporosis: Etiology, Diagnosis and Management. New York: Raven Press, 1988;333–358.

113. Aitken JM, Hart DM, Anderson JB, et al. Osteoporosis after oophorectomy for non-malignant disease in premenopausal women. BMJ 1973;i:325–328.

114. Richelson LS, Wahlner HW, Melton LJ III, et al. Relative contributions of aging and estrogen deficiency to postmenopausal bone loss. N Engl J Med 1984;311:1273–1275.

115. Nilas L, Christiansen C. Bone mass and its relationship to age and the menopause. J Clin Endocrinol Metab 1987;65:697–702.

116. Parfitt AM. Trabecular bone architecture in the pathogenesis and prevention of fracture. Am J Med 1987;82(Suppl B):68–72.

117. Eriksen EF, Mosekilde L, Melsen F. Trabecular bone resorption depth decreases with age: differences between normal males and females. Bone 1985;6:141–146.

118. Heaney RP. Osteoporotic fracture space: an hypothesis. Bone Miner 1989;6:1–13.

119. Kleerekoper M, Villanueva AR, Stanciu J, et al. The role of three-dimensional trabecular microstructure in the pathogenesis of vertebral compression fractures. Calcif Tissue Int 1985;37:594–597.

120. Dempster DW, Shane E, Horbert W, et al. A simple method for correlative

light and scanning electron microscopy of human iliac crest bone biopsies: qualitative observations in normal and osteoporotic subjects. J Bone Miner Res 1986;1:15–21.

121. Heaney RP, Recker RR, Saville PD. Calcium balance and calcium requirements in middle-aged women. Am J Clin Nutr 1977;30:1603–1611.

122. Heaney RP, Recker RR, Saville PD. Menopausal changes in calcium balance performance. J Lab Clin Med 1978;92:953–963.

123. Heaney RP, Recker RR, Saville PD. Menopausal changes in bone remodeling. J Lab Clin Med 1978;92:964–970.

124. Mundy GR, Boyce BF, Yoneda T, et al. Cytokines and Bone Remodeling. In R Marcus, D Feldman, J Kelsey (eds), Osteoporosis. San Diego, CA: Academic Press Publishers, 1986;477–482.

125. Horowitz MC. Cytokines and estrogen in bone: anti-osteoporotic effects. Science 1993;260:626–627.

126. Girasole G, Jilka RL, Passeri G, et al. 17 beta-estradiol inhibits interleukin-6 production by bone marrow derived stromal cells and osteoblasts in vitro: a potential mechanism for the antiosteoporotic effect of estrogens. J Clin Invest 1992;89:883–891.

127. Cheleuitte D, Mizuno S, Glowacki J. In vitro secretion of cytokines by human bone marrow: effects of age and estrogen status. J Clin Endocrinol Metab 1998;83:2043–2051.

128. Cohen-Solal ME, Boitte F, Bernard-Poenaru O, et al. Increased bone resorbing activity of peripheral monocyte culture supernatants in elderly women. J Clin Endocrinol Metab 1998;83:1687–1690.

129. Chen MM, Yeh JK, Aloia JF. Anabolic effect of prostaglandin E_2 in bone is not dependent on pituitary hormones in rats. Calcif Tissue Int 1998;63:236–242.

130. Kodama Y, Takeuchi Y, Suzawa M, et al. Reduced expression of interleukin-11 in bone marrow stroma cells of senescence-accelerated mice (SAMP6): relationship to osteopenia with enhanced adipogenesis. J Bone Miner Res 1998;13:1370–1377.

131. Shimizu T, Mehdi R, Yoshimura Y, et al. Sequential expression of bone morphogenetic protein, tumor necrosis factor, and their receptors in bone-forming reaction after mouse femoral marrow ablation. Bone 1998;23:127–133.

132. Raisz LG. Local and systemic factors in the pathogenesis of osteoporosis. N Engl J Med 1988;318(13):818–828.

133. Pacifici R, Rifas L, Teitelbaum S, et al. Spontaneous release of interleukin 1 from human blood monocytes reflects bone formation in idiopathic osteoporosis. Proc Natl Acad Sci U S A 1987;84:4616–4620.

134. Pacifici R, Brown C, Puscheck E, et al. Effect of surgical menopause and estrogen replacement on cytokine release from human blood mononuclear cells. Proc Natl Acad Sci U S A 1991;88:5134–5138.

135. Gowen M, Wood DD, Ihrie EJ, et al. An interleukin-1 like factor stimulates bone resorption in vitro. Nature 1989;306:378–380.

136. Stock JL, Coderre JA, MacDonald B, Rosenwasser LJ. Effects of estrogen in vivo and in vitro on spontaneous interleukin-1 release by monocytes from postmenopausal women. J Clin Endocrinol Metab 1989;68(2):364–368.

137. Jilka RL, Hangoe G, Girasole G. Increased osteoclast development after estrogen loss: mediation by interleukin-6. Science 1992;257:88–91.

138. Matsuzaki K, Udagawa N, Takahashi N, et al. Biochem Biophys Res Commun 1998;246:199–204.

139. Mizuno A, Amizuka N, Irie K, et al. Severe osteoporosis in mice lacking osteoclastogenesis inhibitory factor/osteoprotegerin. Biochem Biophys Res Commun 1998;247:610–615.

140. Yasuda H, Shima N, Nakagawa N, et al. Proc Natl Acad Sci U S A 1998;95:3597–3602.

141. Nordin BEC, Need AG, Morris HA, et al. Evidence for a renal calcium leak in postmenopausal women. J Clin Endocrinol Metab 1991;72(2):401–407.

142. Heaney RP. A unified concept of osteoporosis. Am J Med 1965;39:377–380.

143. Gallagher JC, Riggs BL, Jerpbak CM, et al. The effect of age on serum immunoreactive parathyroid hormone in normal and osteoporotic women. J Lab Clin Med 1980;95:373–385.

144. Eastell R, Riggs BL. Diagnostic evaluation of osteoporosis. Endocrinol Metab Clin North Am 1988;17:547–571.

145. Reid IR. Pathogenesis and treatment of steroid osteoporosis. Clin Endocrinol (Oxf)1989;30:83–103.

146. Seeman E, Walmer HW, Offord KP, et al. Differential effects of endocrine dysfunction on the axial and the appendicular skeleton. J Clin Invest 1982;69:1302–1309.

147. Hui SL, Epstein S, Johnston CC Jr. A prospective study of bone mass in patients with type I diabetes. J Clin Endocrinol Metab 1985;60:74–80.

148. Devogelaer JP, Crabbe J, De Deuxchaisnes CN. Bone mineral density in Addison's disease: evidence for an effect of adrenal androgens on bone mass. Br Med J 1987;294:798–800.

149. Seeman E, Melton LJ III, O'Fallon WM, et al. Risk factors for spinal osteoporosis in men. Am J Med 1983;75:977–983.

150. Daniell HW. Osteoporosis of the slender smoker: vertebral compression fractures and loss of metacarpal cortex in relation to postmenopausal cigarette smoking and lack of obesity. Arch Intern Med 1976;136:298–304.

151. De Vernejoul MC, Bielakoff J, Herve M, et al. Evidence for defective osteoblastic function: a role for alcohol and tobacco consumption in osteoporosis in middle-aged men. Clin Orthop 1983;179:107–115.

152. Jensen J, Christiansen C, Rodbro P. Cigarette smoking, serum estrogens, and bone loss during hormone-replacement therapy early after menopause. N Engl J Med 1985;313:973–975.

153. Crilly RG, Anderson C, Hogan D, et al. Bone histomorphometry, bone mass, and related parameters in alcoholic males. Calcif Tissue Int 1988;43:269–276.

154. Diamond T, Stiel D, Lunzer M, et al. Ethanol reduces bone formation and may cause osteoporosis. Am J Med 1989;86:282–288.

155. Ettinger B, Winger J. Thyroid supplements: effect on bone mass. West J Med 1982;136:472–476.

156. Fallon MD, Perry HM, Bergfeld M, et al. Exogenous hyperthyroidism with osteoporosis. Arch Intern Med 1983;143:442–444.

157. Hahn TJ. Drug-induced disorders of vitamin D and mineral metabolism. Clin Endocrinol Metab 1980;9:107–129.

158. Melton LJ III, Riggs BL. Clinical Spectrum. In BL Riggs, LJ Melton III (eds), Osteoporosis: Etiology, Diagnosis, and Management. New York: Raven Press, 1988;155–260.

159. Mazanec DJ, Grisanti JM. Drug-induced osteoporosis. Cleve Clin J Med 1989;56:297–303.

160. Nordin BEC. Calcium and osteoporosis. Nutrition 1997;13:664–686.

161. Reid IR, Ames RW, Evans MC, et al. Long-term effects of calcium supplementation on bone loss and fractures in postmenopausal women: a randomized controlled trial. Am J Med 1995; 98(4):331–335.

162. Chevalley T, Rizzoli R. Nydegger V, et

al. Effects of calcium supplements on femoral bone mineral density and vertebral fracture rate in vitamin-D-replete elderly patients. Osteoporosis Int 1994;4(5):245–252.

163. Dawson-Hughes B, Harris SS, Krall EA, et al. Effect of calcium and vitamin D supplementation on bone density in men and women 65 years of age or older. N Engl J Med 1997;337(10):670–676.

164. Chapuy MC, Arlot ME, Duboeuf F, et al. Vitamin D3 and calcium to prevent hip fractures in the elderly women. N Engl J Med 1992;327(23):1637–1642.

165. Heaney RP, Recker RR. Effects of nitrogen, phosphorus, and caffeine on calcium balance in women. J Lab Clin Med 1982;99:46–55.

166. Parfitt AM. Dietary risk factors for age-related bone loss and fractures. Lancet 1983;2:1181–1185.

167. Ruff CB, Hayes WC. Subperiosteal expansion and cortical remodeling of the human femur and tibia with aging. Science 1982;217:945–948.

168. Zagba-Mongalima G, Goret-Nicaise M, Dhem A. Age changes in human bone: a microradiographic and histological study of subperiosteal and periosteal calcifications. Gerontology 1988;34:264–276.

169. Tinetti ME, Speechley M. Prevention of falls among the elderly. N Engl J Med 1989;320:1055–1059.

170. Resnick NM, Greenspan SL. Senile osteoporosis reconsidered. JAMA 1989;261:1025–1029.

171. Baran DT, Faulkner KG, Genant HK, et al. Diagnosis and management of osteoporosis: guidelines for the utilization of bone densitometry. Calcif Tissue Int 1997;61:433–440.

172. O'Brant KJ, Bengner U, Johnell O, et al. Increasing age-adjusted risk of fragility fractures: a sign of increasing osteoporosis in successive generations? Calcif Tissue Int 1989;44:157–167.

173. Melton LJ III, Atkinson EJ, O'Fallon WM, et al. Long-term fracture prediction of bone mineral assessed at different sites. J Bone Miner Res 1993;10:1227–1233.

174. Washnich RD, Ross PD, Heilbrun LK, Vogel JM. Prediction of postmenopausal fracture risk with use of bone mineral measurements. Am J Obstet Gynecol 1985;153:745–751.

175. Nevitt MC, Johnell O, Black DM, et al., for the Study of Osteoporotic Fractures Research Group. Bone mineral density predicts non-spine fractures in very elderly women. Osteoporos Int 1994;4:325–331.

176. Gardsell P, Johnell O, Nilsson BE. Predicting fractures in women by using forearm bone densitometry. Calcif Tissue Int 1989;44:235–242.

177. Hui SL, Slemenda CW, Johnston CC. Baseline measurements of bone mass predict fracture in white women. Ann Intern Med 1989;111:355–361.

178. Garnero P, Hausherr E, Chapuy MC, et al. Markers of bone resorption predict hip fracture in elderly women: the EPIDOS prospective study. J Bone Miner Res 1996;11:1531–1538.

179. Van Daele PLA, Seibel MJ, Burger H, et al. Case-control analysis of bone resorption markers, disability, and hip fracture risk: the Rotterdam study. Br Med J 1996;312:482–483.

180. Akesson K, Ljunghall S, Jonsson B, et al. Assessment of biochemical markers of bone metabolism in relation to the occurrence of fracture: a retrospective and prospective population-based study of women. J Bone Miner Res 1995;10:1823–1829.

181. Ross PD, Wasnich RD, Knowlton WK. Skeletal alkaline phosphatase (Tandem©-R Ostase©) measurements predict vertebral fractures: a prospective study [Abstract]. J Bone Miner Res 1997;12(Suppl 1):SS150.

182. Delmas PD. The role of markers of bone turnover in the assessment of fracture risk in postmenopausal women. Osteoporosis Int 1998;8(Suppl 1):S32–S36.

183. Nagant de Deuxchaisnes C. Calcitonin in the treatment of Paget's disease. Triangle 1983;22:103–128.

184. Graf E, Holser E, Chayen R, et al. Cortisol and endorphin increase produced by calcitonin administration. Isr J Med Sci 1985;21:483–484.

185. Fiore CE, Castorina F, Malatino LS, et al. Antalgic activity of calcitonin: effectiveness of the epidermal and subarachnoid routes in man. Br J Clin Pharmacol Res 1983;3:257–260.

186. Jensen ME, Evans AJ, Mathis JM, et al. Percutaneous polymethylmethacrylate vertebroplasty in the treatment of osteoporotic vertebral body compression fractures: technical aspects. AJNR 1997;18:1897–1904.

187. Aloia JF, Cohn SH, Ostuni JA, et al. Prevention of involutional bone loss by exercise. Ann Intern Med 1978;89:356–358.

188. Dalsky GP, Stocke KS, Ehsani AA, et al. Weight-bearing exercise training and lumbar bone mineral content in very elderly women. Ann Intern Med 1988;108:824–828.

189. Chow R, Harrison JE, Notarius C. Effect of two randomized exercise programmes on bone mass of healthy postmenopausal women. Br Med J 1987;295:1441–1444.

190. Smith EL, Gilligan C, McAdam M, et al. Deterring bone loss by exercise intervention in premenopausal and postmenopausal women. Calcif Tissue Int 1989;44:312–321.

191. Black-Sandler R, Cauley JA, Hom DL, et al. The effects of walking on the cross-sectional dimensions of the radius in postmenopausal women. Calcif Tissue Int 1987;41:65–69.

192. Cavanaugh DJ, Cann CE. Brisk walking does not stop bone loss in postmenopausal women. Bone 1988;9:201–204.

193. Sinaki M, McPhee MC, Hodgson SF, et al. Relationship between bone mineral density of spine and strength of back extensors in healthy postmenopausal women. Mayo Clin Proc 1986;61:116–122.

194. Sinaki M, Grubbs NC. Back-strengthening exercises: quantitative evaluation of their efficacy for women aged 40 to 65 years. Arch Phys Med Rehabil 1989;70:16–20.

195. Huddleston AL, Rockwell D, Kulund DN. Bone mass in lifetime tennis athletes. JAMA 1980;244:1107–1109.

196. MacKinnon JL. Osteoporosis. A review. Phys Ther 1988;68:1533–1540.

197. Krolner B, Toft B, Nielsen SP, et al. Physical exercise as prophylaxis against involutional vertebral bone loss: a controlled trial. Clin Sci 1983;64:541–546.

198. Sinaki M, Mikkelsen BA. Postmenopausal spinal osteoporosis: flexion versus extension exercises. Arch Phys Med Rehabil 1984;65:593–596.

199. Simkin A, Ayalon J, Leichter I. Increased trabecular bone density due to bone-loading exercises in postmenopausal osteoporotic women. Calcif Tissue Int 1987;40:59–63.

200. Linsday R. Estrogen and Osteoporosis. In JC Stevenson, R Lindsay (eds), Osteoporosis. London: Chapman & Hall, 1998.

201. Writing Group for the PEPI. Effects of hormone therapy on bone mineral density: results from the postmenopausal estrogen/progestin interventions (PEPI). JAMA 1996;276(17):1389–1396.

202. Nachtigall LE, Nachtigall RH, Nachtigall RD, Beckman EM. Estrogen

replacement therapy I: a 10-year prospective study in the relationship to osteoporosis. Obstet Gynecol 1979;53:277–281.

203. Lindsay R, Hart DM, Forrest C, Baird C. Prevention of spinal osteoporosis in oophorectomised women. Lancet 1980;2:1151–1154.

204. Lufkin EG, Wahner HW, O'Fallon WM, et al. Treatment of postmenopausal osteoporosis with transdermal estrogen. Ann Intern Med 1992; 117:1–9.

205. Komulainen MH, Kroger H, Tuppurainen MT, et al. HRT and Vit D in prevention of non-vertebral fractures in postmenopausal women: a 5-year randomized trial. Maturitas 1998; 31:45–54.

206. Cauley JA, Seeley DG, Ensrud K, et al., for the Study of Osteoporotic Fractures Research Group. Estrogen replacement therapy and fractures in older women. Ann Intern Med 1995;122:9–16.

207. Greenspan SL, Bell N, Bone H, et al. Differential effects of alendronate and estrogen on the rate of bone loss after discontinuation of treatment. J Bone and Miner Res 1999;14:S160.

208. Haskell SG, Richardson ED, Horwitz RI. The effect of estrogen replacement therapy on cognitive function in women: a critical review of the literature. J Clin Epidemiol 1997;50:1249–1264.

209. Hulley S, Grady D, Bush T, et al., for the Heart and Estrogen/progestin Replacement Study (HERS) Research Group. Randomized trial of estrogen plus progestin for secondary prevention of coronary heart disease in postmenopausal women. JAMA 1998; 280:605–613.

210. The Collaborative Group on Hormonal Factors in Breast Cancer. Breast cancer and hormone replacement therapy: collaborative reanalysis of data from 51 epidemiological studies of 52705 women with breast cancer and 108411 women without breast cancer. Lancet 1997;350:1047–1059.

211. Powles TJ, Hickish T, Kanis JA, et al. Effect of tamoxifen on bone mineral density measured by dual energy x-ray absorptiometry in healthy premenopausal and postmenopausal women. J Clin Oncol 1996;14:78–84.

212. Love RR, Mazess RB, Barden HS, et al. Effects of tamoxifen on bone mineral density in postmenopausal women with breast cancer. N Engl J Med 1992;326;852–856.

213. Fisher B, Costantino, JP, Wickerham DL, et al. Tamoxifen for prevention of breast cancer: report of the National Surgical Adjuvant Breast and Bowel Project P-1 Study. J Natl Can Inst 1998;90:1371–1388.

214. Cosman F, Lindsay R. Selective estrogen receptors modulators: clinical spectrum. Endocr Rev 1999;20(3):418–434.

215. Ettinger B, Black DM, Mitlak BH, et al., for the Multiple Outcomes of Raloxifene Evaluation (MORE) Investigators. Reduction of verterbral fracture risk in postmenpausal women with osteoporosis treated with raloxifene: results from a 3-year randomized clinical trial. JAMA 1999;282(7):637–645.

216. Cummings SR, Eckert S, Krueger KA, et al. The effect of raloxifene on risk of breast cancer in postmenopausal women: results from the MORE randomized trial. JAMA 1999;281(23): 2189–2197.

217. Liberman UA, Weiss SR, Broll J, et al., for the Alendronate Phase III Osteoporosis Treatment Study Group. Effect of oral alendronate on bone mineral density and the incidence of fractures in postmenopausal osteoporosis. N Eng J Med 1995;333(22):1437–1443.

218. Black D, Cummings S, Karpf D, et al., for the Fracture Intervention Trial Research Group. Randomised trial of effect of alendronate on risk of fracture in women with existing vertebral fractures. Lancet 1996;348(9041):1535–1541.

219. Pols HAP, Felsenberg D, Hanley DA, et al., for the Fosamax International Trial Study Group. Multinational, placebo-controlled, randomized trial of the effects of alendronate on bone density and fracture risk in postmenopausal women with low bone mass: results of the FOSIT study. Osteoporos Int 1999;9(5):461–468.

220. Harris ST, Watts NB, Genant HK, et al., for the Vertebral Efficacy with Risedronate Therapy (VERT) Study Group. Effects of risedronate treatment on vertebral and nonvertebral fractures in women with postmenopausal osteoporosis: a randomized controlled trial. JAMA 1999;282(14):1344–1352.

221. Reginster J-Y, Minne HW, Sorenson OH, et al. Randomized trials of the effects of risedronate on vertebral fractures in women with established postmenopausal osteoporosis. Osteoporos Int 2000;11(1):83–91.

222. McClung M, Easteli R, Bensen W, et al. Risedronate reduces hip fracture risk in elderly women with osteoporosis. Osteoporosis Int 2000;11(2) abstract 559:S207.

223. Overgaard K, Riis BJ, Christiansen C. Effect of calcitonin given intranasally on early postmenopausal bone loss. Br Med J 1989;299:477–479.

224. Overgaard K, Hansen MA, Jensen SB, et al. Effect of calcitonin given intranasally on bone mass and fracture rates in a dose response study. BMJ 1992; 305:556–561.

225. Ellerington HC, Hillard TC, and Whitcroft SI. Intranasal salmon calcitonin for the prevention and treatment of postmenopausal osteoporosis. Calcif Tissue Int 1996;59(1):6–11.

226. Silverman SL, Moniz C, Andriano K, et al. Salmon-calcitonin nasal spray prevents vertebral fractures in established osteoporosis. Final worldwide results of the PROOF study. 26th European Symposium on Calcified Tissue, Maastricht, the Netherlands; May 7-11, 1999. [Abstract]:0–26ccc.

227. Lindsay R, Nieves J, Formica C, et al. Randomized controlled study of effect of parathyroid hormone on vertebral-bone mass and fracture incidence among postmenopausal women on estrogen with osteoporosis. Lancet 1997;350:550–555.

228. Finkelstein JS, Klibanski A, Schaefer EH, et al. Parathyroid hormone for the prevention of bone loss induced by estrogen deficiency. N Engl J Med 1994;331:1618–1623.

229. Roe EB, Sanchez SD, del Puerto GA, et al. Parathyroid hormone 1-34 (hPTH 1-34) and estrogen produce dramatic bone density increases in postmenopausal osteoporosis: results from a placebo-controlled randomized trial. J Bone Miner Res 1999;14(abstract 1019)(Suppl 1):pS137.

230. Hodsman AB, Fraher LJ, Ostbye T, et al. An evaluation of several biochemical markers for bone formation and resorption on a protocol utilizing cyclical parathyroid hormone and calcitonin therapy for osteoporosis. J Clin Invest 1993;91:1138–1148.

231. Neer RM, Arnaud C, Zanchetta JR, et al. Recombinant human PTH [rhPTH(1–34)] reduces the risk of spine and non-spine fractures in postmenopausal osteoporosis. Proc 87th Annual Meeting of the Endocrine Society, June 21–24, 2000, Toronto:42(Abstract).

232. Pak CY, Sakhaee K, Adams-Huet B, et al. Treatment of postmenopausal osteoporosis with slow release sodium fluoride. Ann Intern Med 1995;123:401–408.

8

Physiology of Synovial Joints and Articular Cartilage

VAN C. MOW AND MATTHEW T. SUGALSKI

Joints are functional connections between adjoining bones of the skeleton. Three types of joints are found in the human body; the type created during embryogenesis depends on the function they must perform (i.e., the amount of relative motion they must allow and the load they must bear).[1] Diarthrodial or synovial joints, such as elbows, hips, knees, and shoulders, are capable of large range of motion achieved through a combination of rolling and sliding of one articulating surface relative to the other.[2] Synarthroses or fibrous joints, such as the coronal sutures, allow no relative motion. Amphiarthroses or cartilaginous joints, such as the intervertebral disk and symphysis pubis, provide some motion for the required flexibility, but no rolling or sliding relative motion occurs.

Of these three types of joints, diarthrodial joints present many common clinical problems in orthopedics and rehabilitation, and they have been the most thoroughly studied.[3] The primary function of diarthrodial joints is to facilitate the movement of body segments in manipulation and locomotion. All body movements and activities of daily function involve to varying degrees motion of these diarthrodial joints. Under normal physiological conditions, these joints provide efficient bearing systems with excellent engineering characteristics such as friction, lubrication, and wear properties. Under normal conditions, these joints undergo little deterioration throughout an individual's life.[2-5] As it often occurs during dissection of cadaveric hip, knee, or shoulder specimens as old as 90 years of age, no discernible degenerative changes on the articular cartilage, or osteophytes, are observable by the naked eye. This is all the more remarkable when one considers that for the lower extremities, the knee, hip, and ankle must be able to withstand loads of up to six times body weight on a repetitive basis, for up to a million cycles per year,

depending on the specific joint and function.[6-8] However, for a large percentage of the elderly, 65 years or more, degenerative joint disease and osteoarthritis (OA) do occur with characteristic fibrillations over much of the joint surface (usually these lesions start at the high load-bearing areas of articular cartilage surface) followed by a total loss of articular cartilage and bony eburnation, osteophyte formation at the joint periphery, and other bony deformities.[9,10] These changes are usually accompanied by neuromuscular deficiencies that, together with the structural, material, and biological changes occurring within the joint, totally compromise the physiological function of diarthrodial joints resulting in severe limitations in joint function and pain, which impairs the quality of life of the afflicted individual.[9-11]

Adult articular cartilage is the avascular and aneural dense tissue that covers the articulating ends of bones. In the joint, the cartilage serves as the primary load-bearing material of joints, with excellent friction, lubrication, and wear characteristics (Figure 8-1).[2-5] Most OA changes begin with focal lesions on the cartilage surface, eventually leading to complete breakdown and to OA.[9,10] Because this tissue plays a unique role in the function of diarthrodial joints, researchers have made great efforts to understand its biology, molecular structure, biochemistry, and biomechanical properties.[10-15]

Disease and dysfunction of diarthrodial joints, such as in OA and rheumatoid arthritis, are initiated by the destruction of articular cartilage and bony changes such as osteophyte formation.[9-11] OA is a common problem of the aging (e.g., it afflicts more than 50% of women older than 65 years of age).[10] When the joint is considered as an organ, the OA process involves a cascade of metabolic, biochemical, enzymatic, and biomechanical abnormalities. Because the OA process appears to start

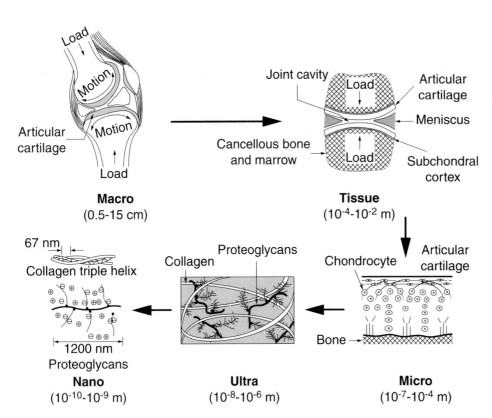

FIGURE 8-1 Important hierarchical structural features in diarthrodial joints starting with collagen and proteoglycan molecules at the nano scale (10^{-10}–10^{-9} m), ultra scale (10^{-8}–10^{-6} m), micro scale (10^{-7}–10^{-4} m), tissue scale (10^{-4}–10^{-2} m), and gross anatomic scale (10^{-3}–10^{-1} m). In diarthrodial joints, articular cartilage serves as the primary load-bearing material of joints, with excellent friction, lubrication, and wear characteristics. (Reprinted with permission from VC Mow, WC Hayes [eds], Basic Orthopaedic Biomechanics. Philadelphia: Lippincott–Raven, 1997.)

with minute lesions on the articular cartilage surface, and once begun, inexorably progresses to frank cartilage degeneration, knowledge of the biochemical and biomechanical properties of articular cartilage is central to understanding the physiology and pathophysiology of diarthrodial joints.[9–11]

In this chapter, we discuss the gross anatomy and ultrastructure of diarthrodial joints and articular cartilage, followed by a more detailed discussion of the mechanical properties of normal and OA articular cartilage. The biochemical and biomechanical response of cartilage in several well-known clinical settings, exercise, immobilization, aging, and OA, are also presented. We conclude with a brief discussion on the pathogenesis of OA. This information will help to provide a valid rationale for the rehabilitation of joints affected by degenerative disease.

JOINT STRUCTURES AND ANATOMY

Two components are common to all diarthrodial joints: synovial fluid and soft connective tissues (see Figure 8-1). The synovial fluid is a concentrated biomacromolecular solution of blood plasma and hyaluronic acid.[2–5] The soft connective tissues include articular car-

tilage, capsule, menisci, and ligaments.[1,13,16] Abnormalities in any of these articular structures can lead to significant pain and loss of joint function.

Synovium

The synovial membrane covers the inner surface of the fibrous capsule of the joint, forming a closed sac called the *synovial cavity* (see Figure 8-1, top left).[1] It is composed of loose connective tissue on which the densely packed surface cells are arranged in an epithelium-like fashion. These synovial lining cells secrete the synovial fluid and nutrients, and absorb the metabolic wastes produced by the chondrocytes and by other soft tissues inside the joint (e.g., ligaments, menisci, labrum). During OA, particularly at the later stages, swelling and pain in the joint result from excessive secretion and inflammation of the thickened synovium.[9,10]

Synovial Fluid

Synovial fluid is a clear, colorless, or slightly yellow liquid that resides in the joint cavity (see Figure 8-1, top right) and for most joints its volume is small.[1,2,17,18] In most joints it measures just 0.2 ml, but for large joints such as the knee, hip, or shoulder it may range up to 5 ml.[17] Under normal conditions, the synovial cavity contains just enough fluid to moisten and lubricate the articular and synovial surfaces with a film layer of approximately 15 μm thick,[4] but in an injured or inflamed joint, the fluid may accumulate in painful amounts.[9,10,17] Biochemically, synovial fluid is a transudate of blood plasma that contains a hyaluronic acid protein complex with a molecular weight of approximately $(0.5-1.0) \times 10^6$ dalton.[18] The presence of this biomacromolecule gives synovial fluid its non-newtonian and viscoelastic flow properties (e.g., the viscosity of the fluid decreases as the rate of shearing increases, and a normal stress effect).[19,20] These flow behaviors play important roles in joint lubrication[4,19] and protect the cartilage from frictional wear.[5,21-23] Synovial fluid samples obtained from osteoarthritic joints show that many of the non-newtonian and viscoelastic properties, and presumably their lubrication and wear protection properties, are diminished; this is even more so for synovial fluids obtained from rheumatoid joints.[4,17-20]

The synovial fluid, secreted by the synovium, is also the conduit for the nutrients necessary for the nourishment of the avascular articular cartilage (see Figure 8-1, top two figures). At skeletal maturation, the physis is closed, and an impermeable calcified cartilage layer is formed separating the vascular marrow space and the uncalcified articular cartilage. Thus, in adult articular cartilage, chondrocytes receive their nutrients only via the synovial fluid route across the articular surface; this route is also the avenue by which the toxic metabolic waste products are carried away from the tissue. Low-molecular-weight solutes, such as glucose, appear to be readily transported through articular cartilage by diffusion and fluid convection; the latter transport mechanism occurs because interstitial fluid flow always accompanies joint motion and loading that results in cartilage deformation.[4,12,13] The transport mechanism of the larger molecules, such as serum albumin, is less clear.[24] It is believed that molecules with molecular weight greater than 20,000 are filtered out by the dense collagen-proteoglycan (PG) networks of articular cartilage.[24,25] However, a new theory has been proposed that suggests that large biomolecules may indeed penetrate the tissue.[26] The proposed rapid macromolecular transport mechanism uses an enhanced concentration buildup across the molecule-size interstices and the entropy of mixing to drive the solute through the microscopic pores.[26]

Articular Cartilage

Anatomic Form

The thickness of the articular cartilage layer and its variation over the joint surface have been of interest to many researchers for decades, including anatomists, bioengineers, biologists, microscopists, orthopedists, pathologists, physical anthropologists, and other interested individuals. However, until relatively recently there were no measuring tools of significant accuracy or methods of analysis available to fully characterize an entire joint surface. With the advent of new and accurate stereophotogrammetry, computed tomography, magnetic resonance imaging, and computer graphics technology, a complete characterization of articular cartilage surface topography and thickness maps have become available.[27-31] In general, under normal physiological conditions, for the smaller joints (wrist, fingers, toes, and facet joints of the spine), articular cartilage is usually within the range of 0.5-1.5 mm thick; for the elbow, hip, and shoulder it is usually within the range of 1.0-2.5 mm; and for the patella, trochlea of the distal femur, and tibial plateau it may be as thick as 7.0 mm. Fine differences in the thickness within these ranges vary with regions of loading, with those habitually loaded being slightly thicker than the less frequently loaded regions.

The shoulder and hip are nearly spherical joints with closely matching radii of curvature between the two mating surfaces.[8,29] The patellar and distal femoral surfaces are quite complex and difficult to describe by simple geometric forms, with many regions of sharp contours (Figure 8-2).[27-30] Nevertheless, the patellofemoral articulation is still quite congruent in the coronal plane to maintain necessary medial-lateral knee stability. But in the sagittal plane, this articulation is altogether incongruent to permit free sliding motion of the patella relative to the femoral trochlea to facilitate knee flexion.[31] The shapes of the distal femoral condyles are best described as geometric involutes of revolution that allow rolling and sliding to occur at the tibiofemoral articulation, producing a complex motion not at all resembling a hinge.[31] The carpal joints of the wrist are smooth and confluent, but the trapeziocarpal joint of the thumb is a saddle-shaped joint and may not become incongruent when the thumb is in pronation; the saddle shape articulation permits a near universal range of motion at the base of the thumb.[32] (For more details on knee geometry and knee motion, please see references 27-30.)

FUNCTION AND LOAD SUPPORT

During locomotion and other activities of daily living, forces of significant magnitude are generated across the articulating surfaces, by virtue of the high muscular forces required to overcome the large moments (because of the long lever arms) of the functional loads.[2,6-8,33-37]

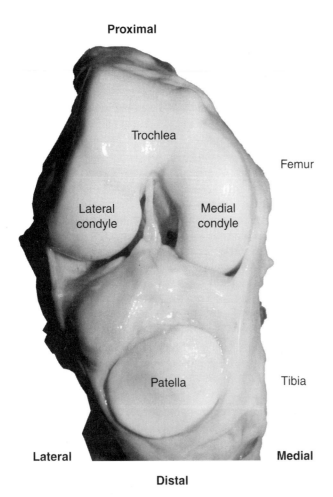

Proximal

Trochlea

Femur

Lateral
condyle

Medial
condyle

Patella

Tibia

Lateral

Medial

Distal

FIGURE 8-2 The patellar and distal femoral surface of a normal human knee joint. They form complex articulating surfaces that are difficult to describe by simple geometric forms. Contrary to visual appearances, mathematical analysis shows that there are many regions of sharp contours.[28,29]

These joint reaction forces are transmitted across limited contact areas, which therefore develop high compressive contact stresses, ranging from 0.5–1.0 MPa* in the fingers and carpal joints,[33,34] 1.0–2.5 MPa in the shoulder and elbow,[35-37] 10–15 MPa in the patellofemoral joint and tibiofemoral contacts in the knee,[6,7,27,28,31,32] to as high as 22 MPa in the hip.[8] Moreover, these high levels of stresses are applied repetitively over a million cycles per year, normally without causing any undue effects or damage to the articulating cartilage. For most biological tissues, this does not pose any problems because vascularized tissues can and do actively repair any microdamage that might have resulted from these high levels of repetitive loading. However, articular cartilage is avascular and aneural, thus it does not sense the high loads it

bears nor does it have any significant capacity for self-repair.[9-11,15,38-40] Thus, the tissue must have a special construction and physical properties that would allow it to resist and survive the high repetitive loads, year in and year out. Indeed, nature has designed a unique bearing material capable of supporting such loads that functions with superb friction, lubrication, and wear characteristics.[4,13,41,42] The secret of how and why articular cartilage functions so well lies in the nature of its multiphasic composition and microstructural organization.

Composition and Microstructure

Multiphasic Nature of Articular Cartilage

Articular cartilage is a multiphasic material consisting of three distinct phases: a solid phase that is charged, porous, and permeable, and is composed of collagen fibers and PGs; a fluid phase composed of water; and an ion phase composed of dissolved electrolytes.[24,43,44] For normal tissues, the pores are 50–60 Angströms† in diameter, thus they offer high frictional resistance to interstitial fluid flow.[45-46] Indeed, it is this fundamental property that gives rise to many of the important material and functional properties that cartilage exhibits.[43-46] Thus, each phase endows the tissue with a set of mechanical, electrical, and physicochemical properties that have now been well studied and reported in the literature and described below.[13,24,41-46]

Chondrocytes

The chondrocytes (cells that reside within cartilage) account for less than 1% of the wet weight of articular cartilage, and therefore they do not contribute in any significant way to the overall mechanical properties of the tissue. They have a distinct pattern of distribution throughout the three zones of the tissue (see Figure 8-1, bottom right). In the superficial zone, they are oblong, with the long axis aligned parallel to the articular surface; in the middle zone, they are ovoid and randomly distributed; and in the deep zone, they are round and often arranged in a columnar fashion perpendicular to the *tidemark* that demarcates the boundary between the uncalcified and calcified cartilage.[13,47]

The cells in the different zones appear to be phenotypically different, secreting different types of collagen and PGs.[15,48,49] The chondrocytes function as the manu-

---

*1.0 MPa in SI units equals approximately 145 pounds per square inch (Psi); 1.0 MPa = 10^6 Pa; 1.0 Pa = N/m²; 1.0 N = 1.0 newton.
†1.0 Å = 0.000,000,000,1 m (10^{-10} m).

facturer and organizer of the extracellular matrix (ECM) that is zone and locale specific.[38–40,48,49] The cells themselves in turn are ensconced and protected within a strong, resilient, and cohesive PG-collagen solid matrix. Within the ECM there is an elaborate layer of pericellular matrix that is rich in PGs and fine collagen fibrils (type VI), forming a structural entity known as the *chondrin* that completely surrounds a chondrocyte, and occasionally two chondrocytes; this pericellular matrix possesses distinctively different mechanical properties than those of the cell.[50,51] This structural unit is then embedded within a strong and architecturally complex territorial and interterritorial matrix that protects these cells from the constant high loads of joint function.[6–8,39,51,52] In this manner, the ECM also serves as the signal transducer for the mechanical, electrical, and physicochemical events that occur within cartilage during loading.[51–53] Indeed, these are the physical signals that chondrocytes perceive and transduce into intracellular biochemical signals required for the regulation of gene expression and thus the production of the macromolecules needed to maintain the ECM in homeostasis.[52–59]

The chondrocytes are terminally differentiated mesenchymal cells.[38] They synthesize, secrete, and maintain the organic components of the ECM, organize its microarchitecture, and respond to the mechanical, electrical, and physicochemical environments that surround them.[15,38–40,48,49,54–59] Basically, the ECM consists of two interacting macromolecular networks: a permanent network of insoluble collagen fibers (mostly type II, with some quantitatively minor types including I, V, VI, IX, X, XI) with slow turnover rates,[60,61] and a network of soluble large PGs ($100–200 \times 10^6$ dalton) that exhibits rapid turnover.[14,15,48,62–64] These two networks are enmeshed within each other, forming a strong, cohesive, fiber-reinforced solid matrix that is charged, porous, and permeable that constitutes the ECM (see Figure 8-1, bottom middle). The interstices of this porous-permeable network are completely filled with water and dissolved electrolytes.

Collagen

In articular cartilage, collagen composes the majority of the organic content: 50–80% of the dry weight or approximately 10–20% of the wet weight of the ECM. The collagen fibers of the ECM are mainly type II collagen and are produced and organized by the tissue chondrocytes.[15,48,60,61] Type II collagen tropocollagen molecules are formed from three identical left-handed helical alpha chains (nomenclature: $\alpha_1[I]$) that are wound in a right-handed helix, similar to a rope, that appears to have been specifically designed to resist ten-

sion. Each alpha chain is composed of a sequence of glycine/proline/X, where X may be either hydroxyproline or another amino acid residue (Figure 8-3, top). These tropocollagen molecules self-aggregate in a quarter-stagger manner to form the collagen fibril in the extracellular space and they are stabilized by intramolecular covalent cross-links. These collagen fibrils possess the characteristic dark and light bands (indicative of the quarter-stagger spacing) that are regularly spaced at 0.1 μm (see Figure 8-3, bottom); this microstructural feature is always seen when examining collagen under electron microscope. These collagen fibrils further aggregate into small-diameter fibrils of 10–25 nm* commonly found in the pericellular matrix and into larger diameter fibrils up to 300 nm that form the territorial matrix. These collagen fibrils are still much smaller than the type I collagen fiber bundles commonly found in ligaments, tendons, and menisci that are 1–2 μm in diameter. Intermolecular covalent cross-links between the collagen fibrils form the insoluble, strong, and cohesive collagen network that provides the load-carrying capacity of the ECM.[48,60,61] Studies have shown that these intracollagen and intercollagen-to-collagen cross-links are important in determining the tensile stiffness and strength of articular cartilage.[65–69]

Proteoglycans

PG aggrecans (in the older literature, it is also known as a *PG monomer* or *PG subunit*) constitute the second largest portion of the organic material of articular cartilage (see Figure 8-1, bottom left), accounting for 5–10% of the wet weight and approximately 25% of the dry weight of the solid matrix.[14,15,48,70] These aggrecans (Figure 8-4A) are sulfated protein-polysaccharide molecules that exist in the ECM generally as PG aggregates linked to a hyaluronan filament (Figure 8-4B). The hyaluronan to which the aggrecans are attached is a nonsulfated disaccharide linear unbranched chain that can be as long as 4 μm, and its molecular weight ranges from $0.5–1.0 \times 10^6$ dalton. Figure 8-4C shows an electron micrograph of a cartilage PG aggregate in solution, confirming the organization of this molecule. The concentration and molecular conformation of PG aggregates in cartilage varies with age and disease[71,72] and the amount of PG present depends on joint loading and motion.[73,74] In general, with aging and disease, the size of the PG aggregates decreases, by either shortening of the hyaluronan chain (i.e., fewer aggrecans may be attached), shortening of the protein core or that of the GAG chains, or all of these factors. Thus, in general,

---

*1.0 nm = 10^{-9} m (a nanometer) or 10^{-3} μm.

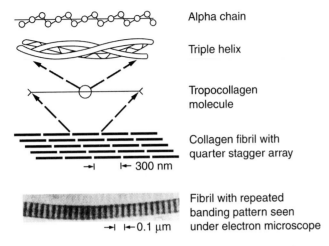

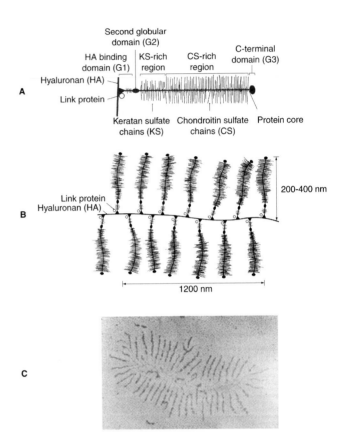

FIGURE 8-3 Hierarchical structures in a collagen fiber, beginning with the amino acid alpha chain that is wound into a left-handed helical triple helix forming the tropocollagen molecule. For articular cartilage type II collagen, the three alpha chains are identical and are composed of a sequence of glycine/proline/X, where X may be either hydroxyproline or another amino acid residue. These tropocollagen molecules self-aggregate in a quarter-stagger manner to form the collagen fibril in the extracellular space, and they are stabilized by intramolecular covalent cross-links. (Reprinted with permission from VC Mow, WC Hayes [eds], Basic Orthopaedic Biomechanics. Philadelphia: Lippincott–Raven, 1997.)

FIGURE 8-4 A. The aggrecans are sulfated protein-polysaccharide molecules; there is a chondroitin sulfate (CS)–rich region, and a keratan sulfate (KS)–rich region near the hyaluronan (HA)-binding region. Each aggrecan can be as large as 10^6 dalton in molecular weight. **B.** The HA chain to which the aggrecans are attached is a nonsulfated disaccharide linear unbranched molecule that can be as long as 4 μm, and its molecular weight ranges from $0.5–1.0 \times 10^6$ dalton. On each HA chain is attached 100–200 aggrecans, making the proteoglycan aggregate a macromolecule with a molecular weight of $100–200 \times 10^6$ dalton. The stability of the association between the HA chain and aggrecan is provided by a link protein.[77,78] **C.** An electron micrograph of a cartilage proteoglycan aggregate in solution is shown, confirming the organization of this molecule. (Reprinted with permission from VC Mow, WC Hayes [eds], Basic Orthopaedic Biomechanics. Philadelphia: Lippincott–Raven, 1997.)

the PG population present in articular cartilage is more heterogeneous in aging and disease, and there is less of it in total. Also, with short-term joint immobilization (< 12 weeks in canine models), the PG content is decreased and its molecular conformation is altered as well, although less defined at present. However, with remobilization, such PG changes and their associated material property changes are partially reversed.[75,76] Indeed, these various in vivo changes in PG are caused by the demonstrated sensitivity of chondrocytes to loading conditions as seen in vitro explant studies.[52,54–59,65] It is stressed that these physiological events may be particularly important to physical therapists who are concerned with restoring the patient's range of motion.

An aggrecan consists of a long protein core to which approximately 150 GAG chains are attached.[14,15,48,70,71] The two sulfated GAGs found in articular cartilage are chondroitin sulfate and keratan sulfate; chondroitin sulfate is composed of repeating disaccharide units of glucuronic acid and galactosamine, and keratan sulfate is composed of repeating disaccharide units of glucosamine and galactose. Chondroitin sulfate may reach a molecular mass of 20,000 dalton, and keratan sulfate may reach 10,000 dalton. In normal adult articular cartilage, the entire PG aggregate may attain a mass of approximately 200×10^6

dalton, whereas those from young chondroepiphyseal cartilage may reach 400×10^6 dalton.[70,71] Most importantly for physiological function of articular cartilage, the sulfate groups on the chondroitin sulfate and keratan sulfate chains are charged in situ, and the carboxyl groups along the chondroitin sulfate and hyaluronan are charged when dissolved in the interstitial water. Thus, there are charged groups every 10–20 nm along the various branches of the PG aggregate molecule. It is known that genetic defects that result in undersulfation (i.e., charged groups) lead to dwarfism and skeletal deformities in mice.[48,77]

There is a heterogeneous distribution of the GAGs along the protein core, consisting of a region rich in keratan sulfate near the hyaluronan-binding region of the protein core, and a region rich in chondroitin sulfate extending away from the binding region (see Figure 8-4A). This structural arrangement gives a *bottle brush* appearance to the aggrecan. The individual aggrecan also varies structurally in length, weight, and composition. A link protein is required to stabilize the noncovalent bond between an aggrecan and the hyaluronan filament.[77,78] This link protein also provides structural rigidity to the aggregate, thus imparting strength to the ECM of cartilage.[63] Loss of this link protein, owing to aging or an arthritic condition, weakens the ECM by decreasing the size of PG aggregate, increasing its rate of loss from the ECM, and thus increasing the propensity of cartilage to develop further mechanical damage.[13,15,77–80]

Water

Water, the most abundant component of articular cartilage, and the most thoroughly studied component, accounts for the remaining 70–75% of the total wet weight in normal articular cartilage.[24,81–86] The water content in the tissue is inhomogeneously distributed throughout the depth, decreasing in a nearly linear fashion, from approximately 80% near the joint surface to 65% at the subchondral bone.[24,83,86] Approximately 70% of the total volume of water is found in the extrafibrillar space available for solvation of the PGs, and 30% in the intrafibrillar and intracellular space that excludes PGs.[24,86–88] The water serves several important functions in the maintenance of the cartilage: (1) It maintains the PGs in solution and allows the PGs to extend to a maximum possible domain within the space provided by the surrounding collagen network.[56,57,89,90] (2) It modulates, together with the PGs, the diameter of the collagen fibrils, allowing the PGs and collagen fibers to form a tightly enmeshed strong network.[48,55,77,88] (3) It supports most of the joint loading acting on the articular surface.[13,41,43,91,92] (4) Its movement from the ECM into the synovial cavity controls the compressibility of the cartilage under loading conditions and contributes to the lubrication of the joint.[3,4,19,41,43] (5) It permits transport of nutrients and waste products between the chondrocytes in the cartilage and the surrounding synovial fluid.[3,13,41,91,92]

Ultrastructure of Articular Cartilage

In addition to the molecular structures of collagen (see Figure 8-3) and PGs (see Figure 8-4), articular cartilage also has an elaborate microscopic organization, with the content and structure of collagen and PG in articular cartilage varying with depth from the articulating surface.[13,24,77,93–96] The most salient organizational feature of cartilage is the layering of its major components (collagen, PGs, and chondrocytes) throughout its depth. This has often been depicted as a four-layer model (Figure 8-5A) and consists of superficial tangential zone, middle zone, deep zone, and the zone of calcified cartilage.[13,15,93–98] The superficial

FIGURE 8-5 A. The generally accepted four-layer model of collagen ultrastructure consisting of superficial tangential zone, middle zone, deep zone, and the zone of calcified cartilage. (Reprinted with permission from VC Mow, WC Hayes [eds], Basic Orthopaedic Biomechanics. Philadelphia: Lippincott-Raven, 1997.) **B.** Scanning electron microscopic view (magnification × 3,000) of the collagen ultrastructure.

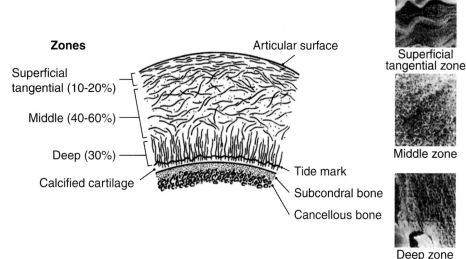

A   B

tangential zone, the thinnest of the four zones of articular cartilage, accounts for 10–20% of the total tissue thickness. It contains sheets of fine densely packed collagen fibers that are randomly woven in planes roughly parallel to the articular surface (Figure 8-5B). This zone provides a strong and resilient membrane that can sustain high tensile stresses and serves to limit the rate of interstitial fluid exudation.[25,66–68,96,97] In the middle zone, which accounts for 40–60% of the total thickness, the distance between the collagen fibers is greater. These fibers are more evenly distributed throughout the middle zone and are optimally distributed to resist the stresses within the tissue from joint loading.[89,90,96] In the deep zone, approximately 30% of the total thickness, the collagen fibers form anastomoses to make larger, radially oriented bundles that cross the tidemark and insert into the calcified cartilage, forming a system that anchors the cartilage to the subchondral bone.[47,98] The zone of the calcified cartilage separates uncalcified, or hyaline cartilage, from the subchondral bone. With aging, even in normal diarthrodial joints, this zone remodels as seen by repetition of the tidemark and thinning of uncalcified articular cartilage.[47,99] Finally, the morphology and arrangement of these cells closely resemble the collagen ultrastructure (Figure 8-6). The chondrocytes in each zone appear to be phenotypically different.[49]

If the surface of the cartilage is punctured with an awl, *split line patterns* are produced that are believed to demonstrate the orientation of the collagen fibers in the superficial tangential zone in the plane of the surface

(Figure 8-7).[100,101] The split line patterns can be important when evaluating the effect of the orientation of collagen fibers on the mechanical properties of the cartilage.[66–68] Microscopically, the appearance of the visually smooth cartilage surface disappears even for normal nonarthritic tissues.[93–95,102] The relatively rough surface has four distinct orders of contours: (1) primary anatomic contours of the articular surfaces; (2) secondary irregularities less than 0.5 mm in diameter; (3) tertiary hollows 20–45 μm in diameter and 0.5–2.0 μm deep; and (4) quaternary ridges 1–4 μm wave crests and 0.1–0.3 μm deep.[102,103] The quaternary ridges first appear in the second decade of life and become more common with age. Knowledge of the surface topography is important in determining the mechanisms involved in joint lubrication because effective lubricant thickness required for fluid film lubrication rarely exceeds 20 μm.[2,4] Scanning electron micrographs of normal and OA cartilage show a wide range of variations in surface topography (Figure 8-8A–C). OA dramatically alters the microstructure of articular cartilage by creating surface fissures and fibrillations (i.e., lesions) and peeling off the most superficial layers as if layer by layer.[103,104] These microstructural aberrations adversely affect the efficacy of the load support mechanisms in cartilage by weakening the superficial tangential zone, permitting more rapid fluid transport and altering the natural lubrication mechanisms in synovial joints, thus accelerating the wear and other microdamage processes within the tissue.[4,13,41,66,89,91,92,97]

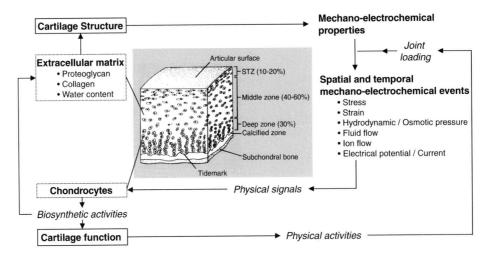

FIGURE 8-6 Morphologic arrangement of these chondrocytes throughout articular cartilage reflects the collagen ultrastructure in the top three zones. Figure also depicts the mechanoelectrochemical events within cartilage that control chondrocyte metabolic activities. (STZ = superficial tangential zone.) (Reprinted with permission from VC Mow, CB Wang, CT Hung. The extracellular matrix, interstitial fluid and ions as a mechanical signal transducer in articular cartilage. Osteoarthritis Cartilage 1999;7:41–58.)

Mechanical Behavior of Articular Cartilage

As the load-bearing material in diarthrodial joints, articular cartilage serves three primary functions: (1) It minimizes contact stresses through deformations that increase the contact area. (2) It provides a hydrostatic load support mechanism via the interstitial water component of the tissue; this load support mechanism minimizes the stresses acting on the collagen-PG solid matrix and thus shields the chondrocytes from excessive loads and deformations. (3) It contributes to the joint lubrication process minimizing friction and wear.[2–5,13,43–45,88,92,105] When an external load is applied across a diarthrodial joint (i.e., the joint reaction force) a complex distribution of tensile, shear, and compressive stresses acts *within* the ECM, and a fluid pressure of significant magnitude is generated *within* the interstitial fluid of articular cartilage. Further, for articular cartilage, a charged, hydrated soft tissue, even in an unloaded state, there is a third type of stress: Donnan's osmotic pressure is generated by the charged groups attached to the PGs of the solid matrix.[13,24,44,46,89,106] This swelling pressure is always balanced by the resisting tensile stress in the collagen network. Thus, there are three types of stresses acting within articular cartilage: (1) the mechanical stresses (tensile, shear, and compressive) that act within the solid ECM; (2) a fluid pressure that acts within the interstitial water; and (3) an osmotic pressure. The mechanical stress acting within the solid matrix is caused by the deformation of the ECM caused by the loading; the fluid pressure acting within the interstitial water is caused by compression and flow effects resulting from joint loading; and the osmotic pressure is caused by the extra number of positively charged particles (e.g., sodium ions) that are required to maintain electroneutrality within the charged (proteoglycans) ECM.[13,24,41–46,107,108]

Stresses and strains in solids, stresses and flow rates in fluids, and osmotic pressure and ion concentrations are related to each other by their mechanical and physical properties. For solids, they are the elastic or viscoelastic moduli, for fluids they are the viscosities and frictional drag coefficients, and for ions they are osmotic and activity coefficients. The mathematical relationships between each pair of these events (e.g., stress and strain) are known as *constitutive laws*, and the coefficients embodied in these laws are the mechanical and physical properties of the material.[13,109,110] These coefficients describe the *intrinsic* properties of the materials themselves, and they depend on its composition, concentration, molecular structure, and ultrastructure (see Figure 8-1). Conse-

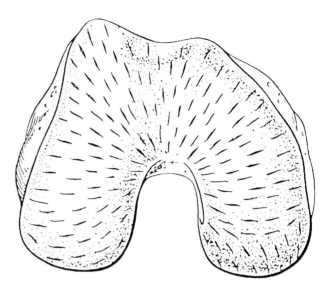

FIGURE 8-7 Split line patterns are produced by a round awl and are believed to demonstrate the orientation of the collagen fibers in the superficial tangential zone in the plane of the surface.[100,101] However, with scanning electron microscope studies, there is no evidence of such strong preferred directions for the collagen network.[93–95]

quently, for a material such as articular cartilage, it is important to understand its response to different loading conditions.[13,24,41–46,66–69,109–113] However, because in vivo experimental measurements of stresses and strains in articular cartilage, meniscus, ligaments, and other tissues of diarthrodial joints are limited and often impossible to obtain, theoretical models must be used to predict some of these quantities. For emphasis, contrary to many misconceptions, one can *never* (i.e., physically impossible) measure the stresses *within* articular cartilage, or for that matter in any material; however, strains may be measured by various optical or electronic methods.[13,109] Indeed, stresses within a material must always be calculated. Clearly, the accuracy of these model-based calculations must necessarily depend on the accuracy of the measured material properties and on the ability of theories to describe the experiment.[13,109,110] In general, the material properties are controlled not only by the components of the tissue (e.g., collagen, PG, and water), but also by their reciprocal interactions. In this section, several theoretical models describing cartilage are presented to illustrate those research methodologies, along with a review of the properties of normal and OA articular cartilages.[13,41–46,66–69,75,91,92,105–116]

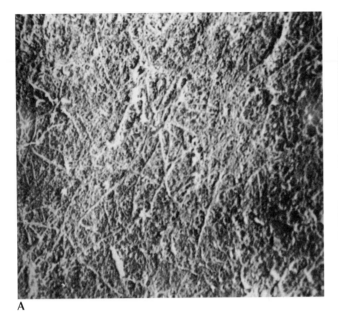

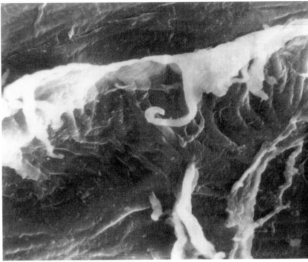

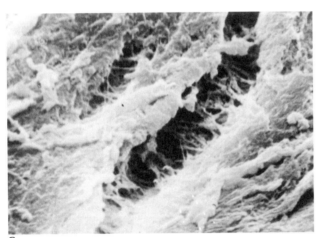

FIGURE 8-8 A. Scanning electron micrograph of a normal articular surface (magnification × 3,000) from a fractured human femoral head removed by surgery. **B, C.** Scanning electron micrographs of two osteoarthritic cartilage surfaces show a wide range of variations in surface topography and damage (**B**, peeling; **C**, fractured surface).

BASIC CONCEPTS IN MATERIAL TESTING

Some basic knowledge of fundamental engineering concepts is necessary to understand the basics of deformation, the constitutive relationships between stresses and strains, and the experiments that are required to obtain the material properties. It is beyond the scope of this chapter to describe all the types of constitutive relationships for materials or experiments that have been used to study articular cartilage. (The reader is cautioned that because of the theoretical difficulties of the subject and the complexity of biological tissue behaviors, many earlier attempts to describe articular cartilage constitutive laws and experiments, in retro-

spect, are grossly in error. This is a natural consequence of scientific progress. Attempts have been made to cite only those references that are theoretically valid and experimentally sound by today's scientific standards. However, some earlier erroneous references have been cited for historical context.) The reader is referred to the references cited in this chapter for more details.[13,41–46,66–69,75,85,91,92,105,109–116]

Relationships between Stresses and Strains

When a material body is subjected to an external force applied on its boundary, the resulting deformation depends on its intrinsic mechanical properties and its

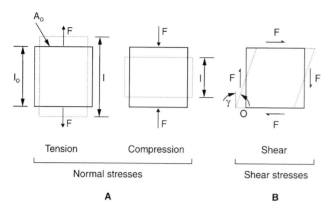

FIGURE 8-9 A. Normal stress $\sigma = F/A_o$ acting on the surfaces of a prismatic bar, where F is the applied force and A_o is the original cross-sectional area: left is tension ($+$); right is compression ($-$). The force F acts *perpendicular* to the surface: l_o is the original of the undeformed object, and l is the deformed (i.e., stretched) length. The lineal strain ε is defined by the ratio $(l_o - l)/l_o$. **B.** Shear stresses $\tau = F/A_o$ acting on the surfaces of a rectangular object. Here the force F acts parallel to the surface. The shear strain γ equals the change in angle from two lines that were (originally) mutually perpendicular to each other at point O.

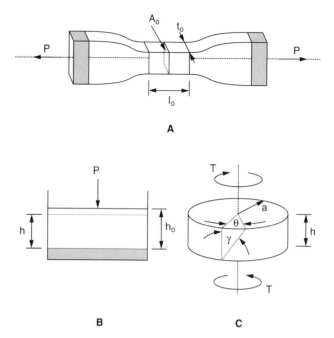

FIGURE 8-10 Typical shapes for tensile (**A**), compressive (**B**), and shear (**C**) test specimens. l_o and t_o are the original length and thickness of the tensile specimens, h_o is the original thickness of a compressive specimen, and a is the radius of a circular shear specimen. (Reprinted with permission from VC Mow, WC Hayes [eds], Basic Orthopaedic Biomechanics. Philadelphia: Lippincott–Raven, 1997.)

geometric shape. In general, there are two types of stresses: normal stress and shear stress (Figure 8-9A and B). Normal stresses act perpendicular to a cross-sectional area A_o and they may be in tension ($+$) or compression ($-$). They elongate or shorten the material in the direction of the applied load. Shear stresses change the angle between two lines in or inscribed on the material that were originally mutually perpendicular to each other from point O.

To remove the geometric influences on the force-deformation behavior of the material, *stress* and *strain* are used to determine its intrinsic material properties. Stress (σ) is defined as the force (F) per unit of original area (A): $\sigma = F/A$. Lineal strain (ε) is defined as the change in length (Δl) per unit of the original length (l_o): $\varepsilon = \Delta l/l_o$, and shear strain γ is defined as a change of the angle between two originally mutually perpendicular line elements emanating from a point in the material. Defined in this manner, the stress-strain relationship of any material is independent of its geometric form, and its stiffness is determined solely by its intrinsic mechanical properties. Six quantities are required to completely define the state of stress (strain) at any point on or inside the object: three normal stresses (lineal strain) that could be tensile, compressive, or both, and three shear stresses (shear strain).

Modulus, Stiffness, and Strength

The intrinsic stiffness of a material is defined by a coefficient (usually a constant) known as a *modulus* in units of force per unit area (pounds per square inch [psi] or newton per square meter [pascal]). Under an arbitrary loading condition of an arbitrarily shaped object made of an arbitrary material(s), the stresses and strains inside the object are quite complex. The objective of a carefully designed material test is to simplify the loading condition, geometry, and material microstructure, so that the resulting stresses and strains may be easily analyzed. For biological materials testing, however, the material cannot be made simpler than its natural state, and there is a limited possibility of changing its shape.

For any material test, it is necessary to have specimens with cross-sectional areas and lengths known *a priori* (Figure 8-10A–C). It is also necessary to apply a specified stress or strain (tensile, compressive, or shear) precisely and predictably onto the specimen. If a slow and constant strain rate is applied onto the test specimen, then a resulting stress-strain relationship is obtained that provides an intrinsic material property. A typical tensile stress-strain graph for a linear ductile material such as

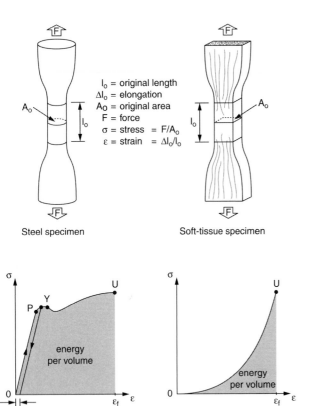

l_0 = original length
Δl_0 = elongation
A_0 = original area
F = force
σ = stress = F/A_0
ε = strain = $\Delta l_0/l_0$

Steel specimen

Soft-tissue specimen

energy per volume

permanent deformation

energy per volume

FIGURE 8-11 (*Left*) Typical stress-strain diagram for a metallic specimen tested in tension. The steel specimen exhibits a linear relationship between stress and strain up to point P (the proportional limit). At Y (the yield point), the specimen does not return to its original length (i.e., plastic deformation has taken place). Beyond Y, the material goes into plastic flow, necks down deforming into a smaller diameter while elongating until failure occurs at U (ultimate stress and strain). The shaded area under this stress-strain curve is the energy per unit volume needed to fracture the specimen. Values of tensile stiffness of steel, aluminum, titanium, and bone are, respectively, 200, 7, 1,100, and 3 GPa. (Reprinted with permission from SR Simon. Orthopaedic Basic Science. Rosemont, IL: American Academy of Orthopaedic Surgeons Press, 1994.) (*Right*) Typical tensile stress-strain diagram for a fibrous biological tissue (such as articular cartilage, ligament, and tendon) tested in tension. The shape of this curve is always convex because of the *fiber-recruitment* phenomenon. The energy per unit volume needed to fracture the specimen is much less than for ductile materials such as steel. Values of tensile stiffness for ligament, tendon, meniscus, and cartilage are, respectively, 500, 500, 100, and 20 MPa.

steel, aluminum, or titanium is shown in Figure 8-11 (left). The slope of the linear proportion of the stress-strain graph (below the yield point Y) defines Young's modulus: $E = \sigma/\varepsilon$ (after Thomas Young, 1773–1829). The ultimate stress (U) is the largest stress that develops

in the material (i.e., strength of material); this is often known as the *failure stress* (i.e., the stress at which the sample fractures). A typical tensile stress-strain behavior for a soft fibrous biological material such as ligament, tendon, meniscus, and cartilage is shown in Figure 8-11 (right). For such materials, there is no proportional limit or yield point, and ultimate limit and U are the failure point. It can be seen that these two types of tensile behaviors are vastly different, representing the macroscopic manifestations of their intrinsic differences in composition and microstructural organization between metals and biological tissues. For material such as steel, Young's modulus is generally 200 GPa; for bone it is of the order of 3 GPa; for ligaments, 500 MPa; and for cartilage, 20 MPa (in tension). For cartilage and meniscus in compression, respectively, the Young's modulus is of the order of 1.0 and 0.5 MPa.[13,41–43,45] If in a shear test, the response of a test specimen is linear, then the shear modulus (G) is defined as the ratio between the shear stress (τ) and the shear strain (γ): $G = \tau/\gamma$. It is also known as the *modulus of rigidity*. For normal articular cartilage, the shear modulus is 0.3 MPa.[13,112–115]

THEORETICAL MODELS OF MATERIAL BEHAVIOR

Linear Elasticity

A material is linearly elastic if (1) the strain is reversible when the stress is removed; (2) the material response is rate insensitive; and (3) the stress and strain are linearly related, as seen in Figure 8-12A. For these materials, following Sir Robert Hooke's law (1635–1703), the deformations produced by forces are *linearly proportional* to each other, while Young defined the relationship between stresses and strains. Isotropic, linearly elastic materials have elastic properties that are independent of orientation. Therefore, from basic theoretical considerations, only two moduli (for example, tension and shear) completely define their stress-strain behaviors.[13,109,110] For anisotropic, linearly elastic materials, which have different mechanical properties in different directions, more elastic constants are required. Examples of anisotropic materials are wood and bone. Wood is orthotropic, requiring nine elastic constants, and bone is transversely isotropic, requiring five elastic constants to define their respective stress-strain behaviors. The complete set of elastic constants for these materials is difficult to obtain. Within certain limits, many engineering materials (steel, aluminum, titanium, and so forth) obey the constitutive law of linear elasticity. An important property exhibited by such metals is that when they are loaded at room temperature, their deformations do not increase with time (i.e., buildings made of steel do not fall down in time). This theory, however, does not explain the time-dependent, stress-strain responses of plastics and most hydrated, soft, fibrous biological materials such as articular cartilage, meniscus, intervertebral disk, ligament, and tendon. These time-dependent properties are attributable to frictional resistance between macromolecules (collagen and PG) that make up the material or between water and the porous-permeable ECM. The time-dependent behaviors are described as *viscoelastic effects*.[13,109,110]

Linear Viscoelasticity

For many materials, including polymers and biological materials, the proportionality between stress and strain is not constant but varies with time. Viscoelastic materials exhibit time-dependent behaviors known as *creep* and *stress relaxation*, and their stress-strain responses are strongly sensitive to strain rate (e.g., how fast the load is being applied). These characteristics result from a combination of the elastic and viscous or frictional elements within the material. An *elastic* material by definition is a material that returns all the mechanical energy required for it to be deformed (e.g., a deformed rubber ball would return all the energy when it is unloaded). Such materials are solids whose deformational behaviors are not time independent. A material that does not return all the energy has internal dissipation mechanisms that convert the mechanical energy to heat; they are said to have internal friction. Classical dissipation mechanisms are *viscosity* or *friction* within fluids or at fluid-solid interfaces. These dissipation mechanisms give rise to time-dependent behaviors. Solids are modeled by springs that are linearly elastic (Figure 8-12A), and fluids are modeled by frictional dashpots that are also linearly viscous (Figure 8-12B). For the solid the proportionality is called the *spring constant k* (see Figure 8-12A, lower left) or *Young's modulus E* (see Figure 8-12A, lower right). For fluids the proportionality is called the *coefficient of friction c* (see Figure 8-12B, lower left) or *coefficient of viscosity η* (see Figure 8-12B, lower right). Thus, a linear viscoelastic material is modeled by linear springs linked together by linear viscous dashpots in a variety of combinations. Figures 8-12C and 8-12D depict the two simplest linear viscoelastic materials, one with the spring and dashpot linked in parallel (see Figure 8-12C), known as a *Kelvin-Voigt solid* (ca. 1855), and the other linked in series (see Figure 8-12D), known as a *Maxwell fluid* (ca. 1870).

The Kelvin-Voigt and Maxwell materials show distinctly different responses to creep and stress-relaxation

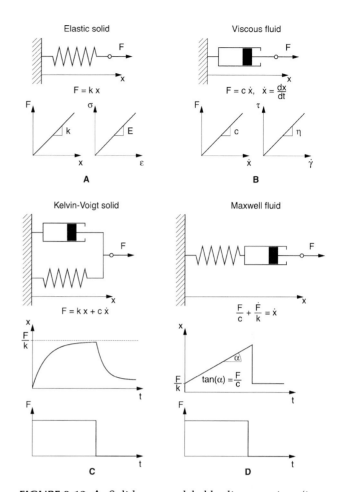

FIGURE 8-12 A. Solids are modeled by linear springs (i.e., the force is directly proportional to the elongation); F = kx, where F is the applied load, k is the spring constant, and x is the stretch. Lower diagrams illustrate the force-deformation relationship (*left*) and stress-strain relationship (*right*). The Young's modulus is designated by E. **B.** Fluids are modeled by frictional dashpots that provide a linear relationship between force and rate of stretch (dx/dt) or speed of stretch (*lower left*). (The dot indicates time derivative.) A Newtonian viscous fluid has a linear relationship between the strain rate (dγ/dt) and shear stress (τ) (*lower right*). The frictional dissipation coefficient is denoted by c, and the viscosity is designated by η. **C.** A Kelvin-Voigt material is a viscoelastic solid defined by a spring and a dashpot linked together in parallel. Under a constant load (*lower diagram*), the deformation (x) increases with time to limit defined by the spring constant (*middle diagram*). **D.** A Maxwell material is a viscoelastic fluid defined by a spring and a dashpot linked together in series. Under constant load (*lower diagram*), the deformation (x) increases linearly without limit (*middle diagram*). (Reprinted with permission from VC Mow, WC Hayes [eds], Basic Orthopaedic Biomechanics. Philadelphia: Lippincott-Raven, 1997.)

tests, because of the way the springs and dashpots are arranged, in parallel or in series. A creep test measures the deformation of the material as a function of time under a *constant* loading condition. A stress-relaxation test measures the force as a function of time under a *constant* strain. Elastic solids exhibit neither creep nor stress relaxation. Figures 8-12C and D show the creep behaviors of these two materials. The specifics of their creep behaviors (i.e., the initial response, the rate of creep, and the equilibrium response) are governed by the manner in which the spring and the dashpot are connected, and by the set of constants (k, c or E, η) that characterize the elements making up the material. The Kelvin-Voigt material does not creep indefinitely, because the spring is in parallel with the dashpot, limiting the creep. This is the essential characteristic of a solid. Therefore, the Kelvin-Voigt material is a viscoelastic solid. The Maxwell material creeps indefinitely, as long as the load is maintained, because of the behavior of the dashpot. This is the essential characteristic of a fluid. Thus, a Maxwell material is a viscoelastic fluid. Figure 8-12C shows the creep behavior of the Kelvin-Voigt solid, and Figure 8-12D shows the stress-relaxation behavior of the Maxwell fluid. More complex behavior of real materials may be described by connecting a number of springs and dashpots in series or parallel.[13,109,110] The most commonly used model for a viscoelastic solid or fluid is one in which the spring and dashpot are connected to a Kelvin-Voigt model. This is known as the *standard* or *three-element viscoelastic material*.

A theoretical model is successful in describing a material if the general trends of the creep and stress-relaxation responses are similar to those obtained from experimental tests. The material coefficients (k, c or E, η) are determined by matching the actual experimental data with a theoretic creep or stress-relaxation curve. Several investigators have proposed such a viscoelastic model to describe the compressive and shear behaviors of cartilage.[111,116] A more comprehensive theory, the quasilinear viscoelastic theory, was developed by Fung to describe the viscoelasticity in tension of biological soft tissues such as ligaments and tendons.[109,110] This theory has been shown to be quite successful for tissues such as tendons and ligaments that predominantly carry tensile stresses.[109,110] However, these constitutive laws are not always consistent with known information about the structure and composition of biological tissues; in particular, they do not address the high water content (70–75%) that always exists within the tissue. In particular, for tissues such as articular cartilage, meniscus, and inter-

vertebral disks, predominantly compressive load-carrying tissues, the influence of the high-degree hydration on the mechanical behaviors of biological tissues must be taken into consideration.[13,41–46]

Multiphasic Theories of Viscoelasticity and Swelling

Both elastic and viscoelastic models treat cartilage as a single-phase material, while ignoring the fluid and ion components in the tissue. Studies have long suggested that water and electrolytes (Na^+, Cl^-, Ca^{++}, and so forth) are essential components to the proper functioning of articular cartilage.[13,24,25,41–46,82–86] To date, the most successful theory for cartilage-compressive behaviors, when ion effects are neglected, is the biphasic theory for creep and stress-relaxation developed by Mow and coworkers in 1980 that account for the influence of interstitial fluid on the mechanical properties of cartilage.[13,41,43,45] When ion effects are included to describe Donnan's osmotic pressure and other electrochemical events, the triphasic theory developed by Lai and coworkers in 1991 must be employed.[24,42,44,46] Thus, the triphasic theory is often referred to as the *mechanoelectrochemical theory* because it includes mechanical, electrical, and chemical phenomenons. When considering only mechanical effects such as high loads acting on the surface of joint cartilage, then only the biphasic theory is needed. Typically, joint loading is in the range of 5–10 MPa, whereas Donnan's osmotic pressure is in the range of 0.1–0.2 MPa, much smaller than joint loads, and therefore physicochemical effects can be neglected. However, when considering osmotic pressure or electrical effects, then the triphasic theory is needed; the osmotic pressure is one of the mechanisms responsible for the maintenance of fluid content in the tissue and the electrical potential or current are important in signal transduction to chondrocytes.[39,52] These multiphasic theories have been developed using basic thermodynamic and mathematical considerations, and therefore they are fundamentally valid. Since 1980, the biphasic theory has been proposed and validated to describe articular cartilage, cornea, meniscus, intervertebral disk, ligaments, and tendons. It has now become the new paradigm for analyzing and testing almost all biological tissues, and therefore, it would be worthwhile to briefly describe the theory for the reader.

The theory begins with a material (e.g., articular cartilage) that is composed of a collagen network and PG gel. The mixture of these two materials forms a porous-permeable matrix that exists in a solid state (i.e., it does not flow). All the physical attributes of this porous-permeable *solid phase* may be prescribed mathematically (e.g., ratio of pore volume to solid volume, frictional drag coefficient, elastic moduli, permeability, and their variations throughout the tissue, and so forth), and ideally they may be experimentally measured. The second phase (i.e., the *fluid phase*) is composed of water; it flows. The biphasic theory further assumes the solid phase and the interstitial fluid phase of the tissue are immiscible, and each phase to be intrinsically incompressible.[43,117] The fact that these two phases are immiscible is obvious; the incompressibility assumption has only been relatively recently experimentally validated.[117] The pores of the solid phase are assumed to be "open and connected," and therefore interstitial fluid may flow through the solid matrix by a pressure gradient or by the *apparent* compression of the solid matrix (i.e., *by reducing the total pore volume*). Although the water content ranges from 70–75% of normal articular cartilage, the average *pore size* from various measurements and calculations has been determined to be approximately 60 nm[24,45] (i.e., water in such tissues exists in microscopic pores). Viscous dissipation in articular cartilage is dominated by the frictional drag of interstitial fluid flow through the micropores of the permeable, collagen-PG solid matrix. Simply, as the water molecules are forced to flow through the microscopic pores, they collide with the collagen network and branches of the dissolved PGs, and in turn there is a transfer of momentum from the water molecules to the solid phase. This exchange of momentum slows down the flow speed of water and by Newton's third law of action and reaction, the collagen-PG solid matrix is compressed. There is also friction between the collagen network and trapped PGs that manifests as an intrinsic viscoelastic effect.[13,26,97,111–113] Generally, however, these intrinsic viscoelasticity effects in articular cartilage are of minor consequence; in tendons and ligaments, however, these intrinsic viscoelasticity effects dominate over the fluid-solid frictional effects described by the biphasic theory.[109–115]

Fundamentally, the principle of partial pressure enables these multiphasic tissues to function in load support. Consider the compressive stress that knee joint cartilage must support. Various calculations and measurements have shown that loads reaching as high as 10 MPa exist in the knee during ordinary activities of daily living (e.g., stair climbing) or 20 MPa in the hip when getting up from a sitting position.[6–8,32] Such pressures can easily crush the ECM and the chondrocytes, because the ECM has a compressive modulus of 1 MPa, and chondrocytes have a compressive modulus of 1 kPa.[39,51] Survival of cartilage under these loading conditions must rely on the principle of partial pressure that derives from its multiphasic nature. When such a material is loaded in compression, both the fluid phase and the solid phase join to support the load. This load-sharing ability protects the ECM and chondrocytes, and the shifting of load from the fluid phase onto the solid phase gives rise to the time-dependent viscoelastic behaviors (creep and stress-relaxation) of articular cartilage. Initially, when the tissue is loaded, the interstitial fluid supports greater than 95% of the applied load and therefore the fluid is pressurized.[13,41,42,105] The remaining portion of the load must be provided by the solid phase. By its nature, fluid flows away from the highly pressurized region, thus diminishing the fluid pressure in that region. However, because the load remains constant, by Newton's laws, the solid phase must make up the load support with greater compression. Eventually, in time, this shifting of load from the fluid phase to the solid phase would be complete when the fluid pressure vanishes; at this point, the solid phase carries all the applied load.[41–43] The time required for this load-transfer process to occur is governed by the law of inverse square of the tissue thickness. Thus, for normal cartilage, typically 2–5 mm thick, it would take from 4,000–20,000 seconds to complete this load-transfer process.[41,43] Clearly, then, under physiological conditions, and for the typical time duration of activities of daily living, the fluid phase would support most of the load most of the time.[41–43,105] Thus, nature has made a marvelous bearing material using the fluid phase to support most of the massive loads of joint function, one that protects the ECM and chondrocytes from being crushed, one that provides lubrication, and one that almost never wears out. Unfortunately, accidents and diseases do occur that damage the tissue and prevent this mechanism from functioning properly. Thus, once damage has occurred in articular cartilage, biochemically or biomechanically induced, because of its aneural and alymphatic nature, low cellularity, lack of blood supply, and the isolated nature of the chondrocytes encased within the strong collagen-PG solid matrix, an inexorable degenerative process occurs that leads to the destruction of cartilage and eventually OA.[9–11,38–40,48–52,118–120]

Mechanical Properties of Articular Cartilage

Compression Tests

Creep A number of experiments have been developed to test the validity of the previously described load-sharing concept and to determine the intrinsic material properties of articular cartilage, compressive modulus, and permeability. The most commonly used experiment is the one-dimensional confined compression test, in which the specimen is restricted to move in only one direction (Figure 8-13).[13,41,43] Both compression creep and stress-relaxation measurements may be taken in this test chamber. Figure 8-14 (top) depicts the biphasic creep phenomenon in this experiment: The left figure denotes a loading curve where the load is suddenly applied at time $t_o = 0$ and held constant thereafter; the right figure denotes an actual creep experiment (experimental data and theoretical prediction).[43,45] The surface of the biphasic cartilage specimen is loaded with a rigid porous-permeable plate compressing the specimen. The porous-permeable plate allows free fluid exudation at the interface with the specimen and thus allows flow into the pores of the filter. The rate of fluid exudation is the rate of volume loss from the tissue, because both the fluid and ECM are intrinsically incompressible; thus the permeability governs the rate of compressive creep. At equilibrium, fluid movement stops, and both internal flow-induced friction and fluid pressure vanish. Load support is then borne entirely by the collagen-PG elastic solid matrix. In this manner, the intrinsic elastic modulus of the solid matrix in compression is determined.[43,45,121] Note that the frictional drag associated with fluid flow produces falsely high values of the compressive modulus if measurements are taken before equilibration occurs (e.g., by the method of 2-second modulus proposed by Kempson and coworkers, or other similar methods).[116] These falsely high moduli of

10–20 MPa in compression have no physical meaning, and they are not to be confused with the intrinsic equilibrium modulus of the ECM, which ranges from 0.5–1.0 MPa. (Note: Clearly, by definition, no valid physical measurement method should depend on the observer. If other observers should choose another time different than 2 seconds, as some have done, then their calculations would produce different results for the compressive modulus, thus invaliding Kempson's method.) By waiting for equilibrium to occur (i.e., when fluid pressurization vanishes) only the solid matrix would support the load and hence the true or intrinsic modulus of the ECM is measured.[13,41,43]

Stress Relaxation Figure 8-14 (bottom) depicts the biphasic stress-relaxation experiment: The left figure denotes a compression curve where the surface-to-surface strain is applied at constant rate to a specified value (e.g., 10%), and thereafter $(t > t_1)$ the compression is held constant; the right figure provides a set of actual stress-relaxation experimental data obtained from bovine articular cartilage and theoretic analysis.[41,43] Again, the surface of the biphasic cartilage specimen is loaded with a rigid porous-permeable plate, and it allows the interstitial fluid to freely drain into the pores of the filter. The significant increase of compressive stress greatly exceeding a direct proportional level between stress and strain is, again, caused by interstitial fluid pressurization and the frictional drag of fluid efflux across the surface. After time t_1 (i.e., when the strain is held constant and when fluid efflux ceases), the stress-relaxation process occurs. The rate of stress-relaxation is governed by the speed at which the strain field inside the ECM can be relieved by a redistribution process between the fluid phase and the solid phase. This redistribution process is governed by a balance of force between the frictional drag caused by the flow of the interstitial fluid through the porous-permeable ECM (i.e., proportional to the permeability coefficient) and the force of compression (i.e., proportional to the intrinsic compressive stiffness of the ECM). At equilibrium, when all frictional drag forces and fluid pressure vanish, the compressive stress and strain become directly proportional, again given by the simple equation $H_A = \sigma_o/\varepsilon_f$. The rate of stress relaxation also provides a means by which tissue permeability may be calculated. The stress-relation data and theoretic analysis provided in Figure 8-14 (bottom right) show the remarkable ability of the biphasic theory to describe such experimental results with high accuracy.[41] Note that the stress-relaxation experiment and the creep experiment are two *independent* tests, and they have been performed on the same pieces of

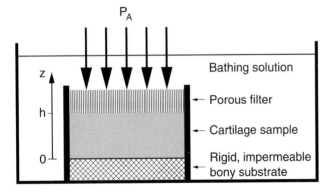

FIGURE 8-13 Schematics of a confined compression test. Load P_A is applied to the cartilage surface via a rigid-porous filter that allows free escape of the interstitial fluid into the pores of the filter. The thickness of cartilage is h, and the compression is in the z direction. Lateral expansion of the specimen is prevented by the confining chamber; all displacements and flows are in the z direction.

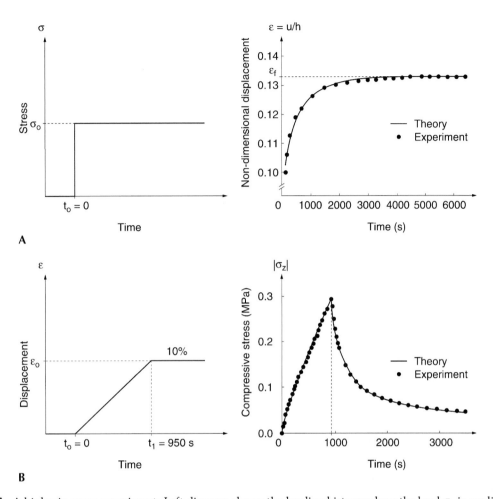

FIGURE 8-14 A. A biphasic creep experiment: Left diagram shows the loading history where the load σ_o is applied at time $t_o = 0$, and held constant thereafter; right diagram shows a typical set of experimental data with biphasic theoretical predictions. By curve fitting the theory to the experimental data, one can calculate the intrinsic material properties of articular cartilage in this manner. The creep rate is dependent on the permeability k of the tissue and the pressure generated within the tissue, and the equilibrium strain ε_f depends on the intrinsic stiffness of the extracellular matrix. The ratio of σ_o/ε_f provides the aggregate modulus H_A, the compressive modulus of the extracellular matrix. (Reprinted with permission from KA Athanasiou, MP Rosenwasser, JA Buckwalter, et al. Interspecies comparison of in situ mechanical properties of distal femoral cartilage. J Orthop Res 1991;9:330–340.) **B.** A biphasic stress-relaxation experiment: Left diagram shows the compression history, where the compression is ramped at a constant rate up to a prescribed value (e.g., 10%) and held constant thereafter ($t_1 = 950$ seconds); right diagram shows a typical set of experimental data with biphasic theoretical predictions. Values of the permeability and aggregate modulus determined by the stress-relaxation test correspond exactly to those determined from the creep test, thus validating the biphasic theory and experimental methods. (Reprinted with permission from GA Ateshian, WH Warden, JJ Kim, et al. Finite deformation biphasic material properties of bovine articular cartilage from confined compression experiments. J Biomechanics 1997;30:1157–1164.)

cartilage specimen. The fact that these tests yield identical results for H_A and k provides an independent validation check on the biphasic theory, as well as the experimental procedure.[13,41–45,75]

The previously described experimental method and theoretic analysis provide, to date, the only means to

obtain the true compressive stiffness and permeability of articular cartilage and other soft hydrated tissues. Over the years, numerous tests have been performed to study the structure-function relationship of normal and OA articular cartilage. Articular cartilage from OA joints generally has an increased water content and a loss of PG

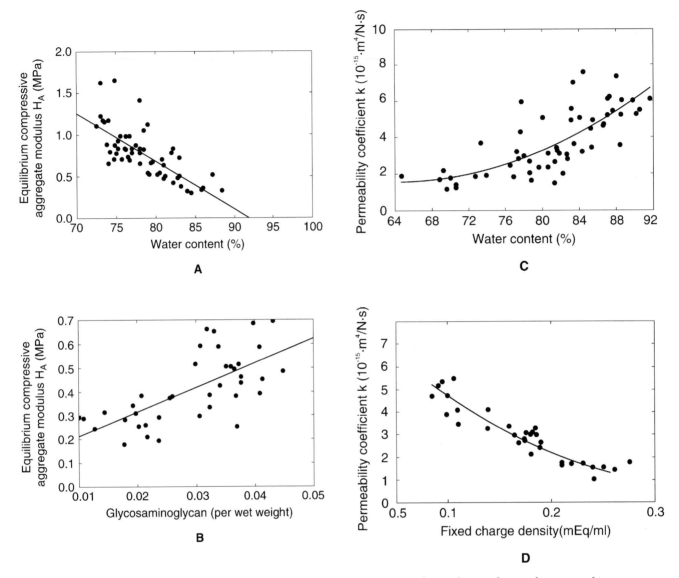

FIGURE 8-15 Variation of the equilibrium compressive aggregate modulus H_A of articular cartilage as functions of its water content (**A**) and proteoglycan content (**B**). Variation of the permeability coefficient k as a function of its water content (**C**) and proteoglycan content (**D**). (Reprinted with permission from **A:** CG Armstrong, VC Mow. Variations in the intrinsic mechanical properties of human articular cartilage with age, degeneration, and water content. J Bone Joint Surg 1982;64A:88–94; **B:** VC Mow, LA Setton, A Ratcliffe, et al. Structure-function relationships for articular cartilage and effects of joint instability and trauma on cartilage function. In KD Brandt [ed], Cartilage Changes in Osteoarthritis. Indianapolis, IA: University of Indiana Press, 1990; **C:** LA Setton, VC Mow, JC Pita, et al. Altered structure-function relationships for articular cartilage in human osteoarthritis and an experimental canine model. In WB van den Berg, PM van der Kraan, PLEM van Lent [eds], Joint Destruction in Arthritis and Osteoarthritis. Basel, Switzerland: Birkhauser Verlag, 1993; **D:** A Maroudas. Physicochemical properties of articular cartilage. In MAR Freeman [ed], Adult Articular Cartilage [2nd ed]. Kent, UK: Pittman Medical Publishing, 1979.)

content.[9–13,24,66,75,81,82,122–125] Figures 8-15A and B provide the equilibrium compressive aggregate modulus H_A of the porous-permeable solid matrix as functions of its water and PG contents. Figures 8-15C and D provide the permeability coefficient k as a function of its water and PG

contents. These trends seem to hold true for all articular cartilage from various joints.[121]

The compressive modulus of cartilage derives two sources: (1) the charge-to-charge electrical repulsive effect associated with the closely spaced charges that is

TABLE 8-1

Compressive Aggregate Modulus H_A, Permeability k, and Thickness h of Normal (i.e., Nonosteoarthritic) Human, Bovine, Canine, Monkey, and Rabbit Knee Joint Cartilage

	H_A (MPa)	$k(10^{-15}.m^4/N\,s)$	h (mm)
Lateral condyle			
Human (n = 4)	0.701 ± 0.228	1.182 ± 0.207	2.31 ± 0.53
Bovine (n =10)	0.894 ± 0.293	0.426 ± 0.197	0.94 ± 0.17
Dog (n = 6)	0.603 ± 0.237	0.774 ± 0.563	0.58 ± 0.20
Monkey (n = 6)	0.778 ± 0.176	4.187 ± 1.545	0.57 ± 0.12
Rabbit (n = 6)	0.537 ± 0.258	1.806 ± 1.049	0.25 ± 0.06
Medial condyle			
Human (n = 4)	0.588 ± 0.114	1.137 ± 0.160	2.21 ± 0.59
Bovine (n = 10)	0.899 ± 0.427	0.455 ± 0.332	1.19 ± 0.24
Dog (n = 6)	0.904 ± 0.218	0.804 ± 0.776	0.90 ± 0.15
Monkey (n = 6)	0.815 ± 0.180	2.442 ± 1.129	0.72 ± 0.09
Rabbit (n = 6)	0.741 ± 0.101	2.019 ± 1.621	0.41 ± 0.10
Patellar groove			
Human (n = 4)	0.530 ± 0.094	2.173 ± 0.730	3.57 ± 1.12
Bovine (n = 10)	0.472 ± 0.147	1.422 ± 0.580	1.38 ± 0.19
Dog (n = 6)	0.555 ± 0.144	0.927 ± 0.844	0.52 ± 0.12
Monkey (n = 6)	0.522 ± 0.159	4.737 ± 2.289	0.41 ± 0.05
Rabbit (n = 6)	0.516 ± 0.202	3.842 ± 3.260	0.20 ± 0.04

Source: Reprinted with permission from KA Athanasiou, MP Rosenwasser, JA Buckwalter, et al. Interspecies comparison of in situ mechanical properties of distal femoral cartilage. J Orthop Res 1991;9:330–340.

fixed on the chondroitin sulfate and keratan sulfate molecules of the PGs[126] or equivalently by Donnan's osmotic pressure associated with the concentration of counterions (e.g., Na^+)[24,44,106]; and (2) by the intrinsic stiffness of the ECM (i.e., not including the fixed charge effects). Using the stress-relaxation test configuration, it has been proven theoretically that under normal physiological conditions, Donnan's osmotic pressure effect and the intrinsic ECM stiffness contribute in nearly equal proportions to the measured compressive stiffness (H_A).[42,127] Thus, the *functional* compressive properties of articular cartilage derive from *three* sources, the two intrinsic mechanisms for matrix stiffness just mentioned, and the hydrodynamic fluid pressure as predicted by the biphasic theory.[41–45]

In a similar fashion, the permeability (i.e., drag force) of the cartilage, or any charged porous-permeable solid matrix, derives from two sources: (1) the fixed charges attract the counterions, thus slowing down the permeation flow[46]; and (2) momentum exchanged caused by the collision of water molecules against the collagen and PGs as they are forced to flow through the fixed porous-permeable solid matrix.[24,25,45,128] With this fundamental understanding, one can easily see why there are strong dependencies of the compressive modulus and permeability on

the tissue's water content and PG content (see Figures 8-15A–D). Table 8-1 provides a summary of the compressive aggregate modulus H_A, permeability k, and thickness h of healthy (i.e., nonosteoarthritic) human, bovine, canine, monkey, and rabbit knee joint cartilage.[121] Table 8-2 provides the contributions of Donnan's osmotic pressure to the biphasic compressive aggregate modulus H_A of articular cartilage.[127] These are given for various known physiological ranges of the fixed charge densities (milliequivalent per milliliter) of healthy and OA articular cartilage, and at 0% and 10% compressive strain. From the triphasic theory, the relationship between the biphasic aggregate modulus H_A and the triphasic aggregate modulus H_a is given by $H_A - H_a = \Delta\pi$ (i.e., the difference of the interstitial Donnan's osmotic pressure between 0% and 5%, and 0% and 10% compressive strains).[42,44,127]

Uniaxial Tension Tests

The collagen network of articular cartilage forms the cohesive fabric that maintains the structural integrity of the ECM.[13,15,66–69] This network is insoluble and strong and has the slow biological turnover rate of 1% per year.[60,61] PGs, on the other hand, are in solution at high concentrations (5–10 mg/ml) within the tissue, although below its saturation point, and form weak elastic net-

TABLE 8-2

Contributions of Donnan's Osmotic Pressure to the Biphasic Compressive Aggregate Modulus H_A of Articular Cartilage for Various Fixed Charge Densities (mEq/ml) at 5% and 10% Compressive Strain*

$c^* = 0.15\,M$ $\varnothing^W_O = 0.85$ $\varepsilon = -0.05$		H_a (MPa)					
		0.1	0.2	0.3	0.4	0.5	0.6
C^F_O (mEq/ml)	0.05	0.126	0.226	0.326	0.426	0.526	0.626
	0.10	0.199	0.299	0.399	0.499	0.599	0.699
	0.15	0.309	0.409	0.509	0.609	0.709	0.809
	0.20	0.445	0.545	0.645	0.745	0.845	0.945
$c^* = 0.15\,M$ $\varnothing^W_O = 0.85$ $\varepsilon = -0.10$		H_a (MPa)					
		0.1	0.2	0.3	0.4	0.5	0.6
C^F_O (mEq/ml)	0.05	0.128	0.228	0.328	0.428	0.528	0.628
	0.10	0.209	0.309	0.409	0.428	0.609	0.709
	0.20	0.329	0.429	0.529	0.509	0.729	0.829
	0.15	0.476	0.576	0.676	0.776	0.876	0.976

*The relationship between the biphasic aggregate modulus H_A and the triphasic modulus H_a is given by $H_A - H_a = \Delta\pi$ (the difference of Donnan's osmotic pressure between 0% and 5%, and 0% and 10% compressive strains).

Source: Reprinted with permission from WM Lai, VC Mow, DN Sun, GA Ateshian. On the electric potentials inside a charged soft hydrated biological tissue: Streaming potential vs. diffusion potential. J Biomech Eng 2000;122(4):336–346.

works among themselves.[62,63,129] Although PGs are relatively labile when compared with the collagen fibers, by virtue of their size and networking abilities, they are trapped by physical entanglements within the collagen network, and thus are immobilized within the ECM.[77,79,90] When the collagen is damaged for whatever reason(s), the trapped PGs expand against the weakened network by drawing more water into the interfibrillar space.[79,90] Indeed, it has long been known that an increase in water content is the first measurable sign of early OA changes in cartilage.[13,81–88] After this increase of water content, PGs gain increased mobility and thus they are lost from the tissue at a greater rate.[25,26,77] Indeed, these events are known to produce a cascade of structure-function changes in articular cartilage that leads to its inexorable degeneration and thus frank OA.[9,10,13,24,66,85,97,114–116,119,122–125]

Because of the importance of the tensile behavior of the collagen network, a number of investigators have examined the tensile behavior of articular cartilage on thin specimens harvested in planes parallel to the articular surface.[66–69,115,116,130–132] In these studies, thin specimens (approximately 200 μm) of the tissue were serially microtomed from various layers of the tissue in directions either parallel or perpendicular to the split lines (see Figure 8-7).[110,111] These tests can be performed at

either a constant strain rate[66,67,130,131] or as creep[69] or stress-relaxation experiments.[132] A slow strain rate experiment[67,68,130,131] or an equilibrium state, reached in either a creep[69] or stress-relaxation experiment,[66,132] is required to defeat the biphasic viscoelastic effect, so that the intrinsic tensile behavior of the collagen-PG solid matrix can be determined. These tests have provided valuable information on the understanding of collagen network properties and the dynamics that exist within the collagen-PG solid matrix.

The tensile stress-strain behavior caused by a constant strain rate exhibits an initial *toe region* that is not linear, followed by a linear stress-strain response. This is the force response that develops from the straightening of the initially *crimped* or *wavy* collagen fibrillar organization in the specimen, and the linear response provides a measure of the true tensile stiffness of the collagen network (Figure 8-16). Many have successfully used an *exponential law* to describe tensile stress-strain behaviors of such fibrous materials.[68,109,110,115] Thus, strictly speaking, Hooke's law is not valid for this material, and Young's modulus cannot be used. However, for simplicity, many investigators have used the proportionality between the linear stress and strain response in the latter portion of the curve as a measure of cartilage tensile stiffness, referring to it as *Young's modulus*. Normal human knee articular cartilage has an intrinsic tensile modulus (sans fluid pressurization effects) that varies with depth, location, and direction; surface specimens from areas of the distal condyle that are habitually loaded have a lower tensile modulus on account of a higher PG content or lower collagen-to-PG ratio (approximately 8 MPa) than tissues from low-weight-bearing areas (approximately 18 MPa) (Figure 8-17).[66] Tensile moduli of specimens taken parallel to the split line are always greater than that of specimens taken perpendicular to the split line.[68,116,130] Comparison of the tensile modulus of healthy human knee cartilage with those of mildly fibrillated human knee cartilage is provided in Figure 8-18; typically pathologists have found that mild fibrillations are the earliest morphologic signs of OA changes on cartilage.[9–11,66,119] Figure 8-18 (left) are results from normal human distal femurs showing layer variations of the tensile modulus; the surface zone is many times stiffer than the subsurface, middle, and middle-deep zones, and specimens tested in deionized water are stiffer than those tested in 0.15 mol/L NaCl. The latter effect is caused by Donnan's osmotic pressure, which acts to stretch the collagen fibers, thus pushing the network to act in the stiffer zone (see Figure 8-16). Figure 8-18 (B) shows results from the mildly fibrillated distal femoral cartilage specimens. Note that although the tensile modulus of the surface specimens is degraded by approximately 40%, the lower zones (subsurface, middle, middle-deep zones) remain undamaged. These data are consistent with the ultrastructural picture presented in Figure 8-8.

Lubrication of Synovial Joints

The major weight-bearing joints of the body, the hips, knees, and ankles, are exposed to large ranges of relative motion in multiple directions as well as loads that are often as great as six times body weight during a normal gait cycle.[2–8] Under normal conditions, these loads must be sustained for seven or eight decades by these and other major joints of the body. As bearing surfaces, these joints must have low friction and wear rates, as well as effective lubrication characteristics that allow effective function in a physically isolated environment. In this section, the biotribologic aspects of joint function are presented. *Tribology* is the study of physics and chemistry of two interacting moving surfaces. The major components of tribology are friction, lubrication, and wear. *Biotribology* is the study of two interacting biological moving surfaces.

Friction Friction is defined as the resistance to sliding motion between two contacting bodies.[2,4] Based on the energy-dissipating mechanisms, there are two types of

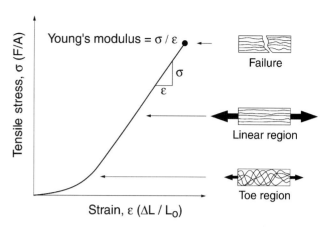

FIGURE 8-16 The nonlinear tensile stress-strain response of articular cartilage demonstrating a toe region caused by the initial straightening of the *crimped* or *wavy* collagen fibrillar organization within the specimen, and a linear response of the true tensile stiffness of the collagen network.

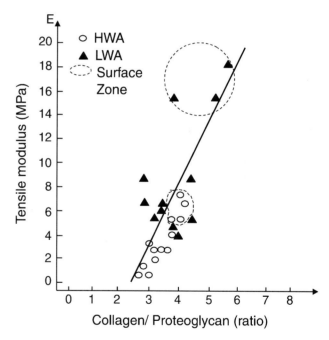

FIGURE 8-17 Intrinsic tensile properties (sans fluid pressurization effects) of normal human knee cartilage that vary with depth and location; surface specimens from areas of the distal condyle that are habitually loaded have lower tensile modulus on account of a higher proteoglycan content or lower collagen-to-proteoglycan ratio. (HWA = high weight–bearing areas; LWA = low weight–bearing areas.) (Reprinted with permission from S Akizuki, VC Mow, F Muller, et al. Tensile properties of knee joint cartilage: I. Influence of ionic conditions, weight bearing, and fibrillation on the tensile modulus. J Orthop Res 1986;4:379–392.)

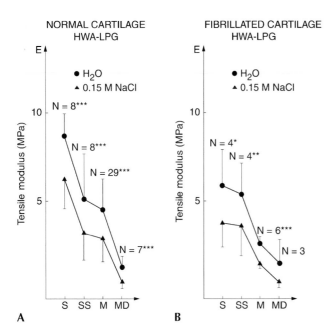

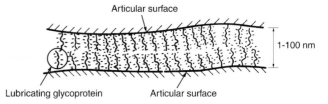

FIGURE 8-19 Schematic depiction of the boundary lubrication mechanism at the articular surface showing an adsorbed monolayer, probably the lubricating glycoprotein, dipalmitoyl phosphatidylcholine, or both. (Reprinted with permission from VC Mow, WC Hayes [eds], Basic Orthopaedic Biomechanics. Philadelphia: Lippincott–Raven, 1997.)

FIGURE 8-18 A. Tensile modulus of normal human distal femoral cartilage showing layer variations for various zones: surface zone (S), subsurface zone (SS), middle zone (M), and middle-deep zone (MD). Note that because of Donnan's osmotic pressure, specimens tested in deionized water are stiffer than those tested in 0.15 mol/L NaCl. **B.** Tensile modulus of mildly fibrillated human distal femoral cartilage specimens. Note that although the tensile modulus of the surface specimens are degraded by approximately 40%, the lower regions (subsurface, middle, middle deep) remain undamaged. (HWA-LPG = high-weight-bearing area–lateral patellar groove.) (Reprinted with permission from S Akizuki, VC Mow, F Muller, et al. Tensile properties of knee joint cartilage: I. Influence of ionic conditions, weight bearing, and fibrillation on the tensile modulus. J Orthop Res 1986;4:379–392.)

friction. The first type is called *surface friction*, where energy dissipation comes from interfacial friction from shear stresses acting to overcome the adhesion of one surface to the other, or viscous dissipation in the lubricant separating the two moving surfaces. The second type of friction is *bulk friction*, and it occurs from the internal energy dissipation within the bulk material or within the lubricant. Surface adhesion is produced most frequently between metal surfaces at the contacting tips of the surfaces' microirregularities. Internal dissipation is caused by the deformations within the bodies in contact. An example of bulk friction is an elastic sphere rolling over a relatively soft viscoelastic material (neglecting air resistance), which eventually comes to rest because the kinetic energy of the rolling ball is dissipated by the internal frictional dissipation within the viscoelastic material. This is

sometimes called *plowing friction*, because harder material (sphere) must plow through the softer material as it moves along. For cartilage, an internal friction is produced by the viscous drag caused when interstitial fluid flows through the porous-permeable solid matrix.[41–45] The coefficient of friction (μ) is commonly used to quantify frictional resistance. It is the ratio of the magnitude of the tangential frictional force (T) that resists the sliding motion, to the magnitude of the normal force (N) that presses the surfaces together ($\mu = T/N$).

Lubrication Two modes of lubrication exist between two sliding contacting surfaces: (1) boundary lubrication and (2) fluid film lubrication.[2–4] Boundary lubrication depends on the thin chemical absorption of a monolayer of lubricant molecules (1–50 nm) on the contacting surfaces (e.g., grease is a common boundary lubricant). During relative sliding motion, the solid surfaces are protected by the lubricant molecules sliding over each other, preventing adhesion and abrasion of the naturally occurring asperities of the surface (Figure 8-19). The molecules thought to be responsible for boundary lubrication in synovial joints have been isolated and are the *lubricating glycoprotein fraction* of synovial fluid or dipalmitoyl phosphatidylcholine (DPPC).[133–135,137] Lubricating glycoprotein consists of a single polypeptide chain containing only oligosaccharides, with a molecular weight of approximately 43,000 dalton, whereas DPPC is much larger at 250,000 dalton.

For fluid film lubrication, a much thicker layer of lubricant is necessary (10–20 μm), as compared with the molecular size of lubricating glycoprotein. This lubricant layer causes relatively wide separation, when compared with the typical surface roughness of normal articular cartilage. The load on the bearing surface is supported by pressure generated in this fluid film. This pressure may be generated in four different ways (Figure 8-20A–D). For *hydrodynamic lubrication*, the noncongruent articulating surfaces move tangentially to

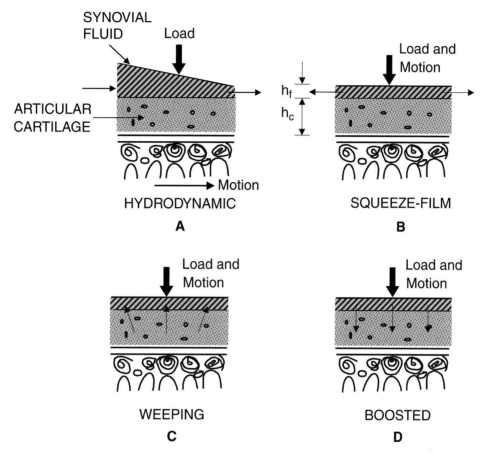

FIGURE 8-20 A. Hydrodynamic lubrication generated by the sliding motion that drags the viscous fluid into a convergent gap. For this mode to be operational, high sliding speed, load, and high viscosity are needed. Theoretical calculations show that synovial fluid film generated by this hydrodynamic action is less than 1 μm (smaller than the typical articular surface irregularities).[2,4] **B.** Squeeze film lubrication occurs when a layer of thin fluid film is squeezed from between the two impinging surfaces. Depending on the force of squeeze action (body weight) and fluid viscosity, for typical cartilage permeability and synovial fluid viscosity, this squeeze film pressure action may only last several seconds before the film is depleted.[137,140,141] **C.** Postulated weeping lubrication[135,136] requires exudation from the cartilage to form a lubricant fluid film. This could be an alternative source of lubricant, although analysis and basic physical considerations do not support this mechanism of film formation.[2,4,137,140,141] **D.** Postulated boosted lubrication[138,139] requires imbibition of fluid by cartilage, leaving a concentrated gel between the two impinging cartilage surfaces. Analyses support this mode of fluid film lubrication.

each other, forming a converging wedge of fluid (see Figure 8-20A); the viscosity of the fluid causes it to be dragged into the converging gap between the surfaces, thus generating a lifting pressure. This mechanism of generating a fluid film is known as *hydrodynamic lubrication*, and it requires high viscosity, low loads, or rapid sliding speeds, none of which is operational in joints. Thus, it is an unlikely candidate for joint lubrication, although it is the dominant mode in man-made machine bearings.[2] If the surfaces are being pressed perpendicularly toward each other, any fluid film that exists in the joint cavity must be squeezed out from the gap between the two surfaces; this squeezing action

also generates a fluid pressure that can support the load (see Figure 8-20B). However, this load-carrying capacity afforded by the squeeze film pressure may only last a few seconds before all the lubricant is squeezed out.[4,136] This mechanism is known as *squeeze film lubrication*, and again for man-made bearing, this is an effective mode of lubrication. The squeeze film lubrication mechanism is particularly effective when there is a large supporting base. It is commonly used to float the large telescopes that need to have precision and frictionless motion. For diarthrodial joints, however, other mechanisms must come into play for fluid to play a viable role in joint lubrication.

If the bearing material is relatively soft, such as articular cartilage, the pressure in the fluid film may cause substantial deformation of the articulating surfaces. These deformations may beneficially alter the fluid film and surface geometries, leading to greater restriction for the joint fluid escape from the contacting area, a longer lasting fluid film, and an increase in its load-carrying capacity. When significant surface deformations are involved in addition to the fluid flow, an *elastohydrodynamic lubrication* mode is said to exist.[2,4,19]

Besides synovial fluid as the lubricant, alternative sources of the lubricant have been postulated. Lubricant fluid film may be generated between the surfaces by the natural compression of the cartilage during joint use, exuding fluid over the articulating surface into the joint cavity (see Figure 8-20C). This has been called *weeping lubrication*.[135,136] This mechanism, however, would require fluid from a low-pressure region in cartilage to flow into a high-pressure region in the synovial fluid. On the other hand, because articular cartilage is porous and permeable, the high pressure in the fluid film could cause the synovial fluid, without the hyaluronate, to flow into the tissue, leaving a concentrated gel in the gap protecting the articulating surfaces (see Figure 8-20D)[2,4,137] This is called *boosted lubrication*.[138–141] Clearly these two hypothetical modes of lubrication are diametrically opposed, and this scientific paradox needed to be resolved. After nearly 40 years, this conundrum was resolved with the publication of three important papers that showed (1) under squeeze film conditions, fluid does indeed flow into the cartilage and may deplete within a few seconds,[136] (2) surface porosity is an important factor determining fluid pressurization at the articular surface,[142] and (3) fluid pressure supports more than 95% of the surface load under dynamic loading conditions.[105] Thus, because fluid pressure supports 95% of the load, the coefficient of friction is expected to be 5% of the normal surface-to-surface contact friction. For many solid-solid contacts, the coefficient of friction is approximately $\mu = 0.3$; thus, for cartilage solid-solid contact (after complete depletion of the synovial fluid) one would expect the coefficient of friction for cartilage-cartilage contact to be $\mu = 0.3 \times 0.05 = 0.015$. Indeed, this value is consistent with all the measured coefficients of friction reported in the literature (Table 8-3).[2,4] These calculations support the concept of boosted lubrication over that proposed for weeping lubrication.

As the articular cartilage surface is not perfectly smooth (see Figure 8-8), and indeed when the thickness of the fluid film is of the same order of magnitude as that of the solid surfaces, then contact between the surface irregularities may be expected to occur (Figure 8-21). These contacts may benefit from the lubrication efficacies of the lubricating glycoprotein, DPPC, and the hyaluronate gel proposed by the boosted lubrication mechanism.[21,133,134,140,141,143] This *mixed lubrication* mechanism may develop during long periods of standing, with the load being carried by both the pressure in the partial fluid film residing in the pockets and at boundary-lubricated contacts.[2,4,140,141]

Measurements of Coefficient of Friction   Friction is a manifestation of dissipation of mechanical energy into heat (e.g., friction from rubbing your hands in cold weather to keep them warm). There are two components that give rise to friction: (1) surface effects, which are shear stresses acting between the two surfaces sliding and breaking adhesive bonds; and (2) bulk effects, plowing (deformation) of the two material bodies, causing internal dissipation. In boundary lubrication, a surface effect, the shear stresses are *independent* of the relative velocity of the two surfaces. If fluid film lubrication exists, changes are observed in the coefficient of friction that *depends* on the changes in either the rela-

TABLE 8-3
Coefficients of Friction for Articular Cartilage in Synovial Joints

Investigator	Coefficient of Friction μ	Joint Tested
Charnley[147]	0.005–0.02	Human ankle
McCutchen[139]	0.02–0.35	Porcine shoulder
Linn[149]	0.005–0.01	Canine ankle
Unsworth et al.[144]	0.01–0.04	Human hip
Malcom[146]	0.002–0.03	Bovine shoulder

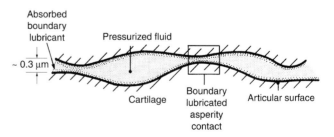

FIGURE 8-21 When the surface irregularities of the articular surfaces ($<50\ \mu m$) are similar in size to the fluid film thickness, contacts between asperities occur, causing a mixed mode of lubrication to develop: boundary lubrication at the contacting asperities and fluid film lubrication over the *pockets* of fluid.

tive velocity of the sliding surfaces or the applied load; this is because of viscous dissipation within the lubricant film. Investigators have employed these basic characteristics (i.e., speed independence or speed dependence) to determine modes of lubrication at the articular surfaces.[2,4,105,140–150] However, if a mixed lubrication mechanism is in place, as is most likely to be the case between articular cartilage contact areas, gross friction measurements alone will not be sufficient to determine the mode of lubrication.[145–150] This had been the long-lasting historical conundrum in the biotribology literature. However, with the advances in understanding boundary lubrication and the load support mechanism at the articular surface, these questions become moot. Indeed, the value of coefficient of friction depends largely on the porosity of the articular surface and the permeability and compressive stiffness of the cartilage; together they dictate the contribution of the interstitial fluid pressure toward load support.

Nevertheless, it is of educational value to review some of the historical methods investigators have used to determine the coefficient of friction in synovial joints and between cartilage surfaces.[133,134,138–141,144–150] First, the coefficient of friction in intact synovial joints has long been known to be extremely low (see Table 8-3). The measurements were originally made on experiments that used a pendulum machine with the joint acting as the fulcrum.[2,4,144–150] Investigators soon learned, however, that such measurements were not sensitive enough to enable them to differentiate between mechanisms of lubrication (boundary or fluid). Some of their results suggested the existence of a fluid film at loads up to body weight. They also noted that in an unlubricated joint, with the synovial fluid removed, the coefficient of friction rapidly returned to normal as load was applied under conditions of plowing friction (Figure 8-22). These results indicate that the friction coefficient decreases with increasing load, and the synovial fluid, above a threshold of load, causes no difference in the frictional properties of joints. This implies that, at physiological load, friction is reduced by either a fluid film generated by the cartilage itself, by the load partition effect at the surface, or by boundary lubrication (lubricating glycoprotein, DPPC, or both).

Another experimental design used for friction testing is one that slides small pieces of cartilage over another surface (Figure 8-23). In these experiments, the entire surface is loaded, eliminating the plowing effect.[139,146] In this type of experiment, researchers found that synovial fluid caused less sliding friction than a buffer lubricant and that there was a much greater reduction in friction coefficient for dynamically applied load than static load

(Figure 8-24). With the advances on the understanding of load partition and support at the articular surface, this second effect is thought to be caused by the increased pressurization of the interstitial fluid at the cartilage surface, and hence increased load partition support by the fluid.[105,142]

In summary, synovial joints are able to withstand a wide range of loading and moving conditions, such as (1) lightly loaded high-speed motions (e.g., the swing phase of gait or throwing motion at the shoulder); (2) loads of large magnitude and short duration (e.g., jumping or other impact loading); and (3) fixed steady loads (e.g., standing for long periods). These joints enjoy remarkable lubricating mechanisms, allowing them to function with almost negligible resistance in any situation. It is unlikely that this can be achieved by a single mode of lubrication. Elastohydrodynamic fluid

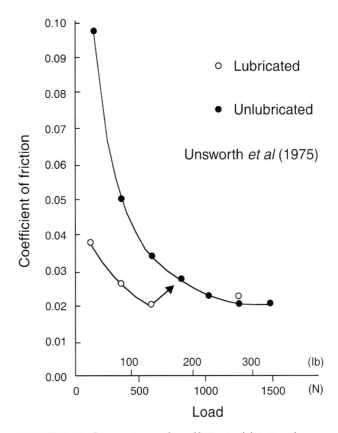

FIGURE 8-22 Comparison of coefficient of friction for an unlubricated hip at various load levels. At physiological load levels, the coefficient of friction of unlubricated hips approaches that of the lubricated hip. (Reprinted with permission fron A Unsworth, D Dowson, V Wright. The frictional behavior of human synovial joints: I. Natural joints. J Lubr Technol 1975;97:360–376.)

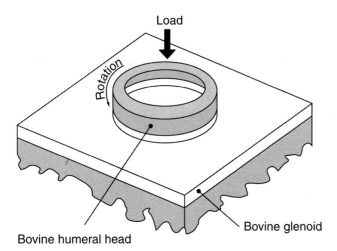

FIGURE 8-23 Surface friction measurements using an annulus of bovine humeral head cartilage sliding in a rotary manner over the surface of a mating glenoid cartilage surface. Both surfaces are nearly spherical and congruent, thus eliminating plowing effects; only surface friction is measured. (Reprinted with permission from LL Malcom. An Experimental Investigation of the Friction and Deformational Responses of Articular Cartilage Interfaces to Static and Dynamic Loading. Thesis, University of California, San Diego, 1976.)

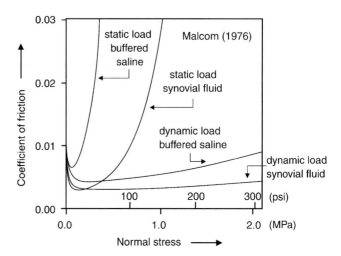

FIGURE 8-24 Surface friction from experiment defined in Figure 8-23 under various loading and lubricating conditions. (Reprinted with permission from LL Malcom. An Experimental Investigation of the Friction and Deformational Responses of Articular Cartilage Interfaces to Static and Dynamic Loading. Thesis, University of California, San Diego, 1976.)

films of both the sliding and squeeze type probably play a vital role in the lubrication of the joint. Surface load partition also plays an important role for loading of long duration. The source of the fluid film appears to come from both synovial fluid and interstitial fluid of the ECM. As the loading conditions become more severe, the fluid flow rate and fluid pressurization slowly decrease. The cartilage, though, can still remain protected through an absorbed layer of boundary lubricant of either lubricating glycoprotein or DPPC. At present, it is impossible, however, to state under which conditions a particular lubrication mechanism may be in effect. It is possible that a combination of mechanisms (mixed mode) will be operating at any time.

RESPONSE OF CARTILAGE TO IMMOBILIZATION AND RUPTURE OF THE ANTERIOR CRUCIATE LIGAMENT IN THE KNEE

Ligamentous injuries and joint immobilization result in altered or lost normal physiological loading conditions of the joint, bone, and cartilage. Atrophic changes of musculoskeletal tissues always occur when function is altered or lost (e.g., loss of bone mass during prolonged

space flight). For articular cartilage there are definable and consistent changes that have been measured and defined. These changes fit well into our total understanding of normal and pathologic physiology of articular cartilage. Clinically, ligamentous injuries result in joint instability, and immobilization involves a loss of motion (e.g., plaster immobilization for fracture healing), altered or loss of normal joint loading from prolonged bed rest, paralysis of a limb or amputation, or a combination of such situations. The lack of clinical specimens has generally precluded detailed studies of cartilage specimens from patients, and the use of cadaveric materials has become common.[9,10,73,85] Therefore, for OA studies on fresh specimens or early in the OA process, a number of animal models have been developed by researchers to examine the effects of joint injury (e.g., impact loading, transection of the cruciate ligaments, or meniscectomy) and immobilization on altered or unloaded articular cartilage.[74–76,151–168] Indeed, many other studies have shown consistent and significant changes in the morphology, biochemistry, and biomechanical properties of the cartilage.[9,10]

The consistency of these research findings is striking, thus the results of only a few are reviewed and discussed here. (The reader is referred to references 9, 10, and 156 for more extended discussions of this subject.) For example, using a rabbit model, Finsterbush and Friedman (1973) showed by both light and electron microscopes that there are early changes in the surface

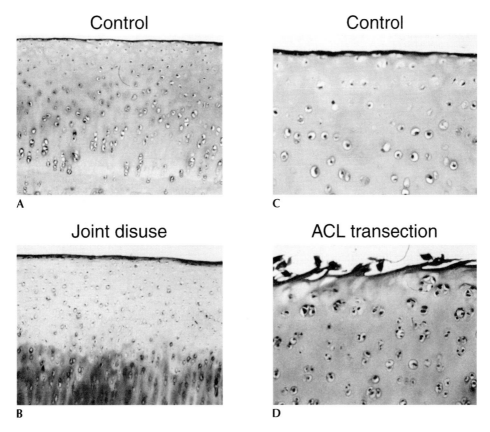

FIGURE 8-25 Comparisons of four histologic sections stained for proteoglycans and collagen. **A.** A control normal canine knee cartilage histologic section showing characteristic chondrocyte morphology and distribution, uniform safranin O staining, dense collagen in the superficial tangential zone, and a smooth articular surface. **B.** A histologic section of a sample of cartilage from an immobilized canine knee. Note the loss of safranin O staining while the articular surface remains smooth and intact. All chondrocytes are alive and maintain their shape. **C.** A control normal canine knee cartilage histologic section showing characteristic chondrocyte morphology and distribution, uniform safranin O staining, dense collagen in the superficial tangential zone, and a smooth articular surface. **D.** A histologic section of a sample of cartilage from a canine knee with its anterior cruciate ligament (ACL) transected. Note that the collagen network of the surfaces is severely damaged and there is a loss of safranin O staining, indicating a significant loss of proteoglycan. Chondrocytes show necrosis (voids) and cloning.

morphology of cartilage from the immobilized rabbit knee joints with 3–6 weeks of immobilization.[151] These surface morphologic changes are quite similar to those found in human hip and knee specimens harvested from surgery and as examined by scanning electron microscopy.[103,104] Later, Caterson and Lowther (1978),[152] using a below-the-knee (stifle joint) amputation sheep model, and Palmoski and coworkers (1979),[153] using a knee immobilization canine model, found that after 6–8 weeks, although the gross appearance of the cartilage remained normal (i.e., white and smooth appearing to the naked eye), the biochemical measures showed that PG concentrations were greatly altered. Figure 8-25 shows a comparison of four histologic sections stained for PGs and collagen. Top left shows a control for a normal canine cartilage histologic section and bottom left shows a cartilage section from a knee that has been immobilized. Top right shows a control for a normal canine cartilage histologic section, and bottom right shows a histologic section of cartilage from a tested knee where the anterior cruciate ligament (ACL) has been transected.

Note that the collagen network of the surfaces of the ACL-transected knee is severely damaged and there is a loss of safranin O staining, indicating a significant loss of PG. Damage to the surface collagen network has been shown to result in increased swelling,[42,44,87,89] diminution of mechanical properties,[114,119,123,124,159] and adverse load carriage characteristics by cartilage with less hydrodynamic load support.[97,105] Over the past 25 years, the canine ACL transection model has been widely used to study the OA initiation and progression processes.[9,10,124,157-159] Today, ACL rupture is a common clinical occurrence in many sports-related activities, particularly skiing. The joint instability after ACL transection results in an altered load transmission process across the joint, which in turn initiates tissue damage biologically and biomechanically that is quite severe and often proceeds to frank OA in the injured joint, including bone remodeling, subchondral eburnation, and osteophyte formation at the joint margins.[9,10,124,158]

Joint immobilization, however, produces quite different, although milder, pathologic changes in cartilage. The bottom left of Figure 8-25 shows a histologic section of cartilage from an immobilized knee.[75] Note that the surface is not damaged from immobilization but there is a significant loss of PGs near the surface. Again, in the context of our understanding of collagen and PG in providing a structure and function to cartilage, one can easily see how these changes can affect all its biomechanical, physicochemical, and electromechanical properties.[11,13,41-46,123,124,159] In those joints that were immobilized there were no synovial effusions and no osteophytes, and the radiographic appearance was normal except for slight bone demineralization. In spite of the grossly normal appearance, there was progressive loss of staining by safranin O (see Figure 8-25, bottom left). This was accompanied by a reduction in PG synthesis and gradual loss of PG aggregation.[10,152,153] These results indicate that changes in the contact area and the absence of weight-bearing forces are both responsible for atrophic changes of the immobilized articular cartilage.[74-76,155-159] These degenerative cartilage changes caused by immobilization or loss of weight bearing may be reversible on remobilization and reloading of the joint and are a major distinguishing factor from those cartilage changes induced by ACL transection where changes have been shown to be progressive and degenerative.[74-76,153,154,158] With remobilization, the chondrocytes are stimulated to increase production of the PG aggrecans and link proteins. With the hyaluronate present, these molecules are assembled into PG aggregates again, tending to restore cartilage to its original form. However, this restoration process is not complete for full recovery.[74-76,154,155] Excessive mechanical loading immediately after prolonged immobilization, such as running after removal of a cast, also inhibits reversal of atrophic changes in knee cartilage.[76,156] In all cases, recovery is stimulated by joint function and loading, but not excessive amounts such as running.

In summary, local mechanical factors, in the form of both joint loading and joint motion, appear to play important physiological roles in the maintenance of normal articular cartilage. The changes described in these models of joint injury bear a striking resemblance to those seen in human osteoarthritic process; changes caused by immobilization appear to be reversible under certain conditions, whereas osteoarthritic changes are progressive with time. Thus, immobilization alone may not be a good OA model. Immobilization, in combination with strenuous exercise, may prove to be a more accurate model of OA, although this model has not been studied extensively.

RESPONSE OF CARTILAGE TO EXERCISE

As discussed previously, both clinical and basic science studies have demonstrated the importance of physiological joint loading on the maintenance of healthy articular cartilage. Moderate exercise is generally believed to enhance and facilitate the beneficial processes of normal cartilage function. Indeed, canine studies on life-long running have shown no deleterious effects on knee cartilage.[160] Also, epidemiologic studies have shown that running does not predispose runners to a higher frequency of OA.[161-163] Conversely, abnormal joint loading from impact may cause irreparable damage to cartilage or contribute to cartilage degeneration.[164-168] In these cases, in which the impact loading is significantly high, as in the case of the *dashboard knee syndrome*, there are subchondral bone microfractures and bone remodeling that accompany the cartilage damage. Damage to the cartilage begins with microfractures of the collagen network at the articular surface and shearing of the cartilage layer off the subchondral bone. The latter leads to the often diagnosed *occult lesions* that are not observable by radiologic or arthroscopic means. The former leads to cartilage swelling (increased water content) and its associated cascade of events discussed previously.

Biochemically, the composition and structure of articular cartilage are maintained through a balance of the anabolic and catabolic activities maintained by the chondrocyte population.[9,10,38-40,48,49,52,80] Chondrocytes are able to perceive and respond to signals generated by the normal load-bearing activities of daily living, such as walking and running. Joint loading produces deformation of the cartilage layer and subsequently changes the mechanoelectrochemical environment of the individual chondrocytes.[39,51,52,132] Chondrocytes respond to spatially and temporally varying tensile, compressive, and shear stresses and strains, as well as fluid pressures and electrical voltage and current by altering their metabolic activity to change the structure and composition of the cartilage in which they reside.[9,10,52] Various models have been developed to evaluate the effects of normal and abnormal joint loading on cartilage in vitro and in vivo. Exercise simulated by cyclic loading has been shown to produce biological responses in articular cartilage opposite to those changes seen in OA degeneration. Cyclic or intermittent compression of in vitro articular cartilage has been shown to increase aggrecan synthesis.[169,170]

It has been well demonstrated that prolonged compressive joint loading is associated with deleterious effects on articular cartilage.[171-173] Static compression of articular cartilage in vitro may be used to model the effects of cast immobilization or underactivity. A study by Sah and coworkers (1990) and Guilak and coworkers (1994) found that low levels of compressive loads suppress PG synthesis[39,174,175]; however, normal PG synthesis returns after the load is released. These studies also showed that release of slightly higher and moderately prolonged loads in fact stimulates increased PG biosynthesis by the chondrocytes; however, a longer recovery time is required before the cartilage is able to withstand normal loads again. This may represent a reparative phase. At the extreme, high levels of compression result in cell death.[38-40]

RESPONSE OF CARTILAGE TO AGING AND OSTEOARTHRITIS

Generally, cartilage degeneration results in the development of fibrillation and fissures at the surface, the appearance of gross ulceration, and partial or complete loss of the full thickness of the tissue. This is also accompanied by an increase in cartilage hydration, subchondral bone changes, osteophytosis, altered chondrocyte activity, and changes in the structure and composition of the PGs, collagen, and other macromolecules in the cartilage (see Figure 8-25). Moreover, at the clinical stage of the disease, changes caused by OA involve not only the cartilage but also the synovial membrane, where an inflammatory reaction is often observed.[9,10] Therefore, OA is considered a group of diseases characterized by degenerative, regenerative, and reparative structural changes in all joint tissues, including articular cartilage, synovium, periarticular connective tissues, and so forth. A definition of OA underscores the concept that OA may not represent a single disease entity[10]:

> OA is a group of overlapping distinct diseases, which may have different etiologies but with similar biologic, morphologic, and clinical outcomes. The disease processes not only affect the articular cartilage, but involve the entire joint, including the

subchondral bone, ligaments, capsule, synovial membrane, and periarticular muscles. Ultimately, the articular cartilage degenerates with fibrillation, fissures, ulceration, and full thickness loss of the joint surface.

The morbidity and economic costs resulting from OA are staggering when measured in terms of loss of function, medical costs, and lost wages. At present, it is estimated that more than 35 million Americans suffer this disabling disease. One survey shows that the annual cost of OA would appear to approach $13,000 per case.[176] With the large prevalence of OA, the overall economic impact of OA is significant.

How does OA develop when there is no obvious antecedent injury to either the joint or the cartilage? This question has been studied extensively, but no clear answers have yet been found. In this section, the changes of articular cartilage during this degenerative process are presented, followed by some thoughts on the etiology of OA.

HISTOLOGIC AND MORPHOLOGIC CHANGES

Macroscopic evidence of OA can be observed on gross examination of the cartilage surface. The earliest findings in OA include flaking and pitting of the surface (see Figure 8-8). As the degenerative process continues, deep fissuring occurs, giving the cartilage a frayed appearance known as *cartilage fibrillation*.[9,10] The final stage of this process is a completely denuded surface exposing the underlying eburnated bone.

Many attempts have been made to quantify the degree of surface damage, both macroscopically and microscopically. Emery and Meachim described and popularized a technique in which the cartilage surface is stained with India ink and then rinsed off lightly with Ringer's solution.[177] Ink particles lodge in any surface irregularities, causing a dark stain. The degree of staining can then be graded as minimal, moderate, or severe, providing a macroscopic view of articular surface damage. Microscopically, cellular injury may be evident, showing only the ghost outlines of the chondrocytes remaining (Figures 8-8 and 8-25). The structural integrity may change microscopically, with clefts and fissures that traverse the ECM. There also may be loss of PGs, as noted on safranin O staining. Finally, there is loss of tidemark integrity as blood vessels cross the tidemark to effect a reparative response. Mankin and coworkers (1971) developed a semiquantitative grading scheme to evaluate the histologic and histochemical changes in the cartilage (Table 8-4).[178] These scores are generally accepted as providing a *semiquantitative measure* of cartilage degeneration during OA when compared with the modern day biochemically and biomechanically measured data.

Microscopic evidence also demonstrates the presence of a reparative process occurring in cartilage during the OA process. This reparative cartilage comes from two sources: (1) the damaged cartilage itself, in the form of cell proliferation and new matrix synthesis; and (2) tissue outside the joint, located on the periphery of the joint, the subchondral bone, or both.[10] Cartilage from the joint margin may be seen as a cellular layer of cartilage extending over, or penetrating into, existing cartilage. From denuded bone, small nodules of fibrocartilage develop.[10,178] Microscopically, fibrocartilage is a fibrous-appearing tissue in which the cells are spindle-like, with a higher density within the tissue. The collagen formed is much more likely type I than type II. In some joints, these

TABLE 8-4
Histologic-Histochemical Grading of Osteoarthritic Change in Cartilage

	Grade
I. Structure	
a. Normal	0
b. Surface irregularities	1
c. Pannus and surface irregularities	2
d. Clefts to transitional zone	3
e. Clefts to radial zone	4
f. Clefts to calcified zone	5
g. Complete disorganization	6
II. Cells	
a. Normal	0
b. Diffuse hypercellularity	1
c. Cloning	2
d. Hypocellularity	3
III. Safranin O staining	
a. Normal	0
b. Slight reduction	1
c. Moderate reduction	2
d. Severe reduction	3
e. No strain noted	4
IV. Tidemark integrity	
a. Intact	0
b. Crossed by blood vessels	1

Source: HJ Mankin, H Dorfman, L Lippiello, et al. Biochemical and metabolic abnormalities in articular cartilage from osteoarthritic human hips. II. Correlation of morphology with biochemical and metabolic data. J Bone Joint Surg 1971;53A:523–537.

nodules of fibrocartilage may form an apparently continuous layer of tissue over the denuded surface.

OA begins in the articular cartilage (see Figure 8-25), but eventually involves the surrounding tissues, bone, and synovium. When the cartilage is absent from the articular surface, the underlying bone is subject to greater local stresses. By Wolff's law of bone remodeling, new bone formation at these areas is expected, resulting in the bony sclerosis that is often seen on radiographs of arthritic joints.[10,179] Subarticular bone cysts are also commonly seen on radiography. They exist only in the absence of overlying cartilage. Bone cysts are a result of the transmission of intra-articular pressure into the marrow spaces of the subchondral bone. The cysts increase in size until the pressure in them is equal to the intra-articular pressure. If the joint becomes covered with reparative cartilage, the cysts may regress.[9,10] Finally, because of the breakdown of both cartilage and bone, a chronic inflammatory response is produced in the synovium of the joint that is generally thought to be the source of pain.

OA is not only a degenerative process, but rather an active, dynamic process including both degeneration and repair. Remodeling of the bone occurs at the joint margins through the formation of osteophytes. Osteophytes form because of enchondral ossification of both the existing cartilage and reparative cartilage from the joint margin. Remodeling of the joint can be considerable. The presence of osteophytes in clinically asymptomatic joints confirms that this reparative process can be effective in increasing joint stability. The new bone formation (osteophytes) and remodeling of the joint might help restoration of tissue loss and better distribution of mechanical forces across the compromised joint.

EFFECTS OF AGING ON BIOMECHANICAL PROPERTIES OF CARTILAGE

The correlation of OA with aging still remains unexplained, because OA often develops parallel with aging, making it difficult to separate the initiation of OA from the effects of age.[9,10] It is, therefore, necessary to characterize the normal age-related changes in cartilage, such that direct comparison between diseased and healthy tissue can be easier. (Effects of OA on biomechanical properties of articular cartilage, in human and animal models, have been discussed previously.) There are many studies on age-related changes in cartilage biomechanical properties, which have shown that OA is not necessarily an inevitable event during the aging process.[9,10]

In a study on aging and maturation, using bovine knee specimens, Roth and Mow (1980) examined the variation of the intrinsic tensile modulus of normal bovine auricular cartilage with skeletal maturity.[68] It is well known that the existence of a physis (growth plate) is an indication of skeletal immaturity; those bones that came from skeletally matured animals did not have a growth plate.[180] The investigators found significant differences in the stiffness and failure stress of cartilage specimens harvested from bones with or without a physis. For cartilage from the skeletally immature group, the failure stress of the surface was 12 MPa and that of the deep zone was 24.5 MPa. For cartilage from the skeletally mature group, these values were 12 MPa for the surface and 3 MPa for the deep zone. No statistical differences were found for the tensile strength of the superficial zone. These findings indicate that, with skeletal maturation, the subsurface zones of the cartilage become mechanically inferior compared with the surface layer; indeed there is a gradual but steady diminution of the tensile stiffness and strength with depth from the surface. These results are entirely consistent with those found in older, normal, human cadaveric knee cartilage (see Figure 8-18).[66] Apparently, after the closure of the physis with skeletal maturation, the physiology of the deep region of cartilage is altered from a region that was nourished by the nearby vascular-rich marrow that resides within the subjacent trabecular bone, to a region that is deep and far away from nutrient sources within the joint space. Moreover, there is a complete closure formed by the impermeable tidemark and the calcified zone after maturation (see Figure 8-6).[47,98,99] This dramatic and sudden change alters the deep zone chondrocyte metabolism, thus affecting both the collagen ultrastructure and PG molecular architecture of the uncalcified cartilage of the deep zone; these changes are also known to change the mechanical properties of the deep zone ECM.[48-50,181-183]

In a more recent study by Kempson (1991), the age-related changes in the tensile property between the femoral head of the hip joint and the talus of the ankle joint were compared.[184] The zone-specific results showed that the tensile failure stress of cartilage from both the superficial and middle zones of the femoral head decreased significantly with increasing age, but this was not seen from both zones of cartilage from the talus of the ankle joint. These results provided a potential explanation of the site-specific prevalence of OA; it commonly occurs in the hip and knee joints with aging, whereas it only rarely occurs in the ankle joint.

SUMMARY

This chapter has provided a thorough discussion on the structure and function relationship of healthy, aging, and OA articular cartilage and joints. Major advances have been made over the past 25 years that defined the details of articular cartilage biochemistry and molecular architecture of type II collagen, PG aggrecans, and aggregates. Equally impressive have been the advances made on chondrocyte biology, the mechanoelectrochemical signal transduction process through the ECM to the cells, and the nature of the signals that might be the regulator of chondrocytes' biosynthetic activities. Finally, in the major emphasis of this chapter, cartilage biomechanics have been presented not only in its present robust form, but also in its historical prospective. During the first 75 years of the twentieth century, basic cartilage biomechanics studies by German anatomists (ca. 1920s), Swedish orthopedic surgeons (ca. 1950s), and English bioengineers (ca. 1960s) led the way, demonstrating the need for more sophisticated theories and experiments in cartilage research. Their results provided the basis for an explosion of new ideas, not only in cartilage biomechanics but also in cartilage biochemistry and physiology that occurred over the past 25 years. One can look confidently into the twenty-first century for even greater gains in scientific advances in these areas; perhaps one may dare to speculate that even a full understanding of the etiology of OA may be developed, with new clinical treatment modalities of care and cure.

Acknowledgments
This work was sponsored by grants from the National Institutes of Health: AR38733, AR41020, and AR41913. Thanks are due to Dr. Alexandre Terrier from the Swiss Federal Institute of Technology in Lausanne, Switzerland, for his helpful assistance in the preparation of this manuscript.

REFERENCES

1. William PL. Gray's Anatomy (38th ed). New York: Churchill and Livingston, 1995;486–510.

2. Dowson D. Basic Tribology. In D Dowson, V Wright (eds), Introduction to the Biomechanics of Joints and Joint Replacement. London: Mechanical Engineering Publications, 1981;49–60.

3. Mow VC, Ateshian GA, Spilker RL.

Biomechanics of diarthrodial joints: a review of twenty years of progress. J Biomech Eng 1993;115:460–467.

4. Mow VC, Ateshian GA. Lubrication and Wear of Diarthrodial Joints. In VC Mow, WC Hayes (eds), Basic Orthopaedic Biomechanics (2nd ed). Philadelphia: Lippincott-Raven, 1997;275–315.

5. Lipshitz H, Glimcher MJ. In-vitro studies of the wear of articular cartilage. II. Characteristics of the wear of articular cartilage when worn against stainless steel plates having characterized surfaces. Wear 1979;52:297–339.

6. Morrison JB. The mechanics of the knee in relation to normal walking. J Biomech 1970;3:164–170.

7. Paul JP. Joint Kinetics. In L Sokoloff (ed), The Joints and Synovial Fluid. Vol 11. New York: Academic Press, 1978;146–176.

8. Hodge WA, Fijan RS, Carlson KL, et al. Contact pressures in the human hip joint measured in vivo. Proc Natl Acad Sci U S A 1986;83:2879–2883.

9. Howell DS, Treadwell BV, Trippel SB. Etiopathogenesis of Osteoarthritis. In RW Moskowitz, DS Howell, VM Goldberg, et al. (eds), Osteoarthritis: Diagnosis and Medical/Surgical Management (2nd ed). Philadelphia: WB Saunders, 1992;233–252.

10. Brandt KD, Doherty M, Lohmander LS (eds). Osteoarthritis. Oxford: Oxford University Press, 1998.

11. Mankin HJ, Mow VC, Buckwalter JA, et al. Structure and Function of Articular Cartilage. In SR Simon (ed), Orthopaedic Basic Science. Rosemont, IL: Amer Acad Orthop Surg Publ, 1994;1–44.

12. Maroudas A, Kuettner KE. Methods in Cartilage Research. San Diego, CA: Academic Press, 1990.

13. Mow VC, Ratcliffe A. Structure and Function of Articular Cartilage and Meniscus. In VC Mow, WC Hayes (eds), Basic Orthopaedic Biomechanics (2nd ed). Philadelphia: Lippincott-Raven, 1997;113–177.

14. Hardingham TE, Fosang A. Proteoglycans: many forms and many functions. FASEB J 1992;6:861–870.

15. Comper WD. Extracellular Matrix. Australia: Harwood Academic Publishers, 1996.

16. Mow VC, Arnoczky SP. Jackson DL (eds). Knee Meniscus: Basic and Clinical Foundations. New York: Raven Press, 1992.

17. Ropes MW, Bauer W. Synovial Fluid Changes in Joint Diseases. Cambridge, MA: Harvard University Press, 1953.

18. Fraser RE, Laurent TC. Hyaluronan. In WD Comper (ed), Extracellular Matrix. Australia: Hardwood Academic Publishers, 1996;141–199.

19. Dintenfass L. Lubrication in synovial joints: a theoretical analysis. J Bone Joint Surg 1963;45A:1241–1256.

20. Lai WM, Kuei SC, Mow VC. Rheological equations for synovial fluids. J Biomech Eng 1978;100:169–186.

21. Swann DA, Radin EL, Hendren RB. The lubrication of articular cartilage by synovial fluid. Arthritis Rheum 1979;22:665–669.

22. Jay GD, Hong BS. Characterization of a bovine synovial fluid lubricating factor. Connect Tissue Res 1992;28:71–98.

23. Wik HB, Wik O. Rheology of Hyaluronan. In TC Laurent (ed), The Chemistry, Biology and Medical Applications of Hyaluronan and Its Derivatives. Wenner-Gren International Series. London: Portland Press, Ltd, 1998;25–32.

24. Maroudas A. Physicochemical Properties of Articular Cartilage. In MAR Freeman (ed), Adult Articular Cartilage (2nd ed). Kent, UK: Pittman Medical Publishing, 1979;215–290.

25. Maroudas A, Bullough P, Swanson SAV, et al. The permeability of articular cartilage. J Bone Joint Surg 1968;50B:166–177.

26. Chou T, Lohse D. Entropy-driven pumping in zeolites and biological channels. Phys Rev Lett 1999;82:3552–3555.

27. Huiskes R, Kreners H, de Lange A, et al. Analytical stereophotogrammetric determination of three-dimensional knee-joint anatomy. J Biomech 1985;18:559–570.

28. Ateshian GA, Soslowsky LJ, Mow VC. Quantitation of articular surface topography and cartilage thickness in knee joints using stereophotogrammetry. J Biomech 1991;24:761–776.

29. Ateshian GA, Soslowsky LJ. Quantitative Anatomy of Diarthrodial Joint Articular Layers. In VC Mow, WC Hayes (eds), Basic Orthopaedic Biomechanics (2nd ed). Philadelphia: Lippincott-Raven, 1997;252–273.

30. Eckstein F, Sittek H, Gavazzeni A, et al. Magnetic resonance chondro-crassometry (MR-CCM): a method for accurate determination of articular cartilage thickness. Magn Reson Med 1996;35:89–96.

31. Blankevoort L, Huiskes R, de Lange A. The envelope of passive knee motion. J Biomech 1988;21:705–720.

32. Andriacchi TP, Natarajan RN, Hurwitz WE. Musculoskeletal Dynamics, Locomotion and Clinical Applications. In VC Mow, WC Hayes (eds), Basic Orthopaedic Biomechanics (2nd ed). Philadelphia: Lippincott-Raven, 1997;37–68.

33. Cooney WP, Chao EYS. Biomechanical analysis of static forces in the thumb during hand function. J Bone Joint Surg 1977;59A:27–36.

34. Xu LF, Strauch RJ, Ateshian GA, et al. Topography of the osteoarthritic thumb carpometacarpal joint and its variation with gender, age, site and osteoarthritic staging. J Hand Surg 1998;23A:454–464.

35. An KN, Chao EYS, Kaufman KR. Analysis of Muscle and Joint Loads. In VC Mow, WC Hayes (eds), Basic Orthopaedic Biomechanics (2nd ed). Philadelphia: Lippincott-Raven, 1997;1–36.

36. Amis AA, Dowson D, Wright V. Elbow joint force predictions for some strenuous isometric actions. J Biomech 1980;13:765–775.

37. Soslowsky LJ, Flatow EL, Bigliani LU, et al. Quantitation of in situ contact areas at the glenohumeral joint: a biomechanical study. J Orthop Res 1992;10:524–534.

38. Stockwell RA. Biology of Cartilage Cells. Cambridege, UK: Cambridge University Press, 1979;7–31.

39. Guilak F, Sah RL, Setton LA. Physical Regulation of Cartilage Metabolism. In VC Mow, WC Hayes (eds), Basic Orthopaedic Biomechanics (2nd ed). Philadelphia: Lippincott-Raven, 1997;179–207.

40. Stockwell RA. The cell density of human articular and costal cartilage. J Anat 1967;101:753–763.

41. Ateshian GA, Warden WH, Kim JJ, et al. Finite deformation biphasic material properties of bovine articular cartilage from confined compression experiments. J Biomech 1997;30:1157–1164.

42. Mow VC, Ateshian GA, Lai WM, Gu WY. Effects of fixed charges on the stress-relaxation behavior of hydrated soft tissues in a confined compression problem. Int J Solids Structures 1998;35:4945–4962.

43. Mow VC, Kuei SC, Lai WM, Armstrong CG. Biphasic creep and stress relaxation of articular cartilage in compression: theory and experiments. J Biomech Eng 1980;102:73–84.

44. Lai WM, Hou JS, Mow VC. A triphasic theory for the swelling and deforma-

tional behaviors of articular cartilage. J Biomech Eng 1991;113:245–258.

45. Mow VC, Holmes MH, Lai WM. Fluid transport and mechanical properties of articular cartilage. J Biomech 1984;17:377–394.

46. Gu WY, Lai WM, Mow VC. A mixture theory for charged hydrated soft tissues containing multi-electrolytes: passive transport and swelling behaviors. J Biomech Eng 1998;120:169–180.

47. Bullough PG, Jasannath P. The morphology of the calcified front in articular cartilage: its significance in joint function. J Bone Joint Surg 1983;65B:72–78.

48. Muir H. Chondrocyte, architect of cartilage: biomechanics, structure, function and molecular biology of cartilage matrix macromolecules. Bioassay 1995;17:1039–1048.

49. Aydelotte MB, Schumacher BL, Kuettner KE. Heterogeneity of Articular Chondrocytes. In KE Kuettner, et al (eds), Articular Cartilage and Osteoarthritis. New York: Raven Press, 1992;237–249.

50. Poole AC. Articular cartilage chondron: form, function, and failure. J Anat 1997;191:1–13.

51. Guilak F, Mow VC. The mechanical environment of the chondrocyte: a biphasic finite element model of cell-matrix interaction in articular cartilage. J Biomech 2000. In review.

52. Mow VC, Wang CB, Hung CT. The extracellular matrix, interstitial fluid and ions as a mechanical signal transducer in articular cartilage. Osteoarthritis Cartilage 1999;7:41–58.

53. Guilak F. Compression-induced changes in the shape and volume of the chondrocyte nucleus. J Biomech 1995;28:1529–1542.

54. Bachrach NM, Valhmu WB, Stazzone E, et al. Changes in proteoglycan synthesis of chondrocytes in articular cartilage are associated with the time dependent changes in their mechanical environment. J Biomech 1996;28:1561–1569.

55. Hall AC, Urban JPG, Gehl KA. The effect of hydrostatic pressure on matrix synthesis in articular cartilage. J Orthop Res 1991;9:1–10.

56. Kim YJ, Bonassar LJ, Grodzinsky AJ. The role of cartilage streaming potential, fluid flow and pressure in the stimulation of chondrocyte biosynthesis during dynamic compression. J Biomech 1995;28:1055–1066.

57. Parkkinen JJ, Lammi MJ, Inkinen R, et al. Influence of short-term hydrostatic pressure on organization of stress fibers in cultured chondrocytes. J Orthop Res 1995;13:495–502.

58. Sah RLY, Kim YJ, Doong J-YH, et al. Biosynthetic response of cartilage explants to dynamic compression. J Orthop Res 1989;7:619–636.

59. Schneiderman R, Keret D, Maroudas A. Effects of mechanical and osmotic pressure on the rate of glycosaminoglycan synthesis in the human adult femoral head cartilage: an in vitro study. J Orthop Res 1986;4:393–408.

60. Eyre DR. Collagen: molecular diversity in the body's protein scaffold. Science 1980;207:1315–1322.

61. Nimni ME, Harkness RD. Molecular Structure and Functions of Collagen. In ME Nimni (ed), Collagen. Boca Raton, FL: CRC Press, 1988;1–78.

62. Hardingham TE, Muir H, Kwan MK, et al. Viscoelastic properties of proteoglycan solutions with varying proportions present as aggregates. J Orthop Res 1987;5:36–46.

63. Mow VC, Zhu WB, Lai WM, et al. The influence of link protein stabilization on the viscometric properties of proteoglycan aggregate solutions. Biochim Biophys Acta 1989;112:201–208.

64. Maroudas A. Determination of the Rate of Glycosaminoglycan Synthesis In Vivo Using Radioactive Sulfate Tracers: Comparison with In Vitro Results. In A Maroudas, KE Kuettner (eds), Methods in Cartilage Research. New York: Academic Press, 1990:143–148.

65. Valhmu WB, Stazzone EJ, Bachrach NM, et al. Load controlled compression of articular cartilage induces a transient stimulation of aggrecan gene expression. Arch Biochem Biophys 1998;353:29–36.

66. Akizuki S, Mow VC, Muller F, et al. Tensile properties of knee joint cartilage: I. Influence of ionic conditions, weight bearing, and fibrillation on the tensile modulus. J Orthop Res 1986;4:379–392.

67. Kempson GE, Tuke MA, Dingle JT, et al. The effects of proteolytic enzymes on the mechanical properties of adult articular cartilage. Biochim Biophys Acta 1976;428:741–760.

68. Roth V, Mow VC. The intrinsic tensile behavior of the matrix of bovine articular cartilage and its variation with age. J Bone Joint Surg 1980;62A:1102–1117.

69. Schmidt MB, Mow VC, Chun LE, Eyre DR. Effects of proteoglycan extraction on the tensile behavior of articular cartilage. J Orthop Res 1990;8:353–363.

70. Heinegard D, Bayliss M, Lorenzo P. Biochemistry and Metabolism of Normal and Osteoarthritic Cartilage. In KD Brandt, M Doherty, LS Lohmander (eds), Osteoarthritis. Oxford, UK: Oxford University Press, 1998;74–84.

71. Buckwalter JA, Rosenberg LC. Structural changes during development in bovine fetal epiphyseal cartilage. Coll Rel Res 1983;3:489–504.

72. Buckwalter JA, Kuettner KE, Thonar EJM. Age-related changes in articular cartilage proteoglycans: electron microscopic studies. J Orthop Res 1985;3:251–257.

73. Perricone E, Palmoski M, Brandt K. The effect of disuse of the joint on proteoglycan (PG) aggregation in articular cartilage. Clin Res 1977;25:616–622.

74. Saamanen AM, Tammi M, Jurvelin J, et al. Proteoglycan alterations following immobilization and remobilization in the articular cartilage of young canine knee (stifle) joint. J Orthop Res 1990;8:863–873.

75. Setton LA, Mow VC, Muller FJ, et al. Mechanical behavior and biochemical composition of canine knee cartilage following periods of joint disuse and disuse with remobilization. Osteoarthritis Cartilage 1997;5:1–16.

76. Haapala J, Arokoski JP, Hyttinen MM, et al. Remobilization dose not fully restore immobilization induced articular cartilage atrophy. Clin Orthop 1999;362:218–229.

77. Muir H. Proteoglycans as organizers of the extracellular matrix. Biochem Soc Trans 1983;11: 613–622.

78. Hardingham TE. Proteoglycans: their structure, interactions and molecular organization in cartilage. Biochem Soc Trans 1981;9:489–497.

79. Pottenger LA, Lyon NB, Hecht JD, et al. Influence of cartilage particle size and proteoglycan aggregation on immobilization of proteoglycans. J Biol Chem 1982;257:11479–11485.

80. Ratcliffe A, Tyler JA, Hardingham TE. Articular cartilage cultured with interleukin 1: increase release of link protein, hyaluronate-binding region, and other proteoglycan fragments. Biochem J 1986;238:571–580.

81. Bollett AJ, Nance JL. Biochemical findings in normal and osteoarthritic articular cartilage. 2. Chondroitin sulfate concentration and chain length, water and ash content. J Clin Invest 1966;45:1170–1177.

82. Jaffe FF, Mankin HJ, Weiss C, et al. Water binding in articular cartilage of rabbits. J Bone Joint Surg 1974; 56A:1031–1039.

83. Lipshitz H, Etheredge R, Glimcher MJ. Changes in the hexosamine content and swelling ratio of articular cartilage as functions of depth from the surface. J Bone Joint Surg 1976;58A:1149–1153.

84. Maroudas A, Venn M. Chemical composition and swelling of normal and osteoarthritic femoral head cartilage. II: swelling. Ann Rheum Dis 1977;36:399–406.

85. Armstrong CG, Mow VC. Variations in the intrinsic mechanical properties of human articular cartilage with age, degeneration, and water content. J Bone Joint Surg 1982;64A:88–94.

86. Torzilli PA, Rose DE, Dethmers DA. Equilibrium water partition in articular cartilage. Biorheology 1982;19:519–537.

87. Maroudas A, Bannon C. Measurement of swelling pressure in cartilage and comparison with the osmotic pressure of constituent proteoglycans. Biorheology 1981;18:619–632.

88. Maroudas A, Wachtel E, Grushko G, et al. The effect of osmotic and mechanical pressures on water partitioning in articular cartilage. Biochim Biophys Acta 1990;1073:285–294.

89. Maroudas A. Balance between swelling pressure and collagen tension in normal and degenerate cartilage. Nature 1976;260:808–809.

90. Pasternack SG, Veis A, Breen M. Solvent-dependent changes in proteoglycan subunit conformation in aqueous guanidine hydrochloride solutions. J Biol Chem 1974;239:2206–2211.

91. Ateshian GA, Lai WM, Zhu WB, Mow VC. An asymptotic solution for two contacting biphasic cartilage layers. J Biomech 1994;27:1347–1360.

92. Ateshian GA, Wang LH. A theoretical solution for the frictionless rollling contact of cylindrical biphasic articular cartilage. J Biomech 1995;28:1341–1355.

93. Clarke IC. Articular cartilage: a review and scanning electron microscope study—1. the interterritorial fibrillar architecture. J Bone Joint Surg 1971;53B:732–750.

94. Lane JM, Weiss C. Review of articular cartilage collagen research. Arthritis Rheum 1975;18:553–562.

95. Clark JM. The organization of collagen in cyrofractured rabbit articular cartilage: a scanning electron microscopy study. J Orthop Res 1985;3:17–29.

96. Askew MJ, Mow VC. The biomechanical function of the collagen ultrastructure of articular cartilage. J Biomech Eng 1978;100:105–115.

97. Setton LA, Zhu WB, Mow VC. The biphasic poroviscoelastic behavior of articular cartilage in compression: role of the surface zone. J Biomech 1993;26:581–592.

98. Redler I, Zimny ML, Mansell J, et al. The ultrastructure and biomechanical significance of the tidemark of articular cartilage. Clin Orthop 1975;112:357–362.

99. Lane LB, Bullough PG. Age-related changes in the thickness of the calcified zone and the number of tidemarks in adult human articular cartilage. J Bone Joint Surg 1980;62B:372–375.

100. Hultkrantz W. Ueber die Spaltrichtungen der Gelenkknorpel. Ver Anat Gesellschaft 1898;12:248–256.

101. Benninghoff A. Form and Bau der Gelenkknorpel in ihren Beziehungen zur Funktion: Zweiter Teil. Der Aufbau des Gelenkknorpels in seinen Bezienhungen zur Funktion. Z Zellforsch Mikrosk Anat 1925;2:783–862.

102. Gardner DL, MacGillivray DC. Living articular cartilage is not smooth. Ann Rheum Dis 1971;30:3–9.

103. Mow VC, Lai WM, Redler I. Some surface characteristics of articular cartilage, part I: a scanning electron microscopy study and a theoretical model for the dynamic interaction of synovial fluid and articular cartilage. J Biomech 1974;7:449–456.

104. Redler I, Mow VC. Biomechanical Theories of Ultrastructural Alterations of Articular Surfaces of the Femoral Head. In WH Harris (ed), Arthritis of the Hip. St/ Louis, MO: CV Mosby Publishers, 1974;23–59.

105. Soltz MA, Ateshian GA. Experimental verification and theoretical prediction of cartilage interstitial fluid pressurization at an impermeable contact interface in confined compression. J Biomech 1998;13:927–934.

106. Donnan FG. The theory of membrane equilibria. Chem Rev 1924;1:73–90.

107. Katchalsky A, Curran PF. Non-Equilibrium Thermodynamics in Biophysics. Cambridge, MA: Harvard University Press, 1975.

108. Schinagl RM, Ting MK, Price J, Sah RL. Video microscopy to quantitate the inhomogeneous equilibrium strain within articular cartilage during confined compression. Ann Biomed Eng 1996;24:500–512.

109. Fung YC. Biomechanics: its scope, history, and some problems of continuum mechanics of physiology. Appl Mech Rev 1968;21:1–20.

110. Fung YC. Biomechanics: Mechanical Properties of Living Tissues. New York: NY Springer-Verlag Publishers, 1981.

111. Hayes WC. Mockros LF. Viscoelastic properties of human articular cartilage. J Appl Physiol 1971;31:562–568.

112. Sprit AA, Mak AF, Wassell RP. Nonlinear viscoelastic properties of articular cartilage in shear. J Orthop Res 1988;7:43–49.

113. Zhu WB, Mow VC, Koob TJ, Eyre DR. Viscoelastic shear properties of articular cartilage and the effects of glycosidase treatment. J Orthop Res 1993;11:771–781.

114. Setton LA, Mow VC, Howell DS. The mechanical behavior of articular cartilage in shear is altered by transection of the anterior cruciate ligament. J Orthop Res 1995;13:473–482.

115. Woo SLY, Mow VC, Lai WM. Biomechanical Properties of Articular Cartilage. In R Skalak, S Chein (eds), Handbook of Bioengineering. New York: McGraw-Hill, 1987;4.1–4.44.

116. Kempson GE. Mechanical Properties of Articular Cartilage. In MAR Freeman (ed), Adult Articular Cartilage (2nd ed). Tunbridge Wells, UK: Pitman Med Pubs, 1979;333–414.

117. Bachrach NM, Mow VC, Guilak F. Incompressibility of the solid matrix of articular cartilage under high hydrostatic pressures. J Biomech 1998; 31:445–451.

118. Pritzker KPH. Pathology of Osteoarthritis. In KD Brandt, M Doherty, LS Lohmander (eds), Osteoarthritis. Oxford: Oxford University Press, 1998;50–61.

119. Mow VC, Setton LA. Mechanical Properties of Normal and Osteoarthritic Articular Cartilage. In KD Brandt, M Doherty, LS Lohmander (eds), Osteoarthritis. Oxford: Oxford University Press, 1998;108–122.

120. Mankin HJ. The response of articular cartilage to mechanical injury. J Bone Joint Surg Am 1982;64(3):460–466.

121. Athanasiou KA, Rosenwasser MP, Buckwalter JA, et al. Interspecies comparison of in situ mechanical properties of distal femoral cartilage. J Orthop Res 1991;9:330–340.

122. Mankin HJ, Thrasher AZ. Water content and binding in normal and osteoarthritic human cartilage. J Bone Joint Surg 1975;57A:76–79.

123. Setton LA, Mow VC, Pita JC, et al. Altered Structure-Function Relationships for Articular Cartilage in Human Osteoarthritis and an Experimental Canine Model. In WB van den Berg,

PM van der Kraan, PLEM van Lent (eds), Joint Destruction in Arthritis and Osteoarthritis. Basel, Switzerland: Birkhauser Verlag, 1993;27–48.

124. Setton LA, Elliot DM, Mow VC. Altered mechanics of cartilage with osteoarthritis: human OA and animal model of joint degeneration. Osteoarthritis Cartilage 1999;7:2–14.

125. Mow VC, Setton LA, Ratcliffe A, et al. Structure-Function Relationships for Articular Cartilage and Effects of Joint Instability and Trauma on Cartilage Function. In KD Brandt (ed), Cartilage Changes in Osteoarthritis. Indianapolis, IN: University of Indiana Press, 1990;22–42.

126. Buschmann MD, Grodzinsky AJ. A molecular model of proteoglycan-associated electrostatic forces in cartilage mechanics. J Biomech Eng 1995; 117:180–192.

127. Lai WM, Mow VC, Sun DN, Ateshian GA. On the electric potentials inside a charged soft hydrated biological tissue: streaming potential vs. diffusion potential. J Biomech Eng 2000; 122:336–346.

128. Lai WM, Mow VC. Drag-induced compression of articular cartilage during a permeation experiment. Biorheology 1980;17:111–123.

129. Zhu WB, Lai WM, Mow VC. The density and strength of proteoglycan-proteoglycan interaction sites in concentrated solutions. J Biomech 1991;24:1007–1018.

130. Woo SLY, Akeson WH, Jemmott GF. Measurement of nonhomogeneous directional mechanical properties of articular cartilage in tension. J Biomech 1976;9:785–791.

131. Kempson GE. Relationship between the tensile properties of articular cartilage from human knee and age. Ann Rheum Dis 1982;41:508–511.

132. Myers ER, Lai WM, Mow VC. A continuum theory and an experiment for the ion-induced swelling behavior of articular cartilage. J Biomech Eng 1984;106:151–158.

133. Radin EL, Swann DA, Weisser PA. Separation of a hyaluronate-free lubricating fraction from synovial fluid. Nature 1970;228:377–378.

134. Swann DA, Silver FH, Slayter HS, et al. The molecular structure and lubricating activity of lubricin from bovine and human synovial fluids. Biochem J 1985;225:195–201.

135. Hill BA. Oligolamellar lubrication of joints by surface active phospholipid. J Rheumatol 1989;16:82–91.

136. Hou JS, Mow VC, Lai WM, Holmes MH. An analysis of the squeeze film lubrication mechanism for articular cartilage. J Biomech 1992;25:247–259.

137. Hill BA, Butler BD. Surfactants indentified in synovial fluid and their ability to act as boundary lubricants. Ann Rheum Dis 1984;43:641–648.

138. Lewis PR, McCutchen CW. Lubrication of mammalian joints. Nature 1960;185:920–921.

139. McCutchen CW. The frictional properties of animal joints. Wear 1962:5:1.

140. Walker PS, Dowson D, Longfield MD, et al. Boosted lubrication in synovial joints by fluid entrapment and enrichment. Ann Rheum Dis 1968:27:512–520.

141. Walker PS, Unsworth A, Dowson D, et al. Mode of aggregation of hyaluronic acid protein complex on the surface of articular cartilage. Ann Rheum Dis 1970:29:591–602.

142. Ateshian GA, Wang H, Lai WM. The role of interstitial fluid pressurization and surface porosity on boundary friction of articular cartilage. J Tribology 1998;20:241–251.

143. Lai WM, Mow VC. Ultrafiltration of synovial fluid by cartilage. J Eng Mech Div 1978;104:79–96.

144. Unsworth A, Dowson D, Wright V. The frictional behavior of human synovial joints: I. natural joints. J Lubr Technol 1975;97:360–376.

145. Unsworth A, Dowson D, Wright V. Some new evidence on human joint lubrication. Ann Rheum Dis 1975;34:277–284.

146. Malcom LL. An Experimental Investigation of the Friction and Deformational Responses of Articular Cartilage Interfaces to Static and Dynamic Loading [Thesis]. San Diego, CA: University of California, 1976.

147. Charnley J. The lubrication of animal joints in relation to surgical reconstruction by arthroplasty. Ann Rheum Dis 1960;19:10–19.

148. Barnett CH, Cobbold AF. Lubrication within living joints. J Bone Joint Surg 1962;44B:662–674.

149. Linn FC. Lubrication of animal joints. I. the arthrotripsometer. J Bone Joint Surg Am 1967;49A:1079–1088.

150. Jones ES. Joint lubrication. Lancet 1936;230:1043–1044.

151. Finsterbush A, Friedman B. Early changes in immobilized rabbit knee joints: a light and electron microscope study. Clin Orthop 1973;92:305–319.

152. Caterson B, Lowther DA. Changes in the metabolism of the proteoglycans from sheep articular cartilage in response to mechanical stress. Biochim Biophys Acta 1978;540:412–422.

153. Palmoski M, Perricone E, Brandt K. Development and reversal of a proteoglycan aggregation defect in normal canine knee cartilage after immobilization. Arthritis Rheum 1979;22:508–517.

154. Palmoski M, Brandt K. Running inhibits the reversal of atrophic changes in knee cartilage after removal of a leg cast. Arthritis Rheum 1981;24:1329–1337.

155. Jurvelin J, Kiviranta I, Tammi M, Helminen JH. Softening of canine articular cartilage after immobilization of the knee joint. Clin Orthop 1986;207:246–252.

156. Tammi M, Paukkonen K, Kiviranta I, et al. Joint Loading-Induced Alterations in Articular Cartilage. In HJ Helminen. Joint Loading. Bristol, UK: Wright Publisher, 1987;64–88.

157. McDevitt CA, Muir H. Biochemical changes in the cartilage of the knee in experimental and natural osteoarthrosis in the dog. J Bone Joint Surg 1976;58B:94–101.

158. Brandt KD, Myers SL, Burr D, Albrecht M. Osteoarthrtic changes in canine articular cartilage, subchondral bone, and synovium fifty-four months after transection of the anterior cruciate ligament. Arthritis Rheum 1991;34:1560–1570.

159. Setton LA, Mow VC, Muller FJ, et al. Mechanical properties of canine articular cartilage are significantly altered following transection of the anterior cruciate ligament. J Orthop Res 1994;12:451–463.

160. Newton PM, Mow VC, Buckwalter JA, Albright JP. The effect of life-long exercise on canine knee articular cartilage. Am J Sports Med 1997;25:282–287.

161. Hannan MT, Felson DT, Anderson JJ, Naimark A. Habitual exercise is not associated with knee osteoarthritis: the Framingham study. J Rheumatol 1993;20(4):704–709.

162. Buckwalter JA, Lane NE. Athletics and osteoarthritis. Am J Sports Med 1997;25:873–881.

163. Lane NE, Michel B, Bjorkengren A, et al. The risk of osteoarthritis with running and aging: a five year longitudinal study. J Rheumatol 1993;20:461–468.

164. Radin EL, Martin RB, Burr DB, et al. Effects of mechanical loading on the tissue of rabbit knee. J Orthop Res 1984;2:221–234.

165. Donohue JM, Buss D, Oegema TR Jr, et al. The effects of indirect blunt trauma on adult canine articular cartilage. J Bone Joint Surg 1983;65A:948–957.

166. Armstrong CG, Mow VC, Wirth CR. Biomechanics of Impact-Induced Microdamage to Articular Cartilage: A Possible Genesis for Chondromalacia Patella. In GAM Finerman (ed), Symposium on Sports Medicine: The Knee. St. Louis, MO: CV Mosby, 1985;70–84.

167. Thompson RC, Oegema TR, Lewis JL, Wallace L. Osteoarthritic changes after acute transarticular load, and animal model. J Bone Joint Surg 1991;73A:990–1001.

168. Verner JM, Thompson RC, Oegema TR, et al. Subchondral damage after acute transarticular loading: an in vivo model of joint injury. J Orthop Res 1992;10:759–765.

169. Kiviranta I, Tammi M, Jurvelin J, et al. Moderate running exercise augments glycosaminoglycans and thickness of articular cartilage in the knee joint of young beagle dogs. J Orthop Res 1988;6:188–195.

170. Parkkinen JJ, Lammi MJ, Helminen HJ, Tammi M. Local stimulation of proteoglycan synthesis in articular cartilage explants by dynamic compression in vitro. J Orthop Res 1992;10:610–620.

171. Enneking WF, Horowitz M. The intra-articular effects of immobilization on the human knee. J Bone Joint Surg 1972;54A:973–985.

172. Kiviranta I, Tammi M, Jurvelin J, et al. Articular cartilage thickness and glycosaminoglycan distribution in the young canine knee joint after remobilization of the immobilized limb. J Orthop Res 1994;12:161–167.

173. Jortikka MO, Inkinen RI, Tammi MI, et al. Immobilisation causes long lasting matrix changes both in the immobilised and contralateral joint cartilage. Ann Rheum Dis 1997;56:255–261.

174. Sah RL, Grodzinsky AJ, Plaas AHK, Sandy JD. Effects of tissue compression on the hyaluronate-binding properties of newly synthesized proteoglycans in cartilage explants. Biochem J 1990;267:803–808.

175. Guilak F, Meyer BC, Ratcliffe A, Mow VC. The effects of matrix compression on proteoglycan metabolism in articular cartilage explants. Osteoarthritis Cartilage 1994;2:91–101.

176. Yelin, E. The Economics of Osteoarthritis. In DK Brandt, M Doherty, and SL Lohmander (eds), Osteoarthritis. Oxford: Oxford University Press, 1998;23–30.

177. Emery IH, Meachim G. Surface morphology and topography of patellofemoral cartilage fibrillation in Liverpool necropsies. J Anat 1973;116:103–120.

178. Mankin HJ, Dorfman H, Lippiello L, et al. Biochemical and metabolic abnormalities in articular cartilage from osteoarthritic human hips. II. Correlation of morphology with biochemical and metabolic data. J Bone Joint Surg 1971;53A:523–537.

179. Wolff I. The Law of Bone Remodeling. P Maquet, R Furlong (trans). Berlin: Springer-Verlag, 1986.

180. Roche AF, Wainer H, Thissen D. Skeletal Maturity: The knee joint as a biological indicator. New York: Plenum Medical Book Co, 1975.

181. Buckwalter JA, Rosenberg LC. Structural changes during development in bovine fetal epiphyseal cartilage. Coll Rel Res 1983;3:489–504.

182. Buckwalter JA, Kuettner KE, Thonar EJM. Age-related changes in articular cartilage proteoglycans: electron microscopic studies. J Orthop Res 1985;3:251–257.

183. Speer DP. Collagenous architecture of the growth plate and perichondrial ossification groove. J Bone Joint Surg 1982;64A:399–407.

184. Kempson GE. Age-related changes in the tensile properties of human articular cartilage: a comparative study between the femoral head of the hip joint and the talus of the ankle joint. Biochim Biophys Acta 1991;1075:223–230.

9

Cardiopulmonary Physiology

JONATHAN R. MOLDOVER, JOEL STEIN,
AND PHYLLIS G. KRUG

Efficient and coordinated functioning of the cardiopulmonary system is essential for supplying oxygen to the tissues of the body and removing carbon dioxide. The central organs (heart and lungs) and the distribution system (blood vessels) must quickly respond to the varying metabolic demands of each of the body's tissues. In this chapter we review the structure and function of each of the system's components, the system's regulation at rest and during exercise, and its adaptation to training.

HEART

Anatomy

The human heart consists of four chambers, two atria and two ventricles, connected in series. Blood is circulated from the left ventricle through the systemic circulation, arterial to venous, then to the right atrium and ventricle and through the pulmonary circulation to return to the left atrium and then the left ventricle, completing its circuit. Unidirectional flow of blood from and to the heart is made possible through a system of valves. Atrial contraction increases the diastolic filling of the ventricles, thus increasing ventricular stroke volume, contributing 15–20% of the cardiac output.[1] The atrial contribution varies with heart rate, being greater at higher heart rates. The atrial contribution also increases in disease states when there is decreased diastolic compliance of the ventricle.

The heart's special metabolic and functional requirements have led to the development of specialized muscular and electrical conduction apparatuses. Cardiac muscle fibers are histologically and functionally distinct from both the skeletal muscle and smooth muscle fibers found elsewhere in the body. Their branched connections allow for propagation of electrical depolarizations, and cardiac muscle fibers are uniquely able to sustain the life-long frequent contractions required of the heart.

The electrical system of the heart is made of specially adapted muscle cells that provide careful coordination of the heart's muscle activity. Electrical impulses normally originate in the sinoatrial node, located in the right atrium. The cells making up the sinoatrial node have the shortest period between spontaneous depolarizations and act as the heart's natural pacemaker. The electrical impulse generated in the sinoatrial node travels through three atrial bundles (internodal pathways) to the atrioventricular node, located in the lower part of the intra-atrial septum. The electrical impulse is then transmitted to the bundle of His, which extends into the ventricular septum where it divides into two main branches, the right and left bundles. The left bundle further divides into anterior and posterior fascicles. Small branches of these major divisions carry the impulses to the myocytes.

A close-fitting fibrous sac, the pericardium, surrounds the heart. It provides some physical protection for the heart and contains a small amount of fluid that provides lubrication for the constantly moving heart. Its resistance to distention prevents rapid changes in cardiac chamber size, although it gradually enlarges to accommodate cardiac dilatation or large pericardial effusions. Surgical removal or congenital absence of the pericardium is generally tolerated well.

Coronary Circulation

The coronary vasculature is of paramount importance; disease of the coronary arteries remains the leading cause of death in the United States. The major epicardial arteries originate in the cusps of Valsalva, at the root of the aorta. The two vessels are the left main coronary artery, and the right coronary artery. The left main artery promptly bifurcates into the left circumflex artery and the left anterior descending artery. The right coronary artery typically supplies the majority of the right ventricular wall as well as the inferior left ventricular wall. The left circumflex artery supplies the lateral wall of the left ventricle. The left anterior descending artery supplies the anterior wall and apex of the left ventricle, as well as most of the interventricular septum. In approximately 60% of persons the right coronary artery gives off the posterior descending artery, which supplies a portion of the interventricular septum. Such persons are said to have right-dominant coronary circulation. In 30%, the posterior descending artery is supplied equally by the right and left circumflex arteries, and in the remaining 10%, the posterior descending artery is given off by the left circumflex artery left-dominant circulation (Figure 9-1).

The venous drainage of the heart consists primarily of the coronary sinus, which runs in the atrioventricular groove. The coronary sinus, a continuation of the great cardiac vein, empties into the right atrium, near the inferior vena cava.

The microcirculation of the heart has been receiving increasing attention, particularly as a cause of the syndrome of microvascular angina.[2] Persons with microvascular angina have objective evidence of ischemia in the absence of angiographically determined stenosis of the epicardial blood vessels. Impaired vasodilator reserve of both the coronary and systemic arterial beds has been found in these persons.[3] Adenosine has been identified as an important mediator of pain in myocardial ischemia.[4]

Myocardial Metabolism

The heart is one of the most metabolically active organs in the body. Oxygen extraction (measured by comparing aortic oxygen content with coronary sinus oxygen content) is approximately 65–70%, as compared with 36% for the brain, and an average of 26% for the entire body.[5] The heart is versatile in its use of substrates for energy metabolism and uses glucose, lactate, ketones, or fatty acids, as available. Normally, carbohydrates contribute approximately 35–40% and the remainder is primarily fatty acids.[6] When adequate oxygen is available, cardiac energy is produced through oxidative metabolism; it shifts to anaerobic metabolism when necessary.

The high oxygen extraction in the resting heart precludes significant increases in extraction with increasing metabolic demand. Therefore, increases in metabolic demand must be met by increased coronary artery flow. Regulation of the coronary circulation is locally controlled. Many substances produce dilatation, including acetylcholine, substance P, serotonin, thrombin, histamine, bradykinin, prostaglandins, and adenosine compounds.[7] Prostacyclin, with a half-life of approximately 3 minutes, exerts a relaxing effect on vascular smooth muscle in addition to inhibiting aggregation of platelets.[8] An important common pathway for vasodilatation of both peripheral and cardiac blood vessels is mediated by nitric oxide,[7,9,10] which is produced from an L-arginine precursor and has a half-life of approximately 3–6 seconds. Its effects are mediated intracellularly by cyclic guanosine-3,5-monophosphate. In addition to the chemical agents that induce its release, flow-induced shear stresses within the vessels stimulate release of nitric oxide. Endothelin is a peptide produced by endothelial cells that causes vasoconstriction.[11] Endothelial dysfunction is one of the earliest manifestations of atherosclerosis, and abnormal endothelial reactivity is a hallmark of atherosclerosis.[12]

Coronary perfusion takes place primarily during diastole, as during systole the increased intramural tension within the myocardial wall prevents, and may even transiently reverse, forward blood flow in the coronary vessels.[13] During early diastole, myocardial wall tension is as its lowest while the perfusion pressure within the aortic root remains high, owing to the elasticity of the aorta, permitting coronary perfusion (Figure 9-2).

Frank-Starling Mechanism

Cardiac output increases in response to increased venous return; this relationship is called the *Frank-Starling mechanism*. It derives from the relationship

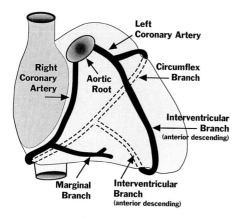

FIGURE 9-1 The coronary arteries of the heart.

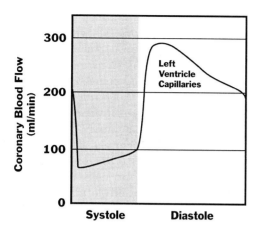

FIGURE 9-2 The relationship of coronary blood flow to the contraction of the left ventricle. (Adapted from AC Guyton. Textbook of Medical Physiology [7th ed]. Philadelphia: WB Saunders, 1986.)

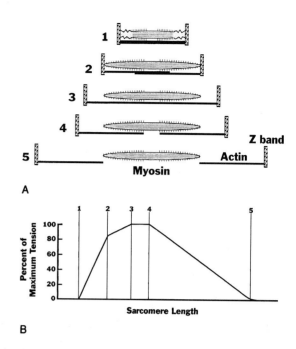

FIGURE 9-3 A. The relationship between the myosin and actin filaments during stretching of myocardial fibers, demonstrating that the number of available cross-bridges increases to a point, but then decreases if the fiber is stretched too far. **B.** The relationship between fiber length and contractile force.

CARDIAC RESPONSE TO EXERCISE

Oxygen Consumption

In reviewing the cardiac response to exercise, it is necessary first to understand the concepts of oxygen consumption ($\dot{V}O_2$) and maximal oxygen consumption

between myocardial fiber length and the force generated with each contraction. At rest there is overlap between the thin actin fibers of the myocardium, reducing the area available for forming cross-bridges with thick myosin fibers. As the sarcomere is stretched, the overlap between the thin fibers is eliminated, and a larger area is available for interaction with the myosin fibers; this allows increased contractile force to be generated. As the sarcomeres are stretched farther, the band of each actin fiber is no longer available to form cross-bridges with the myosin fibers, and the force generated declines (Figure 9-3A). The relationship between fiber length and contractile force is represented graphically in Figure 9-3B.

The relationship between end-diastolic volume and ventricular stroke volume is analogous to (and physiologically based on) the relationship between myocardial fiber length and contractile force. Accordingly, increasing end-diastolic volume causes an increase in ventricular stroke work. The relationship between end-diastolic volume and stroke output may be modified by a decrease in the contractile function of the heart, as in a dilated cardiomyopathy (Figure 9-4).

The Frank-Starling mechanism is an important homeostatic mechanism, as it provides a means of compensating for temporary imbalances in the circulation. For example, if the right ventricle receives increased venous return, it increases its output without a change in heart rate, owing to the increased stroke volume ejected. When the left side of the heart is presented with this same fluid challenge, it too experiences greater diastolic filling, and owing to the Frank-Starling mechanism, a greater stroke volume is ejected.

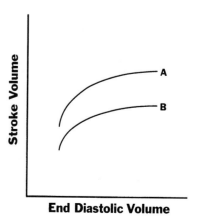

FIGURE 9-4 The relationship between end-diastolic volume and stroke volume in (A) a normal heart and (B) dilated cardiomyopathy.

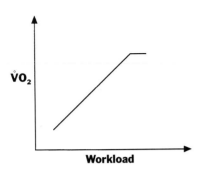

FIGURE 9-5 The relationship between steady-state oxygen consumption ($\dot{V}O_2$) and workload.

($\dot{V}O_2max$), as the intensity of exercise is usually expressed in these terms. $\dot{V}O_2$ is calculated by measuring from the expired air at the mouth, thus representing whole-body oxygen consumption. During exercise there is increased consumption, primarily because of the metabolism of the working skeletal muscle. For any given constant submaximal workload the $\dot{V}O_2$ increases over the first 2–4 minutes and then reaches a steady-state level. With increasing work intensity the steady-state level increases until a point is reached at which increasing the work further does not produce any increase in $\dot{V}O_2$. If the various steady-state levels are plotted against the workloads, the result is a straight line with a short horizontal plateau at the top, representing the $\dot{V}O_2max$ (Figure 9-5). The slope of this line represents the mechanical efficiency of the exercise being performed. Activities that require muscle contraction to stabilize the trunk (e.g., upper extremity ergometry) or activities performed by persons with spastic cocontraction have steeper slopes for the linear increase in oxygen consumption with increasing workload, representing a reduction in mechanical effi-

ciency.[14,15] When plotting various cardiac and pulmonary parameters against increasing work intensity, the independent variable is usually expressed as the percentage of the subject's $\dot{V}O_2max$, although the absolute $\dot{V}O_2$ (e.g., liters of oxygen per minute or milliliters per kilogram body weight per minute) or a mechanical measure of work intensity (e.g., watts or kiloponds) is sometimes used.

Cardiac Output

The cardiac output (expressed in liters of blood per minute) is a function of the heart rate and stroke volume. The relationship between the cardiac output and $\dot{V}O_2$ is linear, at least for nonathletes (Figure 9-6).[16] As we get older the line shifts downward, but there is no significant change in linearity or slope. The relationship of cardiac output to $\dot{V}O_2$ during submaximal work performed in the upright position is parallel to but below the line of work performed when the subject lies supine. Maximum cardiac output in the supine position is less than during upright exercise, as is the $\dot{V}O_2max$.[17] The increasing cardiac output with increasing $\dot{V}O_2$ in the supine position is produced by an increase in heart rate while the stroke volume remains constant. During upright exercise both heart rate and stroke volume increase with increasing exercise intensity. In the presence of a fixed (paced) heart rate, the cardiac output increases by means of increasing stroke volume.[18]

Heart Rate

The relationship between heart rate and $\dot{V}O_2$ is also linear (Figure 9-7). Maximal heart rate is a function of age, whereas the level of physical conditioning determines the slope of the line. The maximal heart rate is approxi-

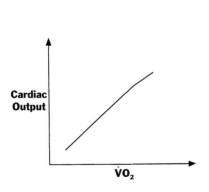

FIGURE 9-6 The relationship between cardiac output and oxygen consumption ($\dot{V}O_2$).

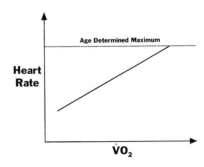

FIGURE 9-7 The relationship between heart rate and oxygen consumption ($\dot{V}O_2$).

mately equal to 220 minus the age in years. The decline in maximal heart rate with age is not related to physical activity.[19] The increase in heart rate with increasing $\dot{V}O_2$ is regulated through the autonomic nervous system (vagal tone versus sympathetic β-adrenergic tone) and by circulating catecholamines.[18,20,21] The vagal tone has impact on the heart rate variability seen at rest and during exercise, with reduced variability being associated with increased cardiac risk. Aging causes impairment of vagal function at rest, whereas the heart rate variability during exercise varies with the individual's level of aerobic fitness.[22]

Stroke Volume

Greater variability occurs in the stroke volume response to exercise than in the response of cardiac output or heart rate. For example, during increasing work in the supine position, the stroke volume may increase, decrease, or stay the same. If there is a change from the resting level, the stroke volume levels out when the $\dot{V}O_2$ reaches 30–40% of $\dot{V}O_2$max.[23] Resting stroke volume in the upright position is approximately 60% of that while supine, and with increasing work the stroke volume increases by 50%, but never to the supine value (Figure 9-8). Older persons demonstrate a smaller increase in stroke volume with exercise in either position.[17,24] Children also demonstrate a lower stroke volume for a given workload when compared with adults. Their stroke volume is a function of left ventricular mass.[25] There is no difference in the cardiac responses of boys and girls.[26]

Myocardial Oxygen Consumption

Although the preceding cardiac parameters form the foundation of most discussions of the cardiac response to exercise, it is myocardial $\dot{V}O_2$ that has the greatest implications for clinical decision making in rehabilitation medicine. Patients with atherosclerotic coronary artery disease develop problems (angina pectoris, arrhythmias, myocardial infarction, sudden death) when the myocardial $\dot{V}O_2$ required by an activity exceeds the maximum oxygen supply that the coronary circulation can deliver. The clinician needs to understand the factors that influence myocardial $\dot{V}O_2$, in order to perform appropriate patient evaluation and program modification.

Indirect Measurement of Myocardial Oxygen Consumption

It is not practicable to measure myocardial $\dot{V}O_2$ directly in most clinical settings, so we must use more easily

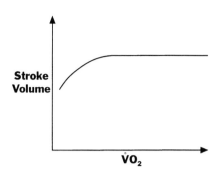

FIGURE 9-8 The relationship between stroke volume and oxygen consumption ($\dot{V}O_2$).

measurable parameters that correlate with it: heart rate, blood pressure, ventricular wall tension, rate of fiber shortening, venous return, and the systemic arterial pressure that the heart must pump against (afterload). It has been shown empirically that only the heart rate and systolic blood pressure need be measured to obtain a reasonable assessment of myocardial $\dot{V}O_2$.[27] The rate-pressure product (RPP) is calculated by multiplying the heart rate by the systolic blood pressure and dividing by 100; this correlates well ($r = 0.85$–0.90) with the directly measured myocardial $\dot{V}O_2$ under a variety of clinical situations.[27-29] The RPP increases in a linear fashion with $\dot{V}O_2$ until the anginal threshold is reached (Figure 9-9). The anginal threshold is the point at which there is evidence of an imbalance between myocardial $\dot{V}O_2$ and the available oxygen supply, as manifested by anginal pain or electrocardiographic abnormality.

Effect of Isometric Muscle Contraction

The cardiovascular response to isometric exercise has been well described by Donald et al.[30] Contractions as

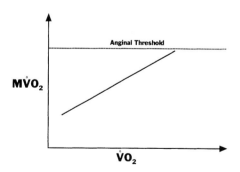

FIGURE 9-9 The relationship between myocardial oxygen consumption ($M\dot{V}O_2$) and total body oxygen consumption ($\dot{V}O_2$).

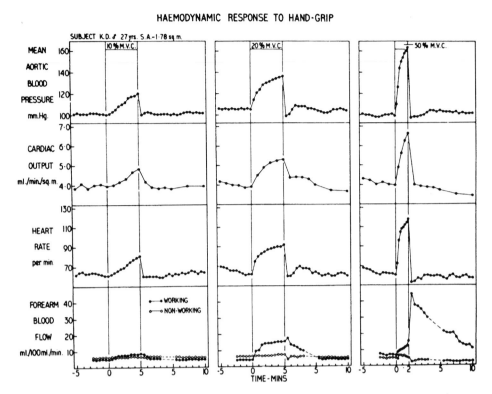

FIGURE 9-10 Increases in blood pressure, cardiac output, heart rate, and forearm blood flow caused by isometric contractions are proportional to the relative intensity of the contraction. (MVC = maximal voluntary contraction.)

small as 10% of the maximal voluntary contraction produce an increase in heart rate that leads to an increase in systolic blood pressure, thus increasing the myocardial $\dot{V}O_2$ out of proportion to the physical work being performed (Figure 9-10). During sustained contractions that are less than 15% of maximum, a steady-state cardiac response is reached, whereas with stronger contractions the RPP continues to increase until fatigue limits the duration of the contraction. This response is proportional to the maximal voluntary contraction for the muscle in use, regardless of the mass of that muscle, and is thought to be a cardioaccelerating reflex initiated by potassium ion flux in the contracting muscle. Stroke volume and total peripheral resistance do not change. It is important to note that the increase in myocardial $\dot{V}O_2$ caused by the isometric contraction is superimposed on the metabolic response to any isotonic work being performed at the same time (Figure 9-11). Thus, a strong hand grip on a cane or walker may create a myocardial oxygen demand out of proportion to the metabolic demands of the slow ambulation of a rehabilitation patient.

Effect of Upper Extremity Exercise

Both the heart rate and the systolic blood pressure are higher for any given submaximal $\dot{V}O_2$ if the work is performed with the upper extremities instead of the lower ones (Figure 9-12).[14,31] The difference between upper and lower extremity work becomes more significant as the workload increases.[14] The values during combined upper and lower extremity exercise are the same as for lower extremity work alone at each submaximal $\dot{V}O_2$.[31] These differences in cardiac response are important for the clinician designing modified exercise testing and testing programs for disabled individuals.[32-35]

Effect of Posture

The effect of upright versus supine posture on the myocardial oxygen consumption (as reflected by the RPP) depends on the relative workload. With lower intensity exercise the RPP is higher for supine than for upright exercise at the same $\dot{V}O_2$.[14,36] At higher intensities the situation is reversed: then, upright exercise produces the higher RPP (Figure 9-13).[31] This distinction is important in rehabilitation when prescribing supine mat exercises for patients who have coexisting coronary artery disease. Such supine exercises may create higher myocardial oxygen demand than ambulation or other upright activities, especially if the exercise contains an isometric component (e.g., bridging). This exaggeration of the cardiac response to low-intensity exercise in the supine posture can be used to increase the range of observable

FIGURE 9-11 Increases in blood pressure and heart rate generated by isometric contractions are superimposed on the increases from aerobic work. (MVC = maximal voluntary contraction.)

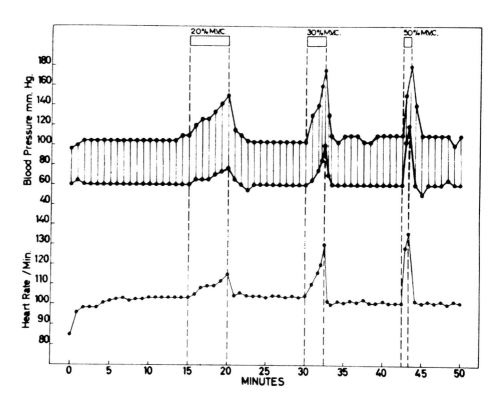

cardiac response during exercise testing of hemiparetic and other patients with limited exercise capacity.[35]

Effect of Bed Rest

Although short periods of bed rest are commonly prescribed for acutely ill and convalescent patients, prolonged bed rest has a deleterious effect on the cardiac response to exercise. Saltin et al. subjected five volunteers to 20 days' strict bed rest and measured various metabolic parameters as well as the cardiopulmonary response to exercise.[37] They found that the average $\dot{V}O_2$max

decreased 27%; the maximum heart rate remained constant, whereas the maximum stroke volume and cardiac output decreased. At a submaximal workload the cardiac output and stroke volume were lower, and the heart rate higher, after the period of bed rest. There was no significant change in mean arterial pressure at rest or during submaximal exercise after bed rest.

Effect of Training

Aerobic training programs modify the cardiac response to exercise. Such programs involve exercising at least

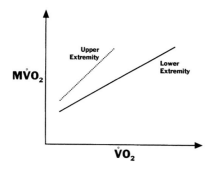

FIGURE 9-12 A comparison of the relationship between myocardial oxygen demand ($M\dot{V}O_2$) and total body oxygen consumption ($\dot{V}O_2$) for upper and lower extremity work.

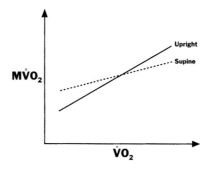

FIGURE 9-13 A comparison of the relationship between myocardial oxygen demand ($M\dot{V}O_2$) and total body oxygen consumption ($\dot{V}O_2$) for upright and supine work.

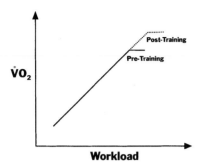

FIGURE 9-14 The effect of training on the relationship between oxygen consumption ($\dot{V}O_2$) and workload.

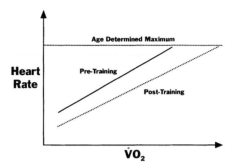

FIGURE 9-16 The effect of training on the relationship between heart rate and oxygen consumption ($\dot{V}O_2$).

three times a week for approximately 30 minutes using large muscle groups in a repetitive fashion, such as running, jogging, swimming, cycling, aerobic calisthenics, rowing, or circuit training with exercise intense enough to produce a heart rate of 60–70% of the maximum heart rate. The changes in the cardiac response to exercise described in the following sections should be evident within 4–6 weeks after the onset of training.

The change in the cardiac response to exercise is most evident when the muscles undergoing training are the same muscles used to generate the cardiac response in testing before and after the training. Thus, if the subject trains with a walking or running program, the cardiac response measured on a treadmill changes significantly, whereas the cardiac response to arm crank ergometry changes little, if at all.

Another key concept for studying the changes in the cardiac response to exercise is that the changes may be different during rest, submaximal exercise, and maximal exercise. Differences during submaximal work are the ones most relevant to rehabilitation.

Effect of Training on Oxygen Consumption

With aerobic training $\dot{V}O_2$max is increased, but the $\dot{V}O_2$ at rest and during any given submaximal load remains unchanged (Figure 9-14). This basic training effect appears to be true for both sexes and different ethnic groups.[38] Although most people, especially those in rehabilitation programs, never exercise to their $\dot{V}O_2$max, the increase is still relevant, because each submaximal activity represents a smaller percentage of the $\dot{V}O_2$max after training, thus generating a smaller increase in the heart rate, systolic blood pressure, and myocardial $\dot{V}O_2$.

Effect of Training on Cardiac Output

The maximal cardiac output increases with training, but there is no change in the cardiac output at rest or at any submaximal workload (Figure 9-15). There is a difference, however, in how the submaximal cardiac output is generated and distributed. (The changes in the heart rate and stroke volume that determine the cardiac output are described in the next two sections.) The distribution of the peripheral blood flow is different in trained subjects. For example, less blood is shunted to the working muscles because they are able to extract and use oxygen more efficiently. This change in distribution produces less of an increase in the total peripheral resistance, and thus less afterload for the heart and a lower systolic blood pressure response to exercise.

Effect of Training on Heart Rate

Training causes the heart rate to be lower at rest and during any submaximal workload, but the maximal heart rate does not change (Figure 9-16). This bradycardia of training is the most noticeable and clinically important change that occurs with aerobic conditioning

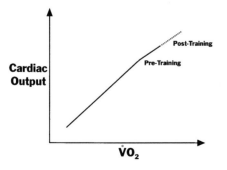

FIGURE 9-15 The effect of training on the relationship between cardiac output and oxygen consumption ($\dot{V}O_2$).

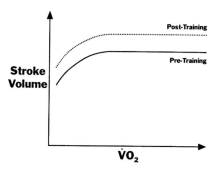

FIGURE 9-17 The effect of training on the relationship between stroke volume and oxygen consumption ($\dot{V}O_2$).

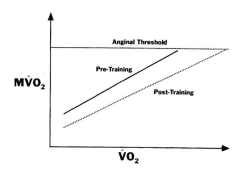

FIGURE 9-18 The effect of training on the relationship between myocardial oxygen demand ($M\dot{V}O_2$) and total body oxygen consumption ($\dot{V}O_2$).

and it is primarily because of an increase in vagal tone combined with a decrease in sympathetic tone and lower levels of circulating catecholamines.[39,40] Aerobic training has been shown to increase heart rate variability.[41] As noted previously, the change in heart rate with exercise is seen only during exercise with the trained muscles. The muscle changes of endurance training are discussed in Chapter 16.

Effect of Training on Stroke Volume

After an aerobic training program, the stroke volume is usually greater at rest and during submaximal and maximal exercise (Figure 9-17). The increase in stroke volume is reciprocal to the decrease in heart rate, maintaining a stable submaximal cardiac output, and is caused by both a longer diastolic filling period resulting from the slower heart rate and increased venous return caused by the exercise-induced increase in blood volume.

Effect of Training on Myocardial Oxygen Consumption

The myocardial $\dot{V}O_2$ is lower at rest and during submaximal exercise after an effective training program, but the anginal threshold is unchanged (Figure 9-18). The decrease in myocardial $\dot{V}O_2$ is caused primarily by the lower heart rate. The systolic blood pressure response to exercise may also be lower, owing to a decrease in peripheral vascular resistance created by less shunting of blood from visceral capillary beds to supply working muscle. The reduced myocardial $\dot{V}O_2$ at submaximal loads explains the effectiveness of properly designed cardiac rehabilitation programs in increasing the work capacity of persons with coronary artery disease, even though short-term exercise does not raise the angina threshold. Continuing exercise training for longer peri-

ods has been shown to increase myocardial perfusion and to increase the peak RPP.[42] More prolonged exercise programs may enhance coronary perfusion because of a combination of reductions in heart rate and improvements in coronary blood flow capacity.[43] This increase in coronary blood flow is multifactorial and includes contributions from metabolic, endothelial, myogenic, and neurohumoral systems. The up-regulation of nitric oxide synthetase production seen with regular exercise contributes to an improved vasodilatory response.[12]

PERIPHERAL CIRCULATION

Anatomy

The blood vessels constitute the *plumbing* of the body, carrying blood to and from all organ systems. Arteries by definition carry blood from the heart to the target organ system, and veins carry blood back to the heart. Arteries contain blood rich with oxygen (with the prominent exception of the pulmonary arteries). Veins carry blood that contains less oxygen and more carbon dioxide, although again the exception is the pulmonary veins. There are several portal systems in the body, in which a portion of the blood supply to an organ derives from venous blood collected from a capillary bed, including the portal systems supplying the liver and the anterior pituitary gland.

Arteries are muscular, thick-walled vessels that are exposed to high pressure. The arteries originate from the aorta and form a branching, and to some degree anastomosing, network. Distally, the smaller arteries branch farther to form arterioles, which give rise to meta-arterioles or directly to capillaries. Gas, nutrient, and waste exchange with the tissues occurs through the

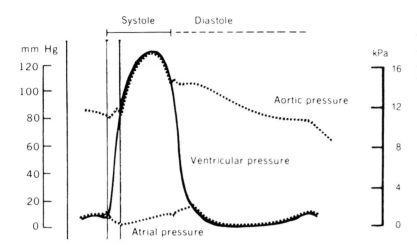

FIGURE 9-19 The maintenance of aortic pressure during diastole is the result of the elasticity of the aortic wall. (Reprinted with permission from P-O Åstrand, K Rodahl. Textbook of Work Physiology [3rd ed]. New York: McGraw-Hill, 1986.)

capillary walls. The effluent from the capillaries goes to the venules, which in turn give rise to the smaller veins, later to join to form the large veins, and then the superior and inferior vena cava.

The wall of the aorta contains a large amount of elastic tissue and a relatively small amount of muscle tissue. Farther down the arterial system this ratio is reversed: There, arterioles contain a high concentration of smooth muscle cells and a small amount of elastic tissue. The elastic aorta serves to buffer and damp the pulsatile pressure of the cardiac output. During systole the aorta expands to accommodate rapid ejection of blood. During diastole, when cardiac output has ceased, the aorta maintains perfusion pressure by contracting by elastic recoil (Figure 9-19). If the arterial system were completely inelastic, the diastolic blood pressure would fall to zero, and, conversely, if the aorta were infinitely distensible, blood pressure would remain at a constant level.

The veins have thinner walls than the arteries, although they are still muscular, and they contain valves to assist in the unidirectional flow of blood. The veins freely form anastomoses and serve as a capacitance reservoir for the circulation. They can contract or expand the volume of blood contained within them to adjust for volume loss or overload. The veins constitute the primary reservoir of blood for the body, normally containing 67% of the intravascular volume*; the arteries contain only 11% and the capillaries 5%. The remaining 17% is contained in the heart (5%) and the pulmonary circulation (12%).*

The valves in the veins allow skeletal muscle to function as an auxiliary pump, particularly in the lower extremities. The contraction of the calf muscles causes compression of the veins in the lower leg, forcing the blood toward the heart. The veins then passively fill during relaxation of the muscles, completing the cycle and preventing the large increases in hydrostatic pressure that would otherwise occur in the legs.[44]

The cross-sectional area of the circulation increases gradually from the aorta to the arterioles, with a large increase at the level of the capillaries. The capillaries, owing to their immense number, have a cross-sectional area on the order of 60 times that of the arterioles and 1,000 times that of the aorta.[45] Autoregulation of the microcirculation limits the effective cross-sectional area of the small blood vessels at any given time, but the effective cross-sectional area remains quite large in comparison with that of the larger blood vessels. Given an essentially closed system in which total capillary blood flow must equal the aortic blood flow, it follows that the velocity of the blood in the capillaries is much slower than in the aorta, allowing more time for exchange of gases and nutrients in the capillary beds.

The arterioles contain a circular band of smooth muscle that enables them to vary the resistance to blood flow within their lumens. The arterioles contribute the bulk of the resistance to blood flow and also function to damp the pulsatile pressure of arterial blood flow, providing the capillaries with a more continuous supply. The ability of the arterioles to vary the resistance they provide allows for regulation of blood flow and redistribution of blood flow to reflect changing metabolic needs (e.g., exercise).

Laplace's law, which describes how an acceptable blood vessel wall stress is maintained throughout the circulation, states that wall tension is proportional to the transluminal pressure and to the radius of the vessel. Calculation of wall stress takes into account wall thickness, with stress being inversely proportional to the

*Values are extrapolated from animal studies.[45]

thickness of the wall. The full equation can be stated thus: S = Pr/v, where S is wall stress, P is transluminal pressure, r is radius, and v is vessel thickness. As vessels become smaller, the wall tension decreases in proportion to the vessel radius. This permits a decrease in vessel wall thickness in smaller vessels without causing an increase in wall stress.

Poiseuille's law states that blood flow through a vessel varies with the fourth power of its radius. Thus, even small decreases in the radius of a vessel from atherosclerosis have a significant effect on its maximal flow. Resistance is defined as the ratio of the change in pressure to flow, and is proportional both to the length of the vessel and to the inverse of the radius to the fourth power.

Turbulence, another important consideration, can be predicted by Reynold's number: N_r = pDV/v, where N_r is Reynold's number, p is density, D is diameter, V is mean velocity, and v is viscosity. Turbulence becomes more likely as N_r increases. N_r varies proportionally with the diameter of a vessel, and inversely with the viscosity of the blood. Atherosclerosis has been shown to have a predilection for areas of high turbulence such as ostia and bifurcations.[46]

The lymphatics are small, thin-walled vessels that carry lymphatic fluid from the periphery to the central circulation. They provide drainage for the interstitial and extravascular spaces. Lymphatics also contain valves to ensure unidirectional flow, and they operate at low pressures. The lymphatics contain some smooth muscle and also use transient increases in local tissue pressure (as during muscle contraction) to pump lymphatic fluid. Lymph passes through one or more lymph nodes before being collected in the larger lymphatics and returning to the circulation via the thoracic duct or the right lymphatic duct.

Circulation at Rest

Tissue Perfusion

The hydrostatic forces present in the capillaries derive from the mean arterial blood pressure, attenuated by the arterioles, which function as the main resistive component of the circulation. The resulting hydrostatic pressure within the capillary ranges from 32 mm Hg at the arteriolar end of the capillary to 15 mm Hg at the venular end. This varies with tissue location: dependent tissues have higher hydrostatic pressure. The counterpressure exerted by the tissue interstitial fluid is small (close to, or perhaps even slightly less than, zero).

Filtration of plasma across the capillary membranes that would result from hydrostatic pressure would cause unacceptable amounts of fluid transudation were it not for the counterpressure or pull exerted by osmotically active substances in the blood. Osmotically active substances are molecules too large to be filtered across the capillary wall (molecular weight approximately 60 kD), the most important being albumin. The osmotic pressure exerted by albumin is greater than would be expected from its concentration and size. This discrepancy can be accounted for by albumin's negative charge, which essentially keeps cations (primarily sodium) in the intravascular compartment, thus increasing the osmotic force generated.

The relationship between the hydrostatic forces and the opposing osmotic forces can be expressed in relation to fluid movement across the capillary walls. Starling's hypothesis can be stated as follows: F = k [Pc + Oi – (Pi + Op)], where F is fluid movement, k the filtration constant of the capillary membrane, Pc the capillary hydrostatic pressure, Oi the osmotic pressure, Pi the interstitial hydrostatic pressure, and Op the osmotic pressure of the capillary fluid.[47] Fluid moves from the capillary to the interstitium when F is positive and from the interstitium to the capillary when F is negative. Only a small fraction (0.02%) of the fluid that passes through the capillaries is filtered. Of this amount, 85% is reabsorbed by the capillaries and venules and the remainder forms the lymphatic fluid.[6]

Control of the Circulation

Blood flow to different organ systems is based both on the size of the organ and its metabolic requirements (Table 9-1); the flow to each organ is regulated by the size of its supplying arteries and by neural, humoral, and local mechanisms. The blood vessels are supplied by autonomic adrenergic, and in some cases cholinergic, fibers. This innervation allows for centrally directed rapid response to changing conditions, such as autonomic sympathetic response seen when a person is confronting danger. Sympathetic adrenergic fibers release norepinephrine at the resistive vessels (arterioles), exerting influence over blood pressure at that site. Sympathetic fibers also provide stimulation to the capacitance vessels (primarily but not exclusively venules) to increase venous return as needed. The α-adrenergic receptors are also present at the arteriolar level; they mediate a vasodilating response to catecholamines and increase blood flow to selected structures such as skeletal muscles.[48]

A secondary means of controlling vascular tone via the sympathetic nervous system involves the sympathetic cholinergic fibers. These fibers cause vasodilata-

TABLE 9-1
Distribution of Blood Flow to Organs at Rest

Organ	Percentage	Volume ml/min	ml/min/ 100 g
Brain	14	700	50
Heart	4	200	70
Bronchi	2	100	25
Kidneys	22	1,100	300
Muscle (inactive)	15	750	4
Liver	27	1,350	95
Bone	5	250	3
Skin (cool weather)	6	300	3
Thyroid gland	1	50	160
Adrenal glands	0.5	25	300
Other tissues	3.5	175	18
Total	**100**	**5,000**	—

tion in the resistance vessels in skeletal muscle, at least in the extremities. Their functional importance in humans remains unclear, but they may play a part in the fight-or-flight response by increasing muscle readiness for action.

The release of catecholamines (epinephrine and norepinephrine) from the adrenal medulla provides a humoral means to influence the peripheral circulation. In small amounts epinephrine produces a vasodilating response, because of the selective stimulation of the α-adrenergic receptors in the arterioles. In larger amounts, epinephrine's α-adrenergic stimulation predominates, causing a pressor response. Norepinephrine, which is much more selective for the α-receptors, produces vasoconstriction at all doses. During normal physiological functioning, however, the physiological significance of circulating catecholamines released from the adrenal medulla is small relative to that released from the sympathetic nerve fibers innervating the vessels.[6]

Reactive hyperemia provides a useful model of local responses of the vasculature to stress. When the blood supply to an extremity is transiently interrupted and then allowed to resume, the tissue increases its blood flow by relaxing the arteriolar sphincters. The degree of reactive hyperemia is related to the length of the occlusion: Longer occlusion causes greater hyperemia. Reactive hyperemia is not neurally mediated, as it is not eliminated by complete denervation or sympathectomy.[49] The mediators of reactive hyperemia are many of the substances that normally mediate local control of vascular tone.

Local control of vascular tone is exerted through several mechanisms. The relative contributions of each mechanism remain somewhat uncertain and vary in different tissues. Among the mediators of this mechanism are prostaglandins, adenosine phosphates, endothelium-derived relaxing factor (nitric oxide), and endothelin, a vasoconstricting factor.

Blood Pressure

Normal blood pressure ranges from 100–120 mm Hg systolic and 60–80 mm Hg diastolic. It is influenced by cardiac output and the peripheral resistance at the level of the arterioles. The mean arterial pressure is approximately equal to the diastolic pressure plus one-third the difference between the systolic and diastolic pressures, based on the (generally accurate) assumption that systole lasts one-third of the cardiac cycle. The mean arterial pressure depends on cardiac output and on peripheral resistance. The pulse pressure, defined as the difference between diastolic and systolic blood pressure, is a function of the stroke volume and of arterial capacitance.

The overall control of blood pressure is complex and involves several components. The fluid component of blood volume is controlled largely through the renin-angiotensin-aldosterone axis. The juxtaglomerular apparatus in the kidney, located adjacent to the afferent arteriole and the glomerulus, is responsible for the secretion of renin into the circulation. Renin converts renin substrate, an α-globulin produced in the liver, to angiotensin I. Angiotensin I is converted in the pulmonary capillary beds to angiotensin II. Angiotensin I is an apparently inactive substance, but angiotensin II is a potent vasoconstrictor and also stimulates secretion of aldosterone by the adrenal cortex. Aldosterone, in turn, is responsible for sodium and water reabsorption in the renal tubules. The increased plasma volume and increased blood pressure resulting from this cascade cause inhibition of the juxtaglomerular apparatus and complete the feedback loop (Figure 9-20).

There are at least three natriuretic peptides found in humans, atrial natriuretic peptide, brain natriuretic peptide, and C-type natriuretic peptide. Atrial natriuretic peptide is found primarily in the atrial wall, brain natriuretic peptide in the ventricular wall, and C-type natriuretic peptide is present primarily in the CNS and is present in the plasma in low concentrations. Both atrial natriuretic peptide and brain natriuretic peptide are released in response to stretch of the atrial or ventricular walls, respectively. These peptides promote loss of sodium and water by increasing the glomerular filtration rate and by decreasing renin secretion. These peptides lower blood pressure through their actions on intravascular volume, the sympathetic nervous system, and direct effects on vascular tone.[50]

The neural control of blood pressure is mediated through the autonomic nervous system and the adrenal medullary catecholamines. The baroreceptors are located in the carotid body and along the arch of the aorta, responding to changing hemodynamic needs. Stimulation of these baroreceptors, as with increased blood pressure, causes a decrease in sympathetic tone and an increase in vagal tone to the heart, to produce bradycardia and a decrease in peripheral resistance. A decrease in blood pressure, as on rising from a supine position, causes a decrease in the tonic firing of the baroreceptors, with an increase in sympathetic vasomotor tone and tachycardia. The baroreceptors accommodate to persistent changes in blood pressure, effectively changing their *set point*. Thus, baroreceptors provide effective moment-to-moment control of blood pressure but have little effect overall on blood pressure, which is controlled primarily through the renal mechanisms already discussed. The regulation of blood pressure during dynamic exercise is mediated by an interplay of CNS activation associated with the inception of muscular activity and the baroreceptors.[51]

Circulatory Response to Exercise

The circulation responds to exercise by shunting blood away from the gut, kidneys, and skin toward the skeletal muscles involved in the exercise. The vasoconstriction in the viscera and skin is accomplished through the sympathetic nervous system. The vasodilatation of the active muscle groups is largely locally mediated, through several factors, including increases in potassium ion concentration, increases in osmolarity, changes in adenosine nucleotide concentrations, and decreasing pH. An increase in muscle blood flow up to 15–20 times the baseline value may accompany the arteriolar dilatation associated with vigorous exercise,[52] and oxygen extraction increases several-fold as well.[53]

The arteriolar dilatation in active muscle groups during vigorous exercise more than offsets the increased resistance in the viscera and skin circulation, and during vigorous exercise causes total peripheral resistance to decrease perhaps to 50% of the resting value. The cardiac output increases even more, primarily through increases in heart rate, which causes an increase in blood pressure despite the decreased total peripheral resistance. The increase in blood pressure is

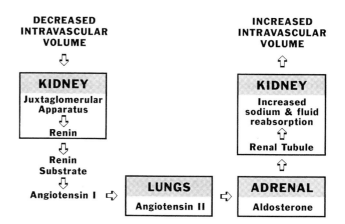

FIGURE 9-20 The role of the renin-angiotensin system in responding to decreased intravascular volume.

both systolic and diastolic, although the systolic increase is greater.

LUNGS

Anatomy

The lungs consist of two sponge-like organs separated by the mediastinal structures. The functional unit of the lung is the alveolus. There are approximately 300 million alveoli in an adult lung, and they provide a surface area on the order of 85 m^2 for gas exchange with the capillaries.[54] The multibranched structure of the bronchial tree makes possible this large surface area in a compact volume. Each alveolus is constructed of thin-walled alveolar cells that are heavily invested with capillaries, allowing for diffusion of gases.

The muscles of respiration consist of the diaphragm, intercostal muscles, sternocleidomastoids, scalene muscles, and abdominal muscles. The diaphragm is a dome-shaped muscle with a tendinous central portion that separates the thoracic and abdominal cavities. It performs most of the work of quiet breathing. The other muscles of respiration become more active during forceful inspiration and expiration (see Mechanics of Respiration, later in this chapter). The crural part of the diaphragm has no attachments to the rib cage and causes abdominal displacement only while inflating the lungs.[55] Because of this different action, as well as its separate embryonic origin and segmental innervation, it may be thought of as a muscle distinct from the rest of the diaphragm.[56]

The surface of the lung is enveloped by the pleura, which is reflected to cover the parietal surface as well. The area between the two pleural surfaces is known as the *pleural space*, although in fact it is primarily a potential space in healthy persons, containing only a small amount of lubricating fluid.

The lungs have a dual blood supply. The pulmonary arteries carry blood with low oxygen tension. A low-pressure system, with normal systolic pressures in the vicinity of 22 mm Hg, it allows gas exchange in the alveoli. The bronchial arteries constitute the secondary blood supply. They originate directly from the aorta and contain blood with a high oxygen tension and at systemic pressures, providing nutrition to the pulmonary tissues.

The lungs are divided into five lobes. The right lung consists of the right upper, right lower, and right middle lobe. The left lung contains only an upper and a lower lobe. The lingula is considered the left lung's anatomic correlate of the right middle lobe. Each lobe is further divided into segments, a total of 19 for the two lungs.

The diaphragm is innervated by the phrenic nerves. Each intercostal muscle is supplied by the corresponding intercostal nerve, which runs in the neurovascular bundle. The parietal pleura, unlike the visceral pleura, is capable of providing sensory information, such as pain or touch, to the brain. It is supplied in part by the intercostal nerves and in part by the phrenic nerves.

The nerve supply to the lungs includes both sympathetic fibers from the sympathetic chain and parasympathetic fibers from the vagus nerve.

Lung Volumes

The normal volume of air exchanged during quiet respiration is termed the *tidal volume*. After a normal expiration, the volume of air that remains in the lung is known as the *functional residual capacity*. On completion of a maximal expiration, the volume remaining in the lungs is called the *residual volume*. The *vital capacity* is the amount of air exhaled after a maximal inspiration and subsequent maximal expiration. *Total lung capacity* consists of the vital capacity plus residual volume (Figure 9-21). Approximately 150 ml of air remains in the nasopharynx, trachea, and bronchial tree during respiration and is thus unavailable for gas exchange in the alveoli. This volume is the anatomic dead space. The volume of air that ventilates alveoli that are not fully perfused by blood is the physiological dead space.

In addition to these static volumes, a number of dynamic volumes are useful in evaluating patients with pulmonary or neuromuscular problems. Forced expiratory volume (FEV) is the volume of air that can be exhaled with maximal effort during a specified unit of time, usually expressed as a percentage of the vital capacity. The time, in seconds, is denoted by a subscript (e.g., FEV_1 is the volume of air exhaled during the first second of a forced expiration). The FEV is particularly useful for evaluating patients with obstructive pulmonary disease. Pulmonary function tests measure the lung capacity based on the expiratory volume, flow, or both measurements. This measurement depends on the maximal effort of the respiratory muscles. Muscle weakness caused by atrophy, poor nutrition, disease, or lack of effort produces poor results. Respiratory muscle strength can be evaluated in the measures of maximal inspiratory and expiratory pressures. Endurance is measured in maximum volume ventilation.

Maximal voluntary ventilation is the volume of air exhaled during a period of time as the patient is told to

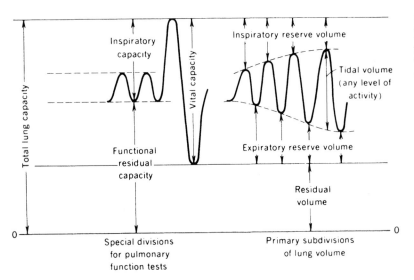

FIGURE 9-21 The relationship of the various lung volumes to the total lung volume. (Reprinted with permission from P-O Åstrand, K Rodahl. Textbook of Work Physiology [3rd ed]. New York: McGraw-Hill, 1986.)

breathe as rapidly and deeply as possible. Data are usually collected for a short time (15 seconds), and the results are extrapolated to the volume per minute. Maximal voluntary ventilation is influenced by the mechanical and neuromuscular status of the chest wall and lungs. Fatigue of the inspiratory muscles limits the ability to sustain a high minute ventilation. There is a characteristic electromyographic pattern that indicates the onset of inspiratory muscle fatigue; this pattern has been recorded from both the intercostal muscles and the diaphragm. Patients with chronic obstructive pulmonary disease demonstrate this pattern of inspiratory muscle fatigue during exercise, as do patients with neuromuscular and skeletal diseases.[57–59] Exercise tolerance in chronic obstructive pulmonary disease is limited by both lung mechanics and respiratory muscle performance.[60]

Mechanics of Respiration

Before inspiration, the intrapleural pressure is approximately –5 cm H_2O. This negative pressure is generated by the elastic recoil of the lungs, and the pressure in the alveoli immediately before inspiration is zero relative to the environment. With inspiration, negative pressure is generated in the pleural space by diaphragmatic contraction. This negative pressure (approximately 8–10 mm Hg) results in a negative pressure in the airways, causing the movement of air into the lungs. Quiet expiration is a passive process, driven by the elastic recoil of the lungs and of the chest wall.

Deeper inspiration is accomplished by the additional use of the external intercostal muscles, which contract and cause the ribs to move upward and forward, increasing both the anteroposterior dimension and side-to-side dimensions of the thoracic cage (Figure 9-22). Maximal inspiratory efforts make use of the sternocleidomastoid and the scalene muscles, which raise the sternum and first two ribs, respectively.

Forced expiration uses the internal intercostal muscles to move the ribs downward and backward, an action opposite to that effected by the external intercostal muscles. This leads to a decrease in both anteroposterior and side-to-side dimensions of the thorax. The abdominal musculature (rectus abdominis, internal and external obliques, and the transversus abdominis) also contribute to forced expiration by increasing intra-abdominal pressure, pushing the diaphragm upward.[61] Expiratory muscles are able to exert the greatest force when the lung volume approaches total lung capacity, by virtue of a favorable length-tension relationship. Conversely, the inspiratory muscles can exert the greatest force at lung volumes approaching residual volume. Maximal expira-

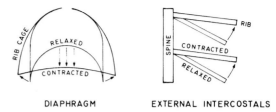

FIGURE 9-22 The effect of the mechanical action of the diaphragm and external intercostal muscles on chest wall dimensions. (Reprinted with permission from A Haas, H Pineda, F Haas, et al. Pulmonary Therapy and Rehabilitation: Principles and Practice. Baltimore: Williams & Wilkins, 1979.)

tory force averages 230 cm H_2O for men aged 20–55 years and 150 cm H_2O for women of the same age. Maximal inspiratory force averages 125 cm H_2O for men aged 20–55, and 90 cm H_2O for women in this age group.[62]

During quiet respiration, the resistance to air flow derives primarily from the medium-sized bronchi. The terminal bronchioles contribute less than one-fifth of the resistance.

The energy requirement, or cost of respiration, is determined by the resistance to flow of air and the elasticity of the lungs and chest wall. The relative contributions of these two vary individually and according to breathing pattern. Breathing deeply increases the elastic work of breathing disproportionately, whereas breathing at faster rates increases the proportion of work caused by airway resistance. The work performed on the lung can be graphically represented by plotting pleural pressure versus lung volume (Figure 9-23).

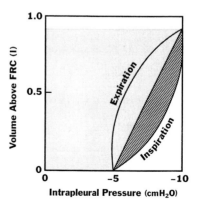

FIGURE 9-23 The pressure-volume curve of the lung demonstrating the work of inspiration overcoming elastic (*shaded area*) and viscous (*cross-hatched area*) forces. (FRC = functional residual capacity.) (Adapted from JB West. Respiratory Physiology—The Essentials [3rd ed]. Baltimore: Williams & Wilkins, 1989.)

In chronic obstructive pulmonary disease the respiratory muscles are subjected to increased loading as airflow obstruction progresses. This increased load results in progressive damage to the musculature and connective tissue. The structure and function of the diaphragm change with the course of disease. In early stages of chronic increased work of breathing the muscle hypertrophies and undergoes changes consistent with strength and endurance training. As the disease progresses, the long-term demand on the musculature ultimately causes overuse atrophy. The additional component of poor nutrition that often coincides with advanced disease further complicates the atrophy. The diaphragm is attached to the lower ribs and T-10 to T-12. As lung disease progresses, with the resulting increase in residual volume and total lung capacity, the increased air trapping causes distortion to the chest wall so that the diaphragm can no longer function as an inspiratory muscle and begins to function as an expiratory muscle.

Impaired ciliary function, irritation of the mucous membranes, and inflammation of the bronchial walls result in increased mucus production. Physiological factors associated with excessive mucus are dehydration, hypoxia, and electrolyte imbalance.[63] Thus, mucus results in reduced airway size, decreased ventilatory space, and increased work of breathing. Removal of secretions through postural drainage can change lung volume consequent on a decrease in airway resistance, improve ventilation and perfusion, and reduce the work of breathing. Reduction of airway secretions is associated with clinical improvement, in addition to the slowing of the downhill course of FEV_1.[64]

The normal energy requirement of quiet breathing through the nose is approximately 1 calorie per minute. This may increase to 20–25 calories per minute with a minute ventilation of 70 L.[65] The oxygen consumption of the respiratory muscles is 0.5–1.0 ml/L of ventilation at rest, representing approximately 1–2% of the body's total oxygen consumption.[46] This increases rapidly with increased ventilation (Figure 9-24), reaching 5 ml/L of ventilation when minute ventilation reaches 180 L.[66] Endurance training can increase maximal oxygen consumption of the respiratory muscles as much as 67%.[66]

Expiration is normally a passive process for a person at rest, but with increased ventilatory demands becomes active and consumes a considerable portion of the energy required by the respiratory muscles. During forced expiration by a normal individual, 80% of the lung volume is exhaled in the first second. Similarly, early inspiration contains the bulk of the inspired volume. These facts allow for considerable increases in respiratory rate without impairing the ability to exchange full tidal volumes with each breath.

Ventilation and perfusion are gravity and posture dependent. Thus, in an upright position, the lower lung fields have better perfusion and thus provide more efficient oxygenation. The expansion of the thorax is three-dimensional and is directly related to the muscle length of the involved musculature. Depending on the effects of various disease processes on the chest wall and its musculature, varying positions have an effect on ventilation and perfusion. Spinal flexion and extension are necessary for full thoracic expansion. Thus, limitation in spinal mobility directly affects full respiratory capability.

Alveolar ventilation is the volume of air that each minute reaches the alveoli for gas exchange and is calculated by subtracting anatomic dead space from tidal volume and multiplying the result by the respiratory rate. Rapid shallow breathing thus provides less effective ventilation for a given volume of air breathed.

The fundamental purpose of the lung is gas exchange. For this to be effective a mechanism for transporting oxygen from the air in the alveoli to the blood, and carbon dioxide in the reverse direction, is needed. Transport of carbon dioxide is facilitated by its higher solubility in blood (20 times greater than oxygen), by formation of bicarbonate in the red blood cells through carbonic anhydrase, and through the formation of carbamino compounds through the nonenzymatic combination of carbon dioxide with the terminal amine groups on proteins, primarily hemoglobin.

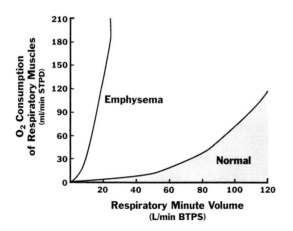

FIGURE 9-24 The work of breathing in a normal individual compared with a patient with emphysema. (BTPS = body temperature, atmospheric pressure, saturated; STPD = standard temperature [37°C], pressure [760 mm HG], dry [0].) (Adapted from VB Mountcastle. Medical Physiology. St. Louis: CV Mosby, 1974.)

The amount of oxygen that can dissolve in blood is quite small, approximately 0.3 ml per 100 ml of arterial blood at a partial pressure of oxygen (PO_2) of 100 mm Hg. Hemoglobin is responsible for the remainder of oxygen transport and can bind 20.8 ml of oxygen per 100 ml of blood.[67] The affinity of hemoglobin for oxygen varies with the PO_2, a relationship described by the hemoglobin-oxygen dissociation curve (Figure 9-25A). The advantages of this curve include allowing for a relatively small decrease in oxygen content per decrement in PO_2 in the upper, flatter part of the curve, and a large release of oxygen during the steep midportion of the curve. Thus, oxygen content of the blood is minimally affected by small changes in ambient PO_2 or mild alveolar hypoventilation, and a large amount of oxygen can be delivered to the body tissues as the blood PO_2 decreases during passage through the periphery.

The hemoglobin-oxygen dissociation curve may be shifted by a number of factors. Acidosis, elevated temperature, and increased PCO_2 all cause the curve to shift to the right, in association with a decrease in the affinity of hemoglobin for oxygen (Figure 9-25B). Hypoxia causes an increase in red blood cell 2,3-diphosphoglycerate, which also causes a shift to the right. These adaptations allow for delivery of more oxygen to the peripheral tissues, especially during times of stress, when tissue oxygen demand may be increased.

Movement of oxygen and carbon dioxide across the alveolar wall takes place through diffusion. The rate of diffusion (V_{gas}) is described by Fick's law and is proportional to the difference in the partial pressures of the gas ($P_1 - P_2$), the surface area available for diffusion, and a diffusion constant. It is inversely proportional to the thickness of the barrier. The solubility and molecular weight of the gas determine the diffusion constant.

Regulation of Respiration

Neural Factors

The control of the basic respiratory pattern appears to be centered in clusters of neurons in the medulla, which form a central pattern generator.[68,69] This center receives inhibitory impulses from the rostral pons as well as from the pulmonary stretch receptors, which send feedback via vagal afferents. The inhibition from the stretch receptors is known as the *Hering-Breuer reflex*. This basic mechanism is influenced by many other factors, including cortical, extrapyramidal, and peripheral neural input, as well as chemical factors. The situation is further complicated by the individual's inability to exert

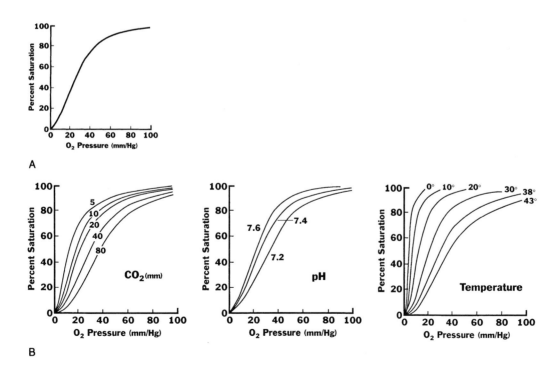

FIGURE 9-25 A. The oxyhemoglobin dissociation curve. **B.** The effect of carbon dioxide, pH, and temperature on the oxyhemoglobin dissociation curve. (Reprinted with permission from P-O Åstrand, K Rodahl. Textbook of Work Physiology [3rd ed]. New York: McGraw-Hill, 1986.)

a significant amount of voluntary control on the process and by the effects of emotional expression.

Central Chemoreceptors

The central chemoreceptors are located on the surface of the medulla. These receptors respond to changes in the pH of the cerebrospinal fluid, which in turn is influenced by the PCO_2 of arterial blood. Activation of these receptors results in an increased rate of firing of the pattern generator as well as an increased threshold for neurons that respond to inhibitory influences, thus increasing the depth of respiration. The minute ventilation is thus increased by a combination of increased ventilatory rate and increased tidal volume in response to an increase in the PCO_2.

Sleep has a physiological influence on respiration, which can have major adverse effects on gas exchange in patients with respiratory insufficiency. These effects relate to a reduction in various stimulant inputs to the brain stem respiratory center. Conditions that may be associated with sleep-related respiratory insufficiency range from pulmonary disorders (such as chronic obstructive pulmonary disease), to central respiratory insufficiency (such as central alveolar hypoventilation), neurologic and neuromuscular disorders (such as polio and muscular dystrophy), and thoracic cage disorders (such as kyphoscoliosis). All these conditions have in common the finding of hypoxemia and hypercapnia, which become more pronounced during sleep. The relative hypoventilation that is common to each condition is caused by varying combinations of an inadequate respiratory drive and an increase in the work of breathing. Management should first be directed at correcting the underlying disorder, then at correcting hypoxemia, use of pharmacologic therapy, and the use of assisted ventilation. Use of assisted ventilation during the night is associated with beneficial effects during the day, par-

ticularly improved awake gas exchange and respiratory muscle strength, in addition to less dyspnea and improved quality of life.[70,71]

Studies have shown that the increase in arterial blood carbon dioxide tension is a predictor of respiratory insufficiency and is probably caused by fatigue and weakness of inspiratory muscles that are working at a mechanical disadvantage. There is also the factor of low compliance of the chest wall that requires increased muscle effort for inspiration.[72,73] Negative pressure ventilation during sleep can reverse chronic hypercapnia and hypoxemia and so alter the natural history of respiratory insufficiency caused by restrictive chest wall disorders.[74]

Medications can alter the respiratory response to activity. For example, salicylates increase the depth and rate of respiration by directly stimulating the medulla, increasing the sensitivity of the central chemoreceptors to carbon dioxide.[75] This greater increased sensitivity interacts with increased carbon dioxide production caused by the uncoupling of oxidative phosphorylation in the skeletal muscles.

Peripheral Chemoreceptors

The peripheral chemoreceptors are located in the carotid and aortic bodies. These clusters of epithelioid cells have a high metabolic rate and are sensitive to decreases in PO_2. The hypoxic drive may be generalized because of hypoxemia or local because of decreased blood flow. Decreased blood flow at the receptors may be caused by either generalized hypotension or a local decrease in blood flow caused by sympathetic activation or circulating catecholamines. It is important to remember that it is the local PO_2 at the receptor sites, not the arterial PO_2 or the oxygen saturation, that determines the activation of these receptors. At least part of the hyperventilation caused by salicylates appears to be related to stimulation of these peripheral chemoreceptors,[76] a phenomenon that is independent of the inhibition of prostaglandin synthesis.[77]

Respiratory Response to Exercise

The stimulation and regulation of respiration during exercise remain controversial; the relative importance of neural and chemical factors are undetermined.[78] The minute ventilation increases in a linear fashion with increasing work intensity up to a point, and then the response becomes much steeper (Figure 9-26). During most of this increase there is no measurable change in PCO_2, PO_2, or pH. With greater loads there is a decrease in the pH that is not proportional to the ventilatory response, and with very high loads PO_2 may decrease.

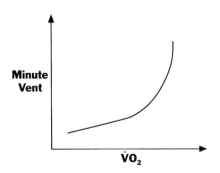

FIGURE 9-26 The relationship between minute ventilation and oxygen consumption ($\dot{V}O_2$).

Both factors are involved, although the precise mechanisms of control still are not clear. There is a rapid ventilatory response to exercise; this is mediated by neural mechanisms, through somatosensory feedback from working muscles and moving joints stimulating the medullary centers. As exercise continues, additional control is exerted by the effect of acidosis on the medullary chemoreceptors and hypoxia on the peripheral chemoreceptors. The hypoxic effect is exaggerated by the activation of the sympathetic nervous system and circulating catecholamines, depending on the relative stress of the exercise (i.e., the fitness of the individual).

The typical ventilatory response to exercise described previously refers to dynamic exercise. The response to isometric exercise is exaggerated in the same way that the cardiac response is exaggerated when an isometric component is superimposed on dynamic exercise.[79] The rapid onset and offset of the increased ventilation, out of proportion to the metabolic demands, suggest a neural reflex. The stimulus for this reflex is not clear.

An increased demand on the respiratory system occurs with upper extremity exercise. The upper extremity has a smaller muscle mass and reduced cross-sectional area, resulting in lower power output. The higher percentage of type II muscle fibers makes the upper extremity musculature less efficient, with an early onset of anaerobic metabolism resulting in an increase in respiratory drive and higher energy cost. The smaller capillary beds lend to higher systemic vascular resistance and early onset of blood lactate.

With the progression of lung disease, there is an increased recruitment of muscles of the neck and chest wall to help in the breathing effort. Accessory respiratory muscles such as the pectoralis major and minor and serratus anterior are activated in the upper extremity exercise and are unable to effectively compensate for increasing the respiratory demand. Lower extremity activity decreases the systemic vascular resistance and increases venous return. There is also an increase in type I fibers, which increases the oxidative capacity of the body, resulting in an increase in aerobic metabolism, decrease in carbon dioxide production, and increase in work efficiency. Lower extremity exercise should be incorporated into an exercise program along with the upper extremity exercise to provide the reduced systemic vascular resistance, allowing for more efficient cardiac work, more oxidative capacity, and decreased carbon dioxide production, thus reducing the ventilatory demand.

Physical training has less of an effect on the ventilatory response to exercise than the cardiac response. In general, the rate of respiration is somewhat slower and the depth greater at any given submaximal load, but the minute ventilation remains essentially unchanged.

REFERENCES

1. Ruskin J, McHale PA, Harley A, et al. Pressure-flow studies in man: effects of atrial systole on left ventricular function. J Clin Invest 1970;49:472–478.
2. Brush JE Jr, Cannon RO III, Schenke WH, et al. Angina due to coronary microvascular disease in hypertensive patients without left ventricular hypertrophy. N Engl J Med 1988;319:1302–1307.
3. Sax FL, Cannon RO III, Hanson C, et al. Impaired forearm vasodilator reserve in patients with microvascular angina, evidence of a generalized disorder of vascular function? N Engl J Med 1987;317:1366–1370.
4. Crea F, Gaspardone A. New look to an old symptom: angina pectoris. Circulation 1997;96(10):3766–3773.
5. Guyton AC. Textbook of Medical Physiology (7th ed). Philadelphia: WB Saunders, 1986.
6. Berne RB, Levy MN. Cardiovascular Physiology. St. Louis: CV Mosby, 1986.
7. Furchgott RF, Vanhoutte PM. Endothelium-derived relaxing and contracting factors. FASEB J 1989;3:2007–2018.
8. Gryglewski RJ, Botting RM, Vane JR. Mediators produced by the endothelial cell. Hypertension 1988;12:530–548.
9. Ignarro LJ. Endothelium-derived nitric oxide: actions and properties. FASEB J 1989;3:31–36.
10. Moncada S, Palmer RM, Higgs EA. The discovery of nitric oxide as the endogenous nitrovasodilator. Hypertension 1988;12:365–372.
11. Rubino A, Loesch A, Burnstock G. Nitric oxide and endothelin-1 in coronary and pulmonary circulation. Int Rev Cytol 1999;189:59–93.
12. Britten MB, Zeiher AM, Schachinger V. Clinical importance of coronary endothelial vasodilator dysfunction and therapeutic options. J Int Med 1999;245:315–327.
13. Klocke FJ, Mates KE, Canty JM Jr, et al. Coronary pressure-flow relationships: continued issues and probable implications. Circ Res 1985;56:310–323.
14. Moldover JR, Downey JA. Cardiac response to exercise: comparison of 3 ergometers. Arch Phys Med Rehabil 1983;64:155–159.
15. Lundberg A. Oxygen consumption in relation to work load in students with cerebral palsy. J App Physiol 1976;40:873–875.
16. Faulkner JA, Heigenhauser GF, Schork MA. The cardiac output-oxygen uptake relationship of men during graded bicycle ergometry. Med Sci Sports 1977;9:148–154.
17. Ekelund LG, Holmgren A. Central hemodynamics during exercise. Circ Res 1967;20(Suppl 1):133–143.

18. Braunwald E, Sonnenblick EH, Ross J, et al. An analysis of the cardiac response to exercise. Circ Res 1967;20(Suppl 1):144–158.

19. Fitzgerald MD, Tanaka H, Tran ZV, Seals DR. Age-related declines in maximal aerobic capacity in regularly exercising vs. sedentary women: a meta-analysis. J Appl Physiol 1997;83(1):160–165.

20. Kotchen TA, Hartley LH, Rice TW, et al. Renin, norepinephrine, and epinephrine responses to graded exercise. J Appl Physiol 1971;31:178–184.

21. von Euler US. Sympatho-adrenal activity in physical exercise. Med Sci Sports Exerc 1974;6:165–173.

22. Tulppo MP, Makikallio TH, Seppanen T, et al. Vagal modulation of heart rate during exercise: effects of age and physical fitness. Am J Physiol 1998;274(2 Pt 2):H424–H429.

23. McLaren PF, Nurhayati Y, Boutcher SH. Stroke volume response to cycle ergometry in trained and untrained older men. Eur J Appl Physiol 1997;75(6):537–542.

24. Bevegård S, Holmgren A, Jonsson B. The effect of body position on the circulation at rest and during exercise, with special reference to the influence on the stroke volume. Acta Physiol Scand 1960;49:279–298.

25. Turley KR, Wilmore JH. Cardiovascular response to treadmill and cycle ergometer exercise in children and adults. J Appl Physiol 1997;83(3):948–957.

26. Turley KR, Wilmore JH. Cardiovascular responses to submaximal exercise in 7 to 9 year old boys and girls. Med Sci Sports Exerc 1997;29(6):824–832.

27. Kitamura K, Jorgensen CR, Gobel FL, et al. Hemodynamic correlates of myocardial oxygen consumption during upright exercise. J Appl Physiol 1972;32:516–522.

28. Jorgensen CR, Wang K, Wang Y, et al. Effect of propranolol on myocardial oxygen consumption and its hemodynamic correlates during upright exercise. Circulation 1973;48:1173–1182.

29. Nelson RR, Gobel FL, Jorgensen CR, et al. Hemodynamic predictors of myocardial oxygen consumption during static and dynamic exercise. Circulation 1974;50:1179–1189.

30. Donald KW, Lind AR, McNicol GW, et al. Cardiovascular responses to sustained (static) contractions. Circulation Res 1967;20(Suppl 1):I15–I30.

31. Stenberg J, Åstrand P-O, Ekblom B, et al. Hemodynamic response to work with different muscle groups, sitting and supine. J Appl Physiol 1967;22(l):61–70.

32. Glaser RM, Sawka MN, Laubach LL, Suryaprasad AG. Metabolic and cardiopulmonary responses to wheelchair and bicycle ergometry. J Appl Physiol 1979;46:1066–1070.

33. Bostom AG, Bates E, Mazzarella N, et al. Ergometer modification for combined arm-leg use by lower extremity amputees in cardiovascular testing and training. Arch Phys Med Rehabil 1987;68:244–247.

34. King ML, Guarracini M, Lennihan L, et al. Adaptive exercise testing for patients with hemiparesis. J Cardiopulm Rehabil 1989;9:237–242.

35. Moldover JR, Daum MC, Downey JA. Cardiac stress testing of hemiparetic patients with a supine bicycle ergometer: preliminary study. Arch Phys Med Rehabil 1984;65:470–473.

36. Lecerof H. Influence of body position on exercise tolerance, heart rate, blood pressure, and respiration rate in coronary insufficiency. Br Heart J 1971;33:78–83.

37. Saltin B, Blomqvist G, Mitchell JH, et al. Response to exercise after bed rest and after training. Circulation 1968;38(Suppl 7):1–50.

38. Duey WJ, O'Brien WL, Crutchfield AB, et al. Effects of exercise training on aerobic fitness in African-American females. Ethn Dis 1998;8(3):306–311.

39. Ekblom B, Lundberg A. Effect of physical training on adolescents with severe motor handicaps. Acta Paediatr Scand 1968;57:17–23.

40. Winder WW, Hagberg JM, Hickson RC, et al. Time course of sympathoadrenal adaptation to endurance exercise training in man. J Appl Physiol 1978;45:370–374.

41. Schuit AJ, vanAmelsvoort LG, Verheij TC, et al. Exercise training and heart rate variability in older people. Med Sci Sports Exerc 1999;31(6):816–821.

42. Linxue L, Nohara R, Makita S, et al. Effect of long-term exercise training on regional myocardial perfusion changes in patients with coronary artery disease. Jpn Circ J 1999;63(2):73–78.

43. Laughlin MH, Oltman CL, Bowles DK. Exercise training-induced adaptations in the coronary circulation. Med Sci Sports Exerc 1998;30:352–360.

44. Guyton AC. The venous system and its role in the circulation. Mod Concepts Cardiovasc Dis 1958;27:483.

45. Milnor WR. Hemodynamics. Baltimore: Williams & Wilkins, 1982.

46. Otis AB. The Work of Breathing. In WO Fenn, H Rhan (eds), Handbook of Physiology. Vol 1, Sec 3: Respiration. Washington: American Physiological Society, 1964;463–476.

47. Starling EH. On the absorption of fluids from the connective tissue spaces. Lymphology 1984;17(4):124–129.

48. Weiner N, Tatlor P. Neurohumoral Transmission: The Autonomic and Somatic Motor Nervous Systems. In AG Gilman, LS Goodman, TW Rall, et al. (eds), The Pharmacological Basis of Therapeutics (7th ed). New York: Macmillan, 1985;72–73.

49. Duff F, Shepard JT. The circulation in the chronically denervated forearm. Clin Sci 1953;12:407–416.

50. Levin ER, Gardner DG, Samson WK. Mechanisms of disease: natriuretic peptides. N Eng J Med 1998;339:321–328.

51. Raven PB, Potts JT, Shi X. Baroreflex regulation of blood pressure during dynamic exercise. Exerc Sport Sci Rev 1997;25:365–389.

52. Shephard RJ. Physiology and Biochemistry of Exercise. New York: Praeger, 1982.

53. Berger RA. Applied Exercise Physiology. Philadelphia: Lea & Febiger, 1982.

54. West JB. Respiratory Physiology—The Essentials (3rd ed). Baltimore: Williams & Wilkins, 1985.

55. De Troyer A, Sampson M, Sigrist S, et al. The diaphragm: two muscles. Science 1981;213:237–238.

56. Roussos CS, Macklem PT. The respiratory muscles. N Engl J Med 1982;307:786–797.

57. Roussos CS. Diaphragmatic fatigue in man. J Appl Physiol 1977;43:189–197.

58. Gross D, Grassino A, Ross WR, Macklem PT. Electromyogram pattern of diaphragmatic fatigue. J Appl Physiol 1979;46:1–7.

59. Grassino A. Inspiratory muscle fatigue as a factor limiting exercise. Bull Eur Physiopathol Respir 1979;15:105–115.

60. Spiro SG. An analysis of physiologic strain of submaximal exercise in patients with chronic obstructive bronchitis. Thorax 1975;30:415–425.

61. Taylor AE, Rehder K, Hyatt RE, et al. Clinical Respiratory Physiology. Philadelphia: WB Saunders, 1989.

62. Black LF, Hyatt RE. Maximal respiratory pressures: normal values and relationship to age and sex. Am Rev Respir Dis 1969;99:646–702.

63. Newhouse MT. Factors affecting sputum clearance. Proceedings of the Thoracic Society. Thorax 1973;28:261.

64. Cherniack RM, Ferguson GT. Manage-

ment of chronic obstructive pulmonary disease. Am Rev Resp Dis 1974;110: 188–192.

65. Roussos CS, Campbell EJM. Respiratory Muscle Energetics. In AP Fishman (ed), Handbook of Physiology. Vol 3: The Respiratory System. Bethesda, MD: American Physiological Association, 1986.

66. Bradley M, Leith D. Ventilatory muscle training and the oxygen cost of sustained hypernea. J Appl Physiol 1978;45:885–892.

67. West JB. In Best and Taylor's Physiological Basis of Medical Practice (12th ed). Baltimore: Williams & Wilkins, 1991;564.

68. von Euler C. On the central pattern generator for the basic breathing rhythmicity. J Appl Physiol 1983; 55:1647–1659.

69. Åstrand P-O, Rodahl K. Textbook of Work Physiology (3rd ed). New York: McGraw-Hill, 1986.

70. McNicholas WT. Impact of sleep in respiratory failure. Eur Respir J 1997;10(4):92–93.

71. Hoeppner VH, Cockcroft DW, Dosman JA, Cotton DJ. Nighttime ventilation improves respiratory failure in secondary kyphoscoliosis. Am Rev Respir Dis 1984;129:240–243.

72. Cooper DM. Respiratory mechanics in adolescents with idiopathic scoliosis. Am Rev Respir Dis 1984;130:16–22.

73. Lisboa C. Inspiratory muscle function in patients with severe kyphoscoliosis. Am Rev Respir Dis 1985;132:48–52.

74. Simonds AK, Branthwaite MA. Efficiency of negative pressure ventilatory equipment. Proceedings of the British Thoracic Society. Thorax 1985;40: 209–240.

75. Cameron IR, Semple SJ. The central respiratory stimulant action of salicylates. Clin Sci 1968;35:391–401.

76. McQueen DS, Ritchie IM, Birrell GJ. Arterial chemoreceptor involvement in salicylate-induced hyperventilation in rats. Br J Pharmacol 1989;98:413–424.

77. Kuna ST, Levine S. Relationship between cyclooxygenase activity (COA) inhibition and stimulation of ventilation by salicylates. J Pharmacol Exp Ther 1981;219:723–730.

78. Cunningham DJC. Regulation of breathing in exercise. Circ Res 1967;20(Suppl 1):1122–1131.

79. Wiley RL, Lind AR. Respiratory responses to simultaneous static and rhythmic exercises in humans. Clin Sci Mol Med 1975;49:427–432.

10

Urogenital Physiology

MARK A. CABELIN, ALEXIS E. TE,
AND STEVEN A. KAPLAN

Two of the most important goals in the rehabilitation of patients with neurologic lesions are restoration of voiding and of sexual function. In this chapter the micturition cycle is divided into its two major phases, storage (filling) and emptying (voiding), and relevant lower urinary tract anatomy and neurophysiology are discussed. The lower urinary tract is well suited for its primary function, the storage and timely expulsion of urine.[1] The storage function of the bladder is performed largely by its ability to increase volume, up to a point, with little or no change in intravesical pressure. The sphincteric action of both the vesical neck and the proximal urethra maintain continence despite the wide range of intravesical pressures that occurs during ordinary physical activity. Micturition is a complex series of finely tuned and integrated neuromuscular events that involve many neurologic pathways. Final integration of these events occurs in the rostral pons in an area known as the *pontine micturition center*.[2] As an important relationship exists between the lower urinary tract and sexual function, pertinent male and female anatomy, and the physiology of both erection and female response, are reviewed. Erectile physiology in men and the engorgement of the external genitalia and vaginal lubrication in women involve a complex series of neurologically mediated vascular phenomena within a hormonal milieu. Supraspinal psychological and neurologic factors play an important role in modifying these essentially reflex phenomena. It should be emphasized that much of the experimental work to date has been done in animals, so exact extrapolation to the human model is not possible. In particular, the human psyche is difficult to evaluate, qualitatively or quantitatively. This chapter, therefore, presents the basic mechanisms underlying the physiology of both micturition and sexual function.

GENITOURINARY ANATOMY

Although no anatomic distinction exists, the lower urinary tract can be thought of as being composed of a bladder and a sphincter. Grossly, the muscle fibers and mucosa of the bladder blend imperceptibly with those of the vesical neck and urethra, and no real *anatomic* sphincter exists that can be seen with the naked eye. Rather, the sphincter is a unique arrangement of smooth and striated muscle interlaced with fibrous and elastic connective tissue that constitutes the *physiological* sphincter. Of note, the mucosal lining of the urethra is characterized by inner wall softness, which keeps the walls coapted and forms a water-tight seal.[3]

The bladder is composed of two main components, the body and the base.[4] The detrusor is composed of interlacing bundles of smooth muscle arranged in a loose network. Individual muscle bundles cross one another; they follow no consistent pattern, but the outer and inner layers tend to be oriented longitudinally, particularly as they approach the vesical neck.[4,5] The detrusor is present in both the body and base and is responsible for the storage and pump functions of the bladder. The base detrusor is generally considered to be nondistendible and relatively fixed as a horizontal plate. In addition, some investigators describe a series of detrusor fibers, termed the *fundal ring*, that originates posteriorly and loops around the trigone and vesical neck.[6] Posteriorly, these fibers are separated from the internal orifice by the trigone. Anteriorly, they are in close approximation to the internal urethral orifice.

Because of this complex arrangement of interlacing detrusor bundles, with loops around the vesical neck, the horizontal configuration of the base detrusor is transformed into a vertical funnel by the action of detrusor contraction.

The trigone proper is a triangular area located in the bladder base and is demarcated superiorly and laterally by the ureteral orifices and inferiorly by the internal urethral orifice. It is superficial to the base detrusor and is composed of smooth muscle extensions from the distal ureteral musculature. As this musculature approaches the bladder, it loses its spiral configuration and assumes a longitudinal one. The ureterovesical junction is marked by an external layer of smooth muscle called *Waldeyer's sheath*, which serves to anchor the ureter to the detrusor body. The intramural ureter traverses the bladder obliquely through a tunnel approximately 2 cm in length. At the ureteral orifice, an internal layer of musculature is composed of ureteral smooth muscle that fans out and meets the musculature from the other side to form the trigone proper. The trigonal muscle continues through the urethra and extends to the verumontanum in male subjects and to the distal third of the urethra in female subjects. Because of the relative thinness of the trigone as compared with the detrusor musculature of the base, it is thought that its only function is to anchor the ureteral orifices so that they are pulled distally and inferiorly during voiding. Because of this dual-sheath concept at the ureteral vesical junction (internal-external layers of musculature) and its oblique course through the intramural tunnel, detrusor contraction during voiding results in compression of the ureteral lumen and prevents vesicoureteral reflux.[5,7,8]

The musculature of the urethra consists of circularly and longitudinally oriented fibers of both striated and smooth muscle, but the proportion and functional significance of each remains a subject of controversy. Important differences exist between male and female anatomy. It is widely agreed that in both sexes there are longitudinal or helical bundles of smooth muscle that extend from the base of the bladder into the prostatic urethra in the man and almost throughout the entire urethra in the woman. In the man there is a rather well-defined, circularly oriented smooth muscle group just below the bladder neck.[7,9] Some researchers believe that this proximal urethral circular smooth muscle is identical to the prostatic capsule and that this structure is the primary involuntary internal sphincter. Dixon and Gosling, however, deny that this is a urinary sphincter; they believe that it is a *genital* sphincter that serves as a barrier to retrograde ejaculation during sexual intercourse.[5]

The intraurethral rhabdosphincter and periurethral musculature of the pelvic diaphragm make up the striated voluntary muscle component of the urethra. The intraurethral portion surrounds the middle third of the female urethra and is composed mostly of slow-twitch muscle fibers.[5] The muscle is even more prominent in the male subject and extends to the vesical neck.[10,11] Some investigators believe this rhabdosphincter constitutes the primary urethral sphincter in both sexes.

In summary, the presence of both circular and longitudinal fibers in both the vesical neck and urethra provide the anatomic substrate for understanding the mechanisms of micturition and urinary continence. Thus, contraction of longitudinal fibers serves to shorten and widen the urethra during voiding, thus opening the urethra for unimpeded flow. Contraction of circular fibers aids in the maintenance of continence; relaxation opens the urethra for micturition.

GENITOURINARY NEUROPHYSIOLOGY

Afferent Pathways

Afferent fibers are projections of dorsal spinal root ganglia axons, and in some species there is evidence that some of the afferent fibers are located in the ventral root as well.[12] Afferent fibers establish many synapses after leaving the posterior root ganglion. Some of these synapses include (1) the pelvic nucleus in the anteromedial area, (2) the dorsal horn, which ascends ipsilaterally, and (3) the dorsal horn, which crosses the midline and ascends the contralateral spinothalamic tract. The afferent fibers of the pelvic nerve are thought to initiate voiding through impulses arising from tension receptors in the bladder wall transmitted via small diameter $A\gamma$ and C fibers.[13] Most bladder afferents contain substance P, vasoactive intestinal polypeptide, and other neuropeptides.

Parasympathetic Nerves

The primary parasympathetic nerve involved in micturition is the pelvic nerve. Its primary neurotransmitter is acetylcholine at both the preganglionic and postganglionic synapses. The pelvic nerve nucleus is located in the anteromedial cell column of the second, third, and fourth segments of the sacral spinal cord.[14,15]

The ventral roots of the second through the fourth sacral segments house the efferent parasympathetic fibers. These fibers merge to form the pelvic nerve (nervi erigentes), but the anatomy of this nerve varies considerably from species to species.[16,17] The pelvic nerve plexus is formed by fibers of both the pelvic nerve and the hypogastric nerve. Although it never forms an identifiable nerve trunk, the pelvic nerve plexus does send *twigs* of fibers to both bladder and urethra, and then the majority of efferent fibers resynapse in the pelvic ganglia in or near the walls of the bladder and urethra. Elbadawi and Schenk called these peripheral ganglia the *urogenital short neuron system*.[18] This system connects extensively with sympathetic fibers, which are similarly situated throughout the bladder and urethral wall.

Detrusor contractions can be caused either by administration of acetylcholine or electrical stimulation of the pelvic nerve[14,16,19-21]; however, the bladder contraction induced by electrical stimulation cannot be completely blocked by atropine, unlike the detrusor contraction elicited by administration of acetylcholine.[22,23] Evidence suggests that this atropine-resistance effect, recognized for many years, may be related to a noncholinergic, nonadrenergic neurotransmitter.[24] The effect of acetylcholine and pelvic nerve stimulation on the muscles of the urethra is even less well understood. Researchers variously reported increased urethral resistance, decreased urethral resistance, or no change.[20,25-28]

The ganglia of the short neuron system are composed predominantly of three types of cells: adrenergic, cholinergic, and small intensely fluorescent neurons.[29,30] The importance of the short neuron system is that it ensures that neurologic lesions do not completely denervate the bladder and urethra. For example, extensive radical surgery, such as abdominoperineal resection of the rectum, does not ablate the short neuronal system. Thus, central or preganglionic neurologic lesions result in decentralization rather than denervation.

Sympathetic Nerves

The importance of the sympathetic nervous system in voiding is controversial, but studies in cats provide new information that may be clinically applicable.[31-34] The cell bodies of the sympathetic nerves lie in the intermedial lateral cell column of T-10 to L-2. After traversing the ventral roots, efferent sympathetic fibers form synapses in the prevertebral ganglia of the lumbar sympathetic chain. At this point, they branch out to form the presacral plexus, which then bifurcates to form the right and left hypogastric nerves. The hypogastric nerve meets the pelvic nerve to form the pelvic plexus. The sympathetic ganglia located in the pelvic plexus and the urethral and bladder wall are part of the urogenital short neuron system. Modulation of reflex activity

affecting micturition is an important function of the intramural neuronal network, and sympathetic activity is mediated at least in part by the vesicosympathetic reflex (pelvic-hypogastric reflex). The vesicosympathetic reflex is a negative feedback mechanism whereby increasing bladder pressure triggers an increase in sympathetic efferent activity, allowing the bladder to accommodate larger volumes of urine at relatively low pressures. Pressure-sensitive mechanoreceptors in the urinary bladder relay information to Aδ afferents traveling within the pelvic nerve that project into dorsal horn of the lumbosacral spinal cord. Information is then relayed rostrocaudally either by direct synaptic transmission or via spinal interneurons to sympathetic preganglionic neurons located in the intermediolateral gray matter of spinal segments T-11 to L-2. Axons of these preganglionic sympathetic neurons pass to the sympathetic chain ganglia and then to prevertebral ganglia in the superior hypogastric and pelvic plexuses as mentioned previously. Sympathetic postganglionic nerves are tonically active during bladder filling, providing excitatory input to the bladder neck, inhibitory input to smooth muscle of the bladder body, and inhibitory input to vesical parasympathetic ganglia abetting low-pressure storage of urine. Different neurotransmitter receptor subtypes affect bladder-urethral function by anatomic site separation and concentration. α-Adrenoreceptors of the sympathetic system mediate storage of urine in two ways. The first action is via closure of both the proximal urethra and the bladder neck; the second action is via inhibition of neuronal transmission between the preganglionic and postganglionic parasympathetic nerve.[34] β-Adrenoreceptors mediate relaxation of the body of the bladder.[35-39] The sympathetic nervous system has little role in sensory function; in fact, in humans presacral neurectomy has no effect on either afferent urethral or bladder function.[40]

Somatic Nerves

The striated muscles of the pelvic floor, as well as the rhabdosphincter, are innervated primarily by the pudendal nerve. Histochemical studies using horseradish peroxidase have demonstrated that the pudendal nerve cell bodies originate in Onuftowicz's (Onuf's) nucleus in the anterior horn of the second through the fourth segments of the sacral spinal cord.[8,41] It is of interest that the cells of Onuf's nucleus are much more resistant to degenerative processes such as amyotrophic lateral sclerosis than other anterior horn cells, although Onuf's nucleus cells are always affected in Shy-Drager syndrome. The pudendal nucleus is located at either S-2 or S-3, which is one segment above the parasympathetic nucleus.[42] Thus, certain neurologic disorders, such as myelodysplasia or multiple sclerosis, may cause disparate lesions of the bladder and striated external urethral sphincter.[43,44]

Somatic efferent pathways to the external urinary sphincter are carried in the pudendal nerve from Onuf's nucleus. Urinary continence is ensured by an increase in efferent pudendal activity to the external sphincter during bladder filling. Afferent information from the urethra, striated sphincter, female sex organs, and also the skin of the genitalia of both sexes travels via the pudendal nerve into the dorsal horn of the sacral spinal cord. Information is then relayed to somatic motor neurons located in the anterior horn. Stimulation of these areas supplied by sensory branches of the pudendal nerve reflexively causes contraction of the muscles supplied by motor fibers of the pudendal nerves. Branches of the pudendal nerve and other sacral somatic nerves also carry efferent impulses to muscles of the pelvic floor, including the levator ani, striated muscle of the urogenital diaphragm, paraurethral striated muscle, superficial perineal muscle, and the anal sphincter, that aid in maintaining fecal continence and preserving the anorectal angle.

PHYSIOLOGY OF VOIDING

Storage of Urine

Physical Principles

The behavior of the normal bladder depends on both its active and passive properties. Collagen, elastin, and resting smooth muscle constitute the main tissues responsible for the passive properties of the bladder. In contrast, the active behavior of the bladder is determined by the contractile elements of smooth muscle. *Elasticity* is that property of a material that determines the tendency of the stressed material to return to its unstressed geometric configuration; viscosity is that property of a material that tends to retard deformation of the stressed material.[45] On the other hand, *plasticity* refers to the ability of a substance to sustain an irreversible deformation that occurs only after a certain threshold of stress is exceeded.[46] Elasticity can be measured by the change in wall tension as the bladder is stretched. Thus, in cystometrography, bladder pressure and volume are measured; when they are plotted against each other, the relationship is not linear and, thus, indicates that physical properties other than elasticity alone are involved.

The low-pressure storage of increasing volumes of urine is primarily a passive phenomenon attributable to the viscoelastic properties of the detrusor. Neural reflexes mediated at the spinal cord level help to ensure low-pressure storage and continence. Tension receptors in the bladder wall send afferent signals to the CNS, most notably via the pelvic nerve. These afferents consist of small myelinated (Aδ) and unmyelinated C fibers. Aδ fibers convey information in a graded manner concerning intravesical pressure. The intravesical pressure threshold for activation of Aδ afferents is approximately 5–15 mm Hg, which is within the range that most human subjects report a first sensation during filling cystometry. C-fiber afferents are activated by chemical irritation of the bladder mucosa or cold intravesical temperature.

The response of the bladder to stretch is dependent on a number of factors, including the duration of stretch, the rate at which the bladder is stretched, and hysteresis.[45,47,48] If the bladder is stretched rapidly, detrusor pressure and wall tension are great, but if it is stretched to a new length and that length is maintained, pressure decreases. Thus, during a cystometrogram, the faster the filling rate, the higher the pressure increase. *Hysteresis* refers to a property of the bladder: The tension-length or pressure-volume relationship is dependent on the conditions that existed before the strain (i.e., the degree of filling). Thus, if the bladder is filled and emptied at a constant rate, each phase has a different pressure-volume curve.

Accommodation is that property of the bladder that allows it to accept increasing volumes of urine without a concomitant increase in intravesical pressure. Usually, the degree of pressure increase during normal bladder filling is no more than 15 cm H_2O. This pressure-volume relationship is defined by Laplace's equation: $P = 2T/R$, where P is detrusor pressure, T is the wall tension in the bladder, and R is the radius of the bladder. Because the bladder radius is the same for any given bladder volume, the equation can be simply reduced to one that says that pressure is dependent on wall tension. Thus, bladder wall tension is dependent on both the active and passive properties and constituents of the bladder (i.e., actin, myosin, collagen, and elastic tissue). As the bladder wall becomes stiffer (thicker or hypertrophic) wall tension increases for a given volume and there is a concomitant increase in detrusor pressure.

Compliance is defined as the change in the volume-pressure relationship. Bladder compliance is difficult to assess in the human bladder, for a number of reasons; it is dependent on the rate of filling, hysteresis, the duration of filling, and smooth muscle activity. In addition, compliance may vary during different parts of the filling curve. The behavior of actin and myosin during bladder filling is not clearly understood, nor is the relative effect of smooth muscle contractions on the volume-pressure curve. Research has demonstrated that some individual smooth muscle cells manifest spontaneous activity during vesical filling and that this may contribute to bladder tone.[49]

For continence to be maintained, urethral pressure must be higher than intravesical pressure, which is the sum of intra-abdominal pressure, inherent detrusor pressure, and the potential (or gravitational) energy that is related to the *height* of urine above the meatus. *Urethral closure pressure* is defined as the difference between intravesical and urethral pressure. The resting urethra has a significantly higher pressure than the bladder, usually in the range of 40–80 cm H_2O. Both passive and active forces play prominent roles in the maintenance of this relatively high intraurethral pressure. Passive forces result from both the elastic and collagen fibers and also inner wall softness.[3] Active pressure changes are caused by periurethral striated muscles of the pelvic floor and also by intraurethral smooth and striated muscle contractions. In contrast to the bladder, the urethra is cylindrical. The pressure-volume relationship in the urethra is defined by Laplace's equation for a cylinder: $P = T/R$. In summary, high intraurethral pressure is caused, in large part, by its small radius and its dynamic high wall tension when compared with that of the bladder.

Expulsion of Urine

Voluntary micturition is accomplished by activation of the micturition reflex, which is integrated in the pontine micturition center (Figure 10-1). This complex coordinated event is initiated by sudden and complete relaxation of the striated muscle of the urethra and pelvic floor.[2,43] Urethral pressure decreases and detrusor pressure increases concomitantly, heralding the detrusor contraction. The reduction in urethral pressure is greatest at the membranous urethra in the male subject and at the distal urethra in the female subject. Both the urethra and the bladder neck gradually open and assume their widest cross-sectional area during peak flow, and bladder and urethra become a single isobaric unit as flow begins.[50-52] The mechanism of the micturition reflex is discussed in the section Neurologic Considerations, later in this chapter.

Physical Principles
The active or dynamic component of the bladder muscle wall consists of both actin and myosin filaments. Actin (thick) filaments are attached to the cell membrane; myosin (thin) filaments are located in the cytoplasm.

FIGURE 10-1 A representation of the neurologic events that occur during storage of urine, bladder emptying, and during sudden interruption of the voiding stream. Note that during micturition, detrusor (bladder) pressure is greater than urethral pressure with electrical silence of the electromyogram (EMG).

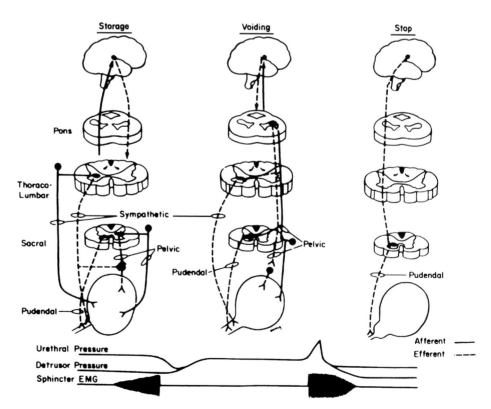

Depolarization of the cell, mediated by calcium influx and phosphorylation of myosin, results in muscle contraction. Muscle shortening is secondary to sliding of actin and myosin filaments past each other.[53] When the detrusor muscle contracts, one of two events occurs: muscle shortening or the development of force. The faster the muscle contracts, the less force it generates.

Some individual smooth muscle cells demonstrate spontaneous activity during filling and may act as pacemakers to regulate bladder activity.[49] In addition, at rest, detrusor smooth muscle cells have spontaneous action potentials. When stretched, the action potentials increase, both in frequency and in amplitude, whereas the resting membrane potential decreases.[54] Thus, as the bladder fills there is a gradual increase in the quantity of spontaneous action potentials, resulting in contraction of individual muscle fibers. At a certain level of firing, the detrusor contracts and voiding ensues.

When the expulsive energy of the bladder overcomes the resistance of the urethra, voiding is accomplished. If one applies hydrodynamic principles to the lower urinary tract, the bladder can be conceptualized as a pump and the urethra as a pipe. Urethral resistance determines the flow rate for any given bladder contraction, but the applicability of this mathematical model is limited because the urethra is distensible. There have been a variety of both mathematical and computer-generated indices of bladder function, but to date none has achieved wide clinical applicability.[55]

A more sophisticated approach to expulsion is to study the energy balance during micturition. The energy that the bladder provides to expel urine is derived from three sources: intra-abdominal pressure, inherent detrusor pressure, and the potential or gravitational energy, which reflects the level of urine above the meatus. Intravesical pressure is the sum of these three components. The energy provided by the bladder is then converted to either heat, which is dissipated in the urethra, or kinetic energy of the urinary stream.

The dissipated heat energy in the urethra plays little role with respect to voiding; however, there are various theories regarding the mechanism of heat dissipation during micturition. One is dissipation secondary to friction. When fluid passes through a tube, the rate of energy lost as friction depends on the characteristics of the fluid (viscosity); the characteristics of the flow (velocity); and the characteristics of the tube (length and cross-sectional area).[56] The dissipation of energy increases as friction as the urethra gets longer, narrower, or more irregular; with urine, dissipation increases velocity. Another theory is dissipation occurs secondary to geometric considerations: The preceding considerations about friction

assume that the urethra is a rigid tube, but the characteristic geometric configuration of the urethra is not static. Thus, during a contraction, two potential scenarios may ensue, based on the relative distensibility of the urethral wall proximal to the contraction. If the urethra is relatively nondistensible, flow is constant throughout the contraction. Because the cross-sectional area of the urethral wall at the site of the contraction is reduced, the velocity of the urine increases. Thus, the kinetic energy of the fluid increases. Similarly, if the urethral wall is more distensible, flow rate across the contraction may diminish as does the kinetic energy.

Neurologic Considerations

As bladder volume and pressure increase, afferent impulses from the bladder and urethra signal the time to void. Voluntary micturition ensues unless it is consciously suppressed.

The micturition reflex (see Figure 10-1) is integrated in the rostral brain stem in an area designated the pontine micturition center, which is connected to the sacral micturition center via spinal pathways in the posterior and lateral columns.[2,57-59] The micturition reflex is a coordinated interaction between the detrusor muscle and the urinary sphincter. No single stimulus appears to initiate the micturition reflex; rather, multiple neural events exert influence via one or more mechanisms and affect the threshold for voiding. Descending neural influences from the cingulate and frontal cortex, hypothalamus, and medial regions of the pons raise the threshold of micturition. In contrast, the threshold for micturition is lowered by increasing activity of the vesical afferents and the dorsolateral pons and mammillary bodies.[58-61] The first event in the micturition reflex is relaxation of the external urethral sphincter caused by cessation of efferent pudendal nerve firing.[2] At the same time, sympathetic activity is suppressed, which results in cessation of the inhibitory effects of sympathetic stimulation. Then the combination of neural impulses across the pelvic ganglion and efferent postganglionic firing results in a detrusor contraction. Finally, inhibition of vesical neck stimulation allows opening of the urethra (see Figure 10-1).

Spinal cord injury, transverse myelitis, multiple sclerosis, or myelodysplasia can interrupt this long routed micturition reflex and usually results in uncoordinated micturition.[2,62,63] Control over the micturition reflex is accomplished by ill-understood neural pathways that connect different parts of the brain with the pontine micturition center. Suprapontine neurologic lesions, such as a cerebrovascular accident, tumor, Parkinson's disease, or normal pressure hydrocephalus, usually result in loss of control over the micturition reflex.[2]

PATHOPHYSIOLOGY OF LOWER URINARY TRACT SYMPTOMS

Based on urinary tract physiology, it is useful to classify lower urinary tract dysfunction into one of three groups: bladder filling and storage problems, bladder emptying problems, or combinations of the two.[1] Accurate diagnosis of a problem depends on careful assessment of the patient's history, physical examination, laboratory studies, and urodynamic assessment. Bladder symptoms are characterized as either irritative or obstructive. Irritative symptoms include urinary frequency, urgency, urge incontinence, nocturia, dysuria, and a constant feeling of suprapubic discomfort, pain, or urge to void. Obstructive symptoms consist of urinary hesitancy, decreased size and force of the stream, a feeling of incomplete bladder emptying, postvoid dribbling, overflow incontinence, and total urine retention. Symptoms elicited from the patient are often unreliable predictors of underlying disease and should serve only as a guide for directing further diagnostic evaluation.

The most remediable cause of urinary bladder symptoms is urinary tract infection, and no patient should be evaluated further until infection has been excluded by urinalysis and appropriate cultures. If hematuria is noted on routine urinalysis when infection has been excluded, radiologic evaluation of the kidneys and upper tracts, via either intravenous pyelography or ultrasonography, and cystoscopy are mandatory to exclude neoplastic conditions and urolithiasis.

Screening urodynamic evaluation should be performed on most uninfected patients whose persistent bladder symptoms do not respond to empiric treatment. For most patients, an accurate diagnosis can be obtained by cystometry, an estimation of urinary flow rate, postvoiding residual urine volume, and, in selected cases, voiding cystourethrography. More sophisticated studies such as sphincter electromyography and synchronous video and urodynamic studies are more accurate, but necessary only for persistent diagnostic and therapeutic problems.[64] Cystometry is performed by filling the bladder with gas or liquid while recording the detrusor pressure, bladder volume, and sensations of first urge and severe urge to void. Cystometry assesses bladder compliance, sensation, capacity, and involuntary bladder contractions (Figure 10-2). Urine flow rate is measured electronically with commercially available flow meters. Reduced urine

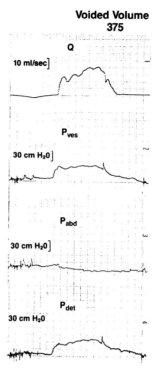

FIGURE 10-2 A typical bladder pressure-urinary flow rate curve. Q represents flow, P_{ves} is total vesical or bladder pressure, P_{abd} is abdominal pressure, and, finally, P_{det} is the subtracted pressure ($P_{ves} - P_{abd}$), which represents inherent bladder pressure. In this patient, the maximal flow rate was 21 ml/second and maximal detrusor pressure 50 cm H_2O.

flow suggests either bladder outlet obstruction or impairment of bladder contractility.[64]

Urinary Filling or Storage Problems

Involuntary Detrusor Contractions
The most common cause of irritative voiding symptoms is involuntary detrusor contractions, defined as a sudden nonvolitional increase in bladder pressure. Their numerous causes include neurologic problems and bladder outlet obstruction, but some are idiopathic. Involuntary bladder contractions caused by neurologic lesions are categorized as detrusor hyperreflexia; in the absence of a neurologic lesion, the condition is termed *detrusor instability*.

Involuntary detrusor contractions are treated according to cause. When involuntary contractions are secondary to bladder outlet obstruction, relief of the obstruction usually results in cessation of the involuntary detrusor contractions. When there is no obstruction, the gold standard of therapy has been anticholinergic medication such as propantheline bromide or oxybutynin; however, these medications are effective for only approximately 50% of patients. Many patients also require intermittent self-catheterization to empty the bladder. Other therapeutic modalities currently being investigated include behavior modification, functional electrical neural stimulation (transcutaneously, percutaneously, or by direct stimulation of nerve roots), and surgical *denervation procedures* such as dorsal root section. Augmentation enterocystoplasty is almost always effective, but usually requires intermittent self-catheterization.

Small Bladder Capacity

Normal bladder capacity is quite variable, but usually is greater than 300 ml. Therefore, irritative voiding symptoms occur if the bladder capacity is smaller (i.e., 200 ml or less). The most common causes of a *pathologically* reduced bladder capacity include infection or involuntary detrusor contractions and low compliance.

It is difficult to distinguish idiopathic sensory urge (i.e., urinary frequency, urgency, in the absence of intrinsic lower urinary tract disease) from a pathologically reduced bladder capacity. Both tuberculosis and interstitial cystitis can have characteristic cystoscopic changes; but they are not present in all patients. Repeating the cystoscopic examination under high spinal (above T-6) or general anesthesia may be useful, as the bladder capacity of patients with detrusor fibrosis remains small, whereas in those with idiopathic sensory urgency it is normal.

Therapy of symptomatic small-capacity bladders is directed at the underlying lesion. All patients with sensory urge should undergo diagnostic cystoscopy, and any suspicious lesions should be investigated by biopsy, because one of the most important diagnostic entities to rule out is transitional cell carcinoma in situ of the bladder. This condition may be overlooked unless bladder biopsy is routinely obtained, even when there are no overt cystoscopic lesions. Surgical augmentation cystoplasty is the primary mode of therapy for high-pressure, small-capacity bladders. A segment of large or small bowel is isolated with its vascular pedicle intact, and an anastomosis to the dome of the bladder is created. In some instances it may be necessary to excise most of the diseased bladder and create the anastomosis of bowel to the remaining trigone. Augmentation cystoplasty results in an increase in bladder capacity as well as low-pressure urine storage. Supravesical diversion with percutaneous nephrostomy should be reserved for patients who are not good candidates for augmentation cystoplasty.

Sensory Urgency

Sensory urgency describes a constellation of symptoms characterized by urinary frequency and urgency, often accompanied by suprapubic pain and discomfort or the feeling of a constant urge to void, all without any overt urodynamic abnormalities. These symptoms can usually be reproduced at relatively low bladder volumes, and while the symptoms are occurring, no bladder contractions are evident on cystometry, and bladder capacity is normal under anesthesia. Diagnostic misnomers for this symptom complex have included urethral syndrome, trigonitis, and interstitial cystitis. Patients with idiopathic sensory urgency void frequently, not because of involuntary detrusor contractions or infection, but simply because it hurts too much if they postpone voiding.

Therapy directed at curing infection or alleviating involuntary bladder contractions is doomed to failure in patients with sensory urgency. In this group of patients other empiric therapy is also unsuccessful, and it may in fact exacerbate the condition. Patients develop secondary psychological symptoms, and their symptoms often are thought to have a primary psychiatric cause. In fact, there is no way conclusively to separate patients with primary psychopathology from those who have developed secondary psychiatric symptoms because of their incurable bladder condition. Regardless of the underlying cause, however, structured behavior modification seems to be the most practical approach for these patients with this difficult condition.

Sphincter Abnormalities

Incontinence that occurs when the patient coughs, sneezes, or strains is stress incontinence. It is caused by either abnormal descent of the proximal urethra when the patient increases intra-abdominal pressure (hypermobility) or to intrinsic sphincter deficiency. In the former, the increased intra-abdominal pressure is transmitted unequally to the bladder and urethra. Leakage occurs when vesical pressure exceeds urethral pressure. The sphincter itself is relatively normal; it is capable of maintaining a water-tight seal but cannot withstand the effects of increased pressure. Therefore, any operation designed to prevent descent of the proximal urethra (the suspension operations) is successful in effecting a cure. Other procedures that have been described include the injection of collagen around the urethra. Preliminary results have been encouraging, but careful patient selection is required.

Intrinsic sphincter deficiency describes a condition in which the sphincter cannot maintain a water-tight seal, and therefore leakage occurs with the slightest provocation. Sphincteric failure can be caused by radiation, trauma, hormonal deprivation, multiple surgeries, or neurologic injury (e.g., meningomyelocele).[64,65] The standard procedures described previously to alleviate stress incontinence have little role in the management of these patients; however, the creation of a pubovaginal sling has met with a high success rate.[65,66] Periurethral injection of collagen or implantation of microballoons has been used to treat intrinsic sphincter deficiency with positive results. In men, sphincteric deficiency is usually caused by radical prostatectomy or transurethral resection of the prostate. Collagen injection represents a conservative option and may improve leakage slightly. However, insertion of an artificial urinary sphincter results in social continence in more than 95% of patients.[67]

Bladder Emptying Problems

Impairment of Bladder Contractility

Poor bladder emptying is secondary to either bladder outlet obstruction or impaired detrusor contractility. Although poor detrusor contractions may be attributable to myogenic, neurogenic, or psychological causes, current tests cannot distinguish between these causes. Most neurologic causes of detrusor abnormalities are associated with other neurologic deficits. For example, a neurologic lesion that affects the second through the fourth segments of the sacral spinal cord usually results not only in detrusor areflexia, but also in perianal anesthesia, poor anal tone, absent voluntary control of the anal sphincter, and absence of the bulbocavernosus reflex.

The most effective therapy for this group of patients, regardless of the cause of impaired contractility, is intermittent clean self-catheterization (CIC), timed to regularly empty the bladder and prevent periods of overdistension. A reasonable regimen is to perform CIC approximately every 6 hours; highest priority is given to accomplishing the catheterization on schedule. Despite their widespread use, parasympathomimetics (bethanechol) and α-sympathetic blocking agents (phenoxybenzamine) have not been shown to be effective for these conditions.

Bladder Outlet Obstruction

Bladder outlet obstruction caused by an enlarged prostate is the most common cause of lower urinary tract symptoms in older men. Approximately 10–15% of men aged 50 years with an enlarged prostate require a definitive procedure for prostatism by age 80 years. The pathognomonic diagnosis for bladder outlet obstruction is poor urine flow (less than 12 ml/second) in the presence of an adequate detrusor contraction (>40 cm H_2O).

Relief of the obstruction usually results in resolution of the patient's symptoms. Transurethral resection of the prostate has traditionally been the primary therapy. The procedure generally is tolerated well (mortality, 0.2%), but there has been an explosion in the urologic literature of alternative methods for relieving bladder outlet obstruction. These include transurethral electrovaporization of the prostate, laser ablation, interstitial laser coagulation, microwave thermotherapy, and endourethral stents. They have met with variable success, and long-term studies are needed to assess their efficacy. In women, bladder outlet obstruction is a rare cause of urinary retention. Some anatomic causes include inflammatory processes, urethral diverticulum, pelvic prolapse, carcinoma, and previous anti-incontinence surgery. It is a difficult diagnosis to make and requires sophisticated fluorourodynamic techniques to delineate precisely both the site and the nature of the obstruction.[65]

Bladder neck obstruction may be primary or secondary. Primary bladder neck contraction most likely results from either abnormal contraction of the vesical neck during voiding or failure of the vesical neck to open. The bladder neck usually appears normal during cystoscopic visualization, so the diagnosis may be missed. Transurethral bladder neck incision is usually curative. α-Sympathetic blocking agents and urethral dilatation each reportedly have been effective, but this has not been our experience. Secondary bladder neck obstruction usually is a complication of surgery for bladder outlet obstruction that resulted in scarring; it must be treated surgically.

Urethral meatal stenosis is an uncommon cause of bladder outlet obstruction and is usually the result of a previous transurethral procedure. Yet, meatal stenosis is overdiagnosed. Most urethral meatal *strictures* diagnosed by calibrating the size of the meatus at urodynamic testing are not found to cause obstruction. Empiric urethral dilatation or meatoplasty is a common resort, even though there is no evidence in the literature of the efficacy of either. More important is the potential harm that these procedures may cause, because by causing fibrosis of the urethra they may result in either bladder outlet obstruction or urinary incontinence. Urethral strictures may develop anywhere along the urethra from scarring from prior transurethral procedures. However, a bulbous urethral stricture suggests prior inflammation and fibrosis from repeated gonococcal infections.

Urine Storage and Emptying Problems

Detrusor-external sphincter dyssynergia describes involuntary contraction of the external urethral sphincter during an involuntary detrusor contraction (Figure 10-3). It is seen almost exclusively in patients with neurologic lesions of the suprasacral spinal cord.[2,62] Despite the outlet obstruction caused by the contracting external sphincter, women with this condition, in contrast to men, are at little risk for developing urologic complications unless they are treated with an indwelling catheter.[65] Their main problem is incontinence, which is difficult to manage. The optimal form of therapy is a combination of relaxation of the detrusor with anticholinergic medication and CIC.

For men who are unable to self-catheterize, the traditional next course of management has been external sphincterotomy. This is done by making a transurethral incision through the obstructing sphincter. The procedure renders the patient incontinent and prevents the high intravesical pressures associated with detrusor-external sphincter dyssynergia. The use of endourethral stents has been studied in patients with detrusor-external sphincter dyssynergia. Preliminary studies have demonstrated decreases in peak voiding pressures and postvoid residual volumes comparable with sphincterotomy.[68] Additionally, stent placement is associated with short operative and hospitalization times. If these

methods fail, augmentation cystoplasty with continent vesicostomy, with or without closure of the vesical neck, probably offers the best alternative to supravesical urinary diversion in patients who can catheterize. In patients who cannot catheterize, ileal conduit urinary diversion represents the best option.

Patients with areflexia or *low compliant* bladder and sphincteric incontinence usually have conditions associated with parasympathetic, sympathetic, or pudendal denervation. This may be caused by a variety of conditions, including spinal cord infarction, myelodysplasia, or prior radical pelvic surgery (abdominoperineal resection of the rectum or radical hysterectomy). Treatment for these patients is difficult. On occasion, CIC suffices if the bladder is emptied often enough so that incontinence does not occur. Patients with bladder neck denervation occasionally respond to α-sympathetic stimulation, either alone or in combination with β-blockade. Once rendered continent, the bladder can be emptied by CIC. On occasion, it is necessary to create a pubovaginal sling and to manage the patient with CIC. Figure 10-4 depicts a treatment algorithm for patients with voiding dysfunction.

PHYSIOLOGY OF SEXUAL FUNCTION

As for voiding dysfunction, it is imperative that the health care professional have a clear understanding of normal sexual function, including both physiological and psychological response, before *disorders* can be treated. Normal genital anatomy and innervation, male and female sexual response, and sexual function in patients with neurologic injury are reviewed.

Genital Anatomy

Men
The physiology of penile erection is dependent on a series of complex interactions involving the vascular, hormonal, and neurogenic systems of the body.[69] The penis is divided into three portions: the root, body, and glans. The root, which lies in the superficial perineal pouch, provides fixation and stability. The body consists of three spongy erectile bodies covered by various layers of fascia and skin. The glans is the distal expansion of the corpora spongiosa, which is one of the aforementioned erectile bodies. The skin covering the penis is thin and loosely connected with underlying penile fascia.

The paired corpora cavernosa lie dorsally and are surrounded by a double layer of dense fibrous connective tissue, Buck's fascia. As the corporal cavernosal

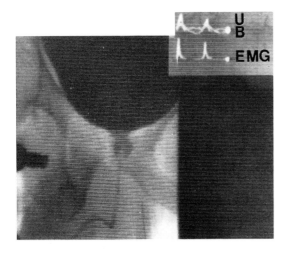

FIGURE 10-3 Urodynamic and radiographic representation of detrusor-external sphincter dyssynergia. Note that during a sustained involuntary bladder contraction (B) there is maximal electromyographic activity. There is minimal passage of contrast beyond the contracted external urethral sphincter. (EMG = electromyogram; U = urethral pressure.)

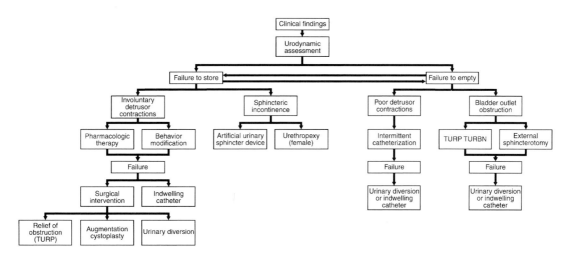

FIGURE 10-4 Treatment algorithm for voiding dysfunction. (TURBN = transurethral resection of bladder neck; TURP = transurethral resection of prostate.)

bodies approach the perineum, they diverge to form the crura of the penis. The corporal bodies are composed of a maze of endothelium-lined spaces invested by smooth muscle. Each crus adheres firmly to the ischial and pubic ramus and is surrounded by the ischiocavernosus muscle. The corpus spongiosum surrounds the urethra and lies ventral and centrally within the penis. Its posterior end is bulbous (the bulbar urethra) and is surrounded by the bulbospongiosus muscle. Its distal end expands conically to form the glans penis and fits over the rounded end of the paired corpora cavernosa. The urethra opens in the most distal aspect of the glans penis. The three masses of erectile tissue that make up the body of the penis expand to become rigid when engorged with blood.

The supporting structures of the penis are the fundiform and suspensory ligaments. The fundiform ligament is superficial and runs in continuity from the abdominal fascia to the penis and finally ends within the septa of the scrotum. The suspensory ligament is deep and attaches at the level of the symphysis pubis. The blood supply to the penis arises from the internal pudendal artery, which is a branch of the internal iliac artery. At the level of the urogenital diaphragm, the perineal segment of the internal pudendal artery divides into four terminal branches: (1) the urethral artery, (2) bulbar artery, (3) deep penile artery, and (4) deep dorsal artery. The urethral artery supplies blood to the corpus spongiosum; the bulbar artery sends branches to the bulbospongiosus and the bulbar urethra; the deep penile artery supplies blood to the paired corpora cavernosa;

and the deep dorsal artery travels between the layers of the suspensory ligament and lies in close continuity between the paired dorsal veins and nerves of the penis. It supplies the glans penis.

The three main channels of venous outflow are the cavernous veins and the superficial and deep dorsal veins. The corpora cavernosum is drained by the cavernous vein. The superficial dorsal vein drains the foreskin and empties directly into the external pudendal vein. Finally, the glans penis and a part of the cavernous bodies are drained by the deep dorsal vein complex, which ends in the prostate venous plexus.

Women

The clitoris is the homologue of the dorsal part of the penis. It consists of two small erectile cavernous bodies. The erectile body consists of two crura clitoridis and the glans clitoridis with overlying skin and prepuce. The glans is situated superiorly at the fused termination of the crura. It is composed of a combination of erectile tissue and a prepuce.

Bartholin's glands lie inferior and medial to the bulbocavernosus muscle. Their secretion is clear, viscid, and alkaline. During sexual activity there is increased secretory activity. In most women the glands become involuted and shrunken after approximately age 30 years. Other glands associated with secretory activity include Skene's glands, whose openings are close to the urethral meatus.

The nerve supply to the female external and internal genitalia includes a complex integration between somatic and autonomic nerve pathways. The innervation of the pudendum (which includes the mons pubis, labia minora and majora, clitoris, and vagina) consists of branches from the iliohypogastric, ilioinguinal, genitofemoral, as well as the sacral plexus. The pudendal nerves carry the somatic sensory fibers. The distribution of nerve endings within the glans clitoris varies from total absence to a rich supply in the prepuce. Obviously, any neurologic injury to the nerve endings to the clitoris takes on clinical significance with respect to potential sexual difficulties during the rehabilitation period.

The neurogenic mediators affecting female genital responses are presently unknown. Preliminary studies implicate nitric oxide and vasoactive intestinal polypeptide as potential agents stimulating vaginal relaxation and secretory processes.[70] As in the male counterpart, nitric oxide has been identified in cavernosal smooth muscle of the clitoris, and phosphodiesterase type V has been isolated in human clitoral smooth muscle culture.[71] In addition, vasoactive intestinal polypeptide as a non-adrenergic, noncholinergic neurotransmitter has been found to cause dose-dependent relaxation of rabbit clitoral cavernosal and vaginal smooth muscle.

Hormones also play an important role in female sexual function. Estradiol levels in animal models affect sensory thresholds of touch receptor zones along the distribution of the pudendal nerve.[72] Postmenopausal declines in circulating estrogen levels have correlated with changes in sexual function. Low testosterone levels in women are also associated with changes in sexual function involving declines in desire, genital sensation, arousal, and orgasm.

The uterus and ovaries are innervated by the autonomic nerves, which include branches of the superior and inferior hypogastric plexus. These plexi contain both sympathetic and parasympathetic (nervi erigentes) components, the nervi erigentes being primarily sensory. Somatic afferent nerves synapse at the T-11 and T-12 segments. The nerve supply of the ovaries arises from the lumbosacral sympathetic chain and passes into the ovary along the ovarian artery.

Neurophysiology of Erection

The hemodynamics of erection can be summarized as an increase in blood flow to the penis with redirection of that blood within the complex and interlacing sinusoids of the cavernosal bodies. Although this statement is simplistic, it does serve as the basic model to describe neurophysiological function. Like the urinary tract, the male genitalia are innervated via both somatic and autonomic nerve fibers. The pudendal nerves mediate penile sensation, and their major role is to provide sensation for the initiation and maintenance of penile erection.[73] The autonomic nervous system provides the major neurologic input to achieve penile erection, specifically the blood vessels in the paired corpora cavernosa. As early as 1863 it was known that electrical stimulation of the pelvic nerve (a parasympathetic nerve) induced an erection in dogs, and it is still thought that the parasympathetic nervous system is the predominant neurostimulator.[74] Neuropeptides may also be important in the initiation or maintenance of erection.

The sympathetic nervous system components that mediate erection originate in the thoracolumbar spinal cord. Investigators noted that ablation of the pelvic parasympathetic nervous system did not totally abolish erectile capability.[75] At present, the role of the adrenergic system in erectile physiology is unclear. Intracavernosal injections of α-adrenergic blocking agents (e.g., papaverine, phentolamine) promote erection. In addition, sympathetic stimulation causes detumescence. It remains to be determined which neurotransmitter modulates this response and at what anatomic site this modulation occurs.

It should be emphasized that there is *higher central* control of penile erection. In monkeys, it has been demonstrated that the anterior medial part of the hypothalamus is a positive locus for erection.[76] In addition, visual stimuli are probably mediated via parts of the subcorticolimbic system (i.e., the mamillary bodies and cingulate gyrus). Electrical stimulation and electroencephalographic studies have demonstrated important centers in the limbic lobe of Broca. Lesions of the medial preoptic lobe of the hypothalamus in rats abolish sexual activity.

The efferent pathway from the cerebral cortex to the sacral spinal cord proceeds from the preoptic hypothalamic region, median forebrain bundle, and substantia nigra of the midbrain.[77] These fibers enter the ventrolateral pons and travel through the spinal cords in the reticulospinal tracts.

Sexual Response Cycle

The sexual response cycle has been divided into four neurophysiological phases by the American Psychiatric Association's *Diagnostic and Statistical Manual of Mental Disorders, Fourth Edition* (Table 10-1).[78] The first phase is the stage of sexual desire or libido that is controlled by a dopamine-sensitive excitatory center and a serotonin-sensitive inhibitory center. In both sexes, testosterone is the hormone that programs these centers during prenatal development. Experiments in feline and

TABLE 10-1
Sexual Response Cycle

Stage	Duration	Response in Women	Response in Men
Desire	Minutes to hours	Psychological interest and arousal	Psychological interest and arousal
Excitement	Minutes to hours	Nipple erection, vaginal lubrication, clitoral erection, vasocongestion, breast engorgement	Penile erection
Orgasm	5–15 seconds	Involuntary contractions of the outer third of the vagina and pelvic muscles	Cowper's gland discharge, ejaculation
Resolution	Minutes to hours	Sense of well-being	Penile detumescence, sense of well-being

Source: Reprinted with permission from IJ Kohn, SA Kaplan. Female sexual dysfunction. Cont Urol 1999;11:54–72.

other mammalian species have located these centers in the hypothalamic and preoptic areas of the limbic system. During the second phase, the stage of excitement, a variety of extragenital and sex-specific genital changes occur (see following discussion). During the third phase, the stage of orgasm, reflex clonic contractions of the levator sling and genital musculature occur mediated by the sympathetic nervous system. Orgasm is a sensory phenomenon occurring in the cerebral cortex in association with the ejaculatory reflex, which involves a complex interplay of somatic and autonomic nervous system pathways. For the orgasmic reflex to occur, physical stimuli of adequate intensity and duration must be applied to sensory nerve endings located around the clitoris in women and the penis in men. Extragenital manifestations during this stage include a maximal sex flush and elevations of blood pressure and respiratory rate. The final phase is resolution, which is of variable duration and results in a cognitive sense of well-being as well as penile detumescence in men.

Male Sexual Response

The sex-specific aspects of the male sexual response consist of penile erection, emission, and finally antegrade ejaculation. During the excitement phase penile erection occurs, which may subside if stimulation is inadequate or ceases. Ejaculation is composed of seminal emission (delivery of semen into the posterior urethra) and propulsion of semen via the glans, with closure of the bladder neck to prevent the entry of seminal fluid into the bladder. The major motor neurologic stimulus to ejaculation is the sympathetic nervous system, mediated via the hypogastric nerve. This includes stimulation of the peristaltic waves of the smooth muscles of the ampulla, seminal vesicles, and prostate. In addition, the bladder neck is closed during ejaculation via α-adrenergic stimulation. The parasympathetic system serves only to provide stimulation of periurethral and prostatic gland secretion. The

somatic nervous system provides penile sensation and contributes to perineal muscle contraction. Finally, cerebral and subcortical centers also influence the ejaculatory reflex with loci identified in the thalamus.[76]

Female Sexual Response

In women, the initial sexual response includes engorgement and swelling of the labia and clitoris as well as lubrication of the vagina. The nipples and breasts also engorge during the excitement phase. The mechanism of this response is a combination of parasympathetic modulation causing vasodilatation, as well as inhibition of sympathetic-mediated vasoconstrictor tone. As stimulation continues, the clitoris becomes increasingly enlarged, and the heart rate and blood pressure increase. Along with enhanced muscle tension, a *sex flush* occurs involving the chest, neck, and face. During orgasm, the clitoris is maximally engorged and the walls of the vagina alternate contraction and relaxation.

In summary, in both men and women, sexual response is a complex interaction of cortical, autonomic, and somatic nervous system events. However, the role of psychosocial phenomena such as performance and orgasmic expression cannot be overemphasized.

Female Sexual Dysfunction after Neurologic Injury

Female sexual dysfunction encompasses disorders affecting all stages of the sexual response cycle. In this chapter, however, we limit our discussion to sexual dysfunctions related to neurologic injury. Although data are limited, studies on sexual function after stroke and spinal cord and traumatic brain injury do exist in the urologic and rehabilitation medicine literature. A marked decline in many aspects of sexual function has been reported in women after a stroke. Common problems include declines in libido, coital frequency, vaginal lubrication, and orgasm. The cause of sexual dysfunction is multifactorial, and major factors involve poor coping skills, psychosocial adjustment issues, fear of recurrent stroke, and effect of sensory and cognitive deficits.[79]

Difficulty with sexuality in women with spinal cord injury is also related to multiple factors. A population-based study in the greater Stockholm area revealed that urinary leakage, spasticity, and positioning problems were the medical problems most significantly interfering with sexual activity.[80] Additionally, women with complete spinal cord injury at T-6 and above have been found to be unable to achieve psychogenic genital responses (vaginal vasocongestion and lubrication). Reflexive genital responses from tactile stimulation are preserved, however.[81] Women with incomplete spinal cord injuries who have preserved T-11 to L-2 pinprick sensation are able to maintain the ability for psychogenic genital vasocongestion.[82]

Management of female sexual dysfunction in the neurologically impaired individual is gradually developing as more basic science and clinical studies are being performed. Sexual counseling is an important aspect of management as well as adequate assessment of medical and functional issues. A comprehensive medical evaluation with pelvic examination is recommended, and when indicated, a hormonal profile may be necessary. Treatment options are also gradually expanding. Estrogen replacement therapy is useful in postmenopausal women and may be administered orally or locally as a topical estrogen cream or vaginal estradiol ring. Improvements in clitoral sensitivity, libido, and dyspareunia are seen with estrogen therapy. The remaining following medical therapies are currently being evaluated in women. Methyl testosterone may improve lack of vaginal lubrication and inhibited desire, and studies have demonstrated usefulness of sildenafil in postmenopausal women.[83] Sildenafil, however, is less effective in spinal cord–injured women. Phentolamine, a nonspecific α-adrenergic blocker that causes smooth muscle relaxation, may improve vaginal blood flow. Finally, apomorphine, a dopamine agonist, may enhance sexual desire.

Male Sexual Dysfunction after Neurologic Injury

Impotence is defined as the inability to achieve or maintain an erection adequate for satisfactory sexual intercourse.[84] The incidence of impotence after spinal cord injury approximates 75%.[85] Only 70% of patients with upper motor neuron lesions attempt intercourse and only one-half of those patients who try are successful.[86]

It is interesting to correlate the level of spinal cord injury with the quality of erectile response. The majority of patients (66%) who are injured above T-12 have erections involving all three corporal bodies, in contrast to patients with injury below T-12, who can achieve erectile engorgement of the corpora cavernosa only. This is most likely because of the lack of sympathetic nervous system effect in patients with injuries below the level of T-12.[87] Erections occur more frequently in patients with lesions of upper motor neuron origin than in those with lower motor neuron lesions. In addition, the likelihood of achieving erections sufficient for vaginal penetration is greater with an incomplete injury than a complete one.

Erections in the spinal cord–injured patient are conveniently classified as either psychogenic or reflex. Psychogenic erections occur because of stimulation mediated at higher cortical levels, whereas reflex erections are mediated through local stimuli. Interruption of supraspinal pathways results in psychogenic erectile dysfunction. However, many of these patients can achieve reflex erections; unfortunately, these are usually of short duration and are poorly sustained. It should be noted that approximately 70% of patients with cauda equina lesions are impotent. Because of impairment of pudendal nerve–mediated sensation, these patients do not have reflex erections. The physiology of psychogenic erections in this group of patients is poorly understood.[73]

The management of erectile dysfunction in spinal cord patients should be directed to one of five treatment regimens or a combination of several. The first involves sexual counseling and behavior therapy. In addition to reassurance and assistance in the *information* process, the physician or counselor can help the patient gradually return to being a sexually functioning adult. Basic concepts of bladder management before sexual stimulation and the prevention of autonomic dysreflexia during intercourse are invaluable to the patient. This alone may be enough to alleviate the anxieties of the rehabilitating patient.[88]

The second treatment regimen involves administration of an oral medication. Sildenafil (Viagra) is a selective inhibitor of type V cyclic guanosine monophosphate phosphodiesterase. During penile erection, nitric oxide is released from autonomic terminal nerve endings and endothelial cells of the arterioles of the penis. Nitric oxide activates guanylate cyclase, which produces the second messenger, cyclic 3′,5′-guanosine monophosphate, which causes smooth muscle relaxation. Corporal tissue has been shown to be composed primarily of type V phosphodiesterase, which breaks down cyclic 3′,5′-guanosine monophosphate. Thus, inhibition of this enzyme enhances penile erection. Both reflexogenic and psychogenic erections have been shown to be improved by sildenafil in spinal cord–injured men. In randomized studies of these patients (American Spinal Injury Association [ASIA] grade A–D) comparing sildenafil with placebo, 75% of patients reported improved erections with sildenafil compared with a placebo rate of 7%.[89,90]

The third treatment regimen includes penile injection of vasoactive substances. The mechanism of erection achieved with intracavernous injection of α-sympatholytic agents (such as papaverine and phentolamine) and prostaglandin E has been researched extensively. Of greatest importance is the finding that men with erectile dysfunction secondary to a neurogenic cause respond to a minimal amount of the drug, so the long-term side effects of penile fibrosis and scarring at the injection site are greatly reduced. The major short-term sequela of intracorporeal injection is priapism. This is easily reversed by intracorporal irrigation with epinephrine. Thus, careful dose titration cannot be overemphasized.

The fourth option for treatment includes the use of a vacuum erection device so that negative pressure allows inflow of blood into the penis. The blood is maintained in situ by placing a band around the base of the penis. Contraindications to the use of a vacuum device include patients who are taking anticoagulants or have blood dyscrasias. Finally, use of this device requires bimanual dexterity, which may be a limiting factor for some patients.[91]

The fifth treatment regimen is a penile prosthesis. Available prostheses include semirigid, self-contained, inflatable, and pump-supported models. Obviously, the likelihood of prosthesis failure is increased with the more exotic prostheses; however, with the advent of intracorporal injections, the need for penile prostheses for spinal cord–injured patients has decreased dramatically. This is fortunate, as these patients have special problems because of their increased incidence of urinary tract infections and skin problems and the potential effects of these on a foreign body. It is not advisable to place a prosthesis in a patient who has a chronic indwelling Foley or suprapubic catheter because of the potential for infection. Other treatment modalities, such as a yohimbine, have not yet been studied adequately to allow us to comment on their overall efficacy.

Male-Factor Infertility and Ejaculatory Dysfunction

Ejaculatory failure is the predominant cause of male-factor infertility in spinal cord–injured patients. Other causes include impaired spermatogenesis and poor semen quality.[92] Poor semen quality has been attributed to stasis of semen, testicular hyperthermia, urinary tract infections, sperm contact with urine, chronic use of various medications, and putative changes in the hypothalamic-pituitary axis and development of sperm antibodies.[93,94] In addition, ejaculatory dysfunction depends on location and degree of neurologic injury. Ejaculations in spinal cord–injured men are reported to occur in 5% with complete upper motor neuron lesions and 18% with complete lower motor neuron lesions. However, in men with incomplete lesions ejaculations occur up to 70% of the time. Patients with cauda equina or conus medullaris injury, especially incomplete lesions, have been found to have preserved ejaculation 60% the time.[73] Because of impairment of pelvic muscles, patients usually have a dribbling type of ejaculation.

A number of treatment modalities address ejaculatory dysfunction in spinal cord–injured men. Pharmacologic manipulation with either subcutaneous physostigmine or intrathecal neostigmine must be carried out in an intensive care unit where blood pressure can be monitored.[85,95] However, vibratory stimulation of the glans penis is considered first-line therapy because of a low investment of time and money.[96] Ejaculation rates are higher with cervical spinal cord–injured patients compared with lower lesions. When performed properly, penile vibratory stimulation is a safe and easy method of semen retrieval, and semen quality is better than when obtained by electroejaculation.

Electrical ejaculation is the next option when penile vibratory stimulation fails. With both modalities employed (penile vibratory stimulation and electroejaculation), up to 100% of patients can be induced to ejaculate (whether in an antegrade or retrograde fashion).[97] During electroejaculation, a large probe is placed into the rectum, and depending on the neurologic status of the patient, anesthesia is used. To prevent autonomic dysreflexia during vibratory stimulation or electroejaculation, 20 mg of nifedipine is administered before the procedure. Better semen quality is obtained when ejaculations are antegrade. To increase the viability of sperm obtained via retrograde ejaculation, the patient is catheterized before electroejaculation and the bladder is instilled with buffers to help alkalinize the urine. Then the patient is stimulated and finally recatheterized to recover sperm. Pregnancy rates using assisted ejaculatory procedures in conjunction with assisted reproductive techniques such as intrauterine insemination and in vitro fertilization average 30%.[97] With the development of intracytoplasmic sperm injection, however, cumulative pregnancy rates can increase as high as 56%.[98]

REFERENCES

1. Wein AJ. Classification of neurogenic voiding dysfunction. J Urol 1981;125:605.

2. Blaivas JG. The neurophysiology of micturition: a clinical study of 550 patients. J Urol 1982;127:958.

3. Zinner NR, Sterling AM, Ritter RC. Role of inner wall softness in urinary continence. Urology 1980;16:115.

4. Woodbourne RT. Anatomy of the Bladder. In S Boyarski (ed), The Neurogenic Bladder. Baltimore: Williams & Wilkins, 1967;3–17.

5. Dixon J, Gosling J. Structure and Innervation in the Human. In M Torrens, JFB Morrison (eds), The Physiology of the Lower Urinary Tract. London: Springer-Verlag, 1987.

6. Uhlenhuth E, Hunter DW Jr, Loechel WF. Problems in the Anatomy of the Pelvis. Philadelphia: JB Lippincott, 1953;1–157.

7. Hutch JA. Anatomy and Physiology of the Bladder, Trigone and Urethra. New York: Appleton-Century-Crofts, 1972.

8. Tanagho EA, Schmidt RA, Araugo CG. Urinary striated sphincter: What is its nerve supply? Urology 1982;24:415.

9. Gil Vernet S. Morphology and Function of Vesico-Prostato-Urethral Musculature. Treviso: Edizioni Canova, 1968.

10. Hanes RW. The striped compressor of the prostatic urethra. Br J Urol 1970;41:481.

11. Oerlich TM. The urethral sphincter muscle in the male. Am J Anat 1980;158:229.

12. Coggehsall RE. Law of separation of function of the spinal roots. Physiol Rev 1980;60:716.

13. deGroat WC, Kawatani M, Hisamitsu T, et al. The role of neuropeptides in the sacral autonomic reflex pathways of the cat. J Auton Nerv Syst 1983;7:339.

14. Kuru M. Nervous control of micturition. Physiol Rev 1965;45:425.

15. Yamamoto T, Satomi H, Ise H, et al. Sacral spinal innervation of the rectal and vesical smooth muscles and the sphincteric striated muscles demonstrated by the horseradish peroxidase method. Neurosci Lett 1978; 7:41.

16. Langworthy OR. Innervation of the pelvic organs of the rat. Investig Urol (Berl) 1965;2:491.

17. Gruber CM. The autonomic innervation of the genitourinary system. Physiol Rev 1933;13:497.

18. Elbadawi A, Schenk EA. A new theory of the innervation of the bladder musculature. IV. Innervation of the vesicourethral junction and external urethral sphincter. J Urol 1974;80:341.

19. Brindley GS. Control of the Bladder and Urethral Sphincters by the Surgically Implantable Electrical Stimulators. In GD Chisolm, DF Williams (eds), Scientific Foundations in Urology. Chicago: Year Book, 1982;464–470.

20. Creed KE, Tulloch AGC. The effect of pelvic nerve stimulation and some drugs on the urethra and bladder of the dog. Br J Urol 1978;50:398.

21. Fagge CH. On the innervation of the urinary passages in dogs. J Physiol 1902;28:304.

22. Ambache N, Zar MA. Noncholinergic transmission by postganglionic motor neurons in the mammalian bladder. J Physiol (Lond) 1970;210:761.

23. Taira N. The autonomic pharmacology of the bladder. Ann Rev Pharmacol 1972;12:197.

24. Elbadawi A. Neuromorphologic basis of vesicourethral function. I. Histochemistry, ultrastructure, and function of intrinsic nerves of the bladder and urethra. Neurourol Urodyn 1982;1:3.

25. Graber P, Tanagho EA. Urethral responses to autonomic nerve stimulation. Urology 1975;6:52.

26. Elliott TR. The innervation of the bladder and urethra. J Physiol 1906–1907;35:367.

27. Girado JM, Campbell JB. The innervation of the urethra of the female cat. Exp Neurol 1959;1:44.

28. McGuire EJ, Wagner FC Jr. The effects of sacral denervation on bladder and urethral function. Surg Gynecol Obstet 1977;144:343.

29. Elbadawi A, Schenk EA. Dual innervation of the mammalian urinary bladder. A histochemical study of the distribution of cholinergic and adrenergic nerves. Am J Anat 1968;119:405.

30. Owman C, Sjostrand NO. Short adrenergic neurons and catecholamine-containing cells in vas deferens and accessory male genital glands of different mammals. Z Zellforsch 1965;66:300.

31. Blaivas JG, Barbalias GA. Characteristics of neural injury after abdominoperineal resection. J Urol 1983;128:84–90.

32. deGroat WC, Lalley PM. Reflex firing in the lumbar sympathetic outflow to activation of vesical afferent fibers. J Physiol 1972;226:289.

33. deGroat WC, Booth AM. Inhibition and facilitation in parasympathetic ganglia of the urinary bladder. Fed Proc 1980;39:2990.

34. deGroat WC, Kawatani M. Neural control of the urinary bladder: possible relationship between peptidergic inhibitory mechanisms and detrusor instability. Neurourol Urodyn 1985;4:285.

35. Benson GS, Wein WJ, Raezer DM, et al. Adrenergic and cholinergic stimulation and blockage of the human bladder base. J Urol 1976;116:174.

36. Downie JW, Dean DM, Carro-Ciampi G, et al. A difference in sensitivity to alpha-adrenergic agonists exhibited by detrusor and bladder neck of the rabbit. Can J Physiol Pharmacol 1975;53:525.

37. Ek A, Alm P, Andersson KE, et al. Adrenergic and cholinergic nerves of the human urethra and urinary bladder: a histochemical study. Acta Physiol Scand 1977;99:34.

38. Nergardh A. The interaction between adrenergic and cholinergic receptor functions in the outlet region of the urinary bladder. Scand Urol Nephrol 1974;8:108.

39. van Buren GA, Anderson GE. Comparison of the urinary bladder base and detrusor to cholinergic and histaminergic receptor activation in the rabbit. Pharmacology 1979;18:136.

40. Learmonth JR. A contribution to the neurophysiology of the urinary bladder in man. Brain 1931;54:147.

41. Morgan C, Nadelhaft L, deGroat WC. The distribution of visceral primary afferents from the pelvic nerve within Lissauer's tract and the spinal gray matter and its relationship to the sacral parasympathetic nucleus. J Comp Neurol 1981;201:415.

42. Rockswold GL, Bradley WE, Chou CM. Innervation of the urinary bladder in higher primates. J Comp Neurol 1980;193:509.

43. Blaivas JG, Labib KB, Bauer SB, et al. A new approach to electromyography of the external urethral sphincter. J Urol 1977;117:773.

44. Blaivas JG, Scott M, Labib KB. Urodynamic evaluation as a test of sacral cord function. Urology 1979;9:692.

45. Coolsaet BRLA. Stepwise Cystometry. A New Method to Investigate Properties of the Urinary Bladder [Dissertation]. Rotterdam: Erasmus University, 1977.

46. van Duyl WA. A model for both the passive and active properties of urinary bladder tissue related to bladder function. Neurourol Urodyn 1985;4:275.

47. Klevmark B. Effects of extrinsic bladder denervation on intramural tension and on intravesical pressure patterns. Acta Physiol Scand 1977;101:176.

48. van Mastrigt R, Coolsaet BLRA, van Duyl WA. The passive properties of the urinary bladder in the collection phase. Med Biol Eng Comput 1978;16:471.

49. Coolsaet BLRA. Bladder compliance and detrusor activity during the collection phase. Neurourol Urodyn 1985;4:263.

50. Griffiths DJ. Urodynamics: The Mechanics and Hydrodynamics of the Lower Urinary Tract. Bristol: Adam Hilger, 1980.

51. Woodside JR. Micturitional static urethral pressure profilometry in women. Neuoradial Urodyn 1982;1:149.

52. Yalla SV, Sharma GVRK, Barsamian EM. Micturitional urethral pressure profile during voiding and the implications. J Urol 1980;124:649.

53. Brading A. Physiology of Smooth Muscle. In M Torrens, JFB Morrison (eds), The Physiology of the Lower Urinary Tract. Berlin: Springer-Verlag, 1987.

54. Ursillo RC. Electrical activity of the isolated nerve urinary bladder strip preparation of the rabbit. Am J Physiol 1961;210:408.

55. Griffiths DJ. The Mechanics of Micturition. In SV Yalla, A Elbadawi, EM McGuire, et al. (eds), The Principles and Practice of Neurology and Urodynamics. New York: Macmillan, 1988.

56. Sterling AM, Ritter RC, Zinner NR, The Physical Basis of Obstructive Uropathy. In F Hinman Jr (ed), Benign Prostatic Hypertrophy. New York: Springer-Verlag, 1983.

57. Barrington FJF. The effect of lesions of the hind and mid-brain on micturition of the cat. Q J Exp Physiol 1925;15:181.

58. Barrington FJF. The localization of the paths sub-serving micturition in the spinal cord of the cat. Brain 1933;56:126.

59. Morrison JFB. Bladder Control: Role of the Higher Levels of Central Nervous System. In M Torrens, JFB Morrison (eds), The Physiology of the Lower Urinary Tract. London: Springer-Verlag, 1987.

60. Barrington FJF. The central nervous control of micturition. Brain 1928;51:209.

61. Barrington FJF. The component reflexes of micturition in the cat. Part III. Brain 1941;64:239.

62. Blaivas JG, Fisher DM. Combined radiographic and urodynamic monitoring: advances in technique. J Urol 1981;125:693–694.

63. McGuire EJ, Brady S. Detrusor-sphincter dyssynergia. J Urol 1979;121:774.

64. Blaivas JG, Salinas J. Type III stress urinary incontinence. The importance of proper diagnosis and treatment. Surg Forum 1984.

65. McGuire EJ, Woodside JR, Borden TA, et al. Prognostic value of urodynamic testing in myelodysplastic patients. J Urol 1981;126:205.

66. McGuire EM, Lytton B, Kohorn EI, et al. Value of urodynamic testing in stress urinary incontinence. J Urol 1980;124:256.

67. Marks JL, Light JK. Management of urinary incontinence after prostatectomy with an artificial urinary sphincter. J Urol 1989;142:302.

68. Chancellor MB, Gajewski J, Ackman CFD, et al. Long-term followup of the North American multicenter UroLume trial for the treatment of external detrusor-sphincter dyssynergia. J Urol 1999;161:1545–1550.

69. Abber JC, Lue TF. Evaluation of impotence. Probl Urol 1987;1:476.

70. Ottesen B, Pedersen B, Nielesen J, et al. Vasoactive intestinal polypeptide provokes vaginal lubrication in normal women. Peptides 1987;8:797–800.

71. Burnett AL, Calvin DC, Silver RI, et al. Immunohistochemical description of nitric oxide synthase isoforms in human clitoris. J Urol 1997;158:75–78.

72. Natoin B, Maclusky NJ, Leranth CZ. The cellular effects of estrogens on neuroendocrine tissues. J Steroid Biochem Mol Biol 1988;30:195–207.

73. Siroky MB. Neurophysiology of male sexual dysfunction in neurologic disorders. Semin Neurol 1988; 8:136.

74. Eckhardt C. Untersuchungen uber die Erektion des Penis beim Hund. Beitr Anat Physiol 1863;13:123.

75. Root WS, Bard P. The mechanism of feline erection through sympathetic pathways with some remarks on sexual behavior after de-afferentation of the genitalia. Am J Physiol 1947;150:80.

76. Maclean PD, Ploog DW. Cerebral representation of penile erection. J Neurophysiol 1962;25:29.

77. Siroky MB, Krane RJ. Physiology of Male Sexual Dysfunction. In RJ Krane, MB Siroky (eds), Clinical Neuro-Urology. Boston: Little, Brown, 1979.

78. American Psychiatric Association. Diagnostic and Statistical Manual of Mental Disorders (4th ed). Washington, DC: American Psychiatric Association, 1994.

79. Korpelainen JT, Kauhanen M-L, Kemola H, et al. Sexual dysfunction in stroke patients. Acta Neurol Scand 1998;98:400–405.

80. Westgren N, Hulting C, Levi R, et al. Sexuality in women with traumatic spinal cord injury. Acta Obstet Gynecol Scand 1997;76:977–983.

81. Sipski ML, Alexander CJ, Rosen RC. Physiological parameters associated with psychogenic sexual arousal in women with complete spinal cord injuries. Arch Phys Med Rehabil 1995;76:811–818.

82. Sipski ML, Alexander CJ, Rosen RC. Physiologic parameters associated with sexual arousal in women with incomplete spinal cord injuries. Arch Phys Med Rehabil 1997;78:305–313.

83. Kaplan SA, Rodolfo RB, Kohn IJ, et al. Safety and efficacy of sildenafil in postmenopausal women with sexual dysfunction. Urology 1999;53:481–486.

84. NIH Consensus Development Panel on Impotence. Impotence. JAMA 1992;270:83–90.

85. Stone AR. The sexual needs of the injured spinal cord patient. Prob Urol 1987;3:529–536.

86. Talbot HS. The sexual functioning paraplegic. J Urol 1973;91:1975.

87. Comarr AE. The Total Care of Spinal Cord Injuries. Boston: Little, Brown, 1977.

88. Strasberg PD, Brady SM. Sexual functioning of persons with neurologic disorders. Sem Neurol 1988;8:141.

89. Maytom MC, Derry FA, Dinsomre WW, et al. A two-part pilot study of sildenafil (VIAGRA™) in men with erectile dysfunction caused by spinal cord injury. Spinal Cord 1999;37:110–116.

90. Guilano F, Hultling C, Masry WSE, et al. Randomized trial of sildenafil for the treatment of erectile dysfunction in spinal cord injury. Ann Neurol 1999;46:15–21.

91. Witherington R. Mitigating impotence with an external vacuum device. Contemp Urol 1990;4:44.

92. Monga M, Bernie J, Rajeskaran M. Male infertility and erectile dysfunction in spinal cord injury: a review. Arch Phys Med Rehabil 1999;80(10):1331–1339.

93. Linsenmeyer TA. Male infertility following spinal cord injury. J Am Paraplegia Soc 1991;14(3):116–121.

94. Linsenmeyer TA, Perkash I. Infertility in men with spinal cord injury. Arch Phys Med Rehabil 1991;72(10):747–754.

95. Le Chapelain L, Nguyen Van Tam P, Dehail P, et al. Ejaculatory stimulation, quality of semen and reproductive aspects in spinal cord injured men. Spinal Cord 1998;36(2):132–136.

96. Brackett NL. Semen retrieval by penile vibratory stimulation in men with spinal cord injury. Hum Reprod Update 1999;5(3):216–222.

97. Sonksen J, Sommer P, Biering-Sorensen F, et al. Pregnancy after assisted ejaculation procedures in men with spinal cord injury. Arch Phys Med Rehabil 1997;78(10):1059–1061.

98. Hultling C, Rosenlund B, Levi R, et al. Assisted ejaculation and in-vitro fertilization in the treatment of infertile spinal cord-injured men: the role of intracytoplasmic sperm injection. Hum Reprod 1997;12(3):499–502.

11

Physiology of the Skin

JANET HILL PRYSTOWSKY

EMBRYONIC DEVELOPMENT

The skin, the body's largest organ, contains the most extensive vascular supply.[1] It maintains body temperature by regulating heat loss, prevents external organisms such as bacteria, fungi, and viruses from entering the body, protects the body against environmental insults such as ultraviolet radiation, and relays diverse information to the central nervous system. This information is mediated by sensory receptors to heat, cold, pain, pressure, and touch.

The skin has three distinct anatomic compartments: epidermis, dermis, and subcutaneous tissue (Figure 11-1). The epidermis has an outer inert keratin layer above a 5- to 10-cell thickness of keratinocytes (Figure 11-2). The epidermal compartment is highly cellular and approximately as thick as a sheet of paper. The acellular nonmetabolizing stratum corneum is 10–20 μm, the cellular epidermis 40–150 μm, and the epidermis ranges 40–150 μm (see Figure 11-1). The cutis is relatively acellular, 10–20 times thicker, and primarily composed of connective tissue fibers. The subcutaneous tissue consists mainly of fat-laden cells divided into lobules by connective tissue septa. It varies considerably in thickness (see Figure 11-1).

The embryonic skin becomes distinct as early as the third week of fetal life, when a single layer of cells, the periderm, constitutes the outer layer. Within days, a second layer, the germinative cell layer, develops. This cell layer is the ancestor of all the appendageal glands as well as the stratified squamous epithelium cells of the epidermis (Figure 11-3). During the second month, connective elements of mesodermal origin are visible; these are noted in a vascular background. The third compartment, the subcutaneous tissue, is not rigidly demarcated, but during the third month of fetal life it contains clearly recognizable lipid-laden cells.

CELLULAR AND GLANDULAR COMPONENTS

Epidermis

Epidermal Cells

The epidermis consists of multiple layers of ectodermal cells, called *keratinocytes* because of their abundant production of the tonofilament keratin. In addition to keratinocytes, made from progenitor cells in the skin, the epidermis normally has immigrant cells, called *Langerhans' cells* (LCs), that are derived from the bone marrow and have a macrophage lineage. During pathologic events, erythrocytes and leukocytes may also be seen in the epidermis. Finally, melanocytes, which are responsible for the formation of melanin pigment, are derived from neuroectodermal elements in neural crest. They, too, migrate to the skin and then locally replicate in the skin.

Differentiation Keratinocytes undergo many changes, known as *differentiation*, during their life cycle. The epidermis has three compartments (see Figure 11-2). The first consists of the basal layer of cells and part of the overlying suprabasal layer. It is also called the *stratum germinativum*, because the cells in the basal and suprabasal layers are mitotically active germinative cells responsible for producing new keratinocytes to replace those shed externally by the epidermis. The second compartment, the *stratum spinosum*, consists of metabolically active cells that have entered into a differentiation process that leads finally to formation of cornified

209

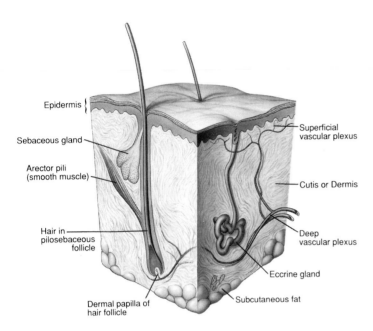

FIGURE 11-1 Constituents and structures of skin: epidermis, cutis, subcutaneous tissue, pilosebaceous units, and appendiceal glands.

cells in the outermost and third compartment, the *stratum corneum.*

The first compartment (germinative cells) and second compartment (differentiating cells) constitute the viable portion of the epidermis. A transitional zone, the stratum granulosum, contains elongated, flattened cells. The third compartment is the outer layer (stratum corneum), consisting of nonviable cellular components that protect the skin from the environment. Shedding of the stratum corneum completes the cellular turnover process of the epidermis (i.e., differentiating cells must constantly replace the shedding stratum corneum to maintain this layer and its protective function). Thus, normally, a germinative cell in the basal or suprabasal compartment gives rise to a differentiating cell, which has lost its proliferative capacity and terminally differ-

entiates into a cornified nonviable component of the stratum corneum.

The precise mechanisms and controls over epidermal proliferation and differentiation remain unclear; however, studies in vivo and in vitro have revealed numerous details of the process. Studies in vitro have shown that proliferation and differentiation are inversely regulated: When proliferation is promoted, differentiation is suppressed, whereas when keratinocytes differentiate they lose the ability to proliferate. The proliferative process has both irreversible and reversible growth arrest states, depending on the composition of the tissue culture medium (e.g., growth factors, amino acid composition).[2]

Furthermore, the concentration of calcium in the medium is a critical regulator of differentiation. Cells in

FIGURE 11-2 Epidermal cell layers.

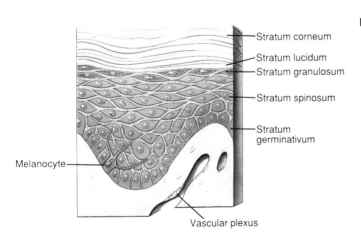

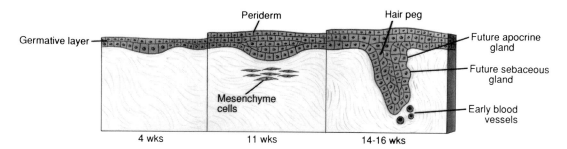

FIGURE 11-3 Embryonic development of the epidermis and adnexal glands.

medium containing 0.1 mmol/liter of calcium remain undifferentiated, proliferate rapidly, and do not stratify, whereas the addition of 1.2–2.0 mmol/liters of calcium is associated with induction of differentiation.[2,3] Differentiation of keratinocytes is demonstrated by colony formation, stratification, and expression of highly organized elements such as specific antigens, involucrin, and keratin tonofilaments. Aberrations in gene regulation and differentiation cause disabling and life-threatening skin diseases.[4] When keratinocytes enter the differentiating process, the synthesis of DNA decreases and is totally inhibited within 24 hours.[3] Other mediators such as retinoids have a marked effect on keratinocyte differentiation, particularly with respect to keratin gene expression.

Keratins are a group of at least 18 proteins referred to as *intermediate filaments* because they function as structural components of the cytoskeleton.[5] They range in molecular weight from approximately 40–70 kD. The keratins synthesized in squamous *keratinizing* epithelium are higher in molecular weight than the keratins found in nonsquamous nonkeratinizing epithelial (mucosal) surfaces.

Differentiation in cultured human epidermal cells is dependent on the absence or presence of retinoids in the medium and on whether the cultures are submerged in medium or grown on a collagen support to allow keratinocyte maturation at an air-water interface.[6] When keratinocytes are grown submerged in medium containing retinoids, the keratins synthesized reflect those found in mucosal surfaces (lower molecular-weight keratins) and the cells do not cornify. The higher molecular-weight keratins associated with terminal differentiation are not made in the presence of retinoic acid. In contrast, cultures grown submerged in retinoid-deficient medium show high-molecular-weight keratin production that reflects what is typically found in vivo in epidermis. Similarly, keratinocytes cultured at an air-water interface with retinoids in the medium below also follow a keratinization process that reflects the situation in vivo

by production of the high-molecular-weight keratins seen in terminal differentiation.[6] Thus, under conditions in vivo, the delivery of retinoids from plasma to the outer layers of the epidermis may be quite limited; terminal differentiation and cornification processes may occur as the keratinocytes progressively become more retinoid deficient in the outer layers of the epidermis. The cornified envelopes are important to provide a barrier against the environment. When the cross-linking of its components is altered from gene mutations in the structural proteins (e.g., transglutaminase 1 and loricrin), keratodermal skin diseases result.[7]

The advances in culturing human keratinocytes in vitro have now made it possible to propagate autologous keratinocytes for grafting onto full-thickness wounds for massive burned areas.[8] Similarly, patients with the inherited disorder epidermolysis bullosa have large areas of denuded skin, owing to defective or absent structural components for the epidermis to adhere to the dermis. These patients can benefit from grafts of autologous epidermis to denuded dermis.

Cell Kinetics Evidence suggests that at any given time, only a fraction of the cells in the germinative compartment are actually cycling, or undergoing mitotic division. The remainder are in a resting phase, called G_0. Cells in G_0 (Figure 11-4) enter the actively cycling pool, G_1, in response to proliferative stimuli.[9] The population of actively dividing cells also appears to be heterogeneous, some cells being more likely than others to undergo cell division.[10,11]

Once cells have entered into the differentiation compartment they are no longer mitotically active. A steady state exists when the production of cells from the germinative compartment is equal to the cell loss through desquamation from the stratum corneum. The time a cell takes to move from the basal layer to a scale sloughed or shed from the stratum corneum is referred to as the *transit* or *epidermal turnover time*. This period has two phases. The first is the time required for a basal cell to

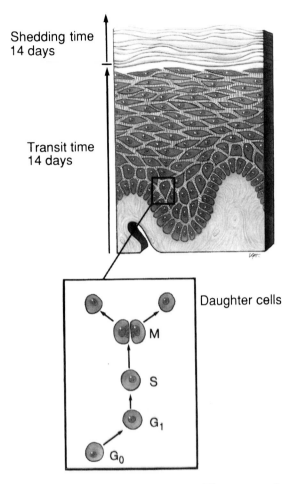

FIGURE 11-4 Epidermal cell kinetics. The stages of cell cycling are composed of the following steps: G_0, resting stage; G_1, cell has entered into cycling process; S, active DNA-synthesizing phase; M, mitotic cell division giving rise to daughter cells.

reach the stratum corneum; the second is the time required for the cellular material that becomes a component of the stratum corneum to be sloughed (Table 11-1).

The thickness of the epidermis depends on the number of keratinocytes between the basal layer and the stratum corneum; it may be altered by changes in the production rate of keratinocytes from the basal layer, epidermal turnover time, or the cell-cycle time. Chronic inflammatory states such as psoriasis may cause significant increases in the epidermal thickness (hyperplasia).

The cell-cycle time is the period required for a basal cell in G_1 (Figure 11-5) to undergo mitosis. As mentioned, at any given time only a fraction of the germinative cells are cycling; many cells remain in the G_0 or resting phase.

TABLE 11-1
Estimated Cellular Kinetics in Normal Skin

Cell Cycle	Time	Reference
S phase	10 hrs	12
Entire cell cycle (G_1–M)	37 hrs	12
Transit time (of basal epidermal cell to stratum corneum)	14–18 days	12
Turnover time (of stratum corneum)	14 days	13

Cell-cycle time cannot be measured directly; mathematical formulae (reviewed by Bauer[12]) are needed to determine these kinetic data. Historically, cell-cycle time has been calculated from autoradiographic studies after incorporation of radioactive DNA precursors into actively cycling cells. More recently, flow cytometry of epidermal cell suspensions has been used to distinguish between diploid (2N DNA content) cells in G_1, G_0, and differentiated cells (no longer cycling), and cells in S, G_2, and M states that contain greater quantities of DNA (between diploid and tetraploid in S and tetraploid in G_2 and M). This is possible because the DNA-specific fluorochrome used emits a signal proportional to the cells' content of DNA. The cell-cycle time and duration of the S phase in normal skin are presented in Table 11-1.

Cell-cycle times, as reported in the literature, show tremendous variability.[12] Probably the largest single responsible factor is the difficulty of accurately assessing the proportion of cells in G_0 (i.e., those not actively cycling). Figure 11-5 illustrates the multiple points at which significant alterations may occur in epidermal cell kinetics in normal cutaneous responses (e.g., irritation, pharmacologically induced changes, and disease states, such as psoriasis).

Cellular kinetic data are useful for understanding skin disease processes and suggesting therapeutic approaches. In psoriasis, for example, the rated cellular turnover of the epidermis is approximately four to six times faster than normal.[12,13] It is not surprising that this results in a hyperplastic epidermis that may be two to five times thicker than normal skin (Figure 11-6). Additionally, the production rate is increased, suggesting that the number of cells cycling is approximately 20 times greater than in normal skin. Thus, cells that would normally be in the resting (G_0) state have been influenced to enter G_1. Predictably, many of the most widely used therapeutic modalities for psoriasis interfere with DNA synthesis (e.g., methotrexate, psoralen plus ultraviolet A phototherapy [PUVA], anthralin, tar) or with recruitment of cells from G_0 into G_1 (corticosteroids).[12] Ultraviolet B, the most commonly used form of photo-

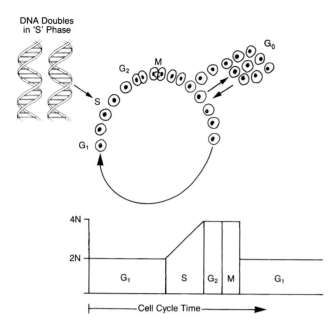

FIGURE 11-5 Epidermal cell cycle. (G_1, cell is in process; S, active DNA synthesis stage; G_2, cell before division containing a diploid quantity of DNA; M, mitotic phase; G_0, cell in resting phase, not undergoing cycling process.)

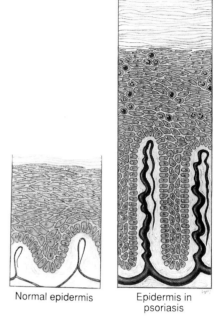

Normal epidermis   Epidermis in psoriasis

FIGURE 11-6 Hyperplastic epidermis, a characteristic feature of psoriasis. The psoriatic skin has a hyperplastic epidermis with marked tortuosity of superficial vasculature within the dermis. Leukocytes are interspersed between epidermal cells in psoriasis.

therapy for skin disease, has been demonstrated to slow the proliferation of cultured normal and immortalized human keratinocytes through inactivation of the epidermal growth factor receptor.[14,15] Inactivation of the epidermal growth factor receptor leads to down-regulation of ornithine decarboxylase, the enzyme that controls synthesis of polyamines, which are necessary for DNA metabolism. Thus, many psoriatic treatments directly or indirectly influence DNA synthesis.

Melanocytes   Melanocytes are normally found interspersed among the basal cells of the epidermis. They are specialized ectodermal cells that embryonically are of a neural crest origin (Figure 11-7A); their biological function is the production of the melanosome, a granular structure shaped like a cucumber. Within this protein structure, a light-opaque high-molecular-weight tyrosine polymer, melanin, is synthesized. The epidermal cell melanin content is primarily responsible for skin color. All races have essentially similar numbers of melanocytes; tyrosine activation is the rate-limiting factor in melanin synthesis. Albinos, whose tyrosinase activity is genetically shut down, synthesize virtually no melanin, whereas the blackest Africans, skin type VI, have approximately 1 g of melanin. Vitiligo, the skin disease characterized by the development of white patches of depigmented skin, is the result of a progressive loss of melanocytes from the epidermis and hair follicles.[16]

The melanocyte's sole function appears to be to manufacture melanin. This dense, opaque polymer is insoluble in aqueous solutions and in most organic solvents and has been demonstrated to have widespread survival value throughout the animal world. The squid's protective behaviors provide a good example. This creature has a contractile sac that ejects melanin in its ink to lay down a *smoke screen* and permit it to escape from a predator. Many animals such as frogs and chameleons use melanin to blend in with their environments. Under neurohormonal control melanin is rapidly synthesized and moved to various locations. Flounders have an extremely well-developed camouflage pattern that employs melanin to mimic a changing sandy background. This is also accomplished by a highly developed ability to rapidly disperse melanin granules.

In humans the major function of melanin is to protect the skin against solar radiation, and the epidermal cells in particular against ultraviolet radiation.[17] Through an adaptive mechanism, the melanocytes, located primarily in the basal cell layer, have developed long dendritic processes that have contact with as many as 30–40 adjacent epidermal cells, often referred to as the *epidermal melanocyte unit* (Figure 11-7B). Through incom-

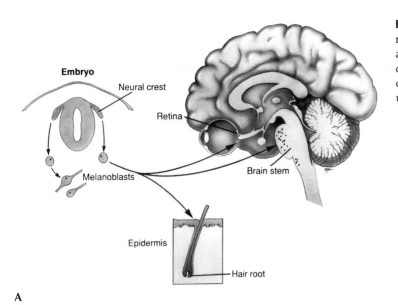

FIGURE 11-7 A. Embryonic development and migratory pattern of melanocytes. **B.** Epidermal melanocyte. The dendritic processes of a single melanocyte may inject melanosomes into 30–40 epidermal cells. This affords a protective mechanism against ultraviolet radiation.

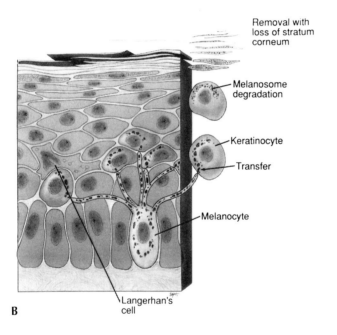

pletely understood mechanisms, they *inject* their pigment granules, melanosomes, into the epidermal cells. These melanosomes, now within epidermal cells, tend to congregate in a supranuclear pattern that, by absorbing and blocking photons of ultraviolet light, affords protection for DNA. Humans exposed to excessive solar radiation show a direct correlation between the amount of melanin and the incidence of basal and squamous cell skin cancer. Severe episodes of acute sunburn in fair-skinned persons are associated with a high incidence of melanoma. The biochemical mechanism of melanin formation in humans is well known, but the hormonal influence on this process needs clarification.[18] A pituitary hormone, melanocyte-stimulating hormone (α-MSH), has been isolated and synthesized. When injected into humans, diffuse pigmentation (except in albinos) is noted within 2 or 3 days. Studies have determined that α-MSH is not produced exclusively in the pituitary but in several sites including skin cells. In melanocyte cultures, α-MSH induces an increase in eumelanin rather than melanin. Adrenocorticotropic hormone, a pituitary hormone biochemically similar to α-MSH, and also made in the skin, has a similar and possibly more potent effect in regulating human pigmentary responses.[18] It is of interest that estrogen, whether administered systemically or applied topically, can cause darkening (melanization) of the nipple and areolar area of the breast. The skin of patients after hypophysectomy or large doses of radiation to the pituitary often becomes lighter in appearance.

In addition to melanin, melanocytes also make a number of melanin-related metabolites that appear to play an important role in protecting epidermal tissues against toxic oxygen radical species.[19] These products may also be important in inflammatory and immune reactions. Little is known regarding pheomelanin, the type of melanin found in red-headed people; it is well known, however, that red-heads have a high incidence of skin cancer. It is well documented that inflammation of the skin associated with heat, trauma, x-ray, and particularly ultraviolet light stimulates melanocytes to synthesize more melanin. Whether or not melanin formation after injury involves a common mechanism is controversial. Although direct neural pathways with melanocytes are present in other species, none has been demonstrated in humans. The melanocyte system and the pigmentary system are intertwined in a complex manner to protect the epidermis from injury. Further research is needed to unravel the numerous mysteries that remain.

Langerhans' Cells Paul Langerhans, as a medical student in 1868, first described the morphology of the unique epidermal dendritic cell that today bears his name. Until relatively recently, the LCs' embryonic origin, uniqueness of structural components, and biological function were controversial.[20]

Paul Langerhans identified LCs by their staining properties with a gold chloride solution that showed their cell structure contained an extensive network of darkly staining dendritic processes. Because it resembled a melanocyte, this feature led to the speculation that the LC was also of neuroectodermal origin and that it had simply lost the capacity to synthesize melanin and thus could be considered an *effete melanocyte*. The fact that LCs, in this vestigial role, constituted close to 4% of all epidermal cells was dismissed as just another anatomic curiosity; however, the LC is now well established as a crucial component of the immune system and is known to be of mesodermal origin, originating from stem cells residing in the bone marrow.

The anatomic observation that led to our present morphologic identification of LC cells was made by Birbeck in 1968 (Figure 11-8). He identified a characteristic cytoplasmic organelle of rod-shaped lamellar appearance with a terminal protuberance that suggested a tennis racket. This ultrastructural unit, Birbeck's granule, was soon found in other sites such as lymph nodes, thymus, tonsils, and histiocytic cells. LCs are also characterized by an irregularly shaped, highly convoluted nucleus and the absence of tonofilaments and melanosomes in the cytoplasm and of desmosomes on the cell membrane. Other properties include intense staining with adenosine triphosphatase (ATPase). A characteristic cell membrane marker known as the Ia antigen can also be detected by fluorescent antibody labeling. This is helpful in distinguishing LCs from normal epidermal cells and melanocytes. Like other members of the mesodermal macrophage series, LC membranes contain receptors for the Fc portion of immunoglobulin G (IgG) and the C3b component of complement.[21]

The origin of these Ia-bearing cells within the epidermis was unclear until 1979, when Katz and coworkers isolated Ia-bearing cells from the bone marrow of donor mice.[22] This was accomplished through the use of isotropically labeled marrow cells injected into the bone marrow of syngeneic recipient animals that had been rendered immunodeficient by lethal doses of x-irradiation. They were therefore devoid of epidermal LCs. The skin of these recipient animals was then shown to contain the labeled Ia-positive cells within 48 hours, indicating that these cells had migrated from the bone marrow compartment and were derived from residual bone marrow cells.[23,24]

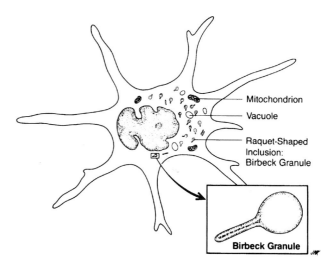

FIGURE 11-8 Langerhans' cell. These dendritic cells are characterized by a convoluted nucleus and cytoplasmic structures (Birbeck's granules) shaped like a tennis racket. The Langerhans' cell, after migrating from the bone marrow, resides in the epidermis and appears crucial for processing antigens.

Silberberg et al.[25] made the initial suggestion that LCs have an immune function. In 1973 they offered a startlingly innovative concept based on studies conducted to compare the cutaneous response to primary irritants and contact allergens in humans previously sensitized to contact allergens.[26] Silberberg and coworkers observed by ultrastructural analysis that in specimens obtained from immunized subjects, LCs and T lymphocytes were closely apposed. In contrast, this type of response was not observed in a primary irritant response. On the basis of these observations, Silberberg et al. postulated that in allergic contact dermatitis a specific interaction occurs between LCs and lymphocytes that is crucial for eliciting the immune response.[25] Further studies showed that LCs could be identified in draining lymph nodes, suggesting that these cells play an important role in the presentation of contact allergens to the immune system.[26] Later studies showed that LCs also had phagocytic properties and could take up ferritin, suggesting the ability to ingest and process antigens.

Toews et al. (1980) provided additional evidence of the crucial role of LCs in allergic contact dermatitis. In an ingenious experiment based on the observation of regional differences in the density of LCs in the dorsal skin and tail of rats,[27] Toews demonstrated that the degree or ability to induce allergic sensitization varied dramatically in these two sites. Indeed, the high degree of sensitization after the application of a hapten to the back correlated directly with the large number of LCs present there, as compared with markedly less sensitization when the tail site, which contained relatively few LCs, was used. Attempts to induce sensitization in tail skin resulted in the induction of immune suppression or tolerance.

Thus, LCs have been shown to be crucial for the induction of allergic contact sensitization in the skin: Conversely, when LCs are reduced or absent, skin exposure to a contact sensitizer tends to result in tolerogenic or suppressor responses rather than sensitization.

The LCs may be one of the major regulators in tumor surveillance.[28] This function may be magnified by the known role of ultraviolet B in skin cancer induction and its emerging effect in depleting the skin of LC.[29] Studies indicate that epidermal LCs play a central role in the immune pathogenesis of contact dermatitis, atopic dermatitis, histiocytosis X, human immunodeficiency virus 1 infection, and skin graft rejection.[30] It is important to appreciate that other dendritic cells reside within the epidermis, as well as the LC. These and other nondendritic antigen-presenting cells in the skin are all considered important in the skin immune system.[31]

Epidermal Appendages and Structures

Skin appendages are important for the skin functioning properly and provide a reservoir of new keratinocytes at times of wounding when the epidermis is removed but the appendages remain (e.g., in a partial-thickness burn wound or in a donor site for a split-thickness skin graft). In contrast, full-thickness wounds are characterized by the absence of appendageal structures at the base of the wound and are capable of healing from the circumference only, which results in a much slower process. Study of the development of the appendages is now amenable to molecular techniques, and this new analysis will help to elucidate the interactions of cells and cytokines that are required to form an appendageal unit.[32]

Sebaceous Glands

Three types of cutaneous adnexal glands derive from epidermal tissue, the sebaceous, apocrine, and eccrine glands. Sebaceous glands (Figure 11-9; see Figure 11-1) vary regionally in density, size, and shape: The face has the most per unit area and the largest gland size.[33] Although their role is still debated, the final destination of the sebaceous gland cells (sebocytes) is the skin surface, where they form an amorphous lipid-rich material called *sebum*. This terminal differentiation or disintegration obliterates all traces of earlier cellular identity. Because of the complete (whole) disappearance of the

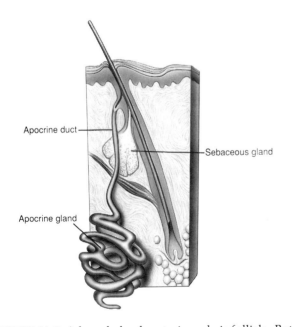

Apocrine duct

Apocrine gland

Sebaceous gland

FIGURE 11-9 Adnexal glands entering a hair follicle. Both apocrine and sebaceous glands enter the pilosebaceous duct, which delivers their contents to the skin surface.

cells, they are often referred to as *holocrine glands.* Sebaceous glands show no neural pattern of innervation; but they are responsive to hormonal stimuli.

The embryonic development of sebaceous glands, like that of other adnexal structures, is ectodermal in origin (see Figure 11-3). As their origin is identical with that of the epidermal cells producing stratum corneum, they retain this function and serve as important components of the wound-healing process. The development of a sebaceous gland can be noted in the epithelium of the hair follicle by the fourteenth week of gestation (see Figure 11-3).[34] It appears as a spherical bud that grows laterally from the hair follicle and develops into a multilobulated gland (see Figure 11-9). In adult life this glandular tissue surrounds more than 50% of the circumference of each hair follicle. The gland's products enter the hair follicle through a short pilosebaceous duct rather than traveling directly to the skin surface.

By the sixth month of gestation a basement membrane surrounds the basal cell layer of sebocytes. As cells are viewed inwardly from the peripheral portion of the gland they become larger and paler and form fat droplets, which increase in size as cellular identity fades. This mechanism is fully operative before term.

Humans have more sebaceous glands than any other mammal. The density ranges from 400–900 glands per square centimeter of skin surface and is greatest on the forehead. Other high-density sites are the scalp, face, and genitalia. The upper chest and back show intermediate sebaceous gland density, and concentrations of 10% or less of the forehead level are found on the wrists and ankles. Sebaceous glands do not occur on the palms and soles. The density distribution of sebaceous glands coincides with the sites at which acne vulgaris lesions most frequently are noted. All sebaceous glands, regardless of size or location, empty into the follicular duct of the hair follicle (see Figure 11-9). This may be related ontologically to their vital importance in protecting aquatic birds' feathers by forming a lipid coating. Their absence is associated with loss of luster and brittleness that affects flight. In mammals the sebum may similarly help protect hair and fur from environmental insults. The proliferation of sebocytes, most pronounced at puberty and accompanied by a massive increase in sebaceous lobule size and accumulation of lipids, is recognized as a growth process initiated, and probably regulated, by direct hormone stimulation.

Increased sebaceous gland proliferation coincides with other signs of puberty such as the emergence of a beard and deep voice in young men and of mammary tissue and body contour in young women. Microscopic examination of the basal cell sebocytes shows a marked increase in mitotic activity during puberty.[35] The historical clinical datum that identified hormonal control of sebocyte proliferation was the observation that sebaceous hyperplasia and acne did not occur in prepubertal castrates and eunuchs, although after testosterone injections hyperplasia and acne developed.[36,37] Additional studies in humans have demonstrated that large doses of estrogen have an inhibitory effect on sebaceous gland hyperplasia. Young women who develop acne probably do so from androgenic hormones elaborated by the adrenal cortex, such as dehydroepiandrosterone. In general, male subjects have higher excretory levels of sebum than female subjects, and older men have lower levels than those of middle age.[38,39] Sebum production correlates with age-related testosterone levels.[40,41]

Although no specific role for sebum on the skin surface of humans is demonstrable at present, many believe that dry skin and winter itch can be minimized by preventing excessive transepidermal water loss. The role of the sebaceous excretory products may be to form a lipid layer on the skin surface that inhibits insensible water loss.[42] Others believe the epidermal cell lipids of the skin are sufficient for this purpose.[43-45] Another possible function of sebum is the production of 7-dehydrocholesterol (provitamin D). The action of ultraviolet B radiation converts this compound to vitamin D, which is important in preventing rickets and osteomalacia in persons whose diet is deficient in vitamin D.

In summary, sebaceous gland activity may aid in maintaining a skin surface lipid level that protects against water loss. Under abnormal hormonal effects, disorders ranging from mild acne to disabling folliculitis may occur.

Apocrine Glands

Apocrine glands (see Figure 11-9) secrete chemical substances related to scent called *pheromones.* Although in many species pheromones elaborate odors that act as sexual attractants or delineate territorial domains, there is no evidence of this in humans. Nevertheless, there continues to be interest in this possibility.[46] Indeed, apocrine glands may well be vestigial sweat glands rather than a scent unit.

The highest concentration of apocrine glands is found in the axillary and genital regions; smaller concentrations are found in the umbilical and perianal zones and the areolar area of the nipples. A modified form of an apocrine gland, the gland of Moll, is found in the eyelids. From an embryonic basis, the glandular tissue of the breast per se can be regarded as an apocrine structure.[47] The embryonic development of the apocrine gland is similar to that of the sebaceous gland and is intimately involved with the hair follicle (see Figure 11-3). Apocrine glands are minute structures that have a ductal connection with hair follicles (see Figure 11-9). The glands can be considered principally as adrenergic response organs, and secretion is stimulated by emotional episodes or by systemic or local injection of epinephrine.[48]

Uncontaminated apocrine sweat is difficult to obtain because of cannulation problems. In pure form it is viscous, milky white fluid that is odorless until residual bacteria in the pilosebaceous apparatus and skin surface act on it. After decomposition by bacterial enzymes a pungent odor, often termed *body odor*, emerges.

The apocrine glands are nonsecretory until puberty; their growth and development are apparently under hormonal control. After development of their glandular structure, apocrine glands can be readily distinguished from eccrine glands. Specifically, the secretory portion of this coiled gland consists of a single layer of palely staining cells with a convex border projecting into a lumen. Contractile myoepithelial cells surround the

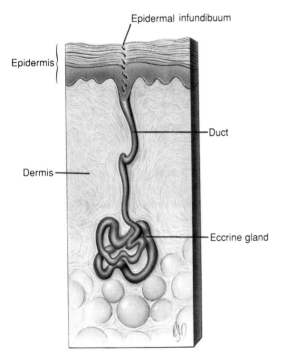

Eccrine Gland

FIGURE 11-10 Eccrine gland. In contrast to sebaceous and apocrine glands, the eccrine gland extends deep into the dermis and has an independent duct that carries its secretions directly to the skin surface.

base of the secretory cells. These contractile cells rhythmically contract, producing a pulsatile secretion.

As noted, the highest concentrations of apocrine glands are in the axillary, perianal, genital, and umbilical areas. Inflammation of the adnexal glands at these sites may be associated with a chronic infection known as *hidradenitis suppurativa*.[49–51] For most patients, apocrine glands serve principally as elaborators of unpleasant odors that can be controlled by appropriate antiperspirant and hygienic procedures.[52,53]

In summary, apocrine glands appear to be vestigial glands in humans. Their hormonal development and adrenergic responsiveness are well documented.

Eccrine Glands

Eccrine glands are appendageal glands that empty directly onto the skin surface (Figure 11-10). They markedly influence body temperature through regulation of water loss, particularly during exercise.[54,55] Age-related differences have been described for sweating and heat dissipation.[56,57]

During routine activities, noneccrine gland mechanisms of water loss include invisible secretion of sweat and respiratory water vapor loss through exhaling. These two physiological processes, often referred to as *insensible water loss*, are continuous and normally play a limited role in temperature control and water regulation. In contrast, eccrine gland activity is crucial for heat regulation. At normal internal and external temperatures, the radiation and convection of the insensible water loss maintain homeostasis.

Under conditions of extreme heat, however, the evaporation of the eccrine gland secretion provides the major cooling effect. Peripheral vasodilatation and hyperpnea augment this cooling process. In hot environments and in response to extreme physical stress, all these cooling mechanisms may prove insufficient and hyperthermia and death may occur.

The average adult human has more than 2 million eccrine glands (see Figure 11-10). They are found in highest concentration on the palms and soles, where they may number more than 300 glands per square centimeter. Approximately one-half this number are found on the forehead, dorsum of the hands, chest, and abdomen. Concentrations are lowest on the buttocks, thighs, medial aspect of the legs, and nape of neck. The actual size of the sweat glands, as measured in biopsy specimens, averages 5×10^{-3} per cubic millimeter (variation 50%). The rate of sweat secretion appears to correlate with gland size.[58] Sweat delivered to the skin surface is a colorless hypotonic solution with a pH of approximately 5.0. Techniques to measure human perspiration have been reviewed.[59]

Embryology

Eccrine gland cells can be identified in the fourth week of fetal life (see Figure 11-3) as the lower cellular layer (germinative) beneath the periderm. These cells are completely distinct from embryo sebaceous and apocrine gland cells. The germinate cells multiply into small buds and migrate downward, but they always maintain direct contact with their original connection to the epidermis. The descent of the glandular cells is completed when they approach the lower portion of the dermis. During this downward migration, which is virtually complete by the fifth to sixth fetal month, the eccrine glands acquire a ductal portion, which communicates directly with the skin surface, as well as vasculature and a nerve supply derived from dermal elements (Figure 11-11). By the eighth month of fetal life the coiled eccrine gland has a double cell layer with a clearly discernible lumen. The ectodermal cells lining the eccrine duct unit retain the ability to regenerate a functional epidermis similar to the pilosebaceous units and are important in wound healing.

Regulation of Thermal Sweating

The major afferent message controlling internal heat is probably the result of warmed blood reaching the hypothalamic center of the brain.[60] Under extreme febrile stress sweat volume may exceed 2 liters per hour. Local heating of any portion of the body from a sufficiently hot external stimulus can also cause sweating by a reflex mechanism.[61,62] However, it is worth remembering that thermoregulatory responses induce dehydration, and this results in a number of interactions between the circulation and body fluid homeostasis.[63]

A modified thermal response occurs in the eccrine glands of the palms, soles, and forehead. Emotional stimuli like anxiety, fear, and pain trigger their maximal response. These same glands are significantly less responsive to thermal stimuli. The glands of the upper lip release acetylcholine in response to *sharp* and spicy foods. This third type of response is often referred to as *localized gustatory sweating*. Hyperhidrosis of the axillae, palms, and for the gustatory type have become amenable to treatment with injections into the affected areas with botulinum toxin. The toxin effectively achieves a chemodenervation of the eccrine sweat glands that lasts for up to a year.[64]

Diseases of the central nervous system have long been recognized to influence eccrine activity. Damage to the cortex of parietal brain tissue is associated with hyper-

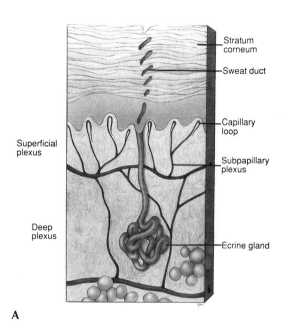

A

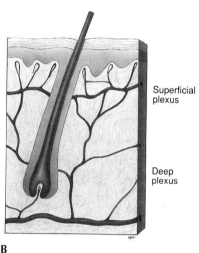

B

FIGURE 11-11 A. Vasculature of the cutis. The cutaneous blood supply is characterized by two parallel branches of vessels connected by communicating branches perpendicular to the skin surface. **B.** Vascular plexus of the cutis. The superficial and deep plexus of vessels provides the blood supply for the cutis.

hidrosis of the contralateral side, where motor paralysis may be observed. Transection of the spinal cord also can be associated with distal hyperhidrosis. This and the parietal lesions suggest a role for an undefined inhibitory substance in eccrine secretion. In contrast, destructive lesions of peripheral nerves (Hansen's disease) are frequently associated with hypohidrosis or anhidrosis.

Pharmacologic (Hormonal) Responses of the Eccrine Gland and Duct

Fibers of the autonomic nervous system that innervate the eccrine gland are sympathetic in anatomic structure, but acetylcholine rather than norepinephrine is released at their nerve endings, with resultant stimulation of eccrine secretion. These postganglionic anatomically adrenergic fibers to the eccrine glands are thus called *sympathetic cholinergic fibers* because of their physiological role. In addition, denervated eccrine sweat glands still secrete when acetylcholine is applied directly. The minimal secretions from the direct glandular effects of norepinephrine are considered secondary to norepinephrine acting on the myoepithelial cells surrounding the gland.[65] Atropine and propantheline (Pro-Banthine), by blocking the receptor site, decrease the response to acetylcholine. Physostigmine blocks acetylcholinesterase and, in so doing, intensifies sweating.[66,67]

The reabsorption of sodium from the eccrine sweat duct is strongly influenced by the adrenal cortical hormone aldosterone. Indeed, the initial secretory product from the gland is hypertonic compared with the plasma; that leaving the duct at the skin surface is hypotonic. Thus, the reabsorption of sodium is an active tubular process. The final eccrine product appears to have lower concentrations of sodium and chloride than serum, whereas sweat has higher concentrations of lactate, potassium, and urea. The increased urea may be a ductal metabolic product rather than a selective secretion effect. Although there are similarities to the renal tubular reabsorption process, this is probably an oversimplification.[58,68]

In summary, thermal regulation, a crucial requirement for human survival, is the major function of this cutaneous appendageal gland. Replacement of the fluid and electrolyte balance after exercise in the heat is important. An excess of the volume of fluid sweated must be ingested together with sufficient electrolytes because of ongoing urine and insensible water losses.[69] However, in debilitated febrile patients sweating increases maceration, particularly in the inframammary and genital areas. If maceration is not adequately controlled, patients may suffer fungal and bacterial infections. One of the most common clinical problems encountered in the eccrine gland is caused by obstruction of the eccrine duct leading to miliaria. This is most commonly seen on the back of hospitalized patients.[70]

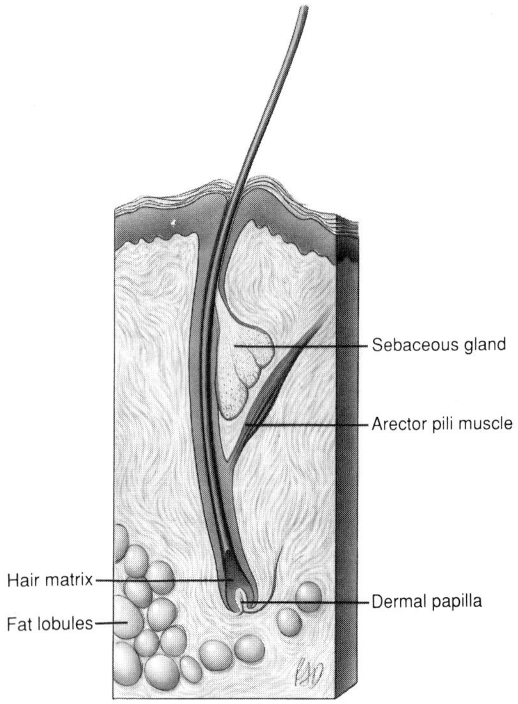

HAIR FOLLICLES AND HAIR

Embryology of Hair Follicle and Hair

Hair follicle cells are derived from ectodermal basal cells (see Figure 11-3).[71] These embryonal basal cells form the hair germ cells, which are bilateral and symmetrically distributed throughout the skin. They descend in a slanted caudal direction and become merged with a mesodermal component that becomes the dermal papilla and the fibrous root sheath (Figure 11-12). Mesodermal cells of the hair germ surrounding the ectodermal follicle cells accomplish this. A cup-like invagination of epithelial cells that they abut forms the dermal papilla. Active hair growth is associated with the union of the matrix cells with an abundant vascular supply. The mesenchyme-derived dermal papilla plays a major regulatory role to the hair follicle and can now be studied in culture to evaluate the key molecules involved in hair biology.[72] Stem cells have been identified in the basal layer of the outer root sheath in an area called the *bulge*. From this reservoir, stem cells, under the control of the dermal papillae, migrate to the hair matrix to proliferate.[73]

Hair represents the end product of highly active hair matrix cells located at the base of the follicle, a site characterized by a high rate of keratin synthesis. Keratin, biochemically a highly insoluble protein, is the basic

FIGURE 11-12 Hair emerging from pilosebaceous duct. The abundant vasculature of the dermal papilla supplies the rapidly dividing ectodermal cells of the hair matrix with sufficient nutrients to produce the keratin product, hair.

Sebaceous gland

Arector pili muscle

Hair matrix

Fat lobules

Dermal papilla

constituent of hair. Only drastic environmental measures, such as a *permanent wave*, alter its structure.

Hair, a terminal protein of epidermal cells, is similar biochemically to nail and is found in all mammals. Hair has several roles in human survival and heat conservation, tactile probing, and physical protection of the skin surface. For humans, hair may serve only a minor sensory tactile function, but it is of considerable aesthetic and cosmetic importance in terms of location, quantity, and quality.

Hairs are best conceived of as nonmetabolizing keratin fibers produced from the hair matrix and discharged from hair follicles. The hair follicle is an epidermal appendage that embryonically descended into the dermis. The hair follicle is characterized by sebaceous glands that proliferate and excrete sebum into their common ducts. The two structures are commonly known as a *pilosebaceous unit* (see Figure 11-12). They are found universally throughout the body, except on the palms and soles. The emerging hair, compact α-keratin, is divided into two groups, terminal and vellus. The terminal hairs make up more than 95% of the hair on the scalp, trunk, and extremities of men. The vellus hairs are much shorter, grow slower, and are more numerous in women.

Hairs do not grow continuously; the matrix cells cycle through anagen and telogen phases, periods of growth with high metabolic activity and periods of rest. Hairs are shed during the telogen phase (Figure 11-13). A shed scalp hair may be 3 years old and have achieved a length of more than 2 feet. Average growth rates depend on metabolic activity of the matrix cells and vary with season; they are greatest in the summer, when scalp hair can grow an inch in 8 weeks. Approximately 90% of terminal hairs on a normal scalp are in the anagen phase. Acute febrile episodes,

typhoid fever, or hormonal changes such as occur after pregnancy may abruptly terminate the anagen phase. The resulting transient hair loss is called *telogen effluvium*. Using recombination and histochemical technology, the growth factors influencing the hair cycle have been under study and their roles are beginning to be elucidated.[74]

The growth of hairs from a given follicle is determined by androgenic hormones,[75] and the responsiveness of a follicle to hormones is genetically determined. Hair follicles from the lower occipital scalp produce hairs when transplanted to the bald midportion. Loss of scalp hair (alopecia) is strongly under polygenic hereditary control and, in men, is referred to as *male pattern baldness* or *androgenetic alopecia*. Women commonly lose hair with age in a thinning pattern rather that a balding pattern; this is referred to as *female pattern alopecia*. Two medical treatments are now available to slow the loss of androgenetic alopecia. In men, both oral finasteride and topical minoxidil are helpful in stimulating some regrowth or slowing of hair loss. In women, only minoxidil has been demonstrated to be helpful in androgenetic alopecia. Treatments of hair loss have been reviewed.[76]

When hairs are visualized in cross section they are usually oval and consist of multiple sections. The major ones are a central medulla and a compact cortex. Interspersed in the cortex is melanin, which adds color to the otherwise translucent hair.

NAILS

The nail, a rigid keratin plate (Figure 11-14), is continuously being produced by rapidly dividing epidermal

FIGURE 11-13 Three stages of hair growth. Under normal conditions more than 90% of scalp hairs are in the actively growing (anagen) stage. A negligible number are in the catagen phase. Fewer than 10% are normally found to be falling out (telogen phase).

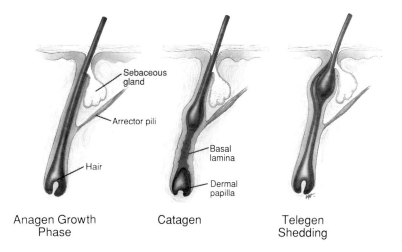

Anagen Growth Phase   Catagen   Telegen Shedding

Sebaceous gland

Arrector pili

Hair

Basal lamina

Dermal papilla

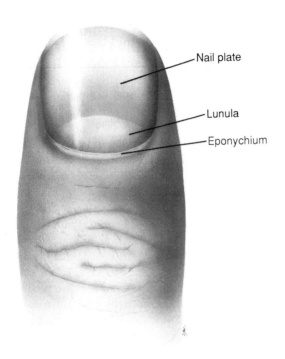

FIGURE 11-14 External appearance of nail. The distal portion of all 10 digits contains a hard nail plate of keratin produced from matrix cells proximal to the lunula.

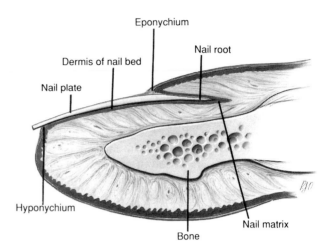

FIGURE 11-15 Longitudinal section of nail unit. The nail, a nonviable, rigid keratin structure, covers the nail bed and protects the dermal vasculature and bone.

cells called the *nail matrix*.[77,78] This relatively small site, proximal to visible nail, under normal conditions, is the only site of nail plate synthesis (Figure 11-15). Fingernails grow at the rate of 0.1 mm a day; in unlikely situations in which no trauma or friction intervened, they have grown to 12 inches or more. Under normal physiological conditions fingernails have a constant thickness of approximately 0.6 mm. Toenails grow significantly more slowly than fingernails, but are approximately 1.2 mm thick.

The embryonic origin of the nail can be detected during the tenth week of fetal life. It consists of a wedge of basal cell–like epithelial cells at the future site of the terminal interphalangeal joint. By the twelfth week, a definite matrix group of proliferating basal cells has produced nail. The distal portion of these keratin-synthesizing cells is the distal portion of the pale lunula of the nail (see Figure 11-14). Changes in the lunula may be an indication of a skin disease or systemic disorder.[79] The nail rests on a nail bed of epidermal cells. After the twentieth week, no granular layer is noted in the nail bed. The lateral margins of the nail plate are encased by lateral nail folds. The nail bed overlies a rich vasculature; however, no subcutaneous tissue develops and underlying bone intimately approximates the nail bed.[80,81]

The hyponychium, the region between the distal portion of the nail bed and the distal nail groove, is another portion of the nail unit. Clinically, the hyponychium appears as a hard, keratinous growth that prevents debris from entering beneath the distal portion of the nail. Although the nail can be considered a relatively vestigial organ, numerous external and systemic agents can affect it. Because it is produced by rapidly dividing cells it is particularly influenced by acute disease states.[82,83] In addition, nail cosmetics may cause allergic contact dermatitis.[84] Nail deformities, either acquired or congenital, may require surgery.[85]

DERMIS

Basement Membrane

The *cutaneous basement membrane* refers to the extracellular structures organized at the interface between the epidermis and dermis. Research has led to a much better understanding of the details of composition, organization, and function in this region.[86]

Congenital defects in the basement membrane may result from either a lack of production of basement membrane constituents or synthesis of defective components. These abnormalities result in poor cohesion between the epidermis and dermis. Clinically, this shows as vesicles, blisters, and bullae after the application of minimal frictional forces.

Fortunately, inherited mechanobullous disorders are uncommon. Commonly encountered processes such as blistering inflammatory dermatoses, autoimmune blis-

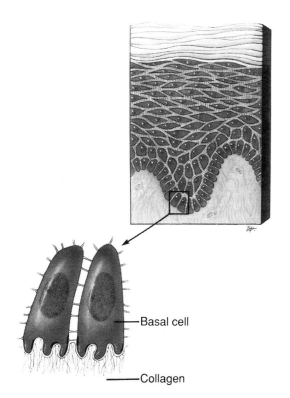

FIGURE 11-16 Basement membrane uniting epidermis and cutis (macro).

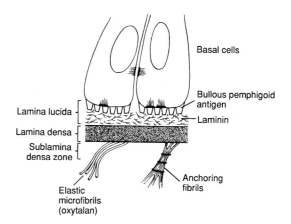

FIGURE 11-17 Basement membrane uniting epidermis and cutis (micro). Cohesion between the epidermis and cutis is well served by a discrete multilayered structure, the basement membrane, which is composed of the lamina lucida, lamina densa, and sublamina densa.

tering disorders, friction blisters, and coma bullae are caused by damage to the basement membrane at the dermoepidermal junction.

The epidermal basement membrane lies between the epidermis and the dermis and is responsible for the bonding of these two layers of the skin (Figure 11-16). The epidermal basement membrane begins at its attachment to the plasma membrane of the basal epidermal cells. These basal cells are predominantly keratinocytes, but Merkel's cells and melanocytes are also found in this cell layer. Electron microscopy shows three morphologically distinct layers of epidermal basement membrane: (1) the lamina lucida, (2) lamina densa, and (3) sublamina densa fibrillar zone (reticular zone; Figure 11-17).

The lamina lucida is located subjacent to the plasma membrane of basal epidermal cells and is 20–40 nm thick. As its name implies, this layer is relatively electron lucent; it contains anchoring filaments, laminin, and fibronectin. The anchoring filaments connect the epidermal cell plasma membranes to deeper structures by traversing this region. The lamina lucida also contains the bullous pemphigoid antigen, a glycoprotein identified by antibodies in the sera of patients with this disorder. Other less well-characterized antigens have been localized to this region by antibodies in the sera of patients with other blistering disorders such as herpes gestationis and scarring pemphigoid.[87]

The lamina densa is an electron-dense band immediately below the lamina lucida that runs parallel to the epidermal cell lower border. It is approximately 30–60 nm thick. The major component of this region is type IV collagen; other components include heparin sulfate and proteoglycan, but the strength of the basement membrane is in large part attributable to type IV collagen. Laminin and type IV collagen bind to each other. Defective isoforms of laminin have been identified in several inborn and acquired diseases, demonstrating their importance in the structural integrity of the skin.[88]

The sublamina densa fibrillar zone lies between the lamina densa above and dermal stroma below. This layer is principally composed of anchoring fibrils and to a lesser extent finer fibrils called *elastic microfibrils* (oxytalan fibers) and interstitial collagen fibrils composed of type III collagen. Two antigens, AF-1 and AF-2, are localized to the sublamina densa as well as the antigens associated with epidermolysis bullosa acquisita.

The anchoring fibrils are cross-banded structures extending from the lamina densa into the dermis. They occasionally form loops linking one portion of the lamina densa to another while anchoring around dermal collagen bundles. The finer fibrils move deeply into the dermis and sometimes are associated with elastic fibers.

The epidermal cells are attached to the basement membrane by hemidesmosomes. The anchoring filaments in the lamina lucida are attached to the basal epidermal cell hemidesmosomes, which are situated along the dermal surface of the basal keratinocytes. Hemidesmosomes are important structures not only for cell adhesion, but also for wound healing and tumor invasion.[89]

RELATIONSHIPS TO DISEASE

Defects in coding for different intracellular and extracellular structural proteins that are responsible for the mechanical strength of the skin have been discovered in a number of diseases characterized by skin fragility. These specific defects influence the level in the skin at which the blistering is observed in these conditions.[90,91] For example, in junctional epidermolysis bullosa, the blistering arises within the lamina lucida and is associated morphologically with rudimentary and sparse hemidesmosomes. In dystrophic epidermolysis bullosa, blistering occurs beneath the lamina densa and morphologically is associated with abnormal anchoring fibrils.

In autoimmune disorders such as bullosa pemphigoid, bullous systemic lupus erythematosus, and dermatitis herpetiformis, deposition of antibodies within the basement membrane zone has been visualized by immunofluorescence and immunoelectron microscopy. Presumably, the presence of the antibodies alters the structural function of the antigenic component of the basement membrane, thus causing dyshesion. Alternatively, or additionally, antigen-antibody complexes may stimulate inflammatory destructive processes (e.g., activation of complement).

The mechanism by which mechanical or frictional bullae develop has not been well characterized, but it appears to involve stress-induced injury to the structural components of the basement membrane. In bullae associated with coma, anoxia of the skin occurs from prolonged periods of pressure caused by the patient's weight while he or she remains in one position. The anoxia presumably results in destruction of the structural integrity of the basement membrane and leads to formation of blisters. In extreme cases, when this occurs over bony prominences, decubitus ulcers form.

VASCULATURE

Compared with other organs, the dermis of the skin has a disproportionately large blood supply. This extensive network of vessels[92] is functionally involved in heat transfer and in serving the metabolic needs of the large numbers of eccrine and sebaceous glands in the cutis.

Embryonically, all three elements of the vasculature (arteries, veins, and lymphatics) are mesodermal in origin and accordingly can regenerate with relative ease. The genetically predetermined extrinsic cues important in the development of the vasculature in embryos are becoming better understood.[93]

Anatomically, the dermis' major vascular network consists of two parallel systems of blood vessels traversing it in a pattern horizontal to the epidermis (see Figure 11-11).[94] These two units are connected vertically by communicating vessels oriented perpendicular to the epidermis. The anatomic origin of the cutaneous vasculature can be traced to perforating vessels emerging from muscular arteries that in turn penetrate through the subcutaneous fascia and then traverse in a direction perpendicular to the skin surface. The vessels that pass directly through the subcutaneous tissue bypass the subcutaneous fat by traversing within the fibrous septa, which separate fat lobules.

The deepest vascular plexus, the transverse one, supplies principally the adnexal glands (sebaceous and eccrine), whereas the more superficial ones form the papillary plexus. This plexus, which is rich in capillaries, is localized in the dermal papillae abutting the epidermis (see Figure 11-11B). The superficial and deep vascular plexus have numerous anastomoses and form an exceedingly abundant blood supply. Blood returns through an almost identical venous pattern of vessels located in close apposition to the arteries. Under most circumstances the arterial venous communications are mediated by a rich capillary network, although the capillary beds may be bypassed by direct shunts between arteries and venules known as *glomus bodies* (Figure 11-18). These are particularly effective in regulating heat loss in these acral areas.

The vascular blood flow is controlled principally by the resistance of arterioles. They constrict after adrenergic stimulation of unmyelinated sympathetic fibers. Hormonal effects on the smooth muscles of arterioles of the skin include a vasopressor action from angiotensin and adrenalin. Histamine, alcohol, prostaglandins, and heat are associated with vasodilatation.

Many vascular anomalies exist in the skin,[95] but the most common concerns for the practitioner are angiogenesis[96] to support wound healing and cutaneous vasculitis,[97,98] which may lead to skin breakdown and delayed healing. Vascular endothelial growth factor has been targeted for gene therapy to overexpress in tissues with poor wound healing or blood flow to stimulate healing.[99,100] Finally, treatment of vascular lesions with lasers has become accepted to effectively destroy

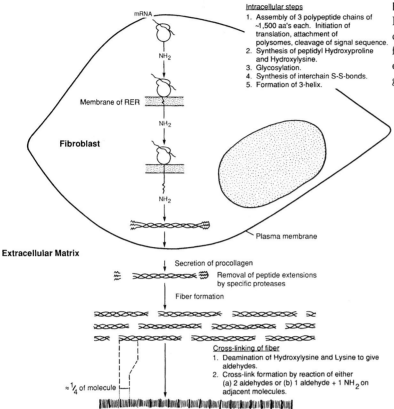

mRNA

NH₂

Membrane of RER

Fibroblast

NH₂

NH₂

Plasma membrane

Extracellular Matrix

Intracellular steps
1. Assembly of 3 polypeptide chains of ~1,500 aa's each. Initiation of translation, attachment of polysomes, cleavage of signal sequence.
2. Synthesis of peptidyl Hydroxyproline and Hydroxylysine.
3. Glycosylation.
4. Synthesis of interchain S-S-bonds.
5. Formation of 3-helix.

Secretion of procollagen

Removal of peptide extensions by specific proteases

Fiber formation

Cross-linking of fiber
1. Deamination of Hydroxylysine and Lysine to give aldehydes.
2. Cross-link formation by reaction of either (a) 2 aldehydes or (b) 1 aldehyde + 1 NH₂ on adjacent molecules.

≈ ¼ of molecule

A

FIGURE 11-18 A. Collagen synthesis and assembly. Procollagen is synthesized and secreted into the extracellular matrix by fibroblasts. Collagen fibers are formed in the extracellular compartment by a specific enzymatic cross-linking process. (mRNA = messenger RNA; RER = rough endoplasmic reticulum.)

certain cosmetically unacceptable lesions in specified locations of the body.

Mast Cells

Mast cells are derived from the bone marrow and distributed via the blood stream to all tissues and organs of the body except solid bone and cartilage. Mast cells contain myriad mediators that are preformed and stored within granules or produced after mast cell activation. The groups that are preformed can be further divided into those that are soluble after mast cell degranulation and those that are insoluble and remain associated with the extruded granules.[101] Table 11-2 lists representative mast cell mediators. Mast cells in humans form two groups, based on their proteinase content. One group contains tryptase; the other, a tryptase and a chymotryptase. In any given anatomic site more than one subpopulation of mast cells may be present, and differences are observable in their mediators.

Although the IgE receptor and the IgE antibody-antigen induction processes have been studied extensively in relation to the activation of the mast cell, a vast array of other mediators and stimuli has also been found to initiate mast cell activation. For example, selected neuropeptides, endogenous opioids, hormones, T-cell factors, complement (C3a, C5a), and interleukin-1 have been found to stimulate histamine secretion. The major rationale for the wide use of antihistamines is to block histamine receptors on target cells and so prevent allergic responses resulting from mast cell histamine release. Corticosteroids inhibit secretion of mast cell mediators and are widely used, systemically and topically, for allergic reactions and for other mast cell disorders such as urticaria pigmentosa.[102]

The mast cell, with its diverse array of mediators, is involved in many biological activities, but the precise role of the mast cell and its mediators in such activities is under investigation and has been reviewed.[101,103–105] Broadly, the mast cell participates in inflammatory responses (both immediate and delayed hypersensitivity), angiogenesis, immunoregulation, and fibrosis. Thus, the skin mast cells are found to accumulate or be activated in the following disorders: (1) normal wound healing,[106] (2) keloids, (3) neurofibromas, (4) mastocytosis, (5) eosinophilic fasciitis, and (6) scleroderma. Mast cells have been implicated as important modulators of hair follicle cycling.[107]

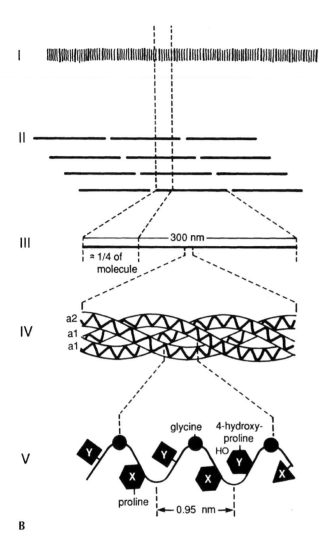

B

FIGURE 11-18 (*continued*) **B.** Collagen structure: I, The banding pattern of collagen seen by electron microscopy; II, the alignment of collagen fibers that accounts for the banding pattern seen in I; III, the 300-nm banding pattern repeats that consist of overlapping collagen fibers; IV, a collagen fiber consists of three collagen chains that are helically arranged; V, the repeating primary amino acid structure of collagen. (Reprinted with permission from J Uitto, et al. Collagen: Its Structure, Function, and Pathology. In Progress in Diseases of the Skin, Vol 1. New York: Grune & Stratton, 1981;103.)

Collagen

Collagen, a protein widely distributed throughout all organs and tissues, makes up 70–80% of the dry weight of human skin.[108] Collagen functions principally in a structural role, maintaining form and limiting deformation. It also participates in blood clotting, inflammation, and tissue repair.

Fifteen distinct types of collagen exist; each has a characteristic tissue distribution. All collagens are composed of three polypeptide chains, referred to as *alpha chains*, which consist of repeating tripeptides gly-X-Y. One-third of the X and Y residues are proline or 4-hydroxyproline. Alpha chains are of 18 different types that combine to form the 15 different types of collagen.[109] Variation between collagen types also depends on the extent of glycosylation of hydroxylysine residues and the hydroxylation of proline.

Type I collagen is the most abundant form and the only collagen type in bone and tendon. The predominant form in adult human skin, type I collagen is composed of two distinct polypeptide chains. Type II, composed of three identical chains, is found in cartilaginous tissues. Type III collagen consists of three identical chains and is distributed widely throughout the body, including the skin. Type IV collagen is a major component of the basement membrane. Type V collagen is present in small amounts throughout the body and can be detected in the dermis. Type VII collagen is present in the skin as part of the anchoring fibril complex.

Granulation tissue contains increased amounts of types I, III, and V collagens. Collagen types I, II, and III form broad, banded, extracellular fibers and are called *interstitial collagens*. Collagen types IV to X are minor collagens that do not form banded fibers.

Collagen has a low rate of cell turnover; the half-life of collagen is estimated to be 2.5 years. The continuous remodeling and degradation of collagen make it a valuable material to study for changes associated with aging. Studies in vitro of the rate of cutaneous collagen synthesis show increases up to age 30–40 years, after which synthesis remains approximately constant.[109]

Collagen is synthesized by fibroblasts in the dermis. Each chain has a distinct gene and corresponding mRNA. A triple helix structure is formed as the collagen chains are released from polysomes. Procollagen is secreted from the cells and is converted to collagen in the extracellular space by the action of neutral endoproteases that remove propeptides (see Figure 11-18).

The largest fibrils of type I collagen are 50–300 nm in diameter. Electron microscopy shows a 67-nm repeating banding pattern caused by the staggered alignment of individual collagen molecules. Aggregates of these collagen molecules form fibrils. Cross-linking between collagen molecules occurs through posttranslational modification of lysine and hydroxylysine residues. Four enzymes are important in these modifications: (1) prolyl-4-hydroxylase, (2) lysyl hydroxylase, (3) galactosyl transferase, and (4) glucosyl transferase. The activity of all these enzymes decreases in human skin with aging.

TABLE 11-2
Mast Cell Mediators

Released in Soluble Form	Stored in Granules Released within Granules (Insoluble)	Synthesized on Mast Cell Activation
Histamine	Proteoglycans	Platelet-activating factors
Serotonin	Proteases	Leukotrienes
Proteases	Inflammatory factors	Prostaglandins
Exoglycosidases	Peroxidase	Adenosine
Chemotactic factors	Superoxide dismutase	—

Source: Reprinted with permission from D Befus, H Fujimaki, TDG Lee, et al. Mast cell polymorphisms. Present concepts, future directions. Dig Dis Sci 1988;33:16S–24S.

The activity of prolyl-4-hydroxylase depends on oxygen and vitamin C intake. Thus, malnutrition or poor circulation would be expected to compromise tissue viability and collagen repair processes.

As collagen matures and stabilizes in the extracellular matrix, it becomes progressively less soluble. Collagen in skin is more susceptible to pepsin digestion than intestinal collagen. Pepsin digestion is inversely related to the extent of cross-linking. The greater solubility of skin collagen may therefore be related to greater turnover of skin collagen. Weight changes alter the need for more skin, and damage resulting from external environmental changes may affect skin collagen and enhance turnover. Many of the factors important in regulating collagen synthesis are only partially understood; however, hydrocortisone and fluorinated corticosteroids applied topically or delivered intradermally inhibit collagen synthesis. This may, in part, explain the dermal atrophy observed with continued use of these agents.[110]

With increasing age, collagen throughout the body shows physical changes that are caused by progressive cross-linking or chemical stabilization. These changes may be responsible for the loss of skin elasticity with age. Collagen is associated with glycosaminoglycans in the dermis. These polymers are lost with aging, and this results in decreased water-binding capacity, or hydration of the skin, leading to a dry, wrinkled appearance.[108]

Elastic Tissue

Elastic tissue, a connective tissue component of the dermis, constitutes approximately 0.6–2.0% of its total dry weight. All elastic tissue components derive from a mesodermal stem cell; the mature fibroblast is the parent of both collagen and elastic fibers. The formation of elastic fibers appears to result from active secretion of a protein-rich microfibril that polymerizes along the cell surface of the fibroblast.[111] This glycoprotein forms tubular bundles that encase an amorphous protein, elastin.

In a mature elastic fiber the elastin component accounts for more than 90% of the total weight. Elastin is an amorphous insoluble protein that, when fully mature, is arranged in sheets. The relative insolubility of elastin is caused principally by covalent linkages of elastin polypeptides by desmosine and isodesmosine, which are unique to elastic fibers. Conclusive data demonstrate that human fibroblasts also synthesize elastin, and, indeed, the presence of a gene controlling elastin synthesis has been demonstrated in fibroblasts by Davidson et al.[111] Elastin messenger RNA has also been identified. An enzyme, lysyl oxidase, which is a crucial initial step in the cross-linking of elastin by deaminating lysyl residues, has been purified. Lysyl oxidase requires copper for biological activity.[112]

Skin turgor or tone (the ability of skin that has been extended by a force to return rapidly to its original position) is the primary function of elastic tissues.[113] Defects in or damage to elastic fibers can alter this property and contribute to old-looking skin.[114–116] The functional and molecular properties of elastin have been reviewed in consideration of it as an elastic biomaterial.[117]

Dermal Matrix

The dermal matrix or ground substance represents the third component of the dermis. It consists primarily of proteoglycan and glycosaminoglycans. Its gross appearance is mucoid, and it contains a high percentage of mucopolysaccharides. Quantitatively, ground substance represents less than 1% of the dry weight of the dermis. It is not a primary source of major cutaneous diseases. The molecular and functional characteristics of matrix proteoglycans have been reviewed.[118]

INNERVATION

More than 1 million afferent nerve fibers located within the skin monitor the external environment for heat, cold, touch, and pain. The terminal endings of these fibers are located principally at the dermoepidermal junction, adnexal structures, or deep cutis (Figure 11-19). They consist of two types of nerve endings: corpuscular, which are in direct contact with cutaneous structures, and free nerve endings, which traverse the cutis. The latter envelop the majority of hair follicles (see Figure 11-19).[119] Specific sensory functions of both the free nerve endings and encapsulated receptors remain controversial. It appears that significant overlap exists in the reception of external stimuli (energies) that are cortically perceived in terms of temperature, touch, and pain (see Figure 11-19).

Corpuscular nerve units were originally (but are no longer) considered as specific for heat, pain, touch, and cold. The types of units may be generally defined as follows: Pacinian corpuscles are ovoid structures that on cross-section are laminar, like an onion (see Figure 11-18). They are found extensively on the soles and, therefore, may subserve pressure. Meissner corpuscles are found in the papillary dermis of glabrous skin. They may be related to tactile sensations. They are found primarily on fingertips, palms, and soles. These lobulated nerve endings are found in all mammals.[120] Merkel's cells may resemble LCs and frequently are located in the epidermal rete ridges. They communicate with nerve fibrils and may be important as specialized cells adapted to touch reception. Ruffini structures are present in heavy concentration in the digits and are connected to myelinated afferent fibers and appear to be related to fine perception.

Somatic Sensory Innervation of the Skin

Free Nerve Endings
Within the papillary dermis an extensive network of ectodermally derived unmyelinated nerve fibers course in a horizontal path. Their external sheath is composed of Schwann's cells in direct contact with the cells of the dermoepidermal junction or enveloping the adnexal glands (see Figure 11-19). A particular group of these fibers, called *thick myelinated Aβ fibers*, appears most receptive to touch and vibration, whereas the thinner Aγ are most sensitive to light touch and pressure. The thinnest, known as Aδ, transmit pain, temperature, and *causal* or physiological itching. A poorly localized sensation of pruritus, often a feature of various chronic dermatologic conditions, appears to be carried by still other nerve fibers that are anatomically deeper and unrelated to pain perception.[121]

Receiving information on the external environment is a prerequisite to human survival and is probably related to the evolutionary development and present overlap of a complex cutaneous sensory network of receptor fibers.

Pruritus (itching) has often been described as a stimulus transmitted to the cortex that elicits a desire to scratch.[122] Although no hard evidence exists, itching may have had survival value in protecting against parasites, fleas, and other insects that were vectors for systemic disease. The mediation of the itch sensation remains controversial. Relatively strong clinical data

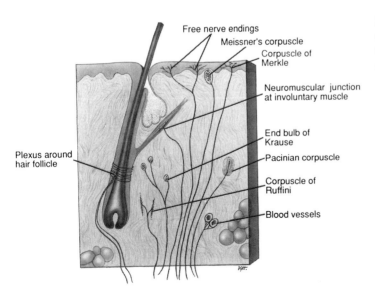

FIGURE 11-19 Corpuscular structure and free nerve endings innervating the skin. Temperature, pressure, touch, and pain are received as afferent stimuli by diverse corpuscular structures and free nerve endings.

indicate that pain and itching are separable sensations; it appears that the papillary dermis has an extensive network of superficial unmyelinated nerve fiber endings, C fibers, that as receptors transmit impulses for both mild cutaneous pain and itching. Indeed, patients with central cord lesions of syringomyelia lose pain sensation but not touch, suggesting that C fibers are polymodal, with varying thresholds of responsiveness.

In chronic, extremely pruritic, widespread skin conditions, the unmyelinated fibers appear to be mediating pruritus solely when minimally excited. In contrast, the sensory fibers of the δ type mediate the mild localized causal itching as well as cutaneous pain in the same fiber. Again, an arbitrary distinction between structure and function in the superficial dermal fibers is difficult if not impossible to make. It is noteworthy that when areas of skin are denuded and devoid of epidermis and dermal papillae itching is not elicited; rather, severe pain is felt. This reinforces the concept that superficial and deep sensory nerve receptors may not be function specific.

What chemical stimuli nerve receptors discharge is also unclear. Current evidence indicates that proteases brought by an inflammatory white blood cell response to an eczematous process provide the stimuli. In other cases, mast cell degranulation liberates several diverse-acting pruritic agents. Studies document that epidermal cells may secrete proteases that they themselves have manufactured. These chemicals or their substrates may be the true initiators of pruritus.

The list of mediators involved in pruritic sensation is constantly expanding. The majority has the chemical structure of peptides. It is probable that each agent has a preferential role in selective sites or situations. Currently under study, in addition to the classical pruritic agent histamine, are serotonin, slow-reacting substance, bradykinins, endorphins, and endopeptidases.[123,124] Mechanisms of pruritus and the latest considerations in treatment have been reviewed.[125]

SUBCUTANEOUS TISSUE

Beneath the dermis is the hypodermis or subcutaneous tissue layer (see Figure 11-1). Its origin in midfetal life derives from mesenchymal cells that give rise to lipocytes and fibrocytes.[43] These, in turn, give rise to a fully mature fibrous tissue and a lobulated adipocyte layer that is in direct apposition to the dermis above and the fascia below (see Figure 11-1). Within the fibrous septa surrounding the lipocytes course nerve fibers, blood vessels, and lymphatics. Under normal conditions the unstained lipocytes have a characteristic clear cyto-plasm, the nucleus being compressed and displaced against the cell membrane. The largest biochemical constituent of lipocytes is triglycerides. Subcutaneous tissue stores energy in the form of fat, provides insulation against heat loss, and cushions internal structures against environmental trauma or pressure.[126]

SELECTED FUNCTIONS

Vitamin D Synthesis

Vitamin D is photosynthesized in keratinocytes after irradiation with ultraviolet B (290–320 nm; Figure 11-20). The synthetic pathway begins with 7-dehydrocholesterol being converted to previtamin D_3 (cholecalciferol) by ultraviolet B. Previtamin D_3 undergoes thermal conversion to vitamin D_3. Vitamin D_3 is released into the blood stream bound to vitamin D–binding protein and is transported to the liver for hydroxylation to form 25-hydroxyvitamin D_3 and then to the kidney to finally form 1,25-dihydroxyvitamin D_3, the most metabolically active form of vitamin D.[127] It has also been demonstrated that, in addition to the kidney, the skin contains the 1-α-hydroxylase and is capable of converting 25-hydroxyvitamin D_3 to the 1,25-dihydroxyvitamin D_3. It is not clear how much of a contribution to vitamin D metabolism there is from the cutaneous synthesis of 1,25-hydroxyvitamin D_3. Circulating 25-hydroxyvitamin D_3 would need to be taken up by the skin to form 1,25-hydroxyvitamin D_3 because the 25-hydroxylase is only found in the liver.

After exposure to intense ultraviolet B, not all of the 7-dehydrocholesterol is converted to previtamin D, because alternative pathways exist for the formation of less active metabolites. These alternative routes of metabolism may be an important mechanism whereby excessive ultraviolet exposure does not lead to hypervitaminosis D.

Vitamin D deficiency results in rickets in children and osteomalacia in adults. It may occur in instances of low dietary intake or inadequate exposure to ultraviolet radiation. Sunscreen lotions with sun protection factor 8 or higher have been shown to block cutaneous synthesis of vitamin D after ultraviolet exposure, presumably by blocking transmission of the 295-nm wavelength necessary for the photochemical synthesis of vitamin D. Because elderly persons are cautious about aging changes and skin cancer as hazards of excessive sun exposure, their vitamin D status is a concern. Their dietary intake of vitamin D is poor, and they often avoid the sun or wear sunscreen.[128]

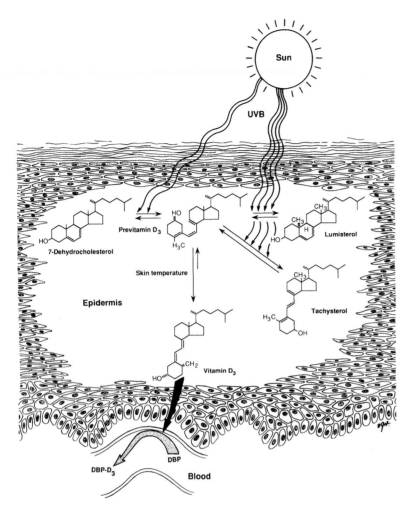

FIGURE 11-20 Synthesis and metabolism of vitamin D in the skin. Previtamin D is formed after the ultraviolet B (UVB) irradiation of 7-dehydrocholesterol. Thermal catalysis converts previtamin D_3 to vitamin D_3. Excessive ultraviolet radiation causes previtamin D_3 to form the less active metabolites, lumisterol and tachysterol. Vitamin D–binding protein (DBP) binds and transports the vitamin D_3 to the liver for hydroxylation.

Vitamin D and its active metabolites form an endocrine system important in the absorption of calcium from the diet, conservation of calcium by the kidney, mineralization of bones, and maintenance of normal plasma levels of calcium (important for normal neuromuscular conduction). These processes were comprehensively reviewed by DeLuca.[127]

The cellular effects of 1,25-dihydroxyvitamin D_3 are mediated through interaction with a nuclear receptor protein of 55,000 kD that belongs to a superfamily of receptors that bind steroid hormones, retinoic acid, and thyroid hormone.[129] The 1,25-dihydroxyvitamin D_3 receptor protein is expressed in practically all tissues, including keratinocytes and fibroblasts from the skin.[129] Autoradiography of frozen tissue sections using labeled 1,25-dihydroxyvitamin D_3 has suggested the presence of the nuclear receptor in tissues that were not previously considered to be target tissues for vitamin D, such as the parathyroid gland, pancreatic islets, some bone marrow cells, and cutaneous keratinocytes. Another finding is that approximately 60% of all cancer cell lines have large amounts of the receptor.

A number of genes have been recognized to be regulated by 1,25-dihydroxyvitamin D_3: calcium metabolism-related proteins (e.g., preproparathyroid hormone, calcitonin, calbindin), oncogenes (c-myc, c-fos, and c-fes), the 1,25-dihydroxyvitamin D_3 receptor, and several others, among them type I collagen, fibronectin, prolactin, IL-1, and IL-2. For each of these genes, levels of mRNA accumulation are either increased or decreased by 1,25-dihydroxyvitamin D_3.[129]

During the past decade, researchers have identified actions of 1,25-dihydroxyvitamin D_3 in addition to its role in mineral metabolism. These actions include influences on differentiation and proliferation of the hematopoietic cells, cancer cells, and epidermal cells (keratinocytes)[129] and thus may be responsible in part for the clinical findings associated with rickets (i.e., increased infections, impaired neutrophil phagocytosis, anemia, decreased cellularity of the marrow, extramedullary hematopoiesis).

Receptors for 1,25-dihydroxyvitamin D_3 are present in a variety of cancer cell lines, including melanoma.[129] Large doses of 1,25-dihydroxyvitamin D_3 have inhibited melanoma xenografts in mice. Also, 1,25-dihydroxyvitamin D_3 stimulates fibronectin production by human cancer cell lines, and it has been suggested that this may mediate an antimetastatic effect for vitamin D. Future studies will evaluate the potential therapeutic use of vitamin D and its analogues for chemoprevention or therapy of human malignancies.

In cultured skin cells 1,25-dihydroxyvitamin D_3 induces antiproliferative changes, such as decreased DNA synthesis, and promotes terminal differentiation toward nonadherent cornified squamous cells. Preliminary studies of orally or topically administered 1,25-dihydroxyvitamin D_3 to patients with psoriasis have shown that the skin lesions improve. Psoriasis, a benign skin disorder characterized by hyperproliferation of keratinocytes resulting in the formation of thickened plaques, remains a therapeutic problem. Flattening of lesions after therapy with 1,25-dihydroxyvitamin D_3 has been reported and is consistent with the antiproliferative effects of 1,25-dihydroxyvitamin D_3 observed in cultured epidermal skin cells. The role of vitamin D and its analogues in the treatment of psoriasis led to the introduction of topically applied calcipotriene, which binds to the nuclear receptor in the skin and evokes 1,25-dihydroxyvitamin D activity.[130,131] Because it is not absorbed well systemically, the potential side effect of hypercalcemia is minimized.

Percutaneous Absorption

A major function of the skin is as a barrier or interface between the rest of the body and the external environment. This barrier is selective, allowing some molecules that come in contact with the skin to penetrate to various levels within the epidermis and dermis and others, most notably moisture, to escape from the epidermis to the ambient environment.

The penetration of compounds through the skin has been intensively studied by researchers evaluating chemicals used in cosmetics and for topical therapy and those encountered in occupational settings. Determination of the rate and degree of penetration of chemicals into the skin is complex and is dependent on (1) concentration, (2) type of vehicle, (3) skin region, (4) skin condition, and (5) extent of occlusion.[132,133]

Chemicals have different skin penetration rates; the differences may exceed four orders of magnitude.[132] When injury or disease alters the structure of the skin,

making it thinner, thicker, or discontinuous, the rate of absorption may be affected significantly. The stratum corneum, or horny layer, normally varies in thickness from less than 0.01 mm in eyelid skin to 1.0 mm in palmar or plantar skin. Nevertheless, the ease with which certain agents penetrate the skin of the palms or soles may be great despite the thickness of the stratum corneum in these areas. The stratum corneum is still considered the rate-limiting barrier in cutaneous absorption, unless it is absent owing to skin disease or injury. Once the agent or drug has penetrated the stratum corneum, it may diffuse transcellularly or through intercellular spaces to reach the basement membrane and dermis. From the dermis, agents or their cutaneous metabolites are taken up into systemic circulation.

The chemical structure, size, polarity, and degree of hydration are important factors in determining the diffusivity of the compound. Small lipophilic compounds lacking polar groups or ionic charges diffuse most readily. When a lipophilic compound is applied to the skin dispersed in a hydrophilic vehicle, it diffuses into the stratum corneum more effectively than when it is applied in a lipophilic vehicle. In addition to penetration of the epidermis, compounds may also enter the skin via the pores associated with skin appendages (i.e., sweat ducts, hair follicles, sebaceous glands; Figure 11-21). Transfollicular drug delivery has been reviewed.[134]

The hazards from percutaneous absorption of noxious chemicals include (1) direct toxic effects on the skin (e.g., caustic agents); (2) systemic toxicity from absorption through the skin; and (3) induction of contact dermatitis, either the allergic or primary irritant type. Tables of compounds that are particularly hazardous for skin exposure have been made in many countries. These lists may be used to establish guidelines for protective skin covering requirements to prevent toxic exposure, especially in the workplace.

In addition to the general process of percutaneous absorption, there is a phenomenon referred to as the reservoir effect. This is best exemplified in the absorption of topical glucocorticosteroids. Topical corticosteroids accumulate in the stratum corneum after initial application. When, long after the last application of the topical corticosteroid, the skin is covered with plastic wrap, the hydration of the stratum corneum and the remainder of the epidermis increases. This results in increased systemic absorption of the topical corticosteroid because more drug can penetrate the epidermis to reach the circulation.

Percutaneous absorption requires special caution in premature and full-term infants. First, the ratio of the surface area to total body weight is much greater in a

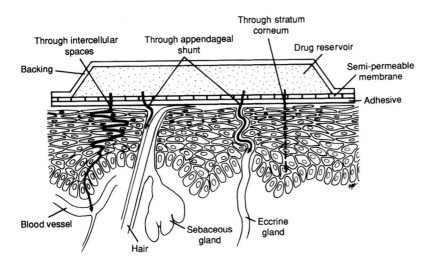

FIGURE 11-21 Absorption of drugs delivered transcutaneously from transdermal patches applied to the skin. This drug delivery system has the following potential routes for transcutaneous absorption of the drug to the blood vessels: (1) intercellular spaces, (2) appendiceal shunts such as the hair follicle or sweat duct, and (3) across cells without partitioning significantly between cells.

newborn than in an adult. Thus, in a newborn a percutaneous dose systemically absorbed is estimated to be approximately 2.7 times greater per kilogram of body weight than the same topical dose per unit area in an adult. The skin of a term infant is considered to be an intact barrier, although because the stratum corneum may be thinner than an adult's, the neonate may absorb more drug. The skin of the premature infant is considered to be an immature barrier that allows greater percutaneous drug absorption and skin water loss. The epidermis matures from weeks 23–33 of gestation.[135] Premature babies born during this period have an incomplete epidermal barrier and characteristically suffer increased transepidermal water loss and increased drug absorption per unit of surface area.[135] After birth,

the premature infant's skin quickly matures, and by postnatal week 2 or 3 its epidermal barrier approximates that of term infants, children, and adults.[135]

Inadvertent drug toxicity has been reported in newborns; often the toxicant is a disinfectant used in nurseries or laundry detergent.[136] Newborn infants have developed cutaneously derived toxic reactions, most commonly from diaper agents, topical antiseptics, and skin preparations. Premature infants are at greatest risk owing to their incomplete epidermal barrier and the greater likelihood of intensive care that requires invasive procedures. In this regard the following observations are offered:

- Routine skin or umbilical care does not require an antiseptic.
- Isopropyl alcohol swabs or aqueous chlorhexidine used sparingly is adequate to prepare the skin for invasive procedures.
- Alcohol solutions, iodine, hexachlorophene, and neomycin-containing sprays are particularly hazardous and should not be used.

Several commonly used dermatologic preparations have associated risks and complications, particularly for newborns (Table 11-3).

Percutaneous Drug Absorption as Therapy

A number of drugs can be delivered effectively and safely transdermally. The drug, dissolved in a suitable vehicle, penetrates a microporous membrane, and the drug is then absorbed through the skin. Nitroglycerine, scopolamine, clonidine, estrogen, and testosterone are among the drugs delivered this way (see Figure 11-21).

The advantages of transdermal drug delivery include (1) avoidance of irregularities in gastrointestinal absorp-

TABLE 11-3
Dermatologic Preparations with High-Risk Potential for Infants

Topical Agent	Toxicity
Corticosteroids	Adrenal suppression, particularly when the epidermal barrier is disrupted
Boric acid	Gastrointestinal, neurologic, dermatologic complications
Lindane	Well documented in animals and may similarly affect infants
Epinephrine	Applied to bleeding sites (e.g., after circumcision) can cause tachycardia and heart failure
Urea cream (10%)	When applied for ichthyosis, blood urea nitrogen level can get high despite normal creatinine value
Estrogens	May produce feminization in boys and pseudoprecocious puberty in girls

tion of drug, avoidance of first-pass metabolism by the liver, and continuous drug delivery. The effective use of transdermal drug delivery is limited to drugs that are active systemically in small quantities, are not irritating or sensitizing to skin, and are absorbed well across the stratum corneum and into the blood stream.

Wound Healing

Wound healing is a dynamic process influenced by multiple factors:

1. Local structural repair elements of the dermis and epidermis
2. Host defenses against external pathogens that gain entry into the wound
3. Inflammatory mediators and growth factors produced locally at the site of injury or delivered via the blood stream
4. Immigrant cells derived from the bone marrow
5. Quality of the regional circulation to a wound
6. Amount of pressure, tension, and movement at the wound surface

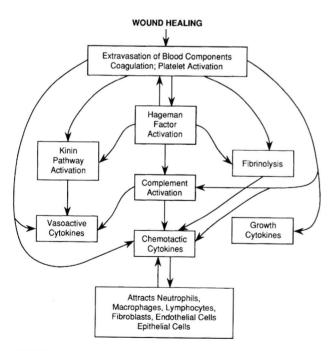

FIGURE 11-22 Wound healing involves a complex process whereby many mediators and cytokines interplay to orchestrate an inflammatory response, removal of debris, and growth of new tissue.

An abnormality in any of these factors impairs the ability of host mechanisms to promote wound healing (Figure 11-22).

Epithelial Repair

Epithelial cells actively divide at the wound edge and roll over each other to re-epithelialize the wound surface. At the same time, the basement membrane to which the epithelial cells become attached is laid down beneath them. Bullous pemphigoid antigen is synthesized first, followed by laminin, and finally type IV collagen. Type IV collagen is synthesized when the entire wound is re-epithelialized (e.g., 4–6 days after wounding).

Epithelial cells migrate only over viable tissue, because they are dependent on underlying tissues for nutrients. Migration has been demonstrated to occur more readily over a moist wound bed. Crusts or eschars impede epithelial migration. It occurs more gradually as the new epithelium fights its way beneath the eschar.

Thus, epithelialization occurs during wound healing by the migration of keratinocytes to the wound site and by their subsequent proliferation. Studies have demonstrated that several mediators (extracellular matrix molecules and soluble peptide factors) modulate cultured keratinocyte motility and proliferation and may be important in vivo (Table 11-4).[137]

Dermal Repair

After tissue injury, perivascular fibroblasts become activated and proliferate. Fibroblasts are responsible for the

TABLE 11-4

Effects of Wound Healing Factors on Keratinocytes

Agent	Keratinocyte Migration	Proliferation
Fibronectin	+ +	
Thrombospondin	+	
Laminin	−	
High calcium	−	
Growth factor-β[a]	+	
Epidermal growth factor[a]	+	+
Somatomedin C[b]		+
Interferon-γ	−	−
Radiation		−

+ = positive effect; + + = strong effect, − = negative effect.
[a]May stimulate migration by induction of fibronectin production.
[b]Stimulates thrombospondin production.
Source: Reprinted with permission from BJ Nickoloff, RS Mitra, BL Riser, et al. Modulation of keratinocyte motility. Am J Pathol 1988;132:543–551.

synthesis of collagen, elastin, glycosaminoglycans, and proteoglycans; all are components of the extracellular matrix.[138] During the early phase of wound repair, fibroblasts synthesize embryonic type III collagen, which as the wound matures is eventually replaced by adult type I collagen. New collagen is present in the wound within the first day after injury. In partial-thickness wounds, collagen synthesis peaks on the second or third day after injury, whereas in full-thickness wounds the rate of collagen synthesis peaks between the fifth and seventh days after injury. Collagen synthesis is accelerated as long as a year after injury, but is accompanied by simultaneous degradation by collagenases as the wound is remodeled. In addition to collagen, the elastin, proteoglycans, and glycosaminoglycans are restored to the connective tissue structure of the dermis. Angiogenesis, the development of new blood vessels, is an important component of wound healing, as it restores nutrient delivery. For example, angiogenesis is needed to bridge the vasculature from grafts to the underlying blood supply, to rejoin vessels across a wound, or to provide new vasculature to a tissue defect. Lymphatics also regenerate, but permanent damage may result in an edematous wound that is susceptible to infection.

Wound Contraction

After full-thickness excision of rodent skin, the defect closes itself by a process referred to as *wound contraction*. The edges of the wound are brought together by a centripetal action attributed to contraction of myofibroblasts at the wound edge. In some areas of human skin (e.g., perineum), this process occurs more readily and is more complete than in other areas. Epithelialization is necessary to achieve complete wound closure. Wound contractures across joints can limit mobility.

TABLE 11-5
Factors That Promote Poor Wound Healing

Local	Systemic
Suboptimal surgical technique	Chronic illness
Drugs (e.g., corticosteroids, antineo- plastics, aspirin)	Malnutrition
Ischemia (arteriosclerosis, pressure occlusion)	Diabetes
Infection	Cushing's syndrome
Trauma	Old age
Skin disease (e.g., psoriasis)	Vasculitis
Foreign body	—
Neuropathy	—

Abnormal Wound Repair

When the modeling of scars is defective, excessive scar tissue may accumulate over time. Some patients form keloids, abnormal tissue growths at the site of tissue injury. They are hypercellular, containing a more concentrated population of fibroblasts and an increased number of mast cells compared with normal dermal tissue. Hypertrophic scars consist of excessive scar tissue, but are less prominent than keloids. Both hypertrophic scars and keloids are more likely to occur in areas of increased skin tension.

Poor healing can also complicate wound repair. It is associated with many local factors as well as multiple systemic conditions, as noted in Table 11-5.

Malnutrition and Wound Healing

Malnutrition causes delayed wound healing and is associated with patients who suffer from malabsorption, inability to receive enteral nutrition, or hypermetabolic or catabolic states. The inability to synthesize wound repair components adequately may result from deficiencies of a vitamin, mineral, protein, carbohydrate, or lipid. Infection may be a major problem secondary to immunodeficiency caused by malnutrition. Finally, edema from hypoalbuminemia poses physical stress on wound edges and can interfere with healing.[139]

Patients with significant wounds should be assessed for nutritional status and requirements. Intervention, as needed, must be a part of the overall approach to the patient with a healing wound.[140]

Vascular Supply and Wound Healing

Oxygen delivery to wounds is often a problem in patients with significant peripheral vascular disease. Determination of transcutaneous oxygen partial pressures has helped identify optimal sites of limb amputation for ischemic arterial disease. Unfortunately, the use of these measurements to predict venous ulcer healing does not distinguish which ulcers will heal. Clearly, many additional factors are involved in wound healing. Although oxygen tension is an important factor, venous ulcers with relatively poor oxygen tension have been shown to be capable of healing.[141]

Wound Dressings

It is now widely accepted that wounds kept moist and free from infections epithelialize faster. Thus, occlusive and semiocclusive dressings are preferred over the formation of a thick eschar that occurs when wounds are kept open to the air. Eschar formation appears to impede keratinocyte migration; however, despite enhanced re-epithelialization, return of the cutaneous barrier functions, as measured by transepidermal water loss, does not return more quickly when these dressings are used (Figure 11-23).[142] Despite the perceived advantages of moist wound healing, there are many instances in which encouraging the wound to form an eschar is preferred. An eschar provides a natural, hard, protective cover for a wound that will heal beneath. These wounds are less likely to become infected and are easier to care for than complicated moist dressing changes. In the elderly with poor tissue, eschar formation can safely be stimulated (1) in draining wounds with calcium alginate products or (2) in drier wounds by leaving the wound open to the air.

New Approaches to Wound Healing

To aid in the healing of deep wounds and to diminish wound contraction, animal models have been developed that demonstrate the feasibility of using synthetic extracellular matrices for regeneration of skin. Extracellular matrices have been synthesized from cross-linked collagen-glycosaminoglycan polymers. Feeding these matrices with fibroblasts and keratinocytes has decreased wound contraction as skin regenerates.[143] To be optimally effective these matrices must be highly porous and show partial resistance to collagenase digestion.

The foregoing approach to wound healing has been extended to incorporate specific growth factors into the collagen matrix, to enhance angiogenesis and epidermal proliferation. For example, heparin-binding growth factor 2 and epidermal growth factor have been covalently bound to biotinylated collagen. This growth factor-enhanced matrix has been shown to sustain accelerated growth rates of human epidermal keratinocytes.[144] Future studies of this modified collagen in synthetic extracellular matrices could potentially enhance our ability to heal deep wounds. In the past several years, a dermal regeneration template (Integra; Integra Life Sciences, Plainsboro, NJ) has been introduced and is approved for the treatment of life-threatening burn wounds. After 2 weeks of the ingrowth of fibroblasts and vessels into the collagen matrix, the artificial silicone epidermis is peeled away and a thin autograft is placed.

Growth factors are also being applied directly to wounds to stimulate wound healing. Epidermal growth factor (10 g/ml) in silver sulfadiazine cream, applied to skin graft donor sites, has been found to accelerate wound healing when compared with control sites treated with silver sulfadiazine cream only.[145] The first commercially available prescription growth factor for wound healing has been introduced. Recombinant platelet-derived growth factor is available for topical application to diabetic foot wounds.[146]

Another advance has been the introduction of a living skin equivalent. Culturing isolated foreskin keratinocytes and fibroblasts and then combining them in a bilaminate sheet provides a living graft for application to venous ulcers. The allografted cells appear to usually disintegrate over the ensuing days to weeks after grafting, but release of important mediators stimulates healing with repeated grafts.[147]

Retinoids   Pretreatment of patients for 2 weeks with topical all-*trans* retinoic acid has been shown to decrease the time required for epithelialization after dermabrasion. Animal studies have further demonstrated that treatment of pig skin with retinoic acid before partial-thickness wounding resulted in enhanced epithelialization.[148] Continuation of the retinoic acid treatment after wounding, however, retarded epithelialization. Priming skin sites with external agents before surgical wounding may increase the capacity of tissues to heal.

Lasers   It has been demonstrated that treatment of skin wounds with low-power laser irradiation enhanced healing.[149]

In summary, advances in wound healing are proceeding at a rapid pace. Improved treatment modalities involving molecular approaches are at present seen at the bedside, as exemplified by the use of recombinant platelet-derived growth factor. Gene therapy holds a lot of promise for the future because it will allow, in theory, the wound tissues to make growth factors continuously over an extended period time, in contrast to periodic topical application of the currently available product.

FIGURE 11-23 Moist wound healing. Occlusive dressings promote more rapid epithelialization than when an eschar is present on dermal wounds.

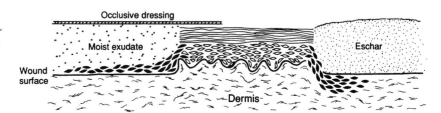

DECUBITUS ULCER

The term *decubitus ulcer* is often used synonymously with the more frequently encountered expressions *bed sores* and *pressure ulcers*. All describe end-stage damage or death of the skin and subcutaneous tissues after ischemia over a bony prominence.[140,150] They vary in severity through a pattern of broad-spectrum tissue destruction that may be arbitrarily divided into the three stages (Figure 11-24).

The first stage is simply sharply demarcated, reversible erythema. In chronic cases there may be diapedesis of red blood cells leading to deposition of hemosiderin. At the end of this stage the central area may be cyanotic, with a periphery of erythema overlying the bony prominence. The affected area is often warm and painful.

When a break in the skin ensues, stage II is operative. It is characterized by a minor abrasion of the epidermis with more extensive damage to connective tissue. Experimental studies[151] indicate that, after pressure, subcutaneous tissue and muscle are more susceptible to

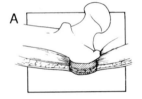

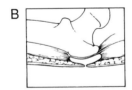

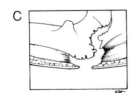

FIGURE 11-24 Decubitus ulcer formation. **A.** Pressure over the greater trochanter results in anoxia of overlying skin and tissue friability. **B.** Continued anoxia results in tissue breakdown and undermining of the ulcer edges, causing wound extension. **C.** Long-standing tissue necrosis permits entry of pathogens into the joint capsule, with attendant osteomyelitis and bone destruction.

necrosis than the epidermis. This contributes to the undermining frequently noted (see Figure 11-24). Small vesicles enlarging to form bullae may be noted in early decubitus ulcers. Secondary bacterial invasion frequently follows. With appropriate therapy and absence of pressure, the ulcer of stage II heals within a few weeks.

When the subcutaneous tissue is involved, the ulcer is rapidly associated with fat necrosis and development of a thick, rigid, black eschar. Continued pressure leads to necrosis of fascia, muscles, and ligaments and involvement of periosteal coverings, stage III. Bacterial infection is invariably present. Under most conditions, healing usually does not occur, even after several months, without extensive surgical intervention.

In the absence of therapy, stage IV rapidly develops. It is characterized by bone necrosis, osteomyelitis, and fistula formation. The mortality for hospital patients with such advanced lesions exceeds 25%.

Decubitus ulcers occur most frequently where external pressure is exerted over bony prominences covered by minimal subcutaneous (adipose) tissue. In order of decreasing frequency these sites are the sacral bone, greater trochanter, ischial tuberosity, and lateral malleolus. As one might anticipate, the incidence of decubitus ulcers is highest in elderly, bedridden patients[150] and next highest among persons with spinal cord injuries that are complicated by urinary and fecal incontinence. Shearing forces such as those incurred when a patient slides in a wheelchair or is pulled across a bed sheet are other major contributing factors. Additional factors that are difficult to rank but that may place patients at increased risk include heavy smoking, hypoalbuminemia, xerotic (dry) skin, and anemia (hemoglobin < 12 g/100 ml). Several factors found in the National Health Survey[140] to be unrelated include obesity, hypertension, and readily palpable femoral and dorsal pedis pulses.[151,152]

Decubitus ulcers can be diagnosed readily by their location and appearance. In selected cases the differential diagnosis includes pyoderma gangrenosum, stasis ulcer, ulceration secondary to ionizing radiation, and vasculitis.

No unique biochemical factors are found in decubitus ulcers, but during the earliest or initial phase of ulcer formation[153] lower pH, decreased PO_2, and increased PCO_2 can be demonstrated. Ferguson-Pell and Hagisawa believe that an increase in the eccrine sweat lactate concentration, demonstrated by pilocarpine administration, may be of some diagnostic aid.[153]

The role of fibrinolysin remains controversial and is based on the following circumstantial evidence: In numerous reports of the histopathologic findings at ulcer margins, fibrin is present in relative abundance. It is particularly noticeable within and without the microvascular system. Fibrin thrombi within dilated capillaries are in turn encircled by a perivascular mononuclear cell infiltrate embedded in a fibrin network. Larger vessels have also been found to contain intraarteriolar fibrin thrombi. Cherry and Ryan[154] believed that a lack of, or defect in, fibrinolytic activity might contribute to the genesis of the decubitus ulcer. Larsson and Risberg[155] have demonstrated experimentally that after prolonged ischemia that had no effect on fibrinolysis, there was marked deposition of fibrin when blood flow was re-established.

During this period, decreased fibrinolytic activity could be demonstrated. It was speculated[154] that pressure ischemia resulted in damage to epidermal cells, which then released an inhibitor of fibrinolysis.[155] The role of fibrin in the pathogenesis would thus be twofold: first as vascular thrombi increasing anoxia, and second as accumulations of perivascular fibrin in amounts large enough to inhibit vascular regrowth and healing of the ulcer, as is routinely observed in classical wounds.

Although this chapter omits consideration of therapy, all therapeutic regimens for decubitus ulcers must include measures to facilitate restitution of the vascular bed and control of the bacterial infection that inevitably ensues. Attention must be paid to the major etiologic factors, which include pressure, shearing forces, friction, and moisture.[156] Active debridement and good nursing facilitate ultimate closure of the ulcer site.[157,158]

REFERENCES

1. Holbrook KA, Wolff K. The Structure and Development of Skin. In TB Fitzpatrick, et al. (eds), Dermatology in General Medicine (3rd ed). New York: McGraw-Hill, 1987.
2. Wilke MS, Hsu BM, Wille JJ Jr, et al. Biologic mechanisms for the regulation of normal human keratinocyte proliferation and differentiation. Am J Pathol 1988;131:171–182.
3. Hennings H, Michael D, Cheng C, et al. Calcium regulation of growth and differentiation of mouse epidermal cells in culture. Cell 1980;19:245–254.
4. Eckert RL, Crish JF, Robinson NA. The epidermal keratinocyte as a model for the study of gene regulation and cell differentiation. Physiol Rev 1997;77:397–424.
5. Fuchs E. Keratins and the skin. Annu Rev Cell Dev Biol 1995;11:123–153.
6. Kopan R, Traska G, Fuchs E. Retinoids as important regulators of terminal differentiation: examining keratin expression in individual epidermal cells at various stages of keratinization. J Cell Biol 1987;105:427–440.
7. Ishida-Yamatoto A, Iizuka H. Structural organization of cornified cell envelopes and alterations in inherited skin disorders. Exp Dermatol 1998;7:1–10.
8. Munster AM. Cultured skin for massive burns: a prospective controlled trial. Ann Surg 1996;224:372–377.
9. Gelfant S. On the existence of noncycling germinative cells in human epidermis in vivo and cell cycle aspects of psoriasis. Cell Tissue Kinet 1982;14:393–397.
10. Lavker RM, Sun TT. Epidermal stem cells. J Invest Dermatol 1983;81(Suppl 1):121–127.
11. Potten CS. Kinetic Organization in Squamous Epithelium. In NA Wright, RS Camplejohn (eds), Psoriasis: Cell Proliferation. Edinburgh: Churchill Livingstone, 1983.
12. Bauer FW. Cell Kinetics. In PD Mier, PCM van de Kerkhof (eds), Textbook of Psoriasis. Edinburgh: Churchill Livingstone, 1986.
13. Rothberg S, Crounse RG, Lee JL. Glycine-^{14}C incorporation into the proteins of normal stratum corneum and the abnormal stratum corneum of psoriasis. J Invest Dermatol 1961;37:497–505.
14. Prystowsky JH, Clevenger CV, Zheng Z-S. Inhibition of ornithine decarboxylase activity and cell proliferation by ultraviolet B radiation in EFG-stimulated cultured human epidermal keratinocytes. J Invest Dermatol 1993; 101:54–58.
15. Zheng ZS, Chen RZ, Prystowsky JH. UVB radiation induces phosphorylation of the epidermal growth factor receptor, decreases EGF binding and blocks EGF induction of ornithine decarboxylase gene expression in SV40-transformed human keratinocytes. Exp Dermatol 1993;2:257–265.
16. Le Poole C, Boissy RE. Vitiligo. Semin Cutan Med Surg 1997;16:3–14.
17. Gilchrest BA. The pathogenesis of melanoma induced by ultraviolet radiation. N Engl J Med 1999;340:1341–1348.
18. Thody AJ, Graham A. Does alpha-MSH have a role in regulating skin pigmentation in humans? Pigment Cell Res 1998;11:265–274.
19. Prota G. Pigment cell research: what directions? Pigment Cell Res 1997;10:5–11.
20. Ebling FJG. Homage to Paul Langerhans. J Invest Dermatol 1980;75:3.
21. Green I, Stingl G, Shevach EM, et al. Antigen presentation and allogeneic stimulation by Langerhans cells. J Invest Dermatol 1980;75:44.
22. Katz SI, Tamaki K, Sachs DH. Epidermal Langerhans cells are derived from cells originating in bone marrow. Nature 1979;282:324–326.
23. Stingl G, Katz SI, Green I, et al. The functional role of Langerhans cells. J Invest Dermatol 1980;74:315.
24. Silberberg I. Apposition of mononuclear cells to Langerhans cells in contact allergic reactions. An ultrastructural study. Acta Derm Venereol 1973; 53:1–12.
25. Silberberg I, Baer RL, Rosenthal SA. The role of Langerhans cells in allergic contact hypersensitivity. A review of findings in man and guinea pigs. J Invest Dermatol 1976;66:210.
26. Thorbecke GJ, Silberberg-Sinakin I, Flotte TJ. Langerhans cells as macrophages in skin and lymphoid organs. J Invest Dermatol 1980;75:32.
27. Toews GB, Bergstresser PR, Streilein JW. Langerhans cells: sentinels of skin associated lymphoid tissue. J Invest Dermatol 1980;75:78.
28. Bickers D, Harber LC, Kripke M. Photo-Immunology. In L Harber, D Bickers (eds), Photosensitivity Diseases. Toronto: BC Decker, 1989.

29. Takashima A. UVB-dependent modulation of epidermal cytokine network: roles in UVB-induced depletion of Langerhans cells and dendritic epidermal T cells. J Dermatol 1995;22:876–887.

30. Hogan AD, Burks AW. Epidermal Langerhans' cells and their function in the skin immune system. Ann Allergy Asthma Immunol 1995;75:5–10.

31. Lappin MB, Kimber I, Norval M. The role of dendritic cells in cutaneous immunity. Arch Dermatol Res 1996;288:109–121.

32. Yin E, Jung HS, Chuong CM. Molecular histology in skin appendage morphogenesis. Microsc Res Tech 1997;38:452–465.

33. Ellis RA, Henrickson RC. The Ultrastructure of the Sebaceous Glands in Man. In WB Montagna (ed), Advances in Biology of Skin. Vol 4. New York: Pergamon Press, 1963.

34. Serri F, Huber WM. The Development of Sebaceous Glands in Man. In WB Montagna (ed), Advances in Biology of Skin. Vol 4. New York: Pergamon Press, 1963.

35. Pochi PE, Strauss JS, Downing DT. Age-related changes in sebaceous gland activity. J Invest Dermatol 1979; 73:108–111.

36. Pochi PE, Strauss JS, Downing DT. Skin surface lipid composition, acne, pubertal development, and urinary excretion of testosterone and 17-ketosteroids in children. J Invest Dermatol 1977;69:485–489.

37. Pochi PE, Strauss JS. Sebaceous gland response in man to the administration of testosterone, delta⁴-androstenedione, and dehydroisoandrosterone. J Invest Dermatol 1969;52:32–36.

38. Pochi PE, Strauss JS. Sebaceous gland suppression with ethinyl estradiol and diethylstilbesterol. Arch Dermatol 1973;108:210–214.

39. Ebling FJ. Hormonal control and methods of measuring sebaceous gland activity. J Invest Dermatol 1974; 62:161.

40. Shuster S, Thody AJ. The control and measurement of sebum secretion. J Invest Dermatol 1974;62:172.

41. Pochi PE, Strauss JS. Endocrinologic control of the development and activity of the human sebaceous gland. J Invest Dermatol 1974;62:191–201.

42. Downing DT, Strauss JS. On the mechanism of sebaceous secretion. Arch Dermatol Res 1982;272:343.

43. Jakubovic HR, Ackerman AB. Development, Morphology and Physiology. In SL Moschella, HJ Hurley (eds), Dermatology (2nd ed). Vol 1. Philadelphia: WB Saunders, 1985.

44. Pochi PE. Sebum: Its Nature and Physiopathologic Responses. In SL Moschella, HJ Hurley (eds), Dermatology (2nd ed). Vol 1. Philadelphia: WB Saunders, 1985.

45. Downey D, Stewart M, Strauss J. Biology of Sebaceous Glands. In TB Fitzpatrick, et al. (eds), Dermatology in General Medicine (3rd ed). New York: McGraw-Hill, 1987.

46. Cohn BA. In search of human skin pheromones. Arch Dermatol 1994;130:1048–1051.

47. Montagna W. The Structure and Function of Skin. New York: Academic Press, 1962.

48. Bell M. Proceedings: the ultrastructure of human axillary apocrine glands after epinephrine injection. J Invest Dermatol 1974;63:147–159.

49. Robertshaw D. Apocrine Sweat Glands. In LA Goldsmith (ed), Biochemistry and Physiology of the Skin. Vol 1. Oxford: Oxford University Press, 1983.

50. Shelley WB. Apocrine sweat. J Invest Dermatol 1951;17:255.

51. Brown TJ, Rosen T, Orengo IF. Hidradenitis suppurativa. South Med J 1998;91:1007–1014.

52. Tani M, Yamamoto K, Mishima Y. Apocrine acrosyringeal complex in human skin. J Invest Dermatol 1980;75:431–435.

53. Robertshaw D. Biology of Apocrine Sweat Glands. In TB Fitzpatrick, et al. (eds), Dermatology in General Medicine (3rd ed). New York: McGraw-Hill, 1987.

54. Armstrong LE, Maresh CM. Effects of training, environment, and host factors on sweating response to exercise. Int J Sports Med 1998;2:S103–S105.

55. Itoh S. Physiological Responses to Heat. In Yoshimura, et al. (eds), Essential Problems in Climatic Physiology. Kyoto: Nankado, 1960.

56. Bar-Or O. Effects of age and gender on sweating pattern during exercise. Int J Sports Med 1998;19:S106–S107.

57. Falk B. Effects of thermal stress during rest and exercise in the paediatric population. Sports Med 1998;25:221–240.

58. Sato K. Biology of Eccrine Sweat Glands. In TB Fitzpatrick, et al. (eds), Dermatology in General Medicine (3rd ed). New York: McGraw-Hill, 1987.

59. Ohhashi T, Sakaguchi M, Tsuda T. Human perspiration measurement. Physiol Meas 1998;19:449–461.

60. Gagge AP, Nishi Y. Heat Exchange Between Human Skin Surface and Thermal Environment. In MJ Fregly, CM Blatteis (eds), Handbook of Physiology. Vol 4: Reactions to environmental agents. Bethesda, MD: American Physiological Society, 1977.

61. Conn JW. The mechanism of acclimatization to heat. Adv Intern Med 1949;3:373–393.

62. Clark G, Magoun HW, Ranson SW. Hypothalamic regulation of body temperature. J Neurophysiol 1939;2:61–80.

63. Morimoto T, Itoh T. Thermoregulation and body fluid osmolality. J Basic Clin Physiol Pharmacol 1998;9:51–72.

64. Odderson IR. Hyperhidrosis treated by botulinum A exotoxin. Dermatol Surg 1998;24:1237–1241.

65. Hyndman OR, Wolkin J. The pilocarpine sweating test. I. A valid indicator in differentiation of preganglionic and postganglionic sympathectomy. Arch Neurol Psychiatry 1941;45:992–1006.

66. Keller A. Descending nerve fibers subserving heat maintenance functions coursing with cerebrospinal tracts through the pons. Am J Physiol 1948; 154:82–86.

67. Myerson A, Loman J, Rinkel M. Human autonomic pharmacology: general and local sweating produced by acetyl-beta-methyl-choline chloride (mecholyl). Am J Med Sci 1937;194:75–79.

68. Bijman J. Transport processes in the eccrine sweat gland. Kidney Int 1987;32:S109–S112.

69. Maughan RJ, Shirreffs SM. Factors influencing the restoration of fluid and electrolyte balance after exercise in the heat. Br J Sports Med 1997;31:175–182.

70. Wenzel FG, Horn TD. Nonneoplastic disorders of the eccrine glands. J Am Acad Dermatol 1998;38:1–17.

71. Ebling FJ. Biology of Hair Follicles. In TB Fitzpatrick, et al. (eds), Dermatology in General Medicine. New York: McGraw-Hill, 1989.

72. Randall VA. The use of dermal papilla cells in studies of normal and abnormal hair follicle biology. Dermatol Clin 1996;14:585–594.

73. Jankovic SM, Jankovic SV. The control of hair growth. Dermatol Online J 1998;4:2.

74. Kealey T, Philpott M, Guy R. The regulatory biology of the human pilosebaceous unit. Baillieres Clin Obstet Gynaecol 1997;11:205–227.

75. Sawaya ME. Biochemical mechanisms regulating human hair growth. Skin Pharmacol 1994;7:5–7.

76. Price VH. Treatment of hair loss. N Engl J Med 1999;341:964–973.

77. Baden H, Zaias N. Biology of Nails. In TB Fitzpatrick, et al. (eds), Dermatology in General Medicine (3rd ed). New York: McGraw-Hill, 1987.

78. Baden HP. The physical properties of nail. J Invest Dermatol 1970;55:115–122.

79. Cohen PR. The lunula. J Am Acad Dermatol 1996;34:943–953.

80. Hashimoto K. Ultrastructure of the human toenail. II. Keratinization and formation of the marginal band. J Ultrastruct Res 1971;36:391–410.

81. Hashimoto K, Gross BG, Nelson R, Lever WF. The ultrastructure of the skin of human embryos. III. The formation of the nail in 16- to 18-week-old embryos. J Invest Dermatol 1966; 47:205–217.

82. Albert SF. Disorders of the nail unit. Clin Podiatr Med Surg 1996;13:1–12.

83. Bodman MA. Miscellaneous nail presentations. Clin Podiatr Med Surg 1995;12:327–346.

84. Kanerva L, Lauerma A, Estlander T, et al. Occupational allergic contact dermatitis caused by photobonded-sculptured nails and a review of (meth) acrylates in nail cosmetics. Am J Contact Dermatitis 1996;7:109–115.

85. Clark RE, Madani S, Bettencourt MS. Nail surgery. Dermatol Clin 1998;16:145–164.

86. Uitto J, Pulkkinen L. Molecular complexity of the cutaneous basement membrane zone. Mol Biol Rep 1996;23:35–46.

87. Ray MC, Gately LE III. Basement membrane zone. Clin Dermatol 1996;14:321–330.

88. Aumailley M, Krieg T. Laminins: a family of diverse multifunctional molecules of basement membranes. J Invest Dermatol 1996;106:209–214.

89. Borradori L, Sonnenberg A. Structure and function of hemidesmosomes: more than simple adhesion complexes. J Invest Dermatol 1999;112:411–418.

90. Korge BP, Krieg T. The molecular basis for inherited bullous diseases. J Mol Med 1996;74:59–70.

91. Uitto J, Pulkkinen L, McLean WH. Epidermolysis bullosa: a spectrum of clinical phenotypes explained by molecular heterogeneity. Mol Med Today 1997;3:457–465.

92. Swerlick RA. The structure and function of the cutaneous vasculature. J Dermatol 1997;24:734–738.

93. Weinstein BM. What guides early embryonic blood vessel formation? Dev Dyn 1999;215:2–11.

94. Braverman IM. The cutaneous microcirculation: ultrastructure and microanatomical organization. Microcirculation 1997;4:329–340.

95. Requena L, Sangueza OP. Cutaneous vascular anomalies. Part I. Hamartomas, malformations, and dilation of preexisting vessels. J Am Acad Dermatol 1997;37:523–549.

96. Arbiser JL. Angiogenesis and the skin: a primer. J Am Acad Dermatol 1996;34:486–497.

97. Gibson LE, Su WP. Cutaneous vasculitis. Rheum Dis Clin North Am 1995;21:1097–1113.

98. Mat C, Yurdakul S, Tuzuner N, Tuzun Y. Small vessel vasculitis and vasculitis confined to the skin. Baillieres Clin Rheumatol 1997;11:237–257.

99. Fan TP, Jaggar R, Bicknell R. Controlling the vasculature: angiogenesis, anti-angiogenesis and vascular targeting of gene therapy. Trends Pharmacol Sci 1995;16:57–66.

100. Achen MG, Stacker SA. The vascular endothelial growth factor family; proteins which guide the development of the vasculature. Int J Exp Pathol 1998;79:255–265.

101. Befus D, Fujimaki H, Lee TDG, et al. Mast cell polymorphisms. Present concepts, future directions. Dig Dis Sci 1988;33:16S–24S.

102. Barton J, Lavker RM, Schechter NM, et al. Treatment of urticaria pigmentosa with corticosteroids. Arch Dermatol 1985;121:1516–1523.

103. Amon U, Nitschke M, Dieckmann D, et al. Activation and inhibition of mediator release from skin mast cells: a review of in vitro experiments. Clin Exp Allergy 1994;24:1098–1104.

104. Schwartz LB. Mediators of human mast cells and human mast cell subsets. Ann Allergy 1987;58:226–235.

105. Peters SP, Schleimer RP, Naclerio RM, et al. Am Rev Repir Dis 1987;135: 1196–1200.

106. Artuc M, Hermes B, Steckelings UM, et al. Mast cells and their mediators in cutaneous wound healing—active participants or innocent bystanders? Exp Dermatol 1999;8:1–16.

107. Maurer M, Paus R, Czarnetzki BM. Mast cells as modulators of hair follicle cycling. Exp Dermatol 1995;4:266–271.

108. Kohn RR, Schnider SL. Collagen Changes in Aging Skin. In AK Balin, AM Kligman (eds), Aging and the Skin. New York: Raven Press, 1989;121–139.

109. Uitto J. Connective tissue biochemistry of the aging dermis. Clin Geriatr Med 1989;5:127–147.

110. Uitto J, Eisen A. Collagen. In TB Fitzpatrick, et al. (eds), Dermatology in General Medicine (3rd ed). New York: McGraw-Hill, 1987;259–287.

111. Davidson JM, et al. Elastin production in human skin fibroblasts: reduced levels in the cells of a patient with atrophoderma. Clin Res 1984;32:147A.

112. Pinnell SR, Martin GR. The cross-linking of collagen and elastin: enzymatic conversion of lysine in peptide linkage to alpha-aminoadipic-delta-semialdehyde (allysine) by an extract from bone. Proc Natl Acad Sci U S A 1968;61:708–716.

113. Sandberg LB. Elastin structure, biosynthesis and its relation to disease states. N Engl J Med 1981;304:566–579.

114. Davidson JM, Smith K, Shibahara S, et al. Regulation of elastin synthesis in developing sheep nuchal ligament by elastin mRNA levels. J Biol Chem 1981;257:747–754.

115. Foster JA. Elastin structure and biosynthesis: an overview. Methods Enzymol 1982;82A:559–570.

116. Uitto J. Biochemistry of the elastic fibers in normal connective tissues and its alterations in diseases. J Invest Dermatol 1979;72:1–10.

117. Debelle L, Tamburro AM. Elastin: molecular description and function. Int J Biochem Cell Biol 1999;31:261–272.

118. Iozzo RV. Matrix proteoglycans: from molecular design to cellular function. Annu Rev Biochem 1998;67:609–652.

119. Montagna W. Morphology of cutaneous sensory receptors. J Invest Dermatol 1977;69:4.

120. Hashimoto K. Fine structure of the Meissner corpuscle of human palmar skin. J Invest Dermatol 1973;60:20.

121. Soden C, Pierson DL, Rodman OG. A classification of cutaneous receptors. J Assoc Milit Dermatol 1981;7:5.

122. Herndon JH. Itching: the pathophysiology of pruritus. Int J Dermatol 1975;14:465–484.

123. Hagermark O, Hokfelt T, Pernow B. Flare and itch induced by substance P in human skin. J Invest Dermatol 1978;71:233–235.

124. Bernstein JE, Hamill JR. Substance P in the skin. J Invest Dermatol 1981; 77:250.

125. Kam PC, Tan KH. Pruritus—itching for a cause and relief? Anaesthesia 1996;51:1133–1138.

126. Braverman IM, Yen AK. Ultrastructure of the human dermal microcirculation III. The vessel in the mid and lower dermis and subcutaneous fat. J Invest Dermatol 1981;77:297.

127. DeLuca HF. The vitamin D story: a collaborative effort of basic science and clinical medicine. FASEB J 1988;2:224–236.

128. Prystowsky JH. Photoprotection and the vitamin D: status of the elderly. Arch Dermatol 1988;124:1844–1848.

129. Reichel H, Koeffler HP, Norman AW. The role of the vitamin D endocrine system in health and disease. N Engl J Med 1989;320:980–991.

130. Kirsner RS, Federman D. Treatment of psoriasis: role of calcipotriene. Am Fam Physician 1995;52:237–240, 243–244.

131. van de Kerkhof PC. An update on vitamin D3 analogues in the treatment of psoriasis. Skin Pharmacol Appl Skin Physiol 1998;11:2–10.

132. Grandjean P, Berlin A, Gilbert M, et al. Preventing percutaneous absorption of industrial chemicals: the "skin" denotation. Am J Ind Med 1988;14:97–107.

133. Mattie DR, Grabau JH, McDougal JN. Significance of the dermal route of exposure to risk assessment. Risk Anal 1994;14:277–284.

134. Lauer AC, Lieb LM, Ramachandran C, et al. Transfollicular drug delivery. Pharm Res 1995;12:179–186.

135. Rutter N. Percutaneous drug absorption in the newborn: hazards and uses. Clin Perinatol 1987;14:911–930.

136. Besunder JB, Reed MD, Blumer JL. Principles of drug biodisposition in the neonate. A critical evaluation of the pharmacokinetic-pharmacodynamic interface (Part I). Clin Pharmacokinet 1988;14:189–216.

137. Nickoloff BJ, Mitra RS, Riser BL, et al. Modulation of keratinocyte motility. Am J Pathol 1988;132:543–551.

138. Alvarez OM, Goslen JB, Eaglstein WH, et al. Wound Healing. In TB Fitzpatrick, et al. (eds), Dermatology in General Medicine (3rd ed). New York: McGraw-Hill, 1987;321–336.

139. Young ME. Malnutrition and wound healing. Heart Lung 1988;17:60–67.

140. Guralnik JM, Harris TB, White LR, et al. Occurrence and predictors of pressure sores in the National Health and Nutrition Examination Survey follow-up. J Am Geratr Soc 1988;36:807–812.

141. Nemeth AJ, Eaglstein WH, Talanga V. Clinical parameters and transcutaneous oxygen measurements for the prognosis of venous ulcers. J Am Acad Dermatol 1989;20:186–190.

142. Silverman RA, Lender J, Elmets CA. Effects of occlusive and semiocclusive dressings on the return of barrier function to transepidermal water loss in standardized human wounds. J Am Acad Dermatol 1989;20:755–760.

143. Yannas IV, Lee E. Orgill DP, et al. Synthesis and characterization of a model extracellular matrix that induces partial regeneration of adult mammalian skin. Proc Natl Acad Sci U S A 1989;86:933–937.

144. Stompro BE, Hansbrough JF, Boyce ST. Attachment of peptide growth factors to implantable collagen. J Surg Res 1989;46:413–421.

145. Brown GL, Nanney LP, Griffen J, et al. Enhancement of wound healing by topical treatment with epidermal growth factor. N Engl J Med 1989;321:76–79.

146. Le Grand EK. Preclinical promise of becaplermin (rhPDGF-BB) in wound healing. Am J Surg 1998;176:48S–54S.

147. Nemecek GM, Dayan AD. Safety evaluation of human living skin equivalents. Toxicol Pathol 1999;27:101–103.

148. Hung VC, Lee JY, Zitelli JA, et al. Topical tretinoin and epithelial wound healing. Arch Dermatol 1989;125:65–69.

149. Rochkind S, Rousso M, Nissare M, et al. Systemic effects of low-power laser irradiation on the peripheral and central nervous system, cutaneous wounds, and burns. Lasers Surg Med 1989;9:174–182.

150. Allman RM. Pressure ulcers among the elderly. N Engl J Med 1989;320:850–853.

151. Daniel RK, Priest DL, Wheatly DC. Etiologic factors in pressure sores: an experimental model. Arch Phys Med Rehabil 1981;62:492–498.

152. Andersen KE, Jensen O, Kvorning SA, et al. Prevention of pressure sores by identifying patients at risk. BMJ 1982;284:1370.

153. Ferguson-Pell M, Hagisawa S. Biochemical changes in sweat following prolonged ischemia. J Rehabil Res Dev 1988;25:57–62.

154. Cherry GW, Ryan TJ. The effects of ischemia and reperfusion on tissue survival. Major Probl Dermatol 1976;7:93–115.

155. Larsson J, Risberg B. Ischemia-induced changes in tissue fibrinolysis in human legs. Bibl Anat 1977;15:556–558.

156. Kanj LF, Wilking SV, Phillips TJ. Pressure ulcers. J Am Acad Dermatol 1998;38:517–536.

157. Petersen NC, Bittman S. The epidemiology of pressure sores. Scand J Plast Reconstr Surg 1971;5:62.

158. Seiler WO, Stahelin HB. Recent findings on decubitus ulcer pathology: implications for care. Geriatrics 1986;41:47–57.

12

Normal Vision Function

KENNETH J. CIUFFREDA, IRWIN B. SUCHOFF,
NEERA KAPOOR, MARY M. JACKOWSKI,
AND STANLEY F. WAINAPEL

Although the importance of adequate visual function in such basic activities as upright stance, ambulation, self-care, and reading cannot be overemphasized, it has been largely overlooked in textbooks and teaching curricula for rehabilitation professionals.[1] This omission is particularly unjustified considering the frequent occurrence of significant vision loss among rehabilitation inpatients,[2] its presence as a comorbidity in patients with stroke[3] or lower extremity amputations,[4,5] and the well-documented effects of vision impairment on falls[6] and deficits in activities of daily living.[7] An understanding of the physiological basis for normal and disordered vision function is thus as crucial to physiatrists and therapists as are the physiological mechanisms underlying volitional movement, sensation, or balance. This chapter provides an overview of the diverse components of normal vision, their anatomic and physiological features, and briefly touches on their clinical significance.

Although vision is conceived as a single entity, in reality, it is the product of a number of subsystems, each of which has its own physiological basis. Furthermore, these subsystems must be elegantly synchronized for optimal visual performance. Consequently, we have chosen to present the visual physiology in terms of a number of these subsystems in which rehabilitation professionals should have a working knowledge to manage their patients optimally.

GROSS ANATOMY OF THE EYE AND VISUAL PATHWAYS

The human eyeball and its neuroanatomic pathways have the following major components and related physiological functions[8,9] (Figure 12-1A).

The *cornea* is the primary refractive component of the eye. It is a transparent tissue covering the eye's anterior surface. The tears that bathe the anterior corneal surface act to maintain a smooth optical surface that optimizes its imaging capability. Peripheral to the cornea and surrounding the remainder of the anterior surface of the eye, as well as lining the inner surface of the eyelid, is the *conjunctiva*, a thin and finely vascularized membrane, which serves mechanical, protective, and nutrient functions.

The *iris* controls the amount of light entering the eye via the variable diameter, circular aperture, the pupil.

The *aqueous humor* fills the space between the cornea and iris (i.e., anterior chamber), and the iris and crystalline lens (i.e., posterior chamber). It is involved in maintenance of the eye's intraocular pressure, as well as serving a nutritional function.

The *crystalline lens* is the secondary refractive component of the eye. Its unique feature is the ability to change curvature and resultant optical power rapidly to focus light on the retina to see objects located at all distances clearly. The alteration in optical power is accomplished by changes in contraction of the ciliary muscle, which in turn alters tension of the crystalline lens zonules. An elastic lens capsule surrounds the crystalline lens and acts to deform it during the process of accommodation (see the section Clinical Assessment of Accommodation).

The large area behind the crystalline lens is the *vitreal chamber*. It is filled with the gelatin-like vitreous humor, which has mechanical, optical, and nutritional functions.

The *retina* is the light-sensitive inner lining of the eye containing two categories of photoreceptors. The cones function to detect fine detail and color, as well as control the focusing function of the eye. They are most densely

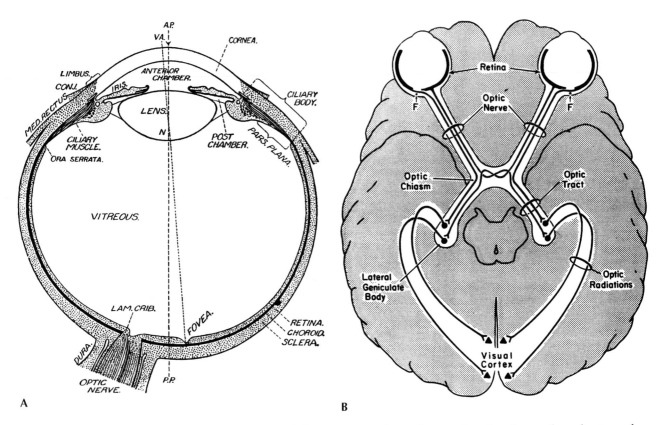

FIGURE 12-1 A. Horizontal section of the human eye. (AP = anterior pole; conj. = conjunctiva; lam. crib. = lamina cribosa; med. rectus = medial rectus; PP = posterior pole; N = nodal point; VA = visual axis.) (Reprinted with permission from RJ Last. Wolff's Anatomy of the Eye and Orbit. Philadelphia: Saunders, 1968.) **B.** Schematic representation of primary neural visual pathways. (F = fovea.) (Reprinted with permission from JD Trobe, JS Glaser. The Visual Fields Manual—A Practical Guide to Testing and Interpretation. Gainesville, FL: Triad Publishing, 1983.)

packed within the central macular region at the high resolution fovea. This retinal region is used to fixate and focus upon an object of interest. Surrounding the fovea is the 5-degree macula area of relatively high resolution, whose fine form and detail-detecting ability progressively decline with increased retinal eccentricity. In contrast, the rods are used to detect low levels of light such as at night, as well as object motion. They are dispersed across the entire retina (except at the central foveal region). The retina is surrounded by the intermediate lining of the eye, the vascular *choroid*, which has a nutritional function. The external lining of the eye, which consists of the tough and collagenous *sclera*, has mechanical and protective functions.

At the rods and cones, the impinging light energy is transformed to electrical energy that then activates the retinal bipolar cells and ganglion cells. There are two distinct types of retinal ganglion cells whose axons form the exiting optic nerve. These are the magno (M) or transient cells, and the parvo (P) or sustained cells. Their axons proceed to the optic chiasm where there is a crossing of

neural fibers from each eye. This crossing, or decussation, ensures that visual information from the right and left sides of the environment are then separated, to be situated in the left and right sides of this pathway, respectively. These fibers then proceed to the optic tract and the lateral geniculate body. At this structure, the basic visual information interacts with nonvisual neural inputs.[10] Some of these fibers proceed to the visual cortex via the optic radiations, whereas others proceed to the tectum and are involved in pupillary behavior. Yet other fibers initially follow the path up to the lateral geniculate body, and then carry information directly to the superior colliculus, where it is used in eye movement and other related behaviors. This constitutes what is referred to as the *primary visual pathway* (Figure 12-1B).

A second level of processing of visual information begins at the extrastriate portion of the visual cortex, or *secondary visual pathway*.[10,11] From here the P-cells communicate with the inferior temporal brain area. This has been shown to be concerned with visual recognition of objects, or the *what* of visual perception. The M-cells proceed first to the middle temporal area, and eventually to the posterior parietal region. True to the physiological characteristics of the M-cells, this pathway is involved in motion and spatial vision, or the *where* aspect of visual perception.

VISUAL ACUITY

Definition and Function

As mentioned earlier, the highest resolving power of the eye providing detailed vision is localized in the central 1 degree of the visual field centered around the fovea. Visual resolution falls off rapidly toward the retinal periphery.

Reasons for this highly localized visual resolution are found in the anatomy of the retina and successive layers of the visual system, each containing a detailed map of the visual world. Although these neural maps preserve the order of the visual world, each emphasizes some regions at the expense of others, thus making each map topographic. One reason for this topographic representation is that the center of the retinal surface has a denser concentration of photoreceptors than does the periphery. In the brain, a major part of the projection of visual space onto the topographic brain maps is devoted to the foveal region. Approximately one-half of the human primary visual cortex is devoted to the foveal and macular region. This representation makes possible the great visual acuity and spatial discrimination humans demonstrate within the central part of their visual field.

Clinical Assessment of Visual Acuity

Visual acuity is a measurement of the resolution capacity of the eye. In the United States, Snellen visual acuity is the most commonly used system of notation. A standard 20/20 notation assumes a minimum angle of resolution of 1 minute of arc; 20/200 acuity assumes a minimum angle of resolution of 10 minutes of arc, and so forth. Snellen visual acuity denotes both the smallest letter size read and the distance at which it can be read (i.e., the test distance). Snellen visual acuity equals test distance divided by letter size. Test distance is the distance of the chart from the observer, typically 20 feet, to eliminate complications from accommodation. Letter size represents the distance at which the letter must be held to have a minimum angle of resolution of 1 minute (i.e., having the same visual angle as a 20/20 letter held at 20 feet). A visual acuity of 20/200 means that the individual can see at 20 feet what a fully sighted and

visually corrected person can see at 200 feet. Beyond the distance indicator of 400 feet, measurements are typically taken in the gross perception of objects (e.g., counting fingers, recorded as CF) at a measured distance, followed by hand motion (recorded as HM) at a certain distance, followed by light perception or projection (recorded as LP), and finally, no light perception (recorded as NLP). Although Snellen visual acuity charts use capital letters, charts with numbers and pictures have been developed as Snellen equivalents (Figures 12-2 and 12-3).

To obtain a quantitative assessment of visual sensory processing from noncommunicative subjects, two strategies, namely behavioral and electrophysiological methods, have been used.

Behavioral Test: Preferential Looking

Visual acuity testing of infants and nonresponsive adults can be accomplished by relying on the *preference* of observers to look at something versus nothing (i.e., to gaze either at a grating pattern or a complex form versus a uniform, blank space). Teller[12] has combined this paradigm with the two-alternative, forced-choice procedure, to estimate an individual's resolution threshold or *grating acuity*. McDonald et al.[13] have also developed an Acuity Card Procedure that uses a subjective judgment on the part of the examiner, and a simplified stimulus presentation protocol, the validity and reliability of

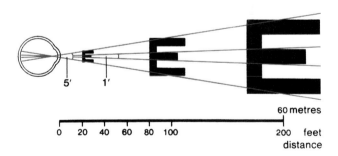

FIGURE 12-2 Letters were constructed so that they would subtend the same visual angle when viewed at distances up to 200 ft. These letters were then mounted on a card and viewed at 20 ft (6 m). The smallest line of letters that can be resolved by the patient is noted. The test distance is then divided by this line to give a fraction. If the patient sees at 20 ft as far as the 40-ft line, the visual acuity is expressed as 20 ft/40 ft = visual acuity of 20/40. This can also be measured in meters 6/12, as a fraction 0.5, or as the angle subtended by the smallest gap of the letter, 2 minutes of arc. Normal visual acuity is 20/20. (Reprinted with permission from DJ Spalton, RA Hitchings, PA Hunter [eds], Atlas of Clinical Ophthalmology. Brookfield, VT: Gower Medical Publishing, Ashgate Publishing Co., 1984.)

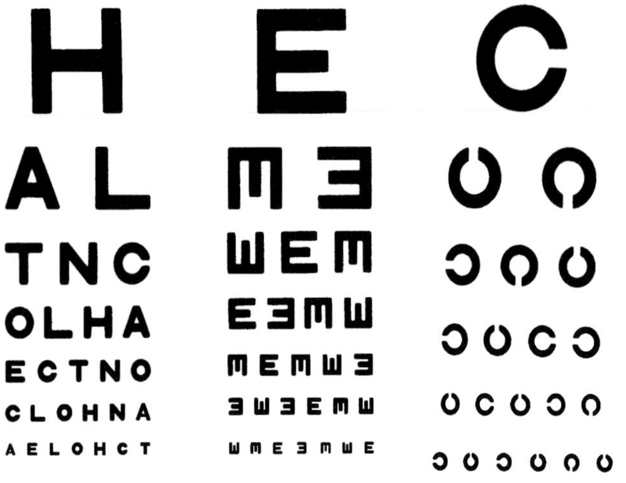

FIGURE 12-3 Snellen test types also rely on factors such as literacy and legibility. For example, an *L* is easier to read than an *A*. To prevent aberration in the visual acuity score, individual letters are matched for difficulty against a Landolt broken ring test, in which the orientation of the gap varies. The score can be compared with that using Snellen letters; any psychological bias can then be eliminated by only using letters of the same Landolt score. Landolt rings can also be used with illiterate patients; alternatively, the patient can be asked to match a cutout letter *E* with the same letter at different orientations. (Reprinted with permission from DJ Spalton, RA Hitchings, PA Hunter [eds], Atlas of Clinical Ophthalmology. Brookfield, VT: Gower Medical Publishing, Ashgate Publishing Co., 1984.)

which have been documented. The finest grating whose spatial location is consistently and correctly responded to provides an estimate of visual acuity (Figure 12-4).

Electrophysiological Testing: Visual-Evoked Potential

The visual-evoked potential is a noninvasive measure of the visual system at the cortical level, which entails recording brain activity that is synchronized with a visual stimulus (see Chapter 15). The integrity of the visual pathway from the retina to the visual cortex is measured by this technique, and, under certain conditions, it can be used to derive an estimate of visual acuity. Stimuli are either flashes of light (generating a *flash* visual-evoked potential) or patterns (generating a *pattern* visual-evoked potential), which is typically used to quantify functional vision. Pattern testing protocols use slow, counterphase, reversing checkerboard patterns. The amplitude and latency of peak responses that occur approximately 100 msec after slow temporal frequency stimuli are presented and are used as a measure of the visual response.[14,15]

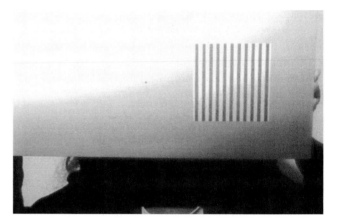

FIGURE 12-4 Assessment of pattern vision with the Preferential Looking Card. The card, which contains a 25.5 × 23 cm area of 2.2-cm wide black-and-white stripes adjacent to a gray homogeneous field, can be presented in various parts of the visual field for an infant with severe visual acuity deficits. (Reprinted with permission from V Dobson. In SJ Isenberg [ed], The Eye in Infancy [2nd ed]. St. Louis: Mosby, 1994.)

VISUAL SENSORY FUNCTIONS

Definition and Function

Two light-dependent functional visual systems exist. The *scotopic system* operates in dim light. It involves the rods with highly convergent neural processing; it does not *see* colors. The *photopic system* is cone mediated. It requires bright light and detailed neural processing, including differential sensitivity to wavelengths. This system supports color perception. At moderate (mesopic) light levels, both systems are operative. The two systems allow one to see over a wide range of illumination intensities (approximately 10^6 log units).

Adaptation

The eye uses different mechanisms to operate over this wide range of ambient light levels. In bright light, the pupil can constrict to allow in approximately $^{1}/_{10}$ the light as in dim illumination. The cone- and rod-mediated systems allow for range fractionation; receptors have either high or low thresholds to light, thus responding to different intensities, with each photoreceptor operating at any given time over a two log unit range (100-fold range). However, the visual receptors can adapt to new levels of illumination by shifting their entire range of responses to operate over a new light level. This adaptation depends on biochemical processes and reorganization of neural activity; it is time dependent. For example, when walking into a dark theater from the bright light, it takes several minutes before some vision is restored. The time courses and overall level of adaptation achieved can be affected by age, ocular disease, drug toxicity, or head injury.[16]

Further processing occurs at the occipital visual cortex. Here there are complex receptive fields responding best to stimuli shaped like elongated bars of particular width, length, orientation, and visual field location, thus creating at higher levels the perception of edges or contours. It is thought that complex shapes may be derived from inputs of neurons detecting simpler shapes, building on each other, in a hierarchical fashion. Most neurons are also *tuned* to a particular spatial frequency that can exist at any level of contrast.[17] To reproduce a complex visual pattern, therefore, all of the spatial frequencies present in a pattern would have to be processed. If the high spatial frequencies are filtered out from an image, the fine details and sharp edges are lost; if the low spatial frequencies are removed, then the large, uniform areas and graded contours are missing. Evidence exists to support the organization of the visual system around many such channels tuned to different frequencies, dealing with only one particular band or class of information from which visual form can be extracted.[18,19] However, recognition of familiar objects requires more than simply accurate perception of forms, as is seen in some stroke patients, who report a perfect visualization of an object, which can be accurately described; however, it cannot be recognized (visual agnosia).

Color

Color perception is a striking aspect of human vision. The first steps involve cone photoreceptors that are specialized to respond to three ranges of visible light, with peaks at (1) 420 nm (short [S] wavelength cones, blue light), (2) 530 nm (middle [M] wavelength cones, green light), and (3) 560 nm (long [L] wavelength cones, yellow/green light). There are roughly equal numbers of M and L receptors, but far fewer S cones; this may explain why visual acuity is much lower with short wavelength illumination than in other parts of the visual spectrum. Genes for the S, M, and L photopigments have been localized in human chromosomes, with genes for the M and L pigments occupying adjacent positions on the X chromosome. These genes can vary among individuals and can produce defects in color vision. Congenital color discrimination defects are much more frequent in human male than female subjects (8% male versus 0.5% female subjects). Because male subjects have one X

chromosome, an M or L pigment mutation can result in color vision impairment. Female subjects, having two X chromosomes, can have defects in genes of one X chromosome with a normal gene copy on the other providing compensation. Persons with hereditary color deficits compensate (i.e., they learn to recognize most colors based on their altered visual color perception using different visual cues, such as luminance, contrast, and so forth). Unlike persons with acquired color deficiencies that are associated with ocular disease, those with hereditary color deficiencies have otherwise normal vision.

Most retinal ganglion cells respond to some wavelengths and are inhibited by others, and target cells in the lateral geniculate body show the same receptive patterns. Four types of spectrally opponent ganglion cells have been identified.[20] Each cell receives input from two types of cones, with one being excitatory and the other inhibitory. The output of the cell is the difference in stimulation that occurs by algebraically summing the positive (+) and negative (–) input signals. Once stimulated, these ganglion cells send their signals to higher synapses for detection of form, depth, movement, and hue. In addition to color detectors, there are also brightness and darkness ganglion cell detectors that receive either stimulation or inhibition from both M and L cones; S cones do not contribute appreciably to our perception of light and dark. In the visual cortex, this color and brightness information is used to segregate forms from their background by differences in hue or intensity.

Besides its aesthetic appeal, the most important role color plays in human vision is in identifying which part of a complex image belongs to one object or another. Color can be used to draw attention to a part of an object or to camouflage it. The visual cortical region V4 is rich in color-sensitive cells. Such cells are perceptually opponent: red versus green, and blue versus yellow. Using positron emission tomography, this area is seen activated when observers view colored objects, but not black and white ones.[21] Brain lesions that include V4 reduce or eliminate color vision specifically. Lack of color vision is called *achromatopsia*. A loss of color vision can also be found in *rod monochromatism*, a congenital deficiency in cone photoreceptors.[22]

Motion

Some retinal ganglion cells respond to image motion, but preferentially to a certain direction of motion. The neurons in the visual cortex area V5 also respond to motion. One report of a patient who lost her ability to perceive motion after a stroke damaging the V5 area of her brain noted that the patient could not perceive continuous motion, but rather only separate successive positions of a moving object.[23] For example, she had trouble pouring liquids, because the fluid appeared to be frozen. Except for her lack of motion perception, visual perception was normal in all other aspects.

Clinical Assessment of Visual Sensory Function

Adaptation

Light Brightness Comparison Test   The subjective impression of the quantity of light perceived during alternating eye stimulation is useful in detecting optic nerve dysfunction. Optic nerve lesions tend to cause a generalized depression in light sensitivity; things look dimmer to the observer. In comparison, even a large macular lesion of the retina does not give this impression.

Dark Adaptation   For individuals with either early ocular disease[22] or traumatic brain injury,[24] loss of light sensitivity in the dark is often marked, despite otherwise normal ocular structures and results of neural imaging. To quantify scotopic sensitivity in these individuals, dark adaptometry is performed.[25] The observer views an intense, bleaching light in a white Ganzfeld apparatus, and is then placed in the dark. Threshold values of light perceived are measured for 30 minutes. Normal observers have a rapid restoration of light sensitivity (2.5–3.0 log units improvement) during the first 5–7 minutes in the dark, which is cone mediated. This is followed by a slower, gradual increase in sensitivity (approximately 2.5–3.0 log units), which is rod mediated.

Color Vision

Pseudoisochromatic Plates   Pseudoisochromatic plates are the most popular clinic color tests, with the Ishihara Series most widely used. It is noted, however, that pseudoisochromatic plates are geared toward the detection of congenital defects of the red/green type. They do not allow assessment of blue/yellow defects. Fortunately, many acquired color defects seen in neuro-ophthalmic diseases are of the red/green type. Testing is done monocularly for acquired defects and can be done binocularly for congenital losses. Although figures in the test plates are large, they are of low contrast, thereby making them difficult for patients with lowered contrast sensitivity (CS). (For example, this would be true in patients with lowered contrast sensitivity due to cataracts, corneal degeneration, optic nerve disease, and so forth.)

Color Sorting Tests   Color sorting tests provide more information in that blue/yellow defects can also be identified.

FARNSWORTH PANEL D-15 TEST   The Farnsworth Panel D-15 test consists of 15 colored caps reflecting 15 points along a specified color circle. The observer arranges the caps in color order, using the reference cap as a starting point. Each type of color vision defect results in a specific anomalous pattern. Acquired defects appear similar to hereditary ones, but are less distinct in interpretation.[26]

FARNSWORTH-MUNSELL 100-HUE TEST   The Farnsworth-Munsell 100-Hue test is an expanded version of the D-15 test, with 85 hues represented. It is a sensitive test that determines the characteristics and severity of both congenital and acquired defects.[27]

Hereditary versus Acquired Color Vision Deficiencies

Hereditary dyschromatopsias are usually seen in male subjects, are a red/green defect, and are typically symmetric and stable. In most cases, visual function is otherwise normal. Test results yield predictable outcomes (i.e., classical color confusions are demonstrated). Acquired color vision deficiencies are seen in both sexes, can be blue/yellow or red/green, are often asymmetric, progressive, and associated with other abnormal visual functions (e.g., reduced acuity, field losses, altered CS, and so forth).[28] Common conditions of the visual system are associated with color defect.[29] Changes in color perception with use of common pharmaceutical agents have been compiled in detail for the clinician.[30,31]

Contrast Sensitivity

Snellen visual acuity has long been the standard for determining the status of the visual system. However, it measures the observer's ability to identify an object at maximum contrast only. Clinicians are often confronted with patients who have subjective complaints of visual disturbance, despite normal visual acuity. CS testing has become recognized as a valuable tool for measuring early functional visual changes and is thought to be a more sensitive and comprehensive measure of visual performance than Snellen visual acuity.[32,33] *Contrast* is defined as the degree of blackness to whiteness of a target or the luminance level of an object when compared with the luminance of its surrounding background. CS testing uses targets made up of sine-wave gratings. The patient's ability to detect these gratings at varying levels of contrast is assessed. By increasing the number of gratings pairs per degree of visual angle (i.e., cycles per degree), CS can be plotted on a graph as a function of test grating spatial frequency (Figure 12-5). The CS curve intersects the x-axis at the spatial frequency at which maximum contrast is needed to see the grating. This point is the equivalent of Snellen acuity, which is represented by a single point on the CS curve. Overall CS can be reduced despite the presence of normal Snellen acuity. CS can be abnormal in patients with multiple sclerosis, compressive optic neuropathy, and cerebral lesions, despite preservation of Snellen visual acuity.[34,35] Up to 70% of optic neuritis patients demonstrate abnormal CS.[36] CS testing has been shown to equal the sensitivity of visual-evoked potentials in patients with optic nerve disease and is more sensitive in detecting visual loss in macular disease.[32]

Contrast Sensitivity Tests Vistech Chart VCTS 6500 (Vistech Consultants, Inc., Dayton, OH) is a wall-mounted chart viewed at 10 m. The test identifies the observer's threshold CS at each of five spatial frequencies (1.5–18.0 cycles per degree). Results are plotted as a CS function curve, which is compared with a normal response range.

Pelli-Robson Letter Sensitivity Chart (Haag-Streit, Bern, Switzerland) uses capital letters instead of sine-wave gratings.[37] The lowest level in which two out of three of the letters is identified correctly is scored as the threshold log CS (Figure 12-6). The chart has proven useful in measuring effects of treatment of patients with traumatic brain injury who complain of photophobia.[38]

VISUAL FIELDS

Definition and Function

The visual field encompasses that portion of visual space in which objects are visible, while an individual steadily fixates a stationary object usually positioned straight ahead.[39] Two primary considerations are necessary to understand the physiology of the visual field. First is its extent, which is not uniform in all directions. The individual projected extents, or limits, are expressed in angular distances from fixation: 60 degrees superiorly, 60 degrees nasally (to the right in the left eye and to the left in the right eye), 75 degrees inferiorly, and 100 degrees temporally (to the left in the left eye and to the right in the right eye).[40] However, physical features such as a protruding frontal bone or deeply set eyes can effectively reduce these limits.

Although the extent gives an indication of the geometric limits of peripheral vision, it does not indicate the functional abilities within the visual field. Traquair[41] conceived of the visual field as an "island of

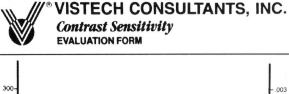

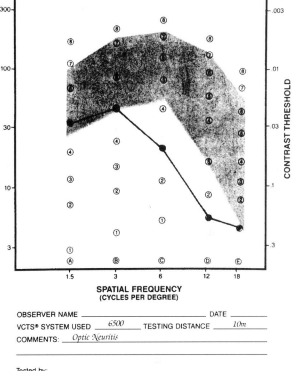

FIGURE 12-5 The normal range of contrast sensitivity is shown in the gray area. It is provided to help aid in the diagnosis of optic, neurologic, or pathologic disorders and should not be used as the sole criterion for diagnosis and treatment. In some cases, depressed contrast sensitivity is caused strictly by normal variation and not to an optic, neurologic, or pathologic problem. For this reason, contrast sensitivity should be used in conjunction with other diagnostic techniques. (Reprinted with permission from BP Rosenthal, RG Cole [eds], Functional Assessment of Low Vision. Philadelphia: Saunders, 1996;54.)

vision." It is conceptualized as a mountain-like configuration, with foveal vision occupying the peak, and the lateral field extent represented by the sloping sides leading to the base. There is a gradual loss of visual resolution (i.e., visual acuity) from the peak to the base. Beyond the base is a "sea of darkness," representing the limits of the peripheral-most retina.

These concepts relate to the psychophysiology of the visual field. They are dependent initially on the distribution and integrity of the rod and cone retinal recep-

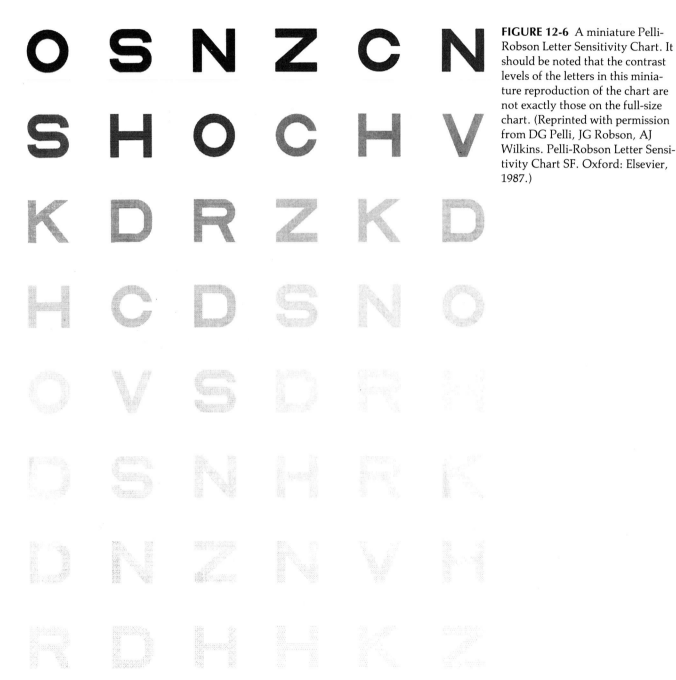

FIGURE 12-6 A miniature Pelli-Robson Letter Sensitivity Chart. It should be noted that the contrast levels of the letters in this miniature reproduction of the chart are not exactly those on the full-size chart. (Reprinted with permission from DG Pelli, JG Robson, AJ Wilkins. Pelli-Robson Letter Sensitivity Chart SF. Oxford: Elsevier, 1987.)

tors. However, as stated earlier, visual information is transmitted from these receptors along the visual pathway to the occipital area. Hence, the visual field is also dependent on the architecture and integrity of the visual pathway from the optic nerve to the occipital area. The clinical value is that deviations from the normal visual field can be indicative of various pathologic processes occurring anywhere along the primary visual pathway. Because visual field defects are common sequelae of

stroke or traumatic brain injury, this basic knowledge is clearly important for the rehabilitation professional.[42]

Clinical Assessment

The term *perimetry* encompasses the various methods to determine and assess the visual field clinically. These methods all rely on the patient monocularly fixating a target that is straight ahead, while stimuli are simultaneously presented at points eccentric to fixation throughout the visual field. The patient indicates when these stimuli are first perceived. The test target can be manually manipulated (kinetic perimetry) or be presented at predetermined positions within the field (static perimetry).[43,44]

Trobe and Glaser[9] have categorized visual field defects in terms of *territories* that reflect the anatomy and physiology of the pathway from the retina to the occipital cortex. These are summarized here.

Territory I: Rods and Cones

The defects are caused by pathology of the outer retina. Thus, even a disease of the surrounding choroid can secondarily affect the underlying rod and cone integrity. This can result in reduced sensitivity in that portion of the visual field corresponding to the location of the compromised retinal receptors.

Territory II: Inner Retina and Optic Nerve

The primary area of the inner retina consists of retinal fibers derived from the macula region and exiting via the optic nerve. This is termed the *papillomacular bundle.* When it is damaged, characteristic defects occur in the visual field corresponding to the specific anatomic location. This is particularly important in the diagnosis and management of glaucoma, which is frequently found in patients with acquired brain injury.

Territory III: Optic Chiasm

As stated earlier in the chapter, there is a decussation or crossing of the nasal retinal fibers of each eye at this structure. Thus, a lesion at the chiasm results in a characteristic bitemporal loss in the visual field (i.e., bitemporal hemianopia); the left half of the world is affected in the left eye, and the right half in the right eye.

Territory IV: Optic Tract to Occipital Lobe

The architectural physiology of the last part of the primary visual pathway explains the visual field defects typically found in patients with acquired brain injury, especially stroke. Insult to the left part of this pathway results in loss of sensitivity in the right visual field of each eye, whereas insult to the right part of this pathway results in loss of sensitivity in the left visual field of each eye. These conditions are termed right (or left) *homonymous hemianopia.* Figures 12-7 and 12-8 present the visual fields of a patient with left homonymous hemianopia.[43]

The previous discussion is limited to the visual field involving the primary visual pathway. However, as mentioned earlier, there is an extended visual pathway that proceeds from the occipital cortex to other higher level regions of the brain. A unique type of visual field defect occurs when a section of this pathway that communicates with the parietal area is involved.[45] The resulting condition is termed *visual neglect.* In contradistinction to field losses from damage to the primary visual pathway, the patient with visual neglect in its truest form is totally unaware of the field loss. Furthermore, it is frequently not documentable by standard methods of perimetry. This condition is particularly prevalent in individuals who have suffered a stroke or traumatic brain injury.[42,46–48]

STEREOPSIS

Definition and Function

Stereopsis refers to the perception of relative depth based on the presence of binocular horizontal retinal-image disparity[49,50] (Figure 12-9). This angular disparity is derived from the lateral anatomic displacement of the eyes, which produces slight differences between the monocular views of an object (i.e., the left eye sees more of the left side of the object, whereas the right eye sees more of the right side of the object). Under binocular viewing conditions, this resultant angular disparity creates the unique three-dimensional percept.

The physiological basis for stereopsis requires the simultaneous stimulation of slightly noncorresponding retinal regions in each eye. This, in turn, stimulates related binocular cells within the visual cortex, which are coded for specific horizontal disparities.[50–55] All targets physically located on the fixation depth plane would have zero horizontal retinal disparity, and therefore, no relative depth with respect to the fixation target (and related surrounding reference depth plane if present, such as found during clinical testing). All targets physically located beyond the fixation plane would have a divergent or uncrossed disparity, and they would be localized farther than the fixation plane. Conversely, all targets physically located in front of the fixation plane would have a convergent or crossed disparity, and they would be localized closer than the fixation plane. As binocular disparity decreases, the sensation of relative depth decreases, until at zero binocular disparity no relative depth is perceived. For example, if target X is moved toward bifixation target T along either dotted line in Figure 12-9, both horizontal retinal disparity and the associated relative depth would decrease proportionately. This fundamental principle is the basis of stereoscopic vision.

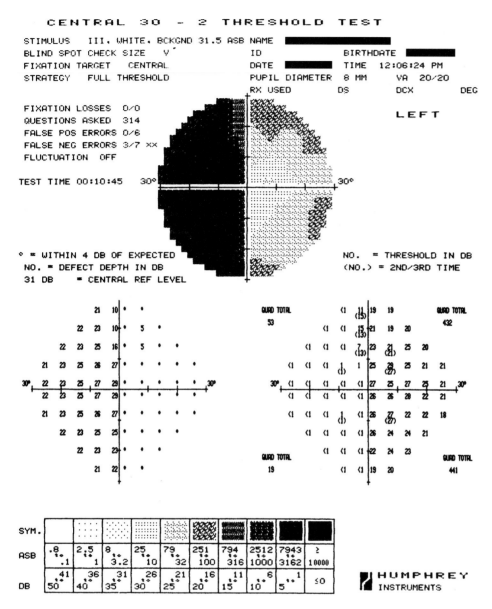

FIGURE 12-7 Central 30-2 Threshold Test of the left eye of a stroke patient. There is a dense left hemianopia shown by the dark areas of the gray-scale display (*center*). The *depth* of the defect is reported in the lower left, where the numbers correspond to deviations from the normative or expected values for the locations tested. Similarly, in the lower right is a numeric display showing the minimal stimulus intensity to which the individual was sensitive. (Reprinted with permission from R Gianutsos, IB Suchoff. Visual Fields after Brain Injury: Management Issues for the Occupational Therapist. In M Scheiman [ed], Understanding and Managing Vision Defects—A Guide for Occupational Therapists. Thorofare, NJ: SLACK Inc, 1996.)

Depth perception, a lay term for stereopsis, is used in many tasks at intermediate and near distances such as parking a car, walking down stairs or along inclines, threading a needle, and picking up small objects on a desk.[52] In reality, depth perception involves the use of stereoscopically derived information, as well as various monocular depth cues such as object overlap, parallax, size, and texture gradient.

Neuroanatomic Pathways

Single-cell recording techniques in animals discovered that stereoscopic abilities were first evident in Brodmann's area 17, also called the *primary visual*

cortex (V1).[54,56] Surrounding V1 is the peristriate cortex, which is associated with further binocular visual processing. It is subdivided into visual areas V2, V3, V4, and V5. Cells in V1 contain visual information from the contralateral hemifield. When binocular visual information is transmitted from the retina via the lateral geniculate body to V1, it is processed by horizontal, vertical, and orientation disparity–detecting cells, some of which exist in V1. Binocular information is further processed in V2, V3, and the medial temporal area (V5), where the number of binocular and disparity-detecting cells is greater than in V1.[51] Although horizontal retinal-image disparity is the primary contributor to stereopsis, vertical and orien-

FIGURE 12-8 Central 30-2 Threshold Test of the right eye of the same patient. Clearly, the pattern of loss corresponds to the left eye. When both eyes have corresponding patterns of loss, the pattern is termed *homonymous*. (Reprinted with permission from R Gianutsos, IB Suchoff. Visual Fields after Brain Injury: Management Issues for the Occupational Therapist. In M Scheiman [ed], Understanding and Managing Vision Defects—A Guide for Occupational Therapists. Thorofare, NJ: SLACK Inc, 1996.)

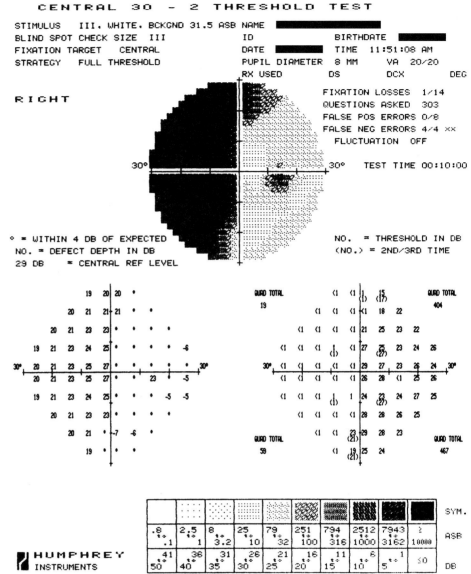

Types of Stereopsis

Clinically, there are two basic stereoscopic stimuli: contour or line stereograms, which assess local stereopsis (i.e., point-to-point disparity detection between the two horizontally disparate retinal images), and random-dot stereograms, which assess global stereopsis (i.e., area-to-area disparity cluster detection between the two horizontally disparate retinal images)[57,58] (Figure 12-10). To perceive random-dot stereograms, one must be bifoveal (i.e., both foveas must aim precisely at the target). However, monocular depth cues present with contour stereograms permit one to determine that one target appears distinct or different from the others under monocular conditions, and this can be misinterpreted as a correct stereoscopic response.

Clinical Assessment

Clinical assessment of stereopsis is twofold: (1) to determine if the individual is bifoveal, thereby ruling out a small-angle constant strabismus (i.e., a condition in which one visual axis does not intersect the target of regard), and (2) to determine the individual's stereoacuity level (i.e., stereoscopic threshold). The global stereograms of the Randot test, with angular binocular

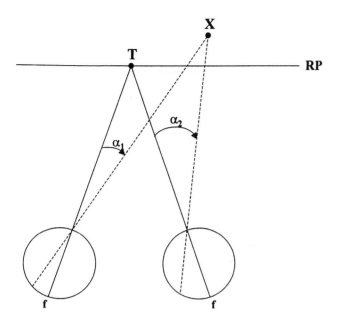

FIGURE 12-9 Geometry of horizontal retinal image disparity. (Angular disparity = $\alpha_2 - \alpha_1$; f = fovea of left and of right eyes; RP = reference plane for disparity; T = bifixation target; and X = an object in the field for which relative depth is assessed.)

disparities of 500-second arc and 250-second arc only, simply serve to determine whether or not an individual is bifoveal. However, it is the contour stereograms, which are more readily available for clinic use, that are used to ascertain the actual stereoscopic threshold (i.e., the minimal angular disparity necessary to elicit the perception of relative depth). Individuals with normal binocular vision, on average, have a stereoscopic threshold of 20 seconds of arc with an upper limit of 40 seconds of arc.[52]

ACCOMMODATION

Definition and Function

Accommodation refers to the process whereby changes in the curvature and hence optical power of the crystalline lens of the eye are made to obtain and maintain clarity of an object of regard on the high-resolution fovea of the eye[59,60] (Figure 12-11). These optical power changes of the eye are expressed in units of diopters (D), which equal 100 divided by the focal distance in centimeters (e.g., an eye focusing at 40 cm has a dioptric power of 2.5D). Blur of the retinal image is the stimulus to accommodation. However, other sources of information such as target size and proximity, optical aberra-

tions, prediction, and volition can influence the accommodative response.

The biomechanical process of accommodation is as follows[59,60] (see Figure 12-1A): (1) the ciliary muscle is innervated and increases its contractile state (for increased accommodation to focus on a near target), and it shifts anteriorly and centripetally in the process; (2) the tension of the lens zonules is reduced, thereby allowing the elastic lens capsule to exert its force on the internal crystalline lens cortical and nuclear moldable lens fiber substance; and (3) the crystalline lens increases its curvature (primarily the anterior surface), thereby increasing its dioptric focusing power and producing a clear retinal image on the fovea. The reverse process is true for reducing the level of accommodation to focus on a more distant target.

There are continuous age-related changes in accommodative ability. The maximum accommodative amplitude, or nearest point of clear vision (i.e., near point of accommodation), progressively declines with increased age from early childhood at a rate of approximately 0.3D per year. Thus, at 10 years of age, it is approximately 13D and at age 52 years it approaches zero.[60] However, at 40–45 years of age, the accommodative amplitude has declined sufficiently, so that the clinical condition of *presbyopia* is attained, thus requiring a bifocal near lens addition to compensate for this normal loss of near focusing ability in middle age. Presbyopia results from a multifaceted, biomechanically based inability to increase crystalline lens curvature.

Neuroanatomic Pathways

The general neurologic sensory and motor sequence of events leading to accommodation is as follows[59,60]: (1) Cones of the retina are stimulated by the defocussed retinal image; (2) summed cone blur signals are transmitted through the magnocellular layer of the lateral geniculate body and then on to cortical area 17; in both anatomic areas, the neurophysiological response to contrast changes is similar to that determined psychophysically in humans; (3) the sensory aspect of the blur signal is formulated based on the summed cortical cell responsivity; (4) a blur-related cortical signal is transmitted to parietotemporal areas for additional processing, informational dissemination, or both; (5) a supranuclear signal is transmitted to the midbrain-oculomotor nucleus complex/Edinger-Westphal nucleus where it is transformed into the correlated motor command; and (6) the motor command is transmitted through the oculomotor

FIGURE 12-10 The three most popular clinical stereo tests are the Titmus stereo test (*lower right*), Randot stereo test (*upper*), and Random Dot E Test (*lower left*). The Titmus stereo test is a line or contour test; the Randot stereo test uses a 660 seconds of arc random-dot stereogram for gross stereopsis and contour stimuli for fine stereopsis; and the Random Dot E Test measures stereoacuity by varying fixation distance. (Reprinted with permission from J Cooper. Stereopsis. In JB Eskridge, J Amos, JD Bartlett [eds], Clinical Procedures in Optometry. Philadelphia: Lippincott, 1991.)

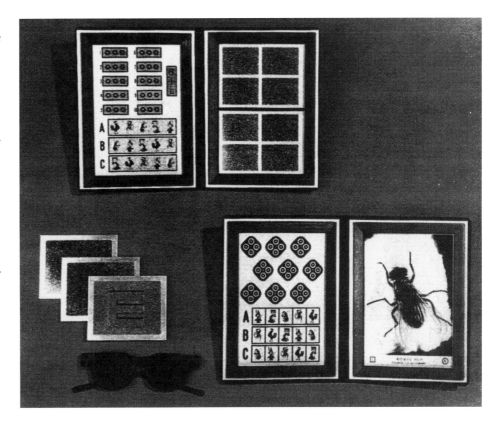

FIGURE 12-11 The eye in sagittal section. Split-field shows anatomic changes related to low (*left*) and high (*right*) levels of accommodation. Important accommodative structures in the anterior third of the eye are shown. (IOD = 10 D of accommodation; OD = zero D of accommodation.) (Reprinted with permission from L Stark. Presbyopia in Light of Accommodation. In L Stark and G Obrecht [eds], Presbyopia. New York: Professional Press Books, 1987.)

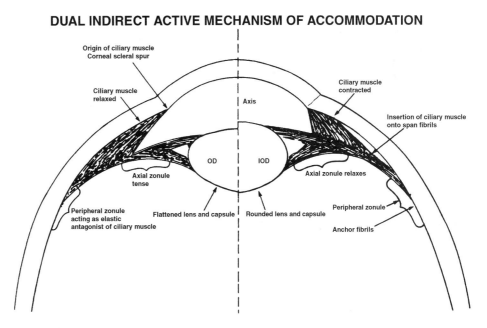

DUAL INDIRECT ACTIVE MECHANISM OF ACCOMMODATION

nerve (III), ciliary ganglion, and then short ciliary nerve to the ciliary muscle, where correlated contraction occurs to deform the crystalline lens to obtain clarity of vision.

The accommodative system is under autonomic control via the parasympathetic and sympathetic systems.[60] The primary drive for dynamic changes of accommodation is mediated by the parasympathetic system, whereas the sympathetic system is mainly involved in optimizing distance focus, as well as sustained near-work tasks.[61] See Figure 12-12 for the related neuroanatomic pathways.

Types of Accommodation

There are two types of accommodation: dynamic and static.[59,60] The dynamic accommodative response takes place when a target changes its distance, or when one shifts attention between targets located at different distances. The response takes approximately 1 second to

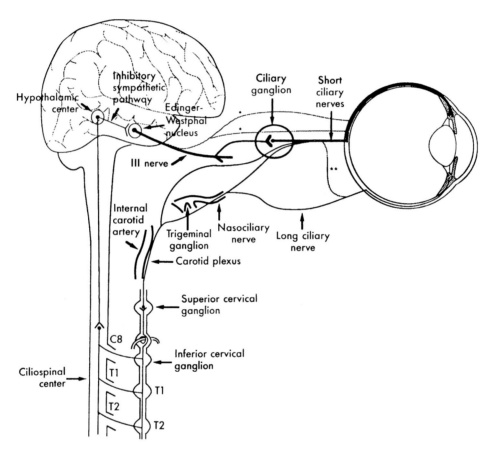

FIGURE 12-12 Parasympathetic and sympathetic pathways to the ciliary muscle. The major innervation to the ciliary muscle is parasympathetic and follows the pathway shown by the thick solid lines. The parasympathetic pathway originates in the Edinger-Westphal nucleus and courses with the third nerve, where the fibers travel to and synapse in the ciliary ganglion. The majority of the postganglionic parasympathetic fibers travels to the ciliary muscle via the short ciliary nerves, but some of them also travel with the long ciliary nerves. There is also evidence for a direct pathway of uncertain functional significance to the internal eye structures from the Edinger-Westphal nucleus. The sympathetic supply to the ciliary muscle (*thin solid lines*) originates in the diencephalon and travels down the spinal cord to the lower cervical and upper thoracic segments, to synapse in the spinociliary center of Budge in the intermediolateral tract of the cord. From there, second-order nerves leave the cord by the last cervical and first two thoracic ventral roots; these preganglionic fibers run up the cervical sympathetic chain to synapse in the superior cervical ganglion. The third-order fibers continue up the sympathetic carotid plexus and enter the orbit, either with the first division of the trigeminal nerve (following the nasociliary division) or independently, where they join the long and short ciliary nerves, in the latter instance passing through the ciliary ganglion without synapsing. (Reprinted with permission from PL Kaufman. Accommodation and Presbyopia. In WM Hart [ed], Adler's Physiology of the Eye [9th ed]. St. Louis: Mosby, 1992.)

complete, which includes the latency (i.e., reaction time) of 400 msec and the actual crystalline lens movement time of 500–800 msec.[62] Once this dynamic phase is completed, the static (or steady-state) response takes place to maintain the newly acquired target in focus. The accuracy of the static response is assessed with respect to the normal, small, residual accommodative error (i.e., the accommodative stimulus level minus the accommodative response in units of diopters) that is typically present.[59,60] The accommodative error progressively increases with decreased target distance (within 1–2 m or closer, i.e., increased dioptric near focusing demand), with the accommodative response being less than the accommodative stimulus.[63] In contrast, for distances greater than 1–2 m, the accommodative response is slightly greater than the accommodative stimulus.

Clinical Assessment of Accommodation

The primary measure of accommodation is the maximum amplitude of accommodation. This is generally measured by the *push-up* technique[60] under both monocular and binocular viewing conditions with full distance refractive correction in place. Under monocular conditions, the primary drive is blur, whereas under binocular conditions, the vergence eye movement drive to accommodation (i.e., vergence accommodation) can add to the blur component. In addition, the amplitude of accommodation, as well as its response at other near distances, can be assessed objectively using dynamic retinoscopy.[59,60]

The overall dynamic accommodative response (i.e., latency plus lens movement time) can be assessed using the lens flipper, *accommodative rock* technique.[60] Essentially, spherical positive and negative lenses (e.g., ±2D) are interposed and alternated in power as rapidly as possible under monocular and binocular viewing conditions as focus is maintained on the near target (40 cm). The number of alterna-

tions in which the individual can rapidly obtain clear vision in 60 seconds is determined. With increased age, this ability progressively declines as presbyopia is approached.

EYE MOVEMENTS

Definition and Function

Eye movements refer to the change in gaze or position of the eyes, typically in response to an object of interest, to maintain the high-resolution fovea on the target.[64] The eyes can move in a horizontal, vertical, or cyclorotary manner, or all three.

Types of Eye Movements

There are two major types of eye movements (Figure 12-13), and these function in a highly coordinated manner. The versional system controls conjugate movement of the eyes (i.e., movement of the eyes in the same direction to see objects positioned in different directions from an individual). In contrast, the vergence system controls disjunctive movement of the eyes (i.e., movement of the eyes in opposing directions to see objects singly at different distances from an individual). Thus, together these two systems precisely and rapidly move the eyes to locate and inspect objects at all distances and directions of gaze. Each system has several subsystems with more detailed and specific functions to perform these special tasks (Tables 12-1 and 12-2).

Neuroanatomic Pathways

Each eye has six extraocular muscles with specific movement functions (Table 12-3), and neural innervation and blood supply (Table 12-4), that are critical for their extremely fine control of gaze. Hence, any damage to the eye muscle, nerve, or blood supply typically results

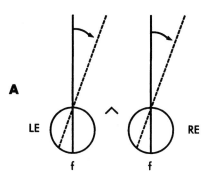 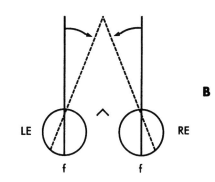

FIGURE 12-13 Schematic drawing of version (**A**) and vergence (**B**) eye movements. (f = fovea; LE = left eye; RE = right eye.) (Reprinted with permission from KJ Ciuffreda, B Tannen. Eye Movement Basics for the Clinician. St. Louis: Mosby, 1995.)

TABLE 12-1
Versional Eye Movements

Subsystem	Stimulus	Function
Fixational	Stationary	To stabilize a target onto the fovea
Saccadic	Step of target displacement	To acquire an eccentric target onto the fovea
Pursuit	Target velocity	To match eye velocity with target velocity to stabilize the retinal image
Optokinetic	Target or field velocity	To maintain a stable image during sustained head movement
Vestibular	Head acceleration	To maintain a stable image with the target on the fovea during transient head movement

Source: Reprinted with permission from KJ Ciuffreda, B Tannen. Eye Movement Basics for the Clinician. Philadelphia: Mosby Year-Book, 1995.

TABLE 12-2
Vergence Eye Movement

Subsystem	Stimulus
Disparity (or fusional)	Target disparity
Accommodative	Target blur
Proximal	Apparent nearness or perceived distance of target
Tonic	Baseline neural innervation

Source: Reprinted with permission from KJ Ciuffreda, B Tannen. Eye Movement Basics for the Clinician. Philadelphia: Mosby Year-Book, 1995.

TABLE 12-3
Primary, Secondary, and Tertiary Actions of the Extraocular Muscles from the Primary Position

Muscle	Primary Action	Secondary Action	Tertiary Action
Medial rectus	Adduction	—	—
Lateral rectus	Abduction	—	—
Inferior rectus	Depression	Excycloduction	Adduction
Superior rectus	Elevation	Incycloduction	Adduction
Inferior oblique	Excycloduction	Elevation	Abduction
Superior oblique	Incycloduction	Depression	Abduction

Source: Reprinted with permission from KJ Ciuffreda, B Tannen. Eye Movement Basics for the Clinician. Philadelphia: Mosby-Year Book, 1995.

TABLE 12-4
Cranial Innervation and Blood Supply to the Extraocular Muscles

Muscle	Cranial Nerve	Blood Supply
Lateral rectus	Abducens (VI)	Lacrimal artery and lateral muscular branch of the ophthalmic artery
Medial rectus	Oculomotor (III)	Medial muscular branch of the ophthalmic artery
Superior rectus	Oculomotor (III)	Lateral muscular branch of the ophthalmic artery
Inferior rectus	Oculomotor (III)	Medial muscular branch of the ophthalmic artery
Superior oblique	Trochlear (IV)	Superior muscular branch of the ophthalmic artery
Inferior oblique	Oculomotor (III)	Infraorbital artery and medial muscular branch of the ophthalmic artery

Source: Reprinted with permission from KJ Ciuffreda, B Tannen. Eye Movement Basics for the Clinician. Philadelphia: Mosby Year-Book, 1995.

in dynamic (e.g., slowed responses), static (e.g., strabismus, paresis, and paralysis), or both kinds of oculomotor dysfunction.

The neural pathways for each eye movement subsystem have considerable differences and relatively complicated interactive network structural arrangements.[64–66] The details are beyond the scope of this chapter. However, some of the brain areas common to many of these eye movement subsystems include the cerebellum, midbrain, frontal eye fields, superior colliculus, parietal cortex, and visual cortex. Hence, damage to any one area might affect multiple eye movement subsystems.

Clinical Assessment of Eye Movements

Each subsystem within the versional and vergence eye movement systems can be examined independently.[64] However, only the following ones are routinely tested in the clinic. With regard to the *fixational* system, the accuracy and presence of any abnormalities (i.e., increased drift, saccadic intrusions, nystagmus, or all three)[67] are determined. With regard to the *saccadic* system, the accuracy and presence of either undershooting or hypometria (i.e., the primary saccade is too small), or overshooting or hypermetria (i.e., the primary saccade is too large), are determined. With regard to the *pursuit* system, the smoothness and presence of any jerky movements (i.e., corrective saccades) are determined. Lastly, with regard to the binocular *vergence* system, the accuracy and maximum amplitude (i.e., the near point of convergence, which does not recede with age as is true for accommodation) are determined.

REFRACTIVE STATUS

Definition and Function

Determination of the eye's refractive status is the basis for the various eye-care professions. It is this entity that is most familiar to the public, and indeed the major reason one seeks vision care.

Refraction refers to the bending of light rays as they pass from one optical medium to another of a different density.[68] The degree of refraction is dependent not only on the difference in density between the optical media interfaces (i.e., the greater the difference, the greater the refraction), but also on the curvature of the surfaces: the greater the curvature, the greater the refraction.

The refractive status of the eye depends on this same optical principle. Light rays from an object are refracted first by the cornea, the primary optical element, then the aqueous humor, crystalline lens, the secondary optical element of the eye, and finally by the vitreous humor.[69]

There are several possible refractive conditions, and these are specified without corrective lenses in place and with accommodation minimal and fully relaxed, while the individual fixates and focuses on a distant object (i.e., at optical infinity)[69] (Figure 12-14). If parallel rays of light from infinity are focused on the retina, then the condition is termed *emmetropia*, and the retinal image is in focus. In contrast, if these rays are not focused on the retina, thus producing a blurred retinal image, then the condition is termed *ametropia*. This results from a mismatch between the total ocular power of the eye and its total axial length. The greater the mismatch, the greater the degree of ametropia, and hence the greater is the resultant retinal blur. There are three basic forms of ametropia. *Myopia* results when the axial length is too long for the ocular power, and the point of focus falls in front of the retina. In contrast, *hyperopia* results when the axial length is too short for the ocular power, and the point of focus falls

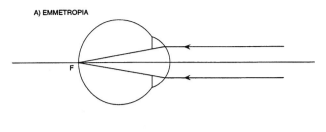

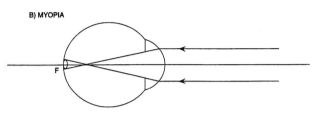

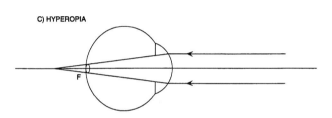

FIGURE 12-14 Diagrammatic representation of the three spherical refractive states. **A.** If the dioptric power of the eye is such that its focal length matches its axial length, the retina is in the correct position to receive focused light from a distant source. This is termed *emmetropia*, or having no refractive error. **B.** When the dioptrics of the eye are too strong for the eye's axial length or the eye is too long and the retina is beyond the eye's focal length, *myopia* results. Images of a distant point source appear as a blurred circle on the retina. **C.** When the dioptrics of the eye are too weak for the eye's axial length or the eye is too short and the retina is beyond the eye's focal length, *hyperopia* results. If the patient does not accommodate to increase the eye's dioptric power, images of a distant point source also appear as a blurred circle on the retina. (f = fovea.) (Reprinted with permission from DO Mutti, K Zadnik. Refractive Error. In Zadnik K [ed], The Ocular Examination. Philadelphia: Saunders, 1997.)

behind the retina. In both cases, there is uniform blur of the retinal image, as it is assumed that the ocular power is the same in all meridians. However, this is frequently not the case. There may be systematic meridional variation primarily in anterior corneal power, and the resulting condition is termed *astigmatism*. There are meridians of maximal and minimal power (separated by 90 degrees), producing two retinal image lines rather than a single point image, with either one or both of these focal lines falling in front of or behind the retina.

Clinical Assessment and Implications

The ametropias are compensated with spectacles, contact lenses, or refractive surgery. Concave, convex, or cylindrical lenses are used in the correction of myopia, hyperopia, and astigmatism, respectively. The lens prescription is determined clinically by subjective, objective, or both kinds of refraction.[70]

These refractive status concepts are important for the rehabilitation professional. For example, relatively small amounts of hyperopia in younger individuals can be overcome by the patient's ability to accommodate. Thus, younger hyperopic patients might see clearly and be asymptomatic without the need for corrective lenses. If as a result of an injury, however, the oculomotor nerve has been damaged, a previously uncorrected 20-year-old patient might now require an optical correction, particularly when engaged in near tasks. The optometrist or ophthalmologist should provide both the rehabilitation team and patient with precise lens-wearing instructions.

OCULAR HEALTH

Definition and Description

Ocular health concerns for brain-injured patients arise secondary to underlying systemic health problems, current medication use, or both. One study investigating ocular and visual conditions in moderate to severe brain-injured patients revealed a significantly higher frequency of dry eye, blepharitis, glaucoma, retinopathy (diabetic and hypertensive), and visual field defects as compared with that found in the non–brain-injured population.[48] Dry eye is a common side effect of antidepressant, tranquilizing, and antianxiety medications.[71] Although it is not visually threatening, a dry eye can produce a gritty sensation and intermittent blurred vision, as well as more general ocular irritation, because of disruption of the tear film layer. Blepharitis arises as a result of poor lid hygiene and, if not treated properly, may lead to infection, inflammation, or both within the eye.[72] Glaucoma encompasses a group of serious vision-threatening diseases involving intraocular pressure, drainage of aqueous fluid, optic nerve head appearance, optic nerve fiber layer appearance, and visual field integrity. The ultimate course of glaucoma may result in marked peripheral visual field loss and, in some cases, total loss of vision. At present, there is no medical cure. However, if diagnosed early in the disease process, the progression may be retarded. Retinopathy, which is usually secondary to uncontrolled or advanced hyper-

tension, diabetes, or both, can be vision threatening if it affects the nerve fiber layer near the optic nerve head or the central macular region. Early intervention allows for retardation, but not cessation, of the disease process. Unless progressive, visual field deficits are not vision threatening. Rather, such defects reduce the field of vision and may require low-vision aids or prismatic spectacle correction to improve the patient's comfort and efficiency during their routine daily activities.

Clinical Assessment and Implications

Pupils

Using a penlight or transilluminator, the pupil shape, size, and symmetry are evaluated, as they reflect basic anatomic and neurologic aspects. Pupils are expected to be round and equal in size and shape. Testing for a relative afferent pupillary defect, which, if present, is indicative of damaged pupillary fibers, space-occupying lesions, tumors, anatomic anomalies of the iris, or degenerative neurologic diseases (i.e., demyelinating diseases, connective tissue disorders, or autoimmune diseases) is also performed. Pupillary responses are mediated by the parasympathetic and sympathetic pathways of the autonomic nervous system.[73]

Anterior Segment

The integrity of the ocular adnexa, including the lids, lashes, tear film, cornea, conjunctiva, aqueous fluid in the anterior chamber and angle, iris, lens, and anterior vitreous, is evaluated using a slit-lamp biomicroscope, which is essentially a low-powered microscope with variable illumination and magnification capabilities. This evaluation is particularly important because of the high frequency of dry eye syndrome and blepharitis in brain-injured patients, as described earlier.

Intraocular Pressure

Intraocular pressure using applanation tonometry is measured on patients to screen for the presence of glaucoma. This potentially serious disease has been found to be more frequent in acquired brain injury patients than in non–brain-injured patients,[42] as mentioned earlier.

The group of diseases falling under the umbrella of glaucoma has four diagnostic criteria[74]: (1) intraocular pressure that is too high for the patient's eye to maintain its normal neuroanatomic and neurophysiological integrity, (2) a narrow anterior angle or impaired drainage of aqueous fluid from the anterior chamber, (3) nasal or arcuate visual field deficits, and (4) optic nerve anomalies. Glaucoma ultimately affects the integrity of the optic nerve and, in turn, reduces the visual field. Optometrists and ophthalmologists screen for and manage glaucoma by evaluating the anterior chamber angle, intraocular pressure, the retina with a dilated fundus examination, and visual field integrity with automated perimetry, as well as provide drug therapy and surgery.

Posterior Segment

Structures in the posterior segment of the eye include the optic nerve head, central fovea and macular region, retinal vasculature, nerve fiber layer, and midretinal periphery. These structures are specifically assessed and most accurately evaluated with a dilated fundus examination. Thus, small elevations can be readily detected because of the binocular, stereoscopic viewing. Alternate methods of evaluating the structures of the posterior segment include direct and monocular indirect ophthalmoscopy, both of which provide monocular, nonstereoscopic views of the fundus.[75]

VISION IN REHABILITATION: A CLINICAL PERSPECTIVE

Vision is more than the sum of its parts as outlined within this chapter. It is a critically important and meaningful sensory function through which we gain much of the information in daily life. Together with proprioception and vestibular function, it is the basis for normal upright stance. Its role in the genesis of falls has been alluded to previously.[6,76] It immeasurably enhances our appreciation of the beauty of our world and the human's artistic contribution to it.

On a more practical level for the rehabilitation professional is the frequency of vision problems as part of disabling diseases of the CNS and the equally common occurrence of vision impairments among patients with unrelated disabilities. Among the latter group are patients with lower extremity amputations,[4,5] whose ambulatory potential despite their double disability is quite good. Similarly, older rehabilitation inpatients frequently display deficits from macular degeneration, cataract, glaucoma, or diabetic retinopathy as comorbidities to their primary reason for rehabilitation hospital stays.[2]

When the CNS is affected by multiple sclerosis, optic neuritis adds challenges to functional independence for individuals who may also have pyramidal, cerebellar, or sensory deficits. Cerebrovascular accidents may produce visual field deficits (e.g., hemianopia, hemineglect), spatial and perceptual distortions, visual agnosia, or even total cortical blindness. Gianutsos and coworkers[77] have documented a greater than 50% rate of visual involvement among patients with severe traumatic brain injury when they receive careful optometric screening.

It should be abundantly clear then that vision impairment is a pervasive issue among patients who are referred to physiatrists, therapists, and rehabilitation medicine departments. A basic knowledge of vision function, the nature and causes of its altered function, and the basic principles of vision rehabilitation should therefore become part of the core knowledge base for rehabilitation personnel.

Acknowledgment

KJC and NK were supported in part during the writing of this chapter by a grant from The Jacob and Valeria Langeloth Foundation.

REFERENCES

1. Wainapel SF. Vision rehabilitation: an overlooked subject in physiatric training and practice. Am J Phys Med Rehabil 1995;74:313–314.
2. Wainapel SF, Kwon YS, Fazzari PJ. Severe visual impairment on a rehabilitation unit: incidence and implications. Arch Phys Med Rehabil 1989;70:439–441.
3. Wainapel SF. Rehabilitation of the blind stroke patient. Arch Phys Med Rehabil 1984;65:382–489.
4. Altner PE, Rusin JJ, DeBoer A. Rehabilitation of blind patients with lower extremity amputations. Arch Phys Med Rehabil 1980;61:82–85.
5. Fisher R. Rehabilitation of the blind amputee: a rewarding experience. Arch Phys Med Rehabil 1987;68:382–383.

6. Tinette M, Inouye S, Gill T, Doucette J. Shared risk factors for falls, incontinence, and functional dependence. JAMA 1995;273:1348–1353.
7. Carabellese C, Appollonio L, Rozzini R, et al. Sensory impairment and quality of life in community elderly population. J Am Geriatr Soc 1993;41:401–407.
8. Last RJ. Wolff's Anatomy of the Eye and Orbit. Philadelphia: WB Saunders, 1968.
9. Trobe JD, Glaser JS. The Visual Fields Manual—A Practical Guide to Testing and Interpretation. Gainesville, FL: Triad Publishing, 1983.
10. Solan HA. Transient and sustained processing: dual subsystem theory of

reading disability. J Behav Optom 1994;5:149–154.
11. Kaas JH. Changing Concepts of Visual Cortex Organization. In JW Brown (ed), Neuropsychology of Visual Perception. Hillsdale, NJ: Erlbaum Publishers, 1989;3–38.
12. Teller DY. The forced-choice preferential looking procedure: a psychophysical technique for use with human infants. Infant Behav Dev 1979;2:135–153.
13. McDonald M, Dobson V, Sebris SL, et al. The acuity card procedure: a rapid test of infant acuity. Invest Ophthalmol Vis Sci 1985;26:1158–1162.
14. Hartman EE. Infant visual development: an overview of studies using

visual evoked potential measures from Harter to the present. Int J Neurosci 1995;80:203–235.

15. Gottlob I, Fendick MG, Guo S, et al. Visual acuity measurements by sweep spatial frequency visual-evoked-cortical-potentials (VECP's). J Pediatr Ophthalmol Strabismus 1990;27:40–47.

16. Jackowski MM, Sturr JF, Turk MA, et al. Clinical indications of altered peripheral field function in patients with traumatic brain injury. Invest Ophthalmol Vis Sci 1999;40(Suppl):32.

17. Campbell FW, Robson JG. Application of Fourier analysis to the visibility of gratings. J Physiol (Lond) 1968;197:551–566.

18. DeValois RL, Albrecht DG, Thorell LG. Spatial Tuning of LGN and Cortical Cells in the Monkey Visual System. In H Spekreijse, H vander Tweel (eds), Spatial Contrast. Amsterdam: Elsevier, 1977;60–63.

19. DeValois RL, DeValois KK. Spatial Vision. New York: Oxford University Press, 1988.

20. DeValois RL, DeValois KK. Neural Coding of Color. In KK DeValois (ed), Handbook of Perception and Cognition: Seeing. Vol 5. New York: Academic Press, 1975;15–35.

21. Zeki S. A Vision of the Brain. London: Blackwell, 1993.

22. Hart WM. Visual Adaptation. In WM Hart (ed), Adler's Physiology of the Eye (9th ed). St. Louis: Mosby, 1992;525–526.

23. Zihl J, von Cramon D, Mai N. Selective disturbance of movement vision after bilateral brain damage. Brain 1983;106:313–340.

24. Jackowski MM, Sturr JF, Turk MA, et al. Altered dark adaptation in patients with traumatic brain injury. Invest Ophthalmol Vis Sci 1998;39(Suppl):401.

25. Records RE, Brown JL. Adaptation. In TD Duane, EA Jaeger (eds), Biomedical Foundations of Ophthalmology. Philadelphia: JB Lippincott, 1988;1–13.

26. Farnsworth D. The Farnsworth Dichotomous Test For Color Blindness-Panel D-15. New York: Psychological Corporation, 1947;1–5.

27. Hart WM. Color Vision. In WM Hart (ed), Adler's Physiology of the Eye (9th ed). St. Louis: Mosby, 1992;720–722.

28. Fischer ML. Clinical Implications of Color Vision Deficiencies. In BP Rosenthal, RG Cole (eds), Functional Assessment of Low Vision. New York: Mosby, 1996;105–127.

29. Pokorny J, Smith VC, Verriest G, et al. Congenital and Acquired Color Vision Difficulties. New York: Grune & Stratton, 1979.

30. Fraunfelder FT. Drug-Induced Ocular Side Effects and Drug Interactions. Philadelphia: Lea & Febiger, 1982.

31. Jaanus SD, Bartlett JD. Adverse Ocular Effects of Systemic Drug Therapy. In JD Bartlett, SD Jaanus (eds), Clinical Ocular Pharmacology. Boston: Butterworth, 1984;917–939.

32. Skalka HW. Comparison of Snellen acuity, VER acuity and Arden grating scores in macular and optic nerve diseases. Br J Ophthalmol 1980;64:24–29.

33. Kupersmith MJ, Nilson JI, Seiple WH, et al. The 20/20 eye in multiple sclerosis. Neurology 1983;33:1015–1020.

34. Kupersmith MJ, Siegel IM, Carr RE. Subtle disturbances of vision with compressive lesions of the anterior visual pathway measured by contrast sensitivity. Ophthalmology 1982;89:68–72.

35. Bodis-Wollner I, Diamond SP. The measurement of spatial contrast sensitivity in cases of blurred vision associated with cerebral lesions. Brain 1976;99:695–710.

36. Fleishman JA, Beck RW, Linares OA, Klein JW. Deficits in visual function after resolution of optic neuritis. Ophthalmology 1987;94:1029–1035.

37. Pelli DG, Robson JG, Wilkins AJ. The design of a new letter chart for measuring contrast sensitivity. Clin Vis Sci 1988;2:187–199.

38. Jackowski MM, Sturr JF, Taub HA, et al. Photophobia in patients with traumatic brain injury: uses of light-filtering lenses to enhance contrast sensitivity and reading rate. Neurol Rehab 1996;6:193–201.

39. Harrington D. The Visual Fields (2nd ed). St. Louis: Mosby, 1964.

40. Anderson DR. Automated Static Perimetry. St. Louis: Mosby, 1992.

41. Traquair HM. An Introduction to Clinical Perimetry. London: Henry Kimpton, 1927.

42. Suchoff IB, Gianutsos R, Ciuffreda KJ, Groffman S. Vision Impairment Related to Acquired Brain Injury. In B Silverston, et al (eds), The Lighthouse Handbook on Vision Impairment and Vision Rehabilitation. Vol 1. New York: Oxford University Press, 2000;517–539.

43. Gianutsos R, Suchoff IB. Visual Fields after Brain Injury: Management Issues for the Occupational Therapist. In M Scheiman (ed), Understanding and Managing Vision Defects—A Guide for Occupational Therapists. Thorofare, NJ: SLACK Inc, 1996;333–358.

44. Johnson CA. Perimetry and Visual Field Testing. In K Zadnik (ed), The Ocular Examination. Philadelphia: WB Saunders, 1997;274–301.

45. Stein JF. Representation of egocentric space in the posterior parietal cortex. J Exper Physiol 1989;74:583–606.

46. Halligan PW, Marshall JC. The History and Clinical Presentation of Neglect. In IH Robertson, JC Marshall (eds), Unilateral Neglect: Clinical and Experimental Studies. Hillsdale, NJ: Erlbaum Assoc, 1993;3–19.

47. Robertson IH, Halligan PW. Spatial Neglect: A Clinical Handbook for Diagnosis and Treatment. Hove, East Sussex, UK: Psychology Press, 1999.

48. Suchoff IB, Kapoor N, Waxman R, et al. The occurrence of ocular and visual dysfunctions in an acquired brain-injured patient sample. J Am Optom Assoc 1999;70:301–308.

49. Bishop PO. Binocular Vision. In RA Moses, WM Hart (eds), Adler's Physiology of the Eye: Clinical Application (8th ed). St. Louis: Mosby, 1987;619–689.

50. Von Noorden GK. Binocular Vision and Ocular Motility: Theory and Management of Strabismus (5th ed). St. Louis: Mosby, 1996;25–30,274–296.

51. Howard IP, Rodgers BJ. Binocular Vision and Stereopsis. New York: Oxford University Press, 1995;105–148.

52. Cooper J. Stereopsis. In JB Eskridge, J Amos, JD Bartlett (eds), Clinical Procedures in Optometry. Philadelphia: Lippincott, 1991;121–134.

53. Hubel DH, Wiesel TN. Stereoscopic vision in macaque monkey: cells sensitive to binocular depth in area 18 of the macaque monkey cortex. Nature 1970;225:41–42.

54. Barlow HB, Blakemore C, Pettigrew JD. The neural mechanism of binocular depth discrimination. J Physiol 1967;193:327–342.

55. Nikara T, Bishop PO, Pettigrew JD. Analysis of retinal correspondence by studying receptive fields of binocular single units in cat striate cortex. Exp Brain Res 1968;6:353–372.

56. Pettigrew JD. The effect of visual experience on the development of stimulus specificity by kitten cortical neurons. J Physiol 1974;237:47–74.

57. Julesz B. Binocular depth perception in computer-generated patterns. Bell System Tech J 1960;39:1125–1162.

58. Julesz B. Foundations of Cyclopean

Perception. Chicago: University of Chicago Press, 1971.

59. Ciuffreda KJ. Accommodation and Its Anomalies. In WN Charman (ed), Vision and Visual Dysfunction. Vol 1. London: Macmillan, 1991;231–279.

60. Ciuffreda KJ. Accommodation, Pupil and Presbyopia. In WJ Benjamin (ed), Borish's Clinical Refraction. Philadelphia: WB Saunders, 1998;77–120.

61. Gilmartin B. A review of the role of sympathetic innervation on the ciliary muscle in ocular accommodation. Ophthalmic Physiol Opt 1986;6:23–37.

62. Campbell FW, Westheimer G. Dynamics of accommodative responses of the human eye. J Physiol 1960;151:285–295.

63. Ciuffreda KJ, Kenyon RV. Accommodative Vergence and Accommodation in Normals, Amblyopes and Strabismics. In CM Schor, KJ Ciuffreda (eds), Vergence Eye Movements: Basic and Clinical Aspects. Boston: Butterworth, 1983;101–173.

64. Ciuffreda KJ, Tannen B. Eye Movement Basics for the Clinician. St. Louis: Mosby, 1995.

65. Leigh RJ, Zee DS. The Neurology of Eye Movements (2nd ed). Philadelphia: FA Davis, 1991.

66. Baloh RW, Honrubia V. Clinical Neurophysiology of the Vestibular System (2nd ed). Philadelphia: FA Davis, 1990.

67. Ciuffreda KJ, Levi DM, Selenow A. Amblyopia: Basic and Clinical Aspects. Boston: Butterworth–Heinemann, 1991.

68. Spraycar M (ed). Steadman's Medical Dictionary (25th ed). Baltimore: Williams & Wilkins, 1990.

69. Rosenfield M. Refractive Status of the Eye. In WJ Benjamin (ed), Borish's Clinical Refraction. Philadelphia: WB Saunders, 1998;2–29.

70. Mutti DO, Zadnik K. Refractive Error. In K Zadnik (ed), The Ocular Examination. Philadelphia: WB Saunders, 1997;87–121.

71. Bartlett JD, Jaanus SD. Clinical Ocular Pharmacology (3rd ed). Boston: Butterworth–Heinemann, 1995;127–617.

72. Catania LJ. Primary Care of the Anterior Segment. Norwalk, CT: Appleton & Lange, 1988.

73. Zinn KM. The Pupil. Springfield, IL: Thomas, 1972.

74. Klopfer J, Paikowsky SJ. Epidemiology and Clinical Impact of the Glaucomas. In M Fingaret, TL Lewis (eds), Primary Care of the Glaucomas. Norwalk, CT: Appleton & Lange, 1993;18–22.

75. Cockburn DM. Tonometry. In JB Eskridge, J Amos, JD Bartlett (eds), Clinical Procedures in Optometry. Philadelphia: Lippincott, 1991;220–230.

76. Tobis JS, Block M, Steinhaus-Donham C, et al. Falling among the sensorially impaired elderly. Arch Phys Med Rehabil 1990;71:144–147.

77. Gianutsos R, Ramsey G, Perlin R. Rehabilitative optometric services for survivors of acquired brain injury. Arch Phys Med Rehabil 1988;69:573–578.

13

Nerve Conduction and Neuromuscular Transmission

NEIL I. SPIELHOLZ AND STANLEY J. MYERS

Nerve conduction studies were introduced into the armamentarium of the clinical neurophysiologist by Hodes et al. (1948).[1] This ground-breaking article described techniques for determining conduction in motor nerves of the upper and lower extremities (by recording from muscles) and presented a wealth of information concerning normal and pathologic conditions. Subsequently, Dawson and Scott (1949) showed that nerve action potentials (APs), although considerably smaller than those evoked from muscles, could also be detected by appropriately placed surface electrodes.[2] These nerve APs, recorded at the elbow in response to stimulation of the median or ulnar at the wrist, contained contributions from sensory fibers, conducting orthodromically, and motor fibers, conducting antidromically. Dawson (1956) then described how conduction in sensory nerves could be studied by simulating the digits through ring electrodes and recording the ascending volley with surface electrodes at the wrist and elbow.[3]

Refinements in technology, and further understanding of normal and abnormal physiology, have advanced the use of these techniques beyond merely determining conduction velocity or evoked amplitudes. It must be remembered, however, that the methods generally employed today only determine activity in a small percent of the total number of fibers present in a peripheral nerve. Motor conduction studies evaluate Aα fibers, whereas sensory studies determine conduction primarily in Aα and Aβ fibers. All these are relatively large and myelinated, but do not represent all the myelinated fibers that are present. Furthermore, the majority of fibers in a peripheral nerve are unmyelinated C fibers,[4] so the information gathered about the *whole* nerve is quite limited. But despite this restriction, conduction studies are helpful indeed, as is described in this chapter. Before going into clinical techniques and their use, pertinent neurophysiology is reviewed.

SOME NEUROPHYSIOLOGY UNDERLYING CONDUCTION STUDIES

Generation of Resting and Action Potentials

Although muscle and nerve fibers perform different functions, they are both enclosed by an *excitable plasma membrane*. For muscle fibers, this membrane is the *sarcolemma*, whereas for nerve fibers it is the *axolemma*. These membranes (1) form the boundary between the cell and the extracellular fluid that surrounds it; (2) generate a potential difference between the inside and outside solutions, the *transmembrane potential*; and (3) can conduct or transmit disturbances in this transmembrane potential along their length, the AP.

Transmembrane potentials are generated across these biological membranes because of their semipermeable characteristics coupled with an uneven distribution of certain ions between the inside and outside solutions. Basically, these membranes are relatively impermeable to large protein anions (A$^-$) that are present inside these cells, while they are differentially permeable to potassium (K$^+$), sodium (Na$^+$), and chloride (Cl$^-$) (Figure 13-1). This differential permeability is such that at rest, K$^+$ is much more permeable than is Na$^+$. As a result, K$^+$, which is more concentrated inside the cell than outside, diffuses out of the cell much faster than Na$^+$, which is more concentrated

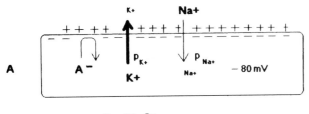

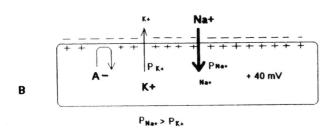

FIGURE 13-1 Representation of a region of an excitable cell at rest (**A**) and while generating an action potential (**B**). The membrane is impermeable to large anions (A⁻, shown by the arrow being reflected at the membrane), whereas it is differentially permeable to the cations K⁺ and Na⁺. The arrows penetrating the membrane indicate the direction these ions diffuse according to their concentration gradients, whereas the thickness of these arrows indicates their relative permeabilities. **A.** Potassium permeability (p_{K+}) is greater than sodium permeability (p_{Na+}). Therefore, K⁺ diffuses out of the cell faster than Na⁺ diffuses in, leaving behind unbalanced negative charges (A⁻). This efflux of K⁺ builds up a corresponding inside negativity that ultimately balances the concentration gradient for K⁺. If no other ion, such as Na⁺, could permeate the membrane, the inside negativity that would retard further net efflux of K⁺ would be the *potassium equilibrium potential* as calculated by the Nernst equation. **B.** Membrane repolarization to threshold causes p_{Na+} to increase well above p_{K+}, so that Na⁺ now diffuses into the cell faster than K⁺ diffuses out. This influx of positive charges makes the inside positive with respect to the outside, reversing the transmembrane potential, thereby generating the action potential in that region. The magnitude of the inside positivity now approximates the *sodium equilibrium potential*.

outside than inside, can diffuse into the cell. This faster efflux of K⁺ leaves behind unbalanced negative charges (A⁻), which cause the inside to become negative with respect to the outside (see Figure 13-1A). But because Na⁺ does enter the cell (albeit slowly), this influx would ultimately neutralize the inside negativity if it were not counteracted by the active transport

of Na⁺ out of the cell, via the adenosine triphosphate–dependent Na⁺-K⁺ pump. For the purpose of this chapter, however, we do not spend any more time on this active transport system.

As K⁺ leaves the cell, the inside becomes increasingly negative until electrostatic attraction halts further net efflux. The semipermeable membrane has therefore acted to separate charges (polarization), which is a voltage. The negativity attained by the faster efflux of K⁺, coupled with the extrusion of Na⁺ by the pump, creates the *resting membrane potential*. However, If K⁺ was the only ion that could permeate the membrane, the transmembrane potential would attain the *potassium equilibrium potential* as calculated by the Nernst equation.[5] However, because Na⁺ does *leak* in slowly, the measured transmembrane potential is a little less negative than the calculated potassium equilibrium potential (Figure 13-2A).[6] The resting membrane potential is the transmembrane potential that is recorded when the cell (nerve or muscle) is not conducting an AP (i.e., the cell is at *rest*). The resting membrane potential, however, is not the same for all cells. For mammalian nerve fibers, the value is approximately –80 mV, for muscle fibers it is closer to –90 mV, and for alpha anterior horn cells it is approximately –60 mV.[7]

Permeability of the membrane to the various ions is not fixed.[8] If a nerve membrane is depolarized quickly by approximately 20 mV, such as from –80 to –60 mV, permeability to Na⁺ begins to increase (*threshold*) and rapidly becomes considerably greater than the permeability to K⁺ (Figure 13-1B). Because Na⁺ is more concentrated outside the fiber than inside, and because the inside is negative with respect to the outside, an *electrochemical gradient* drives Na⁺ into the cell. This influx of positive charges quickly causes (within 1–2 msec) an actual reversal of the transmembrane potential so that the inside of the membrane in that region becomes positive by 30–40 mV. This value approximates the *sodium equilibrium potential*, which is the transmembrane potential calculated by the Nernst equation if Na⁺ was the only permeating ion (see Figure 13-2A). This reversal of the transmembrane potential is the AP, which is the physiological means by which the adjacent region of membrane is subsequently brought to its own threshold, and the sequence repeated.

While the previously mentioned process is occurring, the region that initiated the AP repolarizes. This comes about because of sodium permeability rapidly decreasing accompanied by an increase in potassium permeability.[8] An orchestrated sequence of transmembrane voltage and

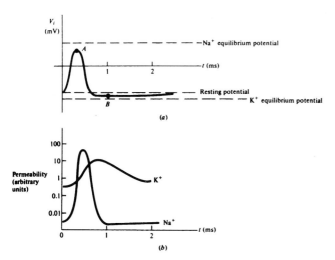

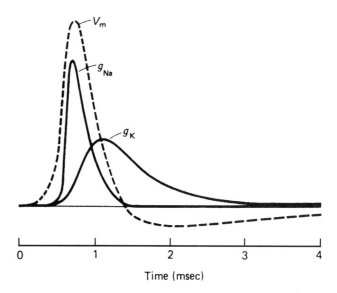

Time (msec)

FIGURE 13-2 **A.** An action potential at a point and its relationship to the sodium equilibrium potential, potassium equilibrium potential, and resting membrane potential. Point A represents the height of the action potential, which approximates the sodium equilibrium potential. Point B represents the maximum repolarization (hyperpolarization) achieved during recovery from the action potential, which approximates the potassium equilibrium potential. Note that the resting potential is a little less negative than the potassium equilibrium potential, which is because of the small influx of sodium. **B.** Representative permeabilities of potassium and sodium. At time zero (before the action potential is generated), K^+ permeability is much higher than Na^+. As the membrane depolarizes to threshold, Na^+ permeability increases sharply and exceeds K^+ permeability. After the height of the action potential is reached, Na^+ permeability drops rapidly and K^+ permeability increases to repolarize the membrane. (Reprinted with permission from JW Kane, MM Sternheim. Physics [formerly Life Science Physics]. New York: Wiley, 1978.)

FIGURE 13-3 Orchestrated sequence of the interaction between the transmembrane potential (V_m), and relative ease with which Na^+ and K^+ pass through the membrane. In this example, g is *conductance* (the reciprocal of resistance), which is an electrical way of measuring permeability. The difference between this figure and Figure 13-2 is that here all the changes are superimposed on a single baseline that represents the resting level for the three measurements. In Figure 13-2, one sees a representation of the relative differences in permeabilities at rest. Also, by superimposing the three traces, one gets a better impression of how the membrane potential starts depolarizing to threshold because of electrotonic spread before the permeability changes. (Reprinted with permission from ER Kandel, JH Schwartz. Principles of Neural Science [2nd ed]. New York: Elsevier, 1985.)

permeability changes thus interact to produce the AP and recovery from it (Figures 13-2B and 13-3). The region of membrane that has gone through this sequence requires approximately 2–5 msec before it can generate another AP. This *refractory period*, which has an *absolutely refractory* and *relatively refractory* component, places an upper limit on the number of APs a membrane can conduct per second. For example, if a membrane's refractory period (ignoring differences between absolutely and relatively refractory) is 5 msec, the highest frequency with which it could conduct APs would be 200 per second. This does not mean that these fibers actually conduct at these frequencies, but that they could if the refractory period was the only factor influencing their behavior.

The electrical stimulation that is used for performing conduction studies brings the axons (motor or sensory)

of the nerve to threshold, and once threshold is reached (or exceeded), the stimulated fibers conduct APs along their length.

Although plasma membranes have been described as "protein sandwiches on lipid bread," this grossly underestimates the constitution and complex physiology of excitable membranes. The permeability phenomena described previously are caused, in part, by dynamic *channels* in these membranes through which the different ions pass. Ions do not simply diffuse randomly through the membranes, but rather through specific channels, whose configurations change depending on the transmembrane voltage. In addition, these channels are not uniformly spaced along the membranes, especially in the case of myelinated fibers. This clustering of channels is described further as we delve deeper into conduction along myelinated and unmyelinated fibers.

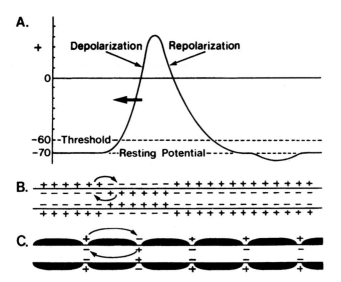

FIGURE 13-4 A. Terms for the various components of the action potential. The arrow indicates the action potential is propagating right to left. **B.** Continuous conduction in an unmyelinated nerve. **C.** Saltatory conduction in a myelinated nerve. In both **B** and **C** the inside region that is conducting the action potential is positive with respect to both the outside and adjacent inside regions. Note how this inside positivity depolarizes by electrotonic spread the adjacent inside region in **B**, whereas it skips to the next node in **C**. (Reprinted with permission from SJ Oh. Clinical Electromyography: Nerve Conduction Studies. Baltimore: University Park Press, 1984;7.)

How Action Potentials Are Conducted

Once an AP is raised in a region, it is conducted from that region to the next (Figure 13-4).[9] Two types of conduction along excitable membranes are recognized. These are *continuous*, a term popularized, although not introduced, by Bostock and Sears,[10] and *saltatory*. Continuous conduction occurs when an AP depolarizes the next, immediately adjacent region of membrane (perhaps 100–200 μm distant), to its own threshold (Figure 13-4B). Continuous conduction occurs in small steps, much like the short, shuffling gait of Parkinson's disease, so that conduction is relatively slow. This is normally the way conduction proceeds along unmyelinated nerves and muscle fibers. Saltatory conduction occurs along myelinated nerve fibers, where an AP generated at one node of Ranvier raises the next node to its threshold (Figure 13-4C). This next node may be 1–3 mm (1,000–3,000 μm) away, which although still a short distance, is considerably further away than the next adjacent region mentioned for continuous conduction. Indeed, this skipping or jumping from node to node (*saltare*, meaning *to jump*) is like taking relatively large

steps during gait, which is faster and more energy efficient than a shuffling gate.

Appreciating the similarities and differences between continuous and saltatory conduction helps one to better understand the consequences of demyelinating conditions, and why they produce either slowing or conduction block (*neurapraxia*).

Continuous Conduction

At the peak of the AP, the interior of the axon at that spot is approximately 40 mV positive with respect to the outside (see Figure 13-2A). This implies an overall transmembrane potential change of approximately 120 mV. However, this region of axoplasm is not only positive with respect to the outside of the membrane, it is also positive with respect to the adjacent inside region of axoplasm (see Figures 13-4B and C). This inside positivity depolarizes the adjacent region to threshold (described later), and the sequence is then repeated on down the fiber. Therefore, the AP, which is a local transmembrane event, becomes propagated via this sequential activation of adjacent regions. How does this activation of the next adjacent region occur?

The positive region of axoplasm influences the adjacent region by a passive mechanism called *local current flow* or *electrotonic spread*, first described by Hodgkin.[11] Two other terms used to describe this type of spread are the *length constant*, symbolized by the Greek letter λ, and the *time constant*, symbolized by the Greek letter τ. These are components of the so-called cable properties of elongated fibers[5] and significantly affect how quickly the fiber conducts from point to point.

Unlike the AP, which is propagated in an all-or-none fashion, electrotonic spread decays exponentially with distance. The length constant (λ) is a measure of how far down the membrane a certain percentage of the potential is *felt*. Similarly, the time constant (τ), is a measure of how fast the transmembrane potential changes because of electrotonic spread. The presence, or absence of myelin, affects both of these constants.

Electrotonic spread can be described, in part, in terms of electronic circuitry.[6] The positive charges that are inside the membrane in the region that has spiked have basically two pathways along which they can move. One is longitudinally along the axoplasm itself (i.e., staying within the axon), and the second is transversely out of the axon, across the adjacent region of membrane, back into the extracellular fluid. These pathways along which current can divide describe a *parallel circuit*. In such an arrangement, current, in this case the movement of positive charges, the Na$^+$ ions, divides between the possible pathways, with more current flowing along the one with the lower resistance. In the case of unmyelinated nerves or muscle fibers, the transmembrane resistance is relatively low, permitting much of the current to leak out relatively close to the region that generated the AP. As a result, the length constant of these fibers is relatively short, and the AP is only capable of depolarizing the next adjacent region to threshold. In other words, the AP's sphere of influence is relatively short.

The interplay of the transmembrane and axoplasmic resistances on a fiber's length constant is approximated mathematically by the formula:

$$\lambda = \sqrt{r_m/r_a}$$

where r_m is the transmembrane resistance, and r_a is the axoplasmic resistance. As seen, λ increases as the ratio of these resistances increases.

In addition to transmembrane resistance, membranes also have *capacitance* that affects how quickly these membrane changes occur.[6]

Saltatory Conduction and the Function of Myelin

Although electrotonic spread also plays a role in how myelinated nerves conduct, the length constant of these nerves is considerably longer than in unmyelinated nerves. This longer length constant is caused by myelin making the fiber's transmembrane resistance much greater than the axoplasmic resistance (as shown by the foregoing equation), thereby shunting the current longitudinally down the axon, instead of letting it leak out across the membrane. As a result, an AP at one node of Ranvier, where the axolemma is bare of myelin, is capable of influencing the next node in the chain, instead of the next immediately adjacent patch of membrane (see Figure 13-4C).

Another benefit associated with myelin and saltatory conduction is that because the AP is generated only at the nodes, sodium channels, which can open or close depending on the membrane potential, can be concentrated at the nodes. They are not necessary along the internode (i.e., along the membrane under the myelin itself). Estimates of sodium channel densities have yielded values ranging from approximately 1,000–12,000/µm^2 of nodal membrane, depending on the assay technique,[12,13] whereas along the internodal membrane, there are just a few sodium channels, estimated as <25/µm^2 by some sources.[12] By contrast, nerves that

are normally unmyelinated (i.e., those that normally propagate impulses by continuous conduction) have approximately 100–200 sodium channels per µm^2 of membrane.[13] The distribution of potassium channels, which is different from sodium channels, is not reviewed.

These findings lead to some interesting hypotheses concerning the etiology of conduction block in conditions that cause acute demyelination. For example, the length constant of the denuded membrane is shortened, meaning that the AP at the last intact node is not *felt* as far down the membrane as it would have been normally. This decrease in λ would lead to more *continuous* conduction, but the now denuded membrane does not have enough sodium channels to generate an AP.[14] Furthermore, the denuded membrane has a higher capacitance than myelin, which leads to a longer time required for the membrane to depolarize to threshold. And the longer it takes for a membrane to depolarize to threshold, the more chance there is for accommodation to take place.[7] The clinical consequence of acute demyelination is conduction block, or neurapraxia.

Recovery from conduction block can occur over time. One mechanism for this is the incorporation of sodium channels into the internodal membrane so that the density of these channels increases to the level needed for continuous conduction to occur. Evidence now exists that this changed distribution of sodium channels is not caused by redistribution of channels from the original node, such as by *lateral diffusion* away from the nodal membrane, but is caused by synthesis of new channels and their incorporation into the demyelinated segments.[15,16] A second mechanism for recovery from conduction block is remyelination of the denuded segments.[17] With either of these mechanisms, however, conduction is slowed until myelination has progressed. However, slow conduction is better than no conduction, similar to the fact that halitosis is better than no breath at all.

Factors Influencing Conduction Velocity

Four factors influence conduction velocity. These are (1) the diameter of the nerve fiber, (2) the thickness of the myelin sheath, (3) temperature, and (4) age.

Diameter of the Nerve Fiber

All other things being equal, the larger the diameter of the fiber, the faster the conduction velocity. Also, large-diameter fibers have a lower threshold to electrical stimulation than small-diameter fibers.

Thickness of the Myelin Sheath

As already described, myelin increases conduction velocity by increasing the nerve's length constant. Up to a certain thickness, myelin is a more efficient means for increasing conduction velocity than is increasing the fiber's diameter. For example, a 20-μm diameter myelinated nerve, which is the diameter of the axon *plus* the encircling myelin, such as found in mammals, conducts much faster than the squid giant axon, which can be as large as 500 μm (or 0.5 mm), but is unmyelinated. Myelin permits *miniaturizing* the nervous system so that speed can be obtained without excessive fiber diameter.

Temperature

Cooling a limb profoundly affects conduction in both sensory and motor fibers. Conduction velocity decreases approximately 2.0–2.4 m per second for each degree Centigrade drop (for in-depth reviews, see other references).[18,19] In general practice, skin temperature is determined at a site between the stimulating and recording electrodes. Dumitru recommends that this tempera-

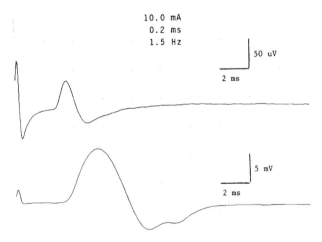

FIGURE 13-5 Median nerve stimulation at the wrist is shown producing an antidromic sensory nerve action potential recorded from index finger (*top*) and orthodromic compound muscle action potential from thenar eminence (*bottom*). Both recordings made simultaneously to 10 mA stimulus. Note the difference in sensitivity between the two channels necessitated by the different amplitudes of sensory nerve action potentials and compound muscle action potentials (as explained in text). Note also the shorter sensory nerve action potential latency despite a longer conduction distance (14 versus 5 cm). This is explained, partially, by the fact that the motor latency includes slower conduction along small-diameter terminal nerve fibers, synaptic delay, and activation of muscle fibers. Palm temperature was 32.5°C.

ture be at least 32°C for the upper extremities and 30°C for the lower extremities.[19] Examining a cold limb may indeed result in a false-positive (abnormal) conduction velocity.

Age

Full-term infants may conduct only approximately one-half of adult values. Velocity then increases and attains adult values by the age of 5. Conduction then decreases again after approximately the age of 60, but does not particularly become *abnormal*. Obviously, clinicians must keep these age factors in mind when interpreting findings.[20–23]

Orthodromic and Antidromic Conduction

When a peripheral nerve fiber is stimulated by an electrical current, such as at the level of the wrist, depolarization occurs under the cathode (negative electrode), and if threshold is reached, the stimulated fiber then generates an AP. This AP conducts away from the point of stimulation *in both directions*. Take, for example, stimulating the median nerve, a mixed nerve, at the wrist using a stimulus amplitude strong enough to excite motor and sensory fibers (Figure 13-5). Looking first at the motor axons, APs that travel away from the point of stimulation into the intrinsic hand muscles are conducting *orthodromically*, whereas APs in these same fibers moving in the other direction from the point of stimulation are traveling *antidromically*. Conversely, in response to the same stimulation at the wrist, but looking now at sensory fibers, APs that conduct into the hand are traveling antidromically, whereas APs that travel up toward the CNS are traveling *orthodromically*. In other words, whether an AP is moving antidromically or orthodromically depends on which direction the APs normally conduct in the nerve under investigation.

Let us now consider what happens when motor axons are stimulated, concentrating on the consequences of the orthodromic impulses.

Neuromuscular Transmission and Muscle Contraction

A single motor axon, the axoplasmic extension of an anterior horn cell, projects within a peripheral nerve, and after entering its target muscle, branches into a number of terminal nerve fibers. Ultimately, each terminal nerve fiber innervates a single muscle fiber, at the muscle fiber's *end-plate*, which is a specialized region of the sarcolemma containing acetylcholine

(ACh) receptors. Because a motor axon gives rise to terminal nerve fibers, one axon actually innervates many muscle fibers. This neuromuscular arrangement is the *motor unit*, and the number of muscle fibers innervated by a single anterior horn cell is the *motor unit ratio*. If the axon conducts an AP, because of either voluntary or reflex activation of the anterior horn cell, or because of artificial activation of the axon, such as by an electrical stimulus, that AP is conducted along the length of the axon, then along each of the terminal nerve fibers, and finally to the distal terminus of these terminal nerves.

The distal end of the terminal nerve fiber is specialized and contains the neuromuscular transmitter ACh. ACh is released in response to the AP, diffuses across the small space separating the nerve's terminus from the end-plate membrane, and combines with ACh receptors in the end-plate membrane, which produces a permeability change of this membrane. If this permeability change is great enough, the end-plate membrane depolarizes to threshold, and another AP is generated along the sarcolemma, moving away from the end-plate. The region where the terminal nerve fiber comes into this close association with the end-plate is the *neuromuscular junction*, and the events just described make up the *neuromuscular transmission*.

Most human skeletal muscle fibers contain a single end-plate that is located approximately midway along the fiber's length. This was originally demonstrated histochemically by Coërs using a cholinesterase *stain*.[24] Therefore, an AP originating at the end-plate spreads away from it in either direction. Furthermore, this AP only has to propagate approximately one-half the length of the fiber, because it originates at the fiber's midpoint, approximately.

Another consequence of end-plates being at about each fiber's middle is that *end-plate zones*, the region in a muscle where the neuromuscular junctions of the skeletal muscle fibers are concentrated, have different configurations depending on the internal architecture of a muscle. For example, muscles that are fusiform, have fibers that run tendon to tendon, parallel to the long axis of the muscle. In these muscles, the end-plate zone runs perpendicular to the muscle's long axis, at about the muscle's middle. Many of the muscles that are routinely recorded in motor nerve conduction studies, such as the abductor pollicis brevis (median nerve), abductor digiti minimi (ulnar nerve), and extensor digitorum brevis (peroneal nerve), have this architecture. The consequences of this are described shortly. Muscles that are pennate, bipennate, or multi-pennate have fibers that are oriented at angles to the long axis of the muscle, and as a result, have different orientations of their end-plate zones.[25]

An AP, originating at an end-plate and then propagating along a muscle fiber, serves as the first step in the sequence called *excitation-contraction coupling*. The specifics of this need not be gone into here, but suffice it to say that the muscle fiber develops tension (i.e., it contracts). It is important to remember that the electrophysiological events recorded from the surface of a muscle when performing a motor conduction study are reflections of the sarcolemmal depolarizations, not the contraction itself.

HOW RECORDINGS ARE MADE

The electrical voltages generated by the membranes of nerves and muscles are approximately 120 mV (0.12 V), give or take a little. This is not a large voltage to begin with, but when recorded by surface electrodes, the amplitudes are even smaller. The fact that voltages can be recorded at distances from these generators is because of the body being a *volume conductor*. This means that in response to a changing voltage (such as an AP), current flows through the electrolyte solution of the body, and this current flow can be detected at a distance. Current flow, however, decreases with distance, so the voltage detected decreases considerably. In addition, the intervening tissue, and the electrode-skin interface, act as *low-pass filters*, further altering the amplitude and shape of these potentials. In essence, waveforms become lower in amplitude, less steep, and more rounded, the greater the distance. Indeed, the potentials recorded by the clinical neurophysiologist are quite different in size and shape from those detected by the basic neurophysiologist using microelectrodes. Despite these differences, however, potentials recorded clinically are quite useful, keeping in mind their strengths and weaknesses.

To detect the biological voltages recorded clinically (i.e., those ranging from 10^{-6} to 10^{-3} V [μV to mV]), *differential amplifiers* are used. These amplifiers perform two major functions. First, they amplify the potential difference (voltage) between two electrodes, thereby making these potentials recordable. Their second function is to reject potentials coming from other sources that might interfere with recording the signals of interest (i.e., they reject *noise*). It is beyond the scope of this chapter to describe how this and other technical requirements are accomplished, but reviews are available.[26,27]

Figure 13-6 depicts schematically how an AP propagating along a membrane is detected and displayed using a differential amplifier.[28] Note in particular the following points:

- The electrodes are outside the membranes of interest, as opposed to microelectrodes, which record inside cells.
- An AP propagating along the surface of a membrane is a region of negativity compared with both the inside of the cell (the transmembrane potential) and with respect to regions outside the membrane that are not active (the longitudinal potential).
- The electrode under which the AP first appears is connected to the negative-up input of the preamplifier. This electrode that *sees* the potential first is sometimes referred to as the *active* electrode, with the distal one being the *reference* electrode. In truth, however, both electrodes are active, because a recording cannot be made with only one electrode (the ground electrode is being ignored for this description).

This figure also shows how a wave of negativity, propagating in one direction, can generate a biphasic (alternating) potential.

Figure 13-7 diagrams how recordings are made clinically.[28] When performing motor nerve conduction studies, electrodes are placed over a muscle. The active electrode is at about the muscle's midpoint, and the other electrode near the tendon of insertion. This is the so-called belly-tendon configuration with the active electrode closer to the muscle's *motor point*, where the nerve enters the muscle, than the distal electrode. Because APs in muscle originate at about each fiber's midpoint (as already described), and because a muscle such as the abductor pollicis brevis is fusiform in structure (as also described previously), the active electrode first becomes negative with respect to the distal electrode. Connecting this proximal electrode to the negative-up input of the preamplifier, usually produces a negative-first potential. Furthermore, because this potential is a summation of all the motor units stimulated, it is called a *compound muscle action potential* (CMAP).

When performing sensory nerve conduction studies, recordings are made from electrodes placed over, or around, sensory nerves. Regardless of whether recording orthodromically or antidromically, the electrode under which the AP first appears is connected to the negative-up input and is again referred to as the *active*

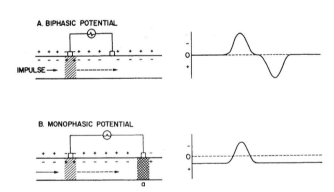

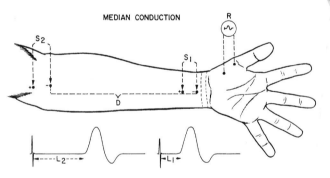

FIGURE 13-7 Procedure for motor conduction study on median nerve. S_1 = stimulus distally (at wrist, between tendons of flexor carpi radialis and palmaris longus); S_2 = stimulus proximally (at elbow, medial side of biceps tendon). For both stimulation sites, the cathode (–) is placed distal to the anode (+). R = recording electrodes over thenar eminence, with proximal (active) electrode connected to negative-up input of preamplifier. L_1 = distal latency (in milliseconds, wrist to muscle) measured to onset of negative phase of compound muscle action potential; L_2 = proximal latency (in milliseconds, elbow to muscle) also measured to onset of negative phase; D = distance (in mm) between cathodes S_1 and S_2. Conduction velocity = $D/(L_2 - L_1)$. Note also that the traces show the compound muscle action potentials originating with negative (upward) phases, as expected.

FIGURE 13-6 A. Representation of how an action potential (*hatched area*), which is a wave of negativity propagating along the outside of an excitable membrane, generates a biphasic waveform when recorded with two electrodes that are also outside of the membrane. The first electrode reached (the *active* electrode) is connected to the *negative-up* input of the preamplifier. Conversely, if the second (or *reference*) electrode becomes negative with respect to the active, the deflection will be down. B. A monophasic potential can be recorded if the reference electrode is over a region of nerve that has been rendered unable to conduct the action potential. In this situation, only the first electrode becomes negative, so no reversal of the recording occurs.

electrode. The waveform recorded is again a summation, but this time of nerve potentials, not muscle potentials. This is the *sensory nerve action potential* (SNAP).

On occasion, a mixed nerve is stimulated distally and recordings made over the same nerve proximally, such as stimulating the median nerve at the wrist and recording over it at the elbow. In this situation, the potential recorded proximally contains contributions from motor fibers conducting antidromically and sensory fibers conducting orthodromically. This mixed nerve potential is sometimes referred to simply as the *nerve action potential*.

Clinical Applications

The clinical neurophysiologist rarely stimulates or records from single nerve fibers. Most clinical studies, especially those routinely performed under the aegis of *electrodiagnosis*, are directed at nerves containing perhaps hundreds of axons. Furthermore, because stimulating and recording electrodes are usually placed on the surface of the body overlying some target nerve, muscle, or both, the stimulation amplitude required to reach threshold for the various fibers depends, in part, on the thickness of the intervening tissues and the electrical characteristics of these tissues (filtering effects, impedances, and so forth). Similarly, the amplitude and configuration of responses recorded by surface electrodes are influenced by these factors. Thus, the laboratory preparation investigated by the clinical neurophysiologist introduces complications not encountered by the basic physiologist.

A basic dictum in neurophysiology is the all-or-none law. In essence, this means that a subthreshold stimulus does not excite a nerve fiber, whereas a stimulus that is either threshold or above threshold causes the fiber to conduct at a velocity and amplitude that is maximum for that fiber (assuming unchanging conditions of temperature, oxygenation, and so forth). A corollary of this is that a single fiber does not produce graded velocities or graded AP amplitudes, all other factors being kept constant. In other words, the fiber either conducts maximally or it does not conduct at all. However, peripheral nerves stimulated in situ are composed of many axons, all of which are situated at slightly different locations from the stimulating electrodes. For these reasons, once threshold for the most sensitive axons has been reached, further increases in stimulating amplitudes cause stepwise increases in recorded responses, until all of the axons making up the nerve have been stimulated (Figure 13-8). When further increases in stimulating amplitude no longer result in corresponding

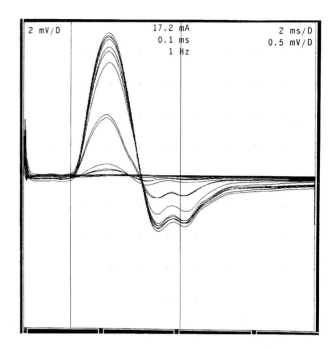

FIGURE 13-8 Increasing stimulus intensities produce increasing compound muscle action potential amplitudes (stimulating median nerve at wrist, recording from thenar eminence). This is not a negation of the all-or-none law, but demonstrates that a peripheral nerve contains many axons that have different thresholds to electrical stimulation. This difference in threshold is caused, in part, by different distances from the stimulating electrodes at the surface of the wrist. Therefore, as explained in the text, stimulation must be high enough to ensure that all fibers are activated.

increases in recorded amplitude, the stimulus is said to be *supramaximal*.

Most motor and sensory conduction studies performed during an electrodiagnostic examination employ supramaximum stimulation. This is done to ensure that all the axons in the target nerve are stimulated. More is said about this below.

MOTOR NERVE CONDUCTION STUDIES

Conduction velocity in motor fibers is determined by stimulating a nerve at two points along its length and recording, for each point of stimulation, the CMAP generated from a distal muscle innervated by that nerve (see Figure 13-7).[28] The arrangement of recording electrodes has already been described.

To calculate the conduction velocity of the fastest conducting fibers to the muscle, supramaximum stimulation is employed. At both the proximal and distal stimulation sites, the *cathode*, or negative electrode, of the stimulator is placed on the nerve distal to the anode. The *latency*, or time to the onset of the initial negative phase of the CMAP, is determined for both the distal and proximal points of stimulation. The distance between the two cathode sites of stimulation is measured and divided by the difference in latency between the proximal and distal points. The formula used is

$$\text{Velocity (m/second)} = \frac{\text{distance (mm)}}{\text{latency difference (msec)}}$$

Note that a single latency is not used to calculate a conduction velocity for motor nerves. This is because a single latency to a CMAP includes factors in addition to conduction along the stimulated axon. As described previously, these other factors must include (1) conduction along terminal nerve fibers, which are smaller diameter than the parent axon and therefore conduct slower; (2) neuromuscular transmission delay, including release of ACh, its diffusion across the space between the nerve and end-plate membrane, and its binding to ACh-receptors; (3) generation of the end-plate potential (EPP); and (4) subsequent conduction along the sarcolemma, which is also slower than along the parent axon. Therefore, when recording from a muscle, a single latency does not accurately reflect conduction along a measured distance between the point of stimulation and the recording electrodes.

To eliminate the extraneous factors enumerated previously, the strategy used to determine conduction velocity along only peripheral motor axons is to subtract the distal latency from the proximal latency. Because both the proximal and distal latencies include the extraneous factors, this subtraction yields a *latency difference* that represents the conduction time along the length of nerve between the two points of stimulation. Note also that these extraneous factors are not a problem when recording directly from a nerve, as opposed to a muscle, because neuromuscular delay, and so forth, is not an issue (see the section Sensory Nerve Conduction Studies).

It should also be noted, however, that there are times when single latencies are useful. The reader, therefore, must not conclude from the previous discussion that distal latencies are only important for their *subtraction value.* Indeed, a prolonged latency across a distal compression site, such as in carpal tunnel syndrome, can yield important localizing information.

A word of caution, however, is required. If stimulus amplitude is too strong, latency can decrease, not because of faster conducting fibers being stimulated, but because of a distal shift of the *effective cathode*.[29,30] In other words, with strong stimulation, the stimulus spreads to a point somewhat distal to where the physical cathode is placed, thereby fictitiously shortening the latency. The moral of this is to *tailor* stimulus amplitude to each patient (e.g., not more than 25% above that needed to produce a maximum evoked response). Do not employ the maximum strength of the stimulator just because it is available.

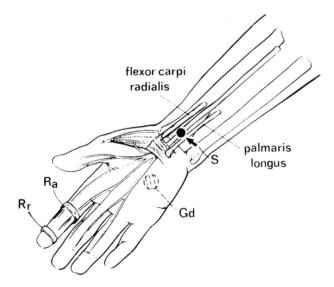

FIGURE 13-9 Technique for performing an antidromic sensory nerve action potential of the median nerve. (Gd = ground; R_a = active recording electrode around interphalangeal joint of digit II; R_r = reference electrode between distal phalanx and tip of finger; S = stimulating cathode at wrist.) (Reprinted with permission from DM Ma, JA Liveson. Nerve Conduction Handbook. Philadelphia: F.A. Davis, 1983.)

SENSORY NERVE CONDUCTION STUDIES

Unlike motor conduction studies that record electrical activity from muscle, sensory techniques record activity generated as the nerves conduct up to, and past, the recording electrodes. Two strategies are available to accomplish this. The *orthodromic* technique stimulates distally, such as with ring electrodes encircling a digit to excite the digital nerves, and record proximally from surface electrodes overlying that nerve, such as at the wrist. The second method, the *antidromic* technique, reverses the stimulating and recording electrodes, so that stimulation is applied proximally and recording is done distally (Figure 13-9).[31] Recall that this is possible because peripheral nerve fibers conduct in both directions when stimulated directly.

TABLE 13-1

Suggested Amplifier Settings for Nerve Conduction Studies

Nerve	Low Frequency (Hz)	High Frequency (Hz)	Sensitivity[a] per Division
Motor nerve	2–5	10,000	2–10 mV[b]
Sensory nerve	5–10	2,000–3,000	10–20 µV[b]
Mixed nerve	5–10	2,000–3,000	10–20 µV[b]

[a]*Sensitivity* is the display resolution of amplified signals, expressed in microvolts (µV) or millivolts (mV) per vertical screen division.[27] Note also that decreasing values, for example going from 20 µV/div to 10 µV/div, means an *increase* in sensitivity. Therefore, sensory nerve action potentials and nerve action potentials, which are low-amplitude potentials, require higher sensitivity than compound muscle action potentials.

[b]Be prepared to adjust up or down depending on amplitude obtained.

Another difference between motor and sensory conduction studies relates to the amplitudes of the recorded potentials. CMAPs represent the summated activity generated by the muscle fibers of the target muscle, and there are many more muscle fibers in a muscle than the number of motor axons innervating it, as described earlier. CMAPs, therefore, are considerably larger than SNAPs, which are generated by a much smaller number of axons. In addition, SNAPs recorded antidromically are larger than SNAPs recorded orthodromically. This is not a negation of the all-or-none law, nor is it evidence that axons conduct differently depending on direction of travel. Anatomically, sensory nerves become more superficial distally. For example, digital nerves are nearer the surface in the digit than they are when at the level of the wrist. Therefore, the antidromic technique detects higher amplitudes than the orthodromic technique.

Table 13-1 presents recommended amplifier filter settings and sensitivity for performing motor, sensory, and mixed nerve studies. Note how the sensitivity values reflect the expected differences described previously. It should also be noted that these are only recommended settings to get started on a study. In any particular patient, settings may need to be changed depending on the responses recorded. Table 13-2 presents suggested stimulator settings.

Clinical Measurements

In the original paper on performing motor nerve conduction velocity determinations in humans, Hodes et al. reported in "several subjects," values ranging from

TABLE 13-2

Suggested Stimulator Settings for Nerve Conduction Studies

Stimulator	Two types of stimulators are available: constant voltage (a measure of *strength* of stimulus), and constant current (a measure of *intensity* of stimulus).
Waveform	Monophasic rectangular (also known as *interrupted DC* or *interrupted galvanic*). The main characteristics describing a waveform are its shape, amplitude (in terms of volts of milliamps), and duration. How strong a stimulus feels is a function of both amplitude and duration.
Polarity	Cathode (negative electrode) positioned closer to recording electrodes than anode (positive electrode).
Duration	0.1 msec (100 µsec), but be prepared to increase if response has not reached maximum. Can go to 1 msec for H-reflex studies.
Strength (V) or intensity (ma)	Most routine studies use supramaximum amplitude (i.e., amplitude of stimulation approximately 25% above that which no longer produces an increasing evoked response). See the section Clinical Applications in the text for more details.
Frequency	Most common is 1/second (1 Hz), but can drop to 0.5/second (1 every 2 seconds) for H-reflex studies and can increase for neuromuscular transmission studies. See the section Clinical Applications in the text for more details.

"46 to 67 meters per second for the various nerves investigated."[1] They found, similar to what is reported today, that nerves of the upper extremities tend to conduct a little faster than nerves of the lower extremities.[32-35] Various explanations have been put forth to account for this finding, including temperature differences between upper and lower extremities, and the distribution of axon diameters in nerves of the upper and lower extremities.[32] Regardless of the cause, however, the clinical neurophysiologist needs to be aware of what the values are normally so that departures from normal are recognized.

Table 13-3 shows representative values for some of the more commonly studied motor and sensory nerves.[33] There are more recent publications that enumerate other nerves and the techniques for studying them,[31,34] but they are beyond the purpose of this chapter, which is to concentrate on the underlying physiology.

It was indicated earlier that motor nerve conduction velocities are determined using the proximal and distal latencies measured to the onset of the CMAP. This technique yields the velocity of the fastest conducting fibers.

TABLE 13-3
Nerve Conduction Measurements and H-Reflex Latency in Control Population of Adult Subjects without Evidence of Neuromuscular Disease

Peripheral Nerve	No. of Nerves	Range (m/second)	Mean (m/second)	Standard Deviation
Peroneal (motor) knee to ankle	49	42.1–63.5	52.1	4.9
Posterior tibial (motor) knee to ankle	30	39.8–66.9	49.9	5.2
Ulnar (motor) elbow to wrist	47	46.5–72.6	59.9	5.7
Median (motor) elbow to wrist	45	46.1–72.1	56.9	5.8
Ulnar (sensory) finger to wrist	52	41.7–59.4	49.4	4.7
Ulnar (sensory) finger to elbow	38	45.3–60.2	55.2	3.5
Median (sensory) finger to wrist	48	36.4–65.4	52.0	36.1
Median (sensory) finger to elbow	36	42.4–61.7	55.9	5.8
H-reflex latency	32	26.5–34.0	29.8	1.8

Source: Reprinted with permission from JAR Lenman. Clinical Electromyography. Philadelphia: Lippincott, 1970;54.

However, there is more information in the recorded CMAP than only how fast the fastest fibers conduct. These other issues are now considered (Figure 13-10).[19]

Although depolarization of motor units innervated by the fastest conducting motor axons generates the onset of the CMAP's initial negative phase, the *amplitude* of the CMAP, usually determined by the maximum height of the negative phase of the potential, is a function of how many motor units in the muscle are innervated, and how synchronously they contribute to the CMAP. For example, a muscle that has recently lost, for example, 90% of its innervating axons, demonstrates a markedly reduced CMAP amplitude. Therefore, the range of normal amplitudes obtained from different muscles is another factor to be considered when interpreting the clinical significance of data.

The *duration*, or *temporal dispersion* of the CMAP, is another parameter that reflects the synchrony of motor unit activation. It is measured from the beginning of the response to the point at which the isoelectric line is re-established. A major determinant of CMAP duration is the spread of conduction velocities among the many axons making up the motor nerve. Differences between the fastest and slowest conducting axons have been reported as 4–7 m per second for the ulnar nerve,[35] whereas for the same nerve, but using a somewhat different calculation, others determined 10–20 m per second.[36] Dumitru[19] references Dorfman as reporting an average of 13 m per second.[37] But whatever the real value, the consequence is that in response to supramaximum stimulation, a volley of nerve APs reaches the muscle and activates the various motor units slightly asynchronously, thus producing a CMAP of a particular amplitude, shape, and duration.

Segmental demyelination, which can slow conduction to different degrees in different fibers, increases the spread of conduction velocities. This, in turn, increases the delay between activation of the various motor units, or desynchronization of the various motor unit potentials, thereby spreading out the overall shape of the CMAP (increasing its temporal dispersion). In addition, this desynchronization frequently decreases the maximum amplitude of the CMAP (Figure 13-11).[38]

Recall also, that another consequence of acute demyelination can be neurapraxia, or conduction block (see Neurapraxia [or Type I Lesion of Seddon], later in this chapter).

The area of the CMAP (measured in terms of mV seconds, which is the integration of the area under the negative and positive phases) is another quantification. Area takes into account both the amplitude and duration variables of the CMAP. Many electrophysiology units today have the software necessary to perform this determination, so the investigator is relieved of doing this manually.

All of the previously mentioned measurements are also performed on SNAPs, keeping in mind though, that the amplitudes are lower (microvolts instead of millivolts).

Clinical Applications

The purpose of an electrodiagnostic examination, of which conduction studies are a component, is to localize the lesion. In the sense being used here, *localize* can have two meanings. One is the usual concept, namely to determine if a focal problem can be identified, such as carpal tunnel syndrome or common peroneal neuropathy at the head of the fibula, or S-1 radiculopathy. In its

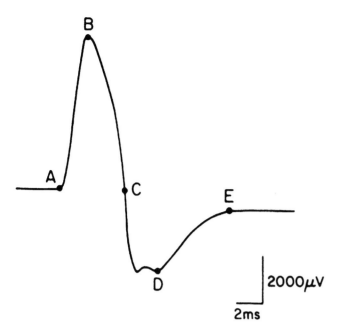

FIGURE 13-10 Example of compound muscle action potential in response to stimulation at wrist. Assuming stimulation occurred at the beginning of the trace, A represents onset latency and B represents peak latency. The time represented by segment A–B is the rise time; A–C is duration of negative phase, and A–E is total duration of the compound muscle action potential. The perpendicular distance from B to a line connecting A–C is the baseline-to-peak amplitude, whereas the perpendicular distance between B and D is peak-to-peak amplitude. (Adapted from D Dumitru. Electrodiagnostic Medicine. Philadelphia: Hanley & Belfus, 1995.)

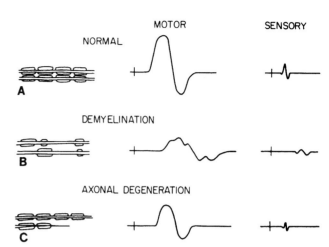

FIGURE 13-11 A. On left is a schematic representation of two normal axons with normal myelin sheaths. Normal evoked motor (compound muscle action potential) and sensory (sensory nerve action potential) responses are demonstrated. The small vertical line preceding the compound muscle action potential and the sensory nerve action potential is the stimulus artifact. Latencies are measured from this artifact to the response. B. In segmental demyelination, axis cylinders are preserved with random loss and attenuation of myelin internodes. The latency to the compound muscle action potential and sensory nerve action potential are increased compared with tracings in A. This increase in latency reflects the slower conduction in these axons. Also note the increased temporal dispersion and lower peak amplitudes of the responses. C. In axonal degeneration, the loss of axons causes reduction in the amplitude of the evoked responses (assuming enough axons have degenerated) and only a slight prolongation of latencies (because of loss of the fastest conducting axons). If all axons had degenerated, then no responses would have been elicited. (Reprinted with permission from G Kraft. Peripheral Neuropathies. In EW Johnson [ed], Practical Electromyography. Baltimore: Williams & Wilkins, 1980.)

second sense, *localize* can also mean localizing, for example, the lesion to the myelin sheath, such as the diffuse demyelination of peripheral nerves, as found in diabetic polyneuropathy, or localizing the lesion to the anterior horn cells, as in polio. Conduction studies are extremely helpful for this purpose, *even when the findings are negative.* Let us look now at the types of nerve lesions and how conduction studies can be used to achieve localization.

Neurapraxia (or Type I Lesion of Seddon)

Neurapraxia is a conduction block, believed to be caused by acute demyelination over a relatively restricted length of nerve.[39] As explained earlier, acute demyelination reduces the length constant of the membrane in that region, and the denuded internodes do not contain sufficient numbers of sodium channels to support even continuous conduction. Depending on how many and which axons in the nerve are affected, motor, sensory, or both motor and sensory loss distal to the site

of the lesion can be partial or complete. As an aside, local anesthetics, such as novocaine, lidocaine (Xylocaine), and so forth, produce a short-lived neurapraxia by chemical blocking of sodium channels, thereby prohibiting the generation of APs past the point of application.

The electrical strategy for identifying neurapraxia is to determine whether a significant difference exists in the size and shape of the CMAP, or SNAP, when stimulating proximal and distal to the site of the lesion. If a neuropraxic lesion is complete (i.e., all fibers are in a state of conduction block), stimulation proximal to the lesion produces no recordable responses distally, whereas stimulation distal to the lesion results in a *normal* response. In an incomplete lesion, however, stimu-

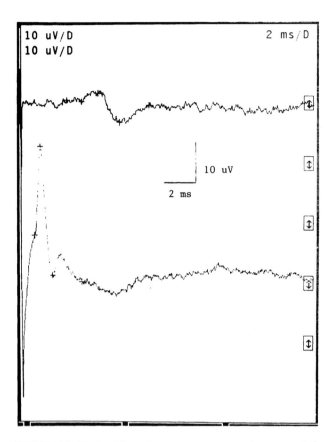

FIGURE 13-12 Antidromic sensory nerve action potentials evoked with stimulation proximal and distal to a presumed site of entrapment producing a partial neurapraxia. Patient was 8 months pregnant with clinical diagnosis of carpal tunnel syndrome. Recording electrodes around index finger. (*Top*) Response to stimulating median nerve at wrist, 14.5 cm proximal to active recording electrode. Sensory nerve action potential is low (7.2 μV), delayed (4.3 msec), and rounded. Initial negative phase is less well defined than the positive phase. (*Bottom*) Response to stimulating median nerve in palm (distal to transverse carpal ligament and presumed site of compression), 7.0 cm proximal to active recording electrode. Sensory nerve action potential has normal amplitude (32 μV), normal latency (1.02 msec), and normal configuration.

lation proximal to the lesion reveals a low-amplitude response compared with stimulation distal to the lesion (Figure 13-12). One caveat is necessary though. It must be remembered that even if a nerve is severed, the segment distal to the lesion retains its ability to respond to direct stimulation for a number of days. Therefore, within say, 4–5 days, both neurapraxia and axonal degeneration give similar findings to stimulation proximal and distal to the lesion. It is only after this time that differences between the two conditions become apparent, namely that conduction distal to the lesion is maintained in neurapraxia, whereas conduction begins to fail and then ceases within approximately 2 weeks, but sometimes sooner or later, with axonal degeneration.

Axonotmesis and Neuronotmesis (Type II and III Lesions of Seddon)

Both of these lesions are associated with axonal degeneration.[39] In the former, all connective tissue sheaths of the nerve (endoneurium, perineurium, and epineurium) remain intact. In other words, axonotmesis is a *lesion in continuity*, in which axons degenerate within their endoneurial sheaths. These endoneurial tubes, however, remain intact and can act as a guidance pathway for regeneration to the tissue normally innervated by the axons. Axonotmesis can occur from severe compression, which goes beyond the neurapraxic stage; diseases affecting the vasa nervosum, such as diabetic mononeuritis multiplex; alcoholic polyneuropathy; uremic polyneuropathy; and diseases of the anterior horn cells. In neuronotmesis, all connective tissue sheaths of the nerve are interrupted. This is a lesion in which nerve continuity is lost; a gap exists between proximal and distal stumps of the nerve. This can occur with penetrating injuries that cut a nerve, fractures that tear a nerve, and of course, amputation, followed by limb salvage.

From the neurophysiological standpoint, axonotmesis and neuronotmesis are indistinguishable. Both produce denervation of muscle and loss of conduction in affected axons. Certain clinical clues, however, can sometimes help in making this distinction. For example, axonotmesis is more likely in compressive rather than penetrating injuries.

For the purposes of this chapter, however, we concentrate on how either of these lesions, which for now we lump together under the heading of *axonal degeneration*, can present in a conduction study:

If the lesion is complete (i.e., all axons have degenerated), and the problem has been present for more than 2–3 weeks, stimulation of the nerve, motor or sensory, results in no responses, either clinically or electrically. If a single nerve is involved, only that nerve will demonstrate these *abnormal* findings, whereas other nerves will produce normal results. Thus, the lesion has been localized to a specific nerve, and indeed, perhaps to a specific region of the nerve. On the other hand, if the lesion is widespread, multiple nerves will be similarly affected.

If the lesion is incomplete (i.e., only some axons have degenerated), the findings then depend on how many, and which axons, are still intact. For example, if only a small percent of axons have degenerated, all conduction findings (latencies, velocities, amplitudes, durations) may still be within normal limits. If a large percent of axons have degenerated, amplitude of the evoked responses is lower than normal and conduction velocity may be a little slower than normal, but not as slow as when demyelination is the major pathology. The mild slowing to approximately 60% of normal noted in axonal lesions is believed to be caused by degeneration of the fastest conducting axons, thus unmasking those that normally conduct a little slower.[40] In other words, these normally slower conducting axons are now the fastest ones present in the nerve (see Figure 13-11).

It should also be noted that if a SNAP is unobtainable using standard methods of detection, *averaging* may reveal that a response is indeed present.[40] Recall that SNAPs are normally low amplitude (microvolts) and can become lost (buried) in the *noise* of the trace if only a few axons remain. When this occurs, the SNAP appears absent. Averaging, however, may reveal that a low-amplitude potential is indeed present, with a normal, or low normal, velocity or latency (Figure 13-13).

Demyelinating Lesions

The hallmark of conditions that produce demyelination or myelin distortion, with or without associated axonal degeneration, is marked slowing of conduction velocity, to less than 60% of normal, with or without evidence of associated conduction block and increased temporal dispersion (see Kimura[41] for a review). Furthermore, the presence of temporal dispersion, conduction block, or both may be accentuated as the distance between the stimulating and recording electrodes increases. This is because the longer conduction distances between stimulating and recording sites offer more chances for differential slowing (desynchronization) and conduction block of APs on their way to the recording site. It has also been reported that increased temporal dispersion and conduction block are more commonly seen in patients with acquired demyelinating neuropathies than in the familial forms.[42] In the latter, slowing of conduction is more uniform throughout the length of the nerve, leading to less drastic changes in waveform with distance.[42]

Mixed Lesions

Mixed lesions are those that contain any combination of conduction block, demyelination, and axonal degeneration.

Late Waves

Two types of late waves are described, the H reflex and the F wave. Both are usually recorded with surface electrodes placed over a target muscle, and both reflect con-

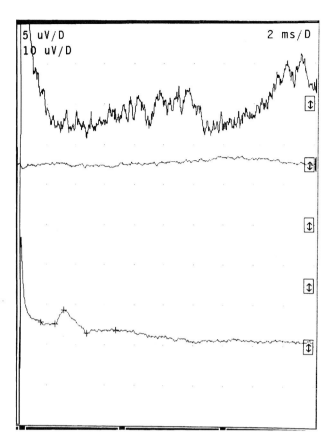

FIGURE 13-13 Ability of averaging to reveal conduction in sensory fibers in a patient with axonal neuropathy. Antidromic technique. (*Top*) No response obtained to single stimulus. (*Middle*) Average of 50 traces *without applying* a stimulus. This demonstrates that averaging 50 traces by itself does not produce a spurious response. (*Bottom*) Average of 50 traces *with stimulation*. Low-amplitude sensory nerve action potential clearly present (2.9 μV) with normal conduction velocity (57.7 m/second). Palm temperature was 33°C.

duction from the point of stimulation up into the spinal cord and then back down into the muscle. However, the pathways into the spinal cord (the afferent limb) are different, as are a number of other characteristics.

H Reflex

Named after Hoffmann,[43] who first described it, this late response requires a sensory input and a motor output, thereby qualifying as true reflex. The afferent limb is provided by Ia fibers, which conduct APs from the nuclear bag fibers of muscle spindles. Nuclear bag fibers are stretch receptors, and it is they that respond to the sudden stretch placed on a muscle when testing the so-called deep tendon reflexes (DTRs). Sudden muscle stretch, such as produced by briskly tapping a tendon, sends impulses into the spinal cord along the Ia fibers. These fibers monosynaptically excite α-anterior horn cells, which then send APs efferently back into the muscle stretched, thereby producing the muscle contraction observed clinically.

The H reflex is basically the electrical correlate of the DTR except for bypassing the muscle spindle.[44] Figure 13-14[45]

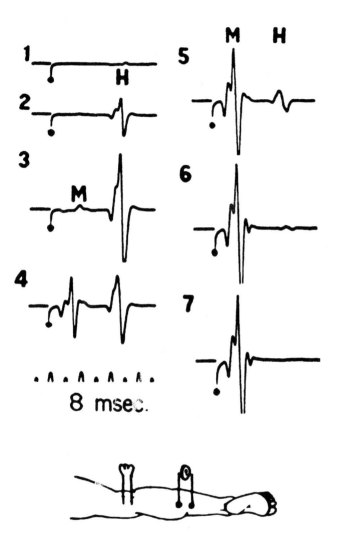

FIGURE 13-14 H-reflex (H) study stimulating posterior tibial nerve in popliteal fossa and recording from soleus muscle. Stimulus is increasing in amplitude from 1 to 7. Small dot indicates stimulus artifact. Note how H is elicited at low-stimulus amplitude and then grows bigger before becoming smaller and finally disappearing when muscle response (M) reaches its maximum. Largest M deflection was approximately 6 mV. (Reprinted with permission from JW Magladery, WE Porter, AM Park, RD Teasdall. Electrophysiological studies of nerve and reflex activity in normal man. IV. The two-neuron reflex and identification of certain action potentials from spinal roots and cord. Bull Johns Hopkins Hosp 1951;88:499–519.)

diagrams the experimental arrangement and the types of recordings obtained. With this arrangement, both the M wave, which is the direct motor response caused by orthodromic conduction in the motor fibers stimulated (the same as the CMAP we have already been talking about), and the H reflex are recorded. The M wave has an average latency of approximately 5 msec because it is traveling only from the popliteal fossa into the muscle. The H reflex, on the other hand, has a considerably longer latency because there is first afferent conduction into the spinal cord, synaptic delay (approximately 1 msec), and then conduction along the efferent axon back to the muscle.

A characteristic of the H reflex is that with increasing stimulus intensity, its amplitude first increases, but then decreases and ultimately disappears (see Figure 13-14). This behavior contrasts with the M wave, whose amplitude increases with increasing stimulus strength, finally reaching a maximum value. Furthermore, the H reflex disappears, or at least becomes remarkably smaller, at approximately the stimulus intensity producing the maximum M wave.

The H reflex is most easily elicited by stimulating the posterior tibial nerve in the popliteal fossa and recording from the soleus or medial gastrocnemius. It can also be obtained from the quadriceps (stimulating the femoral nerve), biceps brachii (stimulating the musculocutaneous nerve), triceps (stimulating the radial nerve), and flexor carpi radialis (stimulating the median nerve). Technically, including the issue of patient comfort, the posterior tibial and median nerves are the easiest to stimulate. Indeed, most, but not all, reported uses of the H reflex have been with these two nerves.

Clinically, the posterior tibial H reflex has been reported helpful for demonstrating S-1 radiculopathy, especially by comparing the latencies on the two sides.[46] This comparison, however, requires using a standardized technique so that the conduction distances on the two sides are comparable. In addition, the technique can result in a false-negative finding if a bilateral radiculopathy is present, because side-to-side differences are looked for.

Prolongation of the H reflex, or even its absence, would not, by itself, distinguish a sciatic nerve lesion from a posterior root lesion or an anterior root lesion. Any of these could affect the H reflex. In addition, metabolic conditions that can cause neuropathy can also affect it, and the ankle DTR itself, making clinical correlation and correlation with other electrophysiological findings absolutely necessary.

F Waves

The F wave also reflects conduction up to the spinal cord and back, but is not a reflex because it has no sensory nerve component. Instead, the F wave arises from antidromic conduction along stimulated motor axons causing backward depolarization of anterior horn cells. This antidromic invasion then causes a small percent of the motor neuron pool to re-excite their axons, sending impulses orthodromically back to the muscle.

At one time, this re-excitation was not thought to occur, because of the refractory period of the axon that had just conducted to the cell body. It is apparent, however, that when using supramaximum stimuli, as when performing a motor conduction study, a small and varying number of these neurons do recover and are capable of conducting back to the muscle (Figure 13-15).[47]

This is one of the major distinguishing electrical characteristics between the H reflex and F wave, namely, that the H reflex is essentially abolished with supramaximum stimulation, whereas the F wave requires supramaximum stimulation to be seen (Table 13-4).

Another feature not shared by these two late responses is that the F wave can be obtained from almost any muscle, whereas the H reflex is more restricted, primarily to muscles in which a DTR is fairly easily obtained. As a result, F waves have been used clinically recording from intrinsic hand and foot muscles, as well as others.[48]

Because the subpopulation of motor neurons that backfire is variable from stimulus to stimulus, there has been considerable discussion concerning the number of recordings to be made. Opinions have ranged from 1–100. If 10–20 are attempted, the parameters measured include minimum latency, mean latency, number of rebounds obtained (persistence), and chronodispersion (the difference between the maximum and minimum latencies). Often, having the subject perform a slight voluntary contraction of the target muscle increases the number of F waves obtained. This presumably occurs because of subthreshold activation of some anterior horn cells, bringing them closer to their firing level. In this facilitated state, the antidromic impulse now completes depolarization to threshold.

F waves have been reported helpful in conditions that affect the more proximal parts of motor axons (i.e., regions of nerve not usually encompassed by routine motor conduction studies).[49,50] However, their full clinical utility is yet to be determined.

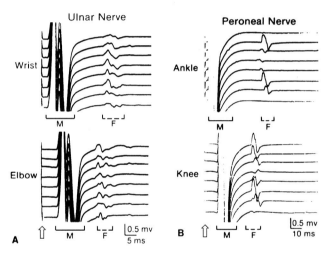

FIGURE 13-15 A. Eight consecutive tracings show normal M responses and F waves recorded from the hypothenar muscles after stimulation of ulnar nerve at wrist and elbow. B. Eight consecutive tracings show normal M responses and F waves recorded from the extensor digitorum brevis after stimulation of peroneal nerve at ankle and knee. Because F waves are relatively low-amplitude potentials, a high sensitivity is needed to see them. This high sensitivity causes the larger M responses, which are caused by orthodromic conduction in motor fibers from the point of stimulation down into the muscle, to be off the screen. Note the following points: (1) the F waves are variable in height, shape, and latency, reflecting different populations of motor neurons that are rebounding; (2) the latency of the M responses are shorter when stimulating at wrist or ankle than they are when stimulating at elbow or knee; however, the reverse is true for the F waves, whose latencies get shorter with the more proximal points of stimulation. This reflects the shorter antidromic conduction distance as the point of stimulation moves proximally. (Reprinted with permission from J Kimura. Electrodiagnosis in Diseases of Nerve and Muscle: Principles and Practice [2nd ed]. Philadelphia: F.A. Davis, 1989.)

TABLE 13-4
Some Comparisons between H Reflex and F Wave

Comparison	H Reflex	F Wave
Abolished by dorsal rhizotomy	Yes	No
Abolished by anterior rhizotomy	Yes	Yes
Abolished by peripheral nerve section	Yes	Yes
Stimulus amplitude to obtain	Low (relatively)	High
Abolished with supramaximum stimulus	Yes	No
Latency when obtained	Stable	Variable
Maximum amplitude*	20–70%	<10%
Muscles from which obtained	Limited	Almost any

*Percent of maximum M wave (compound muscle action potential).

Blink Reflex

The blink reflex is used for assessing peripheral and central facial function by stimulating the trigeminal nerve via its supraorbital branch on one side and recording from the orbicularis oculi, bilaterally.[47,51] Thus, the sensory input is through the trigeminal nerve, and the motor output through the facial. Ipsilateral and contralateral responses are obtained. The ipsilateral early response, whose latency is between 8 and 12 msec, is probably a simple or oligosynaptic reflex, whereas the ipsilateral and contralateral late responses, between 28 and 42 msec after the stimulus, are polysynaptic. The early response is called *R1*, and the late response is *R2*.

In the presence of a facial nerve lesion, both the R1 and R2 responses are absent or delayed on the affected side, whereas the contralateral R2 is normal. When stimulating the side opposite to the lesion, the R1 and R2 responses on that side are normal, but R2 on the affected side is absent or delayed. If the trigeminal nerve is involved, all responses (ipsilateral and contralateral) can be delayed or absent.

Although the blink reflex is normally recorded only from the orbicularis oculi muscle, Kimura et al. reported its presence in the orbicularis oris and/or platysma muscles simultaneously, with the orbicularis oculi in 26 of 29 patients recovering from Bell's palsy.[52] This finding was interpreted as indicating aberrant regeneration of facial nerve axons, wherein some fibers that should have reinnervated the orbicularis oculi are misdirected into the orbicularis oris. Such reinnervation possibly forms the neurologic substrate for the synkinetic movements that occur so often in these patients.

Changes in the blink reflex with the state of arousal[53] and hemispheric lesions[54] have been reported.

A Waves

A waves can be found in neuropathies in which regeneration and reinnervation have occurred. They represent axonal sprouting, usually distal to the nerve lesion.[55] Stimulation, such as at the wrist, using submaximal intensities, produces the expected M wave, followed some time later by a second, usually smaller response, also with a fixed latency. Supramaximum stimulation eliminates the later response. Although this is reminiscent of the H reflex, the latency of the second response is much too short to represent conduction into the spinal cord and then back down. Instead, submaximal stimulation excites one branch that conducts both orthodromically to produce the M wave, and antidromically back to the branch point. At the branch point, the branch not stimulated originally then conducts orthodromically back into the muscle. This late response disappears with supramaximum stimulation because with this high intensity, all axons, branched or not, conduct antidromically, thereby eliminating because of their refractory periods the possibility of conduction back down from the branch point. Note that because there is no afferent nerve involved in this response, it is not a *reflex*. Therefore, the term *A wave* is preferred to the older term *axon reflex*.

Sympathetic Skin Response

The sympathetic skin response is a late response.[56] It appears approximately 1.5 seconds following median nerve stimulation at the wrist, or after 2 seconds after peroneal or tibial nerve stimulation at the ankle. In addition to this prolonged latency, the responses are quite rounded in shape. This combination of features requires sweep speeds of 300–500 msec per division, and low-frequency filters to be set at approximately 0.5 Hz. In addition, these responses habituate easily, so stimuli need to be applied with long rests (e.g., more than 10–15 seconds apart) or randomly. Stimulus durations are 0.1–0.2 msec, and amplitudes are of 15–20 mA.

NEUROMUSCULAR JUNCTION TRANSMISSION STUDIES

As described earlier, the neuromuscular junction is the region where a terminal nerve fiber comes into close approximation with the end-plate membrane of a muscle fiber. Although it is now recognized that a chemical transmitter, ACh, is interposed between the AP depolarizing the distal end of the nerve and generation of the muscle AP, there was a time when it was thought that the nerve AP directly entered the muscle. A raging controversy once existed between the "electrical" school and the "chemical" school. It was finally settled in favor of chemical transmission, based on indirect evidence, by the work of Otto Loewe in the 1920s, in Germany, and Sir Henry Dale and colleagues in the 1930s, in England. We say "based on indirect evidence," because it was not until the advent of the electron microscope in the 1950s that the actual space between the nerve and underlying muscle fiber was visualized. The synaptic cleft, which is only approximately 50 nm wide, is too narrow to be resolved by the light microscope. For a delightful first-hand account of the controversy and the indirect evidence gathered to settle the issue, see Feldberg.[57] Loewe and Dale shared the Nobel Prize in 1936 for their work.

Neuromuscular transmission begins with *excitation-secretion coupling* (reminiscent of *excitation-contraction coupling* mentioned earlier under Neuromuscular Transmission and Muscle Contraction). Basically, depolarization of the nerve terminal permits the passive influx of Ca^{++} from the extracellular fluid. This influx triggers the fusion of synaptic vesicles, which contain ACh, with regions of the terminal's membrane called *release sites* or *active zones*.[58,59] Fusion of vesicles with the membrane releases ACh into the synaptic cleft, an example of *exocytosis*, across which the transmitter diffuses to combine with ACh receptors located in protrusions of the postsynaptic end-plate membrane. Only some of the released ACh reaches the receptors. The diffusion path through the synaptic cleft is a virtual minefield of acetylcholinesterase, which hydrolyzes much of the ACh before it reaches the receptors. Those molecules that make it through the cleft combine with the receptors and cause a permeability change in the end-plate membrane producing an EPP. This EPP, if large enough, generates the sarcolemmal AP that propagates away from the end-plate down the sarcolemma, initiating the first step in excitation-contraction coupling. The ACh molecules that combined with the receptor are also rapidly hydrolyzed, so that repolarization of the muscle membrane occurs before arrival of another AP in the terminal nerve.

It is apparent from the previous discussion that the generation of an EPP depends at least on two factors: the amount of ACh released and the number of ACh receptors available to combine with the transmitter. It has been estimated that in response to depolarization of the presynaptic membrane, approximately 100 synaptic vesicles release their contents into the synaptic cleft,[60] and that each vesicle contains between 6,250 molecules of ACh[61] and "less than 10,000 molecules of ACh."[62,63] The number of ACh receptors available to combine with this transmitter has been estimated as $1-2 \times 10^7$. It is apparent then, that there are more ACh receptors in an end-plate than the number of ACh molecules released by a nerve impulse or that reach an end-plate.

Another intriguing feature of neuromuscular transmission is that it is not a static phenomenon. A number of physical, such as temperature; physiological, such as rate of impulse transmission and duration of activity; pharmacologic, such as curare, succinylcholine, botulinum toxin; and various pathologic conditions can significantly alter what occurs here.

Because the CMAP is a reflection of neuromuscular transmission, we now look at how it is used to study patients with possible neuromuscular transmission defects.

Perhaps the best-known condition affecting the neuromuscular junction is *myasthenia gravis* (MG). In this condition, repetitive use of a muscle results in progressive weakness that recovers after a period of rest.

Historically, the earliest electrophysiological test for MG was reported by Jolly,[64] in which a motor nerve was stimulated and the resulting decrement of force noted. This has been superseded by the more accurate and quantitative method to be described. If the following procedures are to be used in a patient already taking anticholinesterase medication, the drug should be stopped before the test is performed. Otherwise, a false-negative result could occur.

Basically, the procedure is similar to a routine motor nerve conduction study except that now the stimulation is applied to only one site. In addition, these electrodes must be firmly held in place (tapping, strapping, subdermal electrodes), to maintain, as much as possible, consistent activation of the nerve, and the limb immobilized to avoid movement artifact. A supramaximum stimulus amplitude is then found using low-frequency stimulation (1 Hz). Then, after a short rest, trains of 8–10 stimuli at different rates are applied and changes in CMAP amplitude recorded.

Using 2–3 Hz stimulation, subjects with normal neuromuscular transmission show little (<10%) or no decrement of the fifth response compared with the first (Figure 13-16).[65] Patients with MG, on the other hand, may show considerably greater decrement (>10%; Figure 13-17).[65] Note also that in these patients the amplitude of the initial CMAP is within normal limits, contrasted with *myasthenic syndrome*, or *Eaton-Lambert syndrome*. After a few minutes rest, the test should be repeated to show reproducibility.

Furthermore, because not all muscles are affected equally in MG (proximal muscles usually involved more than distal), it is worthwhile to perform this procedure on a number of nerves, using clinical judgment to direct the test toward the most appropriate targets.

Should positive findings be detected with the previously mentioned procedure, further confirmation can be obtained by repeating with intravenous administration of edrophonium chloride (Tensilon), a short-acting anticholinesterase. A positive Tensilon test result is one that shows *repair* of the decrement within the first 1–2 minutes of administration. After another 5 minutes, the decrement should be back. It should be noted, however, that some patients with MG have a negative Tensilon response, but a regional curare challenge may be more helpful.[66,67]

Other corroborating procedures include the patient voluntarily contracting the target muscle for 20 seconds, and then the examiner looking for postexercise facilitation (decrement lessened) followed shortly by postexercise exhaustion (decrement worsened). The physiology of these findings is explained as follows:

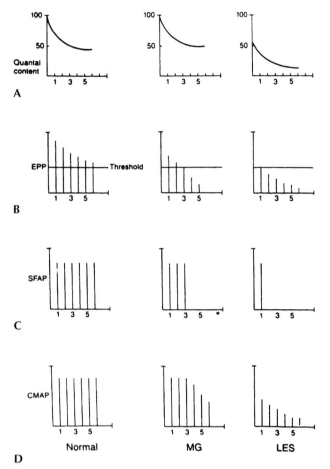

A.

B.

C.

D.

Normal   MG   LES

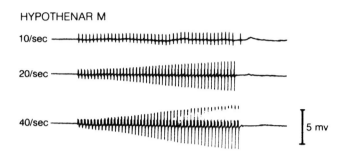

HYPOTHENAR M

10/sec

20/sec

40/sec   ⎱ 5 mv

FIGURE 13-17 Effects of repetitive supramaximal stimulation on compound muscle action potentials recorded from the hypothenar eminence in a patient with Lambert-Eaton syndrome. With increasing frequency (ample rest given between trials), the initially low compound muscle action potential amplitudes increase many-fold, especially with 40/second. (Reprinted with permission from D Elmqvist, EH Lambert. Detailed analysis of neuromuscular transmission in a patient with the myasthenic syndrome sometimes associated with bronchogenic carcinomas. Mayo Clin Proc 1968;43:689–713.)

FIGURE 13-16 Representation of how quantal release changes at individual neuromuscular junctions in response to low-frequency stimulation in normal, myasthenia gravis (MG), and Lambert-Eaton Syndrome (LES, myasthenic syndrome). **A.** Quantal release drops at all three junctions, but starts off smaller in LES. **B.** End-plate potential (EPP) remains above threshold (*horizontal line*) despite being progressively smaller because of decreasing quantal release in the normal neuromuscular junction, but drops below threshold in the MG and LES junctions. **C.** Single fiber action potentials (SFAP) are generated at the normal neuromuscular junction in response to all stimuli, but some fibers do not fire at both the MG and LES junctions. **D.** The resulting compound muscle action potentials (CMAP) do not decrement in the normal state because all fibers have reached threshold and contribute to their CMAP. In MG and LES, however, failure of some fibers to reach threshold causes the resulting CMAPs to decrement, reflecting the decreasing quantal releases. Note that the CMAPs in LES start off at lower amplitudes than either the normal or MG states, and then decrease even further. This response to low-frequency stimulation contrasts dramatically with what happens at LES junctions to high-frequency stimulation. (Reprinted with permission from PL Radecki. Electrodiagnostic Evaluation of Neuromuscular Junction Disorders. In D Dumitru [ed], Clinical Electrophysiology. Philadelphia: Henley & Belfus, 1989.)

A *normal* amplitude CMAP represents the summation of electrical activity generated by the muscle fibers of the motor units that make up the muscle. If for some reason a single end-plate fails to generate a large enough EPP, that muscle fiber does not generate its own AP; it will also not contract, thereby diminishing the force output of that motor unit. As a result, the motor unit AP that the fiber would have contributed to is reduced, and so the CMAP is also reduced. Although the drop out of a single fiber would probably go undetected by the techniques used clinically, if a sufficient number of fibers do not contribute to their respective motor units, then the CMAP amplitude may indeed be reduced.

It is beyond the scope of this chapter to discuss all the possible mechanisms for why a CMAP's amplitude may change and how these mechanisms may be detected electrophysiologically (for an excellent review see Dumitru).[19] However, in two of the most common clinical situations, namely MG and the myasthenic syndrome, the mechanisms and findings are distinctly different.

Theoretically, there are at least three possible causes of an EPP not being large enough to produce an AP along the sarcolemma. Not enough ACh is released, there are not enough ACh receptors with which to bind, or there is a change in the sensitivity of the ACh receptors to the transmitter. Each of these, in turn, can have a number of causes, so the dynamics of the neuromuscular junction are indeed complicated.

With MG, the reason low-frequency stimulation (2–3 Hz) produces a decrement that is not seen in normal junctions is diagrammed in Figure 13-16.[65] As shown, even under normal circumstances, the amount of ACh released at a terminal decreases with 2- to 3-Hz stimulation. The associated EPPs, however, are still large enough to produce sarcolemmal APs in each single fiber, so the CMAPs do not change in amplitude. In MG, on the contrary, the decreasing release of ACh causes the EPPs to fall below the threshold needed to generate an AP, so that by the third, fourth, or fifth repetition, certain single fibers no longer fire, and if enough of these are affected, the CMAP decreases.

So why might the normally reduced release of transmitter cause EPPs to fail in MG, but not in normal junctions? It has been shown that in MG, antibodies to the ACh receptor cause their destruction, thereby reducing the number of receptors available with which the released ACh could bind.[68] Therefore, even though the amount of ACh released is normal in this condition, the combination of a normal reduction in its release and the reduced numbers of receptors results in transmission failure at those junctions. The problem is said to be *postsynaptic*, although historically it was originally thought to be a *presynaptic* defect.

Said differently, normal junctions have enough of a safety factor in terms of numbers of receptors available to the number of receptors needed to produce an adequate EPP not affected by the decrease in ACh. Myasthenic junctions, on the other hand, do not have this luxury, and so failure occurs.

The defect of neuromuscular transmission in MG can also be studied by the technique of *single-fiber electromyography*. This uses a specially constructed needle with a highly restricted pick-up area that permits investigating the individual muscle fiber spikes that contribute to the motor unit potential, as opposed to the motor unit potential itself. This technique measures the variability of the interval between two closely recorded spikes from adjacent muscle fibers of one motor unit. This variability, called *jitter*, is contributed to by conduction over three areas in the neuromuscular mechanism: terminal nerve fiber conduction, neuromuscular transmission, and muscle fiber conduction. Jitter is excessive in disorders such as MG, Lambert-Eaton syndrome, and botulinum. The measurements made include the *mean consecutive difference*, which is the average time, in microseconds, between the two spikes, and the number of times the second potential *blocks*, because of that fiber's end-plate not reaching threshold.

Although the technique is somewhat difficult to master, it is said that the diagnostic sensitivity of electrophysiological tests for MG may double to 80%. Stalberg and Trontelj claim 92% abnormal results.[69]

The most frequently used muscles are the extensor digitorum communis and the frontalis. The latter may be helpful in cranial or purely ocular MG.

Another interesting phenomenon about neuromuscular junctions is that they are not electrically silent at rest. Fatt and Katz first demonstrated the presence of spontaneously occurring *miniature end-plate potentials*, named because their shapes and time courses were similar to full-blown EPPs, but considerably smaller.[70] These potentials are caused by random, spontaneous release of one or just a few packets of ACh, which produces subthreshold depolarizations of the end-plate membrane.

Miniature end-plate potentials, recorded with intracellular microelectrodes, are smaller than normal in MG, although their frequency is unchanged. This smallness is now recognized as reflecting the reduced numbers of ACh receptors in the end-plate membranes of these muscles. Lovelace et al. reported that miniature end-plate potentials can also be recorded extracellularly with electromyography needles, and their amplitudes in patients with MG are correspondingly lower than in normal subjects.[71]

In myasthenic syndrome, first described by Lambert et al.[72] and also known as *Lambert-Eaton syndrome*, weakness is also a complaint, but is different from that in MG. In myasthenic syndrome, weakness is more pronounced after resting and is made temporarily better by exercise. Electrophysiologically, this is manifested by low-amplitude CMAPs at the beginning, which may also decrease with low-frequency stimulation, but with marked facilitation of the amplitude using high-frequency (30–50 Hz) stimulation (see Figure 13-17)[73] or after brief exercise.

In this condition, the problem is *presynaptic* in which not enough vesicles release their ACh into the synaptic cleft, especially after a period of inactivity.

The presumed physiology of the low-frequency decrement but high-frequency increment relates to the aforementioned dynamic nature of neuromuscular transmission. The decrement with low-frequency stimulation is caused by the normal decrease in transmitter release described for MG. In myasthenic syndrome, release is already defective, presumably because of an autoimmune reaction against calcium channels in the nerve endings, so the normal reduction in release with 2- to 3-Hz stimulation accentuates the already low-amplitude CMAP.

With high-frequency stimulation, however, there is normally an increase in the number of vesicles that release their ACh. This *facilitation* of release after high-frequency activity may be caused by accumulation of

Ca^{++} in the terminal nerve endings. Kandell colorfully writes, "Here then is the simplest kind of memory! This neuron remembers that it has generated a train of impulses by increasing the intracellular concentration of Ca^{++} in its terminals, and now each AP in the presynaptic neuron, playing on this memory, produces more transmitter than before."[7] In myasthenic syndrome, this normally occurring phenomenon temporarily improves transmitter release, manifesting as the dramatic increase in CMAPs. Drugs, such as guanidine, exert a similar release-enhancing effect.[74]

To summarize, myasthenic syndrome has the following features: (1) low-amplitude CMAP at beginning of stimulation; (2) decrementing CMAPs with low-frequency stimulation (2–3 Hz), similar to MG, except these CMAPs start off low and become even lower; (3) marked increment in CMAP amplitudes with high-frequency stimulation (30–50 Hz) or immediately after a brief voluntary tetanic contraction.

Before ending this chapter, it should also be noted that some conditions, such as polio and amyotrophic lateral sclerosis, also affect neuromuscular junction transmission,[75,76] as does myotonia congenita,[77] certain antibiotics,[78,79] and botulinum poisoning.[80] Therefore, the clinical significance of these electrophysiological findings, as with all others obtained by these techniques, must be interpreted in light of all other pertinent medical considerations.

REFERENCES

1. Hodes R, Larrabee MC, German W. The human electromyogram in response to nerve stimulation and the conduction velocity of motor axons. Arch Neurol Psychiatry 1948;60:340–365.

2. Dawson GD, Scott JW. The recording of nerve action potentials through skin in man. J Neurol Neurosurg Psychiatry 1949;12:259–267.

3. Dawson GD. The relative excitability and conduction velocity of sensory and motor nerve fibres in man. J Physiol (Lond) 1956;156:336–343.

4. Ochoa J. Microscopic Anatomy of Unmyelinated Nerve Fibers. In PJ Dyck, PK Thomas, EH Lambert (eds), Peripheral Neuropathy. Vol 1. Philadelphia: WB Saunders, 1975;131–150.

5. Woodbury JW. Action Potential: Properties of Excitable Membranes. In TC Ruch, HD Patton, JW Woodbury, AL Towe (eds), Neurophysiology. Philadelphia: WB Saunders, 1965;26–72.

6. Kane JW, Sternheim MM. Physics (Formerly Life Science Physics). New York: Wiley, 1978.

7. Kandell ER, Schwartz JH. Principles of Neural Science (2nd ed). New York: Elsevier, 1985.

8. Hodgkin AL, Huxley AF. A quantitative description of membrane current and its application to conduction and excitation in nerve. J Physiol (Lond) 1952;117:500–544.

9. Oh SJ. Clinical Electromyography: Nerve Conduction Studies. Baltimore: University Park Press, 1984.

10. Bostock H, Sears TA. The internodal axon membrane: electrical excitability and continuous conduction in segmental demyelination. J Physiol (Lond) 1978;280:273–301.

11. Hodgkin AL. Evidence for electrical transmission in nerve. Part I. J Physiol (Lond) 1937;90:183–210.

12. Ritchie JM, Rogart RB. Density of sodium channels in mammalian myelinated nerve fibers and nature of the axonal membrane under the myelin sheath. Proc Natl Acad Sci U S A 1977;74:211–215.

13. Waxman SG, Ritchie JM. Molecular dissection of the myelinated axon. Ann Neurol 1993;33(2):121–136.

14. Waxman SG. Membranes, myelin, and the pathophysiology of multiple sclerosis. N Engl J Med 1982;306:1529–1533.

15. Shrager P. Sodium channels in single demyelinated mammalian axons. Brain Res 1989;483(1):149–154.

16. England JD, Gamboni F, Levinson SR. Increased numbers of sodium channels form along demyelinated axons. Brain Res 1991;548(1–2):334–337.

17. Smith KJ, Hall SM. Nerve conduction during peripheral demyelination and remyelination. J Neurol Sci 1980;48:201–219.

18. Denys EH. AAEM minimonograph #14: the influence of temperature in clinical neurophysiology. Muscle Nerve 1991;14:795–811.

19. Dumitru D. Electrodiagnostic Medicine. Philadelphia: Hanley & Belfus, 1995.

20. Downie AW, Newell DJ. Sensory nerve conduction in patients with diabetes mellitus and controls. Neurology 1961;11:876–882.

21. LaFratta CW. A comparison of sensory and motor NCV as related with age. Arch Phys Med Rehabil 1966;47:286–290.

22. Wagner AL, Buchthal F. Motor and sensory conduction in infancy and childhood: reappraisal. Dev Med Child Neurol 1972;14:189–216.

23. Falco FJE, Hennessey WJ, Goldberg, G, Braddom RL. Standardized nerve conduction studies in the lower limb of the healthy elderly. Am J Phys Med Rehabil 1994;73:168–174.

24. Coërs C. Contribution a l'etude de la jonction neuromusculaire II, Topographie zonale de l'innervation, motrice terminale dans les muscles striés. Arch Biol (Paris) 1953;64:495.

25. Coërs C, Woolf AL. The Innervation of Muscle. Oxford: Blackwell, 1959.

26. Dumitru D, Walsh NE. Practical instrumentation and common sources of error. Am J Phys Med Rehabil 1988;67:55–65.

27. Gitter AJ, Stolov WC. AAEM minimonograph #16: instrumentation and measurement in electrodiagnostic medicine (Pt I). Muscle Nerve 1995;18:799–811.

28. Lovelace RE, Myers SJ. Nerve Conduction and Neuromuscular Transmission. In Downey and Darling's Physiological Basis of Rehabilitation Medicine, (2nd ed). Boston: Butterworth–Heinemann, 1994;215–242.

29. Wiederholt WC. Stimulus intensity and site of excitation in human median nerve sensory fibres. J Neurol Neurosurg Psychiatry 1970;33:438–441.

30. Wiederholt WC. Threshold and conduction velocity in isolated mixed mammalian nerves. Neurology 1970;20:347–352.

31. Ma DM, Liveson JA. Nerve Conduction Handbook. Philadelphia: FA Davis, 1983.

32. Mayer RF. Nerve conduction studies in man. Neurology 1963;13:1021–1030.

33. Lenman JAR, Ritchie AE. Clinical Electromyography. Philadelphia: JB Lippincott, 1970.

34. DeLisa JA, Lee HJ, Baran EM, et al. Manual of Nerve Conduction Velocity and Clinical Neurophysiology, (3rd ed). New York: Raven Press, 1994.

35. Hopf HC. Electromyographic study on so-called mononeuritis. Arch Neurol 1963;9:307–318.

36. Blackstock E, Rushworth G, Gath D. Electrophysiological studies in alcoholism. J Neurol Neurosurg Psychiatry 1972;35:326–334.

37. Dorfman LJ. The distribution of conduction velocities (DCV) in peripheral nerves: a review. Muscle Nerve 1984; 7:2–11.

38. Kraft G. Peripheral Neuropathies. In EW Johnson (ed), Practical Electromyography. Baltimore: Williams & Wilkins, 1980;155–205.

39. Seddon H. Three types of nerve injury. Brain 1943;66:237–288.

40. Behse F, Buchthal F. Alcoholic neuropathy: clinical, electrophysiological, and biopsy findings. Ann Neurol 1977;2:95–110.

41. Kimura J. Facts, fallacies, and fancies of nerve conduction studies: twenty-first annual Edward H. Lambert lecture. Muscle Nerve 1997;20:777–787.

42. Lewis RA, Sumner AJ. The electrodiagnostic distinctions between chronic familial and acquired demyelinative neuropathies. Neurology 1982;32:592–596.

43. Hoffmann P. Uber die beziehungen der sehnenreflexe zur willkurlichen bewegung und zum tonus. Z Biol 1918;68:351–370.

44. Magladery JW, McDougal DB. Electrophysiological studies of nerve and reflex activity in normal man. I. Identification of certain reflexes in the electromyogram and the conduction velocity of peripheral nerve fibres. Bull Johns Hopkins Hosp 1950;86:265–290.

45. Magladery JW, Porter WE, Park AM, Teasdall RD. Electrophysiological studies of nerve and reflex activity in normal man. IV. The two-neurone reflex and identification of certain action potentials from spinal roots and

cord. Bull Johns Hopkins Hosp 1951; 88:499–519.

46. Braddom RI, Johnson EW. Standardization of H reflex and diagnostic use in S1 radiculopathy. Arch Phys Med Rehabil 1974;55:161–166.

47. Kimura J. Electrodiagnosis in Diseases of Nerve and Muscle: Principles and Practice (2nd ed). Philadelphia: FA Davis, 1989.

48. Fisher MA. AAEM minimonograph #13: H reflex and F wave: physiology and clinical indications. Muscle Nerve 1992;15:1223–1233.

49. Kimura J, Butzer JF. F-wave conduction velocity in Guillain-Barre syndrome: assessment of nerve segment between axilla and spinal cord. Arch Neurol 1975;32:524–529.

50. Peioglou-Harmoussi S, Fawcwett PRW, Howel D, Barwick DD. F-response frequency in motor neuron disease and cervical spondylosis. J Neurol Neurosurg Psychiatry 1987;50:593–599.

51. Shahani B. The human blink reflex. J Neurol Neurosur Psychiatry 1970; 33:792–800.

52. Kimura J, Rodnitzky RL, Okawara SH. Electrophysiologic analysis of aberrant regeneration after facial nerve paralysis. Neurology 1975;25(10):989–993.

53. Boelhouwer AJW, Brunia CHM. Blink reflexes and the state of arousal. J Neurol Neurosurg Psychiatry 1977;40:58–63.

54. Kimura J. Effect of hemispheral lesions on the contralateral blink reflex. Neurology 1974;168–174.

55. Fullerton PM, Gilliatt RW. Axon reflexes in human motor nerves. J Neurol Neurosurg Psychiatry 1965;28:1–14.

56. Uncini A, Pullman Sl, Lovelace RE, Gambi D. The sympathetic skin response: normal values, elucidation of afferent components and application limits. J Neurol Sci 1988;87:299–306.

57. Feldberg W. The Early History of Synaptic and Neuromuscular Transmission by Acetylcholine: Reminiscenses of an Eye Witness. In AL Hodgkin, et al. (eds), The Pursuit of Nature: Informal Essays on the History of Physiology. New York: Cambridge University Press, 1977.

58. Dreyer F, Peper K, Akert K, et al. Ultrastructure of the "active zone" in the frog neuromuscular junction. Brain Res 1973;62(2):373–380.

59. Fesce R. The kinetics of nerve-evoked quantal secretion. Philos Trans R Soc

Lond B Biol Sci 1999;354(1381):319–329.

60. Lambert E, Elmquist D. Quantal components of end-plate potentials in the myasthenic syndrome. Ann NY Acad Sci 1971;183:183–199.

61. Fletcher P, Forrester T. The effect of curare on the release of acetylcholine from mammalian motor nerve terminals and an estimate of quantum content. J Physiol (Lond) 1975;251(1):131–144.

62. Kuffler SW, Yoshikami D. The number of transmitter molecules in a quantum: an estimate from the iontophoretic application of acetylcholine at the neuromuscular synapse. J Physiol (Lond) 1975;251:465–482.

63. Hartzell HC, Kuffler SW, Yoshikami D. The number of acetylcholine molecules in a quantum and the interaction between quanta at the subsynaptic membrane of the skeletal neuromuscular synapse. Cold Spring Harb Symp Quant Biol 1976;40:175–186.

64. Jolly F. Myasthenia gravis pseudoparalytica. Berliner Klinische Wochenshrift 1895;32:33–34.

65. Radecki PL. Electrodiagnostic Evaluation of Neuromuscular Junction Disorders. In D Dumitru (ed), Clinical Electrophysiology. Physical Medicine and Rehabilitation: State of the Art Reviews. Philadelphia: Hanley & Belfus, Inc, 1989, 3(4):757–778.

66. Brown JC, Charlton JE. A study of sensitivity to curare in myasthenic disorders using a regional technique. J Neurol Neurosurg Psychiatry 1975;38:27–33.

67. Horowitz S, Genkins G, Kornfeld P, Papatestas AE. Electrophysiologic diagnosis of myasthenia gravis and the regional curare test. Neurology 1976;26(5):410–417.

68. Engel AG, Lindstrom JM, Lambert EH, Lennon VA. Ultrastructural localization of the acetylcholine receptor in myasthenia gravis and its experimental autommimune model. Neurology 1977;27:307–315.

69. Stalberg E, Trontelj JV. Single Fiber Electromyography. Old Woking, Surrey: Miravalle Press, 1979.

70. Fatt P, Katz B. Spontaneous subthreshold activity at motor nerve endings. J Physiol 1952;117:109–128.

71. Lovelace RE, Stone R, Zablow L. A new test for myasthenia gravis: recording of miniature end-plate potentials in situ. Neurology 1970;20:385.

72. Lambert EH, Rooke ED, Eaton LM, Hodgson EH. Myasthenic Syndrome

Occasionally Associated with Bronchial Neoplasm: Neurophysiologic Studies. In HR Viets (ed), Myasthenia Gravis: The Second International Symposium Proceedings. Springfield: Charles C Thomas, 1961;362–410.

73. Elmqvist D, Lambert EH. Detailed analysis of neuromuscular transmission in a patient with the myasthenic syndrome sometimes associated with bronchogenic carcinomas. Mayo Clin Proc 1968;43:689–713.

74. Oh SJ, Kim KW. Guanidine hydrochloride in the Eaton-Lambert syndrome. Neurology 1973;23:1084–1090.

75. Denys EH, Norris FH. Amyotrophic lateral sclerosis—impairment of neuromuscular transmission. Arch Neurol 1979;36:202–205.

76. Daube JR. Electrophysiologic studies in the diagnosis and prognosis of motor neuron disease. Neurol Clin 1985; 3:473–493.

77. Aminoff MJ, Layzer RB, Satya-Muri S, Faden AI. The declining electrical response of muscle to repetitive stimulation in myotonia. Neurology 1977;27:812–816.

78. Kaeser HE. Drug-induced myasthenic syndromes [Review]. Acta Neurol Scand 1984;100(Suppl):39–47.

79. Snavely SR, Hodges GR. The neurotoxicity of antibacterial agents [Review]. Ann Intern Med 1984;101(1): 92–104.

80. Pickett JB. Neuromuscular Transmission. In AJ Sumner (ed), The Physiology of Peripheral Nerve Disease. Philadelphia: WB Saunders, 1980;238–264.

14

The Motor Unit and Electromyography

STANLEY J. MYERS, BHAGWAN T. SHAHANI,
AND FRANS L. BRUYNINCKX

In the broadest sense, *electromyography* (EMG) is the electrophysiological recording and study of nerve conduction and the electrical activity of muscle. It can be more narrowly defined as recording and study of insertional, spontaneous, and voluntary electric activity of muscle.[1] Contemporary practice favors the latter definition; today, the broader description falls under the general heading of clinical neurophysiology. EMG plays a significant role in diagnosis and prognosis and in physiological and kinesiologic research.

Redi postulated in 1666 that electricity was generated from muscle, a fact not demonstrated until 1838, by Matteucci, using an improved galvanometer. DuBois-Reymond confirmed this work and, in 1851, performed the first human EMG study, using jars of liquid as electrodes and recording action currents in a subject's contracting arm. The development of more sophisticated apparatus, especially Einthoven's string galvanometer, made possible further investigations of muscle action potentials and allowed correlation of laboratory findings with normal human muscle potentials. The first extensive clinical EMG study was done in Germany by Piper, who published the first book on EMG in 1912. In 1929, Adrian and Bronk introduced the coaxial (concentric) needle electrode, which made it possible to record potentials from a single motor unit. They also amplified the muscle action potentials through a loudspeaker, as an additional aid in interpreting results. The introduction of the cathode ray oscilloscope by Erlanger and Gasser (1937) freed workers from the limitations of mechanical galvanometers. Later developments in instrumentation, including the use of analog-digital converters, computers, and expanded memory, extended the use of existing recording devices and permitted the development of even more sophisticated systems for data recording, storage, and analysis.

In this chapter we review current understanding of the physiology of the motor unit and how it is affected by internal and external changes resulting from what might be called normal conditions such as aging and temperature, as well as by disease processes.

MOTOR UNIT

Definition

The *motor unit* was defined as the anatomic unit of muscle function by Liddell and Sherrington in 1925. A motor unit consists of a single anterior horn cell (motor neuron), its axon cylinder (including the terminal and subterminal branching within the muscle body), the motor end-plates (neuromuscular junction), and all the muscle fibers innervated by that neuron (Figure 14-1).

Anatomic and Physiological Makeup

The motor axon branches many times to provide end-plates for its multiple muscle fibers. Most of the divisions occur within the terminal intramuscular nerve bundles at the points of branching of the nerve bundles proper at a node of Ranvier.[2] Normally, the divisions form two groups of fibers of approximately equal caliber containing 10–50 nerve fibers each, which, after emerging from the bundle as subterminal nerve fibers, run in isolation across the muscle fibers to terminate in the end-plates. In humans, only 1.5–10.0% of nerve fibers branch after they leave as subterminal nerve fibers.

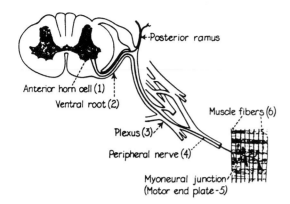

FIGURE 14-1 The motor unit. Terminal and subterminal branching of the nerve fiber occurs between points 4 and 5. (Reprinted with permission from AA Rodriquez, YT Oester. Fundamentals of Electromyography. In S Licht [ed], Electrodiagnosis and Electromyography. New Haven: E. Licht, 1971;321.)

Motor Unit Number Estimation

The number of muscle fibers in each motor unit can be estimated in humans by counting the total number of fibers in a muscle and dividing by the total number of motor nerve fibers.[3,4] The innervation ratio is the ratio of the total number of extrafusal muscle fibers to the number of motor axons supplying a specific muscle, which provides a measure of the average size of the motor unit. Muscles responsible for finer function tend to have a lower ratio than those for coarser movements. Some representative values of the number of muscle fibers per motor unit are opponens pollicis, 13; superior rectus, 23; platysma, 25; biceps brachii, 163; sartorius, 300; rectus femoris, 305; first dorsal interosseus, 340; gracilis, 527; anterior tibial, 610; and gastrocnemius, 2,037. These estimates assume that 60% of the nerve fibers in muscle are motor fibers, as determined from measurements on the nerves to the anterior tibial and gastrocnemius muscles in cats. No correction is made for motor nerve fibers supplying intrafusal muscle fibers. Furthermore, it is unlikely that the proportion of motor nerve fibers is the same in functionally different muscles. Thus, motor unit number estimation (MUNE) is imprecise and is likely to be on the low side. In 1971, McComas and coworkers[5] described a noninvasive MUNE method. By delivering small, graded electrical stimuli to the deep peroneal nerve, they were able to induce an incremental response in the evoked action potential of the extensor digitorum brevis, assuming that each increment of voltage was a result of the excitation of a single motor unit.

By taking the average of approximately 10 motor units and using this to divide into the maximum compound potential amplitude evoked in a muscle by a supramaximal motor nerve stimulus, it was possible to obtain an estimate of the number of motor units in that muscle. This technique has a number of difficulties: Lower threshold (larger) units are preferentially evaluated, the number of motor units sampled is relatively small, and it is not possible to distinguish between two or more motor units that have the same threshold. Over the years, this technique has been modified in a number of ways.[6,7] These methods are best applied to distal muscles. More recently, Brown and colleagues[8] presented a new MUNE technique for use in human subjects. It can also be used with proximal muscles, and it eliminates the error from overlap between thresholds of different motor units. This method combines isometric contraction, intramuscular needle electrode recordings, and spike-triggered averaging techniques to measure the sizes of motor unit potentials as recorded in the innervation zone with surface electrodes. The needle-recorded intramuscular single motor unit spikes serve as the triggering signal. The number of motor units is then estimated by dividing the maximum (M) potential evoked by supermaximal stimulation of the motor nerve recorded with the same surface electrodes by the mean of at least 10 surface-recorded motor unit potentials. This method obviates graded stimulation of motor nerves and can be applied to proximal muscle groups as well as distal ones. The authors used the method to study the biceps brachii, which showed a mean motor unit estimate of 911 ± 254 (1 SD) for subjects younger than 60 years. This spike-triggered averaging-based technique has been further refined by using intramuscular potentials recorded with a macroelectrode. All spike-triggered techniques described, however, are invasive. Shahani et al.[9] introduced a completely noninvasive variant in which the surface-recorded single motor unit action potential (MUAP) is obtained with surface EMG-triggered averaging (Figure 14-2). They compared their method with previous ones and obtained similar MUNE values. In patients with lower motor neuron involvement, their technique showed MUNE counts comparable with the spike-triggered averaging technique. A disadvantage is the slow rising phase of the triggering potential and interference from other EMG activity. This was remedied by aligning the surface signals before averaging. To make sure that enough different motor unit potentials were obtained, the recording electrode was placed over different parts of the muscle, and different (mild to moderate) strengths of contraction were used. Recordings at higher levels of contraction remain a so far unsolved difficulty of all MUNE techniques, however. Another problem with most MUNE techniques is that the total compound muscle action potential amplitude that is used in the calculation does not take into account the phenomenon of phase cancellation, which occurs during summation. This issue was addressed by Fang et al.[10] using spatial and temporal information of every contributing single MUAP. To avoid predisposition toward certain types of motor units they made use of various types of activation. It is likely that none of the MUNE techniques presently in use provides a truly exact MUNE in a muscle.

Motor Unit Territory

Individual muscle fibers extend throughout the length of most muscles and are arranged in parallel, except in the gracilis and sartorius, where they are arranged in series. Most researchers agree that there is intermingling and wide scattering of fibers from different motor units.

If single ventral root fibers innervating the rat anterior tibial muscle are isolated and stimulated repeatedly, the glycogen in the muscle fibers that responds to the stimulation of the single axon is exhausted. Immediately after stimulation, the whole muscle is excised and frozen. Cross sections are cut and stained by the periodic acid–Schiff technique for glycogen, so that the muscle fibers of the stimulated motor unit can be identified. Such preparations show moderate variation in the total number of muscle fibers and motor unit territory and diffuse scattering of the muscle fibers throughout the territory of that motor unit.[11] The vast majority of fibers, approximately 70% of the motor unit, has no contact with other fibers of the same unit. A motor unit occasionally contains groups of muscle fibers, each group consisting usually of two fibers, and rarely more than three.

In humans, Buchthal and coworkers developed indirect methods of analysis using a multilead electrode. They constructed different multielectrode setups of up to 14 leads to study volume conduction of the spike of motor potentials, total muscle cross section, and the territory of the motor unit.[12,13] The spatial spread of action potentials from a given motor unit so obtained indicates the territory occupied by the fibers of a motor unit. With two multielectrodes perpendicular to each other and transverse to the fiber direction and another situated at the periphery of the motor unit field, it is found that the territory of a motor unit is roughly circular (ovoid in some muscles) with an average diameter of 5 mm (range, 2–22 mm).

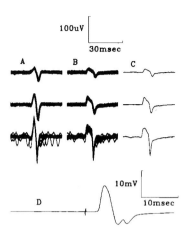

FIGURE 14-2 Motor unit number estimation with surface electromyography–triggered averaging technique. **A.** Superimposed surface electromyography signals recorded from the triggering electrode at three different contraction levels. **B.** Superimposed surface electromyography signals recorded from the recording electrode. **C.** Corresponding averaged results at different contraction levels. **D.** Maximum compound muscle action potential recorded from abductor pollicis brevis muscle after supramaximal stimulation of the median nerve at the wrist. (Reprinted with permission from BT Shahani, J Fang, U Dhand. A new approach to motor unit estimation with surface EMG triggered averaging technique. Muscle Nerve 1995;18:1090.)

Within the same muscle, the territory of different motor units varies by a factor of 4. The area of territory of a single motor unit may encompass fibers of as many as 30 motor units. For example, in the biceps brachii, with an average territory of 4–6 mm, theoretically there is space for the fibers of 10 overlapping motor units. In fact, as many as six different motor units were identified in the same lead, owing to different rates of discharge.[13] These findings agree with the histologic evidence of overlap between fibers of different motor units.

The concept of a subunit arrangement of fibers, with groups of up to 30 muscle fibers from the same unit being adjacent to each other, has been shown to be erroneous. Researchers thought that the clean, smooth spikes of motor unit potentials resulted from contraction of up to 30 perfectly synchronized, tightly packed fibers. This, however, can result from a single fiber.

The spatial distribution of muscle fibers within the territory of a motor unit was studied in the soleus and tibialis anterior of adult cats.[14] Results indicate that a motor unit is distributed over only a portion of the muscle cross-section and that this varies for different muscles and for different parts of an individual muscle, being 25–75% of the muscle cross section for the soleus and 12–26% for the tibialis anterior. Although motor unit fibers were more localized in the tibialis anterior, the absolute areas of the territories were similar in the two muscles. The density of fibers appears to be relatively constant across units, with the size of the motor unit territory varying as a function of the number of motor unit fibers. This study indicates that the spatial distribution of fibers belonging to a motor unit is not randomly scattered or homogeneously dispersed. There is much variation in fiber densities in a single motor unit territory. The high-density areas usually were not located in the center of the territory. There appears to be some subgrouping (not subunits) of fibers within the motor unit territory, together with areas apparently void of motor unit fibers also within the territory. The closely associated motor unit fibers may be a consequence of the branching pattern of a motor axon. These clusters are separated by distances generally shorter than 500 μm and contain many more than 30 fibers. The distribution of fibers within each of the subgroups appears to be random, as determined by adjacency, nearest neighbor, and interfiber distance analysis.

Multiple Innervation

It is not known definitely whether multiple innervation of muscle fibers occurs. There is evidence that it may be present in cats, dogs, and frogs,[15-17] but there is no reliable evidence that it plays any significant role in humans. In the case of the animals mentioned previously, the evidence was obtained mostly indirectly, from the measurement of tensions produced by stimulation of single motor nerve fibers and comparison with the tension produced by stimulation of two or more fibers together. Most muscle fibers do not seem to have more than two motor end-plates, and it has not been determined if these doubly innervated fibers receive their nerve from branches of the same neuron, from separate axons, or from nerve fibers supplied by different cord segments.

Double and multiple innervation has been reported in human gracilis and soleus muscles; the findings are based on histochemical staining of muscle fibers for motor end-plates. Other studies that used the muscles of stillborn infants do not support these conclusions.[3] In most muscles, motor end-plates are found in the middle of the muscle fibers. The gracilis and sartorius are exceptions: In the gracilis, two end-plate bands are noted; in the sartorius the end-plates are disseminated. In the sartorius, the end-plates correspond to the numerous short muscle bundles seen in serial longitudinal sections and are developed from a chain of myoblasts in series, each supplied with only one end-plate. In adult muscles, these longitudinal fiber chains fuse together and create the impression that one is dealing with multiple innervation and multiple end-plates in a single muscle fiber.

The location of the end-plates in the middle portion of the muscle belly affords the fastest activation of all its contractile material, and multiple nerve endings may increase the rate at which tension is developed by the muscle fiber. If nerve impulses reach terminations synchronously at several points along the muscle fiber, impulses are initiated and spread over the length of the muscle fiber in less time than if activity begins at one locus only.

The biceps brachii and opponens pollicis muscles of humans have been demonstrated to have 1.3–1.5 motor end-plates per muscle fiber,[3] and this, too, has been interpreted as indicating multiple innervation of some fibers. The end-plate zone in these muscles is centrally located, as in most other muscles. Therefore, if present, the two end-plates are only a short distance from each other, and multiple innervation can play only a limited role in reducing the activation time.

Excitation and Depolarization

In many ways, muscle fibers and nerve fibers resemble one another in the response of the surface membranes to excitatory stimuli. The physiology of the membrane potential is summarized here and is dealt with in more detail in Chapters 5 and 13.

The differences in potential between the inside and outside of single muscle cells have been measured by microelectrodes. The resulting potential difference between the interior of the muscle cell and the extracellular space is approximately +100 mV in mice and somewhat lower (+60 to +80 mV) in humans.[18] The resting membrane has a high impedance (10 mΩ) and low permeability for most ions. The extracellular concentration of sodium ions is high and of potassium ions low; the opposite is the case inside the cells. Potassium ions are 32–50 times more permeative than sodium ions. However, the continuous flux of sodium ions across the membrane by virtue of a metabolic sodium pump in the cell membrane keeps the ion distribution constant. Because of the higher intracellular concentration, potassium ions diffuse through and accumulate at the outer surface of the membrane, to be held there by the negatively charged impermeable anions at the inner surface. This equilibrium is responsible for the positive polarization of the membrane; its magnitude can be predicted correctly from theoretical laws (Nernst's equation).

Initiation of the excitatory state occurs at the myoneural junction. Small disturbances are rapidly attenuated, but when a stimulus of critical current density is applied to a susceptible membrane area, a propagating electrical potential results. This *action potential* follows an all-or-none law: It travels the length of the muscle fiber with constant velocity and undiminished amplitude. The action potential is caused by a specific increase in the permeability of the membrane to sodium ions (the reverse of the resting situation), as shown by the fact that (1) the absence of sodium in the surrounding fluid renders the muscle nonexcitable and (2) the action potential can be made smaller or larger by altering the extracellular sodium concentration.[19] At the height of excitation, there are more sodium ions (cations) entering than there are potassium ions leaving, so the membrane potential changes from the potassium equilibrium potential (–100 mV inside) through zero when the membrane is depolarized, to an overshoot, the sodium equilibrium potential (+30 mV). Repolarization occurs with the passive outward flux of potassium ions and the restoration of sodium ions by active pumping. The action potential of the muscle fiber differs from that of the nerve fiber, in that the repolarization curve for muscle fiber takes longer because of events in the submembrane tubular structure.

Qualitatively, muscle action potentials are similar to nerve action potentials, as is their mechanism of excitation. Along the membrane, conduction velocity for mammalian skeletal muscle is approximately 3–5 m per second. A refractory period (approximately 2 msec) allows for repolarization before the fiber can be re-excited. Because of shunting of most of the potential difference by nonactive tissue and surrounding fluids, the recorded action potential from muscles is only a fraction of the resting membrane potential. (This is so whether it is from a single fiber, a motor unit, or a group of fibers.) Because, as noted previously, most fibers in the muscle are arranged in parallel, the voltage from a muscle containing many thousands of fibers cannot be greater than the full, unshunted voltage of a single fiber. The muscle action potential initiates the resultant mechanical twitch response. Using the principle of surface EMG spike-triggered averaging, Fang et al.[10] introduced a noninvasive technique for measuring muscle fiber conduction velocity. Apart from being noninvasive, this method has the added advantage that it records conduction of muscle fibers that belong to the same motor unit.

Recording of Muscle Action Potentials

Muscle is a source of electrical activity and is surrounded by a low-resistance conducting medium (the interstitial fluid, blood, and other tissue) usually referred to as a *volume conductor*. This, in turn, is surrounded by skin, the surface of which consists of a layer of horny, dead and dying cells that have a high electrical resistance. EMG is the recording of electrical changes in muscle by electrodes that are either in contact with the skin over the muscle area or inserted into the muscle.

Surface Electrodes

Surface electrodes consist of paired metal (often silver or platinum) plates or pads placed on skin that has been cleaned and prepared with alcohol or lightly abraded to reduce impedance. The electrodes are usually round, but they can be square, rectangular, in strip form, or expandable (e.g., a ring electrode to fit around a digit). Electrode paste or another electrically conductive substance can be used to facilitate recording and minimize artifact. One electrode is usually placed over the motor end-plate area of the muscle to be studied and the other over the electrically inactive tendon or some distance away on the same muscle. A ground electrode must also be used. Although summated electrical potentials are recorded, rapid, low-amplitude potentials are attenuated and fine detail of individual motor units cannot be routinely obtained because of alterations in electrode position, varying degrees of skin and subcutaneous tissue thickness, and the large areas encompassed. Surface electrodes have been used to give a broad survey of action potentials from a whole group of fibers and can be of value in studying kinesiologic patterns such as time relationships and correlation with muscle tension. Clinical applications include muscle re-education and biofeedback.

Needle Electrodes

The two principal types of clinical recording needle electrodes, monopolar (unipolar) and concentric (coaxial), are now available in disposable and reusable forms. Single-fiber needle electrodes and multilead electrodes are also being used clinically and for research (Figure 14-3).

The concentric (coaxial) needle electrode, introduced by Adrian and Bronk in 1929 and still in use today, consists of a steel hypodermic injection-type needle with a centrally mounted insulated wire of stainless steel, silver, or platinum. The tip of the central exploring electrode is exposed flush with the bevel of the cannula. Voltage differences are measured between the center core, whose recording area usually ranges from 0.02 to 0.07 mm^2, and the outer cannula, whose diameter ranges from 0.3 to 0.64 mm. The usual lengths of these needles are from 12 to 75 mm. As with other needle elec-

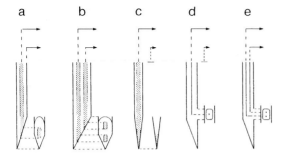

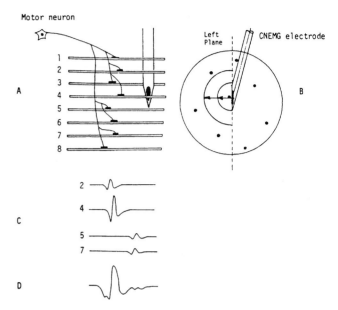

FIGURE 14-3 Schematic illustration of (**A**) concentric or coaxial, (**B**) bipolar, (**C**) monopolar, and (**D, E**) single-fiber needles. Dimensions vary, but the diameters of the outside cannulas shown resemble 26-gauge hypodermic needles (460 μm) for **A**, **D**, and **E**, a 23-gauge needle (640 μm) for **B**, and a 28-gauge needle (360 μm) for **C**. The exposed tip areas measure 150 by 600 μm for a, 150 by 300 μm with spacing between wires of 200 μm center to center for **B**, 0.14 mm² for **C**, and 25 μm in diameter for **D** and **E**. A flat-skin electrode completes the circuit with unipolar electrodes shown in **C** and **D**. (Reprinted with permission from J Kimura. Electrodiagnosis in Diseases of Nerve and Muscle. Philadelphia: F.A. Davis, 1989;39.)

FIGURE 14-4 Schematic of a motor unit action potential recording with a concentric needle (CN) EMG electrode. Longitudinal (**A**) and cross-sectional (**B**) views of the motor unit with recording electrode are shown. Only the action potentials of fibers in the left plane (fibers 2, 4, 5, and 7) are recorded by the active electrode (**C**). The motor unit action potential (**D**) is produced when the potential recorded by the cannula (not shown) is subtracted from the sum of action potentials in **C**. (Reprinted with permission from SD Nandedkar, DB Sanders, EV Stålberg, et al. Simulation of concentric needle electromyography motor unit action potentials. Muscle Nerve 1988;11:152.)

trodes to be discussed, it should be noted that the recording area can vary, depending on the particular manufacturer, whether the needle is reusable or disposable, and on intentional (custom) variations in a particular needle type. The concentric needle selectively records potentials in the direction determined by the bevel, which is approximately a 15-degree angle (Figure 14-4).

The monopolar (unipolar) needle electrode was introduced by Jasper and Ballem in 1949. As used today, it consists of a thin wire, usually stainless steel, insulated with Teflon, except at its tip. The outer diameter is normally 0.35–0.46 mm, and the bare tip has a recording area of 0.15–0.30 mm². Voltage differences are recorded between the needle tip acting as the exploring electrode in the muscle and a more distant reference electrode, usually a metal plate on the skin surface.

The bipolar needle electrode, now less commonly used on a routine basis, may still have some application. This needle electrode consists of two insulated central cores, often of copper or platinum, cemented side by side in a grounded steel cannula. The tips of the electrodes are flush with the bevel of the cannula and can be parallel in the bevel or in tandem. This needle is also known as a *dual concentric needle*. The recording area of the core electrodes is usually between 0.015 and 0.03 mm²; the needle diameter ranges from 0.5 to 0.65 mm. As with the concentric needle electrode, the angle of the bevel determines the recording surface of the core as well as ease of muscle penetration.

Recording Characteristics

Lundervold and Li,[20] using a single needle that could be used for monopolar, concentric, or bipolar recording, observed that the amplitude of motor unit or fibrillation potentials as recorded by the monopolar lead was only slightly larger than that with the concentric but usually considerably larger than that measured with the bipolar electrode. The duration of the negative spike of the action potential was shortest with bipolar and longest with monopolar leads and concentric needle recordings. The electrode records a mean value of the potential, which is spread over the sampling area.[21] The smaller the sampling area, the less the amplitude variation and the higher the amplitude. The amplitude of the potential is also a function of the distance between the recording surface of the electrode and the current source.

With monopolar electrodes the shape and duration of the MUAP are determined by the fact that the muscle acts as a volume conductor, picking up more distant fibers and units, although there is a limit to the recording range, and the absolute duration is still probably representative of a relatively small number of muscle fibers not too distant from the recording electrode. With bipolar electrodes the duration of the potential is considerably shorter because of the short distance between the recording cores. There is partial canceling of the initial and terminal portions of the potentials recorded by each of the inner cores. The advantage of bipolar needle electrodes is that, with maximal interference patterns, it may be possible to analyze individual muscle action potentials. The recording range, however, is too limited for routine clinical EMG. The overall diameter of the bipolar electrode tends to be greater than in monopolar or concentric needle electrodes; this produces more discomfort and trauma for the patient.

Using an automatic method for decomposing complex EMG interference patterns into their constituent MUAPs, Howard and coworkers[22] compared the configurational and firing properties of more than 7,000 MUAPs recorded with either concentric or monopolar needle electrodes from the brachial biceps and anterior tibial muscles of 10 healthy young adults. In both muscles, mean MUAP amplitude, rise rate, and number of turns were significantly greater when recorded with monopolar needle electrodes at three tested levels of isometric contractile force. There was no significant difference between electrode types on measurement of mean MUAP duration or firing rate. Using both concentric and monopolar needle electrodes, Pease and Bowyer[23] examined the extensor digitorum communis muscle of 15 healthy volunteers. They found no significant difference in amplitude or duration of the MUAPs. Although they note that amplitude measurements have been as much as twice as large when taken from monopolar needle electrodes as from concentric needle electrodes, they point out that the technique of manipulating the needle electrode may play a role. Rather than randomly inserting the needle electrode into the muscle, the EMG needle was manipulated so that a maximum peak-to-peak amplitude for the potential was obtained.

Nandedkar and Sanders[24] compared the recording characteristics of concentric needle (reusable) and monopolar needle (disposable) electrodes. They positioned the electrodes within the muscles so that a sharp MUAP was recorded. The MUAPs recorded by the monopolar needle electrode had higher amplitudes and larger areas and were more frequently complex than those seen with the concentric needle electrode. The MUAP duration and area-amplitude ratio were similar for both electrode types. Each monopolar needle electrode was used once, and there was no wearing down of the Teflon coating. The monopolar needle electrode was thought to be more selective: The amplitude of a single

muscle fiber action potential fell more rapidly as the distance from the muscle fiber increased than when recorded by the concentric needle electrode. Nandedkar and Sanders postulate that because the spike component of the MUAP is produced predominantly by the muscle fibers close to the active recording surface of the electrode and because the monopolar needle electrode has a circular recording territory, it registers action potentials from more fibers than the concentric needle electrode, providing for greater MUAP amplitude and area (Figure 14-5). There is also less temporal coincidence, owing to the differences in the action potential propagation velocity and distances between the electrode and the muscle fiber endplates resulting in complex MUAPs. Durations are similar, as there is a greater decline of action potentials with the monopolar electrodes, resulting in distant fibers falling out and not being recorded, counteracting the smaller semicircular recording territory obtained from the beveled concentric needle electrode. Because the monopolar needle electrode has a large recording surface, researchers might, theoretically, expect that the amplitude of the MUAP would be smaller than that recorded with the concentric needle electrode, with which the muscle fiber surface would occupy a proportionately larger surface on the recording electrode. However, Nandedkar and Sanders reason that in a monopolar needle electrode, the current density is likely nonuniform, being greater near the electrode tip, and, therefore, the monopolar electrode behaves as though it had a much smaller recording surface than it actually does.

Thus, most studies do indicate that monopolar needle electrodes tend to record larger amplitude MUAPs than concentric needle electrodes. No significant differences in duration are noted.

Factors to consider in recording characteristics include directionality of beveled needle tips; the wearing down and peeling of insulating coating on monopolar needle electrodes resulting in an enlarged tip area (lower MUAP amplitude); and the distance between the monopolar needle recording electrode and the indifferent recording electrode (reference electrode), which is usually placed over a tendon or other electrically inactive site to minimize interference from surface recording. Variation in electrode impedance, depending on the manufacturer and needle type, is another consideration, although most modern high-input impedance amplifiers can minimize the significance of this. The filter setting is also important. Filtering out low-frequency components results in shorter potential duration and enhanced reproducibility.

Recording and physical characteristics of disposable concentric needle EMG electrodes and reusable ones were compared.[25] MUAPs recorded by the reusable electrodes

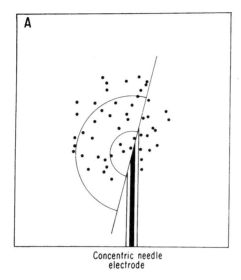
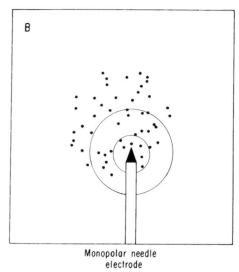

FIGURE 14-5 The distribution of muscle fibers in a motor unit. **A.** The concentric needle electrode has a semicircular recording territory but records action potentials from distant fibers. **B.** The monopolar needle electrode does not record action potentials of distant muscle fibers but has a circular recording territory. The semicircular **(A)** and circular **(B)** boundaries enclose fibers that contribute to the spike component (small radius) and the duration of motor unit action potentials (large radius). The larger boundary encloses similar numbers of muscle fibers for both electrodes; however, the smaller boundary contains more fibers for the monopolar needle electrode. (Reprinted with permission from SV Nandedkar, DB Sanders. Recording characteristics of monopolar EMG electrodes. Muscle Nerve 1991;14:111.)

had greater amplitude and area values. The results obtained might be explained by the fact that it is more difficult to optimize the position of the disposable electrode so that the recording tip is positioned close to the muscle fiber of the motor unit under study. A strong correlation was found between the difference in MUAP amplitudes measured by the two electrode types and the difference in resistance of the needle tips measured in saline, but there was no difference between the duration of the MUAPs. In all, the research confirms that for routine clinical EMG studies, disposable electrodes are quite satisfactory.

Special-Purpose Needle Electrodes

The single-fiber electrode is usually a variant of the concentric needle electrode, which has a small area of recording surface (approximately 25-μm diameter) exposed several millimeters from the tip of the needle. This electrode has limited pick-up area and is obviously directional, enabling single muscle fiber action potentials to be recorded when proper technique is used. Other variations of this electrode use several recording surfaces. When there is only one recording electrode surface on the single-fiber EMG needle, the indifferent recording electrode is usually a skin surface one. The macro EMG electrode is a modified single-fiber EMG electrode; it is discussed later in the section on macro EMG.

Multilead electrodes can contain three or more insulated wires, usually with an exposed surface on the side of the cannula that is considerably larger (1 mm²) than that seen in the multilead single-fiber needle electrode. As many as 14 recording surfaces may be present. One of the wires is the indifferent electrode, and the cannula serves as the ground. Characteristics vary, depending on the distance between the recording electrodes. This type of electrode is used predominantly to measure motor unit territory.

Fine-wire electrodes are most often used for kinesiologic recording. An electrode consisting of two fine, insulated wires, usually platinum and approximately 0.07 mm in diameter, is introduced into the muscle by an injection needle that is subsequently withdrawn.[26] These fine wires cause little discomfort, but their position can be altered only by withdrawing them through the insertion channel created by the needle.

MUSCLE ACTION POTENTIALS: ELECTROMYOGRAPHIC FINDINGS

The electrode registers the average potential over its leading-off area, the recording surface of which is in direct contact with approximately eight muscle fibers, only one or two of which belong to the same motor unit. The sharp spike of the recorded potential is primarily the result of the excitation of a single muscle fiber.[27] This reflects the potential of the motor unit of which it is a part, but it is not the whole motor unit potential.

The amplitude of the action potential depends on several variables, particularly the distance between the recording electrode and the contracting muscle fibers. There is some correlation between the number of muscle fibers per unit and the amplitude of the potential, because summated spikes of contracting fibers near the electrode contribute to the spike component. Buchthal and coworkers[12] have demonstrated the relationship between the leading-off surface area of the electrode and the amplitude recorded. They estimated that eight muscle fibers can be in contact with the surface of a 0.1 by 0.4 mm concentric needle electrode, but at most three of the eight fibers belong to the same unit and contribute to the potential, which totals approximately 4.0 mV. With smaller surface electrodes, such as a multilead electrode, the higher proportion of contracting fiber to surface area produces a larger potential (e.g., 10 mV). Also, muscles that have larger diameter fibers produce potentials of greater amplitude.

The duration of a muscle action potential depends on, but is not proportional to, the mean size of the motor unit.[28] For example, eye muscles, which have small units, produce potentials with a duration of only 1.6–1.8 msec, whereas the potentials of the platysma, with larger units (25 fibers), have an average duration of 4.9 msec. Potentials from the medial head of the gastrocnemius (1,600–2,000 fibers per unit) have a duration of 9.6 msec.

Nerve impulses have been demonstrated to arrive synchronously at all the end-plates of the motor unit under normal circumstances; transmission of the muscle action potentials from different fibers at varying distances from the recording electrode lead to a broadening of the resultant potential curve. Variation in synaptic delay also plays a role in modifying the duration of the action potential. For the human biceps brachii, there is little difference in conduction velocity for the individual muscle fibers of one motor unit (4–5.5 m/second at 36.5°C).[27] This constant velocity has been explained in part by the low external resistance of the extracellular fluid around the muscle fibers, which facilitates mutual interaction between fibers of different diameters.

The shape of the muscle action potential is influenced by factors similar to those that affect amplitude and duration (i.e., the number, distance, and distribution of fibers of the same unit in relation to the recording electrode). A slight temporal dispersion of the component spikes can cause potentials with several phases or humps. The muscle acts as a volume conductor, so the gradual onset and tail of the muscle action potential may be distorted by potentials picked up from more distant motor units.

Thus, it can be seen that the amplitude, duration, and shape of the recorded muscle action potential can vary with the size and type of the electrode and the actual positioning of the electrode within the muscle, amplitude being most dependent on proximity of the electrode to the firing muscle fibers. The *rise time*, the time lag from the initial baseline level or positive peak to the negative peak, provides a guideline to this distance. (By convention, in EMG recording the negative deflection is upward.) The needle electrode should be positioned so that the fastest rise time can be recorded, to obtain most consistent results. A unit accepted for quantitative measurement should have a shorter rise time than 500 μsec, preferably 100–200 μsec.[29]

With monopolar or concentric needle electrodes, biphasic and triphasic potentials make up approximately 80% of all potentials recorded in normal adult subjects (Figure 14-6); a phase is the portion of a wave between the departure from baseline and the return to it.[30] In a complex or serrated action potential, the waveform shows several changes in direction, or turns, that do not cross the baseline.[1] These have a voltage range of 100–3,000 μV and a duration from 2 to 10 msec. The duration of the sharp negative spike is approximately 2 msec. Action potential parameters vary from one muscle to another, as the innervation ratio is not the same. Monophasic and polyphasic potentials are seen in 1–12% of all potentials recorded. Polyphasic potentials, by definition,[1] contain five or more phases and occur with increased frequency in neuropathic and myopathic disorders, although they account for 1–3% of normal potentials (see Figure 14-5).

Spontaneous Activity

Spontaneous activity is recorded from a muscle at rest after insertional activity has subsided and in the absence of a voluntary contraction or external stimuli. The major types of spontaneous activity are fibrillation potentials, end-plate activity, positive sharp waves, fasciculation potentials and repetitive discharges, such as myokymic discharges, complex repetitive discharges, and variations of continuous muscle activity. These last few are not always spontaneous, but can be a form of involuntary activity triggered by a stimulus such as needle insertion or voluntary muscle contraction.

Fibrillation Potential

Fibrillation potentials are muscle action potentials of short duration that result from firing of single muscle

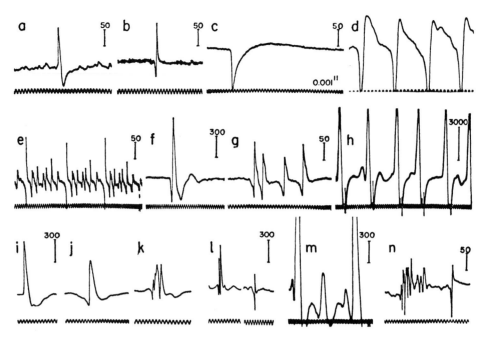

FIGURE 14-6 Motor unit action potentials in electromyography. **(A)** End-plate potential; **(B)** fibrillation potential; **(C)** positive wave from denervated muscle; **(D)** myotonic discharge; **(E)** bizarre high-frequency discharge; **(F)** fasciculation potential, single discharge; **(G)** fasciculation potential, repetitive or grouped discharge; **(H)** synchronized repetitive discharge in muscle cramp; **(I)** diphasic; **(J)** triphasic; **(K)** polyphasic motor unit action potentials from normal muscle; **(L)** short-duration motor unit action potentials in progressive muscular dystrophy; **(M)** large potentials in anterior horn cell disease; and **(N)** reinnervation *nascent* units. Calibration scales are in microvolts; time scales are in milliseconds. An upward deflection indicates a change of potential in the negative direction at the needle electrode. (Reprinted with permission from Mayo Clinic: Clinical Examinations in Neurology [3rd ed]. Philadelphia: Saunders, 1971;276.)

fibers, spontaneously or from mechanical irritation such as needle insertion. They are not visible at the skin surface but may be seen in an exposed muscle or on the tongue. Fibrillation potentials most characteristically have been noted with denervation. When a nerve to a muscle is sectioned, there is a period of wallerian degeneration. Fibrillation potentials are usually observed in human denervated muscle after approximately 1–3 weeks. They are not exclusively indicative of lower motor neuron disease. Some 10–15% of apparently normal subjects have demonstrated a single region of fibrillation potentials.[31] These should not be confused with end-plate potentials (see next section). According to Stöhr,[32] the rhythm of these normal or *benign* fibrillation potentials is almost always irregular. Fibrillation potentials are also noted in some 15–100% of primary myopathic diseases (if carefully sought) such as Duchenne's muscular dystrophy and polymyositis.[33]

Fibrillation potentials recorded with standard monopolar or concentric needle electrodes are most commonly diphasic discharges with an initial positive deflection (see Figure 14-6). The usual amplitude is 50–

150 μV, but potentials up to 3 mV have been recorded. Kraft recorded that the amplitude of fibrillation potentials was largest during the first several months after onset in patients with nerve injury, but a sharp decrease in amplitude occurred during the first 6 months.[34] The amplitude decay then slowed considerably and was gradual over the remaining years, but no fibrillation potentials larger than 100 μV were noted after the first year. Fibrillation potentials can persist as long as several decades following nerve injury, although it is unlikely that the fibrillating muscle fiber is the same. These changes in fibrillation potential amplitude with time after denervation were also demonstrated in a simulation study.[35] The authors show how fibrillation potential amplitude declines depending on muscle fiber size atrophy. They advise that for clinical use the amplitude decline must be carefully evaluated because of the many technical and pathophysiological problems that may interfere. The usual duration of fibrillation potentials is 0.5–2.0 msec. Because of reinnervation or muscle fiber necrosis, with time the overall firing frequency of fibrillation potentials is reduced. Fibrillation potentials most

commonly fire in a regular rhythmic pattern with a frequency of 1–30 Hz. Arrhythmic firing may indicate potentials from more than one muscle fiber, although arrhythmic firing from a single muscle fiber, in the range of 0.1–25 Hz, may also be noted.[36] Studies employing intracellular microelectrode techniques on living white mice have shown that the resting potential remains near the normal level of 100 mV after denervation, until the muscle begins to fibrillate, at which time the potential decreases rapidly, ultimately reaching 77 mV.[37] It is postulated that denervation causes absolute or relative alteration of the sodium pump mechanism, wherein the increased extrusion of sodium caused by the active fibrillatory process results in lowering of the membrane resting potential. Recordings from denervated muscles in vivo showed that spontaneous action potentials in denervated muscles were initiated by biphasic membrane oscillations of increasing amplitude. There is a correlation between membrane potential and the critical level for action potential generation; this relationship is most marked in denervated muscle at levels around the resting membrane potential (–60 to –79 mV).[38] Irregularly firing fibrillation potentials are thought to be triggered by spontaneous oscillations in the decreased resting membrane potential of the denervated muscle.[38] The irregularly discharging fibrillation potentials result from random discrete spontaneous depolarizations of nearly constant amplitude.[36] Hypoxia or cooling decreases the frequency of fibrillation potentials, and ischemia can abolish them. Neostigmine (cholinesterase inhibitors) increases the frequency, as does reduction in extracellular calcium concentration. Kraft,[39] in studies performed on guinea pigs, found that fibrillation potential amplitude is more closely related than any other physical measure of atrophic muscle fibers to the surface area or diameter of type I fibers. Other evidence from studies of rats suggests that fibrillation potentials may not originate in type I fibers.[40]

If the end-plate is excised from actively fibrillating muscle, the fibrillation continues in the strip bearing the end-plate, but ceases in the other sections as soon they are cut off.[41] The membrane at the denervated end-plate zone seems to have properties that are different from the rest of the muscle fiber membrane. Cathodal currents applied to the denervated end-plate area increased fibrillatory frequency, whereas anodal currents decreased the frequency. Currents of a similar magnitude did not change fibrillation frequency when applied to other areas of the muscle fiber. In certain concentrations, acetylcholine and norepinephrine also increase the frequency of fibrillations when applied to the muscle at the denervated end-plate zone, and larger doses of acetyl-

choline depress fibrillation frequency. In spite of the fact that these two agents induce membrane potential changes (depolarization) wherever they are applied, fibrillation frequency is affected only when these agents act on the end-plate area. Thus, the denervated end-plate region acts as a pacemaker site for fibrillation potentials and has chemical and electrical properties different from the rest of the denervated muscle fiber membrane.[42] In light of this information, further studies are necessary to reproduce these findings or to re-evaluate the idea that in patients with myopathies fibrillation potentials can arise from fiber splitting, which may not occur unless there is also incomplete terminal reinnervation of these split-off fibers. Because fibrillation potentials are abolished after ischemia, a circulating substance appears to be involved. Administration of curare does not abolish fibrillation potentials, which suggests that acetylcholine hypersensitivity alone is not responsible. Sensitivity to circulating catecholamine may have a more important role than increased susceptibility to acetylcholine in the production of fibrillation potentials.

Muscle studies in premature infants (before innervation) and in patients with meningomyelocele (in which complete innervation is prevented) showed fibrillation potentials.[43] Muscle fibers of a fetus apparently fibrillate until innervated. This preinnervation activity differs from denervation fibrillations only in its low amplitude (usually <15 µV) and slow frequency (<10 Hz). Fibrillatory activity decreases as the time of normal gestation approaches and innervation is accomplished.

Fibrillation potentials and positive sharp waves may appear in muscles after needling for various procedures, but this is thought to be secondary to local trauma to the muscle membrane.

Spontaneous activity also can be seen within weeks of the onset of an upper motor neuron lesion such as hemiplegia. Although they are not always present, these spontaneous discharges can be noted even in the absence of associated lower motor neuron involvement. The mechanism for this has not been clearly defined; transsynaptic neuronal degeneration remains a possibility (see Upper Motor Neuron Lesions, later in this chapter).

End-Plate Activity
Fibrillation potentials are to be distinguished from potentials recorded in the area of the neuromuscular junction (Figures 14-7 and 14-8).[44,45] These potentials are of two types. Monophasic potentials are spontaneous, localized, nonpropagated potentials of less than 100 µV (usually 10–20 µV), short duration (0.5–1.0 msec), and relatively high frequency (up to 1,000 Hz). These are thought to be miniature end-plate potentials

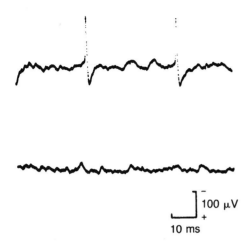

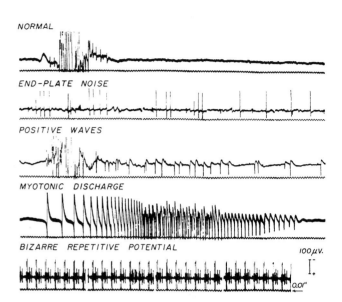

FIGURE 14-8 Insertion potentials evoked by insertion of a needle electrode into muscle. Normally, this consists of a brief discharge of electrical activity lasting a little longer than the movement of the needle. (Reprinted with permission from Mayo Clinic. Clinical Examinations in Neurology [3rd ed]. Philadelphia: Saunders, 1971;279.)

FIGURE 14-7 Spontaneous electrical activity recorded with a needle electrode close to muscle end-plates may be of two forms. (1) Monophasic (both traces): Low-amplitude (10–20 μV), short-duration (0.5–1.0 msec), monophasic (negative) potentials occur in a dense, steady pattern and are restricted to a localized area of the muscle. Because of the multitude of different potentials, the exact frequency, although it appears to be high, cannot be defined. These nonpropagated potentials are probably miniature end-plate potentials recorded extracellularly. This form of end-plate activity has been referred to as *end-plate noise* or *seashell sound* (seashell noise or roar). (2) Biphasic (upper trace): Moderate-amplitude (100–300 μV), short-duration (2–4 msec), biphasic (negative-positive) spike potentials occur irregularly in short bursts with a high frequency (50–100 Hz) restricted to a localized area within the muscle. These propagated potentials are generated by muscle fibers excited by activity in nerve terminals. They have been called *biphasic spike potentials*, *end-plate spikes*, and, incorrectly, *nerve potentials*. (Reprinted with permission from AAEE. Glossary of terms in clinical electromyography. Muscle Nerve 1987;10:G40.)

recorded extracellularly and have also been described as *end-plate noise* or *seashell sound*. These potentials are negative discharges. Biphasic potentials are spontaneous spikes of low amplitude (usually between 100 and 300 μV), usually diphasic with a sharp initial negative deflection, that fire irregularly with a frequency of approximately 50–100 Hz. These propagated potentials are thought to be caused by firing of single muscle fibers in the end-plate area. They resemble fibrillation potentials, except that the initial deflection is negative rather than positive. These potentials have previously been mislabeled *nerve potentials*. If the needle recording electrode is somewhat distant from the end-plate, the initial deflection may be positive, giving the erroneous impression of a fibrillation potential.

Dumitru et al.[46] describe (Figure 14-9) three forms of end-plate potentials in the normal subject: (1) an initially negative biphasic potential that could be seen at the end-plate itself or up to a 0.2 mm distance from it; (2) an initially positive triphasic potential observable anywhere from 0.2 mm from the end-plate and up to 0.5 mm from the muscle-tendon junction; and (3) an initially positive biphasic potential present from the last 0.4 mm of the muscle fiber, but also from mechanical needle-induced impulse blocking. They performed an additional simulation study that confirmed that types of end-plate activity other than the three described previously could result from the summation of two biphasic end-plate potentials. To avoid misinterpretation, special attention should be paid to the irregularity of end-plate potential firing. In general, it is better to avoid examining a muscle in its end-plate zone.

Positive Sharp Waves

Positive sharp waves are spontaneous potentials often seen in association with fibrillation potentials, usually after denervation, that can appear days or weeks before the onset of fibrillation potentials. They may also be associated with myopathy. They are initiated by needle insertion but also fire spontaneously (see Figure 14-8).

FIGURE 14-9 A simulated muscle fiber is shown with an action potential initiated at the neuromuscular junction (NMJ) or end-plate zone. Various recording locations along the muscle fiber (*filled-in circles*) beginning at, and extending from, the end-plate (0.0 mm) are depicted. The computer-generated waveform detected at the electrode recording distance from the end-plate (number in parentheses) is shown. Note that the action potential has only three fundamental morphologies (biphasic initially negative, triphasic initially positive, and biphasic initially positive) directly dependent on the relation between the action potential and recording electrode location. (Reprinted with permission from D Dumitru, JC King, DF Stegeman. End-plate spike morphology: a clinical and simulation study. Arch Phys Med Rehabil 1998;79:637.)

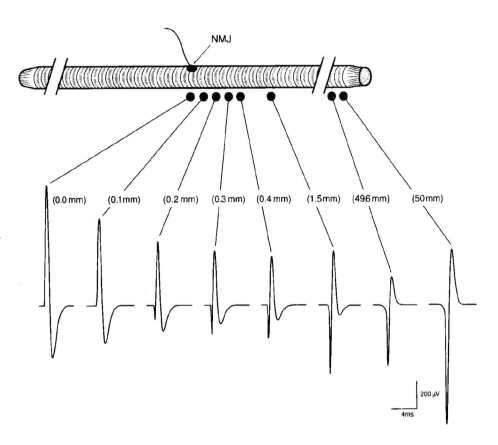

The rhythm is usually regular; frequency ranges from 1 to 50 Hz. Positive sharp waves have an initial rapid positive (downward) deflection that is followed by an exponential negative charge that can continue into a prolonged low-voltage negative phase. The duration of the positive component is usually less than 5 msec and the amplitude up to 1 mV; the negative phase can have a duration of 10–100 msec and lower amplitude (see Figure 14-6). It is thought that positive sharp waves, like fibrillation potentials, arise from single muscle fibers and are caused by the placement of the recording electrode adjacent to a blocked or damaged (depolarized) region of the muscle fiber (Figure 14-10).

Occasionally, a transformation from fibrillation potential to positive sharp wave can be observed during an EMG examination. A clinical and simulation study was published[47] in which the authors report the possible mechanism of this phenomenon. They propose that a transition from fibrillation potential to positive sharp wave can occur when a summation takes place of the waves of two independently but more or less synchronously firing muscle fibers. A role is probably played by the mechanical pressure at the tip of the needle electrode, which deforms several muscle fibers, resulting in partial or total blockade of their action potentials.

Fasciculation Potentials

Fasciculations are involuntary muscle twitches that can often be seen on the surface of the skin or on the tongue. The electrically recorded fasciculation potentials result from spontaneous discharges of a whole or a portion of a motor unit. They are irregular in rhythm (firing frequency <5 Hz), form, voltage, and duration (see Figure 14-6). Fasciculation potentials are noted in many conditions, including benign myokymia, nerve root compression, ischemia, various forms of muscle cramps, and anterior horn cell disease. Although they are characteristically associated with the last condition, in themselves fasciculation potentials are not pathognomonic.

There is some controversy as to the site of origin of fasciculation potentials, but both distal and more proximal sites are likely. Using a collision method, the origin of at least 80% of fasciculations in various lower motor neuron lesions was determined to be the distal extremity of the axon, regardless of the type of lesion, its duration, or the severity of the denervation.[48] Section of the motor nerve in cases of advanced disease of anterior horn cells (amyotrophic lateral sclerosis [ALS]) is followed by the same degree of fasciculation for several days before wallerian degeneration begins,[49] and spontaneous muscle fasciculations may not be affected by

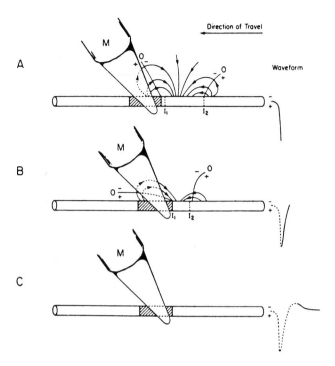

FIGURE 14-10 The generation of a positive sharp wave using volume conduction theory. **A.** A fibrillation potential approaches a monopolar electrode (M) placed next to a denervated muscle fiber. A positive source current is initially detected, and the cathode ray tube records a positive deflection. **B.** As the negative sink approaches the region of the membrane deformed by the needle electrode (*hashed region*), it cannot invade this portion of the membrane. As sodium inactivation and potassium efflux continue, the spatial extent of the negative sink (I_1 and I_2) diminishes. The current distribution and density are subsequently altered. This may be reflected as a decreasing positive or slightly negative potential. If the nonconducting portion of the membrane extends beyond the immediate vicinity of the electrode, a negative phase may not be observed and only a monophasic positive potential is recorded. **C.** With failure of conduction to or beyond the electrode and absence of the negative sink, the cathode ray tube trace returns to baseline. (Reprinted with permission from D Dumitru. Volume Conduction: Theory and Application. In D Dumitru [ed], Physical Medicine and Rehabilitation: State of the Art Reviews, vol 3, no 4. Philadelphia: Hanley & Belfus, 1989;678.)

spinal anesthesia or peripheral nerve block. Neostigmine produces or increases fasciculations, even during spinal anesthesia. Curare abolishes spontaneous fasciculations and prevents induction of fasciculations by neostigmine in healthy subjects. The impulse is presumed to start in the area of the end-plate and to spread antidromically to involve other axon branches, thus accounting for the frequently observed polyphasic nature and prolonged duration of the potentials.[50] Conradi and colleagues[51] studied fasciculation potentials in 10 patients with ALS. EMG recordings of single MUAPs from the extensor digitorum brevis muscle on maximal voluntary effort and on supramaximal electrical stimulation of the peroneal nerve were evaluated. In a series of fasciculations, the shapes of the EMG potentials varied, whereas in a series of voluntary twitch activations of electrical nerve stimulations, EMG potentials were, on the whole, constant. Fasciculations were followed by antidromic impulses in the test unit axon, as judged from collision tests, and they persisted after lidocaine blockade of the nerve to the muscle. These findings are compatible with distal multifocal triggering of fasciculations. Wettstein[52] used collision technique to determine the origin of fasciculations in motor units from patients with ALS and other diseases involving motor neurons. In this study, some 60% of subjects had only fasciculations of proximal origin, approximately 10% only of distal origin, and the rest had mixed origin fasciculations.

Fasciculation potentials may be caused by a central mechanism, as well as a peripheral one.[53] Giant, bizarre, spontaneous potentials are seen in ALS and related diseases, and, unlike other fasciculations, these may be eliminated by nerve block. The anatomic basis for these abnormal potentials may in part be intramuscular axon budding or collateral regeneration from normal to denervated elements. EMG studies of motor unit territory in patients with ALS indicate that the motor units are expanded beyond what can be accounted for by intramuscular sprouting. In some instances, several neural elements at the same spinal level interact to produce synchronous fasciculations in different muscles, which seem to originate from a spinal locus of hyperexcitability. Intraspinal axonal sprouting occurs in ALS patients; it is uncertain whether this sprouting is analogous to the intramuscular collateral regeneration of partially denervated muscle.

After nerve section, fasciculation potentials disappear with the development of wallerian degeneration. Immature terminal and collateral sprouts of motor neurons were found in biopsies from fasciculating muscle regions in patients with ALS.[28] These immature neuromuscular junctions may be more sensitive to humoral agents, and thus fasciculation twitches may be initiated by normal levels of neurohumoral transmitters, such as acetylcholine. Fine, beaded nerve fibers are seen in the intramuscular nerve bundles of patients with motor neuron diseases. These fibers are unmyelinated, and many do not have Schwann cell cover. It is possible that ephaptic transmission across these fibers could produce fasciculatory movements.

Idiopathic *benign* fasciculations and muscle cramps often occur in the calf muscles; they can be associated with salt depletion and often are facilitated by ischemia. The twitches are irregular and variably polyphasic; they can be stopped by voluntary activity. Their polyphasic form seems to indicate that they arise in the terminal branches of the lower motor neuron and have a changing focus of origin. Single or grouped fasciculation potentials can also be present in other normal muscles. The frequency of firing of potentials recorded from normal muscle may be greater (average interval 0.8 seconds, compared with 3.5 seconds in patients with motor neuron disease).[54]

The fasciculation potentials that occur after root compression are often of simple diphasic form and are usually associated with signs of denervation, such as positive sharp waves and fibrillation potentials.

Myokymic Discharges
MUAPs may discharge repeatedly. This is visible on the surface of the skin as a quivering or undulating movement known as *myokymia* (Table 14-1). The firing units have a uniform appearance, and discharge may be brief, repetitive firing of single units for a short period (doublets, triplets, or *multiplets* up to a few seconds) at a uniform rate of 2–60 Hz, followed by 2 or 3 seconds of silence, then repetition of the same sequence for a particular potential. Less commonly, the potential recurs continuously at a fairly uniform firing rate of 1–5 Hz.[1]

Myokymia is more common in facial than in extremity muscles. Myokymic discharges can be present in patients with brain stem tumors, multiple sclerosis, Guillain-Barré syndrome, or radiation plexopathy. Myokymic discharges arise spontaneously at some portion of the motor axon where the axon membrane is hyperexcitable.[55] Hyperventilation (hypocalcemia) enhances the discharges where the hyperexcitable area of the nerve is extramedullary (peripherally), as in Guillain-Barré syndrome.[56]

Complex Repetitive Discharges
Complex repetitive discharges are repetitive discharges of serrated (complex) or polyphasic potentials, which are relatively uniform in appearance, firing at a regular rate, although the frequency of discharge for each particular burst can vary from 5 to 100 Hz (see Figure 14-10). Amplitude ranges from 400 μV to 1 mV. The discharges characteristically start and stop relatively abruptly. They can begin spontaneously or be induced by needle insertion. These discharges have also been called *bizarre high-frequency potentials* or *pseudomyotonia*, but use of these terms is not encouraged. A single fiber in the complex apparently acts as a pacemaker, which then stimulates other fibers ephaptically, continuing the cycle until blocking occurs.[57] These discharges are seen in a number of disorders, including Duchenne's muscular dystrophy, polymyositis, radiculopathies, motor neuron disease, and chronic polyneuropathy.

TABLE 14-1
Electromyographic Characteristics of Repetitive Discharges

Discharge	Induction	Rate of Discharge (Hz)	Motor Unit Action Potential Forms	Run
Myokymia	Spontaneous	a. 2–60 b. 1–5	Uniform appearance	a. Up to several seconds followed by 2–3 seconds of silence b. Continuous
Complex repetitive discharges	Spontaneous or insertional	5–100	Complex, polyphasic, or both	Regular rate of each burst
Neuromyotonic discharges	Spontaneous, insertional, or voluntary contraction	150–300	Motor unit action potentials	Few seconds, often starts and stops abruptly; amplitude usually wanes
Cramp discharges	Spontaneous muscle contraction	Usually high-frequency, up to 150	Motor unit action potentials	Discharge frequency and number of motor unit action potentials increase gradually and then subside gradually
Myotonic discharges	Spontaneous, insertional, or voluntary contraction	20–80	a. Bursts of positive waves 5–20 msec b. Biphasic positive-negative spike potentials usually < 5 msec	Amplitude and frequency of potentials increase or decrease in a waxing and waning form and can last several seconds

Neuromyotonic Discharges

Neuromyotonic discharges are bursts of MUAPs originating in the motor axons and firing at high rates (150–300 Hz) for a few seconds. They often start and stop abruptly. The amplitude of the response typically wanes. Discharges can occur spontaneously or be initiated by needle insertion, voluntary effort, or ischemia.[1] Clinically, continuous muscle fiber activity is manifested as muscle rippling and stiffness.

Cramp Discharges

A cramp discharge consists of involuntary repetitive firing of MUAPs of high frequency (up to 150 Hz) in a large area of muscles, usually associated with painful muscle contraction. Both discharge frequency and the number of MUAPs that are firing increase gradually during development, and both subside gradually with cessation.[1]

Myokymic discharges, complex repetitive discharges, neuromyotonic discharges, and cramp discharges are differentiated one from the other by frequency and firing pattern rather than by the appearance of individual potentials, which are often similar.

Insertional Activity

When the needle is inserted briskly into the muscle, a burst of potentials can be recorded. These potentials are thought to arise from single muscle fibers whose membranes have been injured mechanically by the needle. Obviously, even under normal circumstances, the duration of this insertional activity depends on the speed and duration of the insertion itself. This measurement, therefore, is only semiquantitative. Examiners should attempt to standardize their insertion movements, making them relatively brisk. Under most circumstances, the duration of the burst of normal insertional activity is 50–100 msec.

A careful clinical and simulation study of insertional activity was carried out by Dumitru et al.[58] Even though various distinctive insertional potentials have been described in the literature, they were able to document that there appear to be just two basic insertional potentials, with either a positive or negative waveform. However, these can be combined in different ways and thus produce many differently shaped insertional spikes. In the presence of reduced muscle bulk, as with fibrosis or necrosis, insertional activity is reduced. An increase in insertional activity can be seen when the muscle cell membranes are hyperirritable, as in acute denervation, inflammatory diseases of muscle, and myotonia. The potentials observed after cessation of the needle movement are even more significant from a clinical point of view, as needle insertion can provoke more prolonged runs of fibrillation potentials, positive sharp waves, complex repetitive discharges, and myotonic discharges. Normally, insertional activity lasts only a few milliseconds after needle movement ceases. Because recorded insertional activity is thought to be caused by induced injury to the muscle membrane, several positive waves may be recorded, even in normal subjects immediately after needle insertion. Thus, this alone should not be attributed to a clinically pathologic condition. Increased insertional activity, manifested as brief runs of positive sharp waves or more rarely fibrillation potentials, may appear early in denervation, before the regular spontaneous activity.

Myotonic Discharges

Myotonic discharges occur spontaneously, but can also be produced by needle insertion, voluntary muscle contraction, nerve stimulation, or mechanical stimulation such as muscle percussion. The discharges occur at a rate of approximately 20–80 Hz, and characteristically the amplitude and frequency of the potentials wax and wane (see Figure 14-10). The characteristic audio manifestation is a *dive bomber* sound, although others may describe it as the open and close turning of a motorcycle's gas handle. The myotonic discharges recorded are of two types. (The total duration of the run can be as long as several seconds for both types.) One type consists of bursts of positive waves of 5- to 20-msec duration; the other is biphasic positive-negative spike potentials in which the negative component may predominate, although these potentials can resemble fibrillation potentials and last less than 5 msec. The exact form of the potential recorded is thought to be related to the position of the recording electrode surface relative to the firing muscle fibers.

Myotonic discharges persist after procaine block of the nerve or after curarization, which suggests they originate in muscle. During intracellular recording of human myotonic muscle, Norris[59] found spontaneous slow depolarization of the muscle membrane leading to repetitive spikes or an abortive spike followed by further slow depolarization.

Although myotonic discharges are caused by abnormalities of the muscle fiber membrane, apparently different mechanisms are involved, depending on the underlying disorder (see the section Myotonia). There is also a relation between myotonic discharges and increased serum potassium level.

Myoclonus

Myoclonus is one of the involuntary movements characterized by sudden, jerky, irregular contractions of a muscle or group of muscles not associated with loss of consciousness. There are various causes for this condition, as there are sites of involvement, rhythmicity, and provoking factors. It is thought that most myoclonic disorders are caused by CNS (in particular cortical) involvement. Further discussion, therefore, is not warranted in the context of this section.

Interference Patterns and Recruitment

Needle EMG examination of a normal skeletal muscle at rest reveals an isoelectric baseline (i.e., electrical silence). Recruitment is successive activation of the same and additional motor units with increasing strength of voluntary muscle contraction. With minimal voluntary contraction one or several motor units are activated, usually low-amplitude ones (500 μV). As tension increases, the firing frequency of the individual potential increases. If the amplitude increases at the same time, it is assumed that the number of muscle fibers activated in the motor unit has increased, presumably because all the end-plates of a unit are not in an identical state of physicochemical readiness. Other evidence comes from studies with protected microelectrodes of the human rectus femoris and gastrocnemius muscles in which it was noted that motor unit potentials tended to increase in amplitude with heightened tension during isometric contraction.[60] This increase is attributed to an increase in the number of active muscle fibers involved in successive discharges of a single motor unit.

With increase in tension, additional motor units are recruited, some of higher amplitude. Buchthal and coworkers[21] found the amplitude of the second and third recruited units to be larger than that of the first and attributed this to decreasing distance between the recording electrode and the active unit as the strength of contraction increased. With further increases in tension, even more units are recruited, and temporal and spatial summation of potentials from multiple motor units produces a characteristic interference pattern, so that with monopolar and concentric needle electrodes, muscle action potentials from individual units no longer can be clearly distinguished.

There is an order of recruitment of motor units. At low strength of contraction, only a few motor units are active, and these have a slow rate of discharge and relatively low amplitude. These low-threshold, early-activated units produce relatively small forces used for fine motor control and postural adjustment, and the muscle fibers making up these units are of the S type (slow-fatigue, type I). Increasing tension increases the frequency of discharge by the active motor unit and recruitment of previously inactive units. The higher threshold units have larger force contributions, and muscle fibers are of the FF (fast-fatigue) or FR (fatigue-resistant) types.[61] Motor neuron soma diameter, axon diameter, and conduction velocity are highly correlated.[61] The size principle holds that motor units are recruited in order of size, from small to large. This is most easily demonstrated for slowly developing muscle contraction.[62] In the presence of a normal, smooth, clinically sustained contraction of a muscle, motor units fire at a rate, and in relation to each other, so that fusion of muscle contraction results in a smooth, continuous, nonjerky contraction. In various states of tremor, fatigue, and denervation this relationship breaks down.[61] In the human biceps brachii, the slower firing, low-threshold units tend to be located deep in the muscle, whereas the rapid-firing, higher threshold units are more superficial.[63]

The recruitment interval is the interdischarge interval between two consecutive discharges of a MUAP at the point at which a second motor unit potential is recruited with gradually increasing strength of voluntary muscle contraction (Figure 14-11). The recruitment frequency,

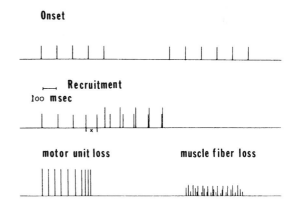

FIGURE 14-11 Essential features of motor unit recruitment are shown in the diagram. Onset level of firing is near threshold for activation, and lapses in firing may occur. Recruitment rate is the rate just before recruitment of a second motor unit during slowly increasing muscle force (innervation). Loss of motor units to disease results in the appearance of individual, easily distinguished single motor unit action potentials firing at a high rate. Loss of muscle fibers results in recruitment of many different motor units at minimal effort. (Reprinted with permission from JH Petajan. Motor unit recruitment. Muscle Nerve 1991;14:494.)

or firing rate, is the firing rate of a MUAP when a different MUAP first appears, with gradually increasing strength of voluntary muscle contraction, and it is the reciprocal of the recruitment interval. These are quantitative measures and are most accurately evaluated when a fixed, low-level percentage of maximal voluntary contraction (MVC) of a particular muscle (25–30%) is maintained, rather than a fixed weight, which can represent a different MVC for different subjects. In neuropathic disease the recruitment interval is shortened because fewer motor units are available. The first unit is usually firing more rapidly at the moment when the second is recruited, shortening the recruitment interval and increasing the recruitment frequency. The converse takes place early in myopathic diseases, as the first unit is firing more slowly at the moment when the second unit is recruited because the first-recruited, slower firing motor unit is not completely knocked out, and each motor unit has fewer functioning muscle fibers and is weaker.[64] Another useful value is the ratio of the average firing rate to the number of active units. In normal subjects it is less than 5:1 (e.g., three units firing at <15 Hz). If two units are firing more than 20 Hz, the ratio exceeds 10:1, indicating loss of motor units.[65]

As noted, when individual motor unit potentials are analyzed during needle EMG examination in healthy subjects, those potentials most readily isolated and clearly distinguished are the low-threshold, type I, low-frequency firing units. This is not necessarily the case in various disease states (e.g., in steroid myopathy with loss of type I fibers, the first-recruited fibers fire more frequently). Under normal circumstances, the principal mechanism for increasing force output is to add more motor units (i.e., spatial recruitment).[61] In different pathologic conditions, further recruitment may not be possible, so motor units fire at much greater than normal rates. This is also seen in rapid force generation. It appears that recruitment has a more important role in grading of activity than does changing the frequency, except at very low and very high contraction strengths. Frequencies of firing of individual MUAPs above 50 Hz are rarely observed. Under most conditions (25–75% MVC), the fastest units respond at frequencies between 25 and 35 Hz. Over the tension range of 5–60% MVC, the firing starts and stops abruptly and the frequency increases, but not in proportion to strength. For example, in one unit observed, the firing commenced at 20 Hz when the tension was 15% of maximum and increased with the tension rise, but only to 30 Hz.[66] Units that are active at tensions below 5% MVC usually have a lower starting frequency (5–7 Hz) and a greater frequency range

and irregular discharge rates, even during constant contraction.

Synchronization

In anterior horn cell diseases such as poliomyelitis, ALS, or syringomyelia, *synchronization* is demonstrated when action potentials are obtained simultaneously from two or more widely separated recording electrodes. The cause of this phenomenon is not clear. One speculation is that there is an intraspinal mechanism for synchronization of discharge rhythm in a number of different motor units supplied by the same spinal segment.[52] Another possibility is that in a given muscle single units of large area (as noted with reinnervated muscle in anterior horn cell disorders) are responsible.

The occurrence of occasional true synchronization of motor units in a number of muscles in human subjects and animals has not received valid confirmation. An electronic model and statistical analysis of EMG records made under a variety of conditions seem to demonstrate the absence of true synchronization of motor neuron activity and voluntary contractions,[67] although grouping of discharges may be seen in the single action potential of the tendon jerk, and partial synchronization and grouping in clonus and various tremors.[68]

Effect of Age

The normal mean duration of the muscle action potential increases with age, so that at age 70–80 years the average duration is as much as 75% longer than in children younger than 4 years.[21] This is explained as a decrease in the propagation velocity of the impulse over the muscle fiber. Peterson and Kugelberg[69] noted that in young persons normal values are obtained from the first-recruited low-threshold muscle action potentials, whereas aging may selectively destroy muscle fibers with the largest calibers and lowest thresholds.

Brown,[70] using the McComas method for counting the number of motor units, studied median innervated thenar muscles and showed a decrease in the number of motor units, especially in subjects older than 60 years. The mean motor unit count of subjects aged 70 years and older was less than one-half that of the subjects 39 years and younger. There was no evidence of denervation in the form of fibrillation potentials, or any evidence for reduction in the size of individual motor units. It was postulated that the reduced motor unit count could be the result of asymptomatic injury to the median nerve, but distal latencies were essentially normal. Using a different method, combining isometric contraction, intramuscular needle electrode recordings, and spike-triggered averaging techniques to measure the sizes of motor unit potentials as recorded in the innervation zone with surface electrodes, the number of motor units in the biceps brachialis muscles of healthy subjects was estimated.[8] Here, too, estimates in subjects older than 60 years were one-half those of subjects in the third decade of life. None of the subjects reported symptoms or had physical findings suggestive of cervical radiculopathy, and EMG did not indicate denervation or reinnervation in the biceps or brachialis muscles. Slawnych and coworkers[71] reviewed a number of studies estimating the number of motor units in elderly subjects and in younger ones; these showed general agreement for reduced motor unit estimates in the extensor digitorum brevis of elderly subjects, although the extensor digitorum brevis and thenar muscles were more severely affected than the hypothenar muscles. Stålberg and Thiele[72] performed a single-fiber EMG study on the extensor digitorum communis muscle in subjects aged 10–89 years and noted that fiber density increases slowly throughout life and progresses faster after age 70 years. There was an indication that impairment of nerve or neuromuscular impulse transmission increases at the same time, suggesting that degenerative loss of motor neurons with aging was compensated for by reinnervation. Motor unit density in the tibialis anterior muscle decreased with age, as measured by macro EMG,[73,74] which could indicate loss of motor units with increasing age. Distal muscles show more extensive changes than proximal ones, and not all muscles are uniformly affected.

Few studies of humans have actually looked at age-related changes in motor neuron numbers in the spinal cord. In one such study[75] spinal cords of 47 subjects aged 13–95 years who died suddenly were examined. There was no evidence for loss of motor neurons up to age 60, but beyond that age, although individual counts varied considerably, there was evidence for a diminishing motor neuron population. After age 60 years, several cases showed counts only 50% those of younger subjects. Cell loss appeared to be uniform throughout all segments and was not accompanied by any other striking morphologic change. There was no history of pre-existing weakness beyond what was "reasonable for age." It is generally accepted, however, that clinical weakness usually is not noted until 40–60% of muscle fibers have been lost. Unfortunately, peripheral nerve and muscle were not examined. In another study[76] of the L-3 to L-5 spinal cord segments of 18 subjects, progressive loss of large motor neurons was noted for all ages examined.

Although the total number of muscle fibers of the rat soleus muscle decreases with age, no difference was found in the number of alpha motor nerve fibers to the muscle.[77] It is possible that there is little or no loss of motor nerve cells in the spinal cord until aging is more advanced (after age 60–70 years in humans) and that peripheral loss of muscle fibers is out of proportion to these findings. Evidence to substantiate this supposition is provided by the random degeneration of the end-plates and some terminal end-plate regeneration. These factors may explain the longer duration of action potentials and the greater number of polyphasic potentials associated with aging in the absence of signs of acute denervation.

Effect of Temperature

As the intramuscular temperature drops, the mean duration of the muscle action potential increases by 10–30% and the mean amplitude decreases by 2–5% for every 1°C reduction. The number of polyphasic potentials can increase as much as 10-fold with a 10°C decrease in temperature.[21] This prolongation of duration is caused by the temperature coefficient of the propagation velocity. The slower propagation velocity of the impulse over the muscle fiber and the terminal nerve fibers can cause temporal dispersion of fibers within the motor unit.

Fatigue

Neuromuscular fatigue can be defined as any reduction in the force-generating capacity of the total neuromuscular system, regardless of the force required in any given situation.[78] In the absence of fatigue, the sum of electrical activity, recorded by surface electrodes of a muscle, bears a simple linear relation to the force developed.[79] The increase in force is caused by the activation of more motor units and, to a lesser degree, to their greater frequency of discharge. In fatiguing muscle, the relative force developed, and the sum of electrical activity, also remain linearly related until the level of mechanical activity cannot be maintained. In the fatigued muscle, however, each increment of physical force requires a larger volume of electrical activity, presumably because of a deficiency in the contractile process rather than changes in electrical propagation. Transmission across the neuromuscular junction may also be modified (especially with high-frequency stimulation), but it probably plays no significant role in normal subjects. The EMG results recorded with surface electrodes reveal increased amplitude of the summated potentials and a decrease in their frequency with fatigue,[80] as a result of grouping of firing units. This disrupts the normal smooth muscle contraction, resulting in a jerky firing pattern. A needle EMG study confirms that discharges of fibers from different motor units tend to group during fatiguing muscle work; there is also an increase in the total number of active motor units. The individual MUAPs are decreased in amplitude, but duration of the potentials is little changed. The number of polyphasic potentials is increased with fatigue,[79] presumably owing to incomplete synchronization between fibers of different motor units[21] or to end-plate alterations, with more irregular firing of individual fibers of the motor unit occurring in the vicinity of the needle electrode tip. Using tungsten microelectrodes, uncontaminated, single-unit potentials from the adductor pollicis of normal human subjects were recorded during MVCs.[81] Their amplitude, duration, and shape showed them to be action potentials from single muscle fibers. In brief, nonfatiguing, maximal contractions, the average firing rate of more than 200 units recorded from five subjects was 29.8 ± 6.4 Hz. During prolonged maximal effort, both force and firing rate always declined. Between 30 and 60 seconds and 60 and 90 seconds after the onset of the contractions, the rates were 18.8 ± 4.6 Hz and 14.3 ± 4.4 Hz, respectively. The percentage of decline in mean motor neuron firing rate paralleled, and appeared to account for, that of the surface EMG recorded simultaneously. These results are direct evidence for a reduction of motor neuron firing rates during this type of fatigue.

After a fatiguing muscle contraction, fewer motor unit spikes per second are needed to maintain a certain low level of force than before the contraction.[82] A significant reduction in spikes per second was found to occur in multiple regions of the biceps muscle examined and in other arm flexors. In addition, surface-rectified, integrated EMG, which measures electrical activity in a larger area of the muscle than the needle electrode, declined in parallel with the decrease in spike counts, indicating that other areas of muscle did not appear to be compensating for a more fatigued portion. These results imply that force can be maintained with a lower level of excitation after fatigue than before. It is thought that fatigue decreases the contraction-relaxation rate of muscle fibers, which lowers the fusion frequency. Thus, lower rates of motor unit activation can result in the maintenance of constant force. A feedback system from muscle to the CNS likely senses this slowing and leads to the spike count reduction.

Effect of Disuse

In muscles with disuse atrophy, polyphasic potentials of more than four phases accounted for 25% of all action potentials, compared with 1–3% in normal muscle.[83] A reduction or increase in duration of the MUAPs occasionally is noted, which may be caused by alteration in fiber conduction velocity. Spontaneous activity has not been reported as being present in disuse atrophy in the absence of superimposed denervation or primary muscle trauma. No significant changes of muscle fiber membrane characteristics have been demonstrated in animals up to a month after disuse was induced by section of the spinal cord at a higher level than the muscle supply and after sectioning of the dorsal roots.[84] In these animals, in which total flaccid paraplegia without lower motor neuron denervation was produced, a reversible decrease of 10 mV in the resting membrane potential was noted in the first week only.

ANALYSIS OF ELECTROMYOGRAPHY AND SPECIAL ELECTROMYOGRAPHIC TECHNIQUES

Single-Fiber Electromyography

Standard EMG records compound action potentials from many muscle fibers making up the motor unit and from multiple motor units. The single-fiber needle electrode permits recording of individual muscle fibers belonging to a single motor unit. Because this technique looks at restricted areas of the motor unit, it is prudent also to use information obtained from routine EMG examination, to allow for valid extrapolation of the functioning of the motor unit and the muscle as a whole. As previously noted, the single-fiber needle electrode, by having a small lead-off surface of approximately 25-μm diameter, can selectively record from single muscle fibers close to it. The recording surface is 3–4 mm along the shaft from the cutting point of the needle tip (see Figure 14-3). There can be a separate indifferent recording electrode, or selectivity can be enhanced by a second electrode on the shaft a short distance (200 μm) from the first. The pick-up area is approximately a hemisphere of 150–300 μm. These electrodes have a high impedance, so the amplifier input impedance must also be quite high (100 mΩ) in order to have a high signal-to-noise ratio and an adequate common mode rejection ratio.[85] Baseline noise and low-frequency discharges from distant potentials must be filtered out, so a low-frequency filter of 500 Hz is used. The amplitude of the single-fiber potential can vary considerably, from 0.2 mV to 100 times that, but a range of 1–7 mV is most common. A triggering device usually set to trigger on the fastest slope of the deflection is necessary, together with a delay line, so that the initial portion of the potential can be recorded. Clinical single-fiber EMG records from voluntary contractions of individual muscle fibers while the patient attempts to maintain minimal contraction with a stable firing rate. The potential is biphasic with an initial positive deflection, and the rise time from positive to negative peak should be less than 300 μsec, and the peak-to-peak amplitude should exceed 200 μV. The shape should be constant with repetitive firing.

Jitter

Ekstedt[27] showed that the difference in arrival time at the electrode of two muscle fiber action potentials from the same motor unit was not constant from discharge to discharge. This jitter phenomenon was on the order of 10–30 μsec in the mutual time interval between the spike components of the composite potentials. This phenomenon can be seen with repetitive nerve stimulation and with voluntary contraction of muscle and can be caused by variability in conduction along the terminal nerve fibers, neuromuscular junctions, and muscle fibers. Variability in transmission time at the neuromuscular junction plays the greatest role in normal subjects. Jitter, therefore, is the variability with consecutive discharges of the interpotential interval between two muscle fiber action potentials belonging to the same motor unit (Figure 14-12).[1] It is usually expressed quantitatively as the mean of the differences between the interpotential intervals of successive discharges (the mean consecutive difference). Newer digital equipment automatically analyzes jitter. Under certain conditions, jitter is expressed as the mean value of the difference between interpotential intervals arranged in order of decreasing interdischarge intervals (the mean sorted difference).[1] Jitter varies, depending on technique (fast sweep speeds are necessary for good resolution), age, and specific muscles tested. The extensor digitorum communis is the muscle most frequently used for single-fiber EMG recording, because it is superficial and easily accessible, does not normally show age-related abnormalities, and can easily be activated, controlled, and supported in a good position. Before the use of computer analysis, 50 potential pairs (10 groups of five or five groups of 10 potentials) were recorded and the mean consecutive difference calculated. Values are abnormal if 10% or more of fiber pairs have jitter that exceeds the upper limit of normal for fiber pairs (55 μs for extensor digitorum communis) or the mean jitter of all

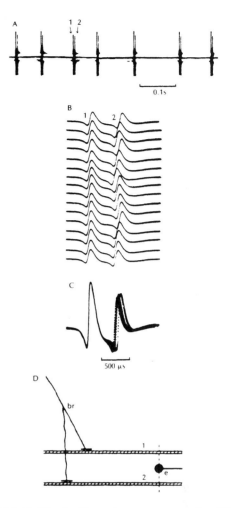

FIGURE 14-12 Single-fiber electromyography (SFEMG) recordings. **A.** At a slow oscilloscope sweep speed, repetitive firing of one pair of potentials can be seen. **B.** At a faster sweep speed, with the sweep triggered by the rising phase of potential 1, the same potential pairs are delayed and displayed rastered. **C.** Ten sweeps are superimposed, demonstrating the variable interpotential intervals (i.e., the neuromuscular jitter). **D.** The recording position of the SFEMG electrode (e). (br = [nerve terminal] branch.) (Reprinted with permission from DB Sanders, LH Phillips. Single fiber electromyography. AAEE Workshop, 1984;2.)

fiber pairs exceeds the upper limit of mean jitter for that muscle (34 μs for extensor digitorum communis). Blocking, failure to fire of the second potential because of failure of end-plate depolarization, is also abnormal when observed (Figure 14-13). In healthy muscles, jitter increases with decreases in temperature or during ischemia (not to be confused with reduced decrement in amplitude of evoked potentials noted with repetitive nerve stimulation). Abnormally increased jitter values

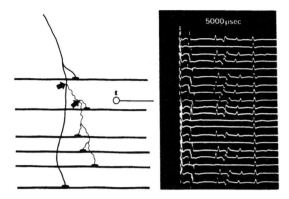

FIGURE 14-13 Concomitant blocking. A recording from six muscle fibers from the same motor unit. The middle four spike components intermittently block together. They also have a large common jitter in relation to the remaining two components. The block is most likely situated in the nerve twig common to the four blocking muscle fibers (i.e., between the arrows in the schematic drawing). (E = electrode position.) (Reprinted with permission from EV Stålberg. In AAEE International Symposium on Peripheral Nerve Regeneration, Washington, DC, 1989;40.)

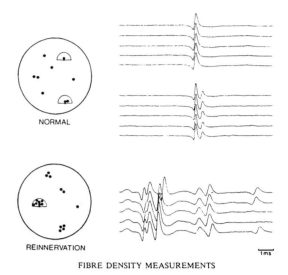

FIBRE DENSITY MEASUREMENTS

FIGURE 14-14 Method for measuring fiber density. In normal muscle, usually one or two single-muscle fiber action potentials from the same motor unit are seen. After reinnervation, the chance to record from many fibers in one motor unit is increased, owing to grouping. (Reprinted with permission from EV Stålberg. In AAEE International Symposium on Peripheral Nerve Regeneration, Washington, DC, 1989;37.)

and blocking are found in patients with myasthenia gravis who have only ocular manifestations and show relative sparing of extremity muscles. More diffuse abnormalities can be present, depending on the severity of the generalized myasthenia gravis. Jitter is abnormal in any condition of impaired neuromuscular transmission, so abnormally increased jitter values and blocking can be found in patients with motor neuron disease, peripheral neuropathy, or myopathy. Some patients with myopathy, such as Duchenne's muscular dystrophy, may have jitter values less than the normal range, possibly resulting from recording of potentials from split muscle fibers with the same innervation.[86] Abnormal jitter values alone should not be used as a criterion for differentiating neurogenic and myopathic diseases. In patients with myasthenia gravis, edrophonium can decrease abnormal jitter and reduce the incidence of blocking. Increased jitter in patients with myopathy could be a result of prolonged propagation time of the muscle fibers or fragmentation of damaged muscle fibers with collateral reinnervation.

Fiber Density

As previously noted, the single-fiber electrode can record from a hemisphere area of approximately 200–300 μm. Random single-fiber EMG electrode insertion in a slightly contracting normal muscle usually records one single-fiber action potential; in approximately 20%

of random insertions two muscle fibers of a single motor unit found are recorded. In fiber density measurement, the electrode is randomly inserted in 20 sites. The amplitude of the triggering potential is maximized, and the number of action potentials that are time locked and meet the criteria for single-fiber potentials (amplitude > 200 μV, rise time less than 300 μs) are counted (Figure 14-14). The fiber density, therefore, provides a measure of the number of muscle fibers from a single motor unit presented as the mean value of the number of spikes recorded at 20 sites. Loss of muscle fiber normally is not detected, because the lowest possible value is 1.0. Normal fiber density varies, depending on the muscle examined, and also increases with age, being most marked after age 70 years. Fiber density is increased in conditions in which collateral sprouting and fiber grouping occur. Therefore, as would be expected, fiber density measurements are a sensitive indicator of chronic motor neuron disease, although increased density is also found in peripheral neuropathies, disorders of neuromuscular transmission, and myopathies.

Macro Electromyography

Macro EMG provides information about the entire motor unit. The macro EMG needle electrode uses a 15-

mm section of the length of the cannula from the tip as the principal recording surface for territorial pickup. Because the territory of most motor units is 5–10 mm, the 15-mm insertion length is both mechanically practical from an insertional point of view and long enough to encompass the area of the motor unit. One channel records the signal between the electrode shaft and a reference electrode (surface or subcutaneous needle electrode); the second channel is a modified single-fiber EMG electrode approximately halfway (7.5 mm) from the tip of the exposed electrode shaft that records a single-fiber EMG signal between the exposed 25-μm diameter platinum wire and the shaft of the same electrode. The sweep is triggered by the single-fiber EMG recording, so that synchronously firing muscle fibers from the same motor unit are time locked to the single-fiber EMG trigger. The signal is averaged until a smooth baseline occurs and the signal parameters do not change (Figure 14-15).[87] An attempt is made to obtain 20 different macro MUAPs recorded at different depths in the muscle, using two to five different skin insertion points. Usually, a voluntary contraction of less than 30% of maximum is used, so that recordings are, therefore, obtained from relatively low-threshold motor units. Technical factors, such as filter settings, proper gain, sweep speed, and triggering, are all important. The presence of jitter and tremor also affects the results; the former causes a more prolonged signal with reduced amplitude and the latter an increase in amplitude as a result of synchronicity between different motor units. The characteristics of the potential are affected by the depth of penetration, as there may be different sizes of superficial and deep motor units, and also by the relationship between the electrode and the center of the motor unit (maximum amplitude being reduced when the electrode is at the periphery of the unit). The distance from the end-plate zone also affects the amplitude, with a diminution in amplitude and area being associated with the temporal dispersion. Because the higher threshold motor units are larger than first-recruited units, this is also reflected in the mean amplitude of the macro EMG potential. Scanning EMG recordings, whereby a concentric needle electrode is pulled in steps of 50 μm through the motor unit, suggest that the peaks seen in macro EMG correspond to fractions of the motor unit, each of which seems to represent muscle fibers innervated by one nerve branch in the nerve tree of the motor unit.[88] Simulation studies show a positive correlation between macro MUAP amplitude and area and the number and size of muscle fibers. The macro MUAP represents the spatial and temporal summation of individual single-fiber action potentials. Mus-

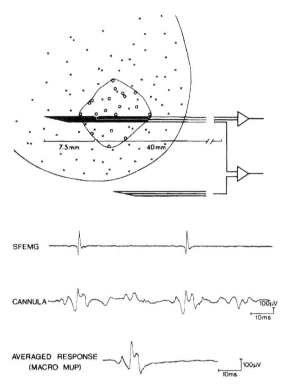

FIGURE 14-15 Principle of macro electromyography recording. The small surface in the macro EMG electrode is positioned to record action potentials from one muscle fiber. This is used to trigger the averager to which the activity recorded with the cannula is fed. (MUP = motor unit potential; SFMG = single-fiber electromyography.) (Reprinted with permission from EV Stålberg. Methods in Clinical Neurophysiology: Macro EMG. Dantec 1990;2.)

cle fiber atrophy decreases the macro MUAP amplitude; however, shrinkage or shortening of distances between individual fibers causes a packing effect and tends to increase the amplitude of the macro MUAP. Both atrophy and shrinkage can occur together, and the net effect, therefore, can vary, depending on the balance between the two. Reinnervation with fiber type grouping can increase amplitude if the total number of fibers is increased (Figure 14-16). The amplitude of macro EMG MUAPs increases with age, especially after age 60.[74] In primary myopathies, the macro EMG amplitude is normal or slightly reduced. In the presence of reinnervation, the macro MUAP usually increases. In many pathologic conditions this situation is dynamic and not stable, and findings can change with time. Information obtained from single-fiber EMG (jitter and fiber density), macro EMG, and conventional EMG provides a better understanding of the anatomic and pathophysiological changes that occur.

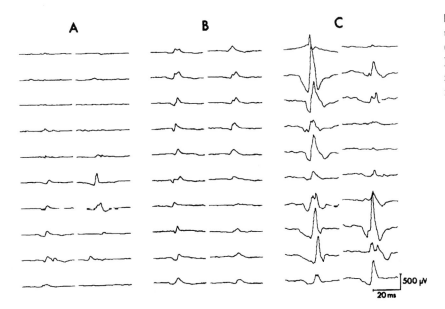

FIGURE 14-16 Examples of macro motor unit potentials in **(A)** limb girdle myopathy, **(B)** normal muscle, and **(C)** amyotrophic lateral sclerogues. (Reprinted with permission from EV Stålberg. Methods in Clinical Neurophysiology: Macro EMG. Dantec 1990;10.)

Quantitative Electromyography and Automatic Analysis

Automatic analysis provides for rapid online readouts, replaces qualitative information with more precise quantitation, and reduces laborious manual computations and sources of human error in interpretation. Quantitative studies of motor unit potential parameters are most often made by manually isolating 20 different motor units in each muscle. Computer analysis then helps plot out histograms of the number of phases, amplitude, duration, and other parameters. A computer can be used to identify and select stable units near the needle tip.

Dorfman and McGill reviewed automatic quantitative EMG,[89] breaking down those properties of interference patterns and MUAPs that lend themselves to measurement (Figure 14-17). The EMG is a dynamically changing signal that is affected by many internal and external factors, including force of contraction, time, position of the recording electrode, and presence of pathology.

As defined by Dorfman and McGill,[89] the lowest level computer-aided approach is to automate only measurement of MUAP properties once the operator has identified the MUAPs. More sophisticated techniques require automatic identification of the MUAP as well as measurements of parameters. Predetermined criteria must be set up for selection of presumed MUAPs on the basis of waveforms and recurrences.

Most methods of automatic motor unit potential analysis rely on template recognition with matching and sorting. The EMG signal from a particular epoch is stored, and recognized potentials are compared and matched with those from subsequent periods. There are differences in techniques, and results can be displayed as histograms, averaged potentials, or individual motor unit potentials, or as a comparison between normal, neuropathic, and myopathic units.[90–93] The various programs have different degrees of sensitivity and selectivity. Stålberg and colleagues [94] have reviewed and compared several different methods and proposed standardized terminology and criteria for measurement, which would have practical value.

The ANOPS computer method bridges the gap between analysis of individual motor unit potentials and the breakdown of more complex interference patterns into component potentials. This technique does not need the signal-processing complexities required for identification and classification, and total recognition may not relate to single motor unit potentials if there is superimposition and noise bursts. MUAPs with faster firing rates are counted more often, so this is called a *frequency-weighted automatic analysis*. This technique traditionally averages 64 potentials at each of 16 sites (1,024 single potentials). Results can be displayed in histograms of amplitude, duration, and phases of potentials. The method is rapid and less precise, but findings have been consistent compared with conventional manual quantitative analysis.[95,96]

Interference Pattern Analysis

Motor unit potential analysis usually requires signals derived from near threshold muscle contractions to visualize individual motor unit potentials.

As the force of the muscle contraction increases, the EMG signal becomes more complex, with superimposi-

FIGURE 14-17 Properties of interference patterns and motor unit action potentials (MUAPs). (Reprinted with permission from LJ Dorfman, KC McGill. AAEE Minimonograph No 29: Automatic quantitative electromyography. Muscle Nerve 1988;11:805.)

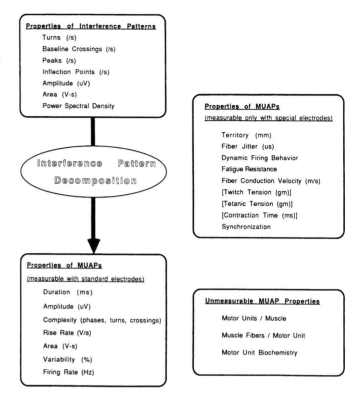

tion of motor unit potentials from different units and ultimate obliteration of the baseline, so that individual motor unit potentials cannot be distinguished. With a submaximal contraction, the interference pattern is less full, but it can be difficult to visually distinguish individual motor unit potentials under normal circumstances, although this can be done with a contraction of relatively low force, such as 5% of MVC.[89] The units seen in such a low-force contraction are the lowest threshold type I units, unless a lesion is present. Ideally, a system of analysis that is capable of breaking down a complex interference pattern into individual motor unit potentials during forceful contraction can also look at the status of higher threshold units.

One of the earliest methods of interference pattern analysis to be described was that of Willison,[97] which attempted to systematize the change in phase of motor unit potentials with reference to a given integer of amplitude and the frequencies arising out of this. Baseline crossings, peaks, and inflection points are related to each other, and one parameter, calibrated amplitude steps (turns), can adequately describe them. During a preselected fixed contraction, the number of notches of the waveform spikes or *turns* (i.e., shifts from positive to negative phase or vice versa) is automatically counted. Using turns of 100 µV, the turn counts per sec-

ond and the mean amplitude are compared with results from healthy controls. This can show whether the recruited potentials are of high amplitude with only a few turns or of low amplitude with numerous turns. A problem with this method is that it does not adequately measure the important parameter of duration of MUAPs, which is useful in defining myopathy, although in primary muscle disease a marked elevation of the turn count was usually noted, as compared with a mean amplitude of more than 2 standard deviations from normal used as the criterion for denervation. Newer computer programs are able to refine this technique. Stålberg and coworkers[98] described the scatter plot or *clouds*, in which mean amplitude per turn is plotted against turns per second, thus eliminating the need to maintain a constant contractile force. In myopathy, excessive turns of low amplitude occur; in neurogenic disease, increased amplitude with a reduced turn count occurs. This comparison technique has been further augmented, providing for automatic measurements of the amplitude of the EMG envelope. When the force of contraction is increased, the interference potential signal contains more MUAP discharges and, therefore, the numerical value of activity increases. The EMG envelope amplitude (ENAMP) increases with the force of contraction and reflects the recruitment of motor

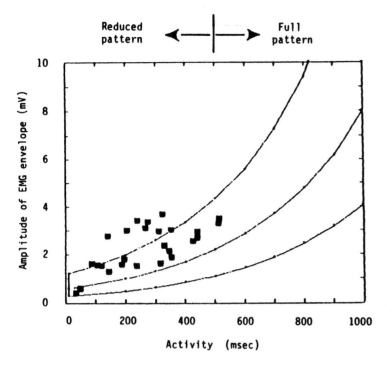

FIGURE 14-18 Analysis of interference pattern (IP) in a patient with neuropathy. All but two epochs had activity values less than 500 msec, indicating reduced IP. The EMG envelope amplitude values are on the upper side of the normal cloud, indicating a neurogenic abnormality. (Reprinted with permission from SD Nandedkar, DB Sanders. Measurement of the amplitude of the EMG envelope. Muscle Nerve 1990;13:937.)

units with large-amplitude MUAPs. Thus, plotting of ENAMP against activity enables one to study the number and size of MUAPs when the force of contraction is increased. When the numerical value of activity is greater than 500 msec, the interference pattern signal appears *full* on visual inspection. Examination of normal clouds show that if the activity values are greater than 500 msec (i.e., if the interference pattern is full) and ENAMP is less than 2 mV, the data point is likely to be outside and below the normal area. This indicates a myopathy. Similarly, when the activity values are less than 500 msec (i.e., reduced interference pattern) and ENAMP values are greater than 6 mV, the data are outside and above the normal cloud, indicating a neurogenic abnormality (Figure 14-18). The shape of the normal turns amplitude is affected by the maximum effort at which recordings are made,[99] so care should be taken to avoid the false interpretation of a neurogenic abnormality when subjects exert near maximum force, although in most clinical settings the clouds described should be adequate and sensitive for EMG analysis.

A number of methods are available for extracting MUAPs from partial interference patterns; however, many of these techniques require complicated computer equipment and are not capable of on-line measurements.[100,101] Automatic decomposition EMG (Figure 14-19)[102] is specifically oriented toward clinical application and can analyze contractile forces corresponding to up to 30% MVC using standard EMG electrodes. The

signal is decomposed into constituent MUAPs in relatively short order, less than 1 minute. Only steady isometric contractions are decomposed, so that MUAP wave shapes and firing rates can be estimated even with incomplete identification. As many as 15 simultaneously active MUAPs can be identified at a single site.

Newer methods were introduced to isolate single MUAPs from an interference pattern. These are accurate and reproducible at up to 50% of maximum voluntary contraction force. Rather than using an approach based on the template-matching technique in the time domain, Fang et al.[103] applied an expansion-matching procedure in the frequency domain to separate superimposed MUAPs in the interference pattern. This procedure is founded on a decomposition principle that is capable of retrieving even greatly superimposed MUAPs. In addition, analysis in the frequency domain is considerably faster than analysis in the time domain. Small MUAPs are hard to isolate from an interference pattern. In the older decomposition systems small MUAPs are excluded. By including *peel-off* schemes to their wavelet transformation technique, Fang et al.[104] were able to accurately identify those smaller MUAPs.

A number of expert systems are now in use. Some of these have been developed by and are in use in small laboratories, others are available as part of the equipment package supplied by commercial manufacturers of electrodiagnostic instruments. Although these expert systems have the potential for providing enhanced accu-

FIGURE 14-19 Decomposition of an interference pattern (IP) using automatic decomposition EMG. In the top portion of the figure, the uppermost trace shows a segment of raw IP signal and just below it the corresponding signals after application of a digital prefilter. The filtered spikes are numbered according to the order in which they were recognized by the automatic decomposition electromyography program. The left lower portion of the figure shows the waveforms of the 14 different motor unit action potentials (MUAPs) identified in the full 10-second EMG record, a segment of which is illustrated above. In the lower right, MUAP 9 is shown magnified, as an example, together with its histogram of interspike intervals (firing rate) and its set of descriptive statistical estimates. (Reprinted with permission from LJ Dorfman, KC McGill. AAEE Minimonograph No 29: Automatic quantitative electromyography. Muscle Nerve 1988;11:813.)

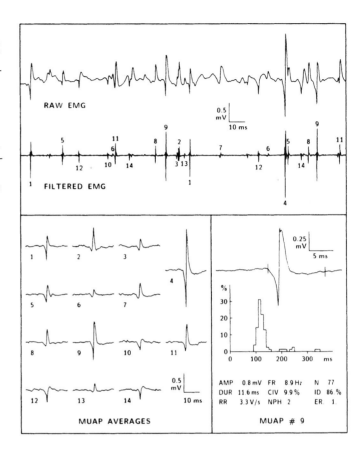

racy of investigation, recording, and reporting, clinicians should be cautious when evaluating results, because standardization and comparisons between systems are not yet readily available.

Power spectrum analysis of the interference pattern, using fast Fourier transformation, can break down an EMG signal for a particular period of time into frequency components. There is a shift from high to low frequency with increasing force. The percentage of low-frequency components also increases as fatigue occurs. For a given percentage of maximum force, the frequency spectrum is shifted toward the higher frequencies in patients with myopathy and toward the lower frequencies in those with neuropathy. When used with other methods of motor unit analysis, such as the turns amplitude analysis and manual measurement of MUAP duration, power spectrum analysis supplemented these methods, increasing diagnostic yield.[105]

CLINICAL APPLICATIONS

This section is not intended to be a clinical manual, and although specific disease entities may produce charac-

teristic EMG findings, these are not discussed in detail except to illustrate pathophysiological changes that apply to a group of disorders as a whole. The general electrodiagnostic texts more than adequately cover the clinical areas,[29,64,106] and there is also a relatively recent specific review.[107]

Diseases that affect the motor unit pathway at any point from the anterior horn cell to the muscle fiber itself can produce an abnormal pattern on EMG. In addition, the higher nervous centers influence the motor neuron apparatus, so that upper motor neuron lesions may alter EMG findings.

Monopolar or concentric needle electrodes are used for routine clinical EMG. The electrical activity produced by the insertion of the needle, any spontaneous activity in the relaxed, resting muscle, the character of the individual MUAPs during weak or submaximal contraction, and the interference pattern in full forceful contraction against resistance are all recorded. More sophisticated quantitative motor unit analysis, single-fiber EMG (SFEMG), and other techniques that can provide additional supplemental information to help establish a diagnosis may be used. A muscle is examined in several locations, and it is often helpful to amplify the sound equivalent of the potentials, as the ear is quite sensitive to variations.

Lower Motor Neuron Disease

The electromyogram in lower motor neuron disease has certain general characteristics. These can include increased insertional activity, fibrillation potentials and positive sharp waves, fasciculation potentials, increased amplitude and average duration of MUAPs together with increased incidence of polyphasic potentials, and decreased number of MUAPs observed during full effort (Figure 14-20). Some of these changes also occur in myopathy, so a single criterion is insufficient to characterize the level of involvement along the motor unit pathway.

Brief comment should be made on collateral and terminal regeneration (Figure 14-21). Collateral regeneration consists of the ingrowth of branches from intact nerve fibers to adjacent denervated muscle fibers. This axonal sprouting has been demonstrated in humans for both sensory and motor nerve fibers. The reinnervated muscle fibers take on the type characteristics of the intact axon. Terminal regeneration occurs in interrupted nerve fibers, whereby new end-plate connections are established by the peripherally regenerating terminal axon branches within the muscle fibers. A normal mean terminal innervation ratio (TIR) of 1.11 ± 0.05 was found for the biceps, palmaris longus, flexor carpi radialis, vastus medialis, and tibialis anterior muscles, with no significant difference in mean TIR between these muscles and no variation with age.[108] TIR was increased in 97% of patients with denervation and weakness and 74% of clinically normal muscles in patients with chronic polyneuropathy. TIR was normal in 82% of patients with muscular dystrophies (100% of patients with Duchenne's muscular dystrophy). TIR was increased in patients with myotonic dystrophy and was normal in those with myasthenia gravis.[109]

Anterior Horn Cell Disorders

The anterior horn cell is involved in disorders such as poliomyelitis, ALS, the progressive spinal muscular atrophies (e.g., Werdnig-Hoffmann disease), and in hereditary degenerative conditions such as Charcot-Marie-Tooth disease. The characteristic features and clinical course vary according to the particular entity, but in general, fibrillation potentials are common and fasciculation potentials may be seen. The degree of spontaneous activity diminishes with chronicity and reinnervation. There is a decrease in total number of motor units but an increase in the number of fibers that make up each individual unit, provided, of course, that the destruction is not so severe that further regeneration cannot occur. Most MUAPs have prolonged duration and increased amplitude that are more pronounced than those associated with impairment of peripheral nerves or roots (Figure 14-22). Early studies showed that motor unit territory may be increased by 80–140%, and the maximum voltage can be five to eight times the normal value in severely involved muscles.[110] As noted, although more recent data confirm that the size of the motor unit is increased (increased fiber density and increased amplitude of macro EMG signal), the overall territory of the motor unit seems to be less enlarged than was previously thought to be the case, and the more dense motor units remain mainly in their original territories.[111]

Findings depend on the rate of progression. In cases that progress rapidly, single-fiber EMG shows increased jitter with a high degree of blocking, whereas fiber density is only moderately increased, but in more chronic conditions, the fiber density increases, as does the total size of the motor unit, with less jitter and blocking. There is extensive collateral regeneration, because the degenerated nerve fibers are scattered over wide areas, and intact and degenerated nerve fibers often lie close together, giving rise to tremendous collateral branching from the surviving fibers. In ALS, polyphasic fasciculations of increased duration may be observed in atrophic muscles and also in muscles that show no weakness or wasting. EMG findings suggest that this is caused by the

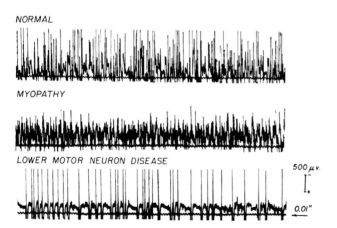

FIGURE 14-20 Motor unit action potentials during maximal voluntary contraction (biceps brachii). (Reprinted with permission from Mayo Clinic. Clinical Examinations in Neurology [3rd ed]. Philadelphia, Saunders, 1971;286.)

firing of a single motor unit rather than the synchronous firing of two or more units, and the fact that the twitching muscle region is larger than that that normally corresponds to a single unit may be explained by the collateral branching that results in a pathologically enlarged motor unit. The action potentials are often polyphasic and of increased duration, again because of temporal dispersion of the enlarged unit together with variable distal conduction in the involved terminal nerve and muscle fibers.

Satellite potentials are small late components of the main MUAP separated by an isoelectric interval and firing in a time-locked relation to the main action potential.[1] These potentials, also called *parasite potentials* or *linked potentials*, usually follow the main action potential (but can precede it) and are caused by slow conduction from a sprouting immature twig. Satellite potentials are found in conditions in which there is chronic reinnervation, such as ALS and other motor neuron diseases. The time-locked relation to the main action potential should prevent confusion with separate low-amplitude units usually associated with myopathies.

Nerve Root and Plexus Lesions

A nerve root or plexus lesion causes denervation in the involved segments, manifested by fibrillation potentials and possibly occasional fasciculations, reduced numbers of MUAPs under voluntary control, and complex polyphasic units, often of increased duration. In the acute phase there may be electrical silence with fibrillation potentials and positive sharp waves appearing only as wallerian degeneration occurs. The peripheral nerve supply to individual muscles is composed of fibers from several spinal cord segments; as a result, normal and diseased motor units may be observed together. When atrophic changes occur in the muscle fibers, spontane-

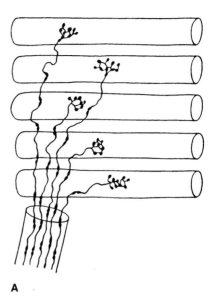

A

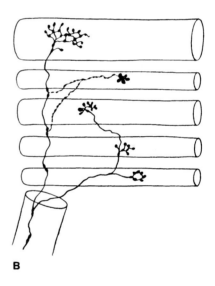

B

FIGURE 14-21 A. Normal arrangement of terminal innervation. Note 1:1:1 relationship (one nerve fiber, one end-plate, one muscle fiber). **B.** Collateral sprouting and reinnervation. Degeneration has taken place in all but one nerve fiber. A sprout has arisen from the intact axon at a node of Ranvier and invaded the Schwann column of a degenerated fiber. One nerve fiber now innervates five muscle fibers, and there is variation in the form of the end-plates. **C.** Probable mechanism of development of changes in terminal innervation in distal neuropathies and also in cases with primary degeneration of muscle fibers. Note tendency for nerve fibers to form several end-plates (more than one on most muscle fibers). (Reprinted with permission from C Coërs, AL Woolf. Innervation of Muscle. Springfield, IL: Thomas, 1959.)

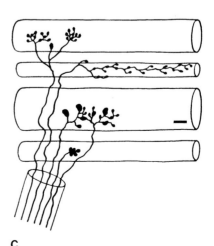

C

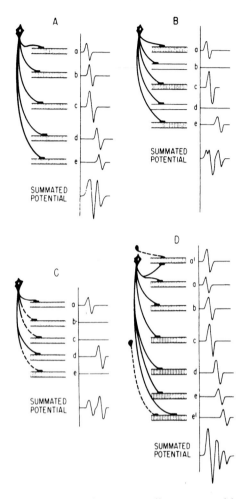

FIGURE 14-22 Simple diagrams to illustrate possible mechanisms for normal and abnormal motor unit potentials. **A.** Normal situation with muscle fiber (c) closest to the electrode. The summated potential differs from any component action potential. **B.** Myopathy with loss of fibers (b, d) causes bizarre alteration of summated potential. **C.** Early terminal regeneration after a nerve lesion. The regenerated axon branches (a, d) excite muscle fibers (a, d) after increased latency; regeneration is incomplete in the other axon branches (*dashed lines*), and the corresponding muscle fibers are not activated. **D.** Motor neuron degeneration with collateral growth from healthy axon branches to innervate muscle fibers (a', e'). This summated potential is a giant potential. (Reprinted with permission from FH Norris. The EMG. New York: Grune & Stratton, 1963.)

ous activity can disappear or the firing and amplitude of fibrillation potentials may be reduced, and evidence of chronic denervation with reinnervation is noted in the muscles supplied by the affected cord segments. Plexus lesions can be differentiated from nerve root lesions by examination of the paraspinal muscles, which are sup-

plied by the posterior primary division of the ventral nerve root proximal to the plexus. In root lesions the paraspinal muscles innervated in part by the involved root manifest signs of denervation. On the other hand, the paraspinal muscles are normal in the more distal plexus lesions.

Peripheral Nerve Disorders

A peripheral nerve damaged by disease or trauma may exhibit temporary loss of conductivity or varying degrees of degeneration.

In physiological block (neuropraxia), continuity of the nerve sheath is maintained without wallerian degeneration, and the condition is characterized by electrical silence at rest. There is no voluntary action potential if the block is complete and a reduced number of normal potentials if the block is partial.

Immediately after the nerve trunk is severed, no voluntary muscle action potentials are seen. The axon cylinder begins to fragment approximately the third day, and at this time nerve conduction velocity distal to the site of injury rapidly decreases. The motor end-plate retains its excitability for another 5–10 days. Not until the end-plate is reduced to the same degree of excitability as the muscle fiber do fibrillation potentials begin to appear. Fibrillation potentials and positive sharp waves (see Figure 14-6) are noted approximately 10 days after the injury and occur in all areas of the muscle receiving their supply distal to the site of injury. Fibrillation potentials last until the regenerating axon arrives at the surface of the muscle fiber and penetrates the end-plate or until the muscle fibers atrophy. Fibrillation potentials have been observed for as long as 18 years,[112] but it can be questioned whether it is the same muscle fibers that are fibrillating or if other fibers break down and show fibrillation potentials or new denervation is occurring. As previously noted, the size of the fibrillation potentials and the rate of firing can be helpful to clinicians seeking to evaluate the chronicity of lesions.

The voluntary motor unit potentials first seen with return of function are of low amplitude, of long duration, and polyphasic. These potentials are called *nascent units*, but the term is not recommended, because the potential configuration is not, in itself, diagnostic. They are caused by early terminal reinnervation of a reduced unit as well as by varying rates of distal conduction. As reinnervation progresses, the motor unit increases in area and number of fibers, so that by 3 months after injury the motor unit territory can be within normal limits and the maximum voltage ranges from normal to 1.8 times normal. Eight months or longer after nerve injury the maximum voltage

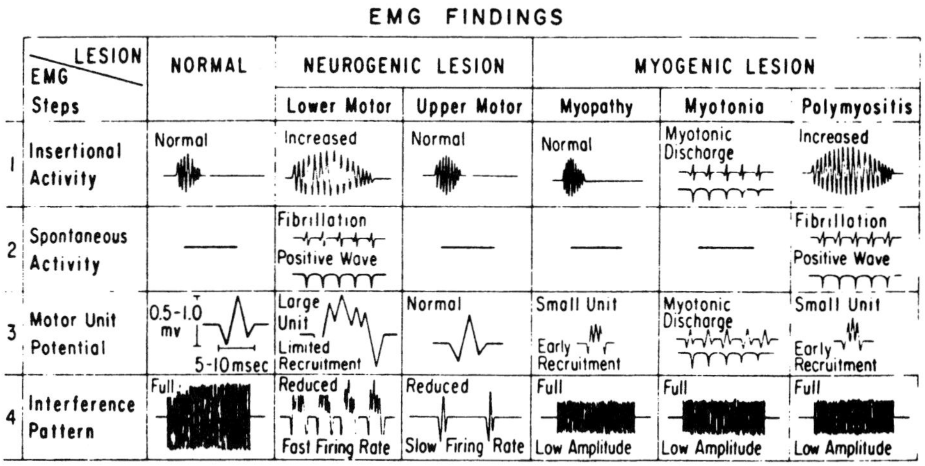

FIGURE 14-23 Typical findings in lower and upper motor neuron disorders and myogenic lesions. (Reprinted with permission from J Kimura. Electrodiagnosis in Diseases of Nerve and Muscle. Philadelphia: F.A. Davis, 1989;252.)

EMG FINDINGS

LESION EMG Steps	NORMAL	NEUROGENIC LESION		MYOGENIC LESION		
		Lower Motor	Upper Motor	Myopathy	Myotonia	Polymyositis
1 Insertional Activity	Normal	Increased	Normal	Normal	Myotonic Discharge	Increased
2 Spontaneous Activity	—	Fibrillation Positive Wave	—	—		Fibrillation Positive Wave
3 Motor Unit Potential	0.5-1.0 mv 5-10 msec	Large Unit Limited Recruitment	Normal	Small Unit Early Recruitment	Myotonic Discharge	Small Unit Early Recruitment
4 Interference Pattern	Full	Reduced Fast Firing Rate	Reduced Slow Firing Rate	Full Low Amplitude	Full Low Amplitude	Full Low Amplitude

is 2.5–3.5 times normal, and the motor unit territory is increased by an average of 15–40%.[109] Single-fiber EMG shows increased fiber density, and macro EMG also reveals that the total number of fibers in the motor unit is increased. The changes in motor unit territory and maximum voltage do not correlate with the degree of paresis as measured by muscle testing. Normal looking action potentials are usually indicative of the return of near synchronous discharge of fibers in the unit. Giant or large-spike potential, up to 15 mV, may be seen 3–5 years after regeneration.[113] Owing to the presence of blocking (increased jitter) in early lesions, the motor unit potential may be unstable, but with reinnervation that is relatively complete, more stable large-amplitude motor unit potentials with no variation in shape or duration are present.

In peripheral neuropathy both axonal degeneration and demyelination can occur. With denervation, fibrillation potentials and positive sharp waves proportional to the severity and extent of the lesion are seen at rest. If progressive degeneration occurs distally before the onset of (or in the absence of) nerve regeneration, there is gradual loss of muscle fibers in the unit, which causes a decrease in amplitude and fragmentation of the action potentials. As the degeneration spreads, there is a reduction of low-voltage initial and terminal deflections of the action potential. This relatively rare EMG picture of distal neuronitis is indistinguishable from that seen with the myopathies. In peripheral neuropathies, with primary axonal degeneration, spontaneous recovery is possible if there is anatomic continuity of the myelin sheaths. The recovery time depends on removal of the pathologic agent, the site of the lesion, and the distance through which regeneration must take place (Figure 14-23).

Recovery occurs by collateral and terminal regeneration. During and after reinnervation, the potentials are complex and of long duration because of temporal dispersion of the motor unit and alterations of conduction velocity along the regenerating distal nerve branches and across the immature end-plates. With time, in stable patients, MUAPs can develop a normal appearance.

Motor End-Plate Disturbances

A defect in transmission across the neuromuscular junction, as in myasthenia gravis, is characterized by a decrease in amplitude of the successively evoked potentials on repeated low-frequency stimulation. Amplitude of single motor units with voluntary contraction varies[114] until, because of fatigue, the unit may fail to respond. A normal pattern may be restored by an injection of neostigmine or edrophonium chloride (cholinesterase inhibitors). The change in amplitude is explained by blocking of excitation at the end-plate to a variable number of muscle fibers supplied by the neuron with fibers recovering at different rates. This may also account for the *myopathic picture* that is sometimes seen of complex polyphasic potentials of normal to decreased amplitude and normal to decreased duration. Myasthenia gravis is thought to be an autoimmune disease in which the defect is at the postsynaptic junction. Defects in neuromuscular transmission have been noted in other conditions, such as ALS and disseminated carcinomatosis.

Myasthenic Syndrome (Lambert-Eaton Myasthenic Syndrome)

In patients with neoplasms, most commonly malignant intrathoracic tumors (and, at times, in patients who have no malignancy), signs suggestive of a neuromuscular transmission defect have been noted. Clinically, the weak, resting patient becomes weaker with continuing muscle contraction or stimulation after an initial period of enhanced strength. Unlike with myasthenia gravis, the initial response to a supramaximal nerve stimulus is only a fraction of normal amplitude, and as contraction continues a period of facilitation occurs that is characterized by increasing responses, but these are often short of normal expected amplitude. The defect in the myasthenic syndrome is in the presynaptic region, as is that associated with botulinum toxin.

Myopathy

Myopathy can be difficult to diagnosis on electrodiagnostic examination. Many of the findings observed are nonspecific, and the EMG may vary, depending on the stage of the disease. Fibrillation potentials have been noted in many myopathies. The mechanism for these abnormal spontaneous muscle potentials is not completely clear. In progressive muscular dystrophy and hyperkalemic periodic paralysis these spontaneous discharges may be related to the increase in excitability resulting from low levels of intracellular potassium.[31] It is also possible that in the dystrophies the degenerating muscle fibers may lose their terminal innervation. In the myositides Coërs and Woolf[2] have demonstrated inflammatory involvement of the subterminal intramuscular nerve endings and end-plate areas. Segmental fiber necrosis and longitudinal fiber splitting may also result in fibrillation potentials. Complex repetitive discharges are often noted in myositis. These are high-frequency runs of similar looking potentials, usually polyphasic, that start and stop abruptly.

In the myopathies, most of the EMG changes in the MUAPs are caused by a reduction in the number of muscle fibers of the individual unit, changes in diameter of muscle fibers affecting conduction, and replacement with fibrous connective tissue. Unless the disease is advanced, the total number of motor unit potentials remains unchanged, so although muscle force and summated voltage are decreased, the number of potentials is maintained with increased frequency of discharge (see Figure 14-20).[115] More electrical activity of action potential spikes is necessary to achieve the amount of force that was attained before the illness. Because of the random degeneration of muscle fibers and of blocking, the smooth summated effect of the normal muscle action potential is lost and complex potentials of low amplitude are noted. The fibers farthest from the recording electrode are likewise decreased, so the duration of the recorded potentials is shortened. Fiber den-

sity is increased and macro MUAP amplitudes are normal or only slightly reduced. Occasionally, long duration, larger amplitude units can be seen together with an increase in macro MUAPs, possibly caused by fiber hypertrophy, splitting, and some collateral reinnervation.[107] This picture is most likely to be observed in patients with polymyositis after several years.[116]

Myotonia

Myotonia is an abnormally sustained contraction and difficulty in relaxation. The EMG shows runs of repetitive high-frequency, waxing and waning discharges, usually of positive waves or biphasic potentials whose initial deflection is positive (see Figure 14-8).

In humans, myotonic discharges may be seen in patients with a dominantly inherited form of muscular dystrophy (myotonia dystrophica), myotonia congenita, associated with periodic paralysis (principally the hyperkalemic type) or with Pompe's disease (glycogenolysis accompanied by acid maltase deficiency of muscle), or paramyotonia congenita. Clinical myotonia, a sustained contraction of muscle after voluntary effort or electrical or mechanical stimulation, can be present in the absence of myotonic discharges, but the reverse is also true. Procainamide and diphenylhydantoin are often used to reduce the intensity of clinical myotonia in patients with myotonic muscular dystrophy, and as these drugs are thought to reduce membrane permeability to ions, their stabilizing effect on the myotonic membrane may indicate a membrane permeability disorder. The slow depolarization of the membrane leading to repetitive spikes and the lower resting membrane potential are also found in denervated striated muscle. With voluntary contraction, the EMG may show short-duration, polyphasic, low-amplitude MUAPs as well as normal looking potentials. High-voltage polyphasic potentials of prolonged duration have also been observed,[117] suggesting denervation with reinnervation. The subterminal nerve fibers have been noted to grow and ramify to form large multiple end-plates. They also can extend parallel to the muscle fibers, giving off short collateral sprouts that terminate in diminutive expansions on the muscle fiber. This, together with the central position of the nuclei in the extrafusal fibers in myotonic dystrophy, suggests conversion of normal extrafusal muscle fiber innervation into the multiple motor innervation characteristic of the intrafusal muscle fibers at the spindles. Thus, the conversion of the innervation of the muscle fibers from an extrafusal to an intrafusal form can lead to hyperexcitable *pseudo–*

muscle spindles that are spread throughout the involved muscles and are accompanied by resultant depolarization and membrane changes. The exact mechanism for the membrane disturbances responsible for the myotonia may not be the same for the different disorders (e.g., myotonia congenita, decreased number of calcium channels; myotonia dystrophica, abnormal sodium channel function; paramyotonia congenita, abnormal temperature dependence of the sodium channel kinetics).[118]

Upper Motor Neuron Lesions

Hoefer and Putnam's[119] classic 1940 study of action potentials in spastic conditions noted that voluntary contraction produced a pattern of decreased frequency and amplitude, but these parameters were proportional to the strength of the contraction. The results of examination of individual discharges were essentially normal. In spastic muscles studied during clonus, there was a strong tendency to synchronization with alternating activity between protagonist and antagonist groups.

More recently, Rodieck et al.[120] introduced the technique of analysis of temporal relationships between consecutive discharges of a single MUAP. The results are easiest to interpret when represented graphically by means of a joint interval histogram (Figures 14-24 and 14-25). In a joint interval histogram the joint distribution of pairs of consecutive discharges of a single MUAP

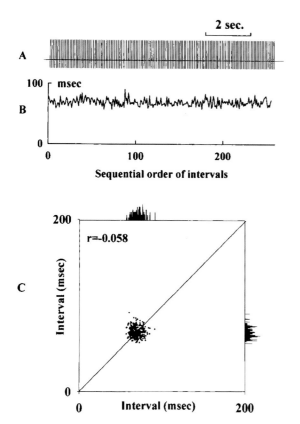

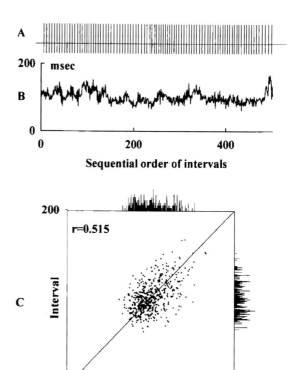

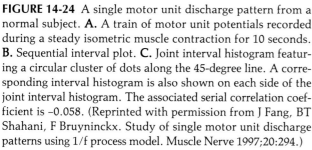

FIGURE 14-24 A single motor unit discharge pattern from a normal subject. **A.** A train of motor unit potentials recorded during a steady isometric muscle contraction for 10 seconds. **B.** Sequential interval plot. **C.** Joint interval histogram featuring a circular cluster of dots along the 45-degree line. A corresponding interval histogram is also shown on each side of the joint interval histogram. The associated serial correlation coefficient is –0.058. (Reprinted with permission from J Fang, BT Shahani, F Bruyninckx. Study of single motor unit discharge patterns using 1/f process model. Muscle Nerve 1997;20:294.)

FIGURE 14-25 A single motor unit discharge pattern from a patient with an upper motor neuron lesion. **A.** A train of motor unit potentials recorded during a steady isometric muscle contraction for 10 seconds. **B.** Sequential interval plot. **C.** Joint interval histogram featuring an elliptical cluster of dots along the 45-degree line. The corresponding serial correlation coefficient is +0.515. (Reprinted with permission from J Fang, BT Shahani, F Bruyninckx. Study of single motor unit discharge patterns using 1/f process model. Muscle Nerve 1997;20:294.)

is measured. In healthy subjects, the joint interval histogram has a circular shape, with a neutral or slightly negative serial correlation coefficient. In patients with an upper motor neuron lesion, the joint interval histogram shows an elliptical shape with a definite positive serial correlation coefficient.

Because the MUAP discharge intervals in upper motor neuron syndromes are rather unstable, they may be better characterized as a 1/f type of stochastical process. This was described by Fang et al.[121] They found that the presence or absence of a 1/f process can be easily concluded from the value of the fractional parameter γ, which was calculated after wavelet transformation of the 1/f process. Wavelet transformation is preferred because of the nonstationary nature of the motor unit discharges. The γ values in upper motor neuron syndromes were definitely above 1, whereas in healthy subjects values below 1 were found.

In a 1998 study[122] Yan et al. reported that discharge properties of single MUAPs (serial correlation coefficient, joint interval histogram, and fractal parameter γ) cannot only be recorded using an intramuscular needle electrode, but also with surface recording electrodes. With this technique, however, it is more difficult to isolate single MUAPs. The main advantage is that the surface recording procedure is noninvasive. It is a painless method, and patients show better compliance during testing. There is also no risk in examining patients with an increased risk of infection or with bleeding disorders.

Yan et al., in another publication,[123] describe that different techniques of analyzing single MUAP discharge patterns (serial correlation coefficient and fractional process parameters) may be useful to document various types of upper motor neuron syndromes, depending, for example, on the degree of positive and negative symptoms those patients show on clinical neurologic examination. Their preliminary results indicate that the fractional process parameter (γ) correlates better than the serial correlation coefficient in patients in whom more pronounced clinical weakness (a negative symptom) is present. More studies are required to further clarify this interesting observation.

In another publication by Yan et al.[124] it was shown that the fractional parameter (γ) correlates well with the functional independence measurement score. This scale is used on a daily basis in rehabilitation medicine. The serial correlation coefficient showed no correlation. Reasons for this may include factors such as muscle fatigue and instability in maintaining contraction. These interfere more with the serial correlation coefficient than with the fractional parameter. Additionally, the serial correlation coefficient reflects only the relationship between pairs of intervals of consecutively firing MUAPs, whereas the fractional parameter characterizes the entire temporal pattern of recorded MUAP discharges. In this study by Yan et al. all categories of the functional independence measurement scale were included with the exception of self-care items. Self-care items did not correlate well with the fractional parameter. Indeed, many patients with, for example, hemiplegic stroke, compensate for difficulties in their self-care by using the unaffected contralateral arm. Also, self-care is not so dependent on muscle strength, a factor that the fractional parameter is especially sensitive to.

EMG findings of positive sharp waves and fibrillation potentials have been reported in some muscles of patients with upper motor neuron lesions who have not shown abnormal nerve conduction studies or findings suggestive of lower motor neuron pathology. One study of hemiplegic patients has shown a 57% prevalence of fibrillation potentials and a 70% prevalence of positive sharp waves.[125] Another study recorded a 73.5% prevalence of spontaneous activity in involved hemiplegic limbs, but a 9% prevalence of fibrillation potentials was also observed on the unaffected side.[126] In patients with high-level spinal cord lesions, fibrillation potentials have been observed in muscles innervated by nerve root segments quite distal to the level of injury. Nepomuceno and colleagues[127] also observed positive sharp waves and fibrillation potentials in patients with upper motor neuron lesions without conditions that involved the lower motor neuron. They studied these potentials to ascertain if there were differences in characteristics between those found in upper motor neuron and lower motor neuron lesions. They found interlesion differences in the mean frequency of occurrence ratio of positive sharp waves to fibrillation potentials: a ratio of 5:1 positive sharp waves to fibrillation potentials in those patients with upper motor neuron lesions and a ratio of 3:1 in those with lower motor neuron lesions. The positive sharp waves associated with lower motor neuron lesions had a longer duration than those seen in patients with upper motor neuron lesions ($p < .015$). The explanation for these differences is not clear at this time.

A number of theories have been proposed to explain the association of fibrillation potentials and positive sharp waves with upper motor neuron lesions. These include transsynaptic neuronal degeneration,[125] membrane instability,[128] and antifibrillation factor.[129]

REFERENCES

1. AAEE Glossary of terms in clinical electromyography. Muscle Nerve 1987;10(8S):G1–G60.
2. Coërs C, Woolf AL. The Innervation of Muscle. Oxford: Blackwell, 1959.
3. Christensen E. Topography of terminal motor innervation in striated muscles from stillborn infants. Am J Phys Med 1959;38:65–77.
4. Feinstein B, Lindegard B, Nyman E, et al. Morphologic studies of motor units normal human muscles. Acta Anat 1955;23:127–142.
5. McComas AJ, Fawcett PRW, Campbell MJ, et al. Electrophysiological estimation of the number of motor units within a human muscle. J Neurol Neurosurg Psychiatry 1971;34:121–131.
6. Ballantyne JP, Hansen S. A new method for the estimation of the number of motor units in a muscle. 1. Control subjects and patients with myasthenia gravis. J Neurol Neurosurg Psychiatry 1974;37:907–915.
7. Milner-Brown HS, Brown WF. New methods of estimating the number of motor units in a muscle. J Neurol Neurosurg Psychiatry 1976;39:258–265.
8. Brown WF, Strong MJ, Snow R. Methods for estimating numbers of motor units in biceps-brachialis muscles and losses of motor units with aging. Muscle Nerve 1988;11:423–432.
9. Shahani BT, Fang J, Dhand U. A new approach to motor unit estimation with the surface triggered averaging technique. Muscle Nerve 1995;18:1088–1092.
10. Fang J, Shahani BT, Graupe D. Motor unit number estimation by spatial-temporal summation of single motor unit potentials. Muscle Nerve 1997;20:461–468.
11. Brandstater ME, Lambert EH. A histological study of the spatial arrangement of muscle fibers in single motor units within rat tibialis anterior muscle. Bull Am Assoc Electromyogr Electrodiagn 1969;16:82.
12. Buchthal F, Guld C, Rosenfalck P. Volume conduction of the spike of the motor unit potential investigated with a new type of multielectrode. Acta Physiol Scand 1957;38:331–354.
13. Buchthal F, Guld C, Rosenfalck P. Multielectrode study of the territory of a motor unit. Acta Physiol Scand 1957;39:83–105.
14. Bodine-Fowler S, Garfinkel A, Roy RR, et al. Spatial distribution of muscle fibers within the territory of a motor unit. Muscle Nerve 1990;13:1133–1145.
15. Brown MC, Matthews PBC. An investigation into the possible existence of polyneuronal innervation of individual skeletal muscle fibers in certain hind limb muscles of the cat. J Physiol 1960;151:436–457.
16. Hunt CC, Kuffler SW. Motor innervation of skeletal muscle: multiple innervation of individual muscle fibers and motor unit function. J Physiol 1954;126:293–303.
17. Walker LB Jr. Multiple motor innervation of individual muscle fibers in the m. tibialis anterior of the dog. Anat Rec 1961;139:1–11.
18. Brooks JE, Hongdalarom T. Intracellular electromyography. Resting and action potentials in normal human muscle. Arch Neurol 1968;18:291–300.
19. Nastuk WL, Hodgkin AL. The electrical activity of single muscle fibers. J Cell Comp Physiol 1950;35:39–73.
20. Lundervold A, Li C. Motor units and fibrillation potentials as recorded with different kinds of needle electrodes. Acta Psych Neurol Scand 1953;28:201–212.
21. Buchthal F, Pinelli P, Rosenfalck P. Action potential parameters in normal human muscle and their physiological determinants. Acta Physiol Scand 1954;32:219–229.
22. Howard JE, McGill KC, Dorfman LJ. Properties of motor unit action potentials recorded with concentric and monopolar needle electrodes: ADEMG analysis. Muscle Nerve 1988;11:1050–1055.
23. Pease WS, Bowyer BL. Motor unit analysis: comparison between concentric and monopolar needle electrodes. Am J Phys Med 1988;67:2–6.
24. Nandedkar SD, Sanders DB. Recording characteristics of monopolar EMG electrodes. Muscle Nerve 1991;14:108–112.
25. Nandedkar SD, Tedman B, Sanders DB. Recording and physical characteristics of disposable concentric needle EMG electrodes. Muscle Nerve 1990;13:909–914.
26. Basmajian JV. Muscles Alive (2nd ed). Baltimore: Williams & Wilkins, 1967.
27. Ekstedt J. Human single muscle fibre action potentials. Acta Physiol Scand 1964;51(Suppl 226):1–96.
28. Wohlfart G. Clinical considerations on innervation of skeletal muscle. Am J Phys Med 1959;38:223–230.
29. Kimura J. Electrodiagnosis in Diseases of Nerve and Muscle: Principles and Practice (2nd ed). Philadelphia: FA Davis, 1989.
30. Buchthal F, Guld C, Rosenfalck P. Action potential parameters in normal human muscle and their dependence on physical variables. Acta Physiol Scand 1954;32:200–218.
31. Buchthal F. Spontaneous and voluntary electrical activity in neuromuscular disorders. Bull NY Acad Med 1966;42:521–550.
32. Stöhr M. Benign fibrillation potentials in normal muscle and their correlation with end-plate and denervation potentials. J Neurol Neurosurg Psychiatry 1977;40:765–768.
33. Wilbourn AJ. The EMG examination with myopathies. AAEE Course A: Myopathies, Floppy Infant and Electrodiagnostic Studies in Children 1987;7–20.
34. Kraft GH. Fibrillation potential amplitude and muscle atrophy following peripheral nerve injury. Muscle Nerve 1990;13:814–821..
35. Dumitru D, King JC. Varied morphology of spontaneous single muscle fiber discharges. Am J Phys Med Rehabil 1998;77:128–139.
36. Buchthal F. Fibrillations: Clinical Electrophysiology. In WJ Culp, J Ochoa (eds), Abnormal Nerves and Muscles as Impulse Generators. Oxford: Oxford University Press, 1982;632–662.
37. Ware F Jr, Bennett AL, McIntyre AR. Membrane resting potential of denervated skeletal muscle measured in vivo. Am J Physiol 1954;177:115–118.
38. Thesleff S, Ward MR. Studies on the mechanism of fibrillation potentials in denervated muscle. J Physiol 1975;244:313–323.
39. Kraft GH. Fibrillation potential amplitude and muscle atrophy following peripheral nerve injury. Muscle Nerve 1990;13:814–821.
40. Tsubahara A, Chino N, Mince, K. Fibrillation potentials and muscle fiber types. Muscle Nerve 1990;13:983.
41. Hayes GJ, Woolsey CN. The unit of fibrillary activity and the site of origin of fibrillary contractions in denervated striated muscle. Fed Proc 1942;1:38.
42. Belmar J, Eyzaguirre C. Pacemaker site of fibrillation potentials in denervated

mammalian muscle. J Neurophysiol 1966;29:425–441.

43. Marinacci AA. Applied Electromyography. Philadelphia: Lea & Febiger, 1968.

44. Goodgold J, Eberstein A. The physiological significance of fibrillation action potentials. Bull NY Acad Med 1967;43:811–818.

45. Wiederholt WC. End-plate noise in electromyography. Neurology 1970; 20:214–224.

46. Dumitru D, King JC, Stegeman DF. Endplate spike morphology: a clinical and simulation study. Arch Phys Med Rehabil 1998;79:634–640.

47. Dumitru D, King JC, McCarter RJM. Single muscle fiber discharge transformation: fibrillation potential to positive sharp wave. Muscle Nerve 1998; 21:1759–1768.

48. Roth G. The origin of fasciculations. Ann Neurol 1982;12:542–547.

49. Forster FM, Alpers BJ. The site of origin of fasciculations in voluntary muscle. Arch Neurol Psychiatry 1944; 51:264–267.

50. Richardson AT. Muscle fasciculation. Arch Phys Med Rehabil 1954;35:281–285.

51. Conradi S, Grimby L, Lundemo G. Pathophysiology of fasciculations in ALS as studied by electromyography of single motor units. Muscle Nerve 1982;5:202–208.

52. Wettstein A. The origin of fasciculations in motoneuron disease. Ann Neurol 1979;5:295–300.

53. Norris FH Jr. Synchronous fasciculation in motor neuron disease. Arch Neurol 1965;13:495–500.

54. Trojaborg W, Buchthal F. Malignant and benign fasciculations. Acta Neurol Scand 1965;41(Suppl 13):251–254.

55. Gutmann L. Facial and limb myokymia. Muscle Nerve 1991;14:1043–1049.

56. Brick JF, Gutmann L, McComas CF. Calcium effect on generation and amplification of myokymic discharges. Neurology 1982;32:618–622.

57. Trontelj J, Stålberg E. Bizarre repetitive discharges recorded with single fiber EMG. J Neurol Neurosurg Psychiatry 1983;46:310–316.

58. Dumitru D, King JC, Stegeman DF. Normal needle electromyographic insertional activity morphology: a clinical and simulation study. Muscle Nerve 1998;21:910–920.

59. Norris FH Jr. Unstable membrane potential in human myotonic muscle.

Electroencephalogr Clin Neurophysiol 1962;14:197–201.

60. Norris FH Jr, Gasteiger EL. Action potentials of single motor units in normal muscle. Electroencephalogr Clin Neurophysiol 1955;7:115–126.

61. Petajan JH. Motor unit recruitment. Muscle Nerve 1991;14:489–502.

62. Henneman E. The Size Principle of Motoneuron Recruitment. In JE Desmedt (ed), Motor Unit Types, Recruitment and Plasticity in Health and Disease: Progress in Clinical Neurophysiology. Basel: S Karger, 1981;26–60.

63. Clamann HP. Activity of single motor units during isometric tension. Neurology 1970;20:254–260.

64. Johnson EW. The EMG Examination. In EW Johnson (ed), Practical Electromyography (2nd ed). Baltimore: Williams & Wilkins, 1988;1–21.

65. Daube JR. Needle examination in clinical electromyography. Muscle Nerve 1991;14:685–700.

66. Bigland B, Lippold OCJ. Motor unit activity in the voluntary contraction of human muscle. J Physiol 1954;125:322–335.

67. Taylor A. The significance of grouping of motor unit activity. J Physiol 1962;162:259–269.

68. Denny-Brown D. Interpretation of the electromyogram. Arch Neurol Psychiatry 1949;61:99–128.

69. Petersen I, Kugelberg E. Duration and form of action potential in the normal human muscle. J Neurol Neurosurg Psychiatry 1949;12:124–128.

70. Brown WF. A method for estimating the number of motor units in thenar muscles and the changes in motor unit count with aging. J Neurol Neurosurg Psychiatry 1972;35:845–852.

71. Slawnych MP, Laszlo CA, Hershler C. A review of techniques employed to estimate the number of motor units in a muscle. Muscle Nerve 1990;13:1050–1064.

72. Stålberg E, Thiele B. Motor unit fiber density in the extensor digitorum communis muscle: Single fiber electromyographic study in normal subjects at different ages. J Neurol Neurosurg Psychiatry 1975;38:874–880.

73. de Koning P, Wieneke GH, van der Most van Spijke D, et al. Estimation of the number of motor units based on macro EMG. J Neurol Neurosurg Psychiatry 1988;51:403–411.

74. Stålberg E, Fawcett PRW. Macro EMG in healthy subjects of different ages. J

Neurol Neurosurg Psychiatry 1982; 45:870–878.

75. Tomlinson BE, Irving D. The number of limb motor neurons in the human lumbosacral cord throughout life. J Neurol Sci 1977;34:213–219.

76. Kawamura Y, O'Brien P, Okazaki H, et al. Lumbar motoneurons of man. J Neuropathol Exp Neurol 1977;36:861–870.

77. Gutmann E, Hanzlikov V. Motor unit in old age. Nature 1966;209:921–922.

78. Bigland-Ritchie B. Changes in EMG and neural control during human muscle fatigue. Am Assoc Electromyogr Electrodiag Didactic 1983;(Program):21–26.

79. Scheffer J, Bourguignon A. Changes in the electromyogram produced by fatigue in man. Am J Phys Med Rehabil 1959;38:148–158.

80. Myers SJ, Sullivan WP. Effect of circulatory occlusion on time to muscular fatigue. J Appl Physiol 1968;24:54–59.

81. Bigland-Ritchie B, Johansson R, Lippold OCJ, et al. Changes in motoneuron firing rate during sustained maximal voluntary contractions. J Physiol 1983;340:335–346.

82. Gooch JL, Newton BY, Petajan JH. Motor unit spike counts before and after maximal voluntary contraction. Muscle Nerve 1990;13:1146–1151.

83. Pinelli P, Buchthal F. Muscle action potentials in myopathies with special regard to progressive muscular dystrophy. Neurology 1953;3:347–359.

84. Brooks JE. Disuse atrophy of muscle. Arch Neurol 1970;22:27–30.

85. Stålberg E, Trontelj J. Single Fibre Electromyography. Surrey: Miraville Press, 1979.

86. Hilton-Brown P, Stålberg E, Trontelj J, et al. Causes of the increased fiber density in muscular dystrophies studied with single fiber EMG during electrical stimulation. Muscle Nerve 1985;8:383–388.

87. Stålberg E. Macro EMG. Methods Clin Neurophysiol 1990;1:1–14.

88. Stålberg E, Antoni L. Electrophysiological cross section of the motor unit. J Neurol Neurosurg Psychiatry 1980; 43:469–474.

89. Dorfman LJ, McGill KC. Automatic quantitative electromyography. Muscle Nerve 1988;11:804–818.

90. Bergmans J. Computer-assisted on-line measurement of motor unit potential parameters in human electromyography. Electromyography 1971;11:161–181.

91. Leifer LJ, Pinelli P. Analysis of motor units by computer aided electromy-

ography. Third International Congress of Electrophysiology and Kinesiology; 1976; Pavia, Italy.

92. Stålberg E, Antoni L. Computer-Aided EMG Analysis. In JE Desmedt (ed), Computer-Aided Electromyography. Basel: S Karger, 1983;186–234.

93. Coatrieux JL. Interference electromyogram processing. Electromyogr Clin Neurophysiol 1983;23:229–242.

94. Stålberg E, Andreassen S, Falck B, et al. Quantitative analysis of individual motor unit potentials: a proposition for standardized terminology and criteria for measurement. J Clin Neurophysiol 1986;3:313–348.

95. Hausmanowa-Petrusewicz I, Kopec J. Quantitative EMG and Its Automation. In JE Desmedt (ed), Computer-Aided Electromyography. Basel: S Karger, 1983;164–185.

96. Kopec J, Hausmanowa-Petrusewicz I. Diagnostic yield of an automated method of quantitative electromyography. Electromyogr Clin Neurophysiol 1985;25:567–577.

97. Willison RG. Analysis of electrical activity in healthy and dystrophic muscles in man. J Neurol Neurosurg Psychiatry 1964;27:386–394.

98. Stålberg E, Chu J, Bril V, et al. Automatic analysis of the EMG interference pattern. EEG Clin Neurophysiol 1983;56:672–681.

99. Nandedkar SD, Sanders DB, Stålberg EV. On the shape of the normal turns-amplitude cloud. Muscle Nerve 1991;14:8–13.

100. LeFever RS, DeLuca CJ. A procedure for decomposing the myoelectric signal into its constituent action potentials. Technique, theory and implementation. IEEE Trans Biomed Eng 1982; 29:149–157.

101. Guiheneuc P, Calamel J, Doncarli C, et al. Automatic Detection and Pattern Recognition of Single Motor Unit Potentials in Needle EMG. In JE Desmedt (ed), Computer-Aided Electromyography. Basel: S Karger, 1983;73–127.

102. McGill KC, Dorfman U. Automatic decomposition electromyography (ADEMG): validation and normative data in brachial biceps. EEG Clin Neurophysiol 1985;61:453–461.

103. Fang J, Ben-Arie J, Wang Z, et al. Separation of superimposed EMG potentials using expansion matching technique. Proceedings of the 19th Annual International Conference of IEEE Engineering in Medicine and Biology; Nov 1997; Chicago, Illinois.

104. Fang J, Agarwal GC, Shahani BT. Decomposition of multi-unit electromyographic signals. IEEE Trans Biomed Eng 1999;46:685–697.

105. Fuglsang-Frederiksen A. Power spectrum of the needle EMG in normal and diseased muscles. Methods Clin Neurophysiol 1990;2:1–8.

106. Dimitri D. Electrodiagnostic Medicine. Hanley and Belfus. Philadelphia, 1995

107. Stålberg E. Electrodiagnostic assessment and monitoring of motor unit changes in disease [Review]. Muscle Nerve 1991;14:293–303.

108. Coërs C, Telerman-Toppet N, Gerrard JM. Terminal innervation ratio in neuromuscular disease: I. Methods and controls. Arch Neurol 1973;29:210–214.

109. Coërs C, Telerman-Toppet N, Gerrard JM. Terminal innervation ratio in neuromuscular disease: II. Disorders of lower motor neuron, peripheral nerve and muscle. Arch Neurol 1973;29:215–222.

110. Ermino F, Buchthal F, Rosenfalck P. Motor unit territory and muscle fiber concentration in paresis due to peripheral nerve injury and anterior horn cell involvement. Neurology 1959;9:657–671.

111. Stålberg EV. Capability of motor unit sprouting in neuromuscular disorders. Am Assoc Electromyogr Electrodiag Didactic 1987;(Program):33–39.

112. Weddell G, Feinstein B, Pattle RE. The electrical activity of voluntary muscle in man under normal and pathological conditions. Brain 1944;67:178–257.

113. Yahr MD, Herz E, Moldover J. Electromyographic patterns in reinnervated muscle. Arch Neurol Psych 1950;63:728–738.

114. Lindsley DB. Myographic and electromyographic studies of myasthenia gravis. Brain 1935;58:470–480.

115. Kugelberg E. Electromyography in muscular dystrophies. J Neurol Neurosurg Psychiatry 1949;12:129–136.

116. Trojaborg W. Quantitative electromyography in polymyositis: a reappraisal. Muscle Nerve 1990;13:964–971.

117. Woolf AL. The theoretical basis of clinical electromyography [Part II]. Am J Phys Med Rehabil 1962;6:241–266.

118. Rudel R. The Pathophysiological Basis of the Myotonias and the Periodic Paralyses. In AG Engel, BQ Banker (eds), Mycology. Vol 1. New York: McGraw-Hill, 1986;1297–1307.

119. Hoefer PFA, Putnam TJ. Action potentials of muscles in spastic conditions. Arch Neurol Psychiatry 1940;43:1–22.

120. Rodieck WW, Kiang NYS, Gerstein GL. Some quantitative methods for the study of spontaneous activity of single neurons. Biophys J 1962;2:351–368.

121. Fang J, Shahani BT, Bruyninckx F. Study of single motor unit discharge patterns using 1/F process model. Muscle Nerve 1997;20:293–298.

122. Yan K, Fang J, Shahani BT. An assessment of motor unit discharge patterns in stroke patients using surface electromyographic technique. Muscle Nerve 1998;21:946–947.

123. Yan K, Fang J, Shahani BT. Motor unit discharge behaviors in stroke patients. Muscle Nerve 1998;21:1502–1506.

124. Yan K, Fang J, Turan B, et al. The use of fractional parameter in analyzing motor unit discharge pattern in stroke patients: a correlation with the functional independence measurement. Electromyogr Clin Neurophysiol 2000; 40:3–9.

125. Goldkamp O. Electromyography and nerve conduction studies in 116 patients with hemiplegia. Arch Phys Med Rehabil 1967;48:59–63.

126. Bhala RP. Electromyographic evidence of lower motor neuron involvement in hemiplegia. Arch Phys Med Rehabil 1969;50:632–637.

127. Nepomuceno C, McCutcheon M, Miller JM III, et al. Differential analyses of EMG findings in motor neuron lesions. Am J Phys Med 1977;56:1–11.

128. Johnson EW, Denny ST, Kelly JP. Sequence of electromyographic abnormalities in stroke syndrome. Arch Phys Med Rehabil 1975;56:468–473.

129. Spielholz NI, Sell GH, Goodgold J, et al. Electrophysiologic studies in patients with spinal cord lesions. Arch Phys Med Rehabil 1972;53:558–562.

15

Evoked Potentials

GARY GOLDBERG

PHYSIOLOGICAL BASIS OF SENSORY- AND MOTOR-EVOKED POTENTIALS

In this chapter, the application of evoked potential (EP) testing is examined and reviewed. Emphasis is placed on the anatomic and physiological basis for the recording and interpretation of these signals. Specific methodologic concerns are not discussed in detail. Issues that relate to the abnormalities seen in specific pathology are generally not addressed here. Common applications of EP testing have been reviewed elsewhere.[1,2] Sensory EPs entail measured electrical, magnetic, or both kinds of fields associated with activation of nervous tissue by a peripheral sensory stimulus. In this chapter, we focus on the electrical field studies. Commonly applied paradigms involve visual, auditory, and somatosensory stimulation. Motor EPs (MEPs) entail measured contraction of limb muscles activated through transcranial stimulation of motor cortex. Transcranial stimulation of motor cortex can be achieved with both electrical and magnetic field stimulation, and we discuss these methods in this chapter. A number of different advantages and disadvantages in the clinical application of the SEP and MEP studies are listed in Table 15-1. An introductory section on the physiological foundation common to all EPs is followed by separate treatments of the specific anatomic and physiological issues related to the generation of visual, auditory, somatosensory, and MEPs. The reader who is interested in learning more about these techniques and performing these studies in a clinical context is encouraged to supplement his or her reading with the several textbook sources available.[3–10] Additional educational material can be obtained from the American Association of Electrodiagnostic Medi-

cine. The American Association of Electrodiagnostic Medicine maintains a catalog of published materials on the World Wide Web at the following address: http://www.aaem.net/publications.html/. Specifically with regard to the somatosensory EPs (SEPs), relevant sections of the *AAEM Guidelines in Electrodiagnostic Medicine*[11,12] are particularly helpful.

Sensory EPs are time-dependent changes in electrical potential recordable at the surface of the body that reflect activation of CNS structures by a discrete sensory stimulus. The potentials are recorded between two different sites with reference to a common ground site using a low-noise differential amplifier with a high common-mode rejection ratio. Most often these potentials are recorded by surface electrodes attached directly to the abraded skin with conductive paste or through subcutaneous needle electrodes. The recorded wave-like signal is evaluated graphically as a plot of voltage versus time referenced to the point of stimulus application. The signal is typically noted to have a series of upward-directed peaks and downward-directed valleys that are referred to as *components*. Measurable component parameters include the peak latency with respect to stimulus onset and the peak amplitude with reference to a baseline value or to some other extreme point of the signal (e.g., the immediately preceding or immediately after peak or valley). Most often, the components are named according to a convention in which the peak is labeled with an *N* for negative or a *P* for positive, according to the polarity of the potential with reference to the baseline. This letter is then followed by the normal median latency of the peak given in milliseconds. A separate standard for component nomenclature that uses Roman numerals has been developed for the brain stem auditory EP (BAEP).

TABLE 15-1
Advantages and Disadvantages of Evoked Potentials

Advantages

  Are reliable clinical tests that yield valid reproducible results with clinical relevance

  Provide an objective, quantitative extension of the clinical examination

  Test sensory and motor function when the clinical examination is not reliable

  Provide objective measure of physiological function with the motor system or a particular sensory system

  Can detect abnormalities that may not be clinically detectable otherwise

  Can be recorded independently of subjective individual state (for short-latency evoked potential components)

  Can be used to localize the anatomic level of impairment

  Can be used to assess prognosis and monitor functional recovery

  Can be used to investigate the organic basis of subjective complaints referable to the central nervous system

  Can be used to monitor the integrity of a critical pathway that is at risk of injury (e.g., as in intraoperative monitoring)

  Are totally noninvasive and can be repeated serially to evaluate physiological change over time

  Can be performed by a well-trained technologist under direct physician supervision

Disadvantages and limitations

  Are prone to artifact (e.g., electromyography, electrooculography, electrocardiography, movement, line interference, and so forth)

  Can be technically challenging because small signals are recovered and analyzed in the presence of a large-amplitude interfering background

  Must use signal averaging; precludes the evaluation of unitary, single-trial responses

  Have significant interindividual variability in measures, especially in the long-latency components

  Require either a cooperative subject or the use of sedation to limit movement and electromyographic artifact

  Have been significantly devaluated through overuse, misuse, and abuse by inadequately qualified personnel

  Do not provide specific pathognomonic information about the underlying etiology producing physiological impairment

  Short-latency components are reliable and reproducible, but provide no information about cognition

  Long-latency components can provide insight into cognitive processing, but are less reliable and less robust

These potentials are often small in amplitude (in the range of 1 µV) and are obscured by ongoing spontaneous fluctuation of large-amplitude surface potentials caused by the activity of a variety of physiological sources. These may be both *targeted* sources in the brain and spinal cord (in the case of the SEP) and *nontargeted* sources, as well as electrical *noise* caused by environmental interference. By targeted sources, we mean those sources whose activity we are interested in evaluating with the study. It is thus often quite technically demanding to recover the sensory EP signal. Most frequently, the signal is extracted from background electrical activity through the process of signal averaging.

The basic transient sensory EP test paradigm involves an idealized conceptual approach that guides the performance of the study and the interpretation of the recorded signals. A discrete, time-limited sensory stimulus is applied repetitively to activate the primary afferent fibers of a specific sensory system at a fixed rate, thus setting up cycles of repeated synchronous action potential volleys in primary sensory afferent nerve fibers. These coherent volleys are expected to produce transient activations of central structures on which they impinge. The rate is chosen to be slow enough so that the time between individual stimuli is sufficient to allow the system to return to a quiescent, resting state. The stimulation can be done through physiological activation of special sensory receptors as occurs in the visual and auditory test paradigms through controlled photic stimulation of the retina or auditory stimulation of the peripheral auditory mechanism and cochlea, respectively. Stimulation can also be done through direct activation of primary afferent fibers with brief transcutaneous electrical current pulses, as is most often done in the SEP. These synchronous input volleys in the primary afferent fibers then trace a path through the more proximal extent of the afferent pathway that enters and traverses the specific sensory system producing sequential transient activation of these central structures. The physiological sequence of events associated with this traversal is the focus of the EP investigation.

Components can be generally classified according to latency into short-, middle-, and long-latency components. Short-latency components are within approximately 15 msec after stimulus onset. These components typically are associated with the activation of the special sensory receptors, primary afferent neuron, and various subcortical sites in the central pathway. They reflect the physiological anatomy of the subcortical pathway and are relatively robust, obligatory responses to the stimulus that are resistant to changes in the conscious state of the subject or the administration of anesthetic agents. They can be viewed as objective manifestations of the physiological activation of the input elements of the sensory pathway. The middle-latency components are generally from 15–150 msec. These components are associated with activation of the primary sensory cortex for the particular sensory modality being evaluated. Middle-latency components can be somewhat dependent on subjective state, and their amplitude can be reduced by certain types of anesthetic agents. The long-latency components that are typically seen at greater than 150 msec after the stimulus are highly variable. Their structural detail can vary significantly between individuals and from one assessment to another. These components can reflect the active information-processing capacity of association cortex directed to stimulus perception and evaluation. Within subjects, they can be enhanced or reduced in amplitude by changes in the attention directed to the stimulus. Long-latency components can vary in amplitude with the amount of context-dependent meaningful information contained within the structure or temporal pattern of the stimulus. In fact, long-latency components can even be produced by the absence of a stimulus, when a stimulus absence at a particular point in time is an unexpected, low-probability, and therefore information-rich, event. They are readily attenuated with changes in level of consciousness or by the administration of anesthetic agents. Paradigms that are specifically constructed to record long-latency components are often used to investigate psychophysiological issues that address cognitive information-processing capacity. Because these paradigms evaluate the systematic variation of long-latency components with the context-dependent relevance of stimulus events, the recorded signals are often referred to as *event-related potentials.* Although these components are interesting research tools for psychophysiological investigation, their variability limits their clinical applicability as compared with the more consistent and predictable earlier EP components. The chapter, therefore, focuses primarily on the short- and middle-latency sensory EP components. It should be recognized that these components assess the input pathway to the cortical level and therefore document the access that exists between the periphery and the primary sensory cortex. They do not, however, evaluate the extent to which the cortex is capable of subsequent active information processing of the stimulus.

Physiological activation of a structure in the pathway is termed *source generation.* The responding structure is defined as the source of a generator potential that then produces current flow through the surrounding tissues, which, in turn, produce a recordable voltage signal at the surface of the body. The underlying physiological phenomenon producing the detectable source-generated signal could be either a traveling wave caused by a synchronous volley of action potentials conducted along a white-matter fiber tract, or a synchronous activation of a population of synapses in a gray-matter deep nucleus or cortical region. In the latter situation, the source signal is a compound postsynaptic potential of either an excitatory or an inhibitory nature. In either situation, the ultimate basis of the physiological source signal is transmembrane ionic current flow across the excitable membrane of the participating neural structures resulting from transient changes in ion channel conduction properties.

For white-matter fiber tract sources, these transmembrane ionic current transients are related to the process of action potential transmission along myelinated fiber tracts. A synchronous, coherent volley of action potentials conducted along parallel fibers in the tract produces currents that summate. An extracellular electrode *sees* the volley coming, arriving, and leaving. This results in a positive-negative-positive triphasic compound action potential (Figure 15-1). If the extracellular

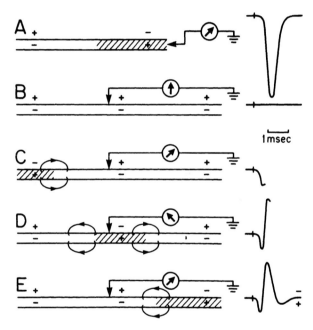

FIGURE 15-1 Extracellular recording of transmitted action potentials (APs). **A.** When the AP is seen to approach the recording site but then stops being transmitted, only a positive deflection is noted. **B.** Before the AP arrives, there is a flat baseline. **C.** As the AP approaches the recording site, there is an initial positive deflection. **D.** As the AP passes beneath the recording electrode, there is a large negative deflection of the recorded potential. **E.** As the AP moves past the recording site, another positive deflection is noted. Thus, a triphasic positive-negative-positive waveform is recorded extracellularly when an AP passes along an axon adjacent to the recording electrode. (Reprinted with permission from J Schlag. Generation of Brain Evoked Potentials. In RF Thompson, MM Patterson [eds], Bioelectric Recording Techniques. Part A: Cellular Processes and Brain Potentials. New York: Academic Press, 1973.)

electrode is positioned beyond the termination of the tract or beyond a point at which the tract changes direction, the electrode only sees the volley coming toward it. The result is a positive deflection only (see Figure 15-1). This monophasic positive deflection can often be recorded at some distance from the point at which the termination of transmission occurs in the context of *far-field* recording.

For gray-matter nuclear and cortical sources, the transmembrane ionic currents are related to the process of postsynaptic potential generation in a synchronously

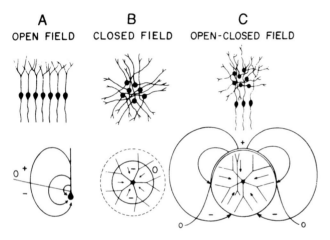

FIGURE 15-2 Lorente de Nò's models of potential field generators in the brain. Indicated fields are those generated by synchronous depolarization of the cell bodies in the structures. **A.** Open field. A schematic representation of pyramidal cells in cerebral cortex. Structural regularity is noted in the parallel alignment of the dendrites and axons. Depolarization of the cell body produces a flow of inward current (sink) at the level of the cell body and an outward current flow (source) from the dendritic extensions. The field at a distance can be picked up because there is additive superposition of the fields generated by each of the cells because of their spatial regularity. **B.** Closed field. A schematic representation of a nuclear structure in which the cell bodies are concentrated in the center of the structure and the dendrites extend radially outward. Somatic depolarization of the cells produces a concentrated field within the structure with maximum amplitude in the center of the nucleus. However, the radially directed inward currents from the dendrites cause the potential gradient to be zero when one records from outside the nucleus. **C.** Open-closed field. This is a hybrid of the two situations that leads to a partially canceled and partially extended field beyond the structure. (Reprinted with permission from Lorente de Nò. Analysis of the distribution of action currents of nerve in volume conductors. Studies from the Rockefeller Institute for Medical Research. New York: Rockefeller Institute for Medical Research. 1947;132:384–477.)

activated population of synapses within a subcortical nucleus or within a cortical neuron population typically localized to a particular cortical layer. The population of synapses could be either inhibitory, with hyperpolarization of the postsynaptic membrane (driven further away from threshold), or excitatory, with depolarization of the postsynaptic membrane (driven closer to threshold). For inhibitory postsynaptic potentials, an extracellular electrode placed nearby would see a negative deflection, whereas the opposite would be noted for excitatory postsynaptic potentials. For gray-matter synaptic population sources, it is important to recognize that the potential recordable at a distance is a compound synaptic potential that depends critically on temporal and spatial summation of transmembrane ionic currents generated at the postsynaptic membrane by individual synaptic transmission events. Therefore, it becomes significantly more difficult to record the associated potential at a distance from the generator if the whole population is not activated synchronously or if the currents caused by the individual synaptic events are not spatially aligned so as to reinforce each other. If the spatial relationship between the recording electrode and the generating population of synapses is not known, as is almost always the case in recording EPs, then it is not possible to directly infer the type of synapse from the polarity of the EP signal. For example, a negative deflection picked up at the surface of the cortex may result from the activation of a population of superficial excitatory postsynaptic potentials in the upper part of the dendritic tree or a population of deep inhibitory postsynaptic potentials near the soma of the same population of cortical pyramidal cells.

For a field to be recorded at a distance, the generator structure must have some internal spatial regularity to allow spatial summation of synaptic currents to occur. A structure that has significant spatial regularity, such as a tract of parallel fibers or a layered population of neurons with parallel dendrites, is labeled an *open-field* generator. This is because the field it generates is open to recording at a distance. A structure in which there is no spatial regularity and in which the individual synaptic currents are directed randomly, is labeled a *closed-field* generator. The field it generates is closed to recording from outside its extent because of a net cancellation of the currents associated with the individual synaptic events (Figure 15-2).

The generator potential is the idealized potential that would be recorded from an electrode placed infinitesimally close to the generator itself with respect to a totally indifferent reference site. It is impossible to record this idealized generator potential typically for two basic reasons: (1) In noninvasive studies one cannot put an electrode directly adjacent to the generator; and (2) as noted previously, there is no totally indifferent reference site available.

The actual potential that can be recovered is recorded at some distance from its generation site. It must, therefore, be conducted through the surrounding tissue that serves as a conducting medium in which currents caused by the generator potential may be induced. In understanding the relationship between the idealized generator potential and the potential actually recorded at a distant site, the surrounding tissue through which the potential is conducted is referred to as a *volume conductor*. The problem of understanding the relationship between the recordable signal recovered at a given location distant to the site of generation, and the activation process of the source itself, is referred to as the *volume conduction* problem. The problem of deriving the currents and potentials recordable at a distance from a given temporally and spatially defined source activity is called the *forward* problem. The problem of deriving spatially localized source activity from a given observed potential field recorded at the skin surface is called the *inverse* problem. Unfortunately, there is no unique solution to the inverse problem. Thus, an infinite number of different source configurations and activities within the volume conductor could lead to the same observed field distribution at the surface. It is, therefore, necessary to constrain the problem by deriving probable source activities from knowledge of the relevant neuroanatomy of the activated pathways and the probable localization of underlying generators. Hypotheses regarding generator localization for different EP components can be checked through clinicopathologic correlation and animal research.

The volume conduction problem is generally addressed through the application of an area of physics called *electromagnetic field theory*. This involves modeling the source activity as a spatially and temporally dynamic electric dipole vector function or electric current source vector function. This source vector has both a time-varying amplitude as well as a spatially defined direction related to the geometry of the source and the net direction of transmembrane source current flows. The source vector then produces an electric and a magnetic field and induces current flows in the surrounding tissues. The electric fields are constrained by the geometry of the volume conductor as well as its spatially distributed electrical conduction properties. Magnetic fields associated with source current activity can also be recorded, but these require the application of a specialized apparatus called a *gradient magnetometer*. The recording of evoked magnetic fields is generally restricted to a limited number of research laboratories

that are currently investigating the use and relative advantage of the magnetic technique as compared with the electric technique. A further discussion of evoked magnetic field recording is beyond the scope of this consideration, and we focus on the recording of electric field potentials. The recorded electric potential at the scalp is thus influenced not only by the source activity but also by the general electromagnetic properties of the medium through which the activity is transmitted. As discussed later, the volume conduction problem involves the electrical properties of the conducting tissue as well as the geometric and spatial factors that influence the structure of the electric potential field produced in the volume conductor by source activity.

Epochs of electrical voltage fluctuations, time locked to the occurrence of the stimulus and recorded from electrodes placed on the skin overlying proximal structures in the sensory pathway, are then captured and averaged together using a computer. In this way, the elements of the signal epochs that are repeatedly correlated in time to the stimulus are enhanced while the uncorrelated noise is suppressed. The signal-to-noise power ratio tends to increase with the square root of the total number of epochs averaged together given certain assumptions about the properties of the noise.

The selection of electrode placement maximizes the amplitude and isolation of the desired signal when one electrode—the *active* electrode—is placed close to the source of the physiological signal, while the other electrode—the *reference* electrode—is placed at a distance over a relatively inactive or *indifferent* site. In reality, no site is truly indifferent or neutral. The distance between the electrodes must be limited because the larger the interelectrode distance, the greater the likelihood of injection of large-amplitude interference from other nontargeted physiological sources spanned by the electrodes (e.g., skeletal muscle or the heart). Therefore, the process of selecting recording sites is necessarily a compromise between maximizing the definition of the source signal and limiting interference from other physiological generators at a distance from the physiological source of interest. When placing electrodes on the scalp, a standardized system for identifying the location of the electrodes, called the *International 10-20 system*, is used (Figure 15-3).

When the electrodes are spaced relatively close to each other with respect to the distance to the source, this is referred to as a *bipolar* recording montage. When the electrodes are spaced further apart so that one electrode is located close to the source of interest, whereas the other electrode is at a relative distance from the source, this is called a *monopolar* recording montage. When the recording electrode locations are placed at a

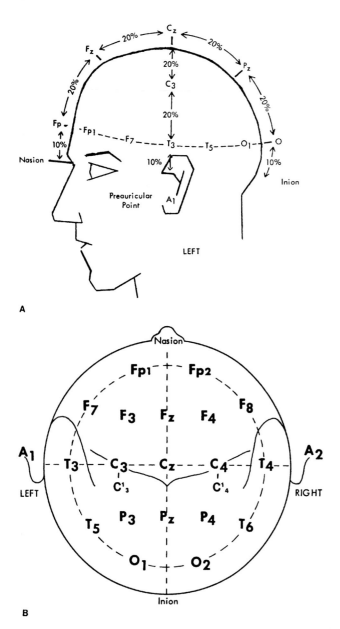

A

B

FIGURE 15-3 The International 10-20 system for identifying scalp sites for electrode placement. **A.** Standard sites for placement: lateral view. **B.** Standard sites for electrode placement including the C3' and C4' sites: view from above. (From G Rinzler. The 10-20 system booklet.)

significant distance from the source location, so that the source-associated volume conducted currents spread widely from the source across the recording surface, this is referred to as a *far-field* recording. Far-field potentials can be recorded on the scalp from deep subcortical structures as widespread positive deflections. Frequently, these are stationary potentials that are pro-

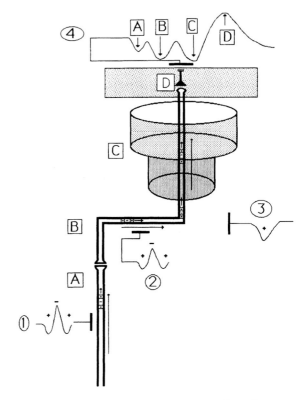

FIGURE 15-4 Schematic representation of mechanisms of evoked potential component generation. A model of a sensory pathway is shown with one synaptic relay (A), a crossing of fibers (B), an abrupt change in the geometry of the volume conductor (C), and an intracortical synapse (D). Recording electrodes that are placed close to the conducting afferent volley record a triphasic waveform (1 and 2). Electrodes located at a distance from the propagation pathway but in the direct line of the pathway see the positive front of the volley coming toward the electrode and pick up far-field positive waves (3 and 4). The positive deflection can be interrupted with a return to baseline by a synaptic gap (A), a change in the direction of conduction of the pathway (B), or a change in the geometry or properties of the volume conductor (C). In this case, the scalp recording site (4) records a sequence of three different far-field positivities, followed by a near-field negative (upward) deflection caused by the postsynaptic activation of the cortical neuron. This model shows that a component recorded on the scalp may result not only from active generators in the pathway, but also from changes in the orientation in space of the conducting pathway and from changes in the volume conductor, which is the electrophysical environment in which the activity is being conducted.

duced when a conducted volley passes across a boundary between volume conductor segments with different conductivity or geometric properties. They can also appear when the tract conveying conducted impulses rapidly switches direction (Figure 15-4).

When the recording electrode locations are located relatively close to the source, small changes in the orientation of the source vector produce significant changes in the spatial distribution and configuration of the recorded potential. This is referred to as a *near-field* recording. Near-field recordings are more readily interpreted in terms of their relationship to the activity of the nearby source. They tend to be larger in amplitude and more sharply localized spatially than are the far-field recordings. The structure and polarity of the field distribution in near-field recording are determined by the orientation of the source dipole relative to the surface as well as the depth below the surface. If the dipole is oriented radially, then the pole that is closest to the surface produces a single maximum point in the field (Figure 15-5A and B). This maximum point directly overlies the source location. If the dipole is oriented tangentially, then there is a polarity reversal produced with positive and negative maxima of approximately equal amplitude located adjacent to each other in the distribution (Figure 15-5C and D). The source is localized between the two maxima near the point of polarity reversal. Most often, the orientation of the dipole is at some oblique angle to the surface. The result is an asymmetric bipolar field. In recording cortically generated EPs at the scalp, the dipole orientation is determined primarily by the orientation of the cortical surface containing the responding zone of sensory cortex, with respect to the scalp surface. On the outer surface of the brain, tangentially oriented dipoles are localized to sites along the walls of cortex in sulci where the cortical surface lies at right angles to the scalp. On the other hand, radially oriented dipoles are oriented at the crowns of the gyri where the cortical surface parallels the scalp. The opposite applies to cortical generators on the medial surface of the hemisphere.

In a simplistic sense, the paradigm for recording the sensory EP can be seen as a proximal extension of the peripheral nerve sensory nerve conduction study. Instead of recording a peripheral afferent neurogram, recordings are viewed as reflecting a sequence of activations from responding structures in the pathway within the CNS. The sensory EP can thus be viewed in a simplistic sense as a *continuity check* of a specific sensory pathway traversing the primary afferent nerve fiber and traveling along an anatomically defined pathway through the CNS. Unfortunately, this *transmission cable* view of conduction through central sensory pathways is highly oversimplified. The appearance of the EP as recorded at the body surface often cannot clearly be directly related in a one-to-one fashion to specific neural

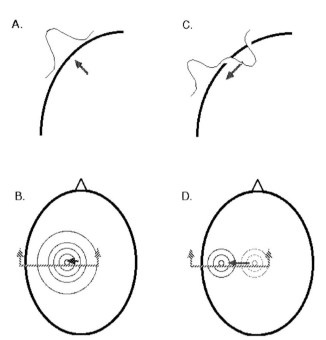

FIGURE 15-5 Near-field distributions produced by cortical generators recorded at the scalp. **A.** Coronal section showing the recorded voltage amplitude along a coronal line on the scalp overlying a radially oriented dipole generator. Note that there is a maximum amplitude noted on the scalp overlying the site of the generator. **B.** View of the scalp from above with the electrical distribution shown in the form of isopotential contour lines showing a single maximum location of voltage overlying the location of the dipole. **C.** Coronal section showing the recorded voltage amplitude along a coronal line along the scalp overlying a tangentially oriented dipole generator. Note that there are now two adjacent maxima, one positive and one negative, lying on either side of the dipole location. **D.** Corresponding view of the scalp from above with the electrical distribution shown in the form of isopotential contour lines. Broken lines indicate a negative voltage, and solid lines indicate a positive voltage. Again, there are two peaks of the distribution, one positive and one negative, located on either side of the dipole location.

elements located along an anatomic pathway. There are a number of different technical reasons for this:

- As noted previously, some neural elements of the pathway (e.g., deep nuclei) may generate internal activity in a closed field configuration that is not recordable at the body surface. This is because of the spatial cancellation of currents that project to outside the region of the neural generator.
- In addition, a variety of factors other than the generation of a source potential can produce recordable far-field components at the body surface (see Figure 15-4).

These include changes in the direction of a conducting pathway, as well as changes in the geometric configuration of the volume conductor.

- A single EP component recorded at the surface may be related to multiple underlying generators that are activated simultaneously through parallel connections or whose sequential activation overlaps in time.
- Phasic subtraction or *cancellation* can occur between difference sources. Activity produced primarily by sources that are located close to one electrode of the differential pair interact with distinct source activity, producing a signal simultaneously picked up primarily at the other electrode.

Another form of EP is the MEP. This study can be viewed as the motor conduction study extended proximally to the primary motor cortex of the precentral gyrus. The motor cortex is stimulated transcranially. This was originally described by Merton and Morton in 1980[13] using a brief, large-amplitude electrical stimulus. However, this approach was painful and not very well tolerated. A relatively painless and better tolerated technique was subsequently described by Barker et al.[14,15] This technique used a large, transient magnetic field to induce currents within the cerebral cortex. A large, brief current was passed through a coiled conductor to produce the stimulus field. When the coil producing the magnetic field was held over the electrically excitable motor cortex, a muscle twitch in the extremities could be produced. The focus of the muscle twitch depended on exactly where the stimulus coil was located with respect to the homuncular map of the motor cortex. The induced currents were sufficient to produce a synchronous activation of pyramidal cells projecting into the corticospinal tract. This activation of motor cortex, in turn, produced a synchronous activation of motor neurons in motor nuclei at the segmental level in the spinal cord and thus a muscle contraction. The muscle contraction can be recorded as a compound muscle action potential using surface electrodes placed over the activated muscle. Onset latency of the compound muscle action potential can be measured and used to infer central motor path conduction times.

BASIC PRINCIPLES OF TECHNIQUE

The most technically demanding aspect of recording EPs involves the extraction of the low-amplitude (0.1–20 μV) EP signal from the background signal mix of electroencephalographic, electrospinographic, electro-oculographic, electrocardiographic, and elec-

tromyographic (EMG) physiological sources, along with various artificial sources of artifact. This background mix can be several times larger in amplitude than the EP signal. Some of these signals may be modifiable with technique. For example, the EMG signal can be reduced by having a properly relaxed or lightly sedated subject. The most common means of extracting the EP signal from the background is signal averaging.

The stimulus is applied repetitively, and sweeps of digitized data points are acquired over an interval that is time locked to the moment of stimulus onset. This process is typically accomplished using computer-based digital data acquisition and processing techniques. Each new sweep of data is added to the average signal that is maintained in computer memory and displayed graphically on the monitor as it is being acquired and updated. The raw input signal data can also be displayed at the same time in order to monitor for the presence of artifactual signals. A special artifact-rejection filtering process can apply a specific criterion to each sweep of data to determine whether it will be accepted for addition to the average signal. Most often, this criterion involves an evaluation of the amplitude of the signal across a selected segment of time. If the amplitude on this segment exceeds a specified level, then the sweep is assumed to contain a large-amplitude artifact and the sweep is automatically rejected and not added to the average. When the averaged signal reaches a stable end point, the averaging process is terminated. The signal can then be inspected and specific components identified with a signal cursor. When these components are marked, the testing system can measure specific latencies and amplitudes of the various components. Latencies may be from the stimulus onset to the peak of the component (absolute latencies) or from the peak of one component to the peak of another (interpeak latencies). Component amplitudes may be defined as either the amplitude above or below a baseline reference, or the amplitude may be defined between specific positive, negative, or positive and negative peaks. Amplitudes have more limited value than latencies, in general, because a variety of different technical factors can influence the amplitude of a component. When amplitude is used, it is usually evaluated in terms of one particular amplitude measure with reference to another, usually by computing an amplitude ratio. Generally, latencies are measured and the presence or absence of normal components is noted. Comparisons of signals between left and right sides are often helpful.

Another important physiological issue in the recording and interpretation of EPs is the need to clearly establish that the stimulus has successfully activated the primary afferent nerve fibers. It is important to obtain evidence that the peripheral structures have been sufficiently activated before concluding that a particular structure in the CNS upstream from the primary afferent neuron has failed to respond because of central pathology. In the visual EP, the presence of a normal retinal EP in the form of an electroretinogram (ERG) helps to verify that the visual stimulus was able to activate receptors in the retina. Any abnormality noted in the visual EP at the cortical level can then be assumed to be caused by a defect in transmission between the retina and the primary visual cortex. In the BAEP, it is not possible to evaluate the quality of transmission through the brain stem auditory pathway unless the initial wave I component is clearly identified. This verifies that the auditory stimulus was transduced to an action potential volley in the primary afferent neurons by the peripheral auditory mechanism and that the volley was delivered to the brain stem–based component of the auditory pathway. Without this verification, it is impossible to determine whether the absence of subsequent components indicates impaired transmission through the brain stem. In the SEP, it is important to record a nerve action potential from the periphery to establish that the peripheral nerve responded to stimulation and was conducting this volley successfully into the CNS. Without this verification, the absence of a response over the spinal cord or over the cerebral cortex cannot be interpreted as indicating abnormalities at these levels.

The major goal of applying EPs to the assessment of CNS disorders is to provide information about underlying pathophysiology. However, before one can conclude that observed changes in the structure of the EP signal reflect pathology, it is important to understand the normal physiology of the responses. A variety of factors can influence the underlying physiological processes. These can be divided into stimulus factors and subject factors. We now turn to a consideration of the physiology of each of the major sensory modalities of EP.

PHYSIOLOGY OF ELECTRORETINOGRAPHY AND VISUAL-EVOKED POTENTIAL

General Considerations

The flow of visual information through the afferent pathways of the visual system traverses structures that are involved in the transduction, transmission, perception, and processing of patterns of visible light. This pathway includes the eyes, optic nerves, optic chiasm, optic tracts, lateral geniculate nuclei of the thalamus, optic radiations, and striate cortex of the occipital lobe (Figure 15-6). Lesions anterior to and including the optic chiasm most often produce altered visual acuity, impairment of color perception, and abnormal central or peripheral vision, which may be monocular if the impairment involves optic nerve fibers on only one side. Retrochiasmatic lesions that are unilateral most often present with visual field defects (hemianopia or quadrantanopia) without visual acuity complaints. Cortical lesions in extrastriate visual association cortex produce impairments of the perception and interpretation of visual information. This includes such problems as object perception and identification, movement perception, color perception, and visual inattention.

Activation of the brain by light stimulation involves the transmission of visual stimulation through the physical structures of the eye. These include the cornea, anterior chamber, lens, and vitreous humor (Figure 15-7). Pupillary size serves as the adjustable aperture of the eye, controlling the total amount of light that passes into the interior. The cornea and lens serve as a focusing mechanism to ensure that a clear representation of the pattern of light crossing a focal plane at a particular distance arrives at the retina. The process of accommodation involves the adjustment of lens shape by the pull of the ciliary muscles so objects at different distances can be brought into focus. In the performance of visual EPs that are driven by alterations in spatial contrast rather than luminance (see the section Electroretinography, later in this chapter), optimal EP recording depends on preserved pupillary control and accommodation, the processes that deliver a focused image of the stimulus to the retina. These processes, in turn, are dependent on a conscious, cooperative, and attentive subject who is able to accurately engage and maintain these processes during gaze fixation. In the evaluation of the system response to a spatial contrast stimulus, it is also important that any refractive error be corrected with external lenses.

Having traversed the ocular media, the photons contained in the stimulation impinge on the retina and the specialized photoreceptors, the rods and cones, that lie in the deepest layer of the retina. The deepest part of these cells adjacent to the retinal pigment epithelium contains the specialized organelles that capture impinging photons. Pigments in the photoreceptors undergo conformational change when they interact with specific types of photons. The activated pigments then stimulate transducin, which then activates cyclic guanosine monophosphate phosphodiesterase. Through a cascade

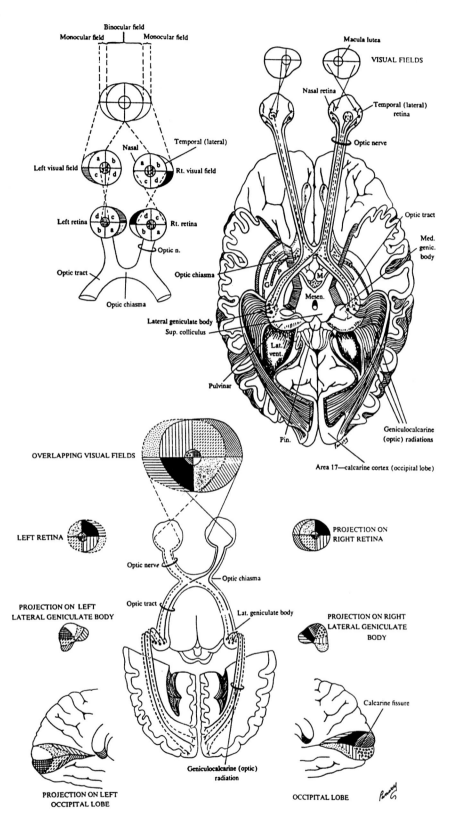

FIGURE 15-6 The anatomy of the visual system. Top left illustration shows how monocular and binocular visual fields are mapped to the retina. Top right illustration shows the general structure of the retinogeniculostriate pathway. The bottom illustration shows how different parts of the visual fields from the left and right retina are mapped to different regions of the lateral geniculate nucleus and the calcarine cortex. Note that the monocular peripheral fields are mapped most anterior whereas the macular fields are mapped most posterior at the cortical level. This gives rise to separate dipole sources at the cortical level generated from stimulation of the peripheral and macular fields. Note also that the inferior retinal fields map to the superior bank of the calcarine fissure and vice versa. (Composite construction of illustrations reprinted with permission from B Pansky, DJ Allen. Review of Neuroscience. New York: Macmillan, 1980;393, 395.)

reaction, cyclic guanosine monophosphate phosphodiesterase activation results in a transient closure of membrane sodium channels and a reduction in the transmembrane sodium current. The end result is a hyperpolarization of the photoreceptor cell.

The visual fields as they are perceived by the subject are mapped in reverse format to the retina by the action of the lens. The nasal hemiretina receives the temporal field, and the temporal hemiretina receives the nasal field. The superior half of the retina receives the lower field, and the inferior half of the retina receives the upper field. This segmentation and transformation of the visual field into neuroanatomic components continues throughout the afferent visual pathway.

The ganglion cells of the retina send their projections that come together to form the optic nerve. The optic nerve has four major segments: intraocular, intraorbital, intracanalicular, and intracranial. The intraocular portion, the optic disk, is composed of the unmyelinated ganglion cell axons and astrocytes. It is located 3–4 mm nasal to the fovea. As it exits the globe, the diameter increases as it becomes myelinated by oligodendrocytes. At this point, the nerve also becomes wrapped with pia, arachnoid, and dura. It is bathed in CSF that is contiguous with the CSF that circulates throughout the CNS. The nerve travels through the orbit and enters the optic canal in the posteromedial part of the sphenoid bone. The nerve courses medially through the bone toward the optic chiasm. The optic nerves join together at the optic chiasm. At the chiasm, the centrally located fibers from the nasal hemiretina cross, whereas the laterally located fibers from the temporal hemiretina remain ipsilateral. The visual afferent fibers then exit posteriorly from the chiasm and diverge to form the left and right optic tracts. The optic tracts travel above the infundibulum, below the third ventricle, and superomedial to the uncal gyri of the temporal lobe. They then turn posterolaterally to the interpeduncular cistern just ventral to the rostral midbrain and the cerebral peduncles. Most of these fibers then synapse in the ipsilateral lateral geniculate nucleus. A few axons peel off to form the accessory optic tract that completes the afferent limb of the pupillary light reflex. The optic radiations exit dorsally from the lateral geniculate nucleus and form two major components. The fibers containing information from the contralateral superior visual field travel in an inferior fascicle that curves in an anteroinferior direction into the anterior pole of the temporal lobe to form Meyer's loop. The fibers containing information from the contralateral inferior visual field travel in a superior fascicle, which lies deep within the parietal lobe. Both fascicles converge on the calcarine cortex of the medial

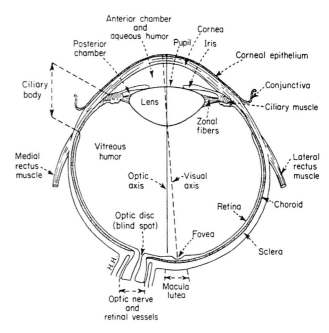

FIGURE 15-7 The anatomy of the eye. This illustration shows the basic structures of the right eyeball viewed from above. (Reprinted with permission from HD Patton, AF Fuchs, B Hille, et al. Textbook of Physiology [21st ed]. Philadelphia: Saunders, 1989;413.)

occipital lobe, with the superior fascicle projecting to the upper bank above the calcarine fissure and the inferior fascicle projecting to the lower bank so that a retinotopic organization is preserved. Thus, the left visual hemifield comes into the right calcarine cortex and vice versa. Within each primary visual cortex region, the fields are mapped in vertically inverted fashion with the lower field to the upper bank and vice versa. The macula is mapped posteriorly toward the optic poles and the more peripheral fields are mapped to the medial cortex adjacent to the calcarine fissure.

Retinal Anatomy and Physiology

The photoreceptors of the human retina are highly active cells. Both rods and cones remain fairly depolarized at rest because of a relatively high baseline membrane permeability to the sodium ion (Na^+). The Na^+ current enters the light-sensitive outer segment of the photoreceptor, and Na^+ ions are actively extruded from the inner segment through a pump mechanism. The retinal pigment epithelium also maintains a steady potential. There is thus a flow of positive current created in the photoreceptor layer directed toward the front of the eye. This produces a voltage difference with the cornea being positive with respect to the back of the eye. This steady potential difference between the front and the back of the eye is the basis of the electro-oculogram.

There are four different photoreceptor types: rods and three different subtypes of cones. The rods are sensitive nocturnal receptors that produce achromatic

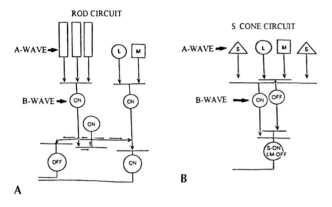

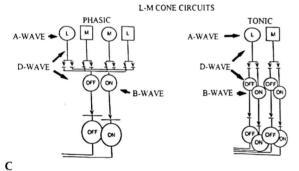

FIGURE 15-8 The anatomy of retinal circuitry. **A.** Rod circuitry. The rods transmit their activity synaptically to on-bipolar cells that synapse on rod amacrine cells. The amacrine cells then transmit their activation to both on- and off-ganglion cells, which the rods share with the L- and M-cones. **B.** S-cone circuitry involved in color-sensitive processing. The S-cone circuit in which the S-cone transmits its activation to S-cone on-bipolar cells. The on-bipolar cell transmits excitatory activity to a unique on/off ganglion cell. L- and M-cone off-bipolar cells also send excitatory signals to the same ganglion cell. **C.** L- and M-cone phasic and tonic circuitry involved in high-spatial-resolution processing. The circuit on the left involves large, fast, phasically responsive ganglion cells. The circuit on the right involves smaller, slow, tonically responsive ganglion cells. In the phasically responsive system, both L- and M-cone outputs are integrated. In the tonically responsive system, the output of the L- and M-cones are maintained separate from each other. (Reprinted with permission from MJ Aminoff. Electrodiagnosis in Clinical Neurology [4th ed]. New York: Churchill Livingstone, 1999;403.)

vision in low ambient light with generally coarse spatial resolution. They outnumber the cones by 20 to 1 and are evenly distributed across the retina. The cones are diurnal receptors that are critical to human functional vision because they mediate high spatial resolution and color vision. They are in highest concentration in the macula, the region of the retina dedicated to central vision. The central part of the macula, the fovea, contains cones only. The cone subtypes include the L and M cones that are involved in high spatial resolution vision and the S cones that are involved in color vision. Each of the different photoreceptor types has a different form of related retinal circuit (Figure 15-8).

When light photons are absorbed in the outer segment specialized organelle of the photoreceptor, the result is a relative hyperpolarization of the cell because of a relative decrease in membrane permeability to Na^+, as discussed previously. This response is true for both rods and cones. The hyperpolarization of the rod produces a disinhibition (i.e., excitation) of the rod bipolar cell. The rod bipolar cell then excites a third-order rod amacrine cell that, in turn, sends a signal to the output cell of the retina, the ganglion cell. The ganglion cells, classified into *on* and *off* cells, indirectly receive input from both rod and cone photoreceptors. The ganglion cells then send their unmyelinated axons along the inner surface of the retina and into the optic nerve.

Cone photoreceptors have a more complicated retinal circuit devoted to them as might be expected from their more complex visual function. Each L and M cone has two different associated types of bipolar cell: an on cell that depolarizes through disinhibition when the cone is activated by light, and an off cell that hyperpolarizes through increased inhibition with light activation of the cone.

Electroretinography

The ERG can be recorded from the eye with specialized electrodes that record potential changes reflecting retinal activation. Two different general types of electrodes can be used. The first type is a contact lens electrode in which the recording electrode is embedded in a specially designed contact lens that is placed on the anesthetized corneal surface. There is a small risk of corneal injury, and the optics of the eye are changed, requiring rere-fraction for the pattern ERG (PERG). The second type is a thin piece of gold foil that is placed deeply into the plane between the lower eyelid and the lower surface of the globe. This type of electrode is suitable for the PERG because the optics of the eye are not altered. A reference electrode is placed on the skin adjacent to the outer canthus of the eye, and a ground electrode can be placed in the midforehead.

The ERG can be done in a number of different ways to selectively activate specific retinal photoreceptor types and related neural circuits. The signal is elicited by a rapid change in the illumination of the photoreceptors produced by a bright flash of light applied uniformly to the retina with the pupils dilated. This is generally done using a special device called a Ganzfeld full-field stimulator. This stimulator helps to distribute illumination more homogeneously across the retina as compared with a stroboscopic flash. The flash illumination initiates a signal that begins with a corneal-negative A-wave that is followed by a slower corneal-positive B-wave. The A-wave of the flash ERG reflects the activation of the cones and rods. The B-wave reflects the synaptic depolarization of the bipolar on cells. The ganglion layer and the optic nerve make no significant contribution to the flash ERG.

The flash ERG can be done under dark-adapted conditions when the retina has no background illumination. Under these conditions, the rods remain sensitive and contribute to the response. This is called a *scotopic* response. The rod response can be isolated by stimulating the dark-adapted retina with low-level blue light. When the retina is light-adapted to bright background illumination, the rods are generally saturated and a *photopic* response is obtained. A bright white or red flash applied to the light-adapted eye generally produces a cone-dominated response. Cones can also be isolated with a 30-Hz flicker stimulation because the rods have a much slower temporal response and are unable to follow illumination that varies at this frequency (Figure 15-9). The flash ERG has been applied to the differential diagnosis of a variety of retinopathies.

The PERG is elicited by a constant luminance high-contrast pattern-shift stimulus similar to that used for the pattern-shift visual EP (PSVEP) (see Figure 15-9). It

FIGURE 15-9 Normal flash electroretinograms and pattern electroretinogram (PERG). **A.** Electroretinogram to single bright white flash. i. Prior to dark adaptation. ii. After 20 minutes in the dark. Higher amplitude caused by enhanced rod response. **B.** Averaged responses to repetitive bright white flashes. iii. White flash at 3 Hz. iv. White flash at 30 Hz (pure cone response). v. Oscillatory potentials. **C.** Scotopic rod responses to dim blue light flashes at increasing intensities. **D.** Pattern electroretinogram with 200 sweeps averaged.

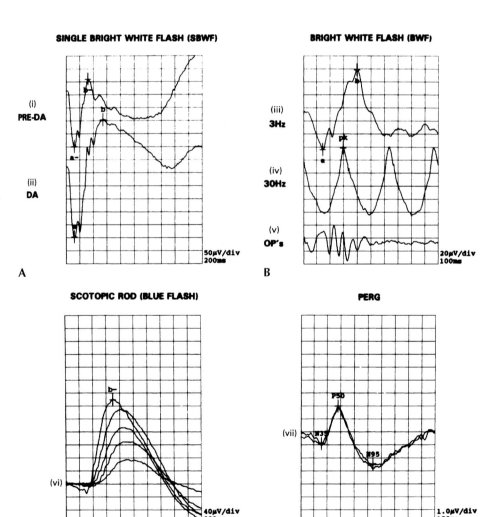

is useful for the evaluation of the ganglion cell layer of the retina because the stimulus causes no net change in retinal luminance, but centers on the response to spatial contrast. Ganglion cells are more responsive to spatial contrast than are the photoreceptors. The amplitude of the PERG is significantly lower than the flash ERG and signal averaging is generally employed. The amplitude increases linearly with contrast so a high-contrast stimulus is recommended for technically adequate studies. The amplitude also varies with the check size of the pattern. Amplitude is maximized with a check size of approximately 35 minutes of arc in stimulus field that subtends 10–15 degrees. The PERG recorded simultaneously with a PSVEP can be helpful as an assessment of the adequacy of gaze fixation in situations in which this may be in question. An abnormal PSVEP result in the presence of a normal PERG result helps to eliminate the possibility of retinal disease or impaired gaze fixation as an explanation for the abnormal PSVEP result. In this case, one can be more confident that the abnormal PSVEP result is an indication of postretinal disease of the optic pathway. The recording of the PERG is only necessary for the purposes of diagnosing postretinal conditions when the monocular PSVEP result is abnormal. This is generally for the purpose of ruling out a primary retinal pathology or poor gaze fixation as an explanation for the abnormal PSVEP result. Binocular stimulation for the recording of the PERG with gold foil electrodes is preferable to monocular recording. It has the advantage of normally showing less intereye amplitude difference and is thus more sensitive in detecting unilateral deficits.

Visual-Evoked Potential Physiology

The basic considerations with respect to visual anatomy have been covered in the previous section. There are two basic ways to activate the visual system: through a diffuse pulse of light energy or through a change in the spatial pattern of a fixed amount of light energy. Corresponding to this, there are two basic types of stimuli that are used to activate the visual system for visual EP testing: flash stimuli and pattern stimuli. The first type of stimulus activates the system through a change in luminance. The second type of stimulus activates the system through spatial contrast with constant luminance. As we have noted with the discussion of the ERG, the flash stimulus can be used to evaluate photoreceptor function by controlling the intensity and spectral content (i.e., color) of the light. Activation of the visual system by a stroboscopic flash does not require gaze fixation or controlled accommodation and can

thus be used in subjects who are unable to maintain a focused image on the retina. However, the flash-elicited visual EP is highly variable in structure with component latency values having standard deviations that are greater than 10% of the mean value.[16] This makes a careful parametric assessment of latency and amplitude difficult and the interpretation less objective. On the other hand, a constant-luminance spatial contrast stimulus, such as the reversal of a black-and-white checkerboard pattern, produces a waveform with a more consistent structure. Peak latency values for the PSVEP using a black-and-white checkerboard stimulus have standard deviations that are approximately 5% of the mean value.[17] Furthermore, the flash-elicited visual EP is significantly less sensitive to pathology than the PSVEP.[18] Another advantage of the pattern stimulus is that one can examine the relationship between PSVEP parameters and spatial frequency (e.g., by varying check size in the checkerboard pattern) as well as temporal frequency (e.g., by varying the rate of pattern reversal) in order to assess visual acuity. Thus, the only times that the flash-elicited visual EP would be used instead of the PSVEP are when one is trying to make a qualitative determination of whether at least part of the visual system remains functional (e.g., after suspected traumatic transection or infarction of the optic nerve), or when one is testing a patient who is unable to cooperate for the PSVEP examination (e.g., in coma, during surgery, or in neonates).

The pattern-shift stimulus can be generated and reversed in a variety of different ways using both mechanical and electronic devices. However, the most commonly employed and most flexible technique involves the display of the pattern on a television monitor, with the formation and control of the projected pattern performed by pattern-generating electronic circuitry. For research purposes, a separate programmable graphics microprocessor controls the display patterns in video memory. In most clinical laboratories, the display is controlled by special purpose electronic circuitry with controls that allow for a limited selection of patterns and check or stripe sizes. Typically, these patterns are displayed on a black-and-white television monitor. The luminance is set with the brightness control, and the contrast can be similarly adjusted. Luminance can be measured and controlled using a photometer.

The PSVEP recorded from the midoccipital site (Oz) to the vertex site (Cz) consists of a triphasic potential. The PSVEP includes a negative peak at approximately 75 msec (N75), a positive peak at approximately 100 msec (P100), and another negative peak at approximately 135 msec (N135). The setup for recording the PSVEP is shown in Figure 15-10. A typical normal study examining left and right eyes independently is shown in Figure 15-11. The major latency measure is that of the primary positive peak, the P100.

The major contribution to the PSVEP comes from the lower half of the visual field corresponding to the upper half of the retina.[19] As we recall from the discussion of anatomy, this component of the visual field is carried by the upper fascicle of the optic radiation that travels deep in the parietal lobe and projects to the upper bank of the calcarine fissure. Presumably, this part of the field produces a source dipole that is oriented in a more radial direction to produce a larger maximum over the occipital scalp. The upper field may also generate a corresponding negative peak over the frontal locations that may be slightly delayed compared with the activity seen over the occipital region. If the phase difference is sufficient, and a midfrontal electrode site (Fz) reference electrode is used, then a bifid or W-shaped response may be seen. This can be resolved by either using a reference at Cz, or by stimulating with only the inferior visual field. In some subjects, the scalp

positivity of the P100 may be shifted upward toward the Pz location in the midline parietal scalp with a low amplitude at the Oz site. This type of variation probably relates to interindividual differences in the location of the calcarine cortex relative to scalp electrode placement sites. This should be kept in mind if the standard Oz-Cz recording does not show a clear waveform. To be sure that such a variant situation is not missed, it has been recommended that additional recordings be obtained from the Pz and Cz sites with reference to a relatively inactive earlobe reference when the response

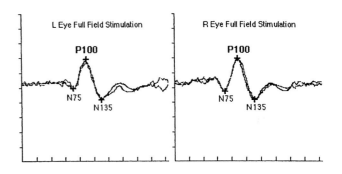

PSVEP - Full Field

LEFT EYE		RIGHT EYE	
Latencies			
N75	72.00	N75	75.00
P100	102.0	P100	105.0
N135	133.8	N135	135.0
Inter-Ocular Latency Difference:	3.0		
Amplitudes			
N75-P100	5.94	N75-P100	6.34
P100-N135	8.06	P100-N135	7.81

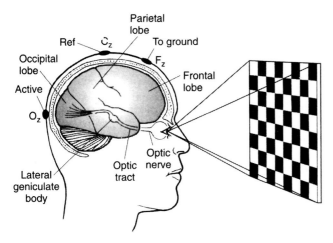

FIGURE 15-10 Setup for the pattern-shift visual-evoked potential. The subject is positioned in front of a television monitor on which a black-and-white checkerboard pattern is displayed. Each eye is tested separately. The subject is instructed to maintain full attention and focus on the pattern on the screen. The recording is obtained from a midoccipital electrode (O$_z$) with reference to the vertex (C$_z$) using the midfrontal electrode site (F$_z$) as a ground. Improved resolution of the distribution of the evoked potential field on the scalp requires additional recording channels. (Reprinted with permission from M Grabois, S Garrison, K Hart, et al [eds], Physical Medicine and Rehabilitation. The Complete Approach. Malden, MA: Blackwell Science, 2000;202.)

FIGURE 15-11 Bilateral normal pattern-shift visual-evoked potential (PSVEP) study. Recordings were obtained from the midoccipital site with reference to the vertex. Stimulation was performed with a reversing black-and-white checkerboard pattern projected on a television monitor such that each check subtended a visual angle of 20 minutes of arc. The full screen stimulus subtended a visual angle of 15 degrees. The major waveform peaks are marked. Note the triphasic structure of the cortical response with a major positive peak located at approximately 100 msec after the stimulus. There is a 10% prestimulus period. Positive deflection at the midoccipital site is displayed upward. Vertical scale: 3 µV per division. Horizontal scale: 30 msec per division. (N = negative peak; P = positive peak.) (Reprinted with permission from M Grabois, S Garrison, K Hart, et al. [eds], Physical Medicine and Rehabilitation. The Complete Approach. Malden, MA: Blackwell Science, 2000;203.)

is not clearly seen in the Oz-Cz recording. Another possible variant caused by changes in the orientation of the source dipole from the calcarine cortex in the horizontal plane is a shift in the peak P100 positivity to the left or right of the midline. This is expected to occur when hemifield stimulation is employed, but may occur in some normal subjects with full-field monocular stimulation. In such subjects it is important to perform a four-channel study with recordings from Oz, Pz, left occipital and right occipital sites with respect to an earlobe. The left occipital and right occipital electrodes can be placed 5 cm to the right and left of the Oz site.

The EP parameters vary significantly with stimulus luminance and contrast. The latency of the response increases significantly with decreasing pattern luminance. Halliday et al.[17] showed that the P100 latency increased approximately 15 msec for each log unit reduction in luminance. The amplitude of the PSVEP also decreases significantly with decreasing pattern brightness. Pupillary size also affects retinal illumination so that gross differences in pupillary size should be noted and taken into account. Pattern contrast is computed by dividing the difference between the luminance of the dark and bright areas of the pattern by the sum of their luminances and multiplying by 100. Reduction in pattern contrast is associated with increased latency of the P100 and decreased amplitude of the PSVEP, but the effect tends to saturate at levels of contrast above 40%. Because most studies are performed with higher levels of pattern contrast, this does not tend to be an important confounding factor.

The amplitude and latency of the PSVEP vary significantly with check size and stimulus field size. With regard to P100 latency, the latency increases and the amplitude decreases as check size increases for a given stimulus field size. However, the smaller the stimulus field, the more rapidly the latency increases and the amplitude decreases for a given check size. The P100 latency remains stable and at a minimum level if the check size is less than 10% of the field size.[20] The amplitude of the P100 drops by approximately 5% as field size decreases from greater than 30 degrees down to 8 degrees and then begins to drop rapidly below a field size of 4 degrees.[20] For a 15-degree stimulus field, the maximum amplitude of the P100 was found at a check size of 15' but the minimum latency was found for a check size of 35' of arc.[5]

The subject is typically positioned in a comfortable chair with the neck supported so that there is a distance of 100 cm from the television monitor to the front of the eyes. The subtended visual angle is computed by dividing the width (or height) of the check or field by 2 and then dividing this by the distance to the screen, using the same units. Using a calculator or trigonometric tables, one uses the inverse tangent (arctan) function to find the angle that has this value as its tangent. For small values, the inverse tangent is approximately equal to its argument, although the value is given in radians and must be converted to degrees by multiplying by a conversion factor of 57.3 degrees per radian. This angle is then multiplied by 2 to give the total subtended visual angle. For example, if a full-field visual display is projected on a 12-inch (30.5 cm) television monitor and the subject is seated 100 cm from the screen, the total subtended visual angle is $2 \times \tan^{-1} [(30.5/2)/100] = 2 \times \tan^{-1} (0.15)$, which is approximately $2 \times 0.15 = 0.3$ radians or 17.2 degrees (0.3×57.3). If this area of display is divided into a checkerboard pattern of 32 by 32 checks, then the subtended angle of each check would be 32.3 degrees. The ratio of check size to field size is 3.1% which is well below the 10% level for optimizing the latency of the P100 component.

All of these stimulus factors that cause significant variations in the PSVEP parameters emphasize the importance of using careful and consistent technique in performing these studies. Care should be taken to control stimulus factors so that test conditions are as similar as possible to the conditions used to collect normative comparison data. This is necessary in order to avoid the mistake of interpreting a parameter deviation caused by different stimulus conditions as an indication of abnormality.

Because of the anatomy reviewed previously, monocular full-field stimulation generates input to both right and left hemispheres with the nasal hemiretina projecting to the contralateral hemisphere and the temporal hemiretina projecting to the ipsilateral hemisphere. In the presence of a unilateral hemispheric lesion, or any retrochiasmatic lesion, monocular stimulation therefore still produces a cortical response. Thus, full-field monocular stimulation is best applied to the detection of retrobulbar, prechiasmatic optic nerve lesions. If one wishes to evaluate retrochiasmatic lesions, it is best to use half-field rather than full-field stimulation. This can be done with binocular stimulation. It is critically important from a technical standpoint that the foveal central field be stimulated consistently when using hemifield stimulation. A larger stimulus field of 30 degrees or greater is therefore recommended for hemifield stimulation. The hemifield response is also more clearly seen with larger checks (40 minutes of arc or greater) that are highly contrasted. This is because the peripheral visual stimulation produces a potential field distribution that is significantly different from that produced by central stimulation. The central field maps to the occipital poles, whereas the peripheral field maps more anteriorly along the medial occipital cortex. In addition, there is significant interindividual variability in the localization and orientation of the calcarine cortex with respect to the scalp as well as significant asymmetry between left and right sides, with the left side having more striate cortex that extends further out onto the lateral surface. All of these factors are responsible for producing significant variability in the potential field distribution of the PSVEP that becomes particularly problematic when attempting to activate one hemisphere with hemifield stimulation. Most often, the P100 positivity is shifted laterally on the scalp toward the side of the hemifield stimulation (Figure 15-12A–C). The topographic field recordings suggest that the hemifield study could best be performed with a three-channel study consisting of the following leads: Oz-Cz, LO-F4, and RO-F3, with LO being a left occipital electrode site and RO being a right occipital electrode site.

FIGURE 15-12 Field distributions for pattern-shift visual-evoked potentials (PSVEPs) with full and hemifield stimulation. **A.** Topographic maps of PSVEP responses to full-field stimulation. Note that the positive peak at approximately 100 msec (P100) response is symmetrically distributed at the back of the head (see lower left map generated at 103.46 msec). Latencies at which each map was generated are given in the upper left corner of each frame. **B.** Topographic maps of PSVEP responses to left hemifield stimulation. Note that the P100 response is now shifted toward the left side (see upper right map generated at 104.92 msec).

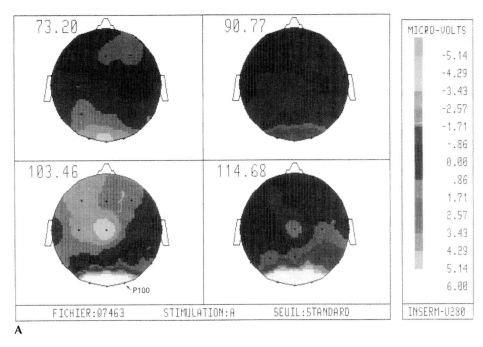
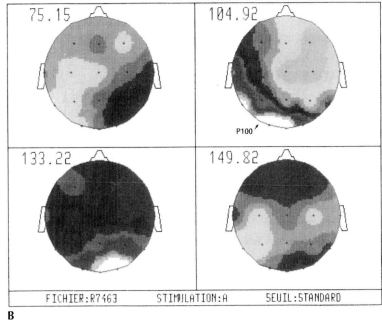
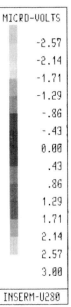

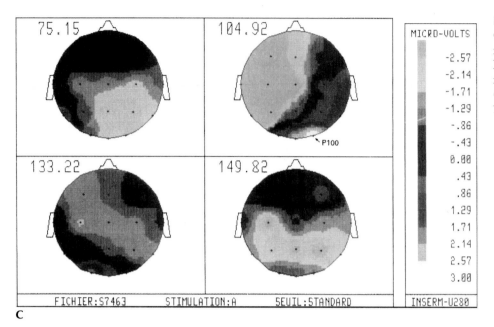

FIGURE 15-12 (*continued*) **C.** Topographic maps of PSVEP responses to right hemifield stimulation. Note that the P100 response is now shifted toward the right side (see upper right map generated at 104.92 msec).

With the use of a progressive occlusion of the central part of the hemifield stimulus field, Blumhardt et al.[21] showed that the hemifield response actually consisted of two different superimposed responses from the stimulated hemisphere (Figure 15-13). The first response generated from the central foveal field was the ipsilateral complex, N75-P100-N145. This complex is seen best over the ipsilateral occipital scalp and is thought to be related to an obliquely oriented dipole generated in the pole and lateral surface of the contralateral occipital lobe where the foveal retina projects. Because of the orientation of the dipole, the P100 component is recorded predominantly over the midline and ipsilateral occipital scalp. The second response is generated on the medial surface of the hemisphere and is best seen contralaterally. It is a P75-N105-P145 complex that is best seen after occlusion of the central 5 degrees of the field and has therefore been referred to as the *paramacular complex*. This complex is likely generated by fibers projecting from the more peripheral parts of the retina. As the central part of the field is occluded, the lateralization becomes more contralateral rather than ipsilateral as the paramacular complex becomes predominant. Under normal circumstances, with both central and peripheral stimulation of the retina, the ipsilateral *macular complex* predominates because of the greater magnification factor (i.e., the ratio of cortical surface area to retinal surface area) for central as compared with peripheral retinal regions.

Several nonpathologic subject-related factors can influence the normal distribution of PSVEP parameters. The mean P100 latency increases with age in the adult, with the actual change with age depending on spatial frequency as well as the luminance of the pattern. After the age of 50, both the mean value and the variance of the P100 latency steadily increase with age. The latency of the P100 tends to be shorter and the amplitude larger in women compared with men on average in the 20–50 age range. This difference was not found to be statistically significant if head circumference was taken into account.[22] When the checkerboard pattern presents relatively small check sizes for foveal stimulation, P100 latency increases steadily and the amplitude decreases when the retinal image defocuses because of visual acuity limitations. It is, therefore, important to check visual acuity and to correct for any refractive errors before performing the PSVEP. Patients who wear glasses should wear them for the study. Patients with decreased visual acuity in an eye because of amblyopia can show low-amplitude, delayed PSVEPs.

There is some concern that subjects who do not maintain a focused image of the pattern on the retina can intentionally reduce the amplitude and latency of the P100. If the subject does not look directly at the stimulus or does not accurately accommodate the lens to focus the stimulus, the P100 measures can be affected. If the subject crosses the eyes and focuses on a nearby point, thus defocusing the more distant stimulus pattern, the PSVEP can be significantly reduced and delayed. This is difficult to maintain with monocular stimulation. Simultaneous recording of the PERG can help to check whether the retina is receiving an adequate stimulus in the more difficult cases. Otherwise,

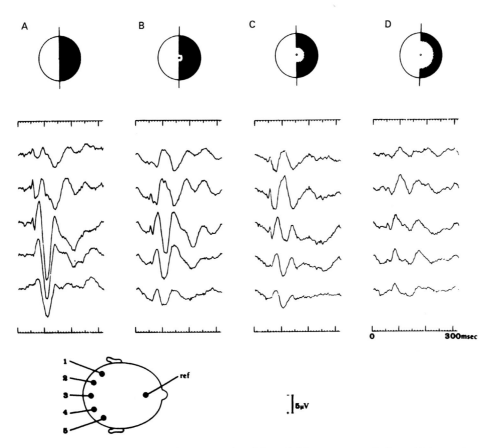

FIGURE 15-13 Pattern-shift visual-evoked potentials associated with hemifield pattern stimulation with increasing central scotomata. **A.** The whole right hemifield is stimulated, and the negative peak at approximately 75 msec, positive peak at approximately 100 msec, and negative peak at approximately 145 msec (N75-P100-N145) complex is shifted toward the right side of the posterior region of the head and is seen best on electrodes 3, 4, and 5. There is also a P75-N105-P135 complex seen over the contralateral occipital region (electrodes 1 and 2). **B, C.** Progressive removal of the central component of the field produces a progressive loss of the ipsilaterally located N75-P100-N145 component. However, there is a relative preservation of the contralaterally located P75-N105-P135 complex. **D.** When the central 10 degrees of the field is removed, the ipsilateral N75-P100-N145 complex is virtually absent, and the contralateral P75-N105-P135 complex is reduced in amplitude. (Reprinted with permission from LD Blumhardt, G Barrett, AM Halliday, A Kriss. The effect of experimental "scotomata" on the ipsilateral and contralateral responses to pattern-reversal in one half-field. Electroencephalogr Clin Neurophysiol 1978;45:376–392.)

careful observation of the patient's behavior during the test along with the use of large stimulus fields and bright, high-contrast checkerboard patterns can help to eliminate this problem. Some of the different clinical applications of the visual EP are listed in Table 15-2. For further discussion of normal vision, see Chapter 12.

PHYSIOLOGY OF THE AUDITORY-EVOKED POTENTIAL

Physiology and Anatomy of Hearing

Mechanical waves of sound pressure are channeled into the external auditory meatus and canal by the external

ear. The pressure waves then travel down the external auditory canal to cause mechanical vibration of the tympanic membrane. The middle ear serves the dual functions of pressure amplification and protection from high-amplitude noise. Lever action of the inner ossicles and a focusing from the area of the tympanic membrane down to the much smaller area of the footplate of the stapes end up concentrating the energy of the mechanical oscillation that converges on the base of the cochlea. Sound protection occurs through a damping mechanism enacted by the muscles (e.g., stapedius) of the middle ear, which are reflexively activated by a sound intensity of greater than 40–50 dB. The cochlea is a round tube that wraps into a spiral of two and a half turns. The circular cross-section of the cochlea is divided into three

TABLE 15-2
Clinical Applications of the Visual-Evoked Potential

Diagnosis in adults
  Optic neuritis
  Multiple sclerosis
  Pseudotumor cerebri
  Tumors (e.g., meningiomas, craniopharyngiomas, chiasmal gliomas)
  Brain trauma
  Parkinsonism
  Spinocerebellar degeneration
  Vitamin deficiencies
  Cortical blindness
  Loss of vision associated with conversion disorder
  Malingering
  Coma assessment
  Optic neuropathy or atrophy
Special applications in pediatrics
  Estimation of visual acuity
  Amblyopia evaluation
  Neonatal asphyxia
  Neurodegenerative diseases
  Hydrocephalus
  Monitoring of neurotoxic effects of medication (e.g., desferrioxamine)
  Congenital malformations
Other applications
  Intraoperative monitoring (e.g., during pituitary tumor excision)

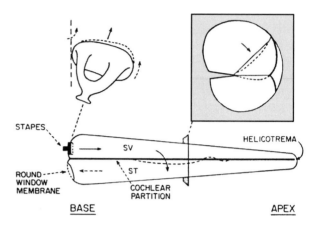

FIGURE 15-14 The generation of pressure gradients in the cochlear tube. The cochlea is drawn uncoiled. Inward movements of the stapes against the oval window cause compensatory outward movements of the round window. With static pressure changes and low-frequency changes, the fluid pressure is transmitted via the helicotrema. For higher frequency pressure changes produced by audible mechanical oscillation, the cochlear partition (the scala media) is displaced in different locations for different frequencies along its length as indicated by the dotted line. (ST = scala tympani; SV = scala vestibuli.) (Reprinted with permission from HD Patton, AF Fuchs, B Hille, et al. Textbook of Physiology [21st ed]. Philadelphia: Saunders, 1989;373.)

fluid-filled compartments by two membranes that run the length of the cochlea. The uppermost compartment is called the *scala vestibuli* and contains perilymph, a fluid similar to CSF. At the basal end of the cochlea, the scala vestibuli opens into a space called the *vestibule*, whose fluid is mechanically vibrated by motion of the stapes footplate against the oval window. The lowermost of the three intracochlear compartments, the scala tympani, also contains perilymph and terminates at the basal end of the cochlea in a membranous section called the *round window*, which is in contact with the air of the middle ear. The middle compartment, the scala media or membranous cochlea, is separated from the other two by two membranes: the basilar membrane below, and Reissner's membrane above. The scala media contains a fluid called *endolymph* that is high in potassium and low in sodium ions (similar to intracellular fluid) and has a high positive potential compared with the perilymph. Sitting on the basilar membrane along the entire length of the cochlea is the organ of Corti, which contains the specialized auditory neuroepi-

thelium. This organ contains the specialized receptor cells and their supporting structures that transduce the mechanical disturbances of the cochlear fluids into electrical signals. The organ of Corti has three rows of outer hair cells and a single row of inner hair cells. The inner hair cells and the outer hair cells are divided by two fibrous structures that come up from the basilar membrane angling toward each other and then fusing together below the tectorial membrane. These are called the *rods of Corti*. The hair cells contact the tectorial membrane, an auxiliary membrane that projects into the scala media above the basilar membrane. Movement of the footplate of the stapes inward against the oval window by a condensation pressure wave against the tympanic membrane moves the base of the basilar membrane inferiorly in the direction of the scala tympani. The pressure wave travels along the length of the cochlea via the perilymph and produces a compensatory outward movement of the round window (Figure 15-14). When the footplate is pulled outward by a rarefaction pressure wave, the basilar membrane is pulled upward toward the scala vestibuli. The frequency of vibration sets up a traveling wave in the basilar membrane and also in the entire organ of Corti sitting on the basilar membrane. The amplitude of this wave increases until it reaches a maximum at the site of optimal frequency activation. Beyond that point, the amplitude decreases. The highest frequencies have their point of maximal amplitude of basilar membrane oscillation near the area of the oval window at the cochlear base. The lowest frequencies set up traveling waves with maxima in the basilar membrane toward the apex of the cochlea. This is because of progressive changes in the mechanical properties of the basilar membrane along its length. The stiffness of the basilar membrane changes by 100-fold, progressively decreasing from the base to the apex of the cochlea. The basilar membrane at the base is narrow and thick and progressively widens and thins along its length toward the apex. This creates a *place code* for frequency representation along the length of the cochlea. Wide-band stimuli, such as an auditory click most often used in BAEPs, produce broad activation along the length of the basilar membrane. The cochlea thus acts as a spectrum analyzer that separates out the different frequencies that make up a complex sound and each different frequency is represented at a different point along the length of the basilar membrane.

The vibration of the basilar membrane sets up a shearing motion between the tectorial membrane and the cilia of the hair cells that activates the hair cells. The stereocilia of the hair cells progress from the shortest at the inner edge of the cell to the tallest at the outer edge. Deflection of the stereocilia of the hair cell from the shortest toward the tallest causes an opening of nonselective cationic channels in the tips of the cilia. This leads to an influx of potassium ions from the endolymph into the hair cell. This depolarizes the cell and causes calcium-mediated release of neurotransmitter (most likely glutamate) from the base of the hair cell, which sets up action potentials in the attached ending of the afferent cochlear nerve fibers. When the stereocilia are deflected in the opposite direction from the tallest toward the shortest, the process is reversed and the cell hyperpolarizes with a relative inhibition of action potentials in the afferent cochlear fibers. As noted previously, there are both inner hair cells and outer hair cells that contact the tectorial membrane. The inner hair cells appear to be responsive to the vibration of the basilar membrane, leading to activation of the afferent fibers of the cochlear nerve whose cell bodies are located in the spiral ganglion that wraps around the cochlea. The outer hair cells appear to be motile and receive input from a smaller number of efferent fibers in the cochlear nerve. The more numerous outer hair cells may be responsible for the dynamic tuning of the receptive mechanism of the cochlea through

an important but poorly understood efferent control system. The nested structure of the auditory mechanism is illustrated in Figure 15-15.

The cochlear nerve then enters the internal auditory meatus and travels through the temporal bone. It then exits from the internal auditory meatus and travels to the brain stem. The cochlear nerve enters the brain stem at the pontomedullary junction where it terminates in the dorsal and ventral cochlear nuclei. Outflow from these input sensory nuclei then travels by way of the trapezoid body to the bilateral superior olivary nuclei. The superior olive then sends output that joins crossed and uncrossed fibers from the cochlear nuclei to form the lateral lemniscus. The lateral lemniscus ascends to the inferior colliculus. The inferior colliculus is a major integrating center for the auditory system and for sound localization in space. Output from the inferior colliculus projects to the medial geniculate body of the thalamus, the thalamic relay nucleus for auditory perception. The medial geniculate sends output to the primary auditory cortex. Tonotopic organization in the projection pattern is maintained throughout the auditory system. The structure of the central auditory pathways is shown in Figure 15-16.

There are four major EPs that have been recorded across different latency ranges after an auditory stimulus: the electrocochleogram (ECochG), the BAEP, the middle-latency auditory EP (MLAEP), and the long-latency auditory EP (LLAEP). In addition, several of the cognitive event-related potentials also incorporate auditory stimuli. These are identified across different time windows after the auditory stimulus and are associated with different aspects of the CNS response to auditory stimulation (Figure 15-17).

Physiology of Electrocochleography

ECochG is the recording of a potential generated by the cochlea and the eighth cranial nerve fibers in the cochlear nerve produced by auditory stimulation. It is best recorded by placing a fine-wire electrode through the tympanic membrane so it lies against the promontory. This is the transtympanic recording technique. The ECochG can also be recorded using an extratympanic technique with placement of an electrode in the external auditory meatus. Extratympanic recording has a lower signal-to-noise ratio than the transtympanic approach. However, this can usually be overcome by averaging more sweeps together. The use of the extratympanic recording technique can also be used to enhance wave I of the BAEP when this component is difficult to identify.

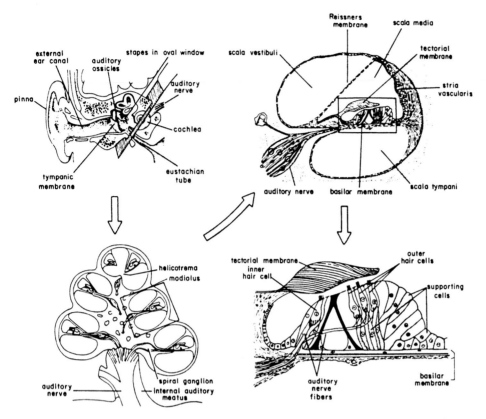

FIGURE 15-15 The nested anatomy of the auditory mechanism. (*Top left*) Overall structure of the outer, middle, and inner ear. (*Bottom left*) Cross-section through the cochlea. (*Top right*) Blowup of a cross-section of the cochlear tube. Note the division of the tube into three sections: the scala vestibuli, the scala media, and the scala tympani. (*Bottom right*) Close-up view of the organ of Corti positioned on the basilar membrane. (Reprinted with permission from G Adelman. Encyclopedia of Neuroscience. Boston: Birkhauser, 1987;90.)

Three different components of the response can be separated by different types of stimulation, stimulus polarities, and the following rates. These are the cochlear microphonic potential, the summating potential, and the compound action potential (Figure 15-18). Each of these components of the ECochG measure activation of the hair cells of the cochlea. The hair cells of the cochlea are the main transducers of the mechanical stimulation of the basilar membrane of the cochlea. The hair cells transform the vibration of the basilar membrane into an electrical waveform transmitted through the auditory division of the eighth cranial nerve. The cochlear microphonic potential is the direct response of the hair cells to a sinusoidal driving stimulus. It is probably produced by the more numerous outer hair cells. The summating potential results from the fact that the basilar membrane has a greater amplitude of oscillation at the scala tympani as compared with the scala vestibuli. It is a stimulus-related slow potential produced by a tone burst stimulus. The compound action potential is the summation of multiple cochlear neurons firing together in response to a click stimulus. It has a sequence of three negative components, N1, N2, and N3, separated by approximately 1 msec. The N1 component of the ECochG corresponds to wave I of the BAEP. The structure and latency of the components of the action potential vary systematically with decreasing click intensity and appear to reflect the response of different populations of hair cells of the middle and basal turns of the cochlea, because the traveling wave moves more quickly along the stiffer basilar membrane at this end of the cochlea, creating greater synchronization of hair cell activation. The ECochG is resistant to the effects of sedatives and anesthetics, but can be abnormal in any condition that produces hair cell or end-organ damage through an ototoxic process.

Physiology of the Brain Stem Auditory-Evoked Potential

In the first 10 msec after the monaural application of a broad-band acoustic stimulus, there is a sequence of waves that can be recorded from the scalp that reflect the sequential activation of different structures in the auditory pathway from the cochlear nerve through the pontine and midbrain elements of the pathway reviewed previously. The waves are far-field potentials that are volume conducted to wide regions of the scalp. This is called the *brain stem auditory-evoked potential*. The signal is robust and resistant to changes

FIGURE 15-16 Auditory pathways in the brain. The pathway is depicted schematically here. The hair cells in the organ of Corti, which transduce the mechanical vibrations of the basilar membrane of the cochlea into neural signals, are connected by a chain of neurons through the brain stem to the medial geniculate body of the thalamus and through to primary auditory cortex of the temporal lobes. (Reprinted with permission from BR Mackenna, R Callander. Illustrated Physiology [6th ed]. Edinburgh: Churchill Livingstone, 1997.)

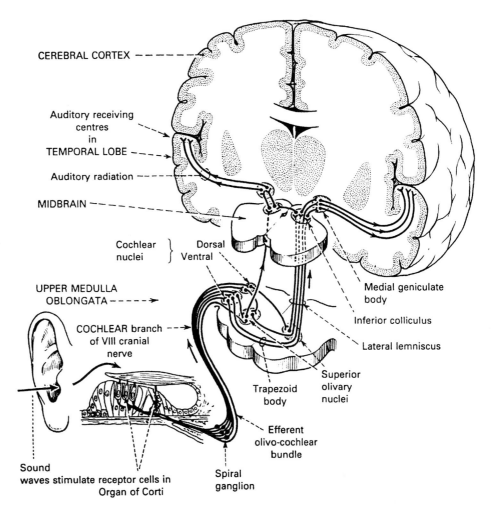

CEREBRAL CORTEX

Auditory receiving centres in TEMPORAL LOBE

Auditory radiation

MIDBRAIN

Cochlear nuclei } Dorsal Ventral

Medial geniculate body

Inferior colliculus

Lateral lemniscus

UPPER MEDULLA OBLONGATA

COCHLEAR branch of VIII cranial nerve

Superior olivary nuclei

Trapezoid body

Efferent olivo-cochlear bundle

Sound waves stimulate receptor cells in Organ of Corti

Spiral ganglion

in conscious state as well as to a variety of sedatives and anesthetics. In addition, there appears to be a relatively reliable correlation between specific components of the response and different elements in the brain stem auditory pathway, giving the study some structural specificity. In fact, there may be a more complex relationship between the different components of the response and the different generators in the pathway.

The recording is typically obtained between the vertex (Cz) and the ipsilateral earlobe (Ai). Additional recordings can be obtained between the contralateral earlobe (Ac) and Ai, and the vertex and Ac. It is displayed so that a vertex positivity is shown as an upward deflection. The sequence of positive components are labeled with Roman numerals following the convention established by Jewett et al.[23] (Figure 15-19).

The first wave in the sequence is wave I and is identified clearly in the Cz-Ai recording. It is also seen in the Ac-Ai recording, but is attenuated or absent in the Cz-Ac recording. The cochlear microphonic may be seen as a series of small waves preceding wave I. The cochlear microphonic reverses polarity when the polarity of the click is changed, but wave I does not reverse polarity although its latency may shift somewhat. A bifid wave I is sometimes present and indicates activation from different parts of the cochlea as do the N1 and N2 components of the ECochG. Wave II is the first clear positive wave seen in the Cz-Ac recording. Wave II may be small or difficult to identify in some healthy subjects. A significant wave III component is identified in the Cz-Ai recording and in the Ac-Ai recording, but may be somewhat small in the Cz-Ac recording. A bifid wave III can sometimes be seen. Waves IV and V are often seen as separate peaks in a single component. This IV/V complex is usually the most prominent component and is often followed by a significant negative trough called the VN component. Wave IV and V can sometimes be more clearly distinguished in the Cz-Ac recording. A reduction in stimulus intensity can also help to reduce the wave IV component and leave the wave V compo-

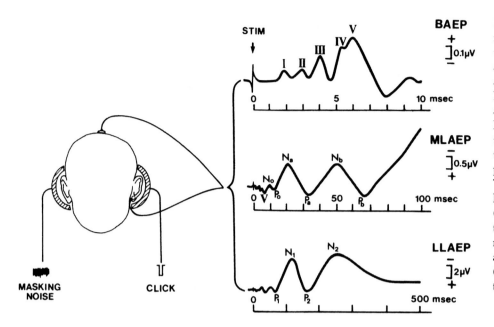

FIGURE 15-17 Basic setup for recording auditory-evoked potentials. The earlobe electrodes (A_1 and A_2) serve as reference sites for an active site at the vertex (C_z). Different components of the overall response to the auditory stimulus are demonstrated on different time bases. The earliest response is the brain stem auditory-evoked potential (BAEP) on the top trace. The next response is the middle-latency auditory-evoked potential (MLAEP) shown on the middle trace. The longest latency components are seen in the long-latency auditory-evoked potential (LLAEP) shown in the bottom trace.

nent intact and isolated. The wave V component is the least sensitive to reductions in stimulus intensity.

The key measures are obtained from the I, III, and V peaks. Absolute latencies are computed, and interpeak latencies between I–III, III–V, and I–V are computed. The left and the right ears are tested separately with monaural stimulation. Masking noise is used on the contralateral ear to prevent contribution from this ear through bone conduction of the stimulus. The interpeak latencies can also be compared between the two sides. The latency of wave I is sometimes called the *peripheral transit time*, whereas the I–V interpeak latency is

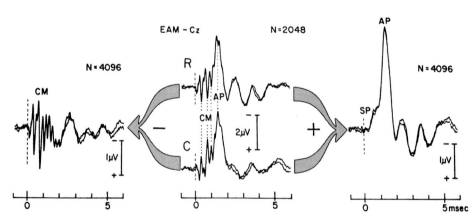

FIGURE 15-18 The components of the electrocochleogram. The electrocochleogram produced exclusively by rarefaction (*middle section, above*) or condensation (*middle section, below*) clicks are composites of the cochlear microphonic (CM), summating potential (SP), and compound action potential (AP). The cochlear microphonic reverses polarity (*dotted lines in middle section*), whereas the summating potential and the AP do not, between rarefaction (R) and condensation (C) clicks. Thus, when the two waveforms in the middle trace are algebraically subtracted (*waveform on the left*), the AP and the summating potential are canceled out and the cochlear microphonic is summated and remains. When the two waveforms (R and C) are algebraically added (*waveform on the right*) the cochlear microphonic is canceled and the AP and the summating potential are summated and appear clearly defined in the waveform. (EAM = external auditory meatus.) (Reprinted with permission from GE Chatrian, AL Wirch, E Lettich, et al. Click-evoked human electrocochleogram. Non-invasive recording method, origin and physiologic significance. Am J EEG Tech 1982;22:151–174.)

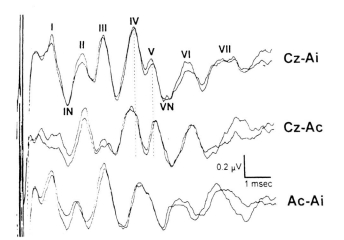

FIGURE 15-19 Brain stem auditory-evoked potentials recorded with three different channels after monaural stimulation. In the top trace, the vertex site (Cz) is linked to the earlobe ipsilateral to the stimulation (Ai). In the middle trace, Cz is linked to the earlobe contralateral to the side stimulated (Ac). In the bottom trace, the two earlobes are linked. Note the separation of the wave IV and V components in the middle trace and the decreased amplitude of wave III in this trace compared with the top trace. Wave III is clearly seen in the bottom trace. (Reprinted with permission from MJ Aminoff [ed]. Electrodiagnosis in Clinical Neurology [4th ed]. New York: Churchill Livingstone, 1999;456.)

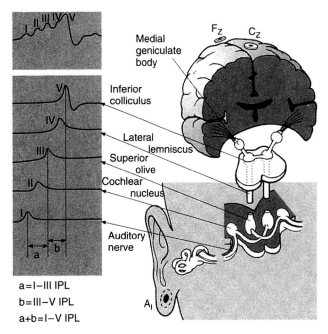

a=I–III IPL
b=III–V IPL
a+b=I–V IPL

FIGURE 15-20 Source generation of the brain stem auditory-evoked potential (BAEP). Note the origin of wave I from the auditory nerve, wave II from the cochlear nucleus, wave III from the superior olive, wave IV from the lateral lemniscus, and wave V from the superior colliculus. For more detailed discussion of specific source relationships, see text. Wave VI may be generated from the medial geniculate nucleus of the thalamus. The BAEP is recorded from the vertex (C_z) with respect to the ipsilateral earlobe (A_i). A ground electrode is placed at the midfrontal site (F_z). (IPL = interpeak latency.) (Reprinted with permission from M Grabois, S Garrison, K Hart, et al [eds]. Physical Medicine and Rehabilitation. The Complete Approach. Malden, MA: Blackwell Science, 2000;205.)

referred to as the *brain stem transit time* or *central auditory transit time*. The amplitude of the wave I component is usually significantly smaller than the amplitude of the wave V component. The ratio of wave I to wave V amplitude can be used as a measure of abnormality. A I/V ratio of greater than 200% is generally considered to be abnormal and indicates an impairment of transmission to the midbrain level.

We now discuss the specific physiological generators of each of the major components of the BAEP. The generation of the BAEP is illustrated schematically in Figure 15-20. Wave I has a latency that is similar to the action potential or N1 of the ECochG and most likely comes from a peripheral segment of the cochlear nerve. It is preserved in isolation in patients with severe deterioration of brain stem function who are thought to be brain dead. It is not recordable in situations in which the cochlea, cochlear nerve, or both are significantly damaged (e.g., when the eighth cranial nerve is infarcted). The negative trough after wave I, the IN component, is generated at the point at which the cochlear nerve emerges from the internal auditory meatus, exiting from a bony canal into a CSF-filled space. Wave II probably reflects activation from the proximal part of the

cochlear nerve, corresponding to N2 of the ECochG, as well as activation of the cochlear nuclei. Wave III is a fairly robust component that is used, along with waves I and V, to compute interpeak latencies. It is probably generated by a horizontal dipole positioned at the level of the trapezoid body or the superior olivary complex in the lower pons. It likely has multiple generators contributing to its formation at this level. Wave IV has generators in the midpons to rostral pons with generators that overlap with but are not identical to those of wave V. It is related to caudal-to-rostral conduction of action potentials in the brain stem auditory pathways at this level and is thus related to transmission in the lateral lemniscus. Lesions involving tissue at the midpons, rostral pons, and mesencephalic levels produce abnormalities of waves IV and V. Wave V reflects the activation of a vertically oriented dipole at the level of the midbrain. It is most likely generated by a combination of

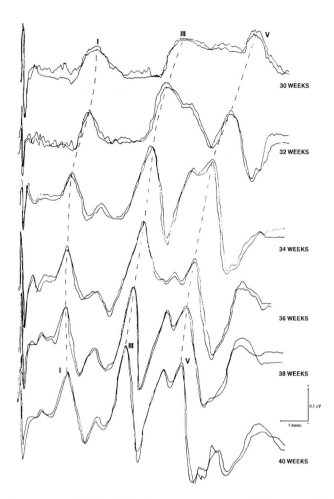

30 WEEKS

32 WEEKS

34 WEEKS

36 WEEKS

38 WEEKS

40 WEEKS

0.1 µV

1 msec

FIGURE 15-21 Serial brain stem auditory-evoked potential studies in an individual preterm infant from 30 through 40 weeks' gestational age. Note the steady decrease in latency and increase in amplitude and definition of the major waves of the response (I, III, and V). (Reprinted with permission from E Niedermeyer, F Lopes Da Silva. Electroencephalography: Basic Principles, Clinical Applications, and Related Fields [4th ed]. Philadelphia: Lippincott Williams & Wilkins, 1998;979.)

action potentials conducted in the lateral lemniscus and postsynaptic potentials generated in the inferior colliculus. Intracranial recordings demonstrate that the wave V component has the largest amplitude adjacent to the inferior colliculus contralateral to the stimulated ear. The large trough after the V component, VN, is also likely related to postsynaptic potentials generated in the inferior colliculus. Waves VI and VII can be identified in the majority of subjects examined but are not easily reproducible. They are generally not used for clinical measurement, and their origin remains unclear.

A number of subject-related factors can influence the BAEP measures. In infants, the first detectable wave is wave I. At birth, waves I, III, and V can usually be identified but the peak latencies and interpeak latencies are normally quite prolonged and the amplitudes decreased compared with adult values, especially in premature infants (Figure 15-21). Initially, the wave I amplitude is noted to be greater than the wave V amplitude, which is the opposite of what is seen in adults. The general structure of the adult BAEP can be identified by 6 months of age. The adult values for interpeak latencies are not reached until 1–3 years of age. There is no significant increase in interpeak latencies noted in adult years. Overall, BAEP component latencies are slightly shorter in female subjects compared with male subjects by approximately 0.1–0.2 msec. This effect is generally washed out when male and female subjects are evenly mixed in normal control groups.

One of the most difficult problems encountered in recording the BAEP is EMG artifact. The reflex response of the postauricular muscle can be problematic at times when it occurs with a latency of less than 10 msec. This reflex amplitude can be significantly reduced by recording from the earlobe rather than the mastoid process.

The great advantage of the BAEP is that it is highly robust and stable. It is generally not changed when the subject is drowsy or sleeping. Little alteration is noted during sleep in the structure of the BAEP. Even during anesthesia or with high doses of barbiturates, the BAEPs are generally stable. Any changes noted can usually be explained by changes in core body temperature. Some of the clinical applications of the BAEP are listed in Table 15-3.

A number of stimulus-related technical factors can affect the recording of the BAEP. There is generally an inverse relationship between wave latency and stimulus intensity. Decreasing click intensity is also associated with progressive changes in BAEP morphology. This is shown in Figure 15-22. Wave V is the most robust component and can be generally identified close to subjective hearing threshold. This feature of the wave V component makes it possible to perform objective testing of hearing threshold by plotting the wave V latency as a function of click intensity. This is the basis of *objective audiometry*. Waves I, II, and IV tend to drop out first with decreasing click intensity and then wave III. The interpeak latencies are relatively unaffected by decreasing click intensities because the latencies of each of the waves shifts outward by approximately the same amount. This makes the interpeak latencies much more stable and reliable measures than the absolute component latencies.

The normal increase in wave V latency and its normal persistence close to hearing threshold can be used to assess auditory acuity. The technique involves monaural stimulation with an *intensity series*. This is a sequence of BAEP studies in which the click intensity is gradually reduced down toward normal hearing threshold levels. When this is done, the wave V latency can be plotted against the click intensity to produce a graph. This plot should lie within a normal region of the graph. If the whole plot is shifted up out of the normal region, but lies generally in parallel with the normal plot so that there is a constant proportionate prolongation of wave V latency at each level of stimulus intensity, a conductive hearing impairment should be suspected. On the other hand, if wave V latency is relatively normal at high stimulus intensities but increases more rapidly than normal with decreasing click intensity, a sensorineural hearing loss caused by cochlear impairment should be suspected (Figure 15-23). This technique is called *evoked response audiometry* or *objective audiometry*. The limitation of the technique is that tone-selective hearing impairment is less readily detected because broad-band click stimulation is used. Techniques have been described to estimate tone responses to clicks by adding filtered masking noise to the click stimulus and evaluating how adding masking noise with different frequency content alters the structure of the wave V component.[24]

The rate of stimulation for neuro-otologic investigation is usually approximately 10–12 clicks per second. However, the BAEP structure stays relatively stable up to rates as high as 30 per second. For this reason, a rate of 31.1 clicks per second can be used to perform evoked response audiometry in order to decrease the time involved in performing the study. Above stimulus rates of approximately 40 per second, the wave V latency begins to gradually increase and the definition of the earlier components of the response decreases.

Physiology of the Middle-Latency Auditory-Evoked Potential

The MLAEP occurs in the range of 10–50 msec after an auditory stimulus. There is a sequence of waves identified that have most often been labeled No, Po, Na, Pa, and Nb (Figure 15-24). There is considerable interindividual variation noted in the structure of the MLAEP, which makes its application more difficult. However, in most subjects, the Na and Pa components can be identified and are thus clinically useful. Initially, because of the overlap in latency with the reflex activation of the postauricular muscle, these waves were thought to be primarily myogenic. However, more recent evidence suggests a significant neurogenic origin with preservation of the components in patients who have been placed under neuromuscular blockade. The distribution

TABLE 15-3
Clinical Applications of the Brain Stem Auditory-Evoked Potential

Diagnosis in adults
  Acoustic neuroma and other cerebellopontine angle tumors
  Multiple sclerosis
  Central pontine myelinolysis
  Leukodystrophy
  Friedreich's ataxia
  Spinocerebellar or brain stem degeneration and inherited ataxias
  Brain stem tumors (e.g., gliomas, pinealoma)
  Brain stem hemorrhage or infarction
  Coma assessment
  Brain death evaluation
  Postconcussion syndrome
  Hearing impairment (investigated with evoked response or *objective* audiometry)
Special applications in pediatrics
  Brain stem gliomas
  Neurodegenerative disorders
  Central nervous system malformations
  Developmental disorders
  Coma assessment
  Hydrocephalus
  Screening for hearing impairment in at-risk neonates (with evoked response audiometry)
  Meningitis
  Monitoring for neurotoxic effects of medications (e.g., aminoglycosides)
Other applications
  Intraoperative monitoring (e.g., posterior fossa and cerebellopontine angle tumor excision)

of the MLAEP on the scalp and its general structure are illustrated in Figure 15-25.

The MLAEP has a sinusoidal structure. When stimulation is applied at a rate of approximately 40 Hz, there is an overlap in sequential generations of the MLAEP that leads to a highly sinusoidal signal because of the superposition of the MLAEPs evoked by each stimulus (Figure 15-26). This response can be readily recorded and has been suggested as a possible objective hearing test.[25] The advantage of the 40-Hz auditory EP is that it can be generated by a wide variety of stimuli including tone bursts at low frequencies and thus can be applied to assess tone-specific impairment. This is less easily addressed with standard evoked response audiometry using the BAEP.

Although there is some controversy regarding the specific origin of each of the components of the MLAEP, there has been general agreement that the Pa component most likely arises in supratemporal primary

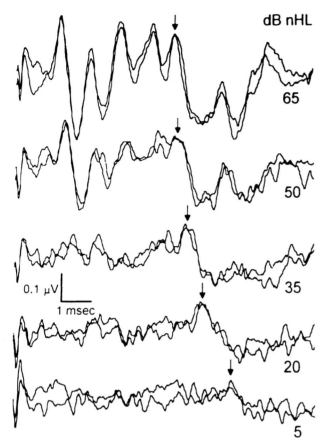

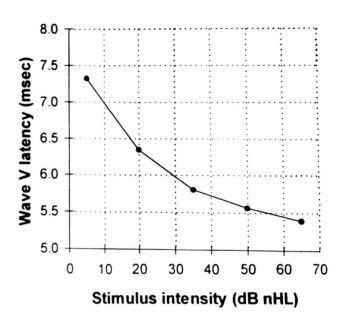

FIGURE 15-22 Brain stem auditory-evoked potentials recorded at progressively lower stimulus intensities are shown in the column on the left. Note the gradual disappearance of all components except for wave V with decreasing click intensity. The wave V latency steadily increases with decreasing click intensity. Wave V latencies can be plotted against stimulus intensity to give the latency-intensity curve on the right side. In a complete study, each ear would be separately tested in a similar fashion. This is a normal study. (Reprinted with permission from MJ Aminoff [ed], Electrodiagnosis in Clinical Neurology [4th ed]. New York: Churchill Livingstone, 1999;460.)

auditory cortex. The Na component appears to come from a subcortical generator because patients with cortical injury affecting the primary auditory cortex lose the Pa component but still have a recordable Na component. For the most part, monaural stimulation is used. Monaural stimulation produces a symmetric pattern on the scalp, suggesting that monaural stimulation activates both hemispheres simultaneously because of crossed and uncrossed pathways. However, in attempts to detect unilateral cortical injury, binaural stimulation can be used to identify the cortical asymmetry.

Physiology of the Long-Latency Auditory-Evoked Potential

At longer latencies after a monaural click or tone pip, there is a large EP consisting of an N100 (or N1) and

P200 (or P2) that is recorded with maximum amplitude at midline frontocentral electrodes. This is the LLAEP. A similar structure of the late vertex-centered response can be seen after both clicks and tone bursts as well as after flash visual stimulation and electrical stimulation (Figure 15-27). These components are quite sensitive to factors such as arousal, cognitive processing, and the effects of drugs. The LLAEP may be abnormal and the BAEP completely normal in patients who have auditory difficulties caused by cortical damage. The LLAEP is best elicited by a loud tone burst with a duration of up to 100 msec. The exact generators of the LLAEP have been difficult to ascertain. There are probably a number of different generators that contribute to the LLAEP. When a coronal montage is used with a nose reference, the N100 potential recorded at the vertex reverses polarity to a P100 component at temporal electrode sites that

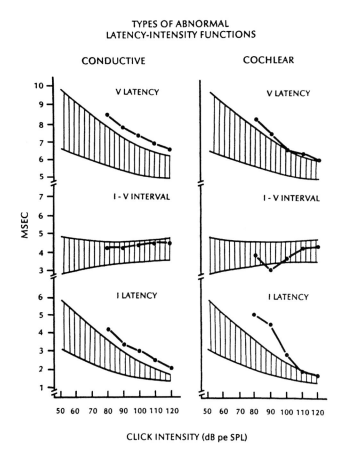

TYPES OF ABNORMAL
LATENCY-INTENSITY FUNCTIONS

CONDUCTIVE   COCHLEAR

CLICK INTENSITY (dB pe SPL)

FIGURE 15-23 Latency-intensity (L-I) curves in objective audiometry for conductive hearing loss (*left*) and cochlear or sensorineural hearing loss (*right*). The hatched areas indicate the bounded areas of normality. Note that the wave V L-I curve is shifted up uniformly for a conductive loss, as is the wave I L-I curve. On the other hand, the wave V and wave I L-I curves are shifted up to a greater degree at lower click intensities than higher click intensities in the presence of a sensorineural impairment. (Reprinted with permission from MJ Aminoff [ed], Electrodiagnosis in Clinical Neurology [4th ed]. New York: Churchill Livingstone, 1999;943.)

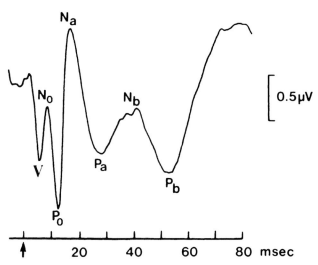

FIGURE 15-24 The middle-latency auditory-evoked potential. This potential is recorded from the vertex (Cz) with reference to the ipsilateral earlobe (A1) using a bandpass filter from 5–500 Hz. The stimulus is at a moderate intensity and may be either a click or a brief tone burst. (Reprinted with permission from R Spehlmann. Evoked Potential Primer. Boston: Butterworth 1985;241.)

are below the sylvian fissure. This suggests that the LLAEP may originate in the primary auditory cortex of each hemisphere.

The LLAEP can be used to obtain estimates of the subject's auditory sensitivity (Figure 15-28). They can also be readily elicited by pure tone stimuli, which makes the assessment of tone-specific auditory impairment more feasible. Low-frequency tone bursts elicit LLAEPs with longer latencies and higher amplitudes than high-frequency tone bursts. The LLAEPs have relatively large-amplitude and low-frequency content and so can be recorded with a limited amplification band-

pass that can help to eliminate various sources of signal artifact and interference. The variability of the response, however, with patient state, makes the reliable use of the LLAEP difficult. In the cooperative adult subject, the LLAEP can be used to assess auditory function. However, it is precisely this type of patient for whom behavioral audiometry can be done with significantly less expense and inconvenience. The LLAEP can be helpful in the adult, however, when one suspects factitious hearing loss that may not be readily detectable with behavioral audiometry. In the neonate or young child, it is not possible to consistently control patient state (e.g., level of arousal), rendering the LLAEP unhelpful for audiometric assessment in these subjects.

Physiology of Cognitive Auditory-Evoked Potentials

Although the variability of the long-latency components of the auditory EP make them difficult to apply clinically, their dependence on subjective state allow them to be employed to examine the active information-processing capacity of the subject. When examined in the context of certain psychophysiological paradigms, these EPs can begin to define a cognitive processing metric that enables an investigation of cognitive capacity. The most extensively studied potential in this class is the

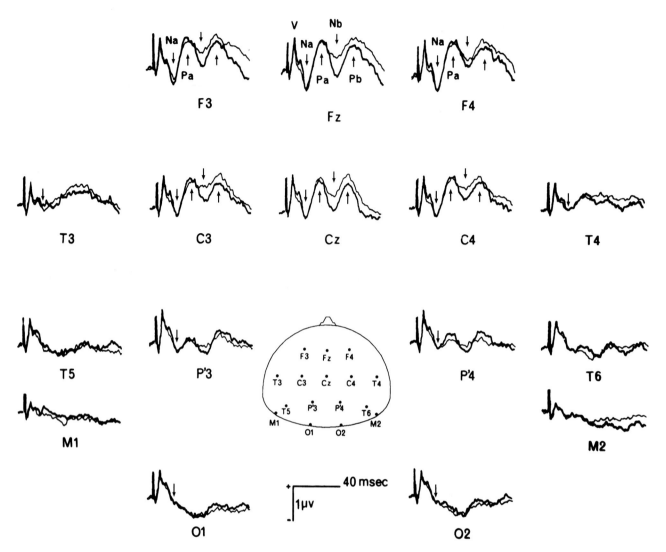

FIGURE 15-25 The scalp distribution of the middle-latency auditory-evoked potential. The middle-latency auditory-evoked potentials were evoked by 100-μsec duration clicks delivered monaurally at an intensity of 80 dB nHL. The thick traces are responses to the right ear and thin traces are the responses to the left ear. A sternovertebral balanced noncephalic reference site was used. The traces are grand averages from nine subjects. No significant lateralization of the scalp distribution according to the stimulated side is noted. (Reprinted with permission from MP Deiber, V Ibañez, C Fischer, et al. Sequential mapping favors the hypothesis of distinct generations for Na and Pa middle latency auditory-evoked potentials. Electroencephalogr Clin Neurophysiol 1998;71:187–197.)

P3, or P300, component. It is elicited by a stimulus that is low probability and to which attention has been directed through an instruction to the subject that makes the stimulus task relevant. Typically, the subject is asked to count the number of rare events in a bivariate sequence. So, for example, a tone of 1.1 kHz occurs with 15% probability randomly interspersed in a train of 1-kHz tones. The auditory EP to the rare *target* tones is separately averaged from the auditory EP to the frequent *nontarget* tones. The subject can be asked to just as easily count the number of stimulus absences in a sequence in which the rare event is the absence of an expected stimulus at that point in time. This would be just as effective in eliciting the P300 component as a rare target stimulus that differed from the frequent nontarget stimulus in some physical characteristic. When a cognitive potential is produced in response to a stimulus absence, this is sometimes referred to as an *emitted* potential.[26] In the response to the frequent stimuli, one sees the typical LLAEP with N100 and P200 components. However, in the response to the rare target stimuli, one sees a large N2 and then a P3 component that

FIGURE 15-26 The process of producing and recording the 40-Hz auditory-evoked potential. **A.** The general setup for recording the response. **B.** (*Top*) The transient middle-latency auditory-evoked potential with vertex-positive shown as a deflection downward. (*Bottom*) A proposed mechanism for the generation of the 40-Hz response, noting that there is significant overlap between the N_a, N_b, and N_c components when the interstimulus interval is 25 msec, corresponding to a stimulation rate of 40 Hz. **C.** The recorded responses to auditory stimuli with increasing click rates. (Reprinted with permission from R Galambos, S Makeig, P Talmachoff. A 40-Hz auditory potential recorded from the human scalp. Proc Natl Acad Sci U S A 1981;78:2643–2647.)

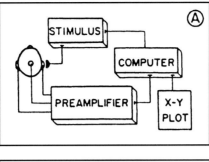

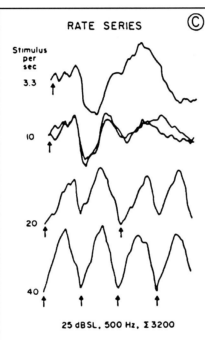

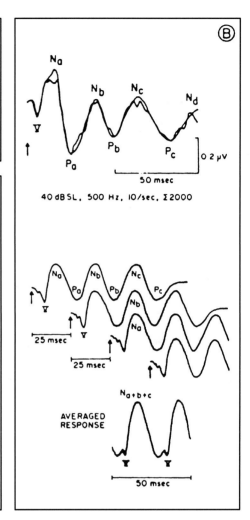

was not present at all in the response to the frequent stimuli (Figure 15-29). A similar structure in which a large positive potential is seen in response to a rare target stimulus can be produced with visual and somatosensory stimulation as well as auditory stimulation (Figure 15-30). The P3 seems to reflect the process of recognizing the rare target stimulus and extracting task-relevant information contained in this stimulus. This study has been applied to evaluate populations with cognitive deficiency and memory loss such as those with progressive dementia[27] or traumatic brain injury.[28,29] Generally, it has been found that cognitive impairment is associated with a P300 with increased latency and decreased amplitude compared with age-matched controls. Unfortunately, measurement of the P300 has not been able to offer much more to the clinician than does a careful mental status and behavioral assessment of the patient, although it does provide a measurable quantitative assessment of change over time. Changes in P300

latency and amplitude are also relatively nonspecific with regard to the underlying disorder so that abnormalities can be seen in progressive dementia, acquired brain disorders such as traumatic brain injury, and in psychiatric conditions such as schizophrenia.

Other cognitive auditory EPs include the contingent negative variation (CNV) and the mismatch negativity (MMN). The CNV is a slow negative potential that develops during the delay between a warning stimulus that prepares the subject for a forthcoming voluntary act (e.g., "Get set!") and the imperative stimulus that signals the performance of the act (e.g., "Go!"). The CNV begins approximately 400 msec after the warning stimulus has occurred and continues until the imperative stimulus occurs. In the original paradigm, described by Walter et al.,[30] the warning stimulus was an auditory tone and the imperative stimulus was the start of stroboscopic pulses of light that could be extinguished by the subject by pushing a button. Thus, the CNV devel-

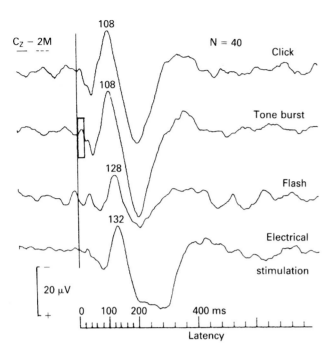

FIGURE 15-27 Long-latency responses to auditory, visual, and somatosensory stimulation. With each modality of stimulation, there is a major negative component with a latency of 108–132 msec followed by a major well-defined positive component with a latency of approximately 200 msec to auditory stimulation. For somatosensory stimulation, the P2 component has a longer latency and is wider. For all recordings, the active electrode is at the vertex (C$_z$) with reference to linked mastoids. The flash and somatosensory responses have somewhat longer latencies than the auditory responses, most likely related to peripheral transduction and conduction delays.

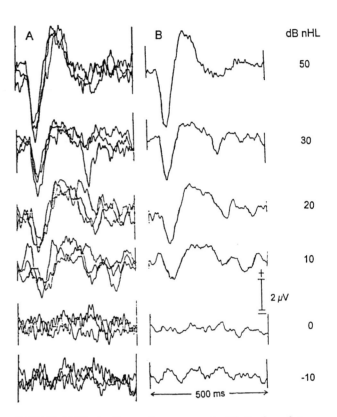

FIGURE 15-28 Audiometric assessment with the long-latency auditory-evoked potential. These are responses to 1,000 Hz tone bursts (10 msec rise and fall times; 10 msec plateau) presented at a rate of 1 Hz. Recording filter passband: 1–70 Hz. **A.** Three replications of 90 trials each with decreasing stimulus intensity from 50 dB nHL down to –10 dB nHL. **B.** Composite averages of the three replications. The tone bursts were reported by the normal-hearing subject to be audible at 10 dB nHL but not at 0 dB nHL and –10 db nHL. (Reprinted with permission from R Goldstein, WM Aldrich. Evoked Potential Audiometry: Fundamentals and Applications. Needham, MA: Allyn & Bacon, 1998;88.)

oped as the subject was expecting the subsequent noxious imperative stimulus to occur and was preparing to perform the motor task as quickly as possible after the beginning of the imperative stimulus in order to limit its noxious effect (Figure 15-31). Because a fixed time interval was set between the warning and the imperative stimulus in a repetitive paradigm, it was possible to anticipate approximately when the imperative stimulus would begin. With longer interstimulus intervals, the CNV appears to have at least two different components: a frontally predominant O-wave or *orientation* component that is a brief negative wave that occurs after the warning stimulus and is presumably related to the recognition of the task-relevant signaling aspect of this stimulus, and a centrally predominant E-wave or *expectancy* component that is a slowly building negativity that precedes and anticipates the occurrence of the imperative stimulus. The origins of these different com-

ponents of the CNV remain somewhat unclear. There is some controversy regarding the degree to which the E-wave is directly linked to the movement-related cortical potential (MRCP; see Physiology of the Movement-Related Cortical Potential and the Motor-Evoked Potential, later in this chapter) versus a separate process associated with task-relevant stimulus contingency and a stimulus-determined preparatory process.

The MMN is a negative component at approximately 200 msec that is elicited by infrequent, physically deviant stimuli buried in a repetitive auditory stimulus sequence with relatively short interstimulus intervals (Figure 15-32). The stimulus paradigm is similar to that which is set up to produce the P300 component, except that the subject is not given any instruction regarding

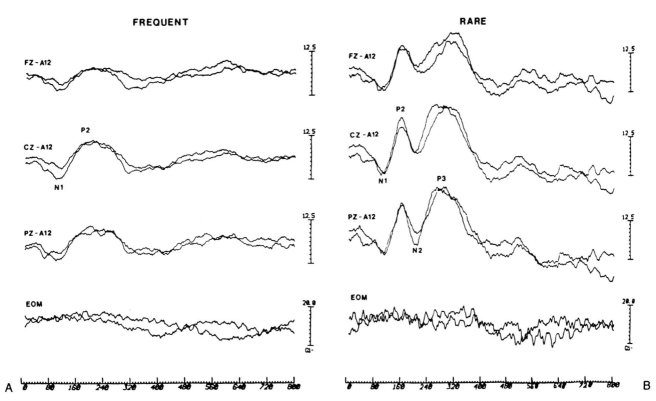

FIGURE 15-29 Long-latency auditory-evoked potentials recorded in a normal subject to frequent 1,000-Hz tone bursts in **A**, on the left side of figure, and to rare 2,000-Hz tone bursts in **B**, on the right side of the figure. The subject was instructed to raise her index finger whenever a rare tone occurred. Three scalp-recorded channels are shown, all with a linked-ear reference. The fourth channel is an eye movement channel to rule out eye movement artifacts. Two replications of the study are shown with traces superimposed. Each trial consisted of a total of 100 tones, 16% of which were rare tones and 84% of which were frequent tones. (Reprinted with permission from KH Chiappa. Evoked Potentials in Clinical Medicine [3rd ed]. Philadelphia: Lippincott–Raven, 1997;531.)

the relevance of the stimuli. It can be recorded in response to any particular discriminating change in physical stimulus properties. It can be seen best when the subject is asked to ignore all the stimuli usually by reading an interesting book. The MMN is thus elicited in a passive context in which there is no conscious effort being made to actively process or differentiate the stimuli. It is thought to be a reflection of a preattentive automatic process that rapidly identifies differences between stimuli or ongoing stimulus change in a rapid stimulus sequence through a process of comparing the most recent stimulus to an internal memory trace that has been built up through the repetition of previous recurrent stimuli.[31,32] The topography of the MMN suggests that it is modality specific and involves participation of both primary and secondary sensory cortical zones. For the auditory modality, the MMN appears to be generated in the supratemporal auditory cortex. Later negative components that generally precede the P300 can be

seen when changes in the physical properties of the stimulus reveal task-relevant information to which the subject is consciously attending. The MMN is dependent primarily on specific physical changes to the stimulus rather than task-related factors such as directed attention or stimulus categorization difficulty. On the other hand, later negative components and the subsequent P300 that reflect active stimulus processing are more dependent on task-specific factors than on differences in the physical properties of the stimuli. The MMN is particularly helpful in determining whether the mechanism that supports preattentive processing of physically deviant stimuli remains intact and functional. It has been applied in a number of clinical contexts including the assessment of language development, the evaluation of patients in coma, and examination of aphasic subjects.[33] It can be used to assess this aspect of cognitive processing under passive conditions and is therefore not dependent on a cooperative and participa-

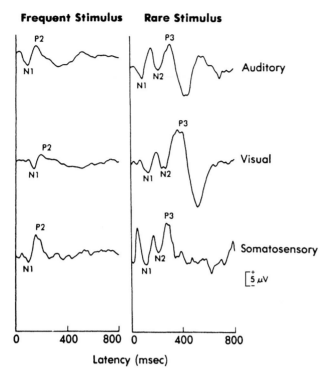

FIGURE 15-30 Long-latency evoked potentials elicited by auditory (*top row*), visual (*middle row*), and somatosensory (*bottom row*) stimuli in which sequences of two types of stimuli within the modality were applied with separate averaging to the two types of stimuli. One stimulus of the two was designated as a *frequent nontarget stimulus*, and the second stimulus of the two was designated as a *rare target stimulus*. The responses to the frequent nontarget stimuli in each modality are shown on the left, and the responses to the rare target stimuli are shown on the right. In each case (as seen in Figure 15-27), the frequent nontarget stimuli elicited a negative (N1)-positive (P2) biphasic response. The rare target stimuli, in addition, elicited a P3 or P300 component. (Reprinted with permission from MJ Aminoff [ed]. Electrodiagnosis in Clinical Neurology [4th ed]. New York: Churchill Livingstone, 1999;571.)

tory subject. For this reason, it can be applied to analyze this cognitive function in young children, as well as unresponsive or aphasic adults.

PHYSIOLOGY OF THE SOMATOSENSORY-EVOKED POTENTIAL

Physiology and Anatomy of the Somatosensory-Evoked Potential

The somatosensory system employs a *labeled-line* approach to conducting a variety of different modali-

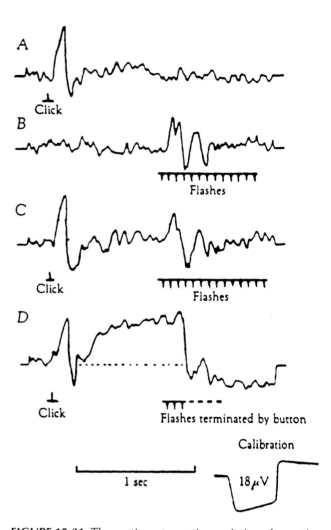

FIGURE 15-31 The contingent negative variation. A negative deflection is shown going upward. **A.** An auditory-evoked potential to a click by itself. **B.** A visual-evoked potential to the onset of a fixed sequence of flashes. **C.** A combination of an auditory-evoked potential to the initial click and a visual-evoked potential to a fixed sequence of visual flashes (the subject is passive). There is a fixed 1-second interval between the click and the flashes. **D.** The subject is given a button that he or she is instructed to press to terminate the sequence of visual flashes. Now a slow increase in negative potential is noted in the interval between the auditory click (the warning stimulus) and the initiation of the visual flashes (the imperative stimulus). This large, sustained, intervening negative potential is termed the *contingent negative variation* and is thought to reflect a temporal contingency between the stimuli that allows the subject to anticipate the generation of an action that will happen at a fixed time interval beyond a point referenced to the warning stimulus. (Reprinted with permission from WG Walter, R Cooper, VJ Aldridge, et al. Contingent negative variation: an electric sign of sensory-motor association and expectancy in the human brain. Nature 1964;203:380–384. Copyright Macmillan Magazines Limited.)

FIGURE 15-32 A. The event-related potential elicited by standard (*thin line*) and deviant (*thick line*) sounds at frontal midline (Fz) and right mastoid (Rm) electrodes. During the recording, the subjects were watching a silent movie with subtitles to direct their attention away from the sounds. The sounds were spectrally rich and standard and deviant differed in pitch by 2.5%. The shaded area indicates the mismatch negativity (MMN). The x-axis displays time in milliseconds and the y-axis the amplitude of response in microvolts. **B.** The subtraction wave obtained by subtracting the evoked-related potential elicited by the standard sound from that of the deviant sound. (Data from M Tervaniemi.)

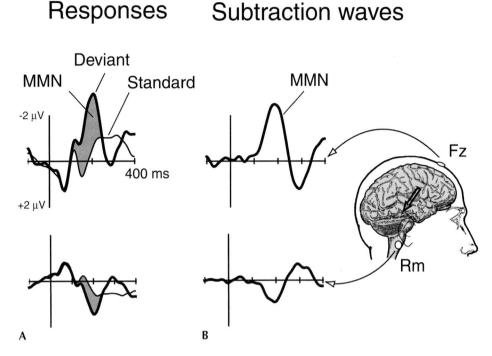

ties of somatic sensation along separate primary afferent fibers with a multitude of different types of specialized receptors. Although it is possible to selectively activate certain classes of somatic receptor with physiological stimulation such as a mechanical tap, skin vibration, joint movement, or somatic pain stimulus, these techniques are technically difficult and are not generally used in the clinical laboratory. Instead, the SEP is most often elicited through the application of a nonphysiological electrical stimulation directly to the skin surface so that the peripheral fibers are depolarized proximal to the sensory receptor. This technique effectively bypasses the peripheral physiological encoding of specific somatosensory information by the receptors. With a submaximal electrical activation of the peripheral nerve, there is selective activation of the low-threshold peripheral fibers that are generally going to be the largest and most heavily myelinated fibers. These fibers are preferentially funneled to the dorsal column lemniscal system. Thus, the typical SEP study selectively examines the large, rapidly conducting afferents that conduct up the dorsal columns and does not evaluate the pain and temperature encoding fibers of the spinothalamic system. In a mixed peripheral nerve, most of the large afferent fibers are muscle afferents from the spindle organs. Large efferent fibers that are primarily alpha motor efferents are also activated, thus producing a brief

muscular twitch. When a cutaneous peripheral nerve is stimulated electrically, the preferentially activated large afferent fibers are mostly conveying discriminative touch and vibration sensation from the skin. In addition to mixed and cutaneous nerves, SEPs have also been recorded with direct electrical stimulation of specific skin regions in a particular dermatome and with stimulation of the motor points from specific muscles.

The anatomy of the dorsal column and lemniscal system is physiologically examined with the SEP. The cell bodies of the primary afferent neurons are in the dorsal root ganglia adjacent to the spinal cord. Their central processes project into the dorsal columns and rostrally to the dorsal column nuclei at the cervicomedullary junction (cuneatus for the upper limb and gracilis for the lower limb fibers). The second-order neurons in the system then project across the midline and up to the somatosensory region of the thalamus in the vicinity of the ventroposterolateral nucleus by way of the medial lemniscus. The third-order neurons in the thalamus then project to the primary somatosensory cortex in the postcentral gyrus area. The anatomy of this system is illustrated in Figure 15-33. The assumption that the SEPs are mediated by this system correlates with the observation that abnormal SEPs are associated with loss of vibration, discriminative touch, and kinesthetic sensation. Additional cor-

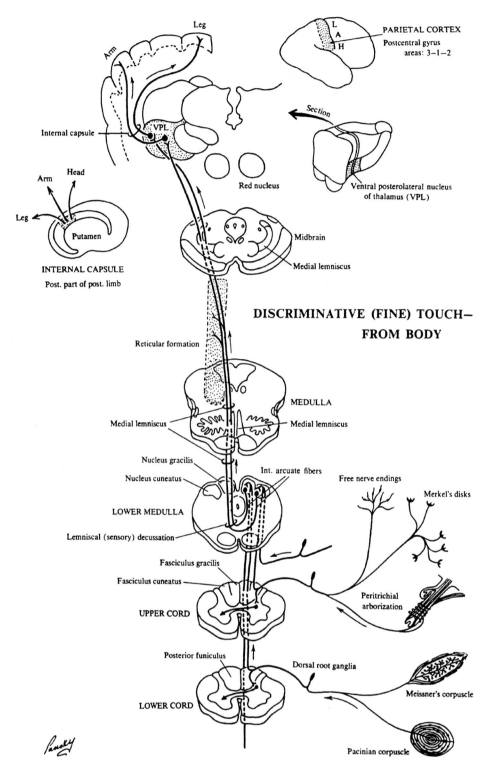

FIGURE 15-33 The dorsal column/lemniscal somatosensory pathway from the periphery to the cortical level. Note the primary afferent neuron is in the dorsal root ganglion, the secondary afferent neuron is in the dorsal column nucleus (gracilis from the leg; cuneatus from the arm), and the tertiary afferent neuron is in the ventroposterolateral (VPL) nucleus of the thalamus. (A = arm; H = head; L = leg.) (Reprinted with permission from B Pansky, DJ Allen. Review of Neuroscience. New York: Macmillan, 1980;177.)

related observations include loss of SEPs after selective destruction of the dorsal columns in subhuman primate experiments,[34] as well as clinicopathologic correlation in patients with hemisection of the spinal cord.[35]

SEPs are typically performed using multichannel recording so that the afferent volley produced by peripheral nerve stimulation can be tracked along the peripheral nerve structures, spinal cord, and cerebrum. The setup for the median nerve SEP is shown in Figure 15-34. A normal four-channel set of signals from a bilateral median nerve study is shown in Figure 15-35. The setup for the tibial nerve SEP is shown in Figure 15-36. A normal four-channel set of signals from a bilateral tibial nerve study is shown in Figure 15-37.

Although there are a variety of different specific testing paradigms that can be applied using the SEP technique, by far the most common and most technically satisfactory studies performed are the mixed nerve stimulation techniques. The most common mixed nerve stimulated in the upper limb is the median nerve, whereas the most common nerve stimulated in the

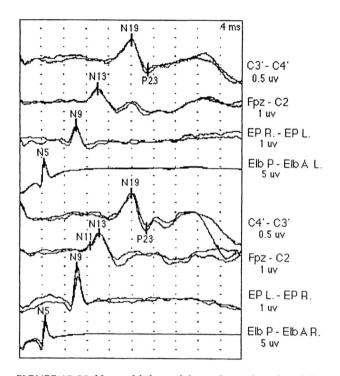

FIGURE 15-35 Normal bilateral four-channel study of the median nerve somatosensory-evoked potential. The recording sites and the vertical scale values for each channel are indicated to the right of the traces. The top four sets of traces were obtained with stimulation of the left median nerve. The bottom four sets of traces were obtained with stimulation of the right median nerve. Major components of the response are marked on each trace. Note the steady progression in latency of the major negative deflection as one proceeds proximally from the site of stimulation. Note the symmetry of amplitude and latency when comparing the responses to left and right median nerves. Abbreviations for electrode sites are as in the International 10-20 System for scalp site identification. Also, C2 = posterior neck midline at the level of the C-2 vertebral body; EP R = Erb's point on the right side; EP L = Erb's point on the left side; Elb P = elbow on the posterior aspect; Elb A = elbow on the anterior aspect overlying the median nerve in the antecubital fossa; L = left; R = right. A relative negative deflection in the second channel at each electrode is displayed upward. Horizontal scale = 4 msec per division. (Reprinted with permission from M Grabois, S Garrison, K Hart, et al [eds], Physical Medicine and Rehabilitation. The Complete Approach. Malden, MA: Blackwell Science, 2000;215.)

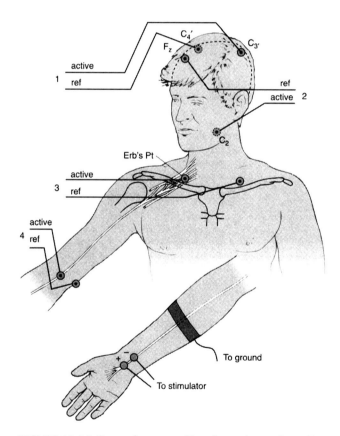

FIGURE 15-34 Setup for recording four-channel median nerve somatosensory-evoked potentials. A similar setup could be used for ulnar nerve studies with stimulation of the ulnar nerve at the wrist and recording from electrodes placed over the ulnar nerve at the elbow. (Erb's pt = Erb's point.) (Reprinted with permission from M Grabois, S Garrison, K Hart, et al [eds], Physical Medicine and Rehabilitation. The Complete Approach. Malden, MA: Blackwell Science, 2000;214.)

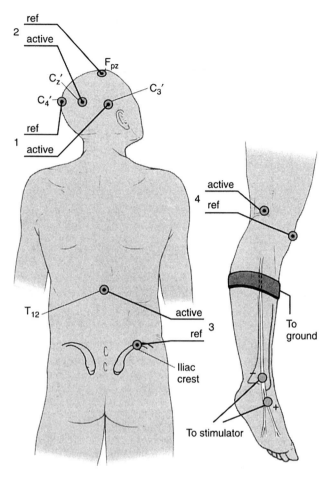

FIGURE 15-36 Setup for recording a four-channel tibial nerve somatosensory-evoked potential. (Reprinted with permission from M Grabois, S Garrison, K Hart, et al [eds], Physical Medicine and Rehabilitation. The Complete Approach. Malden, MA: Blackwell Science, 2000;216.)

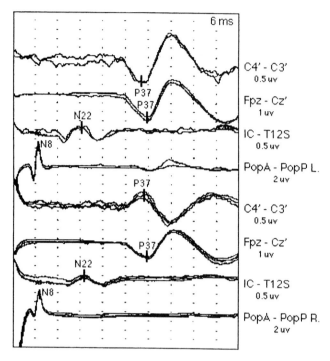

FIGURE 15-37 Normal four-channel study of the tibial nerve somatosensory-evoked potential. The recording sites and vertical scale values for each of the traces are indicated to the right. The top four sets of traces were recorded after stimulation of the left tibial nerve. The bottom four sets of traces were recorded after stimulation of the right tibial nerve. Major components are marked on each set of traces. Note the symmetry of latency and amplitude for the major components when comparing the responses between stimulation of the left and right sides. Abbreviations are as in the International 10-20 System for scalp electrode site identification. (IC = iliac crest; T12S = over the level of the spinous process of the T-12 vertebral body in the posterior midline of the back; PopA = anterior aspect of the knee; PopP = posterior aspect of the popliteal fossa overlying the path of the tibial nerve at this level; L = left; R = right.) A relative negative deflection at the second electrode for each channel is displayed as an upward deflection. Horizontal scale = 6 msec per division. (Reprinted with permission from M Grabois, S Garrison, K Hart, et al [eds], Physical Medicine and Rehabilitation. The Complete Approach. Malden, MA: Blackwell Science, 2000;217.)

lower limb for SEP testing is the tibial nerve. We, therefore, focus on physiological considerations for understanding the components generated in these two specific studies.

Physiology of the Median Nerve Somatosensory-Evoked Potential

In order to establish that an adequate stimulation was applied to the median nerve at the wrist, an afferent neurogram is recorded from the elbow with an active electrode overlying the nerve in the antecubital fossa and a reference electrode applied over the olecranon. This triphasic positive-negative-positive potential reflects conduction of the action potential volley through the nerve at this level. The exact latency is determined by the velocity of peripheral conduction and the distance between the stimulation and recording sites. Absence of this potential indicates either a technical problem with stimulation or recording of the response, or a severe impairment of peripheral nerve conduction.

A diphasic positive-negative potential is recorded at Erb's point with the active electrode at Erb's point on the same side as the stimulation and the reference elec-

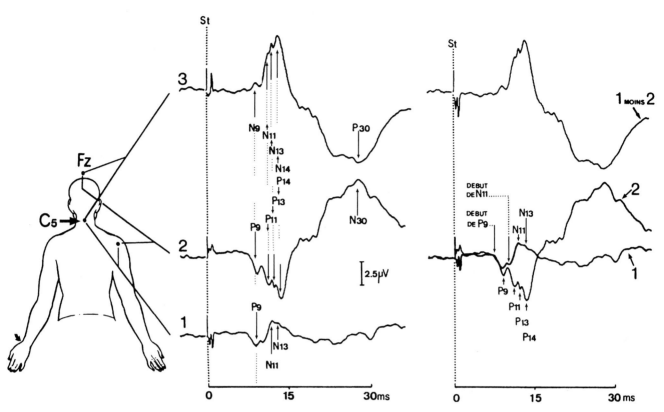

FIGURE 15-38 The cervical to frontal response to median nerve stimulation. Most of the activity recorded in the cervical to frontal (Fz) derivation (trace 3) is picked up at the scalp and consists of the succession of waves P9–P14 far-field positive potentials followed by the frontal cortical N30 component (seen in trace 2 with a noncephalic reference at the opposite shoulder). Note that the contribution of the N13 spinal component identified in trace 1 (C5 referenced to the shoulder) to the waveform recorded with an Fz reference is so small compared with the other scalp-recorded components that its disappearance may not be detected using this recording approach in patients with intramedullary cervical lesions. In patients in whom a cervical spinal cord problem is suspected, the cervical channel should have a noncephalic reference. This can be placed at the front of the neck or on the opposite shoulder. (Reprinted with permission from H Luders. Advanced Evoked Potentials. Foxboro, MA: Martinus Nijhoff, 1989.)

trode at Erb's point on the opposite side. This potential is generated by conduction in both sensory and motor fibers in the ascending volley as it passes through the brachial plexus. Most of the negative peak is generated in the sensory afferent fibers and can be recorded even in the presence of dorsal root avulsions because the dorsal root ganglion remains in continuity with the peripheral nerve. The exact latency of this peak at Erb's point (N9) is related to the length of the arm. Central latencies are often calculated with reference to this latency in order to separate peripheral conduction variability caused by factors such as limb temperature, presence of peripheral neuropathy, height, or arm length, from central conduction times.

There are a sequence of negative components that can be recorded from the back of the neck using a noncephalic reference (Figure 15-38). These include the N11 and N13 components. The N11 component reflects the

ascending volley of action potentials in the dorsal columns. It is not always clearly recordable, especially at the upper cervical levels. The N13 appears on the posterior aspect of the neck with a maximum amplitude from the C5s (C5 spinous process) to the C7s levels. It has a fixed latency when recorded from the C2s to the C6s levels. The N13 recorded posteriorly can be recorded as a P13 with anterior neck leads. This component is thought to be generated by a compound postsynaptic potential generated in the dorsal horn of the spinal cord by the arrival of the action potentials conducted in the large myelinated afferents. Around the same time as the N13, there is a P13 recorded at the scalp that appears to be generated at the level of the dorsal column nuclei. When a montage is used that records the posterior cervical spine with reference to a frontal electrode, these two potentials superimpose and enhance each other, producing a clearly defined negative peak at approximately 13 msec poststimulus. However, this may be confusing because there appear to be separate generators for the neck N13 and the scalp P13 and P14 that are identified at the Fz site with reference to a noncephalic site (see Figure 15-38). In order to avoid the confusion that could arise because of an overlapping of potentials from these two different sources, some investigators have suggested the use of an anterior cervical reference site at the level of the thyroid cartilage for the cervical recording rather than the more frequently used Fz reference site.[36] Similar arguments have been made for the use of an earlobe reference for the recording of the scalp response, rather than the more commonly used Fz cephalic reference site.

The wide distribution on the scalp of a negativity approximately 15 msec after stimulation suggests that the initial elements of this response are conducted up from subcortical sites. Intrathalamic recording in human subjects undergoing neurosurgical interventions shows significant activity in the ventroposterolateral nucleus of the thalamus at approximately the same time as the widespread negativity is developing at the scalp.[37,38] Patients with severe cerebral anoxia can show a recordable N19 component but no subsequent positivity (P23). With more extensive subcortical damage, the N19 component decreases and eventually disappears. Epileptogenic foci in the somatosensory cortex tend to produce enhancement of the P23 but not of the N19 component at the cortical level. It thus appears that the initial negativity produced at the scalp after median nerve stimulation is caused by activation of subcortical structures possibly at the thalamus, whereas the initial positive wave at the scalp, the P23, reflects activation of the primary somatosensory cortex. Differences in the distribution of these components when different fingers of the hand are stimulated suggests that the P23 (or P22) component has a focal structure, whereas the N20 (parietal) and P20 (frontal) components have a much broader structure (Figure 15-39). There is still the possibility of some overlap occurring between subcortical origins that give rise to an earlier broadly distributed negativity and a later dipolar field that is set up by a tangentially oriented dipole in the somatosensory cortex that receives the earliest arriving afferents. A schematic representation for a sequence of dipole activations associated with different components of the median nerve SEP is shown in Figure 15-40. These activations are most likely superimposed on far-field potentials that are transmitted up from subcortical structures during the interval between 16 and 19 msec after stimulation. The overlapping of activation from a variety of different cortical and subcortical sources makes the process quite complex and the exact distribution of the potential fields variable.

The latency of the N19 component increases with age and with body size. Side-to-side differences in N19 latency and in the N13–N19 latency difference, also known as the *central somatosensory conduction time*, do not show any significant age or body size associations. These are, therefore, more reliable measurement parameters. The central somatosensory conduction time is a reliable measure that is closely matched between the two hemispheres under normal conditions. It has a mean value of approximately 5.5 msec and provides an assessment of transmission across the central neuraxis along the somatosensory pathway.[39]

A later negative component in the frontal region, the N30, appears to be generated in the supplementary motor area and is reduced in amplitude when the voluntary movement is performed in the stimulated limb. The reduction in the amplitude of the frontal N30 component may be related to motor programming effects since the reduction in amplitude of the N30 by the intended movement occurs even if the movement is mentally performed but not fully executed.[40]

Physiology of the Tibial Nerve Somatosensory-Evoked Potential

The advantage of the tibial nerve SEP is that it allows evaluation of transmission through the entire length of the spinal cord in addition to testing of the cerebrum. Transmission through the dorsal columns up to the nucleus gracilis is evaluated from the lower limb. In order to establish adequate peripheral stimulation, a compound nerve action potential or afferent neurogram can be recorded from the tibial nerve at the level of the popliteal fossa using a bipolar approach. The negative peak has a latency approximately 8 msec that varies with leg length. This potential is derived from action potentials in both sensory and motor fibers that are activated by stimulation of the nerve at the ankle. A potential can also be recorded at the level of the roots of the cauda equina by placing a surface electrode at the L-5 to S-1 interspace at the base of the spine with reference to a distance site. This, however, is often a small potential that is technically difficult to register. A spinal potential from the lower spinal cord can be recorded with an electrode placed over the\ T-12 vertebrae on the posterior midline with a reference electrode placed over the posterior superior iliac spine. This produces a negative potential with a peak latency of approximately 22 msec. This potential is generated by a horizontally oriented dipolar source at the segmental level and suggests that it is pro-

FIGURE 15-39 Maps of soma-tosensory-evoked potentials with stimulation of different fingers of the right hand. The maps were generated from data gathered from a group of 12 healthy subjects. The orientation of the polarity reversal line of the N20-P20 dipolar field is more vertically oriented for stimulation of the index finger (**A**) than more stimulation of the little finger (**B**). The central P22 component is located close to the central electrode (C3) after stimulation of the index finger and is closer to the midline after stimulation of the little finger (*bottom right map in both upper and lower map sequences*). This somatotopically differentiated distribution of the P22 positivity for the stimulation of different fingers of the hand suggests that the radially oriented dipole generator of the P22 is situated close to the scalp surface, thus generating a scalp field distribution with a highly localized positive field whose position is consistent with somatotopic organization of the cortical map. (Reprinted with permission from MP Deiber, MH Giard, F Mauguière. Separate generators with distinct orientations for N20 and P22 somatosensory evoked potentials to finger stimulation. Electroencephalogr Clin Neurophysiol 1986;65:321–334.)

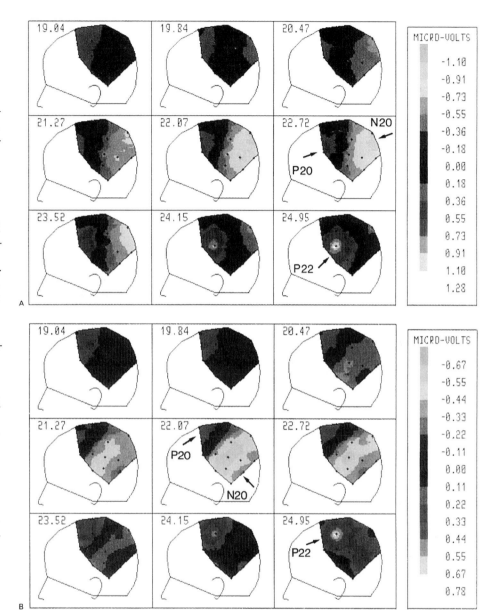

duced by the gray matter of the dorsal horn at the S-1 segment in response to the afferent volley entering the cord at this level.

The cortical responses recorded from the scalp begin with a large positivity, the P37. The positivity is usually seen best with a postcentral midline electrode between the Cz and the Pz sites. The P37 is usually somewhat asymmetric in distribution with greater prominence over the side of the scalp ipsilateral to the stimulated limb.[41] This is probably because of the location of the dipolar source on the medial surface of the hemisphere in the foot region of the primary somatosensory cortex. There is a widespread P30 far-field component seen on

the scalp that can be seen when using the earlobes as a reference electrode. In order to eliminate possible confusion between this component and the cortical P37 component, a scalp reference over the frontal region either at Fpz or at Fz helps to eliminate the P30 from the recording. If the dipole is located in the midline and is horizontally directed, it is possible that a single recording on the scalp from Pz to Fpz or from Cz' (2 cm posterior to Cz) referenced to Fpz or Fz, could miss the P37 component because the recording overlies the point of polarity reversal. In this case, it is helpful to have an additional scalp lead between the left and right central regions of the scalp (e.g., between C4' and C3') that

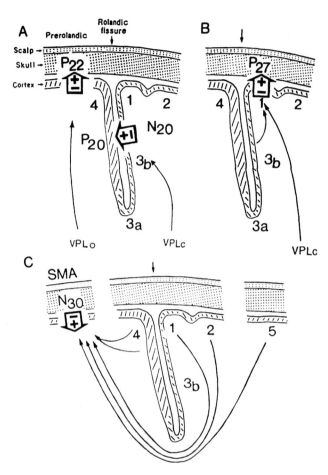

FIGURE 15-40 Schematic representation of the generators for the somatosensory-evoked potentials elicited through stimulation of individual fingers. According to this approach there is a separate activation of a tangential dipole in area 3b on the posterior surface of the central sulcus, and a radial dipole in the precentral gyrus (P22) as well as in the postcentral gyrus (P27). According to this model, the N20, P22, and P27 components are triggered via direct thalamocortical projections originating from the caudal portion of the ventroposterolateral nucleus of the thalamus (VPL$_c$) for the N20 and P27, and the oral part of the same nucleus (VPL$_o$) for the P22 (**A and B**). The N30 is thought to be generated secondarily in the supplementary motor area (SMA) by corticocortical association fibers originating from the precentral and postcentral gyrus (**C**). (Reprinted with permission from JE Desmedt, C Tomberg. Mapping early somatosensory evoked potentials in selective attention: Critical evaluation of control conditions used for titrating by difference the cognitive P30, P40, P100 and N140. Electroencephalogr Clin Neurophysiol 1989;74:321–346.)

identifies lateralized cortical response. In this case, when the side of stimulation is reversed, the polarity of the lateralized cortical recording inverts, whereas the response identified in the midline continues to show an initial positivity (see Figure 15-37).

In most clinical applications of the tibial SEP, the spinal cord transit time is evaluated by measuring the interval between the peak of the wave recorded at the T-12 level (N22) and the peak of the initial cortical potential (P37). The spinal cord transit time tends to have an upper limit of normal of approximately 20 msec in adult subjects.

Physiological Factors Affecting Somatosensory-Evoked Potential Parameters

The effects of two coexisting processes influence SEP parameters during development. These are (1) the myelinogenesis that occurs during maturation of the CNS, and (2) the lengthening of the pathways with head and body growth. With maturation and myelination of the central pathways, the central conduction velocities increase and there is increased synchronization of the conduction process. This tends to decrease conduction times. However, the simultaneous process of growth tends to elongate the pathways, which has the effect of increasing conduction times. During the first 4–5 years of life, the SEP shows evidence of increased synchronization of the somatosensory volley and decreasing latencies of all components. Although peripheral conduction velocities reach normal adult levels within the first 3 years of life, the process of myelination of central pathways proceeds more slowly. Spinal cord conduction times do not reach adult values until 5–6 years of age. However, with continued body growth, the peak latencies then gradually increase until they reach adult levels at approximately 15–17 years of age with stabilization of body height. When evaluating SEP data in children and teenagers, it is helpful to correct the peak latencies by an index, such as limb length or height, which takes path length into account. With corrections for body size as well as brain size using head circumference, it can be shown that the latencies of central SEP components decrease from birth to the age of 10 years and then begin to stabilize from that point on.[42]

Peripheral conduction velocity is reduced with reductions in skin temperature and the central conduction times also increase with decreasing core temperature. This can be seen, for example, during drug-induced hypothermia. Slight changes in the latency, shape, and amplitude of the cortical SEP can be seen during natural sleep in normal subjects. Latency changes are noted to correlate with sleep stages.[43] The main changes are a prolongation of the N19 component latency by approximately 0.4 msec between wakefulness and stage II sleep and a relative reduction of N19 latency of approximately 0.3 msec between stage II sleep and rapid eye movement sleep.

The latencies of the SEP components tend to be fairly stable with a variety of different medications. The interpeak latencies of the SEPs tend to be highly resistant to the effects of a variety of different neuroactive agents. The SEPs can be recorded with stable latencies even in patients who have been placed on high-dose barbiturates for the treatment of raised intracranial pressure and are noted, as a result, to have significant suppression of the electroencephalographic signal. The amplitude of the cortical responses can be reduced when halogenated anesthetics are administered, although the effect is dose dependent. The cervical SEP components tend to be significantly more resistant to the effects of anesthetic agents than the cortical SEP components. This is an important consideration when using the SEP for monitoring purposes in the operating room. Some of the different applications of the SEP are listed in Table 15-4.

As previously noted, the absolute latencies of the major SEP components vary significantly with the length of the path between stimulus site and the component generators. The variability caused by body height or limb length is generally less for interpeak latencies than for absolute latencies and is more pronounced for lower limb SEPs than for upper limb SEPs. For upper limb studies, the variability caused by body size is generally too small to affect interpretation significantly. However, for the lower limb studies, and especially for measurement of the spinal cord transit time, interindividual variability caused by body height is significant and should be considered in the interpretation of the study.[5]

It is possible to record spinal and scalp SEPs after electrical stimulation of the dorsal nerves of the penis or the clitoris. The pudendal nerve is synchronously activated through such stimulation and this produces a corresponding SEP. These potentials are similar in structure and latency to the SEPs that are produced by tibial nerve stimulation at the ankle. The distribution of the cortical potentials is generally symmetric in the midline. The stimulus intensity is generally adjusted to be two to four times the sensory threshold. This produces a strong tapping sensation in the perineal skin distribution that is generally not painful. This technique has been usefully employed to investigate neurogenic impotence and neurogenic bladder disorders.

TABLE 15-4
Clinical Applications of the Somatosensory-Evoked Potential

Diagnosis in adults
  Peripheral nervous system
    Peripheral neuropathy
    Acute inflammatory demyelinating polyradiculoneuritis
      (Guillain-Barré syndrome)
    Plexopathy/root avulsion
    Thoracic outlet syndrome
    Radiculopathy
    Spinal stenosis
  Central nervous system (CNS)
    Multiple sclerosis
    Myelopathy
    Spinocerebellar degenerations or ataxia
    Hereditary spastic paraparesis
    Tumors
  Hemorrhagic or ischemic CNS lesions
    Anoxic encephalopathy
    Traumatic encephalopathy
    Spinal cord trauma
    Coma assessment
    Brain death assessment
    Conversion disorder with anesthesia or weakness
    Myoclonus
    Human immunodeficiency virus–related CNS pathology
    Radiotherapy-induced CNS effects
    Motor neuron disease
    Vitamin deficiencies
    Impotence and neurologic dysfunction (using pudendal
      nerve stimulation)
Other applications
  Intraoperative monitoring (e.g., spinal scoliosis surgery,
    spinal fusion surgery)

PHYSIOLOGY OF THE MOVEMENT-RELATED CORTICAL POTENTIAL AND THE MOTOR-EVOKED POTENTIAL

General Physiological Considerations in the Central Motor System

When considering the CNS response to afferent flow of sensory information, the physiological phenomena that follow the application of sensory stimuli are examined. The reference point is the application of the stimulus, and the physiological activity the stimulus evokes flows subsequent to this event. When considering how motor phenomena are produced by physiological action within the CNS, the flow of time is reversed. The reference point is the occurrence of a muscle contraction. Interest is now focused on those phenomena within the CNS that precede and are causally related to the appearance of an overt motor behavior. In considering the physiology of efferent flow from the cerebral cortex to the periphery, one can distinguish between the more mechanical issue of activation of skeletal muscle by the motor cortex, and the more global executive function of the cerebral cortex in the context of planned, purposive action. In the former, it is possible, as has been previously pointed out, to artificially activate and therefore evaluate transmission in the efferent pathway from cortex to muscle through direct transcranial stimulation of the motor cortex. This is the underlying physiological paradigm for the MEP. In the latter, it is necessary to look back from the point of appearance of the overt motor behavior to see what is happening in the motor systems of the CNS in advance of this appearance. This is the underlying paradigm for the MRCP.

The final common pathway for CNS control of skeletal muscle is the motor unit. The central element of the motor unit is the motor neuron, the specialized neuron that sends its axonal projection out to the periphery via the ventral root and the peripheral nerve to synchronously activate a subset of muscle fibers in a particular muscle by way of a set of neuromuscular junctions. The motor neurons innervating a particular muscle are organized into a spinal motor nucleus in the anterior horn of the spinal gray matter at the spinal segmental level. Several different sources of excitation and inhibition impinge on the motor neuron *pool* supplying a particular muscle. Synaptic drive can arrive by way of direct afferent input (e.g., via the muscle spindle–mediated monosynaptic reflex arc), interneuronal networks in the spinal segmental gray matter, or from suprasegmental inputs from the several descending white matter tracts that originate in different parts of the cerebrum and brain stem. One of these tracts, the corticospinal tract, originates in the motor regions of the frontal and parietal cerebral cortex and provides direct excitatory input into spinal motor nuclei at the cervical and lumbar levels. The anatomy of the corticospinal system is shown in Figure 15-41. It has been known for many years that parts of the human motor cortex, especially the so-called primary motor cortex located in the precentral gyrus, are readily activated by low-level electrical stimulation of the exposed cortical surface. Focal electrical stimulation of motor cortex results in the excitation of large cells in the deep layers of the cortex called *Betz's cells.* These large pyramidally shaped cells give rise to long axons that project down into the corticospinal tract to directly innervate, in some instances by a monosynaptic route, motor neurons in the spinal cord. The closest and most effective connection exists between the precentral motor cortex and motor nuclei in the cervical

and lumbar regions that innervate the more distal muscles of the limbs. Functional studies suggest that the corticospinal tract is particularly involved in the control of high-dexterity, fractionated movement of the hand and foot. When the surface of the exposed motor cortex is electrically excited, a focal limb movement can be elicited. Using stimulation techniques, the surface of the motor cortex can be mapped out in terms of how the topographic organization of the motor cortex relates to the movement of different body regions. This is the basis of the *homunculus,* the distorted human figure drawn along the coronal length of the precentral gyrus to reflect the localization of cortical projection to the periphery and the relative extent of cortical surface that is devoted to movement of a particular region of the body (Figure 15-42).

When a brief low-intensity anodal electrical pulse is applied to the exposed surface of the monkey motor cortex, a single descending volley can be recorded in the corticospinal tract at the level of the pyramids.[44] This major wave has been termed the *D-wave* or *direct wave* because it has a short latency (0.4–0.6 msec in the monkey) that precludes the possibility of interposed synaptic transmission. When the stimulus intensity is increased, a recurrent series of descending bursts of action potentials can be recorded in the corticospinal tract at the level of the pyramids, recurring at intervals of approximately 2 msec. These secondary volleys have been termed *I-waves* or *indirect waves* because they are likely related to reactivation of the projecting cortical neurons by reverberating interneuronal activity within motor cortical circuits. A single D-wave is insufficient to activate motor neurons and produce a visible contraction in the periphery. This occurs through the summation effect of several I-waves descending in sequence. Anodal stimulation is more effective than cathodal stimulation because the direction of current flow with anodal stimulation drives current into the dendrites of the pyramidal tract cells leading to depolarization of the cell and firing of an action potential from the axon hillock. Similar findings have been made in human patients at the time of surgery.

Physiological activation of the motor cortex in the context of the performance of a purposeful movement occurs through a process of sequential activation of circuits within premotor pathways that gradually select out that part of the motor cortex that will be recruited. This occurs through a complex process that involves projections from sensory and associational cortex to the motor and premotor regions of the cerebral cortex. It also involves the participation of *re-entrant* subcortical circuits that include loops that traverse the basal ganglia

FIGURE 15-41 The corticospinal projection system. Note that the pyramidal cell sends its axons all the way down to the segmental level where it can directly and indirectly (via interneurons) impinge on motor neurons located in the anterior horn of the spinal gray matter. Note that 80% of the fibers cross over at the decussation of the pyramids, but 20% of the fibers remain uncrossed and continue in the anterior corticospinal tract. (Reprinted with permission from B Pansky, DJ Allen. Review of Neuroscience. New York: Macmillan, 1980;197.)

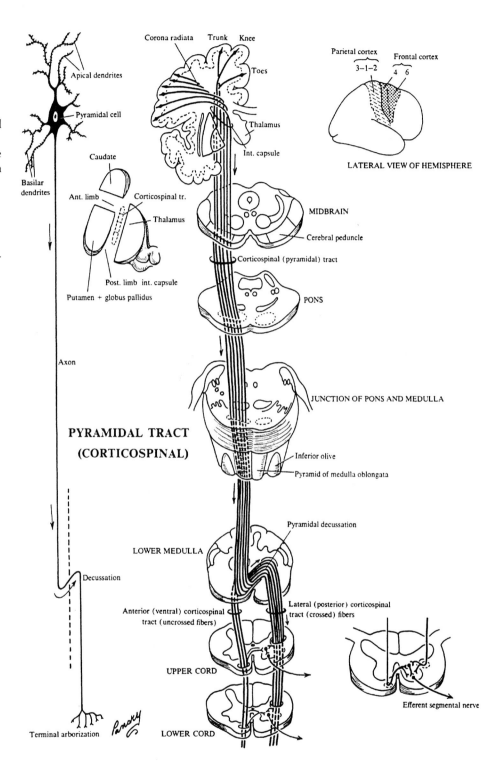

and the cerebellum. Direct somatosensory input from the periphery also can influence the process of recruitment of motor cortex regions through sensorimotor transcortical reflex loops. These processes enable the selection of the appropriate dynamic pattern of muscle activation as well as its online adjustment to conditions in the periphery (e.g., sudden changes in loading circumstances) that may alter the mechanical requirements for successful performance of the movement. Different aspects of these premotor processes may be associated

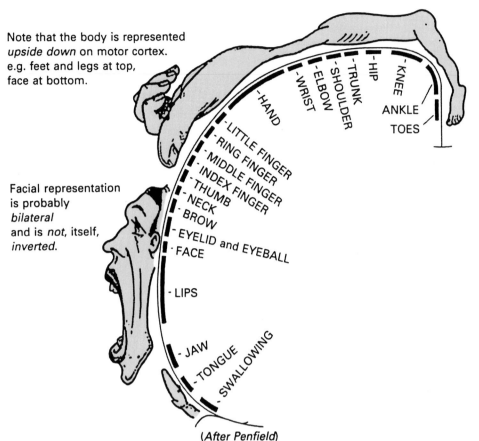

Note that the body is represented *upside down* on motor cortex. e.g. feet and legs at top, face at bottom.

Facial representation is probably *bilateral* and is *not*, itself, *inverted*.

(After Penfield)

FIGURE 15-42 Homunculus describing the somatotopic distribution of cortical control over face, trunk, and limb musculature in primary motor cortex. (Reprinted with permission from BR Mackenna, R Callander. Illustrated Physiology [6th ed]. Edinburgh: Churchill Livingstone, 1997;298.)

with an internal generative aspect that *spontaneously* constructs the desired movement through the application of progressive constraint guided by internal models that permit anticipatory goal-directed executive planning. Other aspects may be associated with the integration of the external context and environmental conditions into the construction process. Under conditions of pathology, a variety of different forms of involuntary movement can appear, each of which may *short-circuit* the normal premovement process in a different way either at the cortical or the subcortical level.

Physiology of the Movement-Related Cortical Potential

Using a technique that enabled the averaging of electroencephalographic signals that preceded a normal spontaneous voluntary movement, Kornhuber and Deecke[45] identified a slowly developing symmetric cortical potential with maximal amplitude at the vertex that began to appear over 1,200 msec before the onset of the EMG in the contracting muscle. This slow potential shift, termed the *Bereitschaftspotential* (BP) or *readiness potential*,

begins to accelerate upward at just under 500 msec before the movement and changes from a symmetric activation over the vertex into a negativity that is more lateralized toward the side opposite to that which is moved. This component has been called the NS′.[46,47] Approximately 50–100 msec before the movement, there is a focused peaking of the potential called the motor potential. These are illustrated in Figure 15-43.

The process associated with the development of the MRCP appears to include activation of supplementary motor area, premotor cortex, and the primary motor cortex, although the exact degree to which activation in each of these areas contributes to different parts of the MRCP over which different time frames remains unclear and somewhat controversial. The closer one gets to the actual overt appearance of the movement, the more focally definite and lateralized is the involvement of the primary motor cortex in the region associated with the body part that is being moved. With subdural recording electrodes, it is possible to identify potentials in the primary motor cortex of the precentral gyrus and the primary somatosensory cortex of the postcentral gyrus that appear 50–100 msec before the

FIGURE 15-43 The movement-related cortical potential. **A.** Nomenclature for different components of the movement-related cortical potential: The Bereitschaftspotential (BP) is the initial slow negative slope. The NS′ is the accelerating segment of the negative premovement slope. The motor potential (MP) is the sharply peaked negative component that occurs shortly after the peripheral onset of movement. **B.** Scalp topography of the movement-related cortical potential using a linked-ear reference. There are two superimposed trials of averaged activity associated with 100–250 repetitions of a self-paced, brisk, voluntary extension of the left middle finger. An averaged electro-oculogram and electromyogram are also shown. Note the greater amplitude over the right central regions compared with the left central regions and the maximum amplitude of the BP at the vertex. (Reprinted with permission R Neshige, H Luders, H Shibasaki. Recording of movement-related potentials from scalp and cortex in man. Brain 1988;111:719–736.)

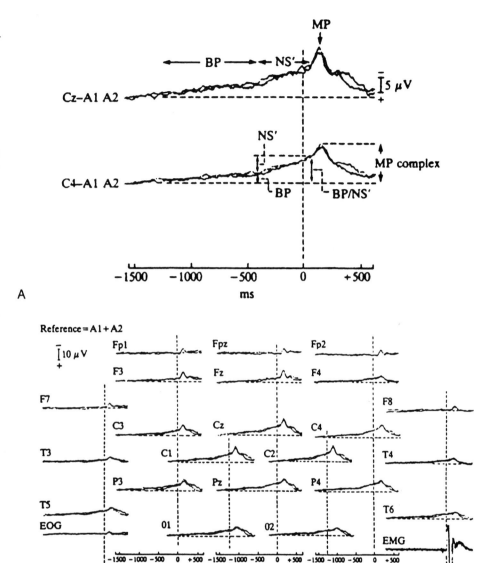

movement and up to 150 msec after the movement.[48,49] This process of localization of activation in the primary motor cortex appears to be linked to preservation of normal function of outflow from the cerebellum. The BP is significantly attenuated or truncated in the presence of lesions of the deep cerebellar nuclei[50] and in damage to outflow from the cerebellum.[51] It is interesting that in problems with cerebellar outflow, the MRCP does not develop, but the CNV continues to be clearly seen.[51] This would suggest that the E-wave of the CNV is not simply an MRCP associated with preparation of the act that is signaled by the imperative stimulus. Development of the MRCP is also impaired in patients with cerebellar atrophy.[52] It is likely that the exact

degree to which different parts of the premotor cortex contribute to the MRCP depends on the extent to which the movement is made in a fully spontaneous and unrestricted way as opposed to a temporally constrained or environmentally dependent manner. It is also clear that a variety of other factors involved in the specific performance of the movement can influence the structure and topography of the MRCP. These factors include the force produced, the complexity of the movement, and the specific temporal dynamics of sequential movements. The MRCP appears before voluntary active movements, but not in advance of passive limb movements. In addition, the degree to which the movement is voluntarily produced can influence the amplitude and structure of the MRCP. So, for example, in patients with Tourette's syndrome who produce involuntary tics, recording of the MRCP before the tics shows that there is little or no significant BP preceding the movement.[53] On the other hand, in subjects who are voluntarily producing tic-like movements or who have functional movement disorders, the movement is preceded by a recordable MRCP.[54] In parkinsonism, the BP component appears to be attenuated and the degree of attenuation can be partially repaired through treatment with L-dopa.[55] In mirror movements, in which voluntary movements are involuntarily linked to other limb movement, the topography of the MRCP is altered.[56] The MRCP technique has been used to investigate the CNS physiological processes that precede different forms of myoclonus. When the electroencephalogram is back-averaged before a myoclonic jerk, some patients have a distinct large-amplitude cortical negative-positive spike that precedes the beginning of the EMG associated with the movement. Other patients with different forms of myoclonus (e.g., subcortical) may show no significant cortical changes that precede the myoclonic jerk. Thus, the MRCP can be used to investigate the cortical antecedents of a movement and can begin to assess the degree to which a movement may have cortical participation in the preparatory process that precedes the overt appearance of the movement. It also has been reported that even under conditions of voluntary production of movement, the physiological activity recordable at the scalp is well under way before the subject is consciously aware that he or she is about to perform a simple spontaneous voluntary movement.[57]

In the context of understanding the physiology of voluntary movement generation in human subjects, the MRCP has proven to be of some value. There is clearly the presence of the extended premovement negativity, or the BP component, before self-initiated movements, but not in advance of movements that are initiated in response to an environmental cue or are performed repetitively.[58,59] Furthermore, the amplitude of the MRCP increases significantly in conjunction with the amount of conscious effort required to perform the movement and also changes systematically as a new motor skill is acquired.[60] This seems to relate to the demands of the task in terms of the precision and complexity of movement timing as well as the degree of interlimb movement synchrony in the moving extremities.[61-63]

The MRCP is recorded using a back-averaging technique in which the most recent data recorded are kept in a circular buffer that can be captured and stored when the EMG that indicates that the movement has occurred is detected. An epoch of data is thus captured around the point of movement onset with up to several seconds of data recorded in a segment that both precedes and follows the reference point of movement onset. The amplifiers must have a bandpass that extends down to $\emptyset$ Hz or close to this point because of the slow development of the BP component. Silver-silver chloride electrodes must be used to avoid problems with artifact caused by electrode polarization at these low recording frequencies. One channel should be used to record the electro-oculogram because this could produce an artifactual signal caused by eye movement that could distort the MRCP signal. Accurate assessment of the structure of the potentials around the time of the movement depends on reproducible triggering of the process at the point of onset of EMG activity. The electrodes that pick up the EMG activity should detect a well-defined burst of EMG activity associated with a brisk voluntary movement so that the onset can be reliably and reproducibly defined. The MRCP can be recorded for finger and thumb movements, foot movements, and saccadic eye movements. Manual identification of the onset of the movement by placement of a cursor at the point at which the data show the beginning of the movement can help to improve the accuracy of the averaging process. For each trial, time-shifting of the data is performed before the average is computed. This is, however, a time-consuming process that is not readily adapted for clinical study application. The use of computer-assisted techniques for identifying onset of movement can be helpful in this regard.[47]

Physiology of the Motor-Evoked Potential

When comparing the processes of transcranial motor cortex stimulation using the electrical and the magnetic techniques, significant differences have been noted.[64,65] Muscle responses to magnetic stimulation tend to have longer latencies and have simpler waveforms, shorter duration, and higher amplitudes. There appear to be different modes of excitation of the motor cortex using these two different techniques. Electrical stimulation appears to activate the pyramidal cells directly by producing a direct excitatory activation followed by several indirect reverberating activations of the outflow from the motor cortex. This produces a rapid onset but prolonged activation. Magnetic stimulation probably does not directly activate the pyramidal cells, but produces activation through transsynaptic excitation of the output cortical neurons. However, the magnetic stimulation appears to be capable of producing a full activation of the underlying cortical region with a coherent activation of the target muscle produced by effectively generating a coherent sequence of descending I-waves. The effectiveness of the magnetic stimulation can be improved with careful positioning of the coil as well as with the use of different coil configurations, such as the butterfly or figure-of-8 coil, that focus the stimulus current more precisely by having two coils wrapped in opposite directions located adjacent to each other. The magnetic field is reinforced at the point at which the two coils are adjacent, and the fields, because of the two coils, tend to cancel each other out away from this point. Using a circular coil, the upper limb muscles are best stimulated with placement of the coil at the vertex. The left hemisphere is better activated with the coil placed so that the current travels in an anticlockwise direction as viewed from above; when the right hemisphere is to be stimulated, the coil can be turned over in order to reverse the direction of current flow. When testing in pathologic states, the amplitude of the response may be low and difficult to differentiate from a tonic contraction background. In this case, it is best to relax the muscle on the target side but to facilitate activation by the magnetically induced stimulation of motor cortex through the contraction of the contralateral homologous muscle. This apparently is able to produce a similar facilitatory effect as actual contraction of the target muscle. This technique enables facilitation of the muscle response without creating the problem of the background EMG activity obscuring the stimulated response from the muscle. The general process of activation and transmission from the motor cortex to muscle that underlies the MEP is illustrated schematically in Figure 15-44.

The amplitude and latency of the evoked muscle response can vary significantly with consecutive stimulation of the motor cortex. This may be explained by a random ongoing background fluctuation of the excitability of the motor cortex in the presence of muscle relaxation in the periphery. In addition, there is a strong facilitation effect of background tone in the muscle. The MEP latency shortens significantly and the amplitude is greatly increased when there is tonic low-level contraction of the target muscle (Figure 15-45). This is known as MEP facilitation. The MEP can be maximally facilitated when the tonic background contraction of the target muscle is approximately 5–15% of the maximal voluntary contraction.[64] This phenomenon is most likely related to a tonic excitation of the motor neuron pool at the spinal segment level by a baseline voluntary contraction that causes the motor neurons to be more receptive to a superimposed phasic series of excitatory volleys from the motor cortex produced by the transcranial magnetic stimulation.

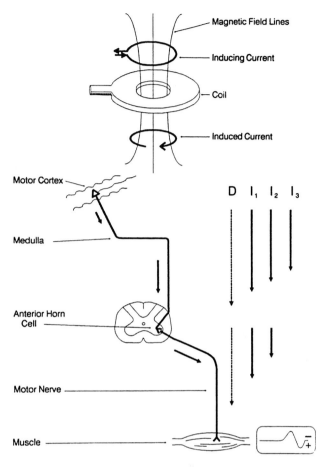

FIGURE 15-44 Schematic representation of the multiple descending volleys of action potentials evoked by a single transcutaneous stimulation of the motor cortex. Anodal electrical stimulation activates the cortical pyramidal cell in the region of the axon hillock, which sets forth an initial D-wave and a subsequent series of I-waves. Magnetic stimulation activates the cortical pyramidal neuron transsynaptically, which produces a series of I-waves but no initial D-wave. A high-intensity stimulation can cause repetitive firing of the anterior horn cell at the segmental level. (Reprinted with permission from MJ Aminoff [ed], Electrodiagnosis in Clinical Neurology [4th ed]. New York: Churchill Livingstone, 1999;551.)

The onset latency of the muscle response can be measured in order to derive a conduction time from cortex to muscle. However, it is helpful to isolate the central component of this pathway in order to derive a central motor conduction time (CMCT). The peripheral part of the pathway can be subtracted out by measuring the conduction time from the root level to the muscle (Figure 15-46). This can be done by placing a large circular magnetic stimulator coil over the back of the neck and stimulating at this point with the subject

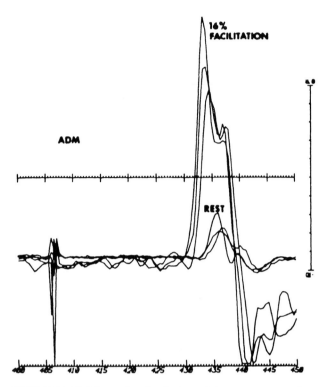

FIGURE 15-45 Magnetic stimulation of the motor cortex in a normal subject with the muscle at rest and during a small background contraction of the target muscle (facilitation). The facilitation has caused the latency to onset of the compound muscle action potential to decrease by approximately 2 msec and the amplitude to increase fivefold. Recording was obtained from the abductor digiti minimi (ADM). Stimulation was produced by a 9-cm mean diameter coil centered at the vertex and set for 80% of maximum stimulation. (Reprinted with permission from KH Chiappa. Evoked Potentials in Clinical Medicine [3rd ed]. Philadelphia: Lippincott–Raven, 1997;482.)

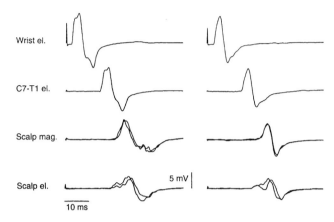

FIGURE 15-46 Responses from the abductor digiti minimi muscle in two healthy subjects with electrical stimulation of the ulnar nerve at the wrist (*Wrist el.*) and at the C-7 to T-1 interspace using a monopolar needle to perform C-8 root stimulation (*C7-T1 el.*). Transcranial magnetic stimulation of motor cortex is performed to activate the muscle (*Scalp mag.*). Finally, anodal electrical stimulation is used to perform transcranial activation of motor cortex (*Scalp el.*). Note that the responses to transcranial magnetic stimulation are larger and more consistent but show a slightly longer latency than the responses to transcranial electrical stimulation. The peripheral motor conduction time is computed between the onsets of the top and second traces, whereas the central motor conduction time can be computed between the onset latencies of the second and third traces down from the top. (Reprinted with permission from MJ Aminoff [ed], Electrodiagnosis in Clinical Neurology [4th ed]. New York: Churchill Livingstone, 1999;552.)

in a seated position and the neck flexed forward to reduce the cervical lordosis.[66] The coil is placed with the stimulus current circulating clockwise for right-sided stimulation and vice versa for left-sided stimulation. This procedure should be avoided in patients with a history of multiple cervical spine fusions, cervical cord compression, cervical spine instability, or tight cervical stenosis. The technique for obtaining the CMCT using a circular stimulus coil is shown in Figure 15-47. Typical recordings from surface electrodes placed over the peripheral muscle are shown in Figure 15-48. The peripheral muscle activation can be recorded from multiple proximal and peripheral muscles in the limb simultaneously. Typically, two muscles in the hand and two muscles in the arm can be sampled. The derivation of the CMCT from these

records is also illustrated. An alternative approach to measurement of the peripheral conduction time is to use F-wave measures from the peripheral hand muscles. The formula $^{1}/_{2}(F + M - 1)$ can be used to estimate the peripheral motor time, where F is the F-wave latency, M is the M-wave latency, and one subtracts 1 msec for the delay in the elicited back-firing activation of the alpha motor neuron by the input volley. The normal CMCT to the intrinsic hand muscles is approximately 6 msec when the target muscle is initially contracted and approximately 8 msec when the baseline condition is complete relaxation of the muscle. The lower limb muscles are best stimulated by positioning a circular stimulus coil approximately 2 or 3 cm anterior to the vertex. Generally, it is easier to get an adequate stimulus of the cervical roots using magnetic stimulation than the lumbar roots. A more reliable approach to stimulation of the lumbar roots when measuring the CMCT for the lower limbs is to use nee-

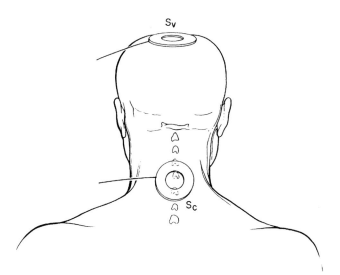

FIGURE 15-47 Basic setup for measuring the central motor conduction time to the upper limb. The stimulator coil is placed at the vertex (S_v), and a peripheral response is obtained. Then the stimulator coil is moved to the posterior cervical spine (S_c). Stimulation at this level activates the cervical nerve roots. Recordings are obtained from a peripheral upper limb muscle such as the abductor digiti minimi. (Reprinted with permission from JA Liveson, DM Ma. Laboratory Reference for Clinical Neurophysiology. Philadelphia: F.A. Davis, 1992;358.)

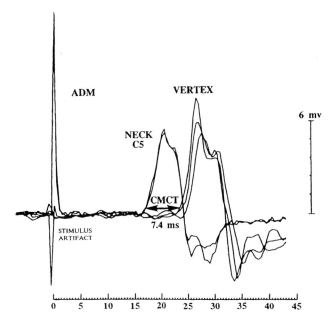

FIGURE 15-48 Normal motor-evoked potential studies recording compound muscle action potentials from the abductor digiti minimi (ADM) after magnetic stimulation of the motor cortex and the cervical spine and nerve roots. The central motor conduction time is the difference in onset latencies between these two compound muscle action potentials. The stimulus that occurred at the point of the recording of the stimulus artifact was delivered during a voluntary low-level contraction of the target muscle. Calibrations are noted in milliseconds on the horizontal scale and millivolts on the vertical scale. The 6-mV mark is for the response from transcranial cortical stimulation. The same calibration bar is 3.1 mV for the response to cervical root stimulation. (Reprinted with permission from D Cros, KH Chiappa. Motor Evoked Potentials. In KH Chiappa [ed]. Evoked Potentials in Clinical Medicine [3rd ed]. Philadelphia: Lippincott–Raven, 1997;488.)

dle stimulation with electrical current pulses with insertion of the needle at the level of the L-1 vertebra in order to stimulate the roots at the level of the conus medullaris. This technique can be used if magnetic stimulation fails to elicit an adequate muscle response in the lower limbs with placement of the stimulus coil over the upper lumbar region. For muscle recording in the lower limb, the tibialis anterior muscle can be used. The CMCT when using the tibialis anterior and evaluating the lower limb is approximately 12 msec. Some clinical applications of the MEP are listed in Table 15-5.

In addition to being applied to the assessment of transmission continuity through the efferent motor pathways, the MEP technique has also been applied in experimental contexts to understand the topographic structure of the motor cortex. By using a figure-of-8 coil applied across a fixed grid on the head, it is possible to map the outflow from the motor cortex to specific regions of the body. Using this approach, it has been possible to show that the topographic representation in the human motor cortex is highly plastic and can be systematically modified under specific conditions such as the learning of a new motor skill.[67] Significant plasticity

of the motor cortex in a variety of different contexts has been revealed through careful evaluation of motor cortex excitability and topographic organization using MEP techniques.[68,69]

SUMMARY

Clinical neurophysiology techniques such as those examined in this chapter are an important subset of the objective evaluation methods available to the medical rehabilitation practitioner. Their careful application and interpretation can, no doubt, be challenging at times. Methods are available to evaluate both sensory afferent and motor efferent function at various different levels within the nervous system.

TABLE 15-5
Clinical Applications of the Motor-Evoked Potential

Diagnosis
    Multiple sclerosis
    Motor neuron disease
    Cervical spondylosis
    Spinal stenosis
    Corticospinal tract degeneration
    Hereditary spastic paraparesis
    Myelopathy/spinal cord trauma/spinal cord ischemia/
        infarction
    Spinocerebellar degeneration/ataxias
    Movement disorders
    Cerebrovascular disease
    Hereditary motor and sensory neuropathy
    Conversion disorder with muscular weakness
    Malingering/factitious paresis
Other applications
    Intraoperative monitoring of the corticospinal pathway
    Evaluation of prognosis for motor recovery in stroke
    Evaluating motor cortex excitability
    Evaluating topographic organization of motor cortex and
        its plasticity

Pathways can be checked from the sensory receptors through to the cortical sensory areas and from the motor cortex back out to the muscle. Several of the techniques that have been reviewed have not yet gained widespread clinical application, although they remain useful research tools. However, clearly, some of the EP methods, such as the SEP, have gained acceptance as valuable and important clinical tools and have been put to use in a variety of settings ranging from the outpatient clinic to the operating room. The successful deployment of EPs in clinical practice depends critically on a thorough knowledge of the basic physiological principles that form the foundation of their use. These principles have been reviewed here. EP techniques can be applied to the problem of obtaining a more complete and objective understanding of the physiological basis of the function of a patient presenting for rehabilitation. This can be a rewarding enterprise if the question to be addressed is prudently formulated, the techniques are applied with thoughtfulness and care, and the results are interpreted knowledgeably.

Acknowledgments

The author would like to thank Dr. Wendy Helkowski for reading the manuscript and providing editorial feedback. The author would also like to recognize the assistance and support of Dr. C. R. Sridhara with whom direction of the Electrodiagnostic Center at MossRehab Hospital was shared during the initial writing of this chapter. Finally, the author would like to acknowledge the assistance and support of colleagues in the new Department of Physical Medicine and Rehabilitation at the University of Pittsburgh during the latter period of writing and assembling this manuscript.

REFERENCES

1. Werner RA, Goldberg G. Clinical application of evoked potential testing. Crit Rev Phys Med Rehabil 1992;4: 105–131.
2. Goldberg G, Toledo S Jr. Update on electrodiagnostic evaluation of central conduction. Techniques and clinical applications. Phys Med Rehabil: State of the Art Reviews 1999;13:347–369.
3. Aminoff MJ (ed). Electrodiagnosis in Clinical Neurology (4th ed). New York: Churchill Livingstone, 1999.
4. Binnie CD, Cooper R, Fowler CH, et al (eds). Clinical Neurophysiology. EMG, Nerve Conduction and Evoked Potentials. Oxford: Butterworth–Heinemann, 1995.
5. Chiappa KH (ed). Evoked Potentials in Clinical Medicine (3rd ed). Philadelphia: Lippincott-Raven, 1997.
6. Delisa JA, Mackenzie K, Baran EM. Manual of Nerve Conduction Velocity and Somatosensory Evoked Potentials (2nd ed). New York: Raven Press, 1987.
7. Goldberg G. Clinical Neurophysiology of the Central Nervous System: Evoked Potentials and Other Neurophysiologic Techniques. In M Grabois, S Garrison, K Hart, D Lehmkuhl (eds), Physical Medicine and Rehabilitation: The Complete Approach. Malden, MA: Blackwell Science, 1999;196–224.
8. Dumitru D. Electrodiagnostic Medicine. Philadelphia: Hanley & Belfus, 1995.
9. Misulis KE. Spehlmann's Evoked Potential Primer: Visual, Auditory and Somatosensory Evoked Potentials in Clinical Diagnosis (2nd ed). Boston: Butterworth–Heinemann, 1994.
10. Maurer K, Lowitzsch K, Stöhr M. Evoked Potentials. Toronto: BC Decker, 1989.
11. American Association of Electrodiagnostic Medicine. Guidelines in somatosensory evoked potentials. Muscle Nerve 1999a;(Suppl 8):S119–S138.
12. American Association of Electrodiagnostic Medicine. Somatosensory evoked potentials: clinical uses. Muscle Nerve 1999b;(Suppl 8):S109–S118.
13. Merton PA, Morton HB. Stimulation of the cerebral cortex in the intact human subject. Nature 1980;285:227.
14. Barker AT, Freeston IL, Jalinous R. Noninvasive magnetic stimulation of human motor cortex. Lancet 1985;2: 1106–1107.
15. Barker AT, Freeston IL, Jalinous R, Jarratt JA. Magnetic stimulation of the human brain and peripheral nervous system: an introduction and the results of an initial clinical evaluation. Neurosurgery 1987;20:100–109.
16. Kooi KA, Guvener AM, Bagchi BK.

Visual evoked responses in lesions of the higher optic pathways. Neurology 1965;15:841–854.

17. Halliday AM, McDonald WI, Mushin J. Visual evoked responses in the diagnosis of multiple sclerosis. BMJ 1973;4:661–664.

18. Halliday AM, Barrett G, Halliday E, Mushin J. A comparison of the flash and pattern-evoked potential in unilateral optic neuritis. Wiss Zeit Ernst-Mortiz-Arndt-Universitat 1979;28:89–95.

19. Kriss A, Halliday AM. A Comparison of Occipital Potentials Evoked by Pattern Onset, Offset and Reversal by Movement. In C Barber (ed), Evoked Potentials. Lancaster: MTP Press, 1980;205–212.

20. Yiannikas C, Walsh JC. The variation of the pattern shift visual evoked response with the size of the stimulus field. Electroencephalogr Clin Neurophysiol 1983;55:427–435.

21. Blumhardt LD, Barrett G, Halliday AM, Kriss A. The effect of experimental "scotomata" on the ipsilateral and contralateral responses to pattern-reversal in one half-field. Electroencephalogr Clin Neurophysiol 1978;45:376–392.

22. Guthkelch AN, Bursick D, Sclabassi RJ. The relationship of the latency of the visual P100 to gender and head size. Electroencephalogr Clin Neurophysiol 1987;68:219–222.

23. Jewett DL, Romano MN, Williston JS. Human auditory evoked potentials: possible brain-stem components detected on the scalp. Science 1970;167:1517–1518.

24. Burkard R, Hecox K. The effect of broad-band noise on the human brainstem auditory evoked response. II. Frequency specificity. J Acoust Soc Am 1983;74:1214–1223.

25. Galambos R, Makeig S, Talmachoff P. A 40-Hz auditory potential recorded from the human scalp. Proc Natl Acad Sci U S A 1981;78:2643–2647.

26. Simson R, Vaughn HG Jr, Ritter W. The scalp topography of potentials associated with missing visual and auditory stimuli. Electroencephalogr Clin Neurophysiol 1976;40:33–42.

27. Polich J. P300 in the evaluation of dementia and aging. Electroencephalogr Clin Neurophysiol 1991;42(Suppl):304–323.

28. Rappaport M, Clifford JO. Comparison of passive P300 brain evoked potentials in normal and severely traumatically brain injured patients. J Head Trauma Rehabil 1994;9:94–104.

29. Keren O, Ben-Dror S, Stern MJ, et al. Event-related potentials as an index of cognitive function during recovery from severe closed head injury. J Head Trauma Rehabil 1998;13:15–30.

30. Walter WG, Cooper R, Aldridge VJ, et al. Contingent negative variation: an electrical sign of sensorimotor association and expectancy in the human brain. Nature 1964;203:380–384.

31. Näätänen R, Michie PT. Early selective attention effects on the evoked potential. A critical review and reinterpretation. Biol Psychol 1979;8:81–136.

32. Näätänen R. Processing negativity: an evoked potential reflection of selective attention. Psychol Bull 1982;92:605–640.

33. Näätänen R. The mismatch negativity: a powerful tool for cognitive neuroscience. Ear Hear 1995;16:6–18.

34. Cusick JF, Myklebust J, Larson SJ, Sances JA. Spinal evoked potentials in the primate: neural substrate. J Neurosurg 1978;49:551–557.

35. Bloom KK, Goldberg G. Tibial nerve somatosensory evoked potentials in spinal cord hemisection. Am J Phys Med Rehabil 1989;68:59–65.

36. Mauguière F. Evoked Potentials. In CD Binnie, R Cooper, CJ Fowler, et al. (eds),Clinical Neurophysiology: EMG, Nerve Conduction and Evoked Potentials. Oxford: Butterworth–Heinemann, 1995;323–563.

37. Morioka T, Shima F, Kato M, Fukui M. Origin and distribution of thalamic somatosensory evoked potentials in humans. Electroencephalogr Clin Neurophysiol 1989;74:186–193.

38. Urasaki E, Wada S, Kadoya C, et al. Origin of scalp far-field N18 of SSEPs in response to median nerve stimulation. Electroencephalogr Clin Neurophysiol 1990;77:39–51.

39. Hume AL, Cant BR. Conduction time in central somatosensory pathways in man. Electroencephalogr Clin Neurophysiol 1978;45:361–375.

40. Cheron G, Borenstein S. Mental movement stimulation affects the N30 frontal component of the somatosensory evoked potential. Electroencephalogr Clin Neurophysiol 1992;84:288–292.

41. Cruse R, Lem G, Lesser RP, Lueders H. Paradoxical lateralization of cortical potentials evoked by stimulation of posterior tibial nerve. Arch Neurol 1982;39:222–225.

42. Tomita Y, Nishimura S, Tanaka T. Short-latency SEPs in infants and children: developmental changes and maturational index of SEPs. Electro-encephalogr Clin Neurophysiol 1986;65:335–343.

43. Yamada T, Kameyama S, Fuchigami Y, et al. Changes of short latency somatosensory evoked potentials in sleep. Electroencephalogr Clin Neurophysiol 1988;70:126–136.

44. Amassian VE, Stewart M, Quirk GJ, Rosenthal JL. Physiological basis of motor effects of a transient stimulus to cerebral cortex. Neurosurgery 1987;20:74–93.

45. Kornhuber HH, Deecke L. Hirnpotentialänderungen bei Willkurbewegungen und passiven Bewegungen des Menschen. Bereitschaftspotential und reafferente Potentiale. Pflügers Archiv für gesampte Physiologie 1965;284:1–17.

46. Shibasaki H, Barrett G, Halliday E, Halliday AM. Components of the movement-related cortical potential and their scalp topography. Electroencephalogr Clin Neurophysiol 1980;49:213–226.

47. Barrett G, Shibasaki H, Neshige R. A computer-assisted method for averaging movement-related cortical potentials with respect to EMG onset. Electroencephalogr Clin Neurophysiol 1985;60:276–281.

48. Lee BI, Luders H, Lesser RP, et al. Cortical potentials related to voluntary and passive finger movements recorded from subdural electrodes in humans. Ann Neurol 1986;20:32–37.

49. Neshige R, Luders H, Shibasaki H. Recording of movement-related potentials from scalp and cortex in man. Brain 1988;111:719–736.

50. Shibasaki H, Barrett G, Neshige R, et al. Volitional movement is not preceded by cortical slow negativity in cerebellar dentate lesion in man. Brain Res 1986;368:361–365.

51. Ikeda A, Shibasaki H, Nagamine T, et al. Dissociation between contingent negative variation and bereitschaftspotential in a patient with cerebellar efferent lesion. Electroencephalogr Clin Neurophysiol 1994;90:359–364.

52. Wessel K, Verleger R, Nazarenus D, et al. Movement-related cortical potentials preceding sequential and goal-directed finger and arm movements in patients with cerebellar atrophy. Electroencephalogr Clin Neurophysiol 1994;92:331–341.

53. Obeso JA, Rothwell JC, Marsden CD. Simple tics in Gilles de la Tourette's syndrome are not prefaced by a normal premovement EEG potential. J Neurol Neurosurg Psychiatry 1981;44:735–738.

54. Toro C, Torres F. Electrophysiologic correlates of a paroxysmal movement disorder. Ann Neurol 1986;20:731–734.

55. Dick JPR, Cantello R, Buruma O, et al. The Bereitschaftspotential, L-DOPA, and Parkinson's disease. Electroencephalogr Clin Neurophysiol 1987; 66:263–274.

56. Shibasaki H, Nagae K. Mirror movement: application of movement-related cortical potentials. Ann Neurol 1984; 15:299–302.

57. Libet B, Gleason CA, Wright EW, Pearl DK. Time of conscious intention-to-act in relation to onset of cerebral activity (readiness potential). The unconscious initiation of a freely voluntary act. Brain 1983;106:623–642.

58. Papa SM, Artieda J, Obeso JA. Cortical activity preceding self-initiated and externally triggered voluntary movement. Mov Disord 1991;6:217–224.

59. Dirnberger G, Fickel U, Lindinger G, et al. The mode of movement selection. Movement-related cortical potentials prior to freely selected and repetitive movements. Exp Brain Res 1998; 120:263–272.

60. Lang W, Beisteiner R, Lindinger G, Deecke L. Changes of cortical activity when executing learned motor sequences. Exp Brain Res 1992;89:435–440.

61. Deecke L, Kornhuber HH, Lang W, et al. Timing function of the frontal cortex in sequential motor and learning tasks. Hum Neurobiol 1985;4:143–154.

62. Lang W, Obrig H, Lindinger G, et al. Supplementary motor area activation while tapping bimanually different rhythms in musicians. Exp Brain Res 1990;79:504–514.

63. Deecke L. Electrophysiological correlates of movement initiation. Revue Neurologique 1990;146:612–619.

64. Hess CW, Mills KR, Murray NMF. Responses in small hand muscles from magnetic stimulation of the human brain. J Physiol 1987;388:397–419.

65. Day BL, Dressler D, Maertens de Noordhout A, et al. Electric and magnetic stimulation of human motor cortex. Surface EMG and single motor unit responses. J Physiol 1989;12: 449–473.

66. Cros D, Chiappa KH. Motor Evoked Potentials. In KH Chiappa (ed), Evoked Potentials in Clinical Medicine (3rd ed). Philadelphia: Lippincott-Raven, 1997;477–507.

67. Classen J, Liepert J, Hallett M, Cohen L. Rapid plasticity of human cortical movement representation induced by practice. J Neurophysiol 1998;79:1117–1123.

68. Hallett M. Motor cortex plasticity. Electroencephalogr Clin Neurophysiol 1999;50(Suppl):85–91.

69. Classen J, Liepert J, Hallett M, Cohen L. Plasticity of movement representation in the human motor cortex. Electroencephalogr Clin Neurophysiol 1999;51(Suppl):162–173.

16

Exercise

WALTER R. FRONTERA, JONATHAN R. MOLDOVER,
JOANNE BORG-STEIN, AND MARY P. WATKINS

Exercise is a cornerstone of rehabilitation medicine's therapeutic armamentarium, but as such it must be well conceived and highly specific. In prescribing exercise, the therapeutic goals must be clear and the recommendations should specifically include the type, frequency, duration, and intensity of the exercise. The rehabilitation medicine clinician must clearly understand the biophysical properties of the tissues involved in exercise, the physiological response to an acute bout of exercise, the nature of the adaptations to exercise training, and the alterations and limitations imposed by the pathomechanics and pathophysiology of various disease states. In this chapter we review the biochemical, physiological, and neuromusculoskeletal response to exercise, with emphasis on clinical applications.

Physical activity has been defined as "any bodily movement produced by skeletal muscles that result in energy expenditure."[1] *Exercise* may be defined as "a subset of physical activity that is planned, structured, and repetitive and has as a final or intermediate objective the improvement or maintenance of physical fitness." In rehabilitation medicine, exercise is prescribed to develop flexibility, strength, endurance, and coordination, in order to restore and to enhance function.

The human body exhibits an elegant and predictable response to the various forms of exercise that are reviewed in this chapter, including the immediate physiological responses to exercise and the longer-term adaptations to regular training that allow the body to enhance its performance. These predictable physiological changes are the rationale for many of our therapeutic programs.

GENERAL PRINCIPLES

Types of Muscle Actions

The nature of the muscle action has a direct effect on the acute response to exercise and on the possible benefits of exercise training programs. In general, muscle actions can be divided into static (isometric) and dynamic (concentric, eccentric, isokinetic) actions.[2]

Static (Isometric)
Static actions occur when the force generated by the active muscle(s) is equal to an externally applied force (e.g., when force is exerted against an immovable or relatively immovable object). Static exercise is defined as muscle action without movement of the joint(s) crossed by the active muscle(s). The intensity of static actions is usually expressed as a percentage of the maximum force.

Dynamic ("Isotonic," Concentric, Eccentric, Isokinetic)
By definition, an isotonic action occurs when the tension or torque generated by the muscle is constant throughout the movement. In reality, this is difficult to accomplish because of the change in the overlapping of myofilaments (responsible for the length-tension relationship) and the mechanical leverage of muscle change throughout the range of motion. Thus, a better term is *dynamic action*. Dynamic actions can be further subdivided into concentric, eccentric, and isokinetic.

Concentric actions are also known as *shortening* or *positive* actions and occur when the force generated by active muscles exceeds the externally applied forces.

Chapter 16

These actions are characterized by joint movements that bring the origin and insertion of the active muscle closer together. The force generated is not uniform throughout the arc of motion. The slower the velocity of shortening, the greater the tension that can be generated.

Eccentric actions are also referred to as *lengthening* or *negative* actions. At any given velocity, the tension produced by an eccentric action is greater than that produced by a concentric action. For this reason, eccentric actions should be used as part of a strengthening program.[3] For a given force level, less energy and a decreased muscle activation (as assessed on electromyography [EMG]) are required during eccentric actions compared with concentric actions. Delayed onset muscle soreness, which commonly occurs 24–48 hours after exercise, is more common with eccentric than with concentric exercise.[4] The possible mechanisms for exercise-induced delayed onset muscle soreness have been reviewed by Fridén and Armstrong.[4,5] Structural damage in the muscle fiber caused by high tension results in disruption of cell membranes and of calcium homeostasis. This process leads to necrosis, which peaks approximately 2 days after exercise. Products of the ensuing macrophage activity and inflammation cause the sensation of soreness.

Isokinetic actions are characterized by constant angular velocities. Torque is generated against a preset device that controls speed of movement.[6] *Torque* is defined as the product of force multiplied by the perpendicular distance between the center of rotation and the point where the force is applied. This form of exercise is defined by the equipment used for the exercise, as such actions do not exist in nature. Most isokinetic devices can use concentric and eccentric actions. The data generated by the devices may be useful for following trends during a rehabilitation program, but caution must be observed in extrapolating from the information to predict function in the real world. Hageman reviewed several issues that may influence the reliability and validity of isokinetic testing.[7] Factors such as positioning in the machine, length of the lever arm, stabilization of the subject, calibration of the machine, speed of contraction, and the effect of gravity are important. In addition, poor correlation among torque values reported by the various currently available machines makes it impossible to compare norms or data of individual patients when they are obtained on different brands of machines. Correlations of printout data with patients' functional outcome has been poor, both for orthopedic and neurologic rehabilitation. The principles of specificity of training and testing suggest that it might be difficult to

estimate functional capacity from the results of isokinetic testing.

Acute Response to Exercise

Energy Metabolism

All forms of exercise require energy. At the cellular level, adenosine triphosphate (ATP), a high-energy phosphate compound, is the major source of available energy. Phosphocreatine (PCr) in the muscle cell is another high-energy compound that is available in limited quantities and serves to regenerate ATP in the following reaction that also involves adenosine diphosphate:

$$\text{Adenosine diphosphate} + \text{PCr} \rightleftarrows \text{ATP} + \text{Creatine}$$

Muscle creatine and PCr can be increased 10–20% with creatine supplementation.[8,9] This results in a reduction of lactate accumulation and enhanced performance during high-intensity repetitive exercise.

Under normal conditions, the available PCr is consumed in seconds[10–12] and depletion of ATP results in rigor. Thus, ATP needs to be regenerated in other ways during continued exercise. This can be done through the glycolytic pathway[13] in the cytoplasm of the cell or aerobically in the mitochondria, through the oxidation of carbohydrate (glycogen), fat (triglycerides and free fatty acids [FFA]), or protein (amino acids) (Figure 16-1).[14]

During glycolysis, glucose is broken down to pyruvate and ATP is generated. In the absence of sufficient oxygen, pyruvate is reduced to lactate (salt of lactic acid) and hydrogen ions.[15] Lactate enters the venous blood and subsequently is reoxidized in the liver, heart, and muscle during the postexercise recovery period, when sufficient oxygen is present. Alternatively, it can be converted to glucose in the liver.[16] The lactate level in blood can be used as a measure of anaerobic metabolism. In the presence of oxygen, pyruvate is converted into acetyl coenzyme A and transported to the mitochondria, where it can continue through Krebs' cycle and the electron transport chain. The metabolism of triglycerides and proteins results in the formation of fatty acids and amino acids, respectively. These can also be converted into acetyl coenzyme A and enter Krebs' cycle.

The activation of the different metabolic pathways that generate ATP is a function of time (Figure 16-2). During the first few seconds of heavy exercise, energy is obtained anaerobically from the already stored high-energy compounds PCr and ATP. This is referred to as the *alactic phase* because it does not result in the pro-

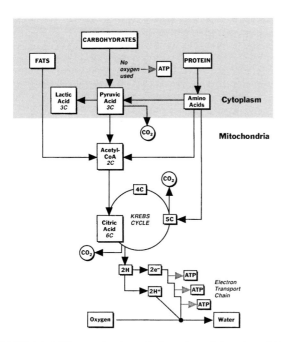

FIGURE 16-1 The production of adenosine triphosphate (ATP) by means of anaerobic metabolism in the cytoplasm or aerobic metabolism in the mitochondria. (CoA = coenzyme A.) (Adapted from P-O Astrand, K Rodahl. Textbook of Work Physiology [3rd ed]. New York: McGraw-Hill, 1986.)

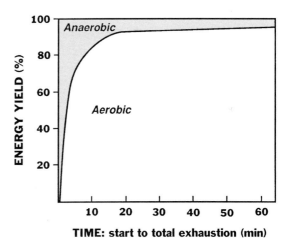

FIGURE 16-2 The temporal relationship of anaerobic and aerobic metabolism during exercise. (Adapted from P-O Astrand, K Rodahl. Textbook of Work Physiology [3rd ed]. New York: McGraw-Hill, 1986.)

duction of lactate. As activity continues over the next 1–2 minutes, stored muscle glycogen and glucose are broken down anaerobically to lactate via glycolysis. This is the anaerobic, or glycolytic, phase. As oxygen becomes available through increased pulmonary ventilation and circulatory changes, ATP can be generated aerobically through the oxidation of carbohydrate, fat, and protein. This is the aerobic phase. During light exercise the aerobic supply may be sufficient to sustain activity, but if the exercise is strenuous the anaerobic contribution may predominate and lactate and hydrogen ions accumulate. During the recovery period, lactate is reoxidized, PCr and ATP are replenished, and oxygen consumption gradually decreases.

The contribution of carbohydrates and triglycerides to the total energy production is related to the intensity and duration of the exercise.[17] During an exercise bout of a given duration (e.g., 30 minutes), the contribution of carbohydrate metabolism to the total energy production increases with the intensity of exercise. The source of carbohydrates is the muscle glycogen stores and the plasma glucose. At a given relative intensity of exercise (e.g., 65% of the maximal aerobic power) triglycerides become the predominant substrate for energy metabolism as the duration of the exercise increases.

The regulation of carbohydrate and fat metabolism during exercise has been explained using the glucose–fatty acid cycle model.[18] This model suggests that an increase in plasma FFAs leads to an elevated oxidation of FFA in active skeletal muscles and a reduction in the use of glucose and muscle glycogen stores. At rest and during low-intensity exercise, lipolysis results in FFA mobilization, increased plasma FFA concentration, and elevated transport and oxidation in active muscles. The transport of FFA into the cell is not only by simple diffusion but also carrier mediated.[19] As the exercise continues, increased FFA oxidation results in elevated acetyl coenzyme A concentrations, which in turn decrease glucose oxidation and uptake.

If the intensity of exercise increases, the proportion of energy derived from carbohydrates increases because of (1) changes in the levels of circulating hormones such as epinephrine, glucagon, and insulin (see following discussion); (2) contraction-mediated glycogenolysis; (3) recruitment of fast twitch fibers; and (4) the demand for a higher energy flux attainable only through glycolysis. This results in inhibition of FFA mobilization and oxidation and increases in hepatic glucose production and uptake and oxidation of glucose in active muscles. At a certain power output (the *cross-over point*), energy derived from carbohydrate metabolism predominates.[20]

Endocrine Response

The metabolic adaptations and changes in fuel use, mainly carbohydrate and fat, required during exercise are regulated by a complex endocrine response.[21,22] Carbohydrates are the main source of energy during many forms of exercise. Three metabolic processes combine to maintain blood glucose concentration and to make more glucose available to the active muscle fibers: (1) muscle glycogenolysis, (2) liver glycogenolysis, and (3) liver gluconeogenesis from amino acids released from muscle as substrates. The effects of several hormones including glucagon, epinephrine, norepinephrine, cortisol, growth hormone, and thyroid hormone together facilitate these processes. A decrease in insulin, which has an antagonistic effect, further contributes to the increased availability of glucose. The reduction in insulin levels is counterbalanced by an increased sensitivity to insulin and increased glucose use by muscle cells, the net result being the maintenance of normal serum glucose concentrations.[23,24]

Fat metabolism is also influenced by various hormones released during exercise. During exercise, triglycerides are reduced to FFAs by the enzyme lipase, which is activated by several hormones including cortisol, epinephrine, norepinephrine, growth hormone, and thyroid hormone to a smaller degree.[22] During prolonged exercise, cortisol peaks after 30–45 minutes and then decreases, while the catecholamines and growth hormone continue to facilitate lipolysis.

Other hormones play a significant role in the maintenance of blood pressure, fluid balance, and thermoregulation during acute exercise. A reduction in plasma volume triggered by a water shift out of the intravascular compartment leads to a reduction in blood pressure. The kidneys respond by activating the renin-angiotensin system resulting in aldosterone release from the adrenal cortex. Aldosterone promotes sodium (and water) reabsorption and maintains fluid balance. Plasma volume and blood pressure are also restored by the actions of antidiuretic hormone. Antidiuretic hormone is released from the posterior pituitary in response to an increase in plasma osmolarity and results in water reabsorption in the kidneys.

Finally, levels of anabolic hormones such as testosterone and progesterone increase during acute exercise, but the significance of this observation is unclear.

Cardiopulmonary Response

During exercise with large muscle groups, significant changes occur in the organs and systems responsible for the transport of oxygen from the atmosphere to the active muscles.[25] Pulmonary minute ventilation increases enhancing oxygen uptake, hemoglobin saturation, and clearance of carbon dioxide. The cardiovascular system responds with increases in heart rate, stroke volume, and cardiac output. Simultaneously,

peripheral vascular resistance is reduced and blood flow is preferentially increased to the exercising muscles as a result of local vasodilatation. Blood is shunted away from nonexercising regions such as the splanchnic and renal beds to the active muscles. Finally, capillaries in active muscles open to allow for a better exchange of nutrients and metabolites. Oxygen extraction by active muscle fibers results in a reduction in the oxygen content of venous blood and a widening of the arteriovenous oxygen difference, the difference between the oxygen content of arterial blood, which remains essentially unchanged during exercise, and the oxygen content of venous blood. The cardiovascular response to exercise is influenced by the amount of muscle mass (arm versus leg exercise) and the type of muscle action (static versus dynamic). Chapter 9 provides a detailed discussion of the cardiopulmonary response to exercise.

Hematologic Response

During exercise there is an acute increase in fibrinolysis as well as an increase in the number of platelets, but platelet function is unchanged.[26,27] A reduction in plasma volume results in hemoconcentration. Plasma volume decreases as a result of fluid shifts into the interstitial space. Increases in capillary hydrostatic pressure and intramuscular osmotic pressure contribute the fluid shift.[28,29] Sweat losses, necessary to dissipate heat and maintain core temperature, also contribute to reductions in plasma volume. Changes in plasma volume during prolonged exercise may compromise efficient temperature regulation and impair performance.

Renal Response

During vigorous exercise, decreases in renal blood flow, glomerular filtration rate, and urine production have been observed. As mentioned previously, the reduction in plasma volume and electrolyte losses in sweat activate the renin-angiotensin system and the release of aldosterone, trigger the release of antidiuretic hormone, and stimulate the electrolyte and water conservation mechanisms.[21] An increase in glomerular membrane permeability, which is more dependent on the intensity than the duration of the exercise, is associated with proteinuria.[30]

Psychological and Analgesic Effects

Aerobic exercise activates different endogenous opioid systems in the CNS including the β-endorphin, dynorphin, and enkephalin systems.[31] The activation of these systems appears to mediate the behavioral, mood (euphoria, sense of well-being, decreased anxiety), and analgesic (an increase in pain threshold) effects of exercise.

Exercise Training

Before considering specific issues clinicians should address in prescribing exercise intended to develop flexibility, strength, or endurance, it is useful to provide a brief review of the basic principles of training that underlie all exercise programs. The specifics vary greatly, depending on the type of training, the patient population, and the desired functional outcome. The term *training effect* refers to a series of predictable biochemical and neurophysiological adaptations to the repetitive performance of exercise.

Specificity

A key concept in training is that the biophysical adaptations and improved performance of muscle are specific to the training stimulus used, both the type of exercise and the specific muscle groups exercised. Furthermore, there is specificity of training, related to motor learning, that enhances the skilled performance of a specific task and is best accomplished by practicing that task.[14] Adaptations to training are greater when testing is conducted using the same training task or device.

Overload

To continue increasing a patient's flexibility, strength, or endurance, the required training stimulus must be increased periodically, in either intensity or duration, to ensure overloading the physiological systems. No training effect occurs unless the appropriate systems are stressed beyond the usual daily requirements or beyond the level to which they have become adapted.

Intensity

Intensity refers to the level at which the exercise will be performed. How intensity is expressed depends on the nature of the exercise being prescribed. When training for endurance (aerobic capacity), intensity may be measured as a percentage of the maximum oxygen consumption or power, maximum heart rate, or perceived rate of exertion. Training for strength may be prescribed in terms of either absolute or relative load (e.g., a percentage of the repetition maximum). These terms are discussed further in appropriate sections of this chapter.

Duration

Duration may be expressed in units of time for aerobic training, anaerobic training, or static holding. When training for muscle strength or endurance, duration can be expressed in terms of the number of sets and repetitions and the duration of the resting periods between them.

Frequency

In prescribing exercise it is important to state the required frequency. Because a training effect often requires overload resulting in a catabolic response in the muscle followed by an anabolic response, daily exercise may not be desirable when the goal is high-intensity strength training. When the goal is achieving optimal health, daily doses of moderate-intensity exercise may be required.[32] On the other hand, for neuromuscular reeducation the frequency of training may have to be more than once a day to produce adaptations and carryover. Stretching exercises usually need to be performed at least once a day to produce a good response. Thus, to decide on the frequency of training required to achieve the desired physiological response in the patient, the clinician needs to consider the goals of the program, type of exercise, its relative intensity, and the duration.

Interval Training

Interval training is exercise, performed intermittently, alternating periods of high-intensity with periods of less intense exercise or rest. This method has several clinical applications. For a deconditioned person with low tolerance, interval training extends the total time and amount of exercise that can be done.[33] Another application is training for short-duration, high-intensity exercise, such as sprint racing, where anaerobic conditioning is desirable. Anaerobic training occurs if relatively high loads are used during short intervals, whereas if the exercise stimulus is of submaximal intensity over longer periods, aerobic energy pathways are used and trained. The intensity and duration of the stimulus ultimately determine which system is preferentially trained.[14]

SPECIFIC TYPES OF EXERCISE

Exercise and Joint Range of Motion

Each joint has a physiological range of motion, and there is some variation among individuals. The clinician may prescribe flexibility exercises to prevent loss of joint range of motion in an immobilized hospital patient, to increase range where limitations already exist, or as stretching for a seasoned athlete. The act of stretching causes tension in both muscle and associated connective tissues. The effects on the connective tissues are detailed in the next section.

Anatomy and Physiology of Connective Tissue

Connective tissue is composed of collagen fibers within a proteoglycan matrix. Loose connective tissue is a relatively disorganized collection of collagen fibers that lines opposing mobile surfaces.[34] It may become fibrotic, contracted, and shortened when subjected to immobilization, resulting in joint capsule contractures and limited range of motion. Tendons and ligaments are made of organized connective tissue and have a linear arrangement of collagen fibers that is determined and maintained by regular deforming forces such as muscle tension. The rate of collagen turnover varies between tissues: Injured tissues have the highest rate of turnover, and tendon and skin relatively slow turnover.[35]

The joint capsule and ligaments provide an important contribution to the stabilization of joints. The capsule consists primarily of collagen and elastin, discounting the 70% that is water.[36] Another large contribution to joint stability derives from the surrounding musculature. Adaptive shortening occurs in muscles as well. A muscle immobilized in a shortened position demonstrates shortening within a week. After 3 weeks in this shortened position, the loose connective tissue in the muscle becomes dense connective tissue, and a fixed muscle contracture develops.[37] During the first 2 weeks of immobilization joint contractures are mainly caused by alterations in muscles and tendons.[38] After 2 weeks, joint changes in bone, cartilage, capsules, and ligaments become more significant.

Synovial fluid bathes the articular cartilage and is necessary to maintain lubrication and mobility of the joint. Boundary lubrication and a hydrostatic mechanism provide lubrication for the articulating cartilaginous surfaces. Boundary lubrication reduces friction by preventing the two articular surfaces from actually coming in contact, and it occurs through the binding of a glycoprotein to the cartilage surfaces.[39] The hydrostatic mechanism functions by squeezing water out of the cartilage by pressure, which coats the cartilage surface, providing lubrication.[40] This mechanism predominates at heavy loads. Hyaluronate provides boundary lubrication for the synovial tissues.[41] Immobility of the normal joint results in reduction in water (up to 6%), hyaluronic acid (40%), and other glycosaminoglycans, with a resultant loss of lubrication efficiency.[42]

Exercise to Maintain Range of Motion

For a healthy person, everyday use is all that is required to maintain a functional range of motion. If illness or surgery interferes with this use, slow, sustained stretch and range-of-motion exercises should be performed two or three times daily. Quick, jerky stretching is to be avoided, as it stimulates the muscle spindle of the intrafusal muscle fibers, causing the muscle to contract reflexively. On the other hand, slower sustained stretching causes firing of the Golgi tendon organs, which lie in series with extrafusal muscle fibers, and results in muscle relaxation.[43] Extra caution must be observed after surgery or in the presence of joint inflammation. Range-of-motion exercises may be performed by the patient actively, with partial assistance, or passively using another extremity, a therapist, or a continuous passive range-of-motion machine. Proper positioning to encourage passive stretching is another important technique in maintaining range of motion.

Stretching   Stretching applies physiological principles similar to those discussed in the preceding section. Tendons demonstrate nonlinear deformation in response to stress (Figure 16-3). In the first phase, little force is required for elongation, as the collagen fibers undergo straightening and the elastic fibers elongate. The second phase of elongation is characterized by breaking cross-links in the tendon and by disruption of some smaller collagen fibers. The second stage requires greater force per increment of elongation. If sufficient force is applied, a third phase of elongation, characterized by tendon failure, ensues when tendons are stretched more than 5–8% their resting length. The deformation of tendons is also time dependent. Application of a smaller force over a prolonged period results in tendon creep or irreversible elongation of the tendon. Application of superficial heat and ultrasound have been shown to facilitate tendon and muscle stretching, and neuromuscular facilitation techniques have been used to relax involved muscles.[44]

Exercise for Strength

Determinants of Strength   Strength may be defined as the maximal force that a muscle can produce. There are several major determinants of strength.

CROSS-SECTIONAL AREA   Strength is proportional to the cross-sectional area of a muscle, which is measured at right angles to the direction of the parallel muscle fibers.[45] Muscle cross-sectional area is related to the number and size of muscle fibers. In pathologic states, fat infiltration of muscle could give false large estimates of muscle cross-sectional area.

MUSCLE FIBER TYPE   The maximum force generated by a muscle is related to the proportions of fiber types that make up the muscle and how this compares with the task being asked of it (see Chapter 5, Table 5-1). Each human

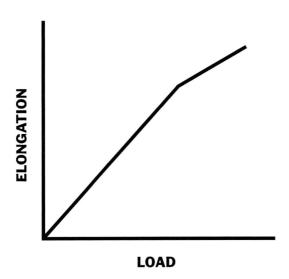

LOAD

FIGURE 16-3 The relationship between load and elongation of a tendon under stretch.

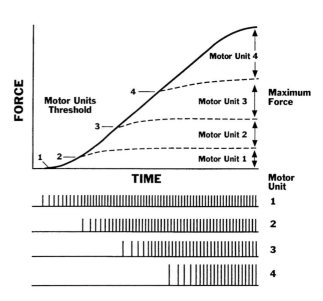

FIGURE 16-4 The sequential recruitment of motor units to provide increasing force of contraction. (Adapted from P-O Astrand, K Rodahl. Textbook of Work Physiology [3rd ed]. New York: McGraw-Hill, 1986.)

muscle is a mosaic of fiber types. The relative proportion of the different fiber types is determined by genetic and environmental influences.[46] Type I fibers are the slow oxidative fibers recruited early and during low-intensity activities. The type II fibers (which have two subtypes, IIa and IIb/IIx) are recruited later and respond to demands requiring higher forces generated over shorter periods. It is now accepted that fiber types represent a continuum rather than discrete fiber groups.[47] Some fibers coexpress more than one myosin heavy chain isoform (e.g., I *and* IIA or IIA *and* IIB) and are known as hybrid fibers. The fiber population of a given muscle is in a dynamic state, constantly adjusting to the current conditions.

RECRUITMENT   Recruitment of motor units in a coordinated, properly sequenced fashion also determines strength. Proper sequencing of agonist and antagonist activity is necessary for maximum voluntary contraction. The number of activated motor units and the degree to which motor units fire simultaneously to produce maximum tension, the synchronization ratio, is one determinant of muscle strength. Another factor in recruitment is the frequency of firing or rate coding.[48] Smaller motor units have a lower threshold for discharge and are recruited with low-force activities. As the need for increased force arises, these smaller motor units increase the frequency of discharge and additional (larger) motor units are recruited (Figure 16-4). These larger motor units in turn increase their discharge rate in response to increasing demand. Thus, both recruitment of new motor units and increasing frequency of firing (rate coding) are determinants of maximal strength.

LENGTH-FORCE AND FORCE-VELOCITY RELATIONSHIPS
The greatest total force that a muscle can develop is the sum of both active and passive force at any given length. In the laboratory, *equilibrium length* is defined as the length of an unstimulated, unattached muscle. Maximal force is generated by a muscle at 120% of its equilibrium length, corresponding ultrastructurally with the length at which there is maximum overlap between actin and myosin and therefore a larger number of cross-bridges.[14] Anatomic limitations of joint motion restrict muscle length to between 70% and 120% of their equilibrium length. In situ we do not know the exact location of the equilibrium length, but maximal force can usually be developed somewhere near the middle of the joint range of motion.

The velocity of muscle actions also affects the maximum strength that can be developed. Rapid concentric actions produce less force than slow concentric actions, whereas rapid eccentric actions produce more force than slow eccentric actions. Accordingly, the greatest force is developed during a rapid eccentric action, and the least force with a rapid concentric action (Figure 16-5).[49] These characteristics can be used in the design of strengthening programs.[50]

PSYCHOLOGICAL FACTORS   Neuropsychological factors play a role in the measurement and development of strength. Motivation at any given time is important as is overall motivation to pursue a training regimen. Astrand and Rodahl discuss the positive and negative effects of psychological stress on athletic performance.[14]

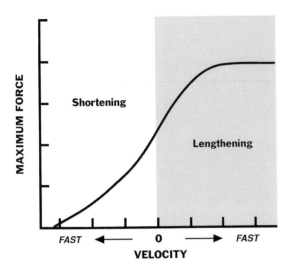

FIGURE 16-5 The relationship between speed of contraction and maximum force generated for shortening (concentric) and lengthening (eccentric) contractions. The 0 velocity point represents an isometric contraction. (Adapted from HG Knuttgen. Neuromuscular Mechanisms for Therapeutic and Conditioning Exercise. Baltimore: University Park Press, 1976.)

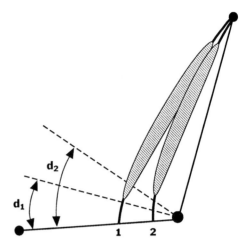

FIGURE 16-6 The relationship between the point of insertion of muscle and the maximum arc of rotation. Insertion closer to the center of rotation allows a greater arc but a lower maximum force. (Adapted from BJ DeLateur. Exercise for Strength and Endurance. In JV Basmajian [ed], Therapeutic Exercise [4th ed]. Baltimore: Williams & Wilkins, 1984.)

Visual input, perceptual ability, and proprioceptive feedback are also necessary for optimal strength.

KINESIOLOGY The geometry of the origin and insertion of the muscle relative to the joint line that will serve as the center of the axis of rotation is important in determining torque. When the muscle inserts close to the center of the axis of rotation, less force can be exerted at the distal end but a larger arc is generated. When the insertion is farther from the center of rotation, the converse is true (i.e., greater force is exerted over a shorter arc) (Figure 16-6).[51] The position of the muscle is also important, as the maximum force is generated at a muscle length approximately 1.2 times the equilibrium length (see Length-Force and Force-Velocity Relationships, earlier in this chapter). The maximum tension that can be generated depends on the lever arm and the relative length at the time of contraction.

Standard Training Programs

Progressive Resistive Exercise

Progressive resistive exercise describes dynamic strengthening exercise that involves using weights or resistance for a specified number of repetitions and sets. As training progresses, resistance is increased. Two techniques of progressive resistive exercise have been popularized in the literature: DeLorme and Oxford.[52,53] In 1945, DeLorme first described his techniques, based on the 10 repetition maximum (10 RM). A *repetition maximum* is

the maximum weight that can be moved through the joint's full range of motion against gravity a given number of times. Thus, the 10 RM is the load that can be lifted 10 times through the full range. Based on a new 10 RM determined each week, the training sessions consist of 10 repetitions each at 50%, 75%, and 100% of the 10 RM. As the patient's strength increases, the 10 RM is increased accordingly. One potential disadvantage of the technique is that the patient may become fatigued toward the end of the session, just when the highest load is to be lifted.

The Oxford technique is similar to the DeLorme technique, except that each session starts with 10 repetitions of 100% 10 RM, followed by 10 repetitions each of 75% and 50% of 10 RM. The fact that patients report less fatigue with the Oxford method may make this a less effective form of training than the traditional DeLorme technique.[54] Another disadvantage of the Oxford technique is that the muscle is not warmed up before maximal effort is exerted. Disadvantages of both techniques are that they are time consuming and may require assistance from a physical therapist or trainer.

Several important issues with any training technique are (1) selection of muscle groups and contraction mode, (2) choice of exercise, (3) order of exercise, (4) number of sets and repetitions, (5) rest periods, and (6) intensity of training.[55,56] To increase the strength of the muscle, the patient may progressively increase the weight lifted or the rate at which a given weight is lifted.

Eccentric Training

Eccentric muscle actions should be part of a strength training routine. The inclusion of eccentric actions can be accomplished using free weights or special devices that variably adjust the resistance or control the angular velocity (isokinetic). In these routines, resistance is provided for both the concentric and eccentric actions of each muscle group. Eccentric actions alone or in combination with concentric actions have been shown to result in larger strength gains, more EMG activity, and larger changes in type II muscle fiber area than concentric actions alone.[3,57,58] Because of the possibility of muscle damage, eccentric actions should be used with caution, especially in untrained subjects.

Isokinetic Training

Isokinetic exercise requires special equipment, now produced by a number of manufacturers, to provide a constant angular velocity (measured in degrees per second) during muscle actions. The machine allows the individual to exert maximum force throughout the range of motion and provides a corresponding resistance to maintain the velocity of the movement. A particularly useful feature of several of these machines is a printout or graphic documentation of a subject's progress. One unique concern of isokinetic training is the specificity of the velocity of training: Optimal training effects are achieved at the velocity at which training occurs; therefore, the velocity chosen for training should correspond to the velocity required for the ultimate (functional) activity.[59] The maximal torque for concentric isokinetic actions decreases with increasing velocity,[60] whereas the reverse is true for eccentric isokinetic actions.[61]

Static (Isometric) Training

Static exercise may be performed for strength training; the recommended duration of each contraction is 6 seconds. Muller described an isometric program with a 1-second maximal contraction per muscle per day.[62] Although this seems attractive in its simplicity and efficiency, most clinicians find that programs of multiple contractions lasting 6 seconds are more effective. The strength gains are specific to the angle at which the exercise is performed, and this limits its general applicability.[55] The major utility of static exercise is for patients whose joint range of motion is either limited or, owing to inflammation or surgery, uncomfortable when the clinician wants to prevent significant atrophy.

Mechanisms of Strength Gain

The two major mechanisms of strength gain that underlie all strengthening programs are peripheral changes in muscle, including hypertrophy of individual muscle fibers, and adaptations in the nervous system.[63] During the first 1–2 weeks of training the major contribution to strength gain is from neural factors.[64] The neural mechanisms underlying the early phase of training are not well understood but appear to include better synchronization and more effective recruitment of motor units, resulting in higher muscle contractile activity.[65] Hypertrophy becomes the dominant factor in increased strength after several weeks. An increase in muscle fiber number has been reported in experimental animals and hyperplasia may also play a role in muscle enlargement in humans.[66,67]

The availability of cellular and molecular techniques has improved our understanding of the mechanism underlying skeletal muscle hypertrophy. An increase in the size of muscle fibers reflects accumulation of contractile and noncontractile proteins.[68,69] This process may be initiated by forces that alter cell shape and generate mechanical signals that influence gene expression and appears to occur in two stages.[70] During the first stage, an increase in protein synthesis is regulated at the translational and posttranslational levels. Later in the time course of muscle enlargement, the levels of myofibrillar protein messenger RNA increase. The increase in mRNA can be achieved by an up-regulation of the given gene (an increase in the transcription rate) or by the activation of satellite cells.[69,71] The fusion of satellite cells with mature muscle fibers provides a source for new myonuclei available for protein synthesis and ensures a tight coupling between the quantity of genetic machinery and the protein requirements of a fiber during hypertrophy.[67,72]

Muscle size and function can be also influenced by the endocrine system and the use of exogenous anabolic steroids. The use of testosterone, growth hormone, and insulin-like growth factor (IGF-1) is known to result in significant fiber hypertrophy and proliferation of satellite cells.[73,74] These agents can interact with resistance exercise and mechanical loading to induce hypertrophy, prevent the effects of disuse, or both. The use of anabolic steroids, in combination with strength training, may enhance the activation of satellite cells.[67]

After strength training, the relative proportion of type I and II fibers remains constant, but considerable changes can occur in the area of each fiber type.[3,75] The mechanism of strength gain does not appear to change with aging: Even nonagenarians have been shown to respond to a strengthening program with increased strength and muscle hypertrophy.[76] Finally, research suggests that genetic factors could influence the magnitude of the response to the strengthening stimulus.[77]

Which type of strengthening exercises to prescribe for a patient depends on the desired goal. Because the expected results are specific to the training modality, it makes the most sense to tailor the training regimen to the patient's needs and the dynamics of the activity. At all times, it must be remembered that the muscle must be *overloaded* and the training tasks must exceed the demands of everyday activity. The clinician must regularly reassess and upgrade the prescription if strength gain is to continue.

Exercise for Endurance

In discussing endurance training, the distinction must first be made between training for muscle endurance and training for total body endurance (cardiovascular or aerobic capacity).

Training Muscle Endurance

Muscle endurance must be defined operationally for each situation. It may refer to the holding time for a static action, the number of repetitions of a brief static action, or the number of repetitions of a dynamic action (concentric, eccentric, or isokinetic). Research shows that static and dynamic endurance can be trained preferentially.[78] It is equally important to consider the force of the action as a percentage of the maximal strength of that muscle. Figure 16-7 demonstrates the relationship between strength and endurance for both dynamic and

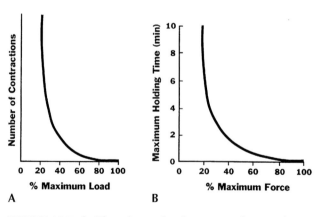

FIGURE 16-7 A. The relationship between endurance (number of contractions) and relative load for dynamic work. (Adapted from HG Knuttgen. Neuromuscular Mechanisms for Therapeutic and Conditioning Exercise. Baltimore: University Park Press, 1976.) **B.** The relationship between endurance (holding time) and relative load for static work. (Adapted from FJ Kottke, GK Stillwell, JF Lehmann [eds], Krusen's Handbook of Physical Medicine and Rehabilitation [3rd ed]. Philadelphia: Saunders, 1987.)

static actions. This relationship clearly indicates that increasing the strength of a muscle increases the endurance for any given absolute submaximal load by making it a smaller percentage of the maximum contraction.

The DeLorme axiom states that muscle endurance can be trained by using relatively low loads for high numbers of repetitions (as opposed to high-load, low-repetition training for strength). This concept was called into question by DeLateur, in a study that demonstrated that loads in a fairly broad range (30–100% of maximum) had similar effects on strength and endurance if the exercises were performed to the point of fatigue.[54] The important role of fatigue in strength training programs has been emphasized by studies in the literature.[79]

Training for Aerobic Capacity

Aerobic training programs increase the ability of the body to transport and use oxygen ($\dot{V}O_2$max).[80] The benefits of aerobic training are caused by a combination of central and peripheral adaptations.[81,82] The changes in the cardiac response to exercise after such a program are discussed in Chapter 9.

An important adaptation to endurance training is an increase in blood volume. The increased blood volume combines with the training-induced bradycardia to produce greater diastolic filling, and thus a larger stroke volume. After training, a higher stroke volume combines with a slightly reduced heart rate to produce a higher maximum cardiac output resulting in an enhanced $\dot{V}O_2$max. An increase in vascular conductance (or reduction in peripheral vascular resistance) facilitates the increase in blood flow needed to deliver the necessary oxygen and nutrients to the active muscle. A reduction in peripheral resistance reduces the afterload on the left ventricle.

Endurance training has a different effect than strength training on the histologic and biochemical properties of skeletal muscle. The adaptations in endurance-trained muscles include an increase in capillarization, an increase in the number and size of mitochondria, and an early (7–10 days) increase in the activity of oxidative enzymes.[83–85] These adaptations enhance the capacity of trained muscles to extract oxygen from arterial blood and to alter fuel metabolism. With prolonged endurance training there may be a decrease in the size of type I fibers. This decrease in the cross-sectional area of the type I fibers, together with the increases in capillary density and in the myoglobin content of the fibers, shortens the diffusion distance for oxygen and nutrients into the cell. Together, these adaptations make each absolute exercise load a smaller percentage of the maximum aerobic capacity.

In the trained state, the metabolic and endocrine responses to exercise are significantly modified. At a given exercise intensity, energy derived from the metabolism of fatty acid metabolism predominates and glycogen stores are spared.[19] This is because of adaptations at different levels including FFA mobilization, transport, uptake, and mitochondrial oxidation. Also, intramuscular triglyceride stores supply a large portion of the increase in oxidized fatty acids.[86] It is interesting that in the trained state resting fatty acid oxidation is increased. This may be an important mechanism for replenishing muscle triglycerides after an acute bout of exercise and for rapidly increasing fatty acid oxidation at the onset of exercise.[87] Finally, the activity of the sympathetic nervous system and the increase in levels of circulating catecholamines at a constant power output associated with the acute response to exercise are depressed with endurance training. This is also true of the growth hormone response to an acute bout of exercise.[88]

Typical aerobic training programs use dynamic exercise of large muscle groups. Owing to the specificity of training it is necessary to include all groups that the patient needs for vocational and avocational uses. The usual exercises include walking, running, swimming, rowing, cycling, aerobic calisthenics, or arm ergometry. The intensity of exercise is usually expressed as a percentage of the maximum heart rate or $\dot{V}O_2$max. Although training at 60–85% of any person's age-determined maximum heart rate (see Chapter 9) is usually considered ideal, training benefits can be achieved with intensities in the range of 40–60% of maximum, if a wider margin of safety is needed because of coronary artery disease or if the patient is too debilitated to tolerate a more strenuous program.

Any exercise training program ought to include warm-up and cool-down phases. During a warm-up of less intense activity, activation of various physiological systems occurs followed by stretching of the soft tissues, making the exercise more efficient and less likely to cause injury.[89] A cool-down phase of gradually decreasing intensity exercise reduces the risk of postural hypotension and cardiac arrhythmia. The duration of training can vary from 20–60 minutes, not including the warm-up and cool-down phases. Frequency of training is usually three to five times a week. A significant increase in aerobic capacity (reflected in lower heart rate at the same submaximal loads) should be evident within 4–6 weeks. At the beginning of the program the patient should be advised that all of the improvements in exercise capacity and cardiac response to exercise will be lost in a short time unless a maintenance program is followed after the end of the formal training period.

Training for Cardiopulmonary Rehabilitation

The changes in the cardiopulmonary response to exercise that occur with aerobic training programs can be used to design rehabilitation programs for cardiac and pulmonary disease patients. Such programs can increase the work capacity of these patients even though there may be no change in the coronary circulation and no change in lung volumes or gas exchange (see Chapter 9).

Cardiac rehabilitation after a myocardial infarction begins in the cardiac care unit. In an uncomplicated case the goal is to provide a gradual increase in exercise intensity, progressing from bed rest to stair climbing over a period of days.[90] After discharge from the hospital the patient usually goes through a 6- to 8-week convalescent phase, during which the intensity of exercise remains constant, but duration is gradually increased. The next phase involves aerobic training (described in Chapter 9). The advantage of training for the cardiac patient is based on the change in myocardial oxygen consumption and the peripheral adaptations. Thus, even though there is no change in the anginal threshold, more exercise can be performed within that limit.

Rehabilitation for pulmonary disease patients has largely the same rationale. (The improved efficiency of ventilation that follows an aerobic training program is also described in Chapter 9.) In addition to the improved ventilatory mechanics, the pulmonary patient who has been inactive for some time may actually realize a decrease in oxygen consumption for submaximal activities, owing to the improved mechanical efficiency that results from improved movement skills.[91] Overall, however, the usual result of training is increased exercise capacity with little or no change in lung volume, flow rate, or arterial blood gases.

Exercise for Neuromuscular Re-Education

For rehabilitation of patients with impaired voluntary motor control caused by CNS disease such as cerebral palsy, cerebrovascular accident, traumatic brain injury, or brain tumor, the focus of the exercise program becomes acquisition or reacquisition of controlled, coordinated voluntary movement rather than of strength or endurance per se. *Control* is the ability to carry out a chosen activity with the proper intensity and to start and stop that activity at will. *Coordination* is the ability to execute a properly timed, sequenced, and manipulated purposeful movement in a smooth manner. In training for coordination, the patient develops a motor engram after many repetitions of the same activity sequence (an *engram* is the neuronal representation in the CNS of a specific preprogrammed pattern of muscle performance). As coordination develops through repetition and practice, the patient can perform the same activity with greater efficiency and fluidity. It has been suggested that millions of repetitions are necessary to develop maximum performance of a new motor activity.[92,93]

The development of an engram requires facilitation of the desired activity and inhibition of undesired movements. All of the various systems for neuromuscular re-education use either facilitative or inhibitory techniques to modify primitive and advanced postural reflexes for the purpose of enhancing movement, increasing coordination, controlling abnormal tone, or enhancing stretching in normal muscles. The clinical applications of neuromuscular re-education programs include pre-exercise stretching, normalization of muscle tone, and enhancement of function in patients with conditions such as cerebral palsy, head injury, stroke, or spinal cord injury. Before discussing the major techniques for neurofacilitation, it is useful to review the underlying neurophysiological reflexes.

Reflexes Used in Neuromuscular Re-Education Programs

The *primitive postural reflexes* are defined as those that are coordinated in the spinal cord or medulla. They include the flexion reflex,[94] the long spinal reflex, and the crossed extension-flexion reflex.[95] With the exception of the stretch reflex, which is normally present in adults, these reflexes are present at birth and normally disappear early in infancy, reappearing only in the presence of abnormal cortical development, as in cerebral palsy, or acquired higher CNS dysfunction such as stroke or head injury.

The stretch reflex (also known as the *myotatic reflex*) is routinely tested during the neurologic examination. It is a simple reflex with the afferent input resulting from change in muscle length received via the muscle spindle and transmitted by the Ia afferents to the spinal cord. Monosynaptic excitement of the alpha motor neurons that supply the stretched muscle results in muscle contraction. Full details are presented in Chapter 6.

Control of Muscle Tone

A certain amount of tone (resistance to passive stretch) is present in normal resting muscle. Diseases that affect the lower motor neuron reduce tone, making the limb floppy. The conditions that are treated with neuromuscular re-education techniques usually involve damage to the upper motor neuron, where there is increased tone or spasticity. The hallmark of spasticity is increased resistance to passive stretch, which becomes greater when the speed of stretching is increased and is associated with increased deep tendon reflexes and clonus. In general terms, spasticity is the result of reduced higher level regulatory influence on the spinal reflexes and decreased inhibition of the Ia motor neurons from descending cortical influence. (For a detailed discussion, see Chapters 1, 2, 3, and 6.) The typical hemiplegic limb demonstrates impaired isolated joint movement; instead, movement patterns are crude and synergistic.[96] There are typical extension and flexion synergy patterns in the lower and upper extremities that become important in the discussion of the different neurofacilitation techniques that follows.

Neurofacilitation and Inhibition Techniques

Next we discuss four commonly used neurofacilitation methods with their physiological rationale and clinical applications. Although all are in common clinical use and most therapists use an eclectic approach, there is little hard evidence that any of these techniques alters the natural history of recovery from the conditions for which they are used. The methods are useful, however, in providing compensatory techniques; making transfers, bed mobility, stretching, and even ambulation safer; and rendering patients better able to perform them with less assistance.

Proprioceptive Neuromuscular Facilitation   Proprioceptive neuromuscular facilitation (PNF) uses resistance to facilitate movement.[97] The therapist provides maximal resistance to the stronger muscle components of specific spiral and diagonal patterns, thus facilitating the pattern's weaker components. The amount of resistance must be limited for patients with spasticity, so as not to further increase the tone. For that reason, PNF is best applied for supraspinal lesions with hypotonia to promote normalization of tone.[98,99]

PNF techniques can be applied to sports medicine. One common application is PNF techniques of stretching, which all use static actions and relaxation of the muscle being stretched.[100] It is not clear that PNF techniques of stretching have any advantage over static stretching techniques in neurologically intact adults. Magnusson et al.[101] studied mechanical and physical responses to stretching with and without prestatic action and found that at a constant angle the viscoelastic and EMG responses were unaffected by the static action. PNF has also been studied to determine possible beneficial effects on reaction time and response time. Surburg[102] compared the effects of three training programs—weight training, PNF without resistance, and PNF with maximum resistance—and found no significant changes between the training groups after 6 weeks.

Brunnstrom Twitchell described six stages of motor recovery, which progress from complete flaccidity and paralysis through the appearance of spasticity and gross synergistic movements to the disappearance of spasticity and the return of isolated joint movements and coordinated activity.[96] The Brunnstrom techniques use resistance, associated reactions, and primitive postural reactions to facilitate gross synergistic movement and return of muscle tone, especially in the early stages of recovery.[103] During later stages of recovery, development of isolated movement and control are emphasized. Like the PNF technique, the Brunnstrom method is advocated to help normalize tone in a hemiplegic patient with persistent flaccidity.

Bobath or Neurodevelopmental Techniques In contradistinction to the PNF and Brunnstrom methods, the neurodevelopmental techniques developed by the Bobaths emphasize normalization of increased tone using certain reflex inhibitory movement patterns.[104] These reflex inhibitory movement patterns are generally opposite to the typical hemiplegia synergy patterns and are performed without resistance. In addition, neurodevelopmental techniques incorporate the use of advanced postural reactions to help stimulate recovery. It has been claimed that neurodevelopmental techniques facilitate motor recovery and reduce hypertonicity.

Rood The Rood method uses tactile stimuli such as fast brushing, quick stroking, or icing of the skin, ostensibly to facilitate specific groups of muscles to promote functional activity.[105,106] The selection of muscle groups depends on which stage of development or recovery the patient has achieved. Rood described four stages of neurophysiological mobility: (1) development of functional mobility, (2) development of stability, (3) development of stability and mobility, and (4) development of skilled movement.[107] Level 1 involves activities such as rolling over. Levels 2 and 3 incorporate the development of stability, which prepares the body for weight bearing, including positions such as quadruped and standing. Last, level 4 involves development of skilled movements, such as walking. The Rood techniques are reversible and can be used either to stimulate activity in a patient with hypotonia or to decrease spasticity in a patient with hypertonia.

Exercise for Development of Proprioception and Coordination

Frenkel's exercises are commonly used for impairment of proprioception caused by CNS pathology or incoordination caused by cerebellar dysfunction. Exercises of progressive complexity begin with the patient in a supine position, followed as the patient improves by sitting and standing. Precise coordination and motion are stressed, as well as accurate performance of each task. Repetition and visual feedback help the patient reinforce the acquired skills.[108]

Plyometric Training

Plyometric exercise harnesses force to store energy using the elastic properties of the myotendinous units. This energy is recovered by a rapid generation of force in the opposite direction to produce an explosive surge of power. A common example of plyometric exercise is vertical jumping. Plyometric exercise is intense and its goal is to optimize the recovery of energy stored in the muscle during an eccentric action by minimizing the time the body has to recover from the force.

Studies analyzing the benefits of plyometric training have demonstrated mixed results. Hewett et al.[109] conducted a study to test the effect of a jump-training program on landing mechanics and lower extremity strength in female athletes involved in jumping sports. After training, female athletes demonstrated lower landing forces, improved hamstring muscle power, and increased mean vertical jump height. It was suggested that this training may have a significant effect on knee stabilization and possibly prevent knee injury in female jump athletes.

In contrast, Kramer et al.[110] found that the addition of plyometric exercise training to the standard training for female rowers did not offer advantages to intercollegiate novice or experienced oarswomen. Cossor et al.[111] examined the effects of a plyometric training program on free-style tumble turns in swimmers. There were equal benefits derived from normal practice time as compared with the group with added plyometric training. Lastly, Heiderscheit et al.[112] analyzed the effects of isokinetic versus plyometric training of the shoulder internal rotators. Isokinetic training of the shoulder internal rotators increased isokinetic power; however, neither form of training resulted in a functional improvement with the softball throw. Although plyometric training may have utility to enhance function in jump athletes, further studies are needed to clarify the efficacy of this approach and determine its most appropriate indications.

FATIGUE

Definition

Fatigue can be defined as the inability to maintain a given force or power output. In a clinical sense, as Dill pointed out, "The various unmistakably disagreeable sensations commonly referred to by the word fatigue are in fact the accompaniments of a great variety of different physiological conditions, which have in common only this, that the physiological equilibrium of the body is somewhere breaking down."[113] Darling has warned against confusing the symptoms of fatigue with fatigue itself.[114] Isolated muscle fatigue is characterized by a diminished response to an unchanging stimulus or requirement of a larger stimulus to produce the same response. Distinctions between generalized fatigue and local muscle fatigue are considered in the following sections.

Generalized Fatigue

For the purposes of this discussion, *generalized fatigue* is defined as the state that occurs when the physiological systems of an organism have been taxed to the degree that the homeostatic mechanisms begin to break down. A preset level of exercise cannot be sustained and objective signs may include decreased speed, accuracy, or coordination. The duration of exercise needed to produce generalized fatigue varies with the relative intensity of the exercise for the individual. Most authorities acknowledge that in the industrial setting an intensity greater than 30–40% of the individual's maximum aerobic capacity cannot be sustained for an 8-hour day without producing generalized fatigue.[14,115] Only well-trained athletes can tolerate exercise at higher intensities (60–80% of $\dot{V}O_2$max) for prolonged (hours) periods. Depending on the type of exercise and its intensity, the limiting factor may be the metabolic alterations associated with products such as lactic acid and hydrogen ions, the depletion of metabolic substrates such as glycogen, or a decrease in CNS input.[116]

The relationship of generalized fatigue to the relative intensity of exercise is extremely important in rehabilitation medicine. People with disabilities must deal with a combination of higher than usual energy requirements for most activities (owing to the poor mechanical efficiency of abnormal gait patterns and assistive devices) and lower than normal aerobic power and endurance (because of underlying pathology and deconditioning). Because they rarely are fit, most people with disabilities avoid generalized fatigue by limiting their activities and lifestyles.

Muscle Fatigue

Muscle fatigue refers to a process that is closer to the original physiological definition of a diminished response to the same stimulus. It may be associated with the subjective symptoms of muscle soreness, stiffness, or pain. Objective signs include decreased rate or rhythm of exercise, substitution of other muscles, and decreased precision of performance. Although the final outcome may be similar, the mechanism of muscular fatigue varies with the type, intensity, and duration of muscle action.[117] Except in myasthenia gravis or dosing with curariform drugs, fatigue is not the result of failure of neuromuscular transmission. With static actions, the limiting factor appears to be local ischemia caused by decreased circulation, which results in significant metabolic alterations in active muscle cells. With dynamic actions there may be a combination of central and peripheral factors, including depletion of intracellular potassium, depletion of glycogen in the muscle, accumulation of lactate and metabolites such as inorganic phosphate, reduced pH (protons can reduce enzyme activity in the muscle fibers or interfere with the contractile elements), reduction of calcium ion release from the sarcoplasmic reticulum, depletion of blood glucose, or undefined CNS factors.[117,118]

The onset and rate of fatigue can be evaluated in the clinical setting or the laboratory by documenting changes in force production and recording EMG indicators. Under dynamic conditions, fatigue has been measured using isokinetic instruments. The reported measures during repeated actions include the average power output over time (*newton-meters per unit time*),[119] the percent decline in force after a preset number of muscle actions,[120] and a fatigue index determined by the percent decline in a specified amount of time such as 15 or 30 seconds of repeated muscle actions.[121] Protocols using sustained static actions have also been described. For example, Kent-Braun recorded the decline in force in 4 minutes of a static maximal action of the ankle dorsiflexors.[122]

Surface EMG has been used extensively to examine the physiological aspects of fatigue onset and development. A major advantage of using EMG is that with careful electrode placement, filtering and signal processing activity of single muscles can be studied. With force or torque measures alone, the contributions of additional or substitute muscles may affect the performance characteristics. Further, changes in force production, occurring at a specific point in time, do not provide insight into the processes that result in the state of fatigue. Integrated EMG, root mean square of compound muscle action potentials generated, frequency spectrum analysis, and total reaction time (premotor time and electromechanical delay) are measures that have been used to describe the physiological events that lead to muscle fatigue. An indicator of the onset of fatigue is an increase in integrated EMG and root mean square, which may reflect recruitment of additional motor units and increased firing rate of active fibers as the force capability of active muscle fibers begins to decline.[123,124] Roy et al. have described a fatigue-related shift in median frequency from high to lower values in healthy subjects and in subjects with low back pain.[125] The firing rate of motor units and the shape of motor unit action potentials are considered important factors that contribute to this spectral shift. Recording the shift in the frequency spectrum allows for documenting the onset and development of the fatigued state, whereas decreases in torque or changes in integrated EMG become obvious when fatigue is already present. Yeung et al. studied the effect of a fatigue protocol of repeated static actions on reaction time.[126] They found that the electromechanical delay time was significantly longer after exercise, which they attribute to a change in peripheral as opposed to central mechanisms.

The use of EMG technology continues to provide information to dissect the physiological elements of muscular fatigue. (See Chapter 14.) Many of the current studies, however, are limited to protocols using static actions in normal, healthy subjects. Although this approach is clinically and scientifically useful, it may be limited when applied to normal daily activities requiring both static and dynamic muscular activity. Future application of this technology to study patients with neuromuscular deficits may aid in the design of more effective therapeutic interventions.

The onset of muscle fatigue with static actions varies with the relative intensity of the exercise. A maximal action can be sustained for a few seconds, 50% maximum for a minute or so, and a 15% maximum contraction for more than 10 minutes. A similar phenomenon is seen with dynamic actions.[14] The decrease in time to fatigue is exponential in relation to the maximum action. Although the exponential increase noted in most studies begins at 10–15% of maximum, there is evidence that this value decreases when applied to a full working day. In the industrial workplace, even loads less than 10% of maximum may produce local muscle fatigue. In the rehabilitation setting, again the emphasis is on relative load for the individual muscles involved. For example, the activity of the upper extremity muscles is higher when a patient walks with an ambulation aid or propels a wheelchair, and if these muscles are not trained they may fatigue prematurely.

Fatigue is reversible with rest. It is a normal phenomenon; indeed, it is necessary for training to occur.[79] Of concern to clinicians is the possibility of irreversible damage resulting from extreme exercise. Although this is most likely to occur in patients with lower motor neuron weakness (best exemplified by the postpolio syndrome), it has also been described in people with apparently normal neuromuscular systems.

OVERTRAINING

The overtraining syndrome has been defined as an imbalance between training and recovery. It is also known as a maladaptive response to the training stimulus resulting from an extended period of overload. This response is not well understood and its diagnosis is elusive. Risk factors for the development of the overtraining syndrome include (1) highly motivated athletes, (2) overly enthusiastic coaches, (3) occupational or social stress, and (4) mistakes in the distribution of the training loads. Commonly reported symptoms are decreased physical performance, fatigue, depressed mood, emotional swings, decreased appetite, sleep disturbances, elevated resting heart rate, and weight loss.

The endocrine system is believed to play a central role in overtraining and alterations in hormonal levels include increases in cortisol and catecholamines and reductions in testosterone and thyroxine.[22,127,128] This combination of hormonal alterations results in a catabolic state. Excessive training may also be associated with an increased incidence of infections.[129] This may be related to a suppression of the immune function manifested by low levels of lymphocytes, antibodies, and complement; especially during the transition between resting and training states. However, not all athletes demonstrate this response during intense training.[130] A reduction in training intensity may be required to eliminate symptoms of overtraining, and cyclic training (periodization) is needed to prevent a recurrence.

CONCLUSION

Therapeutic exercise is likely to remain a cornerstone of the rehabilitation armamentarium. Reasonable, functionally significant goals must be identified before the exercise prescription is selected. Only then can the clinician choose the proper form of exercise and prescribe the proper dose. Suitable rest periods must be considered to avoid the pitfalls of fatigue. Determination of appropriate outcome measures depends on an intelligent understanding of the effects of exercise and the selection of the proper exercise for the established functional goals of patients.

REFERENCES

1. Caspersen CJ, Powell KE, Christenson GM. Physical activity, exercise, and physical fitness: definitions and distinctions for health-related research. Pub Health Rep 1985;100:126–131.

2. Knuttgen HG, Komi PV. Basic Definitions for Exercise. In PV Komi (ed), Strength and Power in Sport. Oxford: Blackwell Scientific Publications, 1992;3–6.

3. Hortobagyi T, Hill JP, Houmard JA, et al. Adaptive responses to muscle lengthening and shortening in humans. J Appl Physiol 1996;80:765–772.

4. Fridén J, Lieber RL. Structural and mechanical basis of exercise-induced muscle injury. Med Sci Sports Exerc 1999;24:521–530.

5. Armstrong RB. Mechanisms of exercise-induced delayed onset muscular soreness: a brief review. Med Sci Sports Exerc 1984;16:529–538.

6. Thistle HG, Hislop HJ, Moffroid M, et al. Isokinetic contraction: a new concept of resistive exercise. Arch Phys Med Rehabil 1967;48:279–282.

7. Hageman PA. Concentric and eccentric isokinetic testing of the extremities. Crit Rev Phys Rehabil Med 1990;2: 49–63.

8. Kamber M, Koster M, Kreis R, et al. Creatine supplementation—Part I: performance, clinical chemistry, and muscle volume. Med Sci Sports Exerc 1999;31:1763–1769.

9. Kreis R, Kamber M, Koster M, et al. Creatine supplementation—Part II: in vivo magnetic resonance spectroscopy. Med Sci Sports Exerc 1999;31:1770–1777.

10. Bogdanis GC, Nevill ME, Boobis LH, et al. Contribution of phosphocreatine and aerobic metabolism to energy supply during repeated sprint exercise. J Appl Physiol 1996;80:876–884.

11. Bogdanis GC, Nevill ME, Lakomy HKA, et al. Power output and muscle metabolism during and following recovery from 10 and 20 s of maximal sprint exercise in humans. Acta Physiol Scand 1998;163:261–272.

12. Walter G, Vandenborne K, McCully KK, et al. Noninvasive measurement of phosphocreatine recovery kinetics in single human muscles. Am J Physiol 1997;41:C525–C534.

13. Conley KE, Blei ML, Richards TL, et al. Activation of glycolysis in human muscle in vivo. Am J Physiol 1997;273:C306–C315.

14. Astrand P-O, Rodahl K. Textbook of Work Physiology (3rd ed). New York: McGraw-Hill, 1986.

15. Wasserman K, Hansen JE, Sue DY. Facilitation of oxygen consumption by lactic acidosis during exercise. NIPS 1991;6:29–34.

16. Péronnet F, Burelle Y, Massicotte D, et al. Respective oxidation of ^{13}C-labeled lactate and glucose ingested simultaneously during exercise. J Appl Physiol 1997;82:440–446.

17. Romijn JA, Coyle EF, Sidossis LS, et al. Regulation of endogenous fat and carbohydrate metabolism in relation to exercise intensity and duration. Am J Physiol 1993;265:E380–E391.

18. Rodgers CD. Fuel metabolism during exercise: the role of the glucose-fatty acid cycle in mediating carbohydrate and fat metabolism. Can J Appl Physiol 1998;23:528–533.

19. Kiens B. Effect of endurance training on fatty acid metabolism: local adaptations. Med Sci Sports Exerc 1997;29:640–645.

20. Brooks GA, Mercier J. Balance of carbohydrate and lipid utilization during exercise: the "crossover" concept. J Appl Physiol 1994;76:2253–2261.

21. Galbo H. Hormonal and Metabolic Adaptations to Exercise. Stuttgart: Georg Thieme Verlag, 1983.

22. Wilmore JH, Costill DL. Physiology of Sport and Exercise. Champaign, IL: Human Kinetics, 1999.

23. Richter EA, Garetto CP, Goodman MN, et al. Muscle glucose metabolism following exercise in the rat: increased sensitivity to insulin. J Clin Invest 1982;69:785.

24. Richter EA, Ruderman NB, Schneider SH. Diabetes and exercise. Am J Med 1981;70:201.

25. Laughlin MH. Cardiovascular response to exercise. Adv Physiol Educ 1999;22: S244–S259.

26. Simon HB. Exercise, Health, and Sports Medicine. In E Rubenstein (ed), Scientific American Medicine. New York: Scientific American, 1988;8.

27. Warlow CP, Ogston D. Effect of exercise on platelet count, adhesion and aggregation. Acta Haematol 1974; 52:47.

28. Oscai LB, Williams BT, Hertig BA. Effect of exercise on blood volume. J Appl Physiol 1968;24:622.

29. Pivarnik JM, Montain SJ, Graves JE, et al. Alterations in plasma volume, electrolytes and protein during incremental exercise at different pedal speeds. Eur J Appl Physiol 1988;57:103.

30. Poortmans JR. Postexercise proteinuria in humans. JAMA 1985;253:236.

31. Hoffmann P, Jonsdottir IH, Thorén P. Activation of different opioid systems by muscle activity and exercise. News Physiol Sci 1996;11:223.

32. Department of Health and Human Services. Physical activity and health: a report of the Surgeon General. Atlanta: National Center for Chronic Disease Prevention and Health Promotion, 1996.

33. Smodlaka VN. Interval training in rehabilitation medicine. Arch Phys Med Rehabil 1973;54:428–431.

34. Kottke FJ. Therapeutic Exercise to Maintain Mobility. In FJ Kottke, GK Stillwell, JF Lehmann (eds), Krusen's Handbook of Physical Medicine and Rehabilitation (3rd ed). Philadelphia: WB Saunders, 1987.

35. Nimni ME. Collagen: structure, function, and metabolism in normal and fibrotic tissues. Semin Arthritis Rheum 1983;13:1–86.

36. McCarty DJ. Arthritis and Allied Conditions (11th ed). Philadelphia: Lea & Febiger, 1989.

37. Halar EM, Bell KR. Contractures and Other Deleterious Effects of Immobility. In JA Delisa (ed), Rehabilitation Medicine: Principles and Practice. Philadelphia: JB Lippincott, 1988.

38. Trudel G, Uhthoff HK. Contractures secondary to immobility: is the restriction articular or muscular? An experimental longitudinal study in the rat knee. Arch Phys Med Rehabil 2000;81:6–13.

39. Swann DA, Radin EL. The molecular basis of articular lubrication I: Purification and properties of a lubricating fraction from bovine synovial fluid. J Biol Chem 1972;274:8069–8083.

40. Linn FC, Sokoloff L. Movement and composition of interstitial fluid of cartilage. Arthritis Rheum 1965;8:481–493.

41. Swann DA, Radin EL, Nazimec M, et al. Role of hyaluronic acid in joint lubrication. Ann Rheum Dis 1974;33:318–326.

42. Akeson WH, Amiel D, Abel MS, et al. Effects of immobilization on joints. Clin Orthop 1987;219:28–35.

43. Wolf SE. Morphological and Functional Considerations for Therapeutic

Exercises. In JV Basmajian (ed), Therapeutic Exercise (4th ed). Baltimore: Williams & Wilkins, 1984.

44. Lehmann JE, DeLateur BJ. Therapeutic Heat. In JF Lehmann (ed), Therapeutic Heat and Cold (3rd ed). Baltimore: Williams & Wilkins, 1982.

45. Maughan RJ, Watson JS, Weir J. Strength and cross-sectional area of human skeletal muscle. J Physiol 1983;338:37–49.

46. Bouchard C, Malina RM, Pérusse L. Genetics of Fitness and Physical Performance. Champaign, IL: Human Kinetics, 1997;221–241.

47. Pette D, Staron RS. Mammalian skeletal muscle fiber type transitions. Int Rev Cytol 1997;170:143–223.

48. Sale DG. Influence of exercise and training on motor unit activities. Exerc Sport Sci Rev 1987;15:95–151.

49. Knuttgen HG. Neuromuscular Mechanisms for Therapeutic and Conditioning Exercise. Baltimore: University Park Press, 1976.

50. Dillingham MF. Strength training. Phys Med Rehabil: State of the Art Reviews 1987;1:555–568.

51. DeLateur BJ. Exercise for Strength and Endurance. In JV Basmajian (ed), Therapeutic Exercise. Baltimore: Williams & Wilkins, 1984;88–109.

52. DeLorme TL, Watkins AL. Technics of progressive resistance exercise. Arch Phys Med 1948;29:263–273.

53. Zinorieff AN. Heavy resistance exercises: the "Oxford technique." Br J Phys Med 1951;14:129–132.

54. DeLateur BJ, Lehmann JF, Fordyce WE. A test of the DeLorme axiom. Arch Phys Med Rehabil 1968;49:245–248.

55. Atha J. Strengthening muscle. Exerc Sport Sci Rev 1981;9:1–73.

56. Fleck SJ, Kraemer WJ. Designing Resistance Training Programs (2nd ed). Champaign, IL: Human Kinetics, 1997.

57. Komi PV, Buskirk ER. Effect of eccentric and concentric muscle conditioning on tension and electrical activity of human muscle. Ergonomics 1972; 15:417–434.

58. Hortobágyi T, Lambert NJ, Hill JP. Greater cross education following training with muscle lengthening than shortening. Med Sci Sports Exerc 1997;29:107–112.

59. Kanehisa H, Miyashita M. Specificity of velocity in strength training. Eur J Appl Physiol 1983;52:104–106.

60. Prietto CA, Caiozzo VJ. The in-vivo force-velocity relationships of the knee flexors and extensors. Am J Sports Med 1989;17:607.

61. Griffen JW. Differences in elbow flexion torque measured concentrically, eccentrically, and isometrically. Phys Ther 1987;67:1205.

62. Muller EA. Influence of training and inactivity on muscle strength. Arch Phys Med Rehabil 1970;51:449–462.

63. Sale DG. Neural adaptation to resistance training. Med Sci Sports Exerc 1988;20(Suppl 5):S135–S145.

64. Moritani T, De Vries HA. Neural factors versus hypertrophy in the time course of muscle strength gain. Am J Phys Med 1979;58:115–130.

65. Akima H, Takahashi H, Kuno SY, et al. Early phase adaptations of muscle use and strength to isokinetic training. Med Sci Sports Exerc 1999;31:588–594.

66. Antonio J, Gonyea WJ. Skeletal muscle fiber hyperplasia. Med Sci Sports Exerc 1993;25:1333–1345.

67. Kadi F, Eriksson A, Holmner S, et al. Effects of anabolic steroids on the muscle cells of strength-trained athletes. Med Sci Sports Exerc 1999;31:1528–1534.

68. Goldspink DF. Exercise related changes in protein turnover in mammalian striated muscle. J Exp Biol 1991;160:127–148.

69. Booth FW, Tseng FW, Flück M, et al. Molecular and cellular adaptation of muscle in response to physical training. Acta Physiol Scand 1998;162:343–350.

70. Goldspink G, Scutt A, Loughna PT, et al. Gene expression in skeletal muscle in response to stretch and force generation. Am J Physiol 1992;262:R356–R363.

71. Schultz E, McCormick KM. Skeletal muscle satellite cells. Rev Physiol Biochem Pharmacol 1994;123:213–257.

72. Roy RR, Monke SR, Allen DL, et al. Modulation of myonuclear number in functionally overloaded and exercised rat plantaris fibers. J Appl Physiol 1999;87:634–642.

73. Bhasin S, Storer TW, Berman N, et al. The effects of supraphysiologic doses of testosterone on muscle size and strength in normal men. N Engl J Med 1996;335:1–7.

74. Florini JR, Ewton DZ, Coolican SA. Growth hormone and the insulin-like growth factor system in myogenesis. Endocr Rev 1996;17:481–516.

75. Seger JY, Arvidsson B, Thorstensson A. Specific effects of eccentric and concentric training on muscle strength and morphology in humans. Eur J Appl Physiol 1998;79:49–57.

76. Fiatarone MA, Marks EC, Ryan ND, et al. High-intensity strength training in nonagenarians. Effects on skeletal muscle. JAMA 1990;263:3029–3034.

77. Thomis MAI, Beunen GP, Maes HH. Strength training: importance of genetic factors. Med Sci Sports Exerc 1998;30:724–731.

78. DeLateur BJ, Lehmann JF, Stonebridge J, Warren CG. Isotonic versus isometric exercise: a double-shift transfer of training study. Arch Phys Med Rehabil 1972;53:212–216.

79. Smith RC, Rutherford OM. The role of metabolites in strength training. I. A comparison of eccentric and concentric contractions. Eur J Appl Physiol 1995;71:332–336.

80. Saltin B, Blomqvist G, Mitchell JH, et al. Response to exercise after bed rest and after training. Circulation 1968;38(Suppl 7):1–50.

81. Paterson DH, Cunningham DA. The gas transporting systems: limits and modifications with age and training. Can J Appl Physiol 1999;24:28–40.

82. Turner DL, Hoppeler H, Claassen H, et al. Effects of endurance training on oxidative capacity and structural composition of human arm and leg muscles. Acta Physiol Scand 1997;161:459–464.

83. Spina RJ, Chi MMY, Hopkins MG, et al. Mitochondrial enzymes increase in muscle in response to 7–10 days of cycle exercise. J Appl Physiol 1996;80:2250–2254.

84. Hoppeler H, Howald H, Conley K, et al. Endurance training in humans: aerobic capacity and structure of skeletal muscle. J Appl Physiol 1985;59:320–327.

85. Taylor AW, Bachman L. The effects of endurance training on muscle fiber types and enzyme activites. Can J Appl Physiol 1999;24:41–53.

86. Martin WH. Effect of endurance training on fatty acid metabolism during whole body exercise. Med Sci Sports Exerc 1997;29:635–639.

87. Romijn JA, Klein S, Coyle EF, et al. Strenous endurance training increases lipolysis and triglyceride-fatty acid cycling at rest. J Appl Physiol 1993;75:108–113.

88. Weltman A, Weltman JY, Womack CJ, et al. Exercise training decreases the growth hormone (GH) response to acute constant-load exercise. Med Sci Sports Exerc 1997;29:669–676.

89. Hartig DE, Henderson JM. Increasing hamstring flexibility decreases lower

extremity overuse injuries in military basic trainees. Am J Sports Med 1999;27:173–176.

90. Wenger NK. Physiological basis for early ambulation after myocardial infarction. Cardiovasc Clin 1978; 9:107–115.

91. Paez PN, Phillipson EA, Masangkay M, et al. The physiologic basis of training patients with emphysema. Am Rev Respir Dis 1967;95:944–953.

92. Kottke FJ. From reflex to skill: the training of coordination. Arch Phys Med Rehabil 1980;61:551–561.

93. Crossman ER. Theory of acquisition of speed-skill. Ergonomics 1959;2:153–166.

94. Marie P, Foix C. Reflexes d'automatisme medullaire et reflexes dits de defense. Le phenomene des raccourcisseurs. Semaine Med 1913;33:505–508.

95. Sherrington CS. The Integrative Action of the Nervous System (2nd ed). New Haven, CT: Yale University Press, 1947.

96. Twitchell TE. The restoration of motor function following hemiplegia. Brain 1951;74:443–480.

97. Knott M, Voss DE. Proprioceptive Neuromuscular Facilitation: Patterns and Techniques (2nd ed). New York: Harper & Row, 1968.

98. Kabat H. Studies on neuromuscular dysfunction, XI. New principles of neuromuscular reeducation. Permanente Found Med Bull 1947;5:111.

99. Kabat H. Proprioceptive Facilitation in Therapeutic Exercise. In SH Licht (ed), Therapeutic Exercise (2nd ed). New Haven, CT: E Licht, 1961.

100. Krivickas LS. Training Flexibility. In WR Frontera, D Dawson, D Slovik (eds), Exercise in Rehabilitation Medicine (1st ed). Champaign, IL: Human Kinetics, 1999.

101. Magnusson SP, Simonsen EB, Aagaard P, et al. Mechanical and physical responses to stretching with and without preisometric contraction in human skeletal muscle. Arch Phys Med Rehabil 1996;77:373–378.

102. Surburg PR. Interactive effects of resistance and facilitation patterning upon reaction and response times. Phys Ther 1979;59:1513–1517.

103. Brunnstrom S. Movement Therapy in Hemiplegia. New York: Harper & Row, 1971.

104. Bobath K, Bobath B. Treatment of cerebral palsy based on analysis of patients' motor behavior. Br J Phys Med 1952;15:107–117.

105. Rood MS. Neurophysiological reactions as a basis for physical therapy. Phys Ther Rev 1954;34:444–449.

106. Stockmeyer SL. An interpretation of the approach of Rood to the treatment of neuromuscular dysfunction. Am J Phys Med 1967;6:900–955.

107. Dewald JP. Sensorimotor Neurophysiology and the Basis of Neurofacilitory Therapeutic Techniques. In ME Brandstater, JV Basmajian (eds), Stroke Rehabilitation. Baltimore: Williams & Wilkins, 1987.

108. Frenkel HS. Treatment of Tabetic Ataxia by Means of Systematic Exercises. Philadelphia: 1902.

109. Hewett TE, Stroupe AL, Nance TA, Noyes FR. Plyometric training in female athletes. Decreased impact forces and increased hamstring torques. Am J Sports Med 1996;24(6):765–773.

110. Kramer JF, Morrow A, Leger A. Changes in rowing ergometer, weight lifting, vertical jump and isokinetic performance in response to standard and standard plus plyometric training programs. Int J Sports Med 1993;14(8):449–454.

111. Cossor JM, Blanks BA, Elliott BC. The influence of plyometric training on the freestyle tumble turn. J Sci Med Sport 1999;2(2):106–116.

112. Heiderscheit BC, McLean KP, Davies GJ. The effects of isokinetic vs. plyometric training on the shoulder internal rotators. J Orthop Sports Phys Ther 1996;23(2):125–133.

113. Dill DB. The Harvard Fatigue Laboratory: its development, contributions, and demise. Circ Res 1967;20(Suppl 1):I161–I170.

114. Darling RC. Fatigue. In JA Downey, RC Darling (eds), Physiological Basis of Rehabilitation Medicine. Philadelphia: WB Saunders, 1971.

115. National Institute for Occupational Safety and Health. Work Practices Guide for Manual Lifting. Num 81–122. Cincinnati, OH: US Department of Health and Human Sciences, 1981.

116. Grandjean E. Fatigue: its physiological and psychological significance. Ergonomics 1968;11(5):427–436.

117. Newsholme EA, Blomstrand E, McAndrew N, et al. Biochemical Causes of Fatigue and Overtraining. In RJ Shephard, PO Astrand (eds), Endurance in Sport. Oxford: Blackwell Scientific Publications, 1992;351–364.

118. Sahlin K. Acid-Base Balance During High Intensity Exercise. In M Harries, C Williams, WD Stanish, et al. (eds), Oxford Textbook of Sports Medicine. Oxford: Oxford University Press, 1994;46–52.

119. Moffroid MP, Whipple RH. Specificity of speed of exercise. J Am Phys Ther Assoc 1970;50:1692–1700.

120. Thorstensson A, Karlsson J. Fatigability and fibre composition of human skeletal muscle. Acta Physiol Scand 1976;98:318–322.

121. Watkins MP, Harris BA. Evaluation of isokinetic muscle performance. Clin Sports Med 1983;2:27–53.

122. Kent-Braun JA. Central and peripheral contributions to muscle fatigue during sustained maximal effort. Eur J Appl Physiol 1999;80:57–63.

123. Bigland B, Lippold OCJ. The relation between force, velocity, and integrated electrical activity in human muscle. J Physiol 1954;123:214.

124. Edwards RG, Lippold OCJ. The relation between force and integrated electrical activity in fatigued muscle. J Physiol 1956;132:677.

125. Roy SH, DeLuca CJ, Emley M, et al. Classification of back muscle impairment based on the surface electromyographic signal. J Rehabil Res Dev 1995;34:405.

126. Yeung SS, Au AL, Chow CC. Effects of fatigue on the temporal neuromuscular control of vastus medialis muscle in humans. Eur J Appl Physiol 1999;80:379–385.

127. Kirwan JP, Costill DL, Flynn MG, et al. Physiological responses to successive days of intense training in competitive swimmers. Med Sci Sports Exerc 1988;20:255–259.

128. Mackinnon LT, Hooper SL, Jones S, et al. Hormonal, immunological, and hematological responses to intensified training in elite swimmers. Med Sci Sports Exerc 1997;29:1637–1645.

129. Nieman DC. Exercise, infection, and immunity. Int J Sports Med 1994;15:S131–S141.

130. Eliakim A, Kodesh E, Gavrieli R, et al. Cellular and humoral immune response to exercise among gymnasts and untrained girls. Int J Sports Med 1997;18:208–212.

17

Gait

D. CASEY KERRIGAN AND JOAN E. EDELSTEIN

Gait, referring to humans walking and running, is one of the most obvious and fundamental actions in life.[1] Without formal training, we are often able to recognize an abnormal gait pattern. A clinician or scientist can learn to identify more subtle gait abnormalities and can learn to describe these patterns. But recognizing and describing gait patterns are just the first steps toward appreciating the complexity of gait physiology. When we try to improve a person's gait pattern, we become acutely aware of the complexity of gait. We attempt to understand the complex relationships between an individual's impairments and the person's gait. Moreover, we attempt to understand the effects of external biomechanical factors such as shoes, orthoses, or prostheses. We realize that gait, although deceptively easy to observe, may be one of the least understood physiological processes. The first goal of this chapter is to enable the reader to describe normal and abnormal gait patterns using standard terminology. The second goal is to familiarize the reader with the tools used to measure various parameters of gait. The third goal is to aid the reader to appreciate the opportunity for improving rehabilitation practice by improving the understanding of gait physiology.

TERMINOLOGY

The basic unit of walking and running is one *gait cycle*, or *stride*. Perry described various temporal and functional parameters within the gait cycle[2] (Figure 17-1) that have formed a standard frame of reference to describe normal and abnormal gait. The classification divides the cycle into the *stance* and *swing* periods. The gait cycle can also be divided into three functional tasks: weight acceptance, single limb support, and limb advancement. *Weight accep-*

tance and *single limb support* are the functional tasks occurring during stance, whereas *limb advancement* is the task occurring primarily during swing. The three functional tasks are further subdivided into eight phases of the gait cycle. The phases of *initial contact* and *loading response* make up the first functional task of weight acceptance, whereas the phases of *midstance* and *terminal stance* make up the second functional task of single limb support. The final phase of stance (preswing) marks the beginning of the last functional task of limb advancement, which continues through the three phases of swing (*initial swing, midswing, and terminal swing*).

Gait velocity is simply the speed of gait. *Stride time* is defined from the time of initial contact of one limb with the ground to the next initial contact of the same limb. *Step time* is the duration of time from initial contact of one limb to the time of initial contact of the contralateral limb. *Stride length* and *step length* refer to the distances covered during their respective times. The *cadence* of gait can be expressed in either strides per minute or steps per minute. At an average walking velocity, the stance period accounts for approximately 60% of the gait cycle, whereas the swing period makes up 40%.

During the stance period of walking, there are two time intervals, termed *double limb support*, when both feet are on the ground. One interval occurs from initial contact into loading response and the other during preswing. *Single limb support* refers to the time interval in stance when the opposite limb is in swing. During normal walking at an average walking speed, each double limb support time makes up approximately 10% of the gait cycle, whereas single limb support makes up approximately 40%. Typical values[2] of temporal gait parameters in able-bodied young adults, walking comfortably on a level surface, are summarized in Table 17-1. At slower walking velocities, the

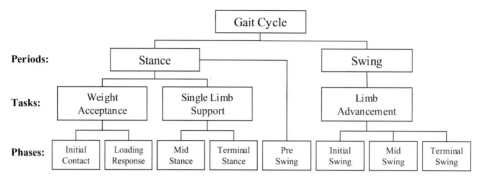

FIGURE 17-1 Periods of the gait cycle. The gait cycle is separated into two distinct periods of stance and swing. Functional tasks include weight acceptance and single limb support during stance and limb advancement during swing. The stance period of the gait cycle includes initial contact, loading response, midstance, terminal stance, and preswing. The swing period includes initial swing, midswing, and terminal swing. (Reprinted with permission from DC Kerrigan, M Schaufele, MN Wen. Gait analysis. In Rehabilitation Medicine: Principles and Practice [3rd ed]. Philadelphia: Lippincott-Raven, 1998.)

double limb support times are greater. Conversely, with increasing walking speeds, the double limb support time intervals decrease. Walking becomes running when there is no longer an interval of time in which both feet are in contact on the ground. The two defining periods of running for each limb are stance and flight; *double float* refers to the interval when both feet are off the ground.

ENERGY CONSERVATION AND THE CONCEPT OF THE DETERMINANTS OF GAIT

In normal gait, it may appear that the body glides smoothly, but, in fact, the body bobs up and down with each step. Bobbing, or more specifically, the lifting of the body with each step, requires energy. In contrast, riding

TABLE 17-1

Typical Temporal Gait Parameters for Comfortable Walking on Level Surfaces in Adult Subjects

Temporal Gait Parameter	Average Value
Velocity (m/min)	80
Cadence (steps/min)	113
Stride length (m)	1.41
Stance (% of gait cycle)	60
Swing (% of gait cycle)	40
Double support (% per leg per gait cycle)	10

Source: Reprinted with permission from J Edelstein. Orthotic assessment and management. In SB O'Sullivan, TJ Schmitz (eds), Physical Rehabilitation Assessment and Treatment [3rd ed]. Philadelphia: F.A. Davis, 1994;677–678.

a bicycle or propelling a wheelchair does not require lifting the body, which might explain why these modes of locomotion require less energy per unit distance. During normal walking, the body's center of mass (COM) travels along both a sinusoidal up and down and sinusoidal side to side path with each step. The up and down path is far more relevant to the energy requirements of gait. The COM, defined as the hypothetical point at which all mass of the body can be considered to be concentrated, reaches its highest point during single limb support and its lowest point during double limb support. Saunders et al.[3] described several mechanisms by which the body minimizes and smoothes the vertical and lateral displacement of the COM during walking as the *determinants of gait*. Since their pioneering description of these determinants, it has been generally believed that minimizing the displacement of the COM during walking is critical to improving the efficiency of walking.[4] Classically, the determinants of gait are listed as follows:

- Pelvic rotation in the transverse plane
- Pelvic obliquity in the coronal plane
- Lateral displacement in the coronal plane
- Interchange between knee, ankle, and foot motion

A hypothetical *compass*, per Saunders et al., assumes what walking would be like without any of these determinants. Per the compass gait model, the legs are represented as rigid levers articulated only at the hip joints, without foot, ankle, or knee components. Pelvic rotation in the transverse plane may reduce the drop in the COM during double limb support. A slight amount of pelvic obliquity (i.e., Trendelenburg) reduces the peak of the COM during single limb support. Diminution of the lateral displacement of the pelvis is influenced by two factors. One, the body is shifted toward the side of the stance limb during loading. Two, the natural valgus between the femur and tibia allows the feet to be relatively close together during forward progression.

The interchange between knee, ankle, and foot motion was described as a mechanism to help alter the pattern of COM motion from a series of arcs as in the hypothetical compass gait situation to the characteristic smooth sinusoidal appearance. Joint motions are described in detail in a later section. For instance, the ankle moves into plantar flexion from initial contact into loading. Also during single limb support, there is progressive ankle dorsiflexion which similarly reduces the peak of COM displacement. The ankle plantar flexes again in double limb support which raises the COM's lowest point. All of these actions occur gradually and in rhythm with foot and knee motion to smooth the curve of COM motion during gait.

If it were not for the combined actions of the determinants of gait, the average total vertical displacement of COM would be approximately twice its actual value of 2 inches.[5] Many impairments and functional limitations can interfere with the determinants and thus theoretically increase the COM displacement and energy cost of walking.[6]

The advent of sophisticated laboratory equipment has challenged the role of several of the determinants in conserving the energy cost of walking. Saunders et al. reported that the second determinant, pelvic obliquity, also known as *pelvic tilt* and *pelvic list*, decreased the vertical excursion of the trunk. A more recent investigation, however,[7] suggests that pelvic tilt occurs before the time when the stance hip reaches its peak elevation during midstance. Pelvic list is nearly neutral during midstance and is maximum shortly after toe-off. Altogether, pelvic list decreases the vertical peaks and the valleys of the trunk's trajectory by approximately 2–4 mm, thus having no notable effect on the vertical excursion of the trunk. Saunders et al. hypothesized that the third determinant, stance phase knee flexion, also contributed to reducing vertical trunk movement, thus aiding energy conservation. Gard and Childress[8] found, however, that the flexion wave occurs before the peak in the trunk's vertical displacement and thus is ineffective in decreasing vertical movement of the body. Knee flexion is greatest at the time of contralateral toe-off, thus probably serving as a shock-absorbing mechanism.

ENERGY COST OF GAIT

At an average comfortable walking velocity, the energy expenditure is approximately four times the basal meta-bolic rate.[9] Interestingly, the velocity that subjects choose as their comfortable speed is also the velocity that requires the least energy per unit distance.[10] Walking slower requires extra energy, probably for balance support, rather than for propelling the body forward.[11] Walking faster also requires more energy, presumably to permit more forceful muscle contraction. Importantly, the rate of energy expended during comfortable walking is consistent across the nondisabled and disabled populations.[9] Thus, although a person with a gait disability tends to walk slower than a person without a disability and may expend more energy to get from point A to point B, both individuals expend the same amount of energy per unit time.[12] For instance, patients with hemiplegia walk slower and expend between 37%[13] and 62%[14] more energy per unit distance than able-bodied subjects; however, the disabled adults expend the same amount of energy per time during comfortable walking as able-bodied subjects.

A major aim of rehabilitation is to reduce the energy required to walk. To this end, the effectiveness of a particular type of treatment can be assessed by evaluating the energy expended during walking. The most direct method to evaluate energy expended is via oxygen-consumption measurements.[9] Alternatively, an estimate of energy expended can be obtained by measuring heart rate before and during walking because the change in heart rate that occurs with walking is linearly correlated with oxygen-consumption measurements.[15] An easier, although more indirect, method to evaluate the energy required to walk is to measure the comfortable walking speed. This measure, which can be performed simply using a stopwatch and a designated walking distance, depends on the fact noted previously that subjects with disability tend to walk at a consistent energy rate, just slower. Thus, comfortable walking speed relates indirectly to the energy required to walk. All of these measures, however, including oxygen consumption, heart rate, and comfortable walking speed, relate to biomechanical aspects of walking and to cardiopulmonary conditioning and psychological factors including mood, as well. A so-called biomechanical efficiency quotient was proposed[5,6] based on the concept of minimizing the COM displacement through the determinants of gait. This measure was introduced as a means to specifically evaluate biomechanical walking efficiency in subjects with gait disability, independent of cardiopulmonary conditioning and psychological factors. The quotient is the measured vertical displacement of the COM divided by the predicted vertical displacement, the latter being a function of the subject's average stride length and height of the pelvis from the ground. Patients with gait disability tend to have higher biomechanical efficiency quotients than nondisabled subjects, and treatments such as an ankle-foot orthosis tend to reduce the biomechanical efficiency quotient.[6]

BIOMECHANICAL CONCEPTS PERTINENT TO GAIT

Standard gait terminology includes the use of several biomechanical terms. *Kinematics* describes the motions

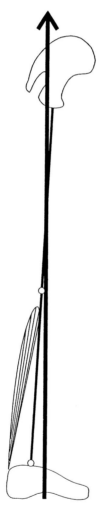

FIGURE 17-2 Quiet standing. The ground reaction force, represented by the solid line with an arrow, is located anterior to the knee and ankle and posterior to the hip. The soleus muscle is active to stabilize the lower limb. (Reprinted with permission from DC Kerrigan, M Schaufele, MN Wen. Gait analysis. In JA Delisa, BM Gans [eds], Rehabilitation Medicine: Principles and Practice [3rd ed]. Philadelphia: Lippincott-Raven, 1998.)

of limb segments and the angular motions of joints. *Kinetics* describes the moments or moments and forces that cause joint and limb motion. *Quantitative gait analysis*, described in a later section, can be used to quantify kinematics and kinetics during the gait cycle.[16–18] Similarly, the firing patterns of muscles can be determined with the aid of dynamic electromyographic (EMG) measurement.

Broadly speaking, the study of kinetics includes the study of muscular activity as well as the study of forces and provides insight into the causes of the observed kinematics. In quantitative gait analysis, we are often interested in computing the moments or net moments acting on muscles, tendons, and ligaments. A moment about a joint occurs when a force is acting at a distance from the joint through a lever, causing acceleration of the joint angle. For instance, a weight placed in the hand produces an externally applied extensor moment about the elbow. In this example, the lever is the forearm and the elbow tends to accelerate uncontrollably into extension. The external moment is the product of the weight of the object and the length of the forearm. The concept of equilibrium dictates that in order that a joint angle remains stable, all the moments acting about the joint must sum to zero. Thus, in our example, for the elbow to be stable, an internal force from the biceps acting through its forearm lever must provide a resisting internal flexor moment to the external extensor moment. Depending on the magnitude of the biceps' force, the elbow joint angle extends in a controlled fashion (eccentric contraction), stays the same (isometric contraction), or flexes (concentric contraction). These basic biomechanical concepts are pertinent to gait analysis.

During walking, the joints and limb segments are in a continuous state of equilibrium. The externally applied forces producing joint moments include gravity, inertial forces from limb segments, and the body's ground reaction force (GRF), defined as the force exerted by the ground at the point of contact (our feet). Internal forces include muscle and ligament forces, inertial forces, and joint forces. During the stance period, the primary external force is the GRF. During swing there is no GRF, only gravitational and inertial forces from the limb segments.

The importance of knowing the direction and magnitude of the GRF and its relationship with muscle behavior and maintenance of equilibrium is best illustrated by the example of quiet standing. In quiet standing, the GRF vector extends from the ground through the foot, passing anterior to the ankles and knees and posterior to the hips (Figure 17-2). At the hip, passive ligamentous forces transmitted through the iliofemoral ligaments usually are sufficient to counteract the external extensor moment. Similarly at the knee, the external knee extensor moment is counteracted by the passive forces transmitted through the posterior ligamentous capsule. At the ankle, the external dorsiflexion moment is usually counteracted with an internal ankle plantar flexor moment provided by the ankle plantar flexors. Thus, the only lower extremity muscles that are consistently active and need to be active during quiet standing are the plantar flexors (primarily the soleus muscle).

When we walk, the GRF is essentially a result of both our body weight and our body's accelerations and decelerations as our COM moves up and down. Knowing where the line of the GRF lies with respect to the hip, knee, and ankle joints gives us a reasonable approximation of the external moments occurring about each of these joints. The GRF can be directly measured with a force plate, described later in the quantitative gait analysis section. Visualizing where the GRF lies with respect to a joint provides a means to approximate what internal moments must be generated in order to stabilize that joint. For instance, if the GRF line lies posterior to the knee, an external knee

flexor moment is produced that is the product of the GRF multiplied by the distance of the GRF line from the axis of the knee joint. In order to maintain stability so that the knee does not collapse into flexion, an internal knee extensor moment must occur. This moment, provided by the knee extensors, is equal in magnitude to the external flexor moment.

During walking, the GRF vector changes position as the body progresses forward (Figure 17-3). During loading response, the vector is anterior to the hip and posterior to the knee and ankle. In midstance, the vector passes through the hip and knee joints and is anterior to the ankle. During terminal stance, the vector moves posterior to the hip, anterior to the knee joint, and maximally anterior to the ankle. With these dynamics in mind, normal gait function is easier to interpret. The muscles fire in response to the need for joint stability. In quantitative gait analysis, whether a muscle group is firing concentrically or eccentrically can be determined by measuring the joint power, which is mathematically the product of the joint moment and the joint angular velocity. A positive joint power implies that the muscle group is firing concentrically, whereas a negative joint power implies that the muscle group is firing eccentrically.

FIGURE 17-3 The eight phases of the gait cycle include initial contact, loading response, midstance, terminal stance, preswing, initial swing, midswing, and terminal swing. The ground reaction force vector is represented by a solid line with an arrow. The active muscles are shown during each phase of the gait cycle. The uninvolved limb is shown as a dotted line. (Reprinted with permission from DC Kerrigan, M Schaufele, MN Wen. Gait analysis. In JA Delisa, BM Gans [eds], Rehabilitation Medicine: Principles and Practice [3rd ed]. Philadelphia: Lippincott-Raven, 1998.)

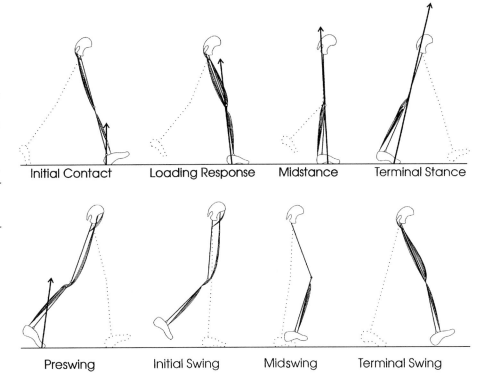

Initial Contact   Loading Response   Midstance   Terminal Stance

Preswing   Initial Swing   Midswing   Terminal Swing

NORMAL KINEMATICS AND KINETICS

The following descriptions of normal kinematics and kinetics are based on data collected from the Spaulding Rehabilitation Hospital Gait Laboratory and are similar to those reported elsewhere. The general patterns of movement are representative of nondisabled adults and children older than 3 years of age.[19]

Sagittal Plane Motion

For each phase, the kinematics and kinetics are described. Figure 17-3 illustrates the chief actions occurring in each phase, with a visual representation of the limb and joint positions, the GRF line, and the muscles that are active during that phase. It may also be useful to refer to Figure 17-4, which graphically demonstrates the joint motion, moments, and powers throughout the gait cycle.

Initial Contact

Initial contact with the ground typically occurs with the heel. The hip is flexed at 30 degrees, the knee is fully extended, and the ankle is in a neutral position. As the GRF is anterior to the hip, the hip extensors (gluteus maximus and hamstrings) are firing to maintain hip stability. At the knee, the GRF creates an external extensor moment, which is counteracted by hamstring activity. The foot is supported in the neutral position by the ankle dorsiflexors.

Loading Response

During this phase, weight acceptance and shock absorption are achieved while maintaining forward progression. The hip extends and continues to extend into the terminal-stance phase. The GRF is anterior to the hip, and the hip extensors must be active to resist uncontrolled hip flexion. Active hip extension implies that the hip extensors are concentrically active. With the location of the GRF now posterior to the knee joint, an external flexor moment is created. This external moment is resisted by an eccentric contraction of the quadriceps, allowing knee flexion to approximately 20 degrees. With the GRF posterior to the ankle, an external plantar flexion moment occurs that rapidly lowers the foot into 10 degrees of plantar flexion. This action is controlled by the ankle dorsiflexors, which fire eccentrically. At the end of loading response, the foot is in full contact with the ground.

Midstance

During midstance, the limb supports the full body weight as the contralateral limb swings forward. The GRF vector passes through the hip joint, eliminating the need for hip extensor activity. At the knee, the GRF moves from a posterior to an anterior position, similarly eliminating the need for quadriceps' activity. Knee extension occurs and is restrained passively by the knee's posterior ligamentous capsule and is possibly actively restrained as well by eccentric popliteus and gastrocnemius action. At the ankle, the GRF is anterior to the ankle, thus producing an external ankle dorsiflexion moment. This moment is counteracted by the ankle plantar flexors, which eccentrically limit the dorsiflexion occurring during this phase.

Terminal Stance

In terminal stance the body's mass continues to progress over the limb as the trunk falls forward. The GRF at the hip is now posterior, creating an extensor moment that is countered passively by the iliofemoral ligaments. The hip is now maximally extended at 10–20 degrees. At the knee, the GRF moves from an anterior to a slightly posterior position. As the heel rises from the ground, the GRF becomes increasingly anterior to the ankle joint, and this dorsiflexion moment continues to be stabilized by ankle plantar flexor activity. During this phase, the ankle is plantar flexing and thus the action of the ankle plantar flexors has switched from eccentric to concentric.

Preswing

During preswing, the limb begins to be propelled forward into swing. This phase is occurring as the contralateral limb now advances through initial contact and loading response. From maximal hip extension, the hip now begins flexing and continues flexing throughout the swing period. The hip flexors (combined activation of the iliopsoas, hip adductors, and rectus femoris) are concentrically active. The knee quickly flexes to 40 degrees as the GRF progresses rapidly posterior to the knee. Knee flexion may be controlled by rectus femoris activity. The ankle continues plantar flexing to approximately 20 degrees with continued concentric activity of the ankle plantar flexors.

Initial Swing

During initial swing, the limb continues to be propelled forward. Hip flexion occurs because of the hip flexion momentum initiated in preswing and because of continued concentric activity of the hip flexors. The rectus femoris and vastus lateralis work independently of each other during initial swing phase, with the rectus femoris activity directly correlated with walking speed.[20] The rectus femoris is active during both loading response and preswing and initial swing phases,

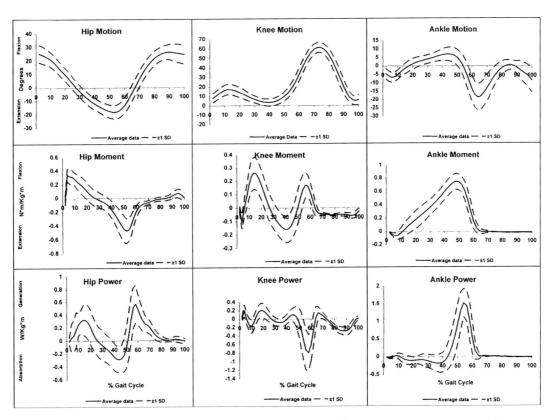

FIGURE 17-4 Kinetics and kinematics at the hip, knee, and ankle. Sagittal joint motion, moments, and powers are shown. (Reprinted with permission from DC Kerrigan, M Schaufele, MN Wen. Gait analysis. In JA Delisa, BM Gans [eds], Rehabilitation Medicine: Principles and Practice [3rd ed]. Philadelphia: Lippincott-Raven, 1998.)

regardless of walking speed, with much variability in patterns of muscular activity. Some subjects exhibit greater activity during late stance, whereas others have higher EMG amplitudes during early stance.[21] The knee continues to flex to approximately 65 degrees. Knee flexion occurs passively as a combined result of hip flexion and the momentum generated from preswing. The ankle dorsiflexors are concentrically active as the ankle dorsiflexes.

Midswing

In midswing the limb continues to advance forward, primarily passively as a pendulum from inertial forces generated in preswing and initial swing. The hip continues to flex, now passively, as a result of the momentum generated in initial swing. The knee begins to extend passively as a result of gravity. The ankle remains in a neutral position with the continued activity of the ankle dorsiflexors.

Terminal Swing

At terminal swing the previously generated momentum is controlled, probably to maintain sufficient stability before the upcoming weight-acceptance phase. At the hip and knee joints, strong eccentric contraction of the hamstrings decelerates hip flexion and controls knee extension. The ankle dorsiflexors remain active, allowing a neutral ankle position at initial contact.

Coronal Plane Motion

Most lower extremity motion during gait occurs in the sagittal plane. Coronal plane motion about the pelvis and hip, and coronal plane kinetics about the hip, knee, and ankle, occur. At initial contact both the pelvis and hip are in neutral positions in the coronal plane. During much of the stance period, the GRF passes medially to the hip, knee, and ankle joint centers as the opposite limb is unloading. This medial GRF about the hip causes an external adductor moment that allows the contralateral side of the pelvis to drop slightly (the slight Trendelenburg's position noted previously as one of the determinants of gait). This motion is controlled by eccentric contraction of the hip abductors. During stance, the GRF position medial to the knee imposes an external varus moment about the knee that must be counteracted by lateral ligament and tendon tension, eccentric muscle activity, or both, as well as by compression forces to the medial compartment of the knee. The presence of a varus moment throughout most of stance explains why osteoarthritis at the knee most typically occurs in the medial compartment of the knee. The varus moment can be affected by external biomechanical factors such as wearing shoes.[22]

Other Normal Considerations

Although most research in gait has been conducted with young adults walking barefoot on a level surface at comfortable, self-selected speed, additional insight is gained by study of walking at various speeds. For example, pelvic list and axial rotation decrease with slower velocity, as does the amplitude of lumbar lateral flexion.[23] Age is another important variable affecting the gait pattern. Gait kinematics of children younger than 5–7 years of age differs from that of able-bodied adults, particularly with regard to the position of the foot at initial contact.[24] Young children strike the floor with the entire sole. By 30 months of age, normal youngsters exhibit heel contact.[24] During preadolescence and adolescence, foot kinematics continues to mature, particularly with decreased intertarsal motion.[25] A number of changes in the biomechanics of gait in the elderly occur, many of which are attributable to a reduced comfortable walking speed.[26,27] The only biomechanical differences between healthy elderly subjects and young adult subjects that persist when elderly subjects walk faster at a speed comparable with young adults are reduced peak hip extension, increased anterior pelvic tilt, reduced ankle plantar flexion, and reduced ankle power generation.[28] Various differences in joint kinetics between healthy elderly and elderly with recurrent falls have been identified[29]; however, the significance of these differences is unclear.

Moreover, subtle gender differences in gait exist.[18] For the same height, women have greater cadence than men.[30] Compared with men, during walking women exhibit greater hip flexion and less knee extension before initial contact, greater knee flexion moment in preswing, and greater peak knee joint power absorption at the knee in preswing.[18] Finally, shoes, orthoses, and assistive devices may alter the gait pattern to a greater or lesser extent. Among healthy children, gait kinematics, kinetics, and temporal-spatial characteristics are not clinically significant when subjects wear tennis shoes as compared with barefoot walking.[31] On the other hand, healthy children and those with cerebral palsy walk differently, with an increased stride length and decreased cadence when fitted with ankle-foot orthoses.[32,33]

NEUROLOGIC CONCEPTS PERTINENT TO GAIT

In addition to biomechanical analysis of gait, consideration of the neurologic basis of walking enhances one's understanding of normal and pathologic walking. The concept of a *central pattern generator* (CPG) refers to a functional network of neurons in various parts of the CNS. The network ultimately determines the pattern of muscular activity. Afferent activation of the CPG occurs primarily at the supraspinal level, particularly during gait initiation and termination. The brain stem has centers that modulate locomotor activity, both with regard to amplitude of muscular activity and timing of muscular contractions.[34] Rhythmic EMG outputs appear related to the CPG phenomenon. The concept of CPG appears to apply to backward, as well as forward, walking.[35] CPG can form the theoretical basis for gait re-education strategies for patients with spinal cord injuries.[36]

GENERAL APPROACH TO EVALUATING A PATIENT WITH AN ATYPICAL GAIT PATTERN

In approaching a patient with an abnormal gait pattern, it should be appreciated that for a given patient, an abnormal gait pattern may not be necessarily functionally significant and should first be evaluated with respect to each of the following: energy requirement, risk of falling, injury, and appearance.

Treatment to change the gait pattern should be prescribed if the pattern is functionally significant with respect to one or more of these four criteria. For instance, knee recurvatum (hyperextension) may or may not be associated with increased forces across the posterior ligamentous capsule of the knee,[37] which would predispose to injury. Another example is equinus during the swing period, which may or may not predispose to tripping depending on the associated compensations. To this end, the associated compensatory gait patterns also need to be evaluated with respect to these four criteria. In the case of equinus in swing, a compensation at the pelvis such as hip hiking would interfere with the pelvic obliquity determinant and thus increase the energy required to walk. Finally, an atypical gait pattern should be evaluated with respect to appearance, and for this assessment, the patient's own perceptions are critical.

Clearly, a comprehensive evaluation of the patient is required. The patient's history, musculoskeletal examination, observational gait analysis, and information from a quantitative gait analysis assist in determining the functional significance of the gait pattern and help identify specific causes for the pattern. Based on these results, a rational treatment plan can be prescribed.

The initial part of a comprehensive gait evaluation should include a focused history and physical examination. It is helpful to anticipate certain gait patterns associated with particular diagnoses as well as to anticipate the need for various components of a quantitative gait analysis. For example, the use of dynamic EMG is particularly useful in detecting inappropriate firing patterns in patients with upper motor neuron (UMN) pathology, but may not be necessary for patients with other diagnoses. The reason for referral should be identified and the patient's chief complaint with regard to walking should be considered. Any previous medications, neurolytic procedures, or surgery, particularly those affecting the lower extremities, should be noted. Also, a detailed history of strengthening and stretching exercises previously and currently being performed should be ascertained. Finally, the use of assistive devices and orthoses should be recorded.

The physical examination should focus on the neurologic and musculoskeletal system and include a static evaluation of the patient's strength, joint range of motion, tone, and proprioception. Although static evaluation is a routine part of a gait consultation and should be included in the assessment of every patient with an atypical gait pattern, it is generally agreed that, especially in the case of UMN pathology, the static evaluation has limited usefulness in determining the underlying mechanisms responsible for the atypical gait pattern.[38–40] Thus, the results from the static evaluation need to be combined with those obtained from quantitative gait analysis to provide dynamically relevant information on which to base treatment.

OBSERVATIONAL GAIT ANALYSIS

Observational, qualitative gait analysis should be the first analysis before consideration of further quantitative testing. The observer describes the gait after watching the patient walk without the aid of any electronic devices. However, it is often difficult to appreciate all limb segment and joint motions throughout the different phases of gait because of the difficulty in concurrently observing multiple body segments and joint motion.[41] Videotaping can be an important part of observational gait analysis because it allows repeated viewing of the patient's gait pattern without causing

undue patient fatigue. The patient should be observed from the side, the front, and from behind. Stride and step length, width, and symmetry should be noted. By concentrating on one joint at a time, including hip, knee, and ankle, atypical motions may be easier to identify. Having the patient walk at faster speed sometimes exaggerates an atypical motion. Observational gait analysis can identify obvious atypical gait patterns, such as excessive ankle plantar flexion or reduced knee flexion in swing. However, in certain cases this approach may not reveal all atypical patterns. For example, an increased lumbar lordosis or anterior pelvic tilt caused by a hip flexion contracture may be apparent only with a quantitative analysis.[42,43] Quantitative gait analysis is also quite helpful in delineating the specific causes for each atypical pattern and thus can help direct the appropriate treatment.[44]

A number of terms are commonly used to characterize various atypical gait patterns that are obvious from observational assessment alone. For instance, *antalgic gait* is a pattern common to patients with pain in one lower extremity. In this pattern, gait is modified to reduce weight bearing on the involved side. The uninvolved limb is rapidly advanced to shorten stance duration on the affected side. Gait is often slow and steps are short to limit the weight-bearing period. *Steppage gait* is a compensatory gait pattern used to describe excessive hip and knee flexion to assist a *functionally long* lower leg to clear the ground in swing. *Festinating gait* has been described as a characteristic pattern of Parkinson's disease in which there is a tendency to take short accelerating steps. *Shuffling gait* is also common in Parkinson's disease and refers to the feet sliding on the floor during swing. *Ataxic gait*, associated with cerebellar and dorsal column pathologies and peripheral neuropathies, is a broad term used to describe a pattern of apparent poor balance, a wide base of support, and variable motions from stride to stride.

Various gait patterns associated with the use of assistive devices are easily noted with observational analysis. A cane essentially increases the base of support by providing an additional point of contact with the ground. When pathology, impairment, or functional limitation involves both lower extremities, two canes or crutches or a walker are occasionally used. In this situation, an *alternating two-point gait* is commonly used in which one cane and the opposite foot are in contact with the ground, alternating with the opposite cane and foot in each successive step. In *three-point gait*, contact with one foot that is fully weight bearing onto the ground alternates with full weight bearing through two crutches that make simultaneous contact with the ground. In *four-point gait*, which provides maximal stability and base of support, usually at the cost of reduced speed of locomotion, there are always three points of support on the ground at all times. It is initiated by forward movement by crutch, followed by forward movement of the contralateral lower limb, then forward movement of the other crutch followed by forward movement of the other lower limb.

QUANTITATIVE GAIT EVALUATION

Current quantitative gait analysis systems usually include measurement of three primary components: kinematics and external and internal kinetics. Quantitative gait analysis can also include other components such as foot switches and oxygen consumption monitoring to measure overall energy expenditure. A variety of equipment are used, including optoelectronic motion analysis systems to measure kinematics, force plates to help measure external kinetics, and a multichannel dynamic EMG apparatus to measure muscle activity. Given the previously described limitations of static evaluations and of observational gait analysis, quantitative gait analysis can be a particularly useful clinical tool for developing a treatment plan.

Systems to Evaluate Temporal Parameters of Gait

Common temporal parameters such as velocity, cadence, and stride length can be measured to monitor a patient's progress outside of a sophisticated gait laboratory. As noted previously, velocity can be measured simply with a stopwatch as a patient traverses a designated distance. Similarly step and stride length can be measured without sophisticated equipment if the soles are marked with adhesive moleskin patches that have been inked. Computerized stride analyzers provide this same information in a more automated fashion.[45] They usually consist of instrumented insoles with foot switches (i.e., pressure-sensitive transducers) typically attached to the heel, toe, and occasionally the metatarsal region. They are connected to data boxes worn by the patient either around the waist or the ankle. These sensors measure the duration of floor contact via opening and closing switches. After acquisition, data transfer and analysis are typically done via a personal computer.

Foot switches are also commonly used to determine the beginning and end of the stance period, allowing calculation of temporal gait parameters such as the duration of the stance and swing periods, single- and double-support time, and cadence. These parameters are useful in interpreting the temporal relationships of kinematic, external kinetic, and particularly dynamic EMG data. Although this same information can be obtained directly from force plate data, foot switches are particularly helpful in the gait laboratory when force plate data cannot be obtained.

Foot switch data also can reveal variations in foot rollover, particularly on the medial side of the foot, especially during late stance.[30]

Foot Pressure Systems

Foot pressure systems are electronic instruments to measure pressure distribution in the soles of the feet. The systems work via a large number of capacitive or force-sensitive sensors in shoe insoles or floor platforms and are linked to a computer by either cable or radio-wave telemetry. Several commercial systems are used clinically and for research. They may help direct shoe and orthotic prescriptions by providing information about abnormal pressure distribution, particularly in patients with structural foot deformities or in patients at risk for developing skin ulcerations because of diabetes mellitus or other vascular and peripheral neuropathy disorders.

Kinematics

Electrogoniometers
Electrogoniometers are computerized versions of the simple goniometer, which is commonly used in clinical practice to assess joint range of motion. An electrogoniometer consists of one or more potentiometers placed between two bars, with one bar strapped to the proximal limb segment and the other strapped to the distal limb segment. The potentiometer, which is placed over the joint, provides a varying electrical impulse, depending on the instantaneous angle between the two limb segments. This electrical impulse information is then transmitted to an analog to digital converter in a computer to plot joint angle information over time. A three potentiometer system allows for measuring rotations between limb segments in all planes. A major disadvantage of electrogoniometers is relatively poor accuracy because they are difficult to apply, particularly about the hip and ankle. Unfortunately, even in the case of good accuracy, the results obtained from electrogoniometers provide only relative, not absolute, positions of the joints of limb segments. Because of these limitations, electrogoniometers cannot be used in conjunction with force plate data to evaluate joint kinetic data.

Optoelectronic Motion Analysis

Quantitative gait analysis involves a sophisticated computerized video camera, referred to as an *optoelectronic motion analysis system*. The system measures the three-dimensional location of an individual marker in a similar fashion as the cinematographic method, but with far greater ease and speed. The system automatically defines the position of each marker from each camera and then automatically triangulates the information to provide a three-dimensional position of each marker at each frame. A layout of a typical laboratory space that includes an optoelectronic motion analysis system is illustrated in Figure 17-5. Most optoelectronic systems can detect the true three-dimensional position of a marker within a few millimeters in each of the three axes. The specific type of camera or lenses, the algorithms used to digitize markers, the size of the markers, and the laboratory environment are all factors that determine the accuracy of a system. Marker position is usually determined at every $1/50$ to $1/200$ of a second, depending on the speed of the cameras used. Multiple markers are affixed to the skin of the pelvis and the lower extremities in relationship to bony landmarks. Occasionally, markers also designate portions of the torso and upper extremities. Similar to the cinematographic method, two cameras are necessary to record each marker to obtain its three-dimensional position. Often a camera cannot visualize a marker during a particular part of a movement because of limb rotation or because another limb segment gets in the way. For this reason, sometimes a laboratory uses more than two cameras to ensure that at every given frame of movement, at least two cameras can visualize each of the markers. In the case in which three or more cameras visualize a marker, an algorithm must be used to determine the true position of the marker because some error invariably occurs such that not all cameras converge on the identical three-dimensional position. Other laboratories strategically position the markers so that the same two cameras can visualize a particular marker throughout the movement.

Two types of optoelectronic systems are used for quantitative gait evaluation: (1) active marker systems in which the markers are actively illuminated by a computer, and (2) passive reflective marker systems. An advantage of an active marker system is that the computer determines which marker it is illuminating at any given frame so that the markers are automatically identified; thus, the lateral femoral epicondyle marker is always differentiated from the lateral malleolus marker. The main disadvantage of active marker systems, however, is that the illuminators require power and thus the multiple wires connected to a power source need to be attached to the subject. The cluster of wires tends to encumber the individual's gait. In con-

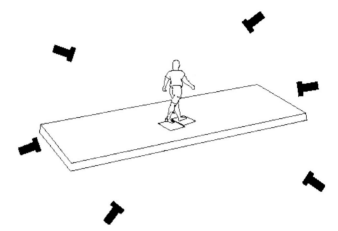

FIGURE 17-5 Optoelectronic motion analysis system. Patient walks along a walkway with reflective markers attached to specific anatomic reference points. Camera pairs record the three-dimensional locations of the reflective markers. Force plates located in the center of the walkway record ground reaction forces. Computer programs combine three-dimensional coordinates and ground reaction forces to calculate joint kinetics and kinematics. (Reprinted with permission from DC Kerrigan, M Schaufele, MN Wen. Gait analysis. In JA Delisa, BM Gans [eds], Rehabilitation Medicine: Principles and Practice [3rd ed]. Philadelphia: Lippincott-Raven, 1998.)

trast, passive marker systems require only that a small reflective piece of material be placed over the desired anatomic landmark. Although passive markers do not encumber the patient, they do require a computer program to determine which marker is which. Fortunately, sophisticated software programs automate this procedure. Thus, passive marker optoelectronic systems are the preferred systems for routine clinical practice.

In order to obtain estimates of joint motion, the optoelectronic system is coupled to a biomechanical model that defines where on the body the markers are optimally placed (Figure 17-6). A simple model to measure knee motion might involve placement of one marker over the greater trochanter, one marker over the lateral femoral epicondyle, and one over the lateral malleolus. The angle formed between the line connecting the greater trochanter with the lateral femoral epicondyle and the line connecting the lateral femoral epicondyle and the lateral malleolus would represent knee flexion. This model, however, would be too simplistic in that knee varus or valgus could easily be misread as true knee flexion. To define sagittal motions such as knee flexion accurately, geometry dictates that three markers (or marker equivalents) be placed on each limb segment, to define the three-dimensional coordinate system

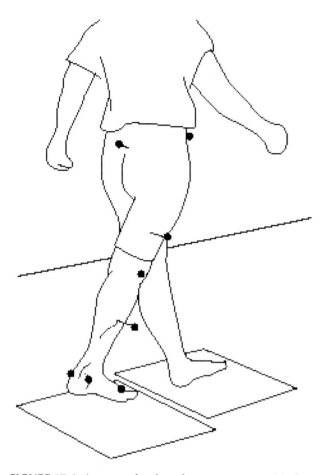

FIGURE 17-6 An example of marker arrangement. Markers are placed on a variety of anatomic landmarks, allowing for the collection of three markers or marker equivalents per rigid body segment. (Reprinted with permission from DC Kerrigan, M Schaufele, MN Wen. Gait analysis. In JA Delisa, BM Gans [eds], Rehabilitation Medicine: Principles and Practice [3rd ed]. Philadelphia: Lippincott-Raven, 1998.)

for that segment. The segment is assumed to be rigid. A marker equivalent could be some imaginary anatomic point calculated on the basis of the position of real markers. For instance, three markers could be used to define a plane in the pelvis. From this plane and the known geometry of the pelvis, the location of the hip joint center can be calculated. The hip joint center then becomes an imaginary marker equivalent and can be used in defining the thigh segment coordinate system. Marker locations are often chosen in order to facilitate estimating joint centers as well as to ensure that the markers can be visualized by the camera system.

Typically, markers are placed over bony landmarks to ensure consistent applications as well as to reduce skin movement artifact. With three markers or marker

equivalents for each body segment, the segment can be represented in the form of a local coordinate system whose orientation is determined with respect to a global coordinate system. The local coordinate system is defined by three mutually perpendicular vectors. Joint angle information then can be ascertained from the proximal and distal limb segment local coordinate systems. Several methods exist for determining joint angle information. Commonly, one axis is chosen to be parallel to the proximal segment local coordinate system axis, and a second axis is chosen to be parallel to the distal segment local coordinate system axis.[46] In this way, a medial and lateral axis is selected from the proximal segment local coordinate system and is considered to be the axis about which joint flexion and extension occur. A longitudinal axis chosen from the distal segment local coordinate system represents the axis about which internal and external rotation occurs. Finally, an axis mutually perpendicular to these two axes is considered as the axis about which abduction and adduction occur.

Kinematic analysis of limb segment motion also may be useful. For instance, kinematic analysis of obstacle clearance illustrates the clinical utility of optoelectronic investigation.[47] In view of the fact that the walking path is often littered with obstacles, particularly outdoors, the walker is at risk for stumbling over the object. Clearance requires modification of the usual swing kinematics. Subjects use four strategies to move the leg, in terms of angular displacement and angular velocity: (1) increase clearance distance with increasing obstacle height; (2) gradual or distinct transition; (3) decrease clearance distance with increasing obstacle height; and (4) interference with obstacle.

Kinetics

Joint moments and power are commonly measured with quantitative gait analysis. The concept of a joint moment has already been described. A joint power, also described previously, represents the net rate of generating or absorbing energy and is the mathematical product of the joint moment and joint angular velocity. A positive joint power implies that the muscle contraction is concentric, because the joint angular velocity and moments are in the same direction. A negative power implies that the muscle contraction is eccentric, as angular velocity and joint moments are in opposite directions. Joint kinetics are calculated, in part, using *inverse dynamic techniques* according to Newton's second law of motion, which essentially calculates the joint moments based on the motion and mass characteristics of the limb segments. Kinetics are typically calculated using a combination of GRF data with inverse dynamic techniques. Thus, kinetic calculations are usually based on (1) knowledge of the position of the joint in relationship to the GRF, (2) estimates of body segment masses and moments of inertia, and (3) knowledge of the body segment positions, velocities, and acceleration.

GRFs are measured using force plates that consist of piezoelectric or strain-gauge transducers. One or more force plates are imbedded in the floor of the walkway (see Figure 17-4). As the subject walks, he or she steps on the force plate(s). To obtain useful GRF data, only one foot must strike the middle of the plate without interference from the other foot or an assistive device. Also, to assess joint kinetics feasibly, kinematic measurements must be collected synchronously with force plate data. The locations of the force plates are predetermined within a calibrated volume in which the kinematic data are measured. A combination of measurements taken on the subject are used in conjunction with reference tables, based on cadaver data, to estimate body segment masses and moments of inertia.[48,49] Clinical gait laboratories report joint moments as either external or internal. An external moment refers to the net external load applied to the joint measured via inverse dynamic techniques. The internal moment, which is equal in magnitude and opposite in sign to the external moment, is the presumed moment caused by the muscle activity, soft tissues, or both to fulfill the requirement that the joint is in equilibrium. For example, an external dorsiflexion moment about the ankle during the stance period of a gait cycle implies that an equal and opposite internal moment provided by the ankle plantar flexors or heel cord is present to maintain joint stability. Similarly, an external flexor moment about the hip during the stance implies that the hip extensors must be active in order to maintain stability. The typical kinetics and kinematics at the hip, knee, and ankle are displayed in Figure 17-4. This type of graphic format is often used for reporting quantitative kinetic and kinematic gait information in the clinical setting.

Dynamic Electromyography

Quantitative gait analysis also includes measurements of muscle activity during walking obtained using dynamic EMG measurement. When combined with kinematic and external kinetic data, dynamic EMG may provide useful information about whether or not a muscle is firing appropriately and if not, how its nonphasic activity may affect gait, particularly in patients with spastic paretic gait. Because muscle activity does not relate linearly to the magnitude of force generated, quantifying the amplitude of activity is not practical.

However, relative normalization to the peak level activity over the gait cycle or the peak level activity, whether it occurs during strength testing or during walking, improves the clinical usefulness of the EMG data.[2]

Muscle activity is measured using either surface electrodes affixed to the skin or fine-wire electrodes inserted in the muscles. Surface electrodes are adequate in studying activity in large superficial muscle groups. In addition to the fact that surface electrodes are not invasive, a major advantage of surface electrodes is that the data obtained are more easily replicated. This latter advantage is undoubtedly because surface electrodes, as compared with fine-wire electrodes, sample data from an inordinately greater number of muscle fibers, representing far more motor units. Because of this fact, fine-wire electrodes are not as prone as superficial electrodes to interference or *cross-talk* from nearby muscles. Fine-wire electrodes are necessary for analyzing activity from smaller, deeper muscles, such as the iliopsoas and posterior tibialis. In addition, fine-wire electrodes are useful for differentiating activity from overlapping muscles such as the rectus femoris and vastus intermedius.

Surface EMG is typically recorded using disposable, gelled electrodes attached to the skin overlying the muscle to be sampled. Commonly, bipolar electrodes are used; the signal recorded is the potential difference between the two electrodes. Fine-wire EMG is often recorded using a wire bipolar electrode consisting of two thin, insulated wires with bared tips. The wires are placed through the shaft of a 25-gauge needle with the two ends bent over the end of the needle and the bared tips staggered so as to avoid contact between them. The needle is inserted through the skin into the muscle and then removed, leaving the wires in place. The bend in the wires provides a means for the electrodes to *catch* on the muscle fascicles. Again, the signal recorded is the potential difference between the two electrode ends. At the end of the study, the wires are removed with a gentle pull.

Preamplified EMG signals, either from fine-wire electrodes or surface electrodes, can be transmitted by cable or radio-wave telemetry to a receiver that is connected to a computer. The EMG signals are usually filtered to remove artifacts created by mechanical movement. The signals are displayed and the gait cycle events identified. Some laboratories report raw EMG signals whereas others report rectified and smoothed EMG activity as well. The timing of the activity is typically what is most important in the assessment. The normal timings of activity of major muscle groups are summarized in Figure 17-7. Muscle timing errors in patients with UMN pathology traditionally are classified into seven catego-

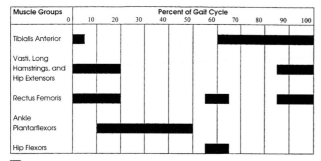

Muscle Groups	Percent of Gait Cycle

FIGURE 17-7 General muscle group activity as a percentage of the gait cycle. (Reprinted with permission from DC Kerrigan, M Schaufele, MN Wen. Gait analysis. In JA Delisa, BM Gans [eds], Rehabilitation Medicine: Principles and Practice [3rd ed]. Philadelphia: Lippincott-Raven, 1998.)

ries: premature onset, delayed onset, curtailed period, prolonged, absent, out of phase, or continuous.[2] Although these categorizations are useful in describing activity in each muscle, it is important to note that they do not necessarily imply pathology about that particular muscle. In some instances, muscle activity differs from that of a nondisabled subject because of compensatory actions. As an example, prolongation of quadriceps activity into the midstance and terminal-stance phases would be compensatory in a patient with an excessive external knee flexor moment. Thus, muscle firing patterns are optimally assessed in conjunction with the external kinetics to help dissociate impairment from compensatory action.

Overall Gait Analysis

The overall gait laboratory analysis procedures take approximately 2 hours for data acquisition and an additional 2 hours for analysis and interpretation. Most of acquisition time is spent applying and confirming placement of the multiple markers and electrodes. The patient is typically evaluated under several conditions (e.g., barefoot, with shoes, and with and without an orthosis or assistive device).

EXAMPLES OF EVALUATION APPROACHES TO SPECIFIC ATYPICAL GAIT PATTERNS

Many atypical gait patterns can be observed in patients with UMN pathology and hemiparetic, paraparetic, or diplegic impairments affecting their gait.[50-56] These atypical patterns include, but are not limited to, reduced knee flexion in swing, also referred to as *stiff-legged gait*; excessive knee flexion in stance, referred to as *crouched gait*; equinus or excessive ankle plantar flexion, occurring during one or more phases in either stance, swing, or both; and knee hyperextension or recurvatum, occurring in one or more phases of stance. Also common, are compensatory atypical gait patterns, including hip hiking, circumduction, or steppage gait.

Spastic Paretic Stiff-Legged Gait

Spastic paretic stiff-legged is a classic atypical gait pattern observed in patients with UMN pathology.[57-59] Stiff-legged gait can be functionally significant for several reasons. From an energy standpoint, lack of knee flexion in swing creates a large moment of inertia that significantly increases the energy required to initiate the swing period of the gait cycle. Additionally, associated compensatory actions to clear the stiff limb, such as vaulting on the unaffected side[60] and excessive pelvic motion,[61] can increase the vertical COM displacement, thereby increasing energy expenditure. From a biomechanical standpoint, the same compensatory actions could place the unaffected knee at risk for posterior capsule damage or the lower back to injury. Finally, lack of knee flexion may cause toe drag during swing, which increases the risk of falling.

One cause of stiff-legged gait is inappropriate activity in one or more bellies of the quadriceps during the preswing, initial swing, or both phases of gait.[57,62-64] Reduced knee flexion may also be caused by weak hip flexors, inappropriate hamstring activity, insufficient ankle plantar flexor muscle action, or all three.[57-59] For many patients with spastic paretic stiff-legged gait who undergo a quantitative gait analysis, the cause of the stiff-legged gait is not obvious from the static or observational gait evaluations. For instance, patients with increased knee extensor tone often can be found to have quiescent quadricep EMG activity during preswing and initial swing. Conversely, a patient with normal knee extensor tone can have inappropriate activity during these phases in one or more of the quadricep muscles. In the latter case, if the inappropriate activity is limited to just one quadricep muscle, an intramuscular neurolytic procedure would be a reasonable treatment to improve the gait pattern. On the other hand, quantitative gait analysis may point to dynamically significant weak hip flexors, indicated by slow progression into hip flexion and poor hip power generation in preswing. These findings commonly are not correlated with hip flexion strength evaluated by static testing. In this case, hip flexion strengthening would be the optimal prescription. In another scenario, a reduced external ankle dorsiflexion moment during stance would imply insufficient ankle plantar flexor muscle action in which case an ankle-foot orthosis with a dorsiflexion stop might be the most appropriate treatment. A quantitative gait analysis also can help provide information about the functional significance of the atypical gait pattern. For instance, the risk for injury to the posterior capsule and ligaments of the unaffected knee can be assessed by measuring the extensor moment during that limb's stance period. Finally, a follow-up quantitative gait assessment may be useful in quantifying the improvement in knee flexion, as well as confirming that the treatment itself did not cause any new problems.

Dynamic Knee Recurvatum

Hyperextension of the knee during the stance period, referred to as *dynamic knee recurvatum*, is a common observation in patients with UMN pathology. This atypical gait pattern may be caused by one or more of the following impairments: quadriceps weakness or spasticity, ankle plantar flexor weakness or spasticity, dorsiflexor weakness, and heel cord contracture.[2,65] A primary functional concern for patients with dynamic knee recurvatum is that the hyperextension may produce an abnormal external extensor moment across the knee, placing the capsular and ligamentous structures of the posterior aspect of the knee at risk for injury. Injury to these tissues may cause pain, ligamentous laxity, and eventual bony deformity. Not all patients have an abnormal knee external moment, in which case the risk for injury is probably less.[37] Knee recurvatum is also important from the standpoint of energy expenditure. The lack of knee flexion can cause a greater displacement of the COM because of the lack of knee flexion during the stance period.

Although multiple factors may contribute to knee recurvatum, it is useful to determine the primary cause in each patient so as to prescribe an optimal treatment plan. In some cases, dynamic recurvatum may be advantageous by providing a control mechanism for an otherwise unstable limb during the stance period of the gait cycle. If the associated knee extensor moment is small, then attempts to improve this atypical pattern may not be the appropriate treatment plan. Thus, quantitative gait analysis provides information that can help assess the functional significance of the atypical gait

pattern as well as information that can help delineate the underlying impairment(s).

Diplegic-Crouched Gait

Crouched gait is defined as excessive knee flexion during the stance period of the gait cycle and most commonly occurs in diplegic gait specific to cerebral palsy.[66–68] Associated gait patterns are adduction and internal rotation at the hips and equinus and forefoot abduction. Reduced knee flexion in swing is also common. Dynamically, hamstring spasticity has been implicated as the principal cause of excessive knee flexion in stance.[66–68] However, clinical experience suggests that tight hip flexors, plantar flexor weakness, and heel cord contracture may also be causative. These potential causes are best evaluated using the combined information obtained from static evaluation and observational and quantitative gait analysis.

Equinus Gait

Excessive ankle plantar flexion occurring in either stance or swing is common in patients with neurologic lesions. As in other atypical gait patterns, the functional significance of the pattern needs to be determined. Kerrigan et al.[69] used biomechanical analyses to show that toe-walking can have biomechanical advantages for individuals with distal lower extremity weakness. Toe-walking can require less knee extensor, ankle plantar flexor, and ankle dorsiflexor strength than walking heel to toe. Thus, for patients with UMN injury who typically have greater distal than proximal weakness, toe-walking may be a more efficient means of ambulation. On the other hand, during swing, excessive plantar flexion may place an individual at increased risk for tripping and falls. Dynamic EMG is useful in identifying the presence of inappropriate soleus, gastrocnemius, or posterior tibialis activity as a cause of the excessive plantar flexion. For equinus in swing, the lack of ankle plantar flexor activity suggests either a heel cord contracture or weak ankle dorsiflexors as a cause. Each patient also deserves evaluation for functionally significant compensatory mechanisms as well such as increased hip flexion and hip hiking in swing.

Gait Patterns Associated with Lower Motor Neuron and Orthopedic Disorders

Unlike that seen in most patients with UMN pathology, the atypical gait patterns associated with specific peripheral nerve injuries cause discrete patterns of muscle weakness and associated characteristic atypical gait patterns. The following examples illustrate atypical gait patterns that arise from weakness of a specific functional muscle group. To determine the underlying impairment and functional limitation responsible for the atypical gait pattern, static evaluation and observational analysis are usually adequate. Kinetic assessment is often useful, however, in helping to determine the functional significance of an atypical gait pattern.

Gait Associated with Femoral Neuropathy

Selected quadriceps weakness, which can occur in femoral neuropathy in diabetes, femoral nerve entrapment, or poliomyelitis, impairs weight-bearing stability during stance. Normally, the quadriceps eccentrically contract to control the rate of knee flexion during the loading response of the limb. With weakness, the knee tends to buckle. The effective compensatory action is to position the lower extremity such that the GRF lies anterior to the knee joint, imparting an extension moment during stance phases. This is first achieved during initial contact by plantar flexing the ankle. Contraction of the hip extensors can also help to hold the knee in hyperextension. As noted previously, quantitative gait analysis may be useful in evaluating the associated knee extensor moment that, if excessive, could place the posterior ligamentous capsule at risk for injury. To compensate, most individuals simply place their ipsilateral hand in front of the thigh to prevent the knee from buckling.

Atypical Gait Patterns Associated with Weak Ankle Dorsiflexors

Dorsiflexor weakness also has a characteristic gait pattern. Clinical conditions in which this is seen are peroneal nerve palsy occurring as a result of entrapment at the fibular head or more proximally as an injury to a branch of the sciatic nerve or in an L-5 radiculopathy. If the ankle dorsiflexors have a grade of 3, 4, or 5, the characteristic clinical sign is *foot slap* occurring soon after initial contact because of the inability of the ankle dorsiflexors to eccentrically contract to control the rate of plantar flexion after heel contact. If the ankle dorsiflexors have less than 3/5 strength, toe drag, a steppage gait pattern, or both with excessive hip flexion in swing are likely. The cause of these patterns can usually be determined with a careful history, physical examination, and standard electrodiagnostic procedures, rather than a dynamic EMG assessment.

Atypical Gait Patterns Associated with Generalized Lower Motor Neuron Lesions

More generalized lower motor neuron lesions commonly involve variable weakness patterns and thus often have unpredictable and often complex associated gait patterns. Poliomyelitis and Guillain-Barré syndrome are examples. For these diagnoses, kinetic assessment can be particularly useful in determining excessive joint moments, implying excessive soft tissue strain or the need for increased compensatory muscle action in another muscle group.

Trendelenburg's Gait

Trendelenburg's gait, also known as *gluteus medius gait*, describes a pattern of either excessive pelvic obliquity during the stance period of the affected side (uncompensated Trendelenburg's gait), excessive lateral truncal lean during the stance period of the affected side (compensated Trendelenburg's gait), or both. Weakness of or reluctance to use the gluteus medius can cause this atypical gait pattern. The most common cause of Trendelenburg's gait is osteoarthritis of the hip or other painful disorder. In this case, the gait pattern, regardless of whether it is compensated or uncompensated, occurs as a compensatory response to reduce the overall forces across the hip during stance. This can be seen as a reduction in the external hip adductor moment, which ordinarily occurs in the stance period. A simple remedy to correct this gait deviation is using a cane, contralateral to the affected side.

Orthotic Influence on Gait

Orthoses are commonly prescribed to improve the gait of patients with orthopedic or neurologic disorders.[70] As Table 17-2 illustrates, a gait deviation or compensation may be caused by anatomic abnormalities or by the orthosis. In some instances, such as circumduction, the orthosis itself can cause the compensation; a knee-ankle-foot orthosis that has a knee lock interferes with the wearer's ability to flex the knee during swing phase. In other cases, a faulty orthosis hampers walking. For example, if the ankle control on an ankle-foot orthosis is eroded or malaligned, the patient may exhibit foot slap during loading response.

Acknowledgments

The work in this chapter was supported in part by grant NIH HD01071-05 from the Public Health Service and by the Ellison Foundation.

TABLE 17-2
Orthotic Gait Analysis

Deviation	Orthotic Causes	Anatomic Causes
Early stance		
Foot slap: forefront slaps the ground	Inadequate dorsiflexion assist Inadequate plantarflexion stop	Weak dorsiflexors
Toes first: tiptoe posture may or may not be maintained throughout stance	Inadequate heel lift Inadequate dorsiflexion assist Inadequate plantarflexion stop Inadequate relief of heel pain	Short leg Pes equinus Extensor spasticity Heel pain
Flat foot contact: entire foot contacts ground initially	Inadequate traction from sole Requires walking aid (e.g., cane) Inadequate dorsiflexion stop	Poor balance Pes calcaneus
Excessive medial (lateral) foot contact: medial (lateral) border contacts floor	Transverse plane malalignment	Weak invertors (evertors) Pes valgus (varus) Genu valgum (varum)
Excessive knee flexion: knee collapses when foot contacts ground	Inadequate knee lock Inadequate dorsiflexion stop Plantarflexion stop Inadequate contralateral shoe lift	Weak quadriceps Short contralateral leg Knee pain Knee and/or hip flexion contracture Flexor synergy Pes calcaneus
Hyperextended knee: knee hyperextends as weight is transferred to leg	Genu recurvatum inadequately controlled by plantarflexion stop Excessively concave calf band Pes equinus uncompensated by contralateral shoe lift Inadequate knee lock	Weak quadriceps Lax knee ligaments Extensor synergy Pes equinus Contralateral knee and/or hip flexion contracture
Anterior trunk bending: patient leans forward as weight is transferred to leg	Inadequate knee lock	Weak quadriceps Hip flexion contracture Knee flexion contracture
Posterior trunk bending: patient leans backward as weight is transferred to leg	Inadequate hip lock Knee lock	Weak gluteus maximus Knee ankylosis
Lateral trunk bending: patient leans toward stance leg as weight is transferred to leg	Excessive height of medial upright KAFO Excessive abduction of hip joint of HKAFO Insufficient shoe lift Requires walking aid (e.g., cane)	Weak gluteus medius Abduction contracture Dislocated hip Hip pain Poor balance Short leg
Wide walking base: heel centers more than 10 cm (4 in.) apart	Excessive height of medial upright KAFO Excessive abduction of hip joint of HKAFO Insufficient lift on contralateral shoe Knee lock Requires walking aid (e.g., cane)	Abduction contracture Poor balance Short contralateral leg
Internal (external) rotation: limb internally (externally) rotated	Uprights incorrectly aligned in transverse plane Requires orthotic control (e.g., rotation control straps, pelvic band)	Internal (external) hip rotators spastic External (internal) hip rotators weak Anteversion (retroversion) Weak quadriceps: external rotation

TABLE 17-2 *(continued)*

Deviation	Orthotic Causes	Anatomic Causes
Late stance		
Inadequate transition: delayed or absent transfer of weight over the forefoot	Plantarflexion stop Inadequate dorsiflexion stop	Weak plantarflexors Achilles tendon sprain or rupture Pes calcaneus Forefoot pain
Swing		
Toe drag: toes maintain contact with the ground	Inadequate dorsiflexion assist Inadequate plantarflexion stop	Weak dorsiflexors Plantarflexor spasticity Pes equinus Weak hip flexors
Circumduction: leg swings outward in a semicircular arc	Knee lock Inadequate dorsiflexion assist Inadequate plantarflexion stop	Weak hip flexors Extensor synergy Knee and/or ankle ankylosis Weak dorsiflexors Pes equinus
Hip hiking: leg elevates at pelvis to enable the limb to swing forward	Knee lock Inadequate dorsiflexion assist Inadequate plantarflexion stop	Short contralateral leg Contralateral knee and/or hip flexion contracture Weak hip flexors Extensor synergy Knee and/or ankle ankylosis Weak dorsiflexors Pes equinus
Vaulting: exaggerated plantarflexion of contralateral leg to enable the limb to swing forward	Knee lock Inadequate dorsiflexion assist Inadequate plantarflexion stop	Weak hip flexors Extensor spasticity Pes equinus Short contralateral leg Contralateral knee and/or hip flexion contracture Knee and/or ankle ankylosis Weak dorsiflexors

HKAFO = hip-knee-ankle-foot orthosis; KAFO = knee-ankle-foot orthosis.

REFERENCES

1. Kerrigan DC, Schaufele M, Wen MN. Gait Analysis. In JA Delisa, BM Gans (eds), Rehabilitation Medicine Principles and Practice (3rd ed). Philadelphia: Lippincott-Raven, 1998;167–187.
2. Perry J. Gait Analysis: Normal and Pathological Function. Thorofare, NJ: SLACK, Inc, 1992.
3. Saunders JBD, Inman VT, Eberhart HD. The major determinants in normal and pathological gait. Am J Bone Joint Surg 1953;35:543–558.
4. Inman VT, Ralston HJ, Todd F. Human Locomotion. In J Rose, JG Gamble (eds), Human Walking (2nd ed). Baltimore: Williams & Wilkins, 1994;1–22.
5. Kerrigan DC, Viramontes BE, Corcoran PJ, LaRaia PJ. Measured versus predicted vertical displacement of the sacrum during gait as a tool to measure biomechanical gait performance. Am J Phys Med Rehabil 1995;74:3–8.
6. Kerrigan DC, Thirunarayan MA, Sheffler LR, et al. A tool to assess biomechanical gait efficiency; a preliminary clinical study. Am J Phys Med Rehabil 1996;75:3–8.
7. Gard SA, Childress DS. The effect of pelvic list on the vertical displacement of the trunk during normal walking. Gait Posture 1997;5:233–238.
8. Gard SA, Childress DS. The influence of stance-phase knee flexion on the vertical displacement of the trunk during normal walking. Arch Phys Med Rehabil 1999;80:26–32.
9. Gonzalez EG, Corcoran PJ. Energy Expenditure During Ambulation. In JA Downey, SJ Myers, EG Gonzalez, JS Lieberman (eds), The Physiological Basis of Rehabilitation Medicine (2nd ed). Stoneham, MA: Butterworth–Heinemann, 1994;413–446.
10. McDonald I. Statistical studies of recorded energy expenditure of man. Part II: Expenditure on walking related to weight, sex, height, speed, and gradient. Nutr Abstr Rev 1961;31:739–762.
11. Duff-Raffaele M, Kerrigan DC, Corco-

ran PJ, Saini M. The proportional work of lifting the center of mass during walking. Am J Phys Med Rehabil 1996;75:375–379.

12. Corcoran PJ. Energy Expenditure During Ambulation. In JA Downey, RD Darling (eds), Physiological Basis of Rehabilitation Medicine (1st ed). Philadelphia: WB Saunders, 1971;185–198.

13. Bard B. Energy expenditure of hemiplegic subjects during walking. Arch Phys Med Rehabil 1963;44:368–370.

14. Corcoran PJ, Brengelmann GL. Oxygen uptake in normal and handicapped subjects, in relation to speed of walking beside velocity-controlled cart. Arch Phys Med Rehabil 1970;51:78–87.

15. Astrand PO, Rodahl K. Textbook on Work Physiology. New York: McGraw-Hill, 1970.

16. Murray MP, Drought AB, Kory RC. Walking patterns of normal men. Am J Bone Joint Surg 1964;46A:335–360.

17. Kadaba MP, Ramakrishnan HK, Wootten ME. Measurement of lower extremity kinematics during level walking. J Orthop Res 1990;8:383–392.

18. Kerrigan DC, Todd MK, Della Croce U. Gender differences in joint biomechanics during walking: normative study in young adults. Am J Phys Med Rehabil 1998;77:2–7.

19. Sutherland DH, Olshen RA, Biden EN, Wyatt MP. The Development of Mature Walking. Philadelphia: Mac Keith Press, 1988.

20. Nene A, Mayagoitia R, Veltink P. Assessment of rectus femoris function during initial swing phase. Gait Posture 1999;9:1–9.

21. Annaswamy TM, Giddings C, Della Croce U, Kerrigan DC. Rectus femoris: its role in normal gait. Arch Phys Med Rehabil 1999;80:930–934.

22. Kerrigan DC, Todd MK, Riley PO. Knee osteoarthritis and high-heeled shoes. Lancet 1998;351:1399–1401.

23. Taylor NF, Goldie PA, Evans OM. Angular movements of the pelvis and lumbar spine during self-selected and slow walking speeds. Gait Posture 1999;9:88–94.

24. Sutherland DH, Olshen R, Cooper L, Woo SL. The development of mature gait. Am J Bone Joint Surg 1980;62: 336–353.

25. Menkveld SR, Knipstein EA, Quinn JR. Analysis of gait patterns in normal school-aged children. J Pediatr Orthop 1988;8:263–267.

26. Murray MP, Kory RC, Clarkson BH. Walking patterns in healthy old men. J Gerontol 1969;24:169–178.

27. Elble RJ, Thomas SS, Higgins C, Colliver J. Stride-dependent changes in gait of older people. J Neurol 1991;238:1–5.

28. Kerrigan DC, Todd MK, Della Croce U, et al. Biomechanical gait alterations independent of speed in the healthy elderly: evidence for specific limiting impairments. Arch Phys Med Rehabil 1998;79:317–322.

29. Lee LW, Kerrigan DC. Identification of kinetic differences between fallers and nonfallers in the elderly. Am J Phys Med Rehabil 1999;78:242–246.

30. Blanc Y, Balmer C, Landis T, Vingerhoets F. Temporal parameters and patterns of the foot roll over during walking: normative data for healthy adults. Gait Posture 1999;10:97–108.

31. Oeffinger D, Brauch B, Cranfill S, et al. Comparison of gait with and without shoes in children. Gait Posture 1999;9:95–100.

32. Brodke DS, Skinner SR, Lamoreux LW, et al. Effects of ankle-foot orthoses on the gait of children. J Pediatr Orthop 1989;9:702–708.

33. Radtka SA, Skinner SR, Dixon DM, Johanson ME. A comparison of gait with solid, dynamic, and no ankle-foot orthoses in children with spastic cerebral palsy. Phys Ther 1997;77:395–409.

34. Duysens J, Van de Crommert HWAA. Neural control of locomotion. Part 1: the central pattern generator from cats to humans. Gait Posture 1998;7:131–141.

35. van Deursen RWM, Flynn TW, McCrory JL, Morag E. Does a single control mechanism exist for both forward and backward walking? Gait Posture 1998;7:214–224.

36. van de Crommert HWAA, Mulder T, Duysens J. Neural control of locomotion: sensory control of the central pattern generator and its relation to treadmill training. Gait Posture 1998;7:251–263.

37. Kerrigan DC, Deming LC, Holden MK. Knee recurvatum in gait: a study of associated knee biomechanics. Arch Phys Med Rehabil 1996;77:645–650.

38. Gage JR. Gait analysis in cerebral palsy. Philadelphia: Mac Keith Press, 1991.

39. Lee EH, Nather A, Goh J, et al. Gait analysis in cerebral palsy. Ann Acad Med Singapore 1985;14:37–43.

40. DeLuca PA. Gait analysis in the treatment of the ambulatory child with cerebral palsy. Clin Orthop 1991:65–75.

41. Saleh M, Murdoch G. In defence of gait analysis. Observation and measurement in gait assessment. J Bone Joint Surg Br 1985;67:237–241.

42. Kerrigan DC, Ehrenthal S. A maladaptive gait abnormality in patients with lumbosacral spinal stenosis. J Back Musculoskel Rehabil 1996;7:53–57.

43. Lee LW, Kerrigan DC, Della Croce U. Dynamic implications of hip flexion contractures. Am J Phys Med Rehabil 1997;76:502–508.

44. Kerrigan DC, Glenn MB. An illustration of clinical gait laboratory use to improve rehabilitation management. Am J Phys Med Rehabil 1994;73:421–427.

45. Hausdorff JM, Ladin Z, Wei JY. Footswitch system for measurement of the temporal parameters of gait. J Biomech 1995;28:347–351.

46. Grood ES, Suntay WJ. A joint coordinate system for the clinical description of three-dimensional motions: applications to the knee. J Biomech Eng 1983;105:136–144.

47. Austin GP, Garrett GE, Bohannon RW. Kinematic analysis of obstacle clearance during locomotion. Gait Posture 1999;10:109–120.

48. Dempster WT. Space Requirements of the Seated Operator. Ann Arbor: University of Michigan, 1955.

49. Zatsiorsky VM, Seluyanov VN. The Mass and Inertia Characteristics of the Main Segments of the Human Body. In H Matsui, K Kobayashi (eds), Human Kinetics. Champaign, IL: Human Kinetics, 1983;1152–1159.

50. Hirschberg GG, Nathanson M. Electromyographic recordings of muscular activity in normal and spastic gaits. Arch Phys Med Rehabil 1947;33:217–224.

51. Peat M, Dubo HI, Winter DA, et al. Electromyographic temporal analysis of gait: hemiplegic locomotion. Arch Phys Med Rehabil 1976;57:421–425.

52. Knutsson E, Richards C. Different types of disturbed motor control in gait of hemiparetic patients. Brain 1979;102:405–430.

53. Shiavi R, Bugle HJ, Limbird T. Electromyographic gait assessment. Part 2: preliminary assessment of hemiparetic synergy patterns. J Rehabil Res Dev 1987;24:24–30.

54. Winters TF Jr, Gage JR, Hicks R. Gait patterns in spastic hemiplegia in children and young adults. Am J Bone Joint Surg 1987;69:437–441.

55. Kerr HD. Silly hematurias: achtung! It's the goose step [Letter]. JAMA 1987;257:1332.

56. Kerrigan DC, Sheffler L. Spastic paretic gait: an approach to evaluation and treatment. Crit Rev Phys Med Rehabil 1995;7:253–268.

57. Kerrigan DC, Gronley J, Perry J. Stiff-legged gait in spastic paresis. A study of quadriceps and hamstrings muscle activity. Am J Phys Med Rehabil 1991;70:294–300.

58. Kerrigan DC, Roth RS, Riley PO. The modelling of spastic paretic stiff-legged gait based on actual kinematic data. Gait Posture 1998;7:117–124.

59. Kerrigan DC, Bang MS, Burke DT. An algorithm to assess stiff-legged gait in traumatic brain injury. J Head Trauma Rehabil 1999;14:136–145.

60. Kerrigan DC, Frates EP, Rogan S, Riley PO. Spastic paretic stiff-legged gait: the biomechanics of the unaffected limb. Am J Phys Med Rehabil 1999;78:354–360.

61. Kerrigan DC, Frates EP, Rogan S, Riley PO. Hip hiking and circumduction: quantitative definitions. Am J Phys Med Rehabil 2000;79:247–252.

62. Waters RL, Garland DE, Perry J, et al. Stiff-legged gait in hemiplegia: surgical correction. Am J Bone Joint Surg 1979;61:927–933.

63. Treanor WJ. The role of physical medicine treatment in stroke rehabilitation. Clin Orthop 1969;63:14–22.

64. Sutherland DH, Santi M, Abel MF. Treatment of stiff-knee gait in cerebral palsy: a comparison by gait analysis of distal rectus femoris transfer versus proximal rectus release. J Pediatr Orthop 1990;10:433–441.

65. Simon SR, Deutsch SD, Nuzzo RM, et al. Genu recurvatum in spastic cerebral palsy. Report on findings by gait analysis. Am J Bone Joint Surg 1978;60:882–894.

66. Gage JR, Perry J, Hicks RR, et al. Rectus femoris transfer to improve knee function of children with cerebral palsy. Dev Med Child Neurol 1987;29:159–166.

67. Sutherland DH, Cooper L. The pathomechanics of progressive crouch gait in spastic diplegia. Orthop Clin North Am 1978;9:143–154.

68. Thometz J, Simon S, Rosenthal R. The effect on gait of lengthening of the medial hamstrings in cerebral palsy. Am J Bone Joint Surg 1989;71:345–353.

69. Kerrigan DC, Riley PO, Rogan S, Burke DT. Compensatory advantages of toe-walking. Arch Phys Med Rehabil 2000;81:38–44.

70. Edelstein JE. Orthotic Assessment and Management. In SB O'Sullivan, TJ Schmitz (eds), Physical Rehabilitation Assessment and Treatment. Philadelphia: FA Davis, 2000.

18

Energy Expenditure during Ambulation

ERWIN G. GONZALEZ AND JOAN E. EDELSTEIN

People with disabilities often consider the ability to walk as the pinnacle of rehabilitation. Yet, the intricacies involved in the seemingly simple act of ambulation are seldom considered until problems occur. As a child attempts to take the first steps, two natural forces, inertia and gravity, make the toddler stumble forward and fall. Eventually, the youngster learns to defy these forces and begins to walk with the fluidity of an adult. Persons with disabilities face similar challenges during the process of learning or regaining the ability to ambulate after an injury or disease that hampers this well-syncopated motion.

NORMAL GAIT

Comprehending the energy requirements of normal and abnormal ambulation requires an understanding of its basic physiology and biomechanics. Recourse can be made to the classic works of Saunders et al.,[1] Inman et al.,[2] and more recent studies by Gard and Childress[3,4] (see Chapter 17). Simply put, the determinants of normal gait appear to minimize inertial changes and the vertical and horizontal displacement of the center of gravity. The net effect is a smooth, sinusoidal translation of the center of gravity through space so the walker requires the least energy expenditure (Ee).

During gait, two main events occur in which energy is consumed. One is in controlling forward movement during deceleration toward the end of swing phase and for shock absorption at heel strike, and the other is in propulsion during pushoff, when the center of gravity is propelled up and forward. Ironically, more energy is expended to control forward movement than to propel forward.

Examination of peak muscle activity during ambulation shows that although muscles generally contract concentrically, the predominant activities in gait occur during eccentric contraction. As examples, the dorsiflexors lengthen to prevent foot slap, the quadriceps absorb shock and allow the knee to bend by contracting eccentrically, and the hamstrings decelerate the limb during the swing phase.

Eccentric contraction is more energy efficient than concentric contraction and demonstrates how the human body has developed kinetically and kinematically to minimize energy cost.[5]

ENERGY SOURCES AND METABOLISM

Physical activity requires expenditure of energy. Oxygen consumption is most commonly used as a measure of Ee during extended activity such as walking, primarily because the principal energy for such types of activities is supplied through aerobic metabolic pathways. After working approximately 2 minutes at a constant submaximal level, the body reaches steady state. At this point, the level of oxygen consumption meets tissue demands, and the heart beat and respiratory rate become constant. The level of oxygen consumption at steady state closely reflects actual energy cost. The only source of energy that the human body can use is the chemical energy contained in complex food molecules. Oxidation of these to simple substances such as water and carbon dioxide is an exothermic reaction.

During activity there is interplay between aerobic and anaerobic mechanisms. In aerobic oxidation (Krebs citric acid cycle), carbohydrates and fats provide the primary fuels. These substrates are oxidized through a series of reactions leading to the production of adenosine triphosphate. Oxygen is the final hydrogen acceptor, and water is formed.

The availability of oxygen is not required in the second type of oxidative reaction. In anaerobic metabolism (glycolytic pathway) glucose is converted to pyruvate and then to lactic acid (lactate).

For activities that require less than 50% of maximal aerobic capacity ($\dot{V}O_2$max), the aerobic mechanisms are usually sufficient to supply the energy. For strenuous exercise, however, both mechanisms are called into play. The anaerobic system yields much less energy per unit of glucose than the aerobic mechanism, and its use is limited by a person's tolerance to the resultant lactic acidosis. In daily life, the anaerobic system is used for sudden and short bursts of activity, making it possible for the body to achieve a higher rate of energy production than can be achieved by aerobic oxidation alone. An understanding of the foregoing concepts is a necessary first step to understanding the energy demands that ambulation places on persons with disabilities (see Chapter 16).

TABLE 18-1
Equivalent Units of Speed, Energy Expenditure (Ee) per Unit of Time, and Distance

Units of speed (1 m/min)
  = 3.28 ft/min
  = 0.037 mph
  = 0.06 km/hr
  = 0.055 ft/sec
  = 0.017 m/sec
Units of Ee/unit distance (work*) (1 kcal [kilocalorie])
  = 1,000 cal (gram calorie)
  = 3,086 ft-lb
  = 427 kg-m
  = 3.988 BTU
  = 0.00156 hp-hr
  = 0.00116 kW-hr
Units of Ee/unit time (power*) (1 kcal/min)
  = 1,000 cal/min
  = 3,086 ft-lb/min
  = 427 kg-m/min
  = 69.733 watts (joules sec)
  = 3.968 BTU/min
  = 0.0935 hp
  = 0.0697 kW

*Although the term is not appropriate for expressing calorie expenditure during ambulation, equivalent values are given for the reader's reference. These units are occasionally used in the literature.

ENERGY MEASUREMENT

Terminology

Work is equal to the product of force and distance. In walking, the forces are primarily gravity and friction, plus the inertia of acceleration and deceleration. The distance is the up-and-down and side-to-side motions of the body's center of gravity and the separate body segments. To diminish the work required, the force may be decreased or the distance may be shortened. *Power*, on the other hand, is the rate of doing work: (force × distance)/time. In handicapped and normal activities, the rate of Ee can be kept tolerable if force, distance, or both are decreased, or if the time spent on the task is increased (i.e., by walking more slowly).[5,6]

Although these concepts are practical, the use of the two terms can be confusing when applied to ambulation. The *work* required for walking is not at all the same as the *Ee per unit distance* of ambulation (kilocalories per meter). Similarly, equating *power* as *Ee per unit time* (kilocalories per minute) is inappropriate, because kilocalories per minute is a measure of energy input per minute of metabolic function, not mechanical force times distance divided by time.[7]

Units of Measurement

Review of the literature is often confusing, because different authors use different units of measurement. Table 18-1 presents conversion factors for some of the more frequently used units of measure. In this chapter, Ee per unit time is expressed as kilocalories per minute per kilogram and Ee per unit distance is analyzed in terms of kilocalories per meter per kilogram. For a 70-kg adult in normal health the basal metabolic rate (BMR) is approximately 1 kcal per minute. This unitary value is convenient for comparing values during various activities for an average-sized adult, which then may be read directly as multiples of the basal rate. The BMR is sometimes referred to as a *metabolic unit* or *MET*. For untrained persons, an Ee greater than 5 kcal per minute or five times the BMR is the maximum that one can sustain for several hours. Anaerobic metabolism starts at this point, leading to oxygen debt and accumulation of lactic acid. This physiological fact probably sets the limit on *light* industrial work or comfortable walking speed (CWS). Table 18-2 lists different types of light activities. Several excellent studies, including those of Passmore and Durnin,[8] Brown and Brengelmann,[9] and Gordon,[10] address energy metabolism and units of measure.

TABLE 18-2

Energy Cost of Light Activities in Adults (kcal/min/70 kg)

Activity	Energy Expenditure (kcal/min/70 kg)
Sleeping	0.9
Lying quietly	1.0
Lying quietly doing mental arithmetic	1.04
Sitting at ease	1.2–1.6
Sitting, writing	1.9–2.2
Standing at ease	1.4–2.0
Walking, 1 mph (27 m/min)	2.3
Standing, washing, and shaving	2.5–2.6
Standing, dressing, and undressing	2.3–3.3
Light housework	1.7–3.0
Office work	1.3–2.5
Typing, electric typewriter	1.13–1.39
Walking 2 mph (54 m/min)	3.1
Light industrial work	2.0–5.0
Walking 3 mph (80 m/min)	4.3

Methods of Measuring Energy Expenditure

Indirect Calorimetry

Atwater introduced estimation of Ee by measurement of oxygen consumption at the end of the nineteenth century. Although precise computation of oxygen consumption and carbon dioxide production is not feasible, the technique is the one method most frequently employed in Ee studies. The procedure rests on the knowledge that, after an average diet, a subject at rest in a postprandial steady state generates approximately 4.83 kcal of energy for every liter of oxygen consumed. This varies slightly, depending on the specific food in question. However, the use of the standard average value of 4.83 kcal/L results in inaccuracies no greater than a few percent in a subject who eats a mixed diet.

Measurement of the oxygen consumption rate under specified resting conditions constitutes the BMR test. At rest, body surface area correlates most accurately with Ee. Surface area is easily predicted from nomograms of height and weight. However, most activities in rehabilitation involve moving all or parts of the body against gravity. During exercise, there is better correlation with the total weight of the subject, plus clothing and adaptive devices worn or carried, than with surface area. Therefore, in this chapter oxygen consumption is expressed per unit of body weight.

In most systems used to measure human oxygen consumption, the expired air is collected and its volume is measured. The concentration of expired oxygen is deter-

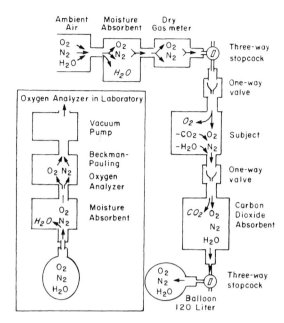

FIGURE 18-1 System used in most oxygen consumption determinations (see the section Indirect Calorimetry). (Reprinted with permission from PJ Corcoran, GL Brengelmann. Oxygen uptake in normal and handicapped subjects, in relation to speed of walking beside velocity-controlled cart. Arch Phys Med Rehabil 1970;51:78–87.)

mined, and the expired volume of oxygen is subtracted from the oxygen in the inspired ambient air, which is 20.93% unless it is altered by environmental changes. The volume is corrected to conditions of standard temperature (37°C), pressure (760 mm Hg), and relative humidity (zero or dry) (Figure 18-1).

The simplest method of collecting expired air is in a large floating bell spirometer if the subject is stationary, or in a rubber-impregnated canvas such as the Douglas bag or a neoprene or other nonporous plastic bag if the patient is moving about. The bell spirometer provides a direct reading of gas volume. If a bag is used, its contents are later passed through a gas meter to determine the expired volume, and the air is analyzed for oxygen content by chemical or physical means. To avoid variation caused by the specific dynamic action of food, metabolic studies are customarily performed on fasting subjects.

Investigators at the Max Planck Institute in Germany in the 1940s developed a small portable respirometer that could be carried on the patient's back like a knapsack. It stored an aliquot of the total expired air in a rubber bladder. This and other similar respirometers permitted many studies of Ee in actual field situations.[11] Speed-controlled and other types of metabolic carts are available to determine oxygen consumption.[12,13] Corcoran and Brengelmann[13] were emphatic about the importance of accurate speed control when studying the metabolic cost of ambulation, because patients use up savings in energy to achieve faster speeds. If speed is not measured accurately or maintained at a constant rate, small variations caused by different sets of conditions may be obscured, as may have happened in some studies.

Carbon dioxide production also correlates with Ee, but the relationship varies more with dietary differences. In addition, the body's bicarbonate buffer system allows significant amounts of carbon dioxide to be stored during exercise or hypoventilation, causing variations in carbon dioxide output that are unrelated to the instantaneous metabolic level. For this reason, oxygen consumption is simpler to use as an indirect measure of Ee than carbon dioxide production.

Heart Rate

Heart rate bears a linear relationship to oxygen consumption and correlates with work measurements such as speed of walking, running, or bicycling in an ergometer. Measurement of heart rate is simple and requires no special equipment. However, the usefulness of heart rate as an index of Ee is limited because data on which the norms are based were derived from studies of high work rates among healthy people, including trained athletes and laborers.

Astrand's nomogram makes possible the prediction of a person's maximum oxygen consumption for lower extremity exercise. Astrand's method is based on heart rate and oxygen consumption during submaximal exercise, multiplied by an age correction factor.[14] In a group of sedentary adults, however, the extrapolation underestimated actual maximum oxygen consumption by 27%.[15] The inaccuracy is more remarkable for the smaller workloads that disabled persons typically bear.

At low work levels, heart rate can vary independently of Ee. Both heart rate and blood pressure show a greater increase when a given rate of work is performed by the upper extremities than with lower extremity activity. This phenomenon probably occurs because when a muscle contracts with a given percentage of its maximum force, the effect on blood pressure is approximately the same as during the same percentage of contraction of any other muscle.[16,17] Thus, the smaller arm muscles contract more markedly and stimulate the cardiovascular system more than the larger leg muscles doing the same work. This should be borne in mind when patients who have cardiovascular disease are considered for

training with hand-held ambulation aids, wheelchairs,[16,17] or any forceful arm and hand exercises. Sustained isometric or static exercise similarly produces a disproportionate cardiovascular response as compared with dynamic or isotonic contraction.[16]

ENERGY EXPENDITURE IN ABLE-BODIED PERSONS

Rest

The BMR is low at birth, reaches its peak around age 2 years, and declines by 30% during the growing years and by another 10% during adulthood. At every age, women tend to have approximately a 10% lower metabolic rate. The metabolic rate also increases approximately 10% for every 1°C increase in body temperature above normal. Cooling the body initiates shivering and also increases BMR, as the body attempts to restore or maintain normal temperature. Extreme shivering can increase the metabolic rate to as much as 6 kcal per minute for short periods.[6]

During sleep, the metabolic rate is 5–10% lower than BMR, or slightly less than 1 kcal per minute for a 70-kg human; sitting and standing at rest require slightly more than 1 kcal per minute (see Table 18-2).

Ambulation

Several studies on the energy cost of walking have produced surprisingly similar data (Table 18-3).[18–22] McDonald's review[18] revealed that the gross Ee at speeds of 60–80 m per minute varied only slightly. The least energy was spent at speeds approximating 80 m per minute, or 3 miles per hour, which is the average self-selected or CWS. Heavy persons use more energy walking at a given speed, but when corrected for their weight plus that of clothing and any equipment carried, their metabolic rate is similar to that of normal-weight subjects. It is of interest to note that after a significant weight loss among obese individuals, the Ee of walking reduced more than expected based on lowered body weight.[23] Height[24] has no effect, but there are conflicting reports regarding the influence of age and gender.[18,20–22,25]

Children (6–12 years) have significantly greater energy consumption (0.073 kcal/min/kg) as compared with teenagers (13–19 years) with average Ee per unit time in the adult range of 0.062 kcal per minute per kg.[25] The Ee per unit distance is likewise higher among children.[25]

The energy cost of walking increases more steeply as speed increases. This relationship is curvilinear (Figure 18-2B). At higher speeds, a given increment in

TABLE 18-3

Energy Expenditure (Ee): Normal Ambulation

Author (Year)	No.	Comment	Speed (m/min) Subject	Speed (m/min) Difference (%) (Normal 80 m/min)	Ee per Unit Time[a] (kcal/min/kg) Subject	Ee per Unit Time[a] (kcal/min/kg) Predicted from Equation at Subject's Speed	Difference (%)	Ee per Unit Distance (kcal × 10⁻³/m/kg) Subject	Ee per Unit Distance (kcal × 10⁻³/m/kg) Difference (%) (NCWS 0.786 kcal × 10⁻³/m/kg)
Ralston (1958)[27]	19	M/F CWS	74	−8	0.058	0.0580	0	0.784	0
Bobbert (1960)[28]	2	M[b]	81	1	0.063	0.0638	−1	0.778	−1
McDonald (1961)[18]	333	Review/M	80	0	0.067	0.0629	6	0.838	7
	58	Review/F	80	0	0.061	0.0629	−3	0.763	−3
Corcoran (1970)[6]	32	M/F CWS	83	4	0.063	0.0655	−4	0.759	−3
Ganguli (1973)[41]	16	M[b]	50	−38	0.044	0.0423	4	0.880	12
McBeath (1974)[120]	10	M/F CWS	72	−10	0.066	0.0565	17	0.917	17
Imms (1976)[124]	8	Servicemen	88	10	0.065	0.0700	−7	0.739	−6
Waters (1976)[37]	25	M/F CWS	82	3	0.063	0.0646	−3	0.768	−2
Blessey (1976)[20]	40	M/F CWS	82	3	0.062	0.0646	−4	0.756	−4
Huang (1979)[45]	25	M/F CWS	80	0	0.074	0.0629	18	0.925	−18

CWS = comfortable walking speed; F = female; M = male; NCWS = normal comfortable walking speed of 80 m per minute.
[a]Equation: Ee (kcal/min/kg) = (29 + 0.0053 V²)/1,000. [V = velocity in m per minute.]
[b]Speed selected by researcher.

speed necessitates a greater increase in oxygen consumption than at slower speeds.

Workman and Armstrong[26] suggested that the requirements of maintaining balance while walking may determine both the CWS and the curvilinearity of the relationship between ground speed and freely chosen step frequency of walking. They have proposed a three-compartment model to present a concept of the way in which the metabolic cost of walking is distributed (Figure 18-3). Compartment 1 is the BMR, which likely continues at the same rate during activity. The size is significant, constituting up to one-third of the total metabolic cost of walking. Most of compartment 2 consists of the metabolic cost of maintaining balance and posture. Because the muscular effort is aimed at preventing unwanted movement rather than producing movement, the activity does not show on force plates or other physical measures. Compartment 3 is the metabolic cost of the walking movement and its size is exponentially speed related.

Ralston[27] derived an equation to calculate Ee per unit time (V = velocity in meters per minute):

$$Ee \ (kcal/min/kg) = \frac{(29 + 0.0053 \ V^2)}{1,000}$$

Given this equation, Ee per unit distance can be easily calculated by dividing the product by the speed in

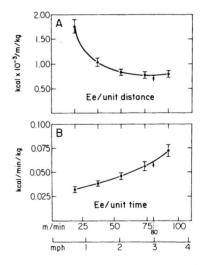

FIGURE 18-2 Energy expenditure (Ee) per unit distance **(A)** decreases to a minimum at approximately 80 m per minute, the normal average comfortable walking speed. However, the energy expenditure per unit time **(B)** increases steadily as walking speed increases. Both curves express the relationship, speed = Ee per unit time/Ee per unit distance. The normal values shown in these curves, and used in this chapter, are derived from the equation (29 + 0.0053 V²)/1,000. The normal values at the comfortable walking speed of 80 m per minute = 0.063 kcal per minute per kg and 0.000786 kcal/m/kg. The dumbbells indicate one standard deviation above and below the mean.

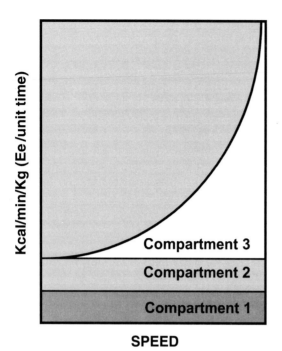

FIGURE 18-3 The three-compartment model of Workman and Armstrong (see the section Energy Expenditure in Able-Bodied Persons). (Ee = energy expenditure.) (Reprinted with permission from JM Workman, BW Armstrong. Metabolic cost of walking: Equation and model. J Appl Physiol 1986;61:1369–1374.)

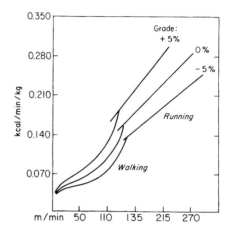

FIGURE 18-4 The energy expenditure per unit time for ordinary walking increases sharply at speeds faster than approximately 135 m per minute, and running becomes less demanding than walking. Note that the relationship of energy expenditure to speed is nearly linear for running. The limit to running speeds is set by the maximum aerobic capacity that the subject can attain. (Adapted from R Margaria, P Cerretelli, P Aghemo, et al. Energy cost of running. J Appl Physiol 1963;18:367–370.)

meters per minute. In this chapter, Ralston's equation is used for comparative purposes; it produces these normal values for Ee at normal CWS of 80 m per minute:

$$Ee/unit\ time = 0.063\ kcal/min/kg$$

$$Ee/unit\ distance = 0.786 \times 10^{-3}\ kcal/m/kg$$

As shown in Table 18-3, various investigators report approximately 80 m per minute as the CWS. The equation closely predicts the Ee per unit time when calculation is based on the speed chosen by the study subjects. Similarly, at the subject's walking speed, the Ee per unit distance varied only slightly from normal CWS. Other second-order regression equations have been published.[13,19,20,26–28]

The Ee per unit distance is greater at slow speeds than at ordinary walking speeds and greater again at faster speeds. Figure 18-2A shows that the calorie cost of walking a given distance is lowest at approximately 80 m per minute, the CWS.

The biomechanical and physiological explanations for the most efficient speed of ambulation are not entirely clear. It seems that human neuromusculoskeletal development has evolved a CWS at which the major determinants of gait are most effective, whereas the metabolic apparatus chooses one with the most economical calorie cost, which does not exceed the 5 kcal per minute limit for sustained work without going into oxygen debt.[5,6] Workman and Armstrong[26] surmise that it is the need to maintain balance and posture while walking that defines CWS, rather than metabolic efficiency.

The upper limit of normal walking speed is 5–6 mph or 135–160 m/min. At speeds in excess of 135 m per minute the energy cost of running is less than that of walking. At slower speeds, walking requires less energy than running.[29] The curve of the energy cost of running at various speeds, if superimposed on the nonlinear curve for walking in Figure 18-2B, intersects the walking curve near the speed of approximately 135 m per minute (Figure 18-4). It costs less energy to run or jog slowly than to walk fast.

The energy cost of walking on a 10–12% grade is approximately twice the Ee of walking on level ground. On a 20–25% upgrade, the cost is tripled. On downgrades the Ee is lowest at a 10% grade and rises again on steeper down slopes.[29]

Adding extra weight, clothing, or adaptive devices to the subject causes a linear increase in the energy cost of

FIGURE 18-5 Relationship between the height of each step (riser), the step frequency, and the energy cost of ascent or descent. The nomogram can be used to predict the energy expenditure for subjects who can use stairs for exercise. (Reprinted with permission from PJ Corcoran, JA Templer. Stair climbing for cardiovascular reconditioning. Presented at the 37th Annual Assembly of the Am Acad Phys Med Rehabil; Nov 19, 1975; Atlanta, Georgia.)

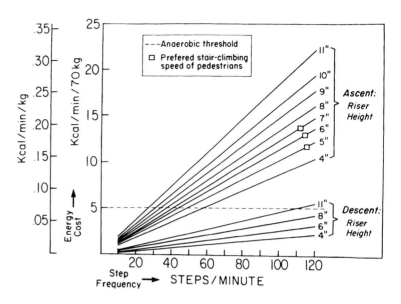

walking. Added loads are carried most efficiently on the head, somewhat less efficiently on the upper back, still less so in the hands, and least efficiently on the feet.[30,31] The addition of 2½ lb to shoe weight can increase the Ee by 5–10%.[6] Wearing heels more than 5 cm high significantly increases Ee.[32]

Effect on Energy Expenditure of Stairs and Ramps

Corcoran and Templer[33] found that both normal and crutch ambulators perform better on stairs than on ramps, in terms of energy cost per vertical rise. The steeper the ramp or stairs, the greater the advantage of stairs in total energy cost; however, if horizontal movement is also considered, the 5% ramp is less taxing. In situations such as those in most transportation terminals, where people need to ascend 10 meters while progressing 200 meters horizontally, stairs require 29% more energy than a 5% ramp, and 45% more time. Fisher and Patterson[34] and Ganguli and Bose[35] also performed experiments on subjects' performance on stairs and noted a nearly twofold increase in the net energy cost for those ambulating with crutches.

The metabolic cost of stair climbing can be predicted from a simple nomogram if the height of step or riser and step frequency are known (Figure 18-5).[33] If a subject's weight and the riser height are known, the nomogram indicates the step frequency needed to achieve any desired rate of Ee. This nomogram makes it possi-

ble to use any stairway as a precise ergometer for aerobic conditioning.

Descending stairs requires only 23% of the energy needed for ascending the same staircase. Because coming down stairs does not exceed light work levels, the process is useless for aerobic conditioning. Ascending one flight of stairs at the usual speed takes only 10–15 seconds but requires a burst of 12–14 kcal per minute per 70 kg. This makes stair climbing the most strenuous activity of the day for most people.

Levels of Activity Measured by Magnitude of Energy Cost

The energy demands placed on a person during different levels of activity and during ambulation require discussion. This topic is important because of the frequent coexistence of deconditioning and cardiovascular disease among people with disabilities who are undertaking rehabilitation. A semiquantitative continuum from light to hard work is useful in rehabilitation.[10] Such a frame of reference for energy consumption for the patients provides the clinician with basic guidelines on which to make decisions on activity levels. Metabolic demands of more than 5 kcal per minute are impossible for an average-sized, untrained adult to sustain without intervals of rest. This level is equivalent to oxygen uptake of 1.0–1.25 L per minute. Table 18-4 lists the grades of work as proposed by Christensen.[36] This classification is based on intermittent work, which is more realistic in real-life situations. Figure 18-6 defines the levels of physical activity as well as the

TABLE 18-4
Work (Intermittent) Classification by Magnitude of Energy Cost

Classification	Ee (kcal/min/70 kg)	Example
Light	2.6–4.9	Mixing cement
Moderate	5.0–7.5	Shoveling 8-kg load
Heavy	7.6–10.0	Splitting wood
Very heavy	10.1–12.5	Carrying 20 lb upstairs
Extraordinarily heavy	12.5	Carrying 60 lb upstairs

Ee = energy expenditure.
Source: Reprinted with permission from EH Christensen. Physiological valuation of work in the Nykroppa Iron Works. Presented at the Ergonomics Society Symposium on Fatigue; 1953; Leeds, London.

functional and therapeutic cardiac classifications plotted against the rate of Ee in normal ambulation, an experience to which most persons can relate to. The graph can be used to plot the Ee of ambulation for different types of disabilities, providing a sensible perception of what patients go through when ambulating. This is particularly relevant because in many disabilities deconditioning and cardiovascular disease are often associated factors.

ENERGY EXPENDITURE WITH DISABILITY

It would be ideal if all the information provided in this section were precise. However, the search of the literature and our experience in the laboratory indicate that, at best, the values quoted are approximations. Clearly, an inherent difficulty lies in studying a large cohort of subjects with disabilities who can ambulate at a constant speed for at least 4 minutes. Most studies are flawed with too many variables that are unaccounted for.

As noted previously, the Ee per unit time for persons with disability walking at their own self-selected CWS is almost equal to a normally capable person walking at a normal CWS of 80 m per minute, with values approximating 0.063 kcal per minute per kg. This implies that a person with a disability compensates by walking slower and thus covering less distance.

There are possible reasons to explain why the Ee per unit time reported in a particular study significantly deviates from the norm of 0.063 kcal per minute per kg.

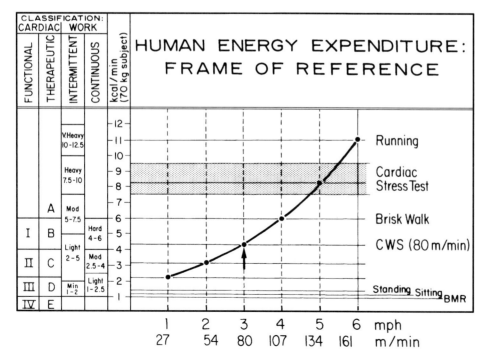

FIGURE 18-6 A frame of reference compares the energy expenditure per unit time among healthy individuals against levels of work and cardiac classification. The diagram can be used to plot the level of energy expenditure of walking and other activities among disabled and nondisabled persons. (BMR = basal metabolic rate; CWS = comfortable walking speed.)

The most likely explanation is that the subjects were not walking at their true self-selected CWS. It is not uncommon for older debilitated subjects to underperform, whereas younger otherwise healthy subjects overachieve in testing situations. In some instances, the researchers have arbitrarily chosen the subjects' speed. In some, the physical status and extent of the disability may be too limiting, and in rare circumstances, it may be because of experimental error.

The Ee per unit time and Ee per unit distance are greater in a disabled person than in a nondisabled individual who is walking at the same speed as a subject is with disability. The harsh reality of life is that the world does not slow down for people with disabilities. It is thus impractical to use this type of comparison between able-bodied persons and persons with disability, although it is sometimes reported.

Most investigators believe that Ee per unit distance walked is the true net energy cost and the best basis for comparing gait efficiency between normal and abnormal ambulation.[34,37,38] This is particularly true if the Ee per unit distance at the speed chosen by a person with disability is matched against the Ee per unit distance at the normal CWS of 80 m per minute. With this approach, the magnitude of difference between abled and disabled walking can be fully appreciated.

In this chapter, the actual values provided in the reference articles are quoted with regard to speed of ambulation and oxygen consumption. *The units of speed and Ee are recalculated as meters per minute, kilocalories per minute per kilogram, and kilocalories per meter per kilogram. Some of the values may have been estimated from graphs. Despite obvious shortcomings, for the sake of uniformity, all comparisons of Ee with normally capable subjects are at the normal CWS of 80 m per minute with Ee per unit time of 0.063 kcal per minute per kg and Ee per unit distance of 0.786 $\times 10^{-3}$ kcal per m per kg.*

Lower Extremity Amputations

More knowledge is available on the energy cost of ambulation with lower extremity amputations than for any other type of disability. Although published data vary in the number of subjects, speed of ambulation, types of prosthesis worn, and technique of Ee determination, adequate information is available to make logical assumptions about the energy demands resulting from amputations.

This disability is unique in the sense that a body part is actually missing and replaced by an external device. Despite innovative approaches in the design of pros-

thetic replacements, the muscles that supply the power and the joints that sense position and load in the limb are no longer present. The higher the level of amputation, the more gait deviations occur, with resultant increase in energy cost.

Syme's Amputation

Waters and coworkers[37] studied 15 vascular Syme's amputees and found their CWS to be 54 m per minute, or 33% slower than normal. The subjects were probably walking slower than they could because the Ee per unit time was less 13% than for normal CWS. The Ee per unit distance was 30% greater at the amputees' slower speed, as compared with normal CWS. These results are not significantly different from those of transtibial (below-knee) amputees.

Transtibial Amputation

Sufficient information exists in the literature to allow reasonable conclusions to be made regarding the energy demands imposed by transtibial amputation (Table 18-5).[37-57] Gonzalez and associates[42] determined oxygen consumption among nine adults with amputations from various causes, whose average age was 58 years. They found a negative correlation between residual limb length and energy cost, but no correlation between limb length and speed of ambulation. The average self-selected CWS was 64 m per minute, 20% slower than normal. At this speed, the Ee per unit time (0.062 kcal/min) was practically equal to normal CWS (Figure 18-7). Similarly, the Ee per unit distance was higher by a factor of 23% than that for normal CWS. Like that of their nondisabled counterparts, the CWS of those with transtibial amputations coincided with the speed of maximum efficiency (Figure 18-8). The research emphasized the importance of preserving residual limb length to minimize the increase in Ee.

In another study, Gailey et al.[43] studied 39 healthy, young men with nonvascular transtibial amputations. The subjects walked 12% slower than normal CWS, whereas Ee per unit distance was higher by 12%. When the subjects were stratified on the basis of long and short residual limb length, the former sustained significantly lower Ee than the latter while walking at comparable pace.

Pagliarulo[44] and Waters[37] et al. investigated 13 vascular amputees and 14 traumatic[37] and 15 nonvascular[44] transtibial amputees. The vascular group, whose average age was 63 years, chose to walk 44% slower; the traumatic and nonvascular transtibial group, who were considerably younger, walked only 11% slower than normal. At their chosen CWS, the rate of oxygen con-

TABLE 18-5
Energy Expenditure (Ee): Transtibial and Syme's Amputation

Author (Year)	No.	Comment	Speed (m/min) Subject	Speed (m/min) Difference(%) (Normal 80 m/min)	Ee per Unit Time* (kcal/min/kg) Subject	Ee per Unit Time* (kcal/min/kg) Difference (%) (NCWS 0.063 kcal/min/kg)	Ee per Unit Distance (kcal × 10⁻³/m/kg) Subject	Ee per Unit Distance (kcal × 10⁻³/m/kg) Difference (%) (NCWS 0.786 kcal × 10⁻³/m/kg)
Reitmeyer (1955)[38]	2	Trauma	60	−25	0.035	−44	0.583	−26
Ralston (1971)[39]	2	—	49	−39	0.055	−13	1.122	43
Molen (1973)[40]	54	Trauma	50	−38	0.066	5	1.320	68
Ganguli (1973)[41]	20	Trauma	50	−38	0.060	−5	1.200	53
Gonzalez (1974)[42]	9	Trauma/PVD	64	−20	0.062	−2	0.969	23
Waters (1976)[37]	13	PVD	45	−44	0.056	−11	1.244	58
	14	Trauma	71	−11	0.074	17	1.042	33
Pagliarulo (1979)[44]	15	Nonvascular	71	−11	0.074	17	1.042	33
Huang (1979)[45]	6	Trauma/PVD	48	−40	0.048	−24	1.000	27
Gailey (1994)[43]	39	Nonvascular	70	−12	0.062	−2	0.885	12
Torbourn (1995)[54]	9	Trauma	82	2	0.085	35	1.036	32
	7	PVD	62	−22	0.063	0	1.032	31
Waters (1976)[37]	15	PVD/Syme's	54	−33	0.055	−13	1.019	30
Prosthetic Components								
Nielsen (1989)[50]	2	Flex-Foot	80	0	0.078	24	0.975	24
Gailey (1997)[56]	10	Regular weight	76	−5	0.062	−2	0.815	4
	10	Heavy weight	76	-5	0.064	3	0.842	7
Lehman (1998)[57]	15	Light weight	88	10	0.075	19	0.857	9
	15	Heavy weight	88	10	0.075	19	0.857	9
	15	Heavy distally	88	10	0.080	27	0.912	16
Casillas (1995)[55]	12	Trauma/SACH	75	−8	0.089	41	1.186	50
	12	Trauma/DER feet	80	0	0.086	36	1.075	36
	12	PVD/SACH	35	−56	0.059	−6	1.168	48
	12	PVD/DER feet	35	−56	0.061	−3	1.174	49

DER = dynamic elastic response; NCWS = normal comfortable walking speed; PVD = peripheral vascular disease; SACH = solid-ankle cushion heel.
*Equation: Ee (kcal/min/kg) = (29 + 0.0053 V²)/1,000. [V = Velocity in m per minute.]

sumption per minute was 11% lower for the vascular subjects and 17% higher for the traumatic group. This implies that the vascular group was walking slower, whereas the trauma subjects were walking faster than their true CWS. The Ee per unit distance rose 58% and 33%, respectively.

Huang et al.[45] also reported findings approximately similar to those of the studies cited previously.

Stair Climbing and Load Carrying with a Transtibial Prosthesis All of the studies previously mentioned were performed on level ground. Ganguli and coworkers[41,46–48] studied a group of young transtibial amputees as they climbed 127 steps with 14.2-cm risers for a vertical ascent of 18 m. Nondisabled control subjects spent 0.0776 kcal per minute per kg; the subjects spent 9% more. The same group applied a similar technique to studying the effect of

load carrying on a cohort of five left-side below-knee amputees. The subject and control groups carried loads of 7.5 kg on level ground and up stairs. As expected, the subjects with amputations consumed more energy than the controls, 47% more. Contrary to what might be expected, the side on which the load was carried did not make any statistically significant difference in Ee. The effect of asymmetry, however, appears to be a factor in the increase in energy cost: Transtibial subjects fare better dividing the load and carrying an equal amount in each hand. The results of stair climbing were difficult to assess in view of the varying rates of ascent. However, this study is important in demonstrating that transtibial amputees can perform work levels of up to 6.5 kcal per minute, a moderate level of intermittent work. This information is useful in vocational rehabilitation.

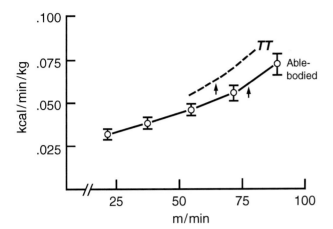

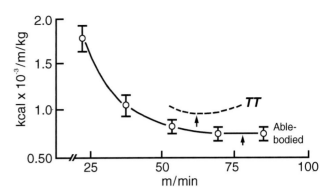

FIGURE 18-7 A comparison of curves of energy expenditure per unit time between able-bodied subjects and transtibial (TT) amputees. The dumbbells indicate one standard deviation. The arrows indicate comfortable walking speed. Note that the energy cost at these two speeds are approximately equal, meaning that a transtibial amputee spends as much energy walking at a slower speed as normal subjects do at the comfortable walking speed of 80 m per minute. (Redrawn with permission from EG Gonzalez, PJ Corcoran, RL Reyes. Energy expenditure in below-knee amputees: correlation with stump length. Arch Phys Med Rehabil 1974;55:111–118.)

FIGURE 18-8 Comparison of energy expenditure per unit distance between able-bodied and transtibial (TT) amputees. The dumbbells indicate one standard deviation. The arrows indicate comfortable walking speeds, which coincide with speed of maximum efficiency for both able-bodied subjects and amputees. (Redrawn with permission from EG Gonzalez, PJ Corcoran, RL Reyes. Energy expenditure in below-knee amputees: correlation with stump length. Arch Phys Med Rehabil 1974;55:111–118.)

Prosthesis Design Despite myriad traditional as well as technologically advanced designs in prosthetic components, their effectiveness in lowering the energy cost of ambulation remains in question. Cummings and coauthors[49] found no difference in Ee between the use of supracondylar cuff suspension and the thigh corset, disproving the commonly held notion that the lighter weight of the cuff suspension or the more secure suspension provided by the thigh corset reduces the energy demand.

Nielsen and coworkers[50] compared the energy cost and gait efficiency during ambulation in two transtibial amputees using the SACH (Kingsley Manufacturing Company, Costa Mesa, CA) and the Flex-Foot (Flex-Foot, Inc., Laguna Hills, CA). A lower Ee was observed with higher walking velocities using the Flex-Foot. The decrease was most noticeable at speeds of 70–80 m per minute and was negligible at slower speeds. It should be noted that 80 m per minute may be an overexertion on the part of the subjects. At this speed, the Ee per unit time is 24% higher than normal CWS. The Ee per unit distance is no different from those reported by Gonzalez et al.,[42] whose subjects used SACH and single-axis feet. The dynamic foot is believed to increase the time subjects are willing to

spend in single support. The result is a smoother vertical trunk motion, greater biomechanical efficiency, and protection of the sound limb against excessive vertical forces.[51–53]

Studies comparing the Ee between the SACH and various dynamic elastic response feet such as the Flex-Foot, Carbon Copy II (Ohio Willow Wood Co., Mt. Sterling, OH), Seattle Lite (Model & Instrument Development, Seattle, WA), Quantum[54] (Hosmer-Porrance Corp., Campbell, CA), and Proteor[55] failed to show reduction in energy cost. The dynamic elastic response feet are designed for active amputees to improve forward progression and pushoff and theoretically reduce energy cost. Unfortunately, the peak energy cost mechanics occur elsewhere in the gait cycle.[54]

Since the 1980s an explosion in the development of light-weight materials and components aimed to reduce prosthetic weight has been seen. These advancements have not lowered the energy cost of walking among transtibial amputees.[43,56,57] Although light-weight distal components may be desirable for other reasons, it is questionable whether ultralight-weight prostheses are cost effective for level walking, particularly among those who are not physically active.[57]

It appears that prosthetic innovations have failed to reduce the energy cost of ambulation, albeit while engendering greater patient acceptance and enthusiasm among clinicians. The literature suggests that basal $\dot{V}O_2$ alone explains 30–40% of the variance in determining the energy cost of ambulation.[5,26] Other variables include speed of ambulation, residual limb length, maintenance of posture and balance and the actual energy cost of walking movement.[5,20–22,26,42,43]

Transfemoral Amputation

Surgeons who are less willing to risk the morbidity of delayed wound healing often opt for transfemoral (above-knee) amputation. Although this may prove most efficacious in the short-term, the long-term ambulatory consequence is poorer, particularly for aged and more debilitated patients.

Encouraging reports were published between the 1950s and early 1970s on the walking speed and energy cost of ambulation among transfemoral amputees. They reported that at slower speeds, the net energy cost was lower than normal.[58–60] This would lead to the spurious conclusion that it becomes easier to walk after losing a leg. However, other studies [37,45,61–66] show that although the Ee per unit time fell within the normal range, the Ee per unit distance, the index of efficiency, increased up to 116% or more (Table 18-6). The results of the studies by Traugh et al.,[63] Otis et al.,[65] and Jaegers et al.[66] suggest that above-knee amputation subjects are not able to walk fast enough to achieve the most metabolically efficient speed.

Locked versus Unlocked Prosthetic Knee   Traugh and coworkers[63] studied transfemoral amputees in an effort

TABLE 18-6

Energy Expenditure (Ee): Transfemoral Amputation

Author (Year)	No.	Comment	Speed (m/min) Subject	Difference(%) (Normal 80/min)	Ee per Unit Time* (kcal/min/kg) Subject	Difference (%) (NCWS 0.063 kcal/min/kg)	Ee per Unit Distance (kcal × 10⁻³/m/kg) Subject	Difference (%) (NCWS 0.786 kcal × 10⁻³/m/kg)
Muller (1952)[58]	2	—	70	–13	0.053	–16	0.757	–4
Muller (1952)[58]	1	—	40	–50	0.023	–63	0.575	–27
Bard (1959)[61]	6	—	68	–15	0.061	–3	0.897	14
Erdman (1960)[59]	9	—	47	–41	0.035	–44	0.745	–5
Inman (1961)[60]	1	—	62	–23	0.017	–73	0.274	–65
Ralston (1971)[39]	1	—	49	–39	0.049	–22	1.000	27
James (1973)[64]	37	Trauma	51	–36	0.061	–3	1.196	52
Ganguli (1974)[62]	6	—	50	–38	0.088	40	1.760	124
Waters (1976)[37]	13	PVD	36	–55	0.061	–3	1.694	116
	15	Trauma	52	–35	0.062	–2	1.192	52
Huang (1979)[45]	6	—	47	–41	0.062	–2	1.319	68
Otis (1985)[65]	5	Tumor	52	–35	0.069	10	1.327	69
Jaegers (1993)[66]	5	Nonvascular	50	–38	0.052	–12	1.108	40
Czerniecki (1994)[68]	8	Nonvascular	70	–13	0.063	0	0.903	15
Prosthetic Design								
Traugh (1975)[63]	9	Lock/free knee	39	–51	0.061	–3	1.564	99
Isakov (1985)[67]	3	Free knee	66	–18	0.088	40	1.333	70
	3	Lock knee	61	–24	0.081	29	1.328	69
Gailey (1993)[69]	10	CAT-CAM	33	–58	0.050	–20	1.492	89
	10	QUAD	33	–58	0.056	–11	1.692	115
	10	CAT-CAM	67	–16	0.075	19	1.132	44
	10	QUAD	67	–16	0.091	44	1.368	74
Boomstra (1995)[79]	13	Otto Bock knee	50	–38	0.049	–22	0.980	25
	14	Pneumatic knee	50	–38	0.052	–17	1.040	32
Buckley (1997)[73]	3	Microchip knee	46	–42	0.062	–2	1.347	71
	3	Pneumatic knee	46	–42	0.062	–2	1.347	71

CAT-CAM = contoured adducted trochanteric-controlled alignment method; NCWS = normal comfortable walking speed; PVD = peripheral vascular disease; QUAD = quadrilateral socket.
*Equation: Ee (kcal/min/kg) = (29 + 0.0053 V²)/1,000. [V = Velocity in m per minute.]

to determine the mode of ambulation that required the least energy. They found the CWS among the amputees to be 51% slower. Like other disabled ambulators, the subjects chose to walk more slowly to keep their rate of Ee close to the normal CWS of 0.063 kcal per minute per kg (Figure 18-9). Compared with normal CWS, the Ee per unit distance rose by 99%, and subjects were unable to reach the most efficient speed (Figure 18-10). Values obtained using crutches without prosthesis were about the same, although heart rate was faster. No statistical difference was found between ambulating with a locked and an unlocked knee; however, a significant reduction (7%) was noted when subjects walked with the knee setting they customarily preferred. On the other hand, wheelchair propulsion imposed an increase above nondisabled values by only 9%.

Isakov and colleagues[67] elaborated further on the differences in Ee between locked and unlocked knees. The older group walked faster with the locked knee, whereas the younger group fared better with the unlocked knee. Oxygen consumption was determined only among the younger group. The increase in Ee was practically the same.

Vascular versus Nonvascular Amputation Young, physically fit nonvascular transfemoral amputees walked at speeds of 45–70 m per minute. At their own self-selected CWS, the Ee per unit time fell within normal, whereas Ee per unit distance rose from 15% to 70%.[37,45,64–70]

Waters and colleagues,[37] in their study of 13 older dysvascular amputees, showed that speed slowed to 36 m per minute, or 55% slower, whereas the Ee per unit distance rose 116% relative to normal CWS. They also calculated the relative energy cost (rate of oxygen uptake divided by the subject's maximum aerobic capacity). The relative cost among the vascular amputees was found to be 63%, in contrast to 35% among the younger subjects. The authors emphasized that activity requiring greater than 50% of maximum aerobic capacity results in anaerobic metabolism and resulting loss of endurance. They noted that this finding is corroborated by their clinical experience that fewer than 10% of dysvascular transfemoral patients were initially fitted with prostheses because of related physical problems. Less than 50% of those fitted walk enough to qualify for their study.

Prosthetic Design More recent prosthetic designs are aimed at improving the biomechanical function and reducing the energy cost of walking. Although there is considerable effort in manufacturing light-weight pros-

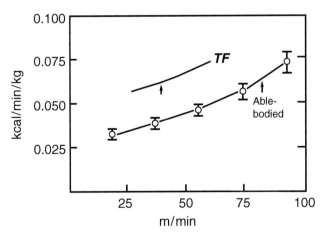

FIGURE 18-9 Comparative curves of energy expenditure per unit time between able-bodied and transfemoral (TF) subjects. The dumbbells indicate one standard deviation. The arrows indicate comfortable walking speeds. The energy costs at these comfortable walking speeds are approximately equal, meaning that a transfemoral amputee spends as much energy walking at a slow pace as able-bodied subjects do at the comfortable walking speed of 80 m per minute. (Redrawn with permission from G Traugh, PJ Corcoran, RL Reyes. Energy expenditure of ambulation in patients with above-knee amputation. Arch Phys Med Rehabil 1975;56:67–71.)

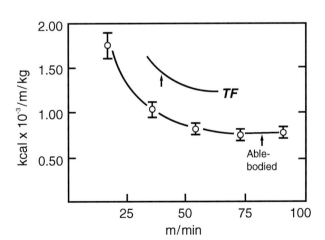

FIGURE 18-10 Energy expenditure per unit distance for normal subjects and transfemoral (TF) amputees. The dumbbells indicate one standard deviation. The arrows indicate comfortable walking speeds, which coincide with speed of maximum efficiency for able-bodied persons. Note that the amputees could not comfortably walk fast enough to reach their most efficient speed. (Redrawn with permission from G Traugh, PJ Corcoran, RL Reyes. Energy expenditure of ambulation in patients with above-knee amputation. Arch Phys Med Rehabil 1975;56:67–71.)

theses, little is known about the effect of shank mass on metabolic cost of ambulation among transfemoral amputees. The theory that lighter weight lowers muscle work in both acceleration and deceleration has not been confirmed. Czerniecki et al.[68] found no difference in the Ee between weighted and unweighted prostheses in eight young transfemoral amputees. This study raises questions as to the rationale for prescribing lighter weight prostheses.

The Contoured Adducted Trochanteric-Controlled Alignment Method (CAT-CAM) was developed by Sabolich[71] to provide a narrower mediolateral dimension than the quadrilateral (QUAD) socket. It claims to improve muscle function, provide better femoral alignment, reduce pelvic motion, and lower energy cost. Flandry et al.[72] reported lower energy cost and faster speed among five transfemoral subjects using the CAT-CAM versus the QUAD socket. Gailey and collaborators[69] in their study of 10 nonvascular transfemoral amputees using the CAT-CAM and 10 subjects using the QUAD socket reaffirmed this initial report. When instructed to walk at 67 m per minute, the CAT-CAM group required 30% less energy per unit distance than the QUAD group. There was no difference in Ee at the slower speed of 33 m per minute.

Despite the popularity of pneumatic and hydraulic knee units, little has been written about the energy cost when using these units as compared with sliding friction knee joints. Boomstra and colleagues[70] studied 28 nonvascular transfemoral amputees. Although most of the subjects preferred the pneumatic swing phase control, the energy cost was actually higher than the sliding friction knee unit. A more recent innovation is the microprocessor-controlled prosthesis that allows the swing speed of the prosthetic shin to adjust automatically as the walking speed changes. Two studies[73,74] involving a small number of subjects showed a slight reduction in energy cost as compared with the pneumatic or hydraulic units, but only at speeds other than the subjects' CWS.

Resection En Bloc and Knee Replacement versus Transfemoral Amputation   Emphasis on the importance of restoring lower extremity function in patients with tumor about the knee has been enhanced by the 80% 3-year disease-free survival rate for patients with osteogenic sarcoma.[65] Otis and coworkers[65] examined 14 patients treated with complete surgical resection of the sarcomatous knee (en bloc resection) and endoprosthetic knee replacement, as well as 12 who underwent transfemoral amputation for osteogenic sarcoma. Those with en bloc resection walked significantly faster (14%) than their transfemoral counterparts. The en bloc resection group also did better than the transfemoral ampu-

tees with regard to Ee per unit distance. Five subjects from each group were tested early (6–12 months postoperatively) and again later (18–30 months postoperatively). The en bloc patients reached an early plateau of maximum performance after 6 months; the transfemoral subjects improved slowly for up to 2.5 years, perhaps as a result of continued experience and training in the use of the prosthesis. At their best, the en bloc resection group had a 50% increase in Ee per unit distance, as compared with 69% increase among the transfemoral amputees. The difference between this group of young amputees and those with traumatic amputation is their lower maximal aerobic capacity (and, thus, higher relative energy cost), which is perhaps attributable to the effect chemotherapy has on the myocardium. The study advocated the en bloc procedure, in view of the short-term superior performance along with the psychological and cosmetic advantages over transfemoral amputation. A later study from the same group made possible the prediction of net energy cost among knee-salvage patients derived from the overall functional score and the percentage of the femur that has been resected.[75]

Load Carrying   In a study of six young trauma amputees, Roy and collaborators[76] tested their subjects walking on level ground at a speed of 50 m per minute, with and without loads on their shoulders of 5, 10, and 15 kg. As expected, oxygen consumption, peak heart rate, and pulmonary ventilation values were higher in the test group. From an ergonomic viewpoint, the authors found what might ordinarily be considered as light work becomes hard or very hard work among transfemoral amputees and encroached much on their physical reserves. For instance, a load of 5 kg caused a mean Ee of 0.089 kcal per minute per kg, or 6.23 kcal per minute for a 70-kg man; this falls in the category of moderately hard intermittent work. A load of 15 kg increases the Ee to 0.118 kcal per minute per kg (8.26 kcal/min for an average-sized person), which falls in the classification of heavy intermittent work. The energy cost for the same task for nonamputees was within the category of light intermittent work. The vocational implications are self-evident.

Bilateral Amputations and Other Levels

Hip Disarticulation and Hemipelvectomy Amputation   Eight patients with hip disarticulation and 10 with hemipelvectomy were investigated by Nowroozi and coworkers.[77] The hip disarticulation group walked 41% slower than nondisabled subjects and the hemipelvectomy amputees walked 51% slower. The Ee per unit distance rose 43% and 75% for hip disarticulation and hemipelvectomy, respectively, as compared with normal CWS. The study also demonstrated that for this group of patients, prosthesis use was more demanding than the use of axillary crutches without a prosthesis. The relatively fine performance of this group of patients, as compared with the transfemoral subjects in the study of Otis and colleagues[65] could be attributed to their physical fitness and to the fact that none had been receiving chemotherapy or radiotherapy for at least 6 months before the study.

Bilateral Transtibial Amputation Meager information is available on Ee among bilateral amputees (Table 18-7). In an unpublished work, Corcoran and associates[78] (cited by Gonzalez's group[42]) reported a 20% reduction in speed of ambulation (64 m/minute) and a 41% increase in Ee per unit distance among a group of bilateral transtibial amputees. Like the unilateral transtibial subjects, they chose the most efficient CWS. At this CWS, the bilateral transtibial subjects spent slightly more Ee per unit time than normal CWS.

DuBow and others[79] investigated six elderly bilateral transtibial amputees. Their subjects chose a CWS of 40 m per minute, a 50% reduction from the norm. The increase in Ee per unit distance, compared with their normal controls' CWS of 62.5 m per minute, was reported at 123%. If comparison were made against normal values obtained from Ralston's equation,[27] the increase in Ee per unit distance would have been 18%; however, this value is unusually low. The authors commented on the poor physical status of their test group,

reporting that most died or became nonambulatory within a year of the study. They also noted technical difficulties with their automated equipment.

Transfemoral-Transtibial Amputation Corcoran et al.[78] reported on two transfemoral-transtibial subjects and found their CWS to be 35 m per minute or 56% slower than able-bodied adults, and they observed a 118% increase in net cost of walking. There are no published papers on transfemoral-transtibial amputation to verify the information.

Bilateral Transfemoral Amputation Huang's group[45] reported findings on three bilateral transfemoral amputees. The speed chosen by the subjects was 23 m per minute, 71% slower than normal CWS. At this speed, the Ee per unit distance is 260% higher than for normal CWS. Findings of this study compare favorably with those of Corcoran et al.[78]

A single bilateral transfemoral amputee subject was examined by Crouse and others[80] to determine the cardiac and metabolic response in ambulating with regular long-leg prostheses as opposed to short-leg prostheses (*stubbies*). The subject and three nondisabled control subjects exercised on a treadmill. The amputee subject was able to exercise for a longer period (27%) while using the short-leg prosthesis. The mean energy cost was 23% higher for the long-leg prostheses than for the short-leg prosthesis, and 80% higher than the cost recorded for the able-bodied controls. Despite metabolic advantages of the short-leg prostheses, the patient

TABLE 18-7
Energy Expenditure (Ee): Bilateral Amputation and Other Levels

| Author (Year) | No. | Comment | Speed (m/min) | | Ee per Unit Time* (kcal/min/kg) | | Ee per Unit Distance (kcal × 10⁻³/m/kg) | |
			Subject	Difference(%) (Normal 80/min)	Subject	Difference(%) (NCWS 0.063 kcal/min/kg)	Subject	Difference(%) (NCWS 0.786 kcal × 10⁻³/m/kg)
Gonzalez (1974)[42]	5	TT-TT	64	−20	0.071	13	1.109	41
Dubow (1983)[79]	6	TT-TT	40	−50	0.037	−41	0.925	18
Huang (1979)[45]	4	TF-TF	23	−71	0.065	3	2.826	260
Corcoran (1971)[78]	2	TF-TF	32	−60	0.072	14	2.250	186
Hoffman (1997)[81]	5	TF-TF	49	−40	0.073	15	1.489	91
Corcoran (1971)[78]	2	TF-TT	35	−56	0.060	−5	1.714	118
Nowroozi (1983)[77]	8	Hip disarticulation, tumor	47	−41	0.053	−16	1.128	43
Nowroozi (1983)[77]	10	Hemipelvectomy, tumor	40	−50	0.055	−13	1.375	75

NCWS = normal comfortable walking speed; TF-TF = bilateral transfemoral; TF-TT = transfemoral-transtibial; TT-TT = bilateral transtibial.
*Equation: Ee (kcal/min/kg) = (29 + 0.0053 V^2)/1,000. [V = Velocity in m per minute.]

preferred the long-leg prostheses because they offered greater social acceptance.

Hoffman et al.[81] studied five young bilateral transfemoral amputees and five able-bodied matched controls. The amputee subjects walked 40% slower and spent 91% higher Ee per unit distance compared with normal CWS. The bilateral transfemoral subjects' CWS did not coincide with the most metabolically efficient speed. The study applied the three-compartment model of Workman and Armstrong[26] to suggest that the higher metabolic costs for the amputee subjects resulted from greater demands for maintenance of balance and posture and for performing the walking movements.

Crutch Walking for Amputees

The question often arises as to why an amputee should walk with a prosthesis when crutches are available as an alternative. Several studies[37,59,61,63,77,82] have compared the metabolic demands of using crutches with and without a prosthesis to those of normal ambulation (Table 18-8). In general, these authors found that amputees walking with crutches but without a prosthesis chose to walk slower than normal (39–71 m/min) but the energy consumption per unit time was more or less equal or somewhat lower when compared with the rate of expenditure at normal CWS. As expected, at the amputees' slower speed, the Ee per unit distance was less efficient than normal. A group of young traumatic transtibial amputees in the study by Waters et al.,[37] walked the fastest at 71 m per minute, but spent considerably more energy per unit time than other groups.

Interesting insights come to light when crutch walking without prosthesis is compared with walking with prosthesis. Waters and colleagues[37] found that crutch walking led to a significant increase in the heart rate and the rate of oxygen consumption in all groups except dysvascular transfemoral amputees, as compared with using a prosthesis. All transfemoral amputee subjects

TABLE 18-8
Energy Expenditure (Ee): Crutch Ambulation in Amputation

Author (Year)	No.	Comment	Speed (m/min)		Ee per Unit Time* (kcal/min/kg)		Ee per Unit Distance (kcal × 10⁻³/m/kg)	
			Subject	Difference(%) (Normal 80/min)	Subject	Difference (%) (NCWS 0.063 kcal/min/kg)	Subject	Difference (%) (NCWS 0.786 kcal ×10⁻³/m/kg)
Bard (1959)[61]	6	TF, forearm	58	−28	0.069	10	1.190	51
Inman (1961)[60]	?	TF, forearm	45	−44	0.065	3	1.444	84
Erdman (1960)[59]	9	TF, axillary	47	−41	0.038	−40	0.809	3
Ganguli (1974)[62]	10	TF, axillary	50	−38	0.065	3	1.300	65
Traugh (1975)[63]	9	TF, axillary	39	−51	0.059	−6	1.513	92
Waters (1976)[37]	13	TF, PVD, axillary	48	−40	0.072	14	1.500	91
	15	TF, trauma, axillary	65	−19	0.076	21	1.169	49
	13	TT, PVD, axillary	39	−51	0.070	11	1.795	128
	14	TT, trauma, axillary	71	−11	0.108	71	1.521	94
	15	Syme's, PVD, axillary	39	−51	0.062	−2	1.590	102
Nowroozi (1983)[77]	8	Hip disarticulation, tumor, axillary	56	−30	0.052	−17	0.929	18
Nowroozi (1983)[77]	10	Hemipelvectomy, tumor, axillary	53	−34	0.050	−21	0.943	20

Forearm = forearm/Lofstrand crutches; NCWS = normal comfortable walking speed; PVD, peripheral vascular disease; TF = transfemoral; TT = transtibial.
*Equation 4: Ee (kcal/min/kg) = (29 + 0.0053 V^2)/1,000. [V= Velocity in m per minute.]

walked faster with crutches alone, whereas the reverse was true for the transtibial amputees, except the traumatic transtibial amputees, who walked at the same speed with either crutches or prostheses.

Traugh and colleagues[63] reported 7% less Ee while walking with crutches, when compared with the energy consumption of those using a prosthesis with the preferred knee setting. Erdman and coworkers[59] did not report any difference in either mode of ambulation, although the heart rate was consistently faster and took longer to recover to baseline when subjects walked with crutches alone. Available research does not indicate with any consistency regarding what mode of ambulation the amputees preferred. Factors such as upper extremity maximum aerobic capacity, general fitness, and motivation all play a role, but these investigations confirm that crutch walking is an effective alternative to using a prosthesis. Additionally, the dictum that the ability to crutch walk is a good indicator that the same patient can walk with a prosthesis seems to hold true. The reverse is, however, not necessarily supported. A summary of our experience in the laboratory is presented in Figure 18-11.

Hemiplegia

The variations in gait characteristics among hemiplegics depend on the extent of neurologic deficit. The degree of gait deviation reflects directly on the metabolic demands of walking (Table 18-9). The earliest study that attempted to quantify the energy requirements of hemiplegic ambulation was published by Bard and Ralston,[61,83] who reported a nearly normal Ee rate per unit time, and a 37% increase in Ee per unit distance compared with normal CWS.

Corcoran and others[84] studied the effects of plastic and metal leg orthoses on speed and energy cost of hemiparetic ambulation. With no brace, the CWS was 42 m per minute, 48% slower than the norm, and averaged 88% greater Ee per unit distance. The use of either the metal articulated ankle-foot orthosis or the plastic solid ankle-foot orthosis resulted in a significant increase in speed (49 m/min) and reduction in Ee, over ambulation with no device. There was, however, no statistically significant difference between Ee per unit distance with the two types of orthoses, which was 74% higher than in normal CWS. At the subjects' CWS, the slope of oxygen consumption was greater than normal, indicating the higher price they have to pay to achieve small increments in speed. At their CWS, the rate of oxygen consumption per unit time was approximately the same as normal CWS (Figure 18-12). When energy cost was expressed per unit distance, it was found that hemiparetic patients

could not comfortably walk fast enough to achieve minimum oxygen consumption per meter walked (Figure 18-13). Wearing either type of orthosis, the subjects' ability to ascend and descend stairs was significantly better than when they wore no device at all.

Gersten and Orr[85] measured the external work of walking in 15 hemiparetic patients at the slow speed of 17 m per minute. They compared the results of a rigid ankle metal brace and one that allowed some dorsiflexion and plantar flexion. They found no significant difference in work per unit distance but indicated that whenever the difference was greater than 7% the subjects invariably chose the orthosis with lower energy cost.

Lehneis and colleagues[86] analyzed the effect of the spiral and hemispiral orthoses and that of conventional metal braces. The study noted a reduction in Ee per unit distance of 12% when the advanced orthoses were used.

Paraplegia

Loss of the major determinants of gait is more pronounced in paraplegia than in amputation or hemiplegia. From a pragmatic point of view, it is immediately

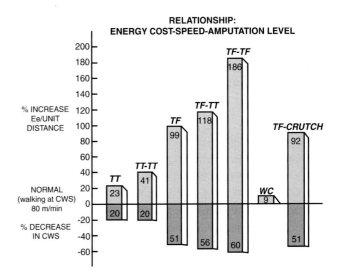

FIGURE 18-11 Summary of increase in energy expenditure (Ee) per unit distance and reduction of velocity among amputees as compared with able-bodied subjects at comfortable walking speeds (CWSs) of 80 m per minute. The values have been derived from various studies performed at Columbia University, College of Physicians and Surgeons, Department of Rehabilitation Medicine, New York, New York.[5,6,42,63,78] (TF = transfemoral; TF-TF = bilateral transfemoral; TF-TT = transfemoral-transtibial; TT = transtibial; TT-TT = bilateral transtibial; WC = wheelchair.)

TABLE 18-9
Energy Expenditure (Ee): Hemiplegia

Author (Year)	No.	Comment	Speed (m/min) Subject	Difference (%) (Normal 80/min)	Ee per Unit Time* (kcal/min/kg) Subject	Difference (%) (NCWS 0.063 kcal/min/kg)	Ee per Unit Distance (kcal × 10⁻³/m/kg) Subject	Difference (%) (NCWS 0.786 kcal × 10⁻³/m/kg)
Bard (1963)[83]	15	Cerebrovascular accident	41	−49	0.044	−30	1.073	37
Corcoran (1970)[84]	15	No orthosis	42	−48	0.062	−2	1.476	88
	15	Plastic AFO	49	−39	0.067	6	1.367	74
	15	Metal AFO	49	−39	0.067	6	1.367	74
Lehneis (1976)[86]	2	Metal AFO	22	−73	0.056	−11	2.545	224
	2	Spiral and hemispiral AFO	22	−73	0.054	−14	2.455	212
Gersten (1971)[85]	15	Articulating ankle	17	−79	0.041	−35	2.412	207
	15	Solid ankle	17	−79	0.042	−33	2.471	214

AFO = ankle-foot orthosis; NCWS = normal comfortable walking speed.
*Equation: Ee (kcal/min/kg) = $(29 + 0.0053\ V^2)/1{,}000$. [V = Velocity in m per minute.]

apparent that the patient with spinal cord injury or impairment that leads to loss of locomotor capability must expend an enormous amount of energy to regain some semblance of walking. It is generally held that patients with lesions at T-1 to T-11 do not become functional ambulators, whereas those with lesions at T-12 and below usually succeed.[87] Spinal cord injury patients and clinicians alike face the emotional tug-of-war in deciding whether to invest considerable time and effort in an activity that may eventually prove expensive and functionally unproductive. To this end, in search of a rational approach, several researchers have evaluated the energy requirements of ambulation for paraplegics (Table 18-10).

Standard Knee-Ankle-Foot Orthosis

The pioneering work, led by Gordon,[88,89] set the direction for subsequent studies on the Ee of paraplegic walking. In his study of 11 subjects with paraplegia of various causes, he found the speed of ambulation to be 66% slower than normal. The Ee per unit distance was more than 300% of normal CWS. He concluded that ambulation seemed to be an impractical solution and offered the wheelchair as an alternative for most, but not all, patients. He demonstrated that continuous paraplegic crutch walking with a swing-through gait was as exhausting as a 400-m run. Clinkingbeard's group[90] reported similarly dismal findings.

Waters et al.[91,92] provided an extensive look at energy requirement in a large cohort of young paraplegic patients. The average CWS was 27 m per minute, or 66% slower than the norm, whereas the Ee per unit time was within normal. When analyzed against normal CWS, the Ee per unit distance was 230% higher. The results indicate that the test group walked slower to keep their Ee down to tolerable levels, but as a result, they were unable to cover much distance. The study also looked into the effects produced by high- and low-level lesions. As expected, the lower the level of the lesion, the faster the speed, and the lower the increase in metabolic requirement.

Advanced Orthotic Designs

Researchers have turned to a variety of orthotic designs and materials in search of ways to lower the metabolic demands of ambulation. The hope was to bring walking within the reach of most paraplegics.

Knee-Ankle-Foot Orthosis Lehman and coworkers[93] noted that the double-ankle stop type of joint requires significantly less vertical lifting of the center of gravity, thus requiring less acceleration to carry the center of gravity forward, which in turn results in less mechanical work. Merkel and coworkers[94] studied eight complete motor paraplegic subjects with lesions at T-10 and below to determine the efficiency of the conventional single-stopped knee-ankle-foot orthosis (KAFO) as

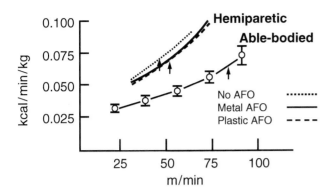

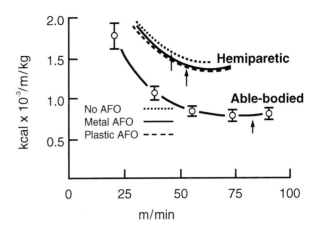

FIGURE 18-12 Polynomial regression curves of average energy cost at various walking speeds for hemiparetic and able-bodied subjects. The dumbbells indicate one standard deviation. Energy expenditure per unit time for both groups is approximately equal at their comfortable walking speeds, as indicated by an arrow. (AFO = ankle-foot orthosis.) (Redrawn with permission from PJ Corcoran, RH Jebsen, GL Brengelmann, et al. Effects of plastic and metal leg braces on speed and energy cost of hemiparetic ambulation. Arch Phys Med Rehabil 1970;51:69–77.)

FIGURE 18-13 Energy expenditure per unit distance among hemiparetic and able-bodied subjects. The dumbbells indicate one standard deviation. Note that, unlike able-bodied subjects, the hemiparetic group falls short of the theoretically optimal speed at which calorie expenditure would be minimal. (AFO = ankle-foot orthosis.) (Redrawn with permission from PJ Corcoran, RH Jebsen, GL Brengelmann, et al. Effects of plastic and metal leg braces on speed and energy cost of hemiparetic ambulation. Arch Phys Med Rehabil 1970;51:69–77.)

opposed to the Scott-Craig KAFO. The latter orthosis is a double upright, with offset knee joint, bail lock, adjustable anterior and posterior ankle pin stops, a crossbar at the level of the ankle joint, and sole plate extending beyond the metatarsal heads. They found no significant difference in Ee for a standing subject between the two types of orthoses. When subjects ambulated with a walker, the Scott-Craig KAFO was more energy efficient than the single-stopped KAFO, but the difference between the two was not statistically significant. While crutch walking, however, the Scott-Craig KAFO required significantly less energy per unit distance than the single-stopped KAFO (Figure 18-14). The fact remains, however, that the energy required for ambulation remains as much as 374% more per meter compared with normal CWS. Miller et al.[95] made similar comparisons during the subjects' negotiation of architectural barriers such as stairs, turns, and ramps and found no significant difference between the two devices in terms of Ee. Huang's group[96] likewise looked into the energy cost of ambulation among spinal cord injury patients using the Scott-Craig KAFO. The rate of ambulation reflected the patients' preferred CWS, which averaged 14 m per minute, or 83% slower than normal CWS. At that speed, the energy cost was roughly equivalent to that of normal persons ambulating at their own CWS, but the Ee per unit distance was 382% more.

Pneumatic In the hope that a light-weight device would increase the use of orthoses, researchers developed the pneumatic orthosis. Ragnarsson and colleagues[97] studied 14 paraplegics, two of whom were in the pediatric age group. When using the pneumatic orthosis, the subjects covered more ground at a CWS of 27 m per minute. The Ee per unit distance was statistically less than with use of standard metal KAFO. The article did not specify the results per kilogram, but assuming an average weight of 70 kg, the subjects demonstrated approximately the same Ee per unit time as normal CWS, but 216% higher Ee per unit distance. The authors expressed doubts if use of the pneumatic orthosis alters the fact that only the most exceptional patients will continue to pursue the exhausting task of ambulating with orthoses.

Mechanical Linkage Hip-Knee-Ankle-Foot Orthosis More recent developments provide a variety of options including mechanical hip-KAFO with linkage coupling, functional electrical stimulation (FES), and a hybrid system, which is a combination of both designs.

Nene and coinvestigators[98] studied 10 subjects with paraplegia ambulating with a hip guidance orthosis.[99] In comparing their results with those in the literature, Nene's group[98] were encouraged to find that the device resulted in more efficient walking than did conventional KAFO. Their subjects, however, walked slowly (13 m/minute) and spent 321% higher energy per unit distance, almost the same as conventional KAFO.

TABLE 18-10
Energy Expenditure (Ee): Paraplegia

Author (Year)	No.	Comment	Speed (m/min) Subject	Difference (%) (Normal 80/min)	Ee per Unit Time* (kcal/min/kg) Subject	Difference (%) (NCWS 0.063 kcal/min/kg)	Ee per Unit Distance (kcal × 10⁻³/m/kg) Subject	Difference (%) (NCWS 0.786 kcal × 10⁻³/m/kg)
General								
Gordon (1956)[88]	11	Various causes	27	–66	0.086	37	3.185	305
	3	Thoracic	27	–66	0.090	43	3.333	324
Clinkingbeard (1974)[90]	4	Thoracic	4	–95	0.043	–32	10.750	1,268
	3	Lumbar	20	–75	0.048	–24	2.400	205
Cerney (1980)[109]	11	T-12 to L-2	32	–60	0.098	56	3.063	290
Chantraine (1984)[107]	3	Parallel bars	15	–81	0.043	–32	2.867	265
	3	Crutches	23	–71	0.079	25	3.435	337
Waters (1985)[91]	67	All levels	27	–66	0.070	11	2.593	230
	10	T-1 to T-9	18	–78	0.058	–8	3.222	310
	57	T-10 and below	28	–65	0.072	14	2.571	227
	36	Spinal cord injury ambulators	41	–49	0.072	14	1.756	123
Yakura (1990)[110]	10	All levels	59	–26	0.075	19	1.271	62
Orthosis types								
Merkel (1984)[94]	8	SC walker	9	–89	0.059	–6	6.556	734
	8	SS KAFO, walker	6	–93	0.061	–3	10.167	1,193
	8	SC crutches	18	–78	0.067	6	3.722	374
	8	SS KAFO, crutch	15	–81	0.089	41	5.933	655
Huang (1979)[96]	8	SC crutches	14	–83	0.053	–16	3.786	382
Ragnarsson (1975)[97]	11	Metal KAFO	21	–74	0.064	2	3.048	288
	14	Pneumatic	27	–66	0.067	6	2.481	216
Nene (1989)[98]	10	Hip guidance orthosis	13	–84	0.043	–32	3.308	321
Ijzerman (1997)[101]	6	Advanced RGO	14	–83	0.104	65	1.486	952
Massucci (1998)[102]	6	Advanced RGO	10	–88	0.066	–5	6.660	747
Harvey (1998)[103]	10	Isocentric RGO	12	–85	0.094	50	8.200	1,043
Marsolais (1988)[104]	2	Functional electrical stimulation	15	–81	0.095	51	6.333	706
Hirokawa (1990)[100]	6	RGO, functional electrical stimulation	12	–85	0.065	3	5.213	663

KAFO = knee-ankle-foot orthosis; NCWS = normal comfortable walking speed; RGO = reciprocating gait orthosis; SC = Scott-Craig orthosis; SS = single-stop.
*Equation: Ee (kcal/min/kg) = (29 + 0.0053 V²)/1,000. [V = Velocity in m per minute.]

The energy costs using the reciprocating gait orthosis (RGO) and its modifications were analyzed in various studies. Hirokawa et al.[100] reported on six subjects who walked at less than 13 m per minute and spent more than 650% Ee per unit distance. Ijzerman and colleagues[101] compared the advanced RGO with a non-RGO and drew inconclusive findings. Massucci's group[102] also studied the effects of advanced RGO in thoracic paraplegic subjects and concluded that its use is not a valid alternative to wheelchair propulsion. Although Harvey and coworkers[103] found the isocentric RGO to be superior to a KAFO joined medially by a hinge mechanism but without the thoracolumbar corset. However, the energy cost remained staggering.

Functional Electrical Stimulation and Hybrid Systems The increased oxygen consumption of patients while ambulating with long-leg braces occurs primarily during the swing phase and is disproportionately less

FIGURE 18-14 Energy efficiency cost per meter of ambulation among paraplegic subjects using either Scott-Craig or single-stopped knee-ankle-foot orthosis and either walker or crutches. Subjects walked at their own comfortable walking speed. (Adapted from KD Merkel, NE Miller, PR Westbrook, et al. Energy expenditure of paraplegic patients standing and walking with two knee-ankle-foot orthoses. Arch Phys Med Rehabil 1984;65:121–124.)

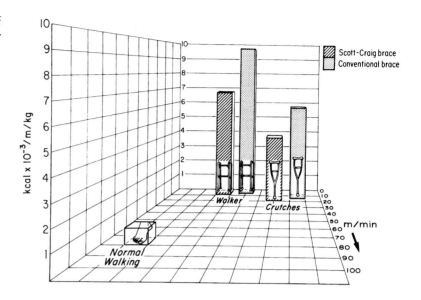

during the stance phase. In addition, the nonreciprocating gait pattern is dynamically discontinuous and loses the advantage provided by momentum as the speed increases. As a consequence, the patient is required to lift all of the body weight with each step or swing-through. The technique of FES is now being applied to respond to these shortcomings (see Chapter 31). Marsolais and Edwards[104,105] reported on the energy cost of ambulation using FES. In an initial inquiry,[104] they studied four paraplegics, reported the results from two subjects, and compared the values with those reported in other studies. The mean Ee per unit time was 0.095 kcal per minute per kg, compared with 0.058 kcal per minute per kg reported for the conventional KAFO.[91] Despite this, however, the authors were encouraged because of an accompanying 75% increase in working muscle mass because of inclusion of the hip and leg muscles. The net result was a decrease in the intensity of energy use relative to working muscle mass. The anaerobic component of FES also appeared to be less. Unlike KAFO and normal walking, the Ee per unit time theoretically decreases as the FES walking speed increases. Unfortunately, the fastest speed a subject achieved with FES was 34 m per minute, and no subject was able to walk more than 300 m because of fatigue or perceived exertion. This is understandable, as the aerobic cost of the activity is approximately six times a patient's BMR. Whereas normal sedentary persons are able to sustain muscle activity at or below 50% of maximum aerobic capacity, the FES anaerobic component probably occurs at or below that level, owing to the synchronized stimulation of motor neurons and muscle fibers. Additionally, FES tends to recruit the large superficial motor neurons (fast twitch) more than the deeper, smaller (slow twitch) motor neurons. In a follow-up report[105] on four complete paraplegic patients, two of whom also participated in the first study, they again measured the metabolic requirement of FES ambulation. They also sought to determine whether the use of an open-loop FES could significantly increase the maximum aerobic capacity and tolerance to lactic acid accumulation when combined with arm ergometry training. Their data suggest that paraplegic subjects could develop sufficient aerobic and anaerobic capacity to walk several hundred meters with FES and a rolling walker, while maintaining a cardiopulmonary reserve. The problem of local muscle fatigue (probably caused by ischemia) continued to plague the subjects. With modern technology and experience, FES holds the potential to advance beyond its present status and offers future possibilities.

The effects of hybrid systems that combine the advantages of passive mechanical orthosis such as the RGO and the active FES are subjects of a few investigations. Hirokawa et al.[100] made comparisons between RGO and FES-powered RGO. The authors noted that additional calculations were necessary to make direct comparisons between the two devices because FES-powered RGO requires Ee from both upper and lower extremities as well as some trunk muscles. Using the standard practice in exercise physiology, the Ee data from RGO were divided by 0.7 to compensate for the noninvolvement of the lower extremity muscles. This was based on the fact that $\dot{V}O_2$max of arm exercise is approximately 70% $\dot{V}O_2$max of lower limb exercise. Their results showed a 16% reduction in energy cost with the FES-powered RGO at speeds of 6.0–12.5 m per minute, but none at higher speeds. A study by Sykes and others[106] argued against the validity of using the correction factor and failed to show any improvement in energy cost while using the hybrid system.

Effects of Long-Term Use of Orthotics

Chantraine[107] and Yakura[108] and their coworkers have studied the effects of long-term orthotic use and the changes in ambulation parameters. Chantraine et al.[107] collected data on seven male paraplegic subjects with complete lesions at T-9 to L-1. Of these, four patients had recently undergone rehabilitation, while three were seasoned walkers. The cost of walking on a treadmill with a swing-through gait between parallel bars was 50% less for trained subjects than for new ambulators. Yakura's group[108] performed a longitudinal study among 10 spinal cord injury volunteers. At 1-year follow-up, the subjects walked significantly faster and more efficiently, had lower heart rate, and required less axial load on their upper extremities. The authors concluded, however, that despite the significant training effect of continued brace walking, the cardiovascular stress and energy demands of walking remain considerable.

Wheelchair Propulsion

Clinicians as well as paraplegic patients and their families all perceive walking as a worthy goal, or even as the sine qua non of successful rehabilitation. Crutch walking often does play a useful role in the initial rehabilitation of a paraplegic patient: It strengthens the upper body, develops balance and aerobic capacity, and imparts a sense of accomplishment, of having made a comeback. Few successful paraplegic ambulators maintain the demanding, and sometimes dangerous, skill for long; and its principal value may be in building a positive attitude toward the wheelchair as a liberating rather than confining device.

If humans had wheels instead of legs and feet, the efficiency of ambulation would be much improved. The horizontal and vertical excursions of the center of gravity would follow a straight line; thus less work. As academic as this notion may appear, the following discussion validates the argument.

Several articles have been published regarding patients engaged in wheeling (Table 18-11). One study[91] showed that the speed of wheeling was only slightly slower than normal CWS and the energy consumed was within the normal range. The elevated heart rate associated with wheeling, in comparison with normal walking, was attributed to the fact that the great majority of the work is done by the upper extremities. Another[109] investigation concluded that wheeling was significantly less difficult

than walking with orthoses. On level ground, their subjects were able to keep up with able-bodied persons as they wheeled at 75 m per minute. They spent no more Ee per unit time and consumed only 9% more Ee per unit distance than normal CWS. The data suggested that the wheelchair is destined to be the primary mode of ambulation for those who require two KAFOs, unless they are willing to work under anaerobic conditions and are able to achieve a velocity of 54 m per minute or faster.

Factors influencing the performance of wheelchairs are illustrated in Figure 18-15. Hildebrandt and colleagues[110] found that steering accuracy, net energy cost, and load on the circulatory system were significantly less with standard rear-wheel-drive chairs than with front-wheel-drive chairs. Hilbers and White[111] compared the sports chair with conventionally designed wheelchairs and found that the energy cost of propelling the former was approximately 17% less than for the latter, and they attributed the greater efficiency of the sports chair to its design rather than its lighter total mass. Wolfe et al.[112] and Glasser et al.[113] examined the effects of floor carpeting and the type of tires on wheelchairs used. The velocity of wheeling was significantly slower on carpeted floors than on tiled surfaces. Among the paraplegic subjects, the speed was almost equal with pneumatic and with hard tires. All subjects had higher oxygen consumption on carpeting than on hard floors, but the difference was not statistically significant except among paraplegic subjects who used pneumatic tires, when the Ee per unit distance on carpeted floors was significantly higher than on concrete floors. These findings should be borne in mind by designers of homes and institutions where wheelchairs will be in common use.

To provide independent mobility at normal CWS for patients with restricted cardiopulmonary reserve, clinicians should not be reluctant to prescribe electrically powered wheelchairs or scooters. Table 18-2 data suggest that the energy cost of using a power wheelchair is similar to that of "sitting at ease" (1.2–1.6 kcal/min/70 kg). The energy cost of using a scooter, which provides less back and arm support, is probably similar to that of "sitting, writing" (1.9–2.2 kcal/min/70 kg). The effect of increasing speed is probably negligible, although comparative data are lacking and research is needed.

Persons with disabilities who walk short distances with great difficulty, or who propel a manual wheelchair slowly and laboriously, can enhance their lifestyles by using a power wheelchair or scooter. Clinicians may advocate withholding power mobility aids from any patient who can propel a manual wheelchair, however awkwardly, in the belief that their stamina would regress if a powered wheelchair were provided. We found no data

TABLE 18-11
Energy Expenditure (Ee): Wheelchair Propulsion

Author (Year)	No.	Comment	Speed (m/min)		Ee per Unit Time* (kcal/min/kg)		Ee per Unit Distance (kcal × 10⁻³/m/kg)	
			Subject	Difference (%) (Normal 80/ min)	Subject	Difference (%) (NCWS 0.063 kcal/min/kg)	Subject	Difference (%) (NCWS 0.786 kcal × 10⁻³/m/kg)
Hildebrandt (1978)[110]	29	Front/rear wheel	67	−16	0.037	−41	0.552	−30
Cerny (1980)[109]	8	Paraplegia	75	−6	0.064	2	0.853	9
Wolfe (1978)[112]	10	Normal, tile	57	−29	0.056	−11	0.982	25
	10	Deconditioned, tile	53	−34	0.062	−2	1.170	49
	15	SCI, tile, firm tire	83	4	0.075	19	0.904	15
	15	SCI, tile, pneumatic tire	80	0	0.075	19	0.938	19
	10	Normal, carpet	43	−46	0.060	−5	1.395	78
	10	Deconditioned, carpet	37	−54	0.067	6	1.811	130
	15	SCI, carpet, firm tire	65	−19	0.081	29	1.246	59
	15	SCI, carpet, pneumatic	64	−20	0.082	30	1.281	63
Waters (1985)[91]	124	SCI, all levels	72	−10	0.055	−13	0.764	−3
	55	T-1 to T-9	68	−15	0.053	−16	0.779	−1
	69	T-10 and below	76	−5	0.057	−10	0.750	−5
Hilbers (1987)[112]	9	Sports chair	67	−16	0.044	−30	0.657	−16
	9	Regular chair	67	−16	0.053	−16	0.791	1

NCWS = normal comfortable walking speed; SCI = spinal cord injury.
*Equation: Ee (kcal/min/kg) = $(29 + 0.0053 \, V^2)/1,000$. [V = Velocity in m per minute.]

to support this notion, but the question requires careful research.

Immobilization of Body Segments

Immobilization and deformity of the joints of the trunk and lower extremities interfere with the harmonious movements of gait. Ralston[114] studied the effects of immobilizing various body segments. The Ee per unit time increased by 6% when one ankle was immobilized. When both ankle and arms were immobilized and the subject walked at a CWS of 73 m per minute, the Ee rose by 9%. The major role played by the knee joint is emphasized by the disproportionate increase of 37% in Ee when the knee was restricted at 135 degrees. Keeping the joint at 180 degrees resulted in 13% increase in Ee. In the optimal angle of immobilization of 165 degrees, the added demands rose by only 10%. Immobilization

of the hip at 180 degrees also resulted in a 13% increase in Ee, but at 150 degrees this dropped to 6%. Torso immobilization caused an increase of 10% over a wide range of speeds.

Waters and coworkers[115] immobilized 20 young, healthy subjects with a plaster cast on the predominant limb. All were placed in a long-leg cast, and 10 each in a cylinder or a short-leg cast. Although no significant increases in the average rate of Ee were noted between types of casts when the subjects walked with full weight bearing without crutches, the velocity of ambulation significantly decreased in proportion to the extent of immobilization. Although the Ee per unit time became progressively higher in proportion to the level of immobilization, the differences were not statistically significant. The net energy cost was consistently higher than normal CWS. The increase in heart rate with all types of casts was also significantly higher than would be expected in

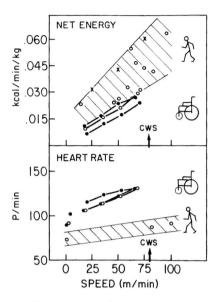

FIGURE 18-15 Energy expenditure per unit time and heart rate during level wheelchair driving compared with corresponding values for walking drawn from the literature. Although this particular study shows lower energy expenditure for propelling a wheelchair on a smooth, level surface than for normal walking, different sets of variables could increase the rate of expenditure. (CWS = comfortable walking speed.) (Redrawn with permission from G Hildenbrant, ED Voight, D Bahn, et al. Energy cost of propelling wheelchairs at various speeds: Cardiac response and effect on steering accuracy. Arch Phys Med Rehabil 1970;51:131–136.)

normal walking. Immobilization with short-leg walking cast and prefabricated lower leg orthoses required significantly more energy than normal, but no significant increase when using the rigid sole surgical shoes.[116] An unstable ankle causes a 10% increase in Ee.[117] By the same token, using a 1-in. shoe lift contralateral to an immobilized knee results in a 10% reduction in Ee.[118]

Crutch Ambulation

Many patients require assistive devices such as crutches during and after rehabilitation, and clinicians are always concerned to ensure that prescribed devices meet the patient's needs. Crutch walking alters the natural movement of the extremities and requires greater lift of the body to swing the legs through. Muscle groups that ordinarily play little or no role in walking are recruited, contributing further to the increased Ee (Table 18-12). Many factors, therefore, must be considered in mobility aids as basic as crutches. Crutch walking as an alternative for amputees has already been discussed (see Table 18-8).

Crutch Walking among Healthy Volunteers

Several studies have reported what happens when an otherwise healthy person is forced to walk with crutches. Shoup et al.[119] and Wells[120] studied the kinematics and energy variation of the swing-through gait and found them to depend on speed and degree of disablement. The trunk serves to conserve approximately one-half the energy that could be expended. Thys et al.[121] reported two to three times higher energy cost with swing-through gait as compared with normal walking, but only 1.3–1.5 times increased mechanical work, indicating a reduction of efficiency of positive work production. McBeath and colleagues[122] tested a group of 10 young volunteers. The subjects used axillary as well as forearm crutches as they walked with the following gait patterns: partial and non–weight bearing, two-point, and swing-through. The self-selected velocity was less than for normal walking, and the energy used was greater than for normal gait for either type of crutch. Walking with two-point alternating and three-point partial weight-bearing (PWB) gaits with either cane or crutches required approximately 18–36% more energy per unit distance than normal CWS. Swing-through and three-point non–weight-bearing gaits required an increase of 41–61% in net energy cost.

No difference in Ee was found while crutch walking, using the standard axillary crutches versus rocker bottom axillary crutch[123] or the ortho crutch.[124]

Fisher and Patterson[34] tested normal volunteers as they ambulated with axillary and forearm crutches and likewise found no difference in Ee with either type of crutches. Oxygen consumption rose twofold (Figure 18-16). The high energy cost of crutch walking was underscored with the finding that, even at the slow speed of 30 m per minute, oxygen consumption was 40% of that for the maximum upper extremity stress test. At 80 m per minute, Ee per unit distance increased to 88%, which is clearly above the anaerobic threshold. Although the investigation did not clarify the most efficient speed, crutch walking at 40–50 m per minute was suggested as being tolerable. The Ee per unit time at this speed is approximately the same as the normal Ee at normal CWS (see Figure 18-16). The authors provided further insights into the cardiovascular stress of crutch walking.[125] Heart rate for crutch walking was significantly higher than that for walking, and the slope versus oxygen consumption for crutch walking parallels that of an upper extremity stress test.

Waters and colleagues[115] immobilized their subjects in long-leg casts, cylinder casts, and short-leg casts and asked them to use crutches with a non–weight-bearing swing-through gait. The degree of oxygen consumption and the physical exertion recorded during crutch walking was above the anaerobic threshold and could be categorized as continuous hard or intermittent moderate work.

TABLE 18-12
Energy Expenditure (Ee): Crutch Walking

Author (Year)	No.	Comment	Speed (m/min)		Ee per Unit Time* (kcal/min/kg)		Ee per Unit Distance (kcal × 10⁻³/m/kg)	
			Subject	Difference (%) (Normal 80/min)	Subject	Difference (%) (NCWS 0.063 kcal/ min/kg)	Subject	Difference (%) (NCWS 0.786 kcal × 10⁻³/m/kg)
Healthy subjects								
McBeath (1974)[122]	10	Cane	60	−25	0.062	−2	1.033	31
	10	PWB, axillary	55	−31	0.051	−19	0.927	18
	10	Two point, axillary	57	−29	0.061	−3	1.070	36
	10	ST, axillary	58	−28	0.070	11	1.207	54
	10	PWB, forearm	55	−31	0.054	−14	0.982	25
	10	Two point, forearm	59	−26	0.058	−8	0.983	25
	10	ST, forearm	55	−31	0.061	−3	1.109	41
	10	NWB, forearm	53	−34	0.067	6	1.264	61
Fisher (1981)[34]	8	3 pt, NWB, axillary	30	−63	0.052	−17	1.733	121
	8	3 pt, NWB, axillary	40	−50	0.066	5	1.650	110
	8	3 pt, NWB, axillary	50	−38	0.071	13	1.420	81
	8	3 pt, NWB, axillary	60	−25	0.087	38	1.450	84
	8	3 pt, NWB, axillary	70	−13	0.095	51	1.357	73
	8	3 pt, NWB, axillary	80	0	0.118	87	1.475	88
Hinton (1982)[124]	15	NWB, axillary	42	−47	0.077	22	1.0784	126
	15	NWB, Ortho crutch	43	−46	0.074	17	1.0720	118
Nielsen (1990)[123]	24	NWB, rocker	60	−25	0.094	45	1.569	99
	24	NWB, axillary	60	−25	0.096	52	1.610	104
Postfracture and cast								
Imms (1976)[126]	3	Fx, long-leg cast, crutch	57	−29	0.082	30	1.439	83
	11	Fx, crutches	65	−19	0.074	17	1.138	45
	10	Fx, two canes	69	−14	0.072	14	1.043	33
Waters (1982)[115]	20	Normal, long-leg cast, ST	51	−36	0.096	52	1.882	139
	10	Normal, cylinder cast, ST	52	−35	0.098	56	1.885	140
	10	Normal, short-leg cast, ST	61	−24	0.104	65	1.705	117

Forearm = forearm/Lofstrand crutches; Fx = fracture; NCWS = normal comfortable walking speed; NWB = non–weight bearing; PWB = partial weight bearing; ST = swing-through gait; 3 pt = three-point gait.
*Equation: Ee (kcal/min/kg) = (29 + 0.0053 V^2)/1,000. [V = Velocity in m per minute.]

Crutch Walking after Fracture and Hip Replacement

Imms and colleagues[126] followed the energy cost of ambulation among 13 patients who were recovering from fractures. Those who ambulated with long-leg cast and crutches spent considerably more energy than persons who walked normally. These patients recovered efficient ambulation as they progressed from crutches to canes and finally to no assistive device, but they ambulated only at slower speeds. Pugh[127] noted a similar sequence of events as he followed the course of one patient after hip replacement. Brown et al.[128] studied the energetics of walking preoperatively and postoperatively in a group of

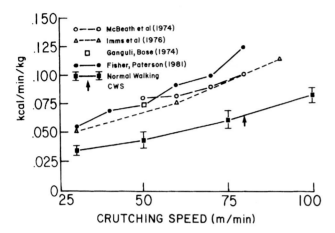

FIGURE 18-16 Relationship between crutch-walking speed and energy expenditure among normal subjects as drawn from the literature. (CWS = comfortable walking speed.) (Redrawn with permission from S Fisher, R Paterson. Energy cost of ambulation with crutches. Arch Phys Med Rehabil 1981;62:250–256.)

patients who had undergone total hip replacement. Those who had unilateral hip disease did quite well and improved their speed of ambulation with a concomitant decrease in Ee per unit distance. Of the patients with bilateral hip disease, those with two hip replacements fared considerably better than those with only one. The evidence presented confirms that it is prudent to ensure that patients engage in upper extremity endurance training before they begin to ambulate with crutches.

Other Disabilities

Olgiati and colleagues[129] found a twofold increase in the energy cost of walking among patients with multiple sclerosis. These patients had a slow pace and frequently experienced dyspnea and leg fatigue. In an effort to define the roles of spasticity, ataxia, and weakness, the same authors studied 33 patients with multiple sclerosis who did not suffer from cardiopulmonary disease.[130] Their findings showed a 65% increase in Ee per unit distance and indicated that lower extremity spasticity, rather than weakness, accounted for at least 40% of the variability.

The effects of a progressive activity program on the physiological work performance of chronic low back pain patients was examined by Thomas et al.[131] Fifteen chronic low back pain sufferers participated twice daily in mat exercises, bicycling, and walking. Before treat-

ment, the average CWS was 55 m per minute, with an expenditure rate of 0.056 kcal per minute per kg; after the program, the CWS increased to 74 m per minute, with an Ee of 0.064 kcal per minute per kg. The small posttreatment increase in rate of oxygen consumption, coupled with a faster CWS, resulted in enhanced efficiency. The authors pointed out that patients with low back pain frequently regress to a lifestyle that eventually reduces their fitness level and stressed the importance of reversing the phenomenon with a proper exercise regimen.

ENERGY EXPENDITURE BY CHILDREN

Children are underrepresented in studies of Ee, possibly because of the dynamic changes that occur in their gait pattern, the metabolic differences between them and adults, and the inherent difficulty of engaging them in experiments. Several investigators have addressed the last problem by proposing innovative ways of measuring energy consumption. The traditional equipment is too cumbersome for some children, particularly those with disabilities; results from a light-weight telemetric oxygen analysis system correlated well with that from a breath-by-breath analyzer used while subjects walked on a treadmill.[132,133] Johnson and associates[134] reported that an accelerometer was not as accurate a predictor of physical activity–related Ee in preadolescent children as compared with subtracting postprandial resting metabolic rate from total daily Ee derived from the doubly labeled water method. They reported that activity Ee was related to gender and fat mass. Rowland and colleagues,[135] however, found no gender-related differences in use of energy during submaximal exercise in children. Eston and coworkers[136] compared the accuracy of heart rate monitoring, pedometry, triaxial accelerometry, and uniaxial accelerometry for estimating oxygen consumption among 30 children who walked, ran, played catch, and engaged in other pastimes; triaxial accelerometry provided the best assessment of activity, whereas pedometry was more appropriate for studying large populations. Treuth and coinvestigators[137] also used heart rate to predict Ee; they compared activity against respiration calorimetry in 20 children during rest, sleep, and exercise and concluded that the combination of heart rate and activity can determine Ee for groups of children and for individuals.

Measurement of Ee of infants is particularly daunting. Thureen and colleagues[138] developed a force plate that they used in conjunction with indirect calorimetry to measure total Ee and energy cost of physical activity in preterm neonates. Expenditure was lowest during quiet sleep and highest when the babies were crying. Wells and Davies[139] conducted a longitudinal study of 124 healthy infants; activity Ee increased from 5% of energy intake at 1.5 months to 34% at 12 months.

Adolescents expend relatively high energy when walking and running, regardless of gender, age, and height.[140] Cureton and associates[141] determined energy consumption of 145 boys and girls, 7–17 years of age in a 1-mile run/walk treadmill task and concluded that age-related improvement in efficiency is caused primarily by an increase in the percent $\dot{V}O_2$ peak and improvement in $\dot{V}O_2$ economy. Wergel-Kolmert and Wohlfart[142] noted day-to-day variations in Ee among 20 female adolescents who walked on a treadmill at two speeds.

Cerebral Palsy

Rose and his group[143] reported that among healthy children, the relationship between heart rate and oxygen uptake was linear throughout a wide range of walking speeds. The same relationship was found in children with cerebral palsy, which offers the possibility of using this parameter as a simple means of evaluating energy costs in pediatric rehabilitation. As with adults, however, the caveat remains that heart rate varies considerably, particularly at lower work intensities. The same research team examined 18 able-bodied children and 13 children with cerebral palsy. The most efficient speed among able-bodied children approximated the adult velocity of 80 m per minute, whereas cerebral palsied children's velocity averaged 51 m per minute. The energy cost of walking for those with hemiplegic cerebral palsy compared favorably with that of their nondisabled counterparts. Children with diplegia expended 200% more energy.[144] Bowen and colleagues[145] concluded that oxygen cost was a more reliable measurement of oxygen use during walking than the physiological cost index for children with cerebral palsy. According to Stallings and coinvestigators,[146] children with spastic quadriplegia who had low body fat stores had a lower resting Ee than those with adequate fat stores.

Seeking an explanation of the higher energy cost, Unnithan and associates[147] compared nine children with cerebral palsy with nondisabled peers during treadmill walking. Electromyographic data and oxygen cost indicated that cocontraction of thigh and lower leg muscles accounted for approximately one-half of the higher energy cost of walking. Duffy and coworkers[148] examined able-bodied children fitted with knee orthoses set in vari-

ous flexion angles, to test the theory that flexed knee walking, common in cerebral palsy, accounts for the increased energy cost; they found that flexed-knee gait does not of itself cause an increase in energy cost. The same group also compared energy consumption of children with cerebral palsy with those having spina bifida; the latter subjects' consumption was significantly lower and more comparable with nondisabled children.[149] Bowen and coinvestigators[150] compared energy use of eight children with cerebral palsy with eight diagnosed with muscular dystrophy; again, cerebral palsy accounted for significantly more consumption. They concluded that measurements may show that a patient can have normal oxygen cost and consumption while walking and yet be functionally limited because of weakness.

A few scientists have used energy consumption as a means of comparing various interventions in the management of cerebral palsy. McGibbon and coworkers[151] evaluated an 8-week program of equine movement therapy on five children having spastic cerebral palsy. All subjects showed significant decrease in Ee during walking, decreased cadence, and increased stride length. Mattson and Andersson[152] examined 10 children with either spastic or ataxic diplegia as they walked with anterior and posterior walkers; although most children preferred the posterior walker, they exhibited no difference in oxygen cost, perceived exertion, or walking speed.

Amputation

Engsberg and colleagues reported two investigations that compared oxygen uptake and other physiological measures of three children, 7–10 years of age with transtibial (below-knee) amputation with healthy age mates. Children with amputation walked at the freely chosen speed and exhibited heart rate and $\dot{V}O_2$ values comparable with those reported for adults with similar disability.[153] The young subjects who wore the SACH foot consumed slightly more oxygen than did the individual fitted with a Flex-Foot. Reporting on 10 children, ranging from 6–18 years of age, the same research team found no significant difference in oxygen uptake for children with amputation as compared with able-bodied control subjects, although the latter had much less vertical displacement while walking on a treadmill.[154] Van der Windt and coworkers[155] compared Ee among children with tibial rotationplasty, transfemoral amputation, and hip disarticulation and found no significant difference among the groups with regard to Ee per unit time or per unit distance, although those with rotationplasty walked fastest.

CONCLUSION

Rehabilitative therapy can have a dramatic effect on the physiological responses of persons with disabilities, just as a potent pharmacologic agent can. The multiplicity of factors that affect the ultimate outcome can be carefully sorted if the process is based on scientific data. Much remains to be learned. The prescription of ambulation aids demands knowledge that is more far reaching than is commonly appreciated. Persons with disabilities walk slower to minimize the rate of calorie expenditure, but at the price of increased net cost and reduced efficiency. The choices between types of ambulatory aids, devices, and gait patterns should be based not on a predetermined protocol but rather on analysis of each individual's unique abilities or disabilities.

REFERENCES

1. Saunders JB, Inman VT, Eberhart HD. The major determinants in normal and pathological gait. J Bone Joint Surg 1953;35A:543–558.

2. Inman VT, Ralston HJ, Todd F. Human Walking. Baltimore: Williams & Wilkins, 1981.

3. Gard SA, Childress DS. The influence of stance-phase knee flexion on the vertical displacement of the trunk during normal walking. Arch Phys Med Rehabil 1999;80:26–32.

4. Gard SA, Childress DS. The effect of pelvic list on the vertical displacement of the trunk during normal walking. Gait Posture 1997;5:233–238.

5. Gonzalez, EG, Corcoran PJ. Energy Expenditure During Ambulation. In JA Downey, SJ Myers, EG Gonzalez, et al. (eds), Physiological Basis of Rehabilitation Medicine (2nd ed). Boston: Butterworth–Heinemann, 1994;413–446.

6. Corcoran PJ. Energy Expenditure During Ambulation. In JA Downey, RD Darling (eds), Physiological Basis of Rehabilitation Medicine. Philadelphia: WB Saunders, 1971;185–198.

7. Fisher SV, Gullickson G Jr. Energy cost of ambulation in health and disability: a literature review. Arch Phys Med Rehabil 1978;59:124–133.

8. Passmore R, Durnin JVGA. Human energy expenditure. Physiol Rev 1955;35:801–840.

9. Brown AC, Brengelmann G. Energy Metabolism. In TC Ruch, HD Patton (eds), Physiology and Biophysics (19th ed). Philadelphia: WB Saunders, 1965;1030–1049.

10. Gordon E. Energy costs of activities in health and disease. Arch Intern Med 1958;101:702–713.

11. Muller EA, Hettinger T. Effect of the speed of gait on the energy transformation in walking with artificial legs. Germ Ztrschr Orthop 1953;83:620–627.

12. Linnarsson D, Mattson E, Broman EL, et al. Determintion of oxygen cost of level walking. Clin Physiol 1989;9:1–10.

13. Corcoran PJ, Brengelmann GL. Oxygen uptake in normal and handicapped subjects, in relation to speed of walking beside velocity-controlled cart. Arch Phys Med Rehabil 1970;51:78–87.

14. Astrand P-O, Rodahl K. Textbook on Work Physiology. New York: McGraw-Hill, 1970.

15. Rowell LB, Taylor HL, Wang Y. Limitations to prediction of maximal oxygen intake. J Appl Physiol 1964; 19:919–927.

16. Darling RC. Exercise. In JA Downey, RD Darling (eds), Physiological Basis of Rehabilitation Medicine. Philadelphia: WB Saunders, 1971;167–183.

17. Moldover JR, Borg-Stein J. Exercise and Fatigue. In JA Downey, SJ Myers, EG Gonzalez, et al. (eds), Physiological Basis of Rehabilitation Medicine (2nd ed). Boston: Butterworth–Heinemann, 1994;393–411.

18. McDonald I. Statistical studies of recorded energy expenditure of man. Part II: expenditure on walking related to weight, sex, height, speed and gradient. Nutr Abstr Rev 1961;31:739–762.

19. Waters RL, Hislop HJ, Perry J, et al. Energetics: application to the study and management of locomotor disabilities energy cost of normal and pathologic gait. Orthop Clin North Am 1978;9:351–377.

20. Blessey RL, Hislop HJ, Waters RL, et al. Metabolic energy cost of unrestrained walking. Phys Ther 1976;56:1019–1024.

21. Waters RL, Hislop HJ, Perry J, et al. Comparative cost of walking in young and old adults. J Orthop Res 1983;1:73–76.

22. Waters RL, Lunsford BR, Perry J, et al. Energy-speed relationship of walking: standard tables. J Orthop Res 1988;6:215–222.

23. Foster GD, Wadden TA, Kendrick ZV, et al. The energy cost of walking before and after significant weight loss. Med Sci Sports Exerc 1995;27:888–894.

24. Censi L, Toti E, Pastore G, et al. The basal metaboic rate and energy cost of standardised walking of short and tall men. Eur J Clin Nutr 1998;52:441–446.

25. Waters RL, Hislop HJ, Thomas L, et al. Energy cost of walking in normal children and teenagers. Dev Med Child Neurol 1983;25:184–188.

26. Workman JM, Armstrong BW. Metabolic cost of walking: equation and model. J Appl Physiol 1986;61:1369–1374.

27. Ralston HJ. Energy-speed relation and optimal speed during level walking. Int Z Angew Physiol Einschl Arbeitsphysiol 1958;17:277–283.

28. Bobbert AC. Energy expenditure in level and grade walking. J Appl Physiol 1960;15:1015–1021.

29. Margaria R, Cerretelli P, Aghemo P, et al. Energy cost of running. J Appl Physiol 1963;18:367–370.

30. Soule RG, Goldman RF. Energy cost of loads carried on the head, hands or feet. J Appl Physiol 1969;27:687.

31. Duggan A, Haisman MF. Prediction of the metabolic cost of walking with and without loads. Ergonomics 1992; 35:417–426.

32. Ebbeling CJ, Hamill J, Crussemeyer JA. Lower extremity mechanics and energy cost of walking in high-heeled shoes. J Sport Phys Ther 1994;19:190–196.

33. Corcoran PJ, Templer JA. Stair climbing for cardiovascular reconditioning. Presented at the 37th Annual Assembly of the Am Acad Phys Med Rehabil; Nov 19, 1975; Atlanta, Georgia.

34. Fisher S, Patterson R. Energy cost of ambulation with crutches. Arch Phys Med Rehabil 1981;62:250–256.

35. Ganguli S, Bose KS. Biomechanical approach to functional assessment of use of crutches for ambulation. Ergonomics 1974;17:365–374.

36. Christensen EH. Physiological valuation of work in the Nykroppa Iron Works. Presented at the Ergonomics Society Symposium on Fatigue; 1953; Leeds, London.

37. Waters RL, Perry J, Antonelli D, et al. Energy cost of walking of amputees: influence of level of amputation. J Bone Joint Surg 1976;58A:42–46.

38. Reitmeyer H. Energy consumption and gait characteristics in walking and bicycling in unilateral below-knee amputees. Z Orthop 1955;86:571–589.

39. Ralston HJ. Dynamics of the human body during locomotion: the efficiency of walking in normal and amputee subjects. Final Report, SRS Grant RD 2849-M, Aug 1971. Berkeley: Biomechanics Laboratory, University of California, 1971.

40. Molen NH. Energy/speed relation of below-knee amputees walking on motor-driven treadmill. Int Z Angew Physiol 1973;31:173–185.

41. Ganguli S, Datta SR, Chatterjee BB, et al. Performance evaluation of amputee-prosthesis system in below-knee amputees. Ergonomics 1973;16:797–810.

42. Gonzalez EG, Corcoran PJ, Reyes RL. Energy expenditure in below-knee amputees: correlation with stump length. Arch Phys Med Rehabil 1974;55:111–119.

43. Gailey RS, Wenger MA, Raya M, Kirk N. Energy expenditure of trans-tibial amputees during ambulation at self-selected pace. Prosthet Orthot Int 1994;18:84–91.

44. Pagliarulo MA, Waters RL, Hislop HJ. Energy cost of walking of below-knee amputees having no vascular disease. Phys Ther 1979;59:538–542.

45. Huang C-T, Jackson JR, Moore NB, et al. Amputation: energy cost of ambulation. Arch Phys Med Rehabil 1979;60:18–24.

46. Ganguli S, Datta SR. Studies in load carrying in below-knee amputees with a PTB prosthesis system. J Med Eng Tech 1977;57:151–154.

47. Roy AK, Ganguli S, Datta SR, et al. Performance evaluation of BK amputees through graded load carrying test. Acta Orthop Scand 1977;48:691–695.

48. Ganguli S, Datta SR, Chatterjee BB, et al. Performance evaluation of amputee-prosthesis system in below-knee amputees. Ergonomics 1973;16:797–810.

49. Cummings V, March H, Steve L, et al. Energy costs of below-knee prostheses using two types of suspension. Arch Phys Med Rehabil 1979;60:293–297.

50. Nielsen PH, Schurr DG, Golden JC, et al. Comparison of energy cost and gait efficiency during ambulation in below-knee amputees using different prosthetic feet. A preliminary report. J Prosthet Orthot 1989;1:24–31.

51. MacFarlane PA, Nielsen DN, Schurr DG, et al. Gait comparison for below-knee amputees using a Flex-Foot versus a conventional prosthetic foot. J Prosthet Orthot 1991;3:150–161.

52. Snyder RD, Powers CM, Fontaine C, et al. The effects of five prosthetic feet on the gait and loading of the sound limb in dysvascular below knee amputees. J Rehabil Res Dev 1995;32:309–315.

53. Wagner J, Sienko S, Supan T, et al. Motion analysis of SACH vs Flex-Foot in moderately active below-knee amputees. Clin Prosthet Orthot 1987;11:55–62.

54. Torburn L, Powers CM, Gutierrez R, et al. Energy expenditure during ambulation in dysvascular and traumatic below-knee amputees: a comparison of five prosthetic feet. J Rehabil Res Dev 1995;32:111–119.

55. Casillas JM, Dulieu V, Cohen M, et al. Bioenergetic comparison of a new energy-storing foot and SACH foot in traumatic below-knee vascular amputations. Arch Phys Med Rehabil 1995;76:39–44.

56. Gailey RS, Nash MS, Atchley TA, et al. The effects of prosthesis mass on metabolic cost of ambulation in non-vascular trans-tibial amputees. Prosthet Orthot Int 1997;21:9–16.

57. Lehmann JF, Price R, Okumura R, et al. Mass and mass distribution of below-knee prostheses: effects on gait efficiency and self-selected walking speed. Arch Phys Med Rehabil 1998;79:162–168.

58. Muller EA, Hettinger TH. Arbeitsphysiologische Untersuchungen verschiedener Oberschenkel-Kunstbeine. Z Orthop 1952;81:525–545.

59. Erdman WJH, Hettinger TH, Saez F. Comparative work stress for above-knee amputees using artificial legs or crutches. Am J Phys Med 1960;39:225–232.

60. Inman VT, Bames GH, Levy SW, et al. Medical problems of amputees. Calif Med 1961;94:132–138.

61. Bard G, Ralston HJ. Measurement of energy expenditure during ambulation, with special reference to evaluation of assistive devices. Arch Phys Med Rehabil 1959;40:415–420.

62. Ganguli S, Bose KS, Datta SR, et al. Ergonomics evaluation of above-knee amputee-prosthesis combinations. Ergonomics 1974;17:199–210.

63. Traugh GH, Corcoran PJ, Reyes RL. Energy expenditure of ambulation in patients with above-knee amputations. Arch Phys Med Rehabil 1975;56:67–71.

64. James U. Oxygen uptake and heart rate during prosthetic walking in healthy male unilateral above-knee amputees. Scand J Rehabil 1973;5:71–80.

65. Otis JC, Lane JM, Kroll MA. Energy cost during gait in osteosarcoma patients after resection and knee replacement and above-knee amputation. J Bone Joint Surg 1985;67A:606–611.

66. Jaegers SM, Vos LD, Rispens P, et al. The relationship between comfortable and most metabolically efficient walking speed in persons with unilateral above knee amptutation. Arch Phys Med Rehabil 1993;74:521–525.

67. Isakov E, Susakz, Becker E. Energy expenditure and cardiac response in above-knee amputee while using prosthesis with open and locked knee mechanisms. Scand J Rehab Med 1985;12(Suppl):108–111.

68. Czerniecki JM, Gitter A, Weaver K. Effects of alterations in prosthetic shank mass on the metabolic cost of ambulation in above-knee amputees. Arch Phys Med Rehabil 1994;73:348–352.

69. Gailey RS, Lawrence D, Barditt C. The CAT-CAM socket and quadrilateral socket: a comparison of energy cost during ambulation. Prosthet Orthot Int 1993;17:95–100.

70. Boomstra AM, Schrama J, Fidler V, Eisma WH. Energy cost during ambulation in transfemoral amputees: a knee joint with a mechanical swing phase control vs a knee joint with pneumatic swing phase control. Scand J Rehabil Med 1995;27:77–81.

71. Sabolich J. Contoured adducted trochanteric- controlled alignment method (CAT-CAM): introduction and basic principles. Orthot Prosthet 1985;9:15–26.

72. Flandry E, Beskin J, Chambers R, et al. The effects of the CAT-CAM above-knee prosthesis on functional rehabilitation. Clin Orthop 1989;239:249–262.

73. Buckley JG, Spence WD, Solomonidis SE. Energy cost of walking: comparison of intelligent prosthesis with conventional mechanism. Arch Phys Med Rehabil 1997;78:330–333.

74. Taylor MB, Clark E, Offord EA, Baxter C. A comparison of energy expenditure by a high level trans-femoral amputee using the intelligent prosthesis and conventionally damped prosthetic limbs. Prosthet Orthot Int 1996;20:116–121.

75. Kawal A, Backus SI, Otis JC, et al. Interrelationship of clinical outcome, prosthetic knee replacement following resection of a malignant tumor of the

distal aspect of the femur. J Bone Joint Surg 1998;80A:822–831.

76. Roy AK, Datta SR, Chatterjec BB, et al. Ergonomic study on above-knee prosthetic rehabilitees carrying graded loads. Ergonomics 1976;19:431–440.

77. Nowroozi F, Saronelli ML, Gerber LH. Energy expenditure in hip disarticulation and hemipelvectomy. Arch Phys Med Rehabil 1983;64:300–303.

78. Corcoran PJ, Reyes RL, Gonzalez EG. Energy cost of ambulation in bilateral leg amputees. Presented at the 48th Annual Session of the American Congress of Rehabilitation Medicine; Nov 10, 1971; San Juan, Puerto Rico.

79. DuBow LL, Witt PL, Kadaba MP, et al. Oxygen consumption of elderly persons with bilateral below-knee amputations: amputation vs wheelchair propulsion. Arch Phys Med Rehabil 1983;64:255–259.

80. Crouse SF, Lessard CS, Rhodes J, et al. Oxygen consumption and cardiac response of short-leg and long-leg prosthetic ambulation in a patient with bilateral above-knee amputation: comparisons with able-bodied men. Arch Phys Med Rehabil 1990;71:313–317.

81. Hoffman MD, Sheldahl LM, Buley KJ, Sanford PR. Physiological comparison of walking among bilateral above-knee amputee and able-bodied subjects, and a model to account for the differences in metabolic cost. Arch Phys Med Rehabil 1997;78:385–392.

82. Ganguli S, Bose KS, Datta SR, et al. Biomechanical approach to functional assessment of use of crutches for ambulation. Ergonomics 1974;17:365–374.

83. Bard B. Energy expenditure of hemiplegic subjects during walking. Arch Phys Med Rehabil 1963;44:368–370.

84. Corcoran PJ, Jebsen RH, Brengelmann GL, et al. Effects of plastic and metal leg braces on speed and energy cost of hemiparetic ambulation. Arch Phys Med Rehabil 1970;51:69–77.

85. Gersten JW, Orr W. External work of walking in hemiparetic patients. Scand J Rehabil Med 1971;3:85–88.

86. Lehneis HR, Bergofsky E, Frisina W. Energy expenditure with advanced lower limb orthoses and with conventional braces. Arch Phys Med Rehabil 1976;57:20–24.

87. Long CH, Lawton EB. Functional significance of spinal cord lesion level. Arch Phys Med Rehabil 1955;36:249–255.

88. Gordon EE. Physiological approach to ambulation in paraplegia. JAMA 1956;161:686–688.

89. Gordon EE, Vanderwalde H. Energy requirements in paraplegic ambulation. Arch Phys Med Rehabil 1956;37:276–285.

90. Clinkingbeard JR, Gersten JW, Hoehn D. Energy cost of ambulation in traumatic paraplegic. Am J Phys Med 1964;43:157–165.

91. Waters RL, Lunsford BR. Energy cost of paraplegic locomotion. J Bone Joint Surg 1985;67A:1245–1250.

92. Waters RL, Yakura JS, Adkins R, et al. Determinants of gait performance following spinal cord injury. Arch Phys Med Rehabil 1989;70:811–818.

93. Lehmann JF, DeLateur BJ, Warren CG, et al. Biomechanical evaluation of braces for paraplegics. Arch Phys Med Rehabil 1969;50:179–188.

94. Merkel KD, Miller NE, Westbrook PR, et al. Energy expenditure of paraplegic patients standing and walking with two knee-ankle-foot orthoses. Arch Phys Med Rehabil 1984;65:121–124.

95. Miller NE, Merritt JL, Merkel KD, et al. Paraplegic energy expenditure during negotiation of architectural barriers. Arch Phys Med Rehabil 1984;65:778–779.

96. Huang C-T, Kuhlemeier KV, Moore NB, et al. Energy cost of ambulation in paraplegic patients using Craig-Scott braces. Arch Phys Med Rehabil 1979;60:595–600.

97. Ragnarsson KT, Sell GH, McGarrity M, et al. Pneumatic orthosis for paraplegic patients: functional evaluation and prescription considerations. Arch Phys Med Rehabil 1975;56:479–483.

98. Nene AV, Patrick JH. Energy cost of paraplegic locomotion with the ORLAU ParaWalker. Paraplegia 1989;27:5–18.

99. Patrick JH, McClelland MR. Low-energy cost reciprocal walking for adult paraplegic. Paraplegia 1985; 23:113–117.

100. Hirokawa S, Grimm M, Le T, Solomonow M. Energy consumption in paraplegic ambulation using the reciprocating gait orthosis and electrical stimulation of the thigh muscles. Arch Phys Med Rehabil 1990;71:687–694.

101. Ijzerman MJ, Baardman G, Hermens HJ, et al. The influence of the reciprocal cable linkage in the advanced reciprocating gait orthoses on paraplegic gait performance. Prosthet Orthot Int 1997;21:52–61.

102. Massucci M, Brunetti G, Piperno R, et al. Walking with the advanced reciprocating gait orthosis in thoracic paraplegic patients: energy expenditure and cardiorespiratory performance. Spinal Cord 1998;36:223–227.

103. Harvey LA, Davis GM, Smith MB, Engel S. Energy expenditure during gait using the walkabout and isocentric reciprocal gait orthoses in persons with paraplegia. Arch Phys Med Rehabil 1998;79:945–949.

104. Marsolais EB, Edwards BG. Energy costs of walking and standing with functional neuromuscular stimulation and long leg braces. Arch Phys Med Rehabil 1988;69:243–249.

105. Edwards BG, Marsolais EB. Metabolic responses to arm ergometry and functional neuromuscular stimulation. J Rehab Res Rev 1990;27:107–114.

106. Sykes L, Campbell IG, Powell ES, et al. Energy expenditure of walking for adult patients with spinal cord lesions using the reciprocating gait orthosis and functional electrical stimulation. Spinal Cord 1996;34:659–665.

107. Chantraine A, Crielarrd JM, Onkelinx A, et al. Energy expenditure of ambulation in paraplegics: Effects of long-term use of bracing. Paraplegia 1984;22:173–181.

108. Yakura JS, Waters RL, Adkins RH. Changes in ambulation parameters in spinal cord injury individuals following rehabilitation. Paraplegia 1990;28: 364–370.

109. Cerney K, Waters R, Perry J. Walking and wheelchair energetics in persons with paraplegia. Phys Ther 1980; 60:1133–1139.

110. Hildenbrandt G, Voigt E-D, Bahn D, et al. Energy costs of propelling wheelchair at various speeds: cardiac response and effect on steering accuracy. Arch Phys Med Rehabil 1970; 51:131–136.

111. Hilbers PA, White TP. Effects of wheelchair design on metabolic and heart rate responses during propulsion by persons with paraplegia. Phys Ther 1987;67:1355–1358.

112. Wolfe GA, Waters R, Hislop HJ. Influence of floor space on the energy cost of wheelchair propulsion. Phys Ther 1977;57:1022–1026.

113. Glaser RM, Sawka MN, Woodrow BK, et al. Energy cost and cardiopulmonary responses for wheelchair locomotion on tile and carpet. Paraplegia 1981;19:220–226.

114. Ralston HJ. Effects of immobilization of various body segments on energy cost of human locomotion. Proceedings of the Second International Congress on Ergonomics, Dortmund, 1964. Ergonomics 1965;12(Suppl):53–60.

115. Waters RL, Campbell J, Thomas L, et al. Energy cost of walking in lower-extremity plaster cast. J Bone Joint Surg 1982;64A:896–899.

116. Fowler PT, Botte MJ, Mathewson JW,

et al. Energy cost of ambulation with different methods of foot and ankle immobilization. J Orthop Res 1993; 11:416–421.

117. Mattson E, Brostrom LA. The increase in energy cost of walking with an immobilized knee or unstable ankle. Scand J Rehabil Med 1990;22:51–53.

118. Abdulhadi HM, Kerrigan C, LaRaia PJ. Contralateral shoe-lift: effect on oxygen cost of walking with an immobilized knee. Arch Phys Med Rehabil 1996;77:670–672.

119. Shoup TE, Fletcher LS, Merrill BR. Biomechanics of crutch locomotion. J Biomech 1974;7:11–20.

120. Wells RP. The kinemetrics and energy variations of swing-through crutch gait. Biomechanics 1979;12:579–585.

121. Thys H, Willems PA, Saels P. Energy cost, mechanical work and muscular efficiency in swing through gait with elbow crutches. J Biomechanics 1996;29:1473–1482.

122. McBeath AA, Bahrke M, Balke B. Efficiency of assisted ambulation determined by oxygen consumption measurement. J Bone Joint Surg 1974:56A:994–1000.

123. Nielsen DH, Harris JM, Minton YM, Motley NS. Energy cost, exercise intensity, and gait efficiency of standard versus rocker-bottom axillary crutch walking. Phys Ther 1990;70:487–493.

124. Hinton CA, Cullen KE. Energy expenditure during ambulation with ortho crutches and axillary crutches. Phys Ther 1982;62:813–819.

125. Patterson R, Fisher SV. Cardiovascular stress of crutch walking. Arch Phys Med Rehabil 1981;62:257–260.

126. Imms FJ, MacDonald ID, Prestidge SP. Energy expenditure during walking in patients recovering from fractures of the leg. Scand J Rehabil Med 1976;8:1–9.

127. Pugh LG. The oxygen intake and energy cost of walking before and after unilateral hip replacement, with some observations on the use of crutches. J Bone Joint Surg 1973;55B:742–745.

128. Brown MB, Batten C, Porell D. Efficiency of walking after total hip replacement. Orthop Clin North Am 1978;9:364–367.

129. Olgiati R, Jacquet J, di Prampero PE. Energy cost of walking and exertional dyspnea in multiple sclerosis. Am Rev Respir Dis 1986;134:1005–1010.

130. Olgiati R, Burgunder J-M, Mumenthaler M. Increased energy cost of walking in multiple sclerosis: effect of spasticity, ataxia, and weakness. Arch Phys Med Rehabil 1988;69:846–849.

131. Thomas LF, Hislop HJ, Waters RL. Physiological work performance in chronic low back disability. Phys Ther 1980;60:407–411.

132. Corry IS, Duffy CM, Cosgrave AP, Graham HK. Measurement of oxygen consumption in disabled children by the Cosmed K2 portable telemetry system. Dev Med Child Neurol 1996; 38;585–593.

133. Bowen TR, Cooley SR, Castagno PW, et al. A method for normalization of oxygen cost and consumption in normal children while walking. J Pediatr Orthop 1998;18:589–593.

134. Johnson RK, Russ J, Goran JI. Physical activity related energy expenditure in children by doubly labeled water as compared with the Caltrac accelerometer. Int J Obes Relat Metab Disord 1998;22:1046–1052.

135. Rowland T, Cunningham L, Martel L, et al. Gender effects on submaximal energy expenditure in children. Int J Sports Med 1997;18:420–425.

136. Eston RG, Rowlands V, Ingledew DK. Validity of heart rate, pedometry, and accelerometry for predicting the energy cost of children's activities. J Appl Physiol 1998;84:362–371.

137. Treuth MS, Adolph AL, Butte NF. Energy expenditure in children predicted from heart rate and activity calibrated against respiration calorimetry. Am J Physiol 1998;275:E12–E18.

138. Thureen PJ, Phillips RE, Baron KA, et al. Direct measurement of the energy expenditure of physical activity in preterm infants. J Appl Physiol 1998; 85:223–230.

139. Wells JC, Davies PS. Estimation of the energy cost of physical activity in infancy. Arch Dis Child 1998;78:131–136.

140. Walker JL, Murray TD, Jackson AS, et al. The energy cost of horizontal walking and running in adolescents. Med Sci Sports Exer 1999;31:311–322.

141. Cureton KJ, Sloniger MA, Black DM, et al. Metabolic determinants of the age-related improvements in one-mile run/walk performance in youth. Med Sci Sports Exer 1997;29:259–267.

142. Wergel-Kolmert U, Wohlfart B. Day-to-day variation in oxygen consumption and energy expenditure during sub maximal treadmill walking in female adolescents. Clin Physiol 1999;19:161–168.

143. Rose J, Gamble J, Medieros J, et al. Energy cost of walking in normal children and in those with cerebral palsy: comparison of heart rate and oxygen uptake. J Ped Orthop 1989;9:276–279.

144. Rose J, Gamble JG, Burgos A, et al. Energy expenditure index of walking

for normal children and for children with cerebral palsy. Dev Med Child Neurol 1990;32:333–340.

145. Bowen TR, Lennon N, Castagno P, et al. Variability of energy-consumption measures in children with cerebral palsy. J Pediatr Orthop 1998;18:738–742.

146. Stallings VA, Zemel BS, Davies JC, et al. Energy expenditure of children and adolescents with severe disabilities: a cerebral palsy model. Am J Clin Nutrition 1996;64:627–634.

147. Unnithan VB, Dowling JJ, Frost G, Bar-Or O. Role of cocontraction in the O2 cost of walking in children with cerebral palsy. Med Sci Sports Exer 1996;28:1498–1504.

148. Duffy CM, Hill AE, Graham HK. The influence of flexed-knee gait on the energy cost of walking in children. Dev Med Child Neurol 1997;39:234–238.

149. Duffy CM, Hill AE, Cosgrove AP, et al. Energy consumption in children with spina bifida and cerebral palsy: a comparative study. Dev Med Child Neurol 1996;38:238–243.

150. Bowen TR, Miller F, Mackenzie W. Comparison of oxygen consumption measurements in children with cerebral palsy to children with muscular dystrophy. J Pediatr Orthop 1999;19:133–136.

151. McGibbon NH, Andrade CK, Widener G, Cintas HL. Effect of an equine-movement therapy program on gait, energy expenditure, and motor function in children with spastic cerebral palsy: a pilot study. Dev Med Child Neurol 1998;40:754–762.

152. Mattsson E, Andersson C. Oxygen cost, walking speed, and perceived exertion in children with cerebral palsy when walking with anterior and posterior walkers. Dev Med Child Neurol 1997;39:671–676.

153. Engsberg JR, MacIntosh BR, Harder JA. Comparison of effort between below-knee amputee and normal children. J Assoc Child Prosthet Orthot Clin 1991;26:46–52.

154. Engsberg JR, Herbert LM, Grimston SK, et al. Relation among indices of effort and oxygen uptake in below-knee amputee and able-bodied children. Arch Phys Med Rehabil 1994;75:1335–1341.

155. van der Windt AWM, Pieterson I, van der Eijken JW, et al. Energy expenditure during walking in subjects with tibial rotationplasty, above-knee amputation, or hip disarticulation. Arch Phys Med Rehabil 1992;73:1174–1180.

19

Physiological Changes Associated with Bed Rest and Major Body Injury

ROBERT J. DOWNEY AND CHARLES WEISSMAN

Despite the variety of pathologies and procedures seen on a surgical service, experience teaches that the course of postoperative recovery often follows a predictable trajectory. Common to operative and accidental trauma, and recovery from other disease processes, is a period of recovery marked by mobilization of the body's resources to effect healing. The physiology of the body's response to injury has been extensively researched and is reviewed in the second half of this chapter. What has been less well recognized is how the alterations in physiology that occur as part of the body's attempt to heal itself are superimposed on another abnormal physiological state (i.e., the alterations in physiology caused by a period of reduced activity and recumbency). Bed rest has been routinely and often casually prescribed for a wide variety of pathophysiological states, with the rationale of reducing functional demands on a diseased body. Earlier in this century, prolonged bed rest was much more widely recommended than today, particularly after myocardial infarction.[1,2] With recognition of the unfavorable effects of prolonged inactivity, emphasis shifted toward more rapid remobilization, particularly in the early postoperative period. However, almost all hospitalized patients undergo a period of reduced activity. Therefore, the physiological alterations that occur as a result of decreased activity and changes in posture form the substrate on which all of the other processes of illness and healing are superimposed. Bed rest needs to be understood as a distinct component of the alterations in physiology seen during a period of injury and recovery. In this chapter, we review the alterations in each bodily system that accompany inactivity, recumbency, or both in the absence of injury. It will become clear that bed rest alone, even without other associated injury, causes a generalized deconditioning of the healthy subject involving most of the physiological systems of the body, including the cardiovascular, pulmonary, gastrointestinal, hormonal, and skeletal systems. When the patient is not only at bed rest but has been injured or has a serious medical or surgical intervention, the consequences can be severe. Certainly, it is unlikely that bed rest should be considered therapeutic for any condition when compared with efforts to resume normal activity. One report[3] reviewed all randomized controlled trials investigating the benefits of bed rest after a medical procedure or the benefits of bed rest as primary treatment for a medical disorder. Of 24 trials investigating the benefits of bed rest after a medical procedure (such as lumbar puncture or cardiac catheterization), no outcomes improved significantly, and eight worsened significantly. In 15 trials investigating bed rest as a primary treatment for specific medical problems (such as acute back pain or myocardial infarction), no outcomes improved significantly, and nine worsened.

CARDIOVASCULAR AND FLUID ALTERATIONS

The many studies that have been undertaken to examine the cardiovascular effects of prolonged immobilization have used a wide variety of experimental subjects and protocols. For example, Dietrick et al.[4] examined physiological and metabolic changes in four healthy young men immobilized in pelvic and leg casts for 6 weeks. Graveline and Barnard[5] examined primarily hemodynamic parameters in four men subjected for up to 24 hours of water immersion to simulate weightlessness.

449

Miller et al.[6] and Vogt et al.[7] focused primarily on the fluid shifts accompanying bed rest in groups of young men for 28 and 10 days, respectively. Saltin et al.[8] measured exercise tolerance in five young men by following maximal oxygen uptake during 21 days of bed rest followed by 8 weeks of recuperative activity. The only two studies using subjects other than young men were performed by Gaffney et al.,[9] who examined short-term effects of head-down tilt in middle-aged men, and Convertino et al.,[10] who examined the hemodynamic alterations associated with exercise after 10 days of bed rest in twelve 50-year-old men. Combining elements of several such studies provides an overview of the cardiovascular changes accompanying bed rest.

The veins of the lower extremity are part of the postcapillary blood pool, which makes up approximately 70% of the overall intravascular volume. Contraction of the gastrocnemius and soleus muscles during normal ambulation compresses sinusoids contained within each muscle and propels venous blood toward the heart. Reflux during muscular relaxation is prevented by the presence of delicate but strong bicuspid valves within the veins below the common iliac vein. These mechanisms are imperfect; on standing, approximately 500 ml of blood shifts from the upper body to the lower and venous pressures stabilize at approximately 80–100 mm Hg.[11] *Modest* levels of lower extremity activity transiently lower this pressure head to approximately 25 mm Hg, but the shift of blood out of the thorax largely persists. When a person is lying down, the blood can more readily leave the lower extremity. This blood acts to augment venous return centrally causing increased stretching of baroreceptors located in the right atrium, the walls of the carotid artery, and the aortic arch, which, in turn, initiates vasodepressor responses consisting of decreased heart rate and contractility, peripheral vasodilatation, increased renal blood flow, and diuresis.

Blomqvist et al.[12] studied the effects of a head-down tilt over 24 hours in 10 healthy men, noting a marked central fluid shift leading to an elevation in the central venous pressure and increase in the left ventricular end-diastolic volume and stroke volume. Because of reflex compensatory decrease in heart rate, there was no increase in cardiac output. These changes were transient, with all values returning to levels similar to the upright position after 24 hours. However, these subjects did demonstrate diminished orthostatic tolerance, increased heart rate, and decreased stroke volume during submaximal exercise and overall decreased maximal exercise capacity if returned to the upright position. More recently, and in some conflict with the results cited previously, Lathers et al.[13] measured cardiovascular responses to degrees of tilt down to –5 degrees and found, during the first 2–3 hours, increased intrathoracic fluid, primarily by sequestration of blood in the lungs,[9] leading to decreased heart rate, stroke volume, pulse pressure, and cardiac output.

With this central fluid shift while lying down and increased effective intravascular volume, an initial diuresis occurs with an average decrease in plasma volume of 5% after 24 hours. This continues and reaches 10% in 6 days and 20% after 14 days.[14] The volume loss exceeds the net return in fluid from the lower extremities and may occur by mechanisms other than renal response to central volume receptors, such as alterations in atrial natriuretic factor. Maillet et al.[15] found that bed rest caused a transient elevation of atrial natriuretic peptide to levels 50% above baseline, accompanied by decreases in plasma noradrenaline and renin activity. Overall the authors suggested that initial changes in these hormones do not last beyond approximately 12 hours, with a new homeostasis being established at 24 hours.

Many investigators have noted orthostatic intolerance after prolonged bed rest. They attributed this, in part at least, to the intravascular volume depletion noted previously, possibly compounded by an increase in venous pooling in the lower extremities because of increased venous compliance after bed rest.[16] In addition to the changes in intravascular volume and venous tone, prolonged recumbency blunts cardiac responsiveness to rapid changes in posture.[17] Bed rest increases the resting pulse from 4–15 beats per minute, and after bed rest there is more pronounced increase in heart rate with exercise. For example, normal volunteers experienced an increase in pulse to approximately 129 beats per minute during submaximal exercise, whereas after bed rest the same exercise demand drove the heart rate to approximately 165 beats per minute.[8,18] Similarly, Chobanian et al.[19] found that bed rest exaggerated the increase in heart rate in response to movement from supine to upright: Controls experienced an increased heart rate of 13%, whereas experimental subjects demonstrated increases of 32% after 3 days of bed rest, 62% after 7 days, and 89% after 21 days. This exaggerated increase in heart rate does not seem to translate into increased cardiac output: In fact, the increases in both stroke volume and cardiac output on maximal exercise are reduced by approximately 25% after prolonged bed rest, perhaps suggesting a poorly defined myocardial depressant factor.[8,19,20] Further, ten Harkel et al.[21] noted an increased variability in hemodynamics after prolonged head-down tilt. Six healthy men underwent 10 days of head-down tilt and were found to almost double the variability in orthostatic blood pressure.

On the basis of echocardiographic studies, Hung et al.[22] suggested that left ventricular ejection fraction increased normally during both supine and upright exercise, but the resting left ventricular end-diastolic volume decreased by 16%, consistent with a decrease in venous return rather than depressed myocardial function.

The observed alterations in the cardiovascular system's ability to accommodate changes in body position and distribution in intravascular volume may be caused by alterations in autonomic function. It has been suggested[23] that the tachycardia seen after bed rest was related either to a decrease in vagal tone, a decreased sensitivity to vagal stimulation, an increase in sympathetic tone, or enhanced sensitivity to sympathetic stimulation. Subjects given atropine to block vagal tone had significantly higher heart rates after bed rest than during control periods, and Robinson et al.[24] and Melada et al.[25] attributed the vasovagal manifestations of orthostatic intolerance after bed rest to increased β-adrenergic activity as these symptoms could be blocked by propranolol. However, Maass et al.[26] measured the density of α_2-receptors on platelets, β_2-receptors on lymphocytes, and the responsiveness of β_2-receptors after a period of bed rest and were unable to demonstrate a significant change in receptor characteristics specifically attributable to head-down tilt.

Bed rest alters peripheral vascular responses. First, after a period of recumbency, calf vein compliance increased by approximately 50%, reflected as an increased calf volume as measured by strain gauge plethysmography.[27] However, this increased venous compliance does not lead to an increased sequestering of infused volume in the vascular space: Gaffney et al.[28] found that rapid infusion of intravenous saline led to a transient blood volume increase of 18% in subjects both at normal activity and after a period of bed rest. Second, Convertino et al.[29] noted an enhanced forearm vascular resistance to graded intravascular volume depletion after 7 days of bed rest, with forearm vascular resistance measured per unit change in central venous pressure doubling after bed rest.

Respiration

Oxygen uptake and carbon dioxide elimination occur through the ventilation of alveoli in contact with circulating blood. A certain inefficiency is built into the system as portions of the airway are ventilated but not perfused (*dead space*) and portions are perfused but

not well ventilated (*shunt*). These mismatches are small in the normal adult but in postoperative and bed-ridden patients, ventilation to perfusion may be badly mismatched.

The normal respiratory cycle of inspiration and expiration occurs as a balance of the opposing tendencies of the elastic lung parenchyma to collapse and the stiffer chest wall to expand. The volume of the lung at rest, after a normal expiration when these forces are balanced, is called the *functional residual capacity* (FRC). In the healthy erect man, there is an uneven distribution of ventilation and blood flow during a spontaneous breath. The amount of perfusion of blood to each area of the lung is a function of the perfusion pressure (pulmonary arterial minus venous pressures) and the pressures in the surrounding tissues (airway pressure and hydrostatic pressures caused by gravity). Based on the varying relationship between these pressures, the isolated lung can be divided into three regions: zone I (apical) in which the alveolar pressure exceeds both pulmonary arterial and venous pressure so that perfusion theoretically does not occur; zone II (middle) in which the alveolar pressure is less than pulmonary arterial pressure but still more than pulmonary venous pressure, so that blood flow is dependent on the pulmonary artery-to-alveolar pressure gradient; and zone III (basilar) in which pulmonary venous pressure exceeds alveolar pressure and blood flow is dependent on the pulmonary artery-to-venous pressure gradient.[30] Any body position other than upright increases the proportion of the lung subject to zone III conditions. The supine position causes posterior lung segments from base to apex to become increasingly zone III, whereas either lateral position increases the extent of zone III in the dependent lung.[31] In zone III areas there is a tendency to increasing distension of the pulmonary vasculature and the accumulation of pulmonary interstitial fluid. Superimposed on the alterations of distribution in pulmonary blood volumes is an increase in overall pulmonary vascular volume with recumbency. A 20-minute head-down tilt leads to a 22% increase in pulmonary blood flow; this increase is not sustained, but decreases by 16% over 10 further days of bed rest.[32]

Gravity causes pleural pressure to become progressively more negative from the lung base to its apex, primarily because of the weight of the basilar lung tissue pulling down on the tissue in the apex. Thus, the airway-distending pressure is most effective at the apex, and at rest, the apical alveoli is more distended than the basilar alveoli. If a breath is initiated from the FRC, the change in transpulmonary pressure is equal at the apices and the base, but because the apical alveoli are already distended and higher on the alveoli pressure-volume curve, the volume change in the lung with each unit pressure of change is less at the apices, and therefore the basilar lung segments are preferentially ventilated.[33,34]

At some point during expiration, as lung volumes are reduced, alveoli close while being perfused and are not available for ventilation. The point at which these alveolar closures begin to occur is called the *closing volume* and normally is below the FRC, meaning that at the end of expiration the alveoli have not yet begun to close.[35] However, in certain circumstances this may not be true. (e.g., In obesity there is a decrease of the expiratory reserve volume, whereas in smokers there is an increase in the closing volume. In each situation, alveolar closure begins to occur at a point above the end-tidal point, causing alveoli to be perfused with blood but not ventilated, rendering them ineffective for gaseous exchange.)

The closing volume has been shown to be relatively independent of posture; however, the FRC decreases by approximately 20% in the supine position.[36] This may be sufficient to place the closing volume above the end-tidal point with subsequent closure of basilar alveoli. These alveoli remain closed for the initial portions of the next inhalation, and the ventilation is shunted to the open apical alveoli. Blood continues to flow through the poorly or nonventilated basilar segments, and the apical segments receive ventilation in excess of blood flow, tending to decrease arterial oxygenation.

Placing a normal patient in a recumbent position leads to changes in all lung volumes except the tidal volume. Craig et al.[37] found that changing a normal human from upright to a supine position resulted in a loss of 2% of the vital capacity, 7% of the total lung capacity, 10% of the closing volume, 19% of the residual volume, 46% of the expiratory reserve volume, and 30% of the FRC. Changes to positions other than the supine lead to smaller losses of volume. Healthy subjects had a decrease in FRC of only 17% when moved from the upright to the lateral decubitus position.[38] Interestingly, these changes might be *less* in patients with chronic pulmonary disease. Marini et al.[38] also reported that patients with chronic airflow obstruction had only a 3.5% change in FRC on moving from an upright to a supine position and a decrease of only 1.9% on moving to a lateral decubitus position. Furthermore, this study reported a significant decrease in arterial oxygen saturation in supine healthy subjects, but not in patients with significant airflow obstruction.

The effects of prolonged periods of recumbency on pulmonary function have been studied by Beckett and coworkers.[39] They assessed pulmonary function in supine subjects before, during, and after three separate bed-rest periods of 11–12 days' duration and compared with an ambulatory control group. Forced vital capacity and total lung capacity both increased during the period of bed rest, whereas residual volume and FRC did not change. Maintaining plasma volume at baseline levels did not prevent an increase in forced vital capacity in recumbent patients, and decreasing plasma volume by diuresis in ambulatory control subjects did not lead to an increase in forced vital capacity. This led the authors to suggest that the alterations seen in respiratory function were independent of the plasma volume changes associated with prolonged recumbency. Supporting data have been provided by Hillebrecht et al.,[40] who examined the hypothesis that fluid shifts affect pulmonary gas exchange. The authors superimposed acute changes in intravascular volume distribution by applying lower body negative pressure and intravenous saline loading to patients after a 10-day period of 6 degrees head-down tilt and found that although lower body negative pressure and intravenous saline loading caused significant alterations in pulmonary blood flow and diffusing capacity, these changes were not significantly different before and after prolonged bed rest.

The actual degree to which the described physiological changes affect respiration has not been completely studied. Cardus[41] found in normal young men that after 10 days of bed rest there was a mean decrease in PaO_2 of 9 mm Hg, an increase of 10 mm Hg in $P(A-a)O_2$, but no change in the mean arterial CO_2 concentration. Such changes would probably not be important in these subjects.

MUSCLE DISUSE

Multiple studies have demonstrated that muscle strength, size, and stamina are all affected by a lack of activity and that this weakening process affects all aspects of muscle function and structure. Booth[42] provides a comprehensive discussion of muscle disuse. Disuse causes a progressive decrease in muscle strength paralleled by a decrease in cross-sectional area of the muscle fibers. In healthy humans, MacDougall et al.[43] described a 5% decrease in arm circumference with a 35% decrease in elbow extension strength after 5 weeks of immobilization. Witzmann et al.[44] demonstrated in rats that both twitch and tetanic tension (expressed as either the product of whole muscle or unit cross-sectional area) was diminished in chronically shortened soleus or extensor digitorum muscle and that this occurs whether the immobilized muscle was on acute stretch, neutral, or shortened.[45]

The decline in maximal attainable tension[42] and loss of muscle weight[35] occurs rapidly, reaching a new steady state by 5–10 days after immobilization. Booth and Seider[46] found that after an initial lag period of slow weight loss during the first day or two, 50% of the eventual loss had occurred by the eighth to tenth day. The muscle wasting is thought to be the result of decreased muscle protein synthesis rather than increased protein breakdown.[47] A detailed analysis by Ferrando and coauthors[48] of the rates of protein synthesis measured by arteriovenous differences after infusion of phenylalanine suggested a 50% decrease in muscle protein synthesis after 14 days of simulated inactivity. Because the cellular content of mRNA for actin remained unchanged for 3 days while the synthesis of actin had decreased by the sixth hour,[45] the level of control was thought to be exerted at some step in the translation or elongation sequence. Muscular collagen synthesis is also reduced, although the rate of decrease in formation is less than that of the noncollagen proteins, resulting in a transient increase in collagen concentration despite a decrease in absolute collagen content.[49] The change in contractile properties may also be caused by qualitative changes in muscle protein composition as well as the quantitative changes in protein levels. Reiser et al.[50] noted a 30% increase in the mean maximal shortening velocity of fibers of immobilized rat soleus muscles, which they attributed to a relative increase in the amount of fast-to-slow myosin isoenzymes. The catabolic effects of bed rest are probably amplified by the hypercortisolemia associated with trauma. Ferrando et al.[51] found that subjects placed at bed rest and receiving infusions of hydrocortisone to mimic the blood cortisol levels seen with severe injury had threefold increases in the rate of amino acid efflux from muscles, compared with subjects at bed rest alone, which suggested that inactivity sensitizes skeletal muscle to the catabolic effects of elevated cortisol levels.

As mass and maximal attainable tension decrease, fatigability during work increases. The peak tension from electrical pulse train stimulation is diminished in the soleus muscle of rats immobilized for 6 weeks compared with controls; before the stimulation exercise the immobilized muscles were found to have decreased levels of adenosine triphosphate (ATP) and glycogen stores[42,46] and more rapid depletion of ATP and glycogen stores and accumulation of lactic acid during exercise than in nonmobilized muscles.[43] Also contributing to rapid fatigability is an apparent decreased ability on the part of the immobilized muscle to use fatty acids[52] in contrast to the trained state in which the muscle uses fat more rapidly and carbohydrates more slowly.[53]

Efforts to offset the loss of muscle mass seen with bed rest have included the use of resistance exercises that can be performed in bed. Ferrando et al.[54] demonstrated that healthy subjects on bed rest who perform leg resistance exercises every other day have muscle protein synthesis that is essentially unchanged from that of subjects with normal activity.

CALCIUM METABOLISM

Maintenance of a skeleton capable of resisting the mechanical forces applied during activity is dependent on the intermittent application of these same forces. When a stress is applied to a bone, as in normal activity or exercise, the strain is sensed, with subsequent changes in osteoclast and osteoblast cellular activity.[55,56] If no force is applied to the skeleton, either because of plaster immobilization, strict bed rest, paralysis, or the weightlessness of space flight, bone mineral is lost because the rate of bone formation falls below the rate of bone mineral absorption. A review of the literature shows that decreased mobility is associated with an early rapid bone mineral loss that later leads to a stable but lesser bone mass.

Bone mineral loss was measured first in convalescing patients,[4] but similar losses occur in healthy patients placed either at prolonged bed rest[57] or under conditions of weightlessness.[58] After 84 days of weightlessness aboard Skylab 4, daily stool and urinary calcium losses averaged 18 g for the three crewmen. A higher rate of loss was recorded from the calcaneus (3.9%) than from the radius, suggesting that the calcaneus is more susceptible possibly because of a proportionately greater reduction in weight bearing or because it is composed of trabecular bone.

In a study of five healthy men at bed rest for up to 36 weeks,[59] a consistent pattern of change was seen: Urinary calcium increased at a rate of 12% per week until a peak level of excretion was reached at 100 mg per day above control levels after approximately 16 weeks. Net losses of total body calcium in urine, sweat, and feces averaged 0.5% per month. There were parallel losses in phosphorus and hydroxyproline, and total body phosphorus declined an average of 150 mg per day below controls. Urinary hydroxyproline excretion was also increased to a level of 10 mg per day above baseline controls by the sixth week. The rate of calcium loss is unequal for different bones of the body: The rate of loss from the calcaneus averaged 5% per month, 10 times the rate of loss from the body as a whole, and the mineral content of the radius revealed no change throughout the 10-week study, suggesting that during bed rest, mineral loss occurs only from bones that are normally weight bearing.[59] During the first days after initiation of bed rest, this is probably not caused by activation in osteoclast and osteoblast activity[60] because excretion of deoxypyridinoline (a marker of bone matrix resorption) increases without elevations in either alkaline or tartrate-resistant acid phosphatase (markers of osteoclast and osteoblast activity). Studies[61] following patients for 12 weeks suggest that, eventually, bed rest does lead to increased osteoclastic and decreased osteoblastic activity. Although one study reported the bone mineral loss from the vertebral bodies of normal men put at strict bed rest was not significant over a 5-week period,[62] it is likely that even short periods of bed rest are associated with significant loss of bone. Takata et al.[63] found that 1 week of continuous bed rest in patients with femoral neck fractures treated with traction led to increases in excretion of urinary calcium of approximately 40% over baseline and in urinary phosphorus of 16% over baseline.

When healthy subjects resumed ambulation, calcium and phosphorus balances begin to return toward positive but slowly, becoming positive only after 4 weeks.[57] The increase in phosphorus balance was much more rapid, suggesting phosphate uptake into tissues other than bone, such as muscle. This study found that the rate of remineralization with ambulation occurred at a rate similar to the rate of loss with immobility and that all subjects had reached or exceeded initial values by the 36th week. Other studies[64] examining disuse osteopenia in patients with fractures have suggested that bone mineral content might not be completely regained with as long as 14 years of activity.

Illness or disease enhances the rate of bone mineral loss beyond that of immobilization alone. The rate of loss in 139 patients confined to bed because of either fractured legs or herniated disks was found to approximate 2% of total calcium per month.[65] Spinal cord injury with paralysis causes osteopenia in the bones below the level of the lesion, with total bone volume decreasing rapidly over the first months after an injury, stabilizing at approximately 70% of baseline, a rate of decrease approximately 100 times greater than that seen with aging.[66]

Current efforts to suppress the bone resorption associated with bed rest and inactivity have focused on the efficacy of intranasal calcitonin and an aminobiphosphonate, alendronate. Calcitonin, given twice a day, counteracted the early increase in bone resorption as measured by a decrease in the urinary hydroxyproline and calcium levels, as well as being associated with a smaller decline in the serum level of 1,25-dihydroxyvitamin D.[67] Alendronate similarly decreased the rise in urinary excretion of calcium seen with bed rest when compared with untreated bed rest controls.[68]

GASTROINTESTINAL ALTERATIONS

Gastrointestinal function is altered with bed rest.[69] Nonviscous boluses, but not viscous materials, pass through the esophagus more rapidly when the subject is upright rather than supine.[70] This increased rate in transit in the upright position is associated with an increased velocity of the esophageal wave and a shortening of the lower esophageal sphincter relaxation time. The transit time of a bolus through the stomach is slowed by up to 66% in the lying position compared with the standing; however,[71,72] gastric acidity is increased because of activation of the sympathetic system inhibition of gastric bicarbonate secretion.[73] Small bowel motility is reduced by inactivity,[74] and defecation is certainly altered by a change in body position. For example, even the apparently minor change in leg support afforded by defecation in a sitting rather than a squatting position is significant. The forces generated during straining after stool in the sitting position are threefold those generated when squatting.[75] Absorptive function is also altered. As noted previously, bed rest is associated with bone loss and urinary excretion of calcium: Stool calcium levels are also increased from a mean of 797 mg per day with normal activity to 911 mg per day with bed rest, and intestinal absorption decreased from 31% of intake with normal activity to 24% with bed rest.[76]

HORMONAL ALTERATIONS

Bed rest causes multiple alterations to occur within the endocrine system, mostly caused by the decreased level of activity and, to a lesser extent, to changes in posture. The affected hormones, other than those related to the changes in intravascular volume discussed previously, are of two axes: insulin and glucose and adrenocortical steroids. Blotner[77] first noted that ill patients whose treatment included prolonged bed rest demonstrated a reduced glucose tolerance, and Deitrick et al.[4] demonstrated that this decreased tolerance was in part caused by bed rest, independent of concurrent disease. Hyperinsulinemia accompanied this hyperglycemia[78] with reduction in peripheral glucose uptake.[79] Because of inactivity, muscle develops insulin resistance, and exogenous insulin administered to subjects on bed rest results in significantly smaller decreases in blood glucose levels when compared with pre–bed rest controls.[80] This intolerance occurs as soon as 3 days after immobilization, with peripheral glucose uptake decreasing by 20% and by 50% by 14 days. There does not seem to be an accompanying alteration in hepatic glucose production,[81] or in the insulin responsiveness of muscle protein breakdown,[82] suggesting that the defect in insulin action is not generalized. Changes in the rhythmicity and levels of multiple hormones closely related to the changes in insulin levels and responsiveness have been observed. Vernikos-Danellis et al.[83] showed that circadian rhythmicity of cortisol blood levels persists, but the amplitude of the cycle diminishes. Samel and coauthors[84] also examined the effect of bed rest on hormonal rhythmicity by studying eight healthy subjects undergoing 12 days consisting of 3 days of baseline studies, 7 days of 6-degree head-down bed rest, and 2 days for recovery; the authors found that only minor changes occurred in circadian acrophases, but that bed rest altered the daily means and amplitudes for multiple physiological functions. Bed rest also destabilizes thyroid hormone rhythms with an accompanying elevation in T_3 levels and, as noted in a separate study,[83] circulating growth hormone (GH) levels decreased after 10 days of inactivity, with a subsequent increase by day 20. Catecholamine and methoxamine (dopamine) levels appear to be unchanged by bed rest[85]; the effect of inactivity on glucagon levels is not known. Taken together these studies suggest that the alteration in glucose homeostasis that occurs with bed rest may result from both decreased muscle responsiveness and alterations in hypothalamic-pituitary axis function.

BED REST AND VENOUS THROMBOSIS

Thrombosis may occur in all venous tracts of the body, but is most frequent in the veins of the legs and pelvis, especially in the deep veins of the calf.[86] Estimates of the incidence of deep venous thrombosis (DVT) range from 29% for the postoperative general surgical patient to 44% after surgery for hip fractures.[87] Schlosser[88] performed meta-analysis of publications attempting to estimate the incidence of postoperative fatal pulmonary embolism; he found the incidence to be approximately 0.2–1.2%. Approximately 600,000 cases of pulmonary embolism occur annually among medical and surgical patients in the United States, with one-third proving fatal.[89] In one autopsy series, Havig[90] reported that pulmonary embolism contributed to death in approximately 20% of cases. The natural history of a

thrombosed vein is eventual recanalization. However, in some patients, thrombosis may result in the destruction of the venous valvular system and, particularly if the thrombosis involves the popliteal veins[91] and the ankle-perforating veins,[92] may lead over a period of years to severe chronic edema and ulcerations.

Since the time of Virchow, clinicians have appreciated that decreased venous blood flow contributes to the creation of thrombus. However, stasis alone is not enough. In fact, Hewson[93] described blood static between two ligatures on a dog's jugular vein remaining uncoagulated for up to 3 hours. Stasis, therefore, is a permissive factor, promoting, but not sufficient to cause, thrombosis. There are many theories to explain the additional factors that cause a static pool of blood to thrombose. Thrombi probably arise simultaneously from several sites within a single venous system, usually valve cusps. Sevitt[94] showed the nidus of origin to be located in the valve pocket near the normal endothelium of the vein wall and to be composed primarily of red blood cells and fibrin, with platelets being restricted to the growing portion of the thrombi. Karino and Motomiya[95] found a stagnant area in the deepest portion of the valve pocket. Stasis may generate local areas of hypoxia that may damage the underlying endothelium, rendering the area thrombogenic.[96]

Even in the absence of direct vessel wall damage, stasis alone probably leads to the generation of the enzyme thrombin, which can lead to platelet aggregation and thrombin deposition.[97] Thrombin may also lead to damage of the endothelial surface.[98] Alterations in fibrinolysis may also play a role. Most surgical procedures seem to be followed by a period of depressed fibrinolytic activity lasting more than a week.[99] It is likely, therefore, that no single factor is responsible for venous thrombosis, but that decreased flow in the deep veins of the legs secondary to inactivity allows the factors responsible for intravascular coagulation to have maximal effect on a concentrated area. Flow in the iliac vein is reduced by approximately 50% during a period of anesthesia in the supine position,[100] and this decrease may be caused in part by a decrease in arterial inflow. Bird[101] demonstrated that calf arterial flow was only 58% of normal after a period of general anesthesia. The profound effect of inactivity on the incidence of DVT is confirmed by observation of its increased incidence in the paralyzed extremities of hemiplegics.[102] Similarly, Marik et al.[103] examined the incidence of DVT in the high-risk group of patients within an intensive care setting. One hundred two patients were studied, of whom 94 (92%) received prophylaxis, and of whom 12 (12%) were documented as having DVT by venous duplex scans. Four (4%) had high-probability ventilation-perfusion scans. Resumption of ambulation and anticoagulation rapidly leads to amelioration of symptoms, with pain and swelling often resolving or absent within even 2 days of increased activity.[104] However, the risk of pulmonary embolus is real, and estimated as being 7%, 5%, and 3% at 10 days after diagnosis for patients with iliofemoral, femoropopliteal, and lower leg DVTs, respectively.[105]

IMMUNE ALTERATIONS

Alterations in body position clearly alter immune function. Ten days of head-down tilt bed rest are not associated with changes in absolute lymphocyte number, or with delayed-type hypersensitivity, but decreases in levels of natural killer cells (although not in levels of other lymphocyte subpopulations) and in measures of lymphocyte responsiveness are seen.[106] This effect is possibly attributable to elevations in plasma cortisol levels as discussed previously.[106] Klokker et al.[107] examined the effect of head-up tilt, and symmetric elevations in lymphocyte levels, and in natural killer cell activity; interestingly, the authors found that the administration of propranolol (β_1 and β_2 blockade) but not metoprolol (β_1 blockade) obliterated the transient lymphocytosis seen, which led the authors to suggest that the effects seen were mediated by epinephrine through activation of β-receptors on the cell surfaces of the lymphocytes.

OVERVIEW OF THE RESPONSE TO INJURY

Major surgical and accidental injury, along with sepsis, causes significant metabolic, hormonal, and hemodynamic responses (Table 19-1).[108] The classic description of this *response to stress* involves the outpouring of the endocrine hormones: glucagon, cortisol, and catecholamines. GH,[109,110] aldosterone,[111] and vasopressin[112] concentrations are also increased. These endocrine effects, augmented by the actions of cytokines such as interleukin-1 (IL-1), tumor necrosis factor-α (TNF-α), and IL-6, produce a response characterized by catabolism, increased synthesis of acute phase proteins,[113] hypermetabolism,[114] altered carbohydrate metabolism,[115] sodium and water retention,[116] and increased lipolysis.[117] The abnormal carbohydrate metabolism includes increased endogenous hepatic glucose production (gluconeogenesis; Figure 19-1) and reduced glucose clearance (insulin resistance), which results in hyperglycemia. Plasma concentrations of insulin are usually elevated, but not sufficiently to prevent hyperglycemia.[118] The major body fuel becomes fat; therefore, lipolysis is increased while lipogenesis is retarded.[119] Protein abnormalities are manifested by negative nitrogen balance, reflecting accelerated net protein breakdown (catabolism).[120] The magnitude of these changes is essentially proportional to the extent of injury,[121,122] whereas their duration is related to the magnitude and duration of the initial stimulus. Therefore, disruption of homeostatic mechanisms is greater after extensive burns than after minor extremity surgery. Traumatic injury causes a large, short-term response, whereas contin-

TABLE 19-1
Alterations That Follow Injury

Ebb (Initial) Phase	Flow (Subsequent) Phase
Blood glucose elevated	Glucose normal to elevated
Normal glucose production	Glucose production increased
Free fatty acids elevated	Free fatty acid flux increased
Serum insulin low	Serum insulin normal to elevated
Catecholamines elevated	Catecholamines normal to elevated
Glucagon elevated	Glucagon elevated
Blood lactate elevated	Blood lactate normal
O_2 consumption depressed	O_2 consumption normal
Cardiac output low	Cardiac output increased
Core temperature decreased	Core temperature elevated

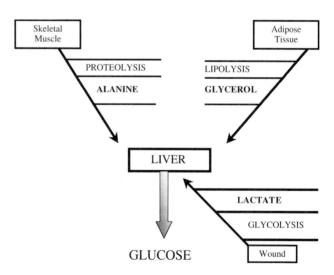

FIGURE 19-1 The substrate for hepatic gluconeogenesis originates from three major sources as shown in the figure.

uous mental stress and chronic disease cause smaller, prolonged responses.

MEDIATORS OF THE RESPONSE

Neuroendocrine Axis

The response to stress can be initiated by afferent neuronal input from an area of injury, emotional activity centered in the limbic system, and humoral factors, including the cytokines TNF-α, IL-1, and IL-6.[123] Afferent impulses stimulate secretion of hypothalamic releasing factors (e.g., corticotropin-releasing factor [CRF][124] and vasoactive intestinal peptide[125]) that, in turn, stimulate the pituitary to release prolactin,[126,127] vasopressin,[112] proopiomelanocortin, and GH.[110,127] The release of prolactin is inhibited by dopamine, whose secretion in turn is inhibited by nitric oxide.[128] Hypothalamic stimulation also results in stimulation of the sympathetic nervous system and fever. Plasma vasopressin concentrations are elevated after a variety of stresses, including surgery,[112,129–131] pneumonia,[132] myocardial infarction with or without left ventricular failure,[133,134] and electroconvulsive therapy.[135] Plasma vasopressin concentrations increase after the start of surgery and often remain elevated for days after its completion. The magnitude and duration of the plasma vasopressin level increases are proportional to the degree of stress.[112,131,132,136,137] Glucocorticoids, especially those administered exogenously, constitute a negative feedback system by suppressing hypothalamic corticotropin-releasing hormone (CRH) and arginine vasopressin (AVP) secretions.[138]

CRF, acting synergistically with vasopressin, stimulates secretion of proopiomelanocortin from the pituitary gland.[135,139,140] Proopiomelanocortin is cleaved to adrenocorticotropic hormone (ACTH), β-endorphin, and α-melanocyte-stimulating hormone (α-MSH), thus, the link between the endogenous opioid and the hypothalamic-pituitary-adrenal (HPA) axis.[141]

Subarachnoid and epidural local anesthetic blockade of the neurogenic stimuli from the area of surgery can attenuate the increases in plasma concentrations of catecholamines,[142] ACTH,[143] aldosterone,[143] cortisol,[144] renin,[143] GH,[145] prolactin,[143] and vasopressin.[146] Large doses of narcotics (4 mg/kg of morphine, 100 μg/kg of fentanyl) can also attenuate the increase in the levels of cortisol and catecholamines, presumably by suppressing CNS output.[147,148]

Catecholamines

The serum levels of the catecholamines norepinephrine,[149] epinephrine,[150] and dopamine[149] increase after a variety of stresses, including anxiety, hypotension,[151] hypothermia, hypercarbia, and accidental injury.[152] Catecholamines exist in the circulation both free and as the sulfur conjugate; the latter accounts for 60–90% of the total catecholamines.[153,154] In most critical illnesses the proportions of free and total (free plus conjugated) catecholamines remain constant.[153] Yet, in postoperative cardiac surgery patients receiving exogenous dopamine, there was a progressive increase in conjugation of endogenous epinephrine and norepinephrine. It is possible that sulfur conjugation is a mechanism regulating free plasma catecholamine concentration.[155]

Epinephrine is secreted in the blood stream by the adrenal medulla in response to sympathetic nervous system activation, whereas norepinephrine is released from the sympathetic nerve endings. Plasma levels of epinephrine and norepinephrine do not necessarily increase concurrently.[156] A study of major accidental injury found that plasma epinephrine concentrations increased for only approximately 48 hours, whereas norepinephrine levels remained elevated for as long as 8–10 days.[157] Abdominal[158] and cardiac[159] surgery produced increases in both hormones, whereas pelvic surgery increased mainly epinephrine.[157] Importantly, in both abdominal[160] and pelvic[144,157] surgery, the greatest plasma epinephrine concentration was observed in the immediate postsurgery period. Halter and colleagues[160] found that during abdominal surgery the initial adrenergic activation occurred during the time of the actual surgery and not between the induction of anesthesia and the skin incision.

Plasma epinephrine concentrations reflect adrenomedullary secretion, whereas plasma norepinephrine levels are an index of sympathetic nervous system activity. Most of the norepinephrine released by sympathetic ganglia is removed from the synapse by reuptake into the nerve ending.[161] Therefore, only the norepinephrine that *spills* over into the plasma is assayed.[162] Plasma levels are determined by the relationship between spillover rate and plasma clearance rate. After cholecystectomy plasma norepinephrine increased considerably because of an increase in the appearance (spillover) rate, whereas neither plasma clearance[163] nor forearm extraction of norepinephrine differed from preoperative values.[164] There was greater norepinephrine spillover and clearance during than after recovery from abdominal sepsis, despite normal plasma norepinephrine concentrations during both periods.[165] Christiansen and colleagues[164] noted that, despite elevated postoperative plasma norepinephrine levels, there was no change in blood pressure, probably reflecting decreased sensitivity to norepinephrine.

Catecholamines, via β-adrenergic stimulation, induce hepatic gluconeogenesis, glycogenolysis, and glucagon release.[166-168] Lipolysis is increased by β$_2$- and β$_3$-adrenergic stimulation and inhibited by α$_2$ stimulation. Epinephrine is a potent stimulator of gluconeogenesis. During starvation, the ability of epinephrine to stimulate gluconeogenesis decreases, in contradistinction to glucagon, whose gluconeogenic ability is less in starved subjects than in fed ones.[169] Epinephrine infusion in normal subjects does not affect protein metabolism.[168,170,171]

Glucocorticoids

Cortisol is a major stress hormone that, when present in elevated plasma concentrations, stimulates gluconeogenesis,[172] increases proteolysis,[173] and sensitizes adipose tissue to the action of lipolytic hormones (GH and catecholamines[174,175]). Cortisol causes insulin resistance by decreasing the rate at which insulin activates the glucose uptake system, probably because of post–insulin receptor block. Glucocorticoids also block the antiproteolytic actions of insulin.[176] Additionally, cortisol has anti-inflammatory and immunosuppressive actions[177] and has a negative feedback effect on ACTH and proinflammatory cytokine production. These dual permissive and suppressive actions are thought to prevent stress-activated defense mechanisms from overshooting and damaging the organism.[178] Unlike elevated concentrations, basal concentrations of cortisol are antilipolytic[179] and probably facilitate normal immune responses.[180]

The increased cortisol secretions after injury are major mediators of the stress response. Adrenalectomized animals and patients provide evidence for this, with Addison's syndrome faring poorly when stressed. This was well demonstrated by the increased mortality observed when etomidate was used to sedate critically ill patients.[181] It was later found that etomidate blocks adrenal steroidogenesis by inhibiting 11-β-hydroxylation and 17-α-hydroxylation.[182,183] Cortisol is a vital hormone because it facilitates catecholamine action and secretion, thus helping to maintain cardiovascular stability during surgical stress.[184] In general, the magnitude and duration of both intraoperative and postoperative ACTH and cortisol levels correlate well with the degree of surgical trauma.[185] After major surgery, during sepsis, and after burn injury, free cortisol concentrations are elevated because of both increased total cortisol concentrations and reduced cortisol-binding globulin (CBG).[186-188] The decrease in CBG may be caused by inhibition of CBG production by IL-6, increased CBG

degradation caused by elevated neutrophil-released esterase, or both.[189] Barton and Passingham[190] found a constant but nonlinear relationship between free and total plasma cortisol and concluded that measurement of total plasma cortisol was an adequate measure of cortisol response in surgical and trauma patients.

During surgery CRH, ACTH, and cortisol are increasingly released in pulsatile fashion so that there are steady increases in plasma cortisol levels.[191] The circadian rhythm of cortisol excretion (maximum levels at 6:00–8:00 AM with a subsequent decrease) is altered but not abolished after surgery.[192,193] After major surgery the rhythm can be shifted in time by as much as 6 hours. Cortisol levels may remain elevated for up to 2 weeks after femur fracture[194] and burns.[195] The increase in ACTH secretion during surgery is often far greater than that required to produce a maximal adrenocortical response.[146] This was demonstrated by the observation that administration of exogenous ACTH during surgery did not increase plasma cortisol concentration.[146]

Other Steroids

The response to injury is characterized by hypogonadotropic hypogonadism. The mechanism appears to be a reduced response of the pituitary gland to hypothalamically secreted gonadotropin-releasing hormone, resulting in decreased release of luteinizing hormone (LH) and follicle-stimulating hormone.[121] Concentrations of follicle-stimulating hormone and LH change little during surgery,[130] but LH and follicle-stimulating hormone decrease on the first postoperative day.[147] Elevated concentrations of CRH and cortisol may also suppress reproductive function.[196-197] In men, testosterone concentrations are markedly decreased in direct relationship to illness severity.[198] In burn patients this was caused by lowered biological activity of LH and suppressed response to the peaks in the pulsatile LH secretion.[199] In premenopausal women, decreased estrogen concentrations during stress are associated with amenorrhea. Adrenal androgens, dehydroepiandrosterone and its sulfate, are suppressed after surgery in male subjects.[200] However, in postmenopausal women, dehydroepiandesterole and its sulfate were increased after cholecystectomy. This is an interesting finding because adrenal androgen concentrations are in decline after menopause.[201]

Glucagon and Insulin

Glucagon and insulin are both secreted by the pancreas, the former by alpha cells and the latter by beta cells.

These endocrine secretions enter the portal vein, so the liver is exposed to high concentrations of both. The principal action of glucagon is to stimulate hepatic glycogenolysis and gluconeogenesis, with lower doses stimulating mainly the former and higher doses both mechanisms.[202] Glucagon increases hepatocyte cyclic adenosine monophosphate (cAMP) and promotes gluconeogenesis.[203] Insulin has the opposite effect: It decreases intracellular cAMP concentration and prevents gluconeogenesis. The receptor mechanism that increases cAMP levels is not the same as that used by adrenergic mediators. In addition, glucagon increases glycogenolysis and ketogenesis in the liver during starvation and diabetic ketoacidosis. There is debate as to whether glucagon also stimulates lipolysis.[204-206] Stimulators of glucagon secretion include hypoglycemia, protein ingestion, amino acid infusion, endorphins, exercise, GH, epinephrine, and glucocorticoids.[207,208] Suppression of glucagon secretion can be achieved by infusion or ingestion of glucose, somatostatin, and insulin.[209]

Insulin is an anabolic hormone with a multitude of effects. In addition to its role in increasing glucose transport across the cell membranes of adipose tissue and muscle, it stimulates glycogen production; promotes glucose oxidation[210]; inhibits lipolysis in adipose tissue and skeletal muscle[211]; inhibits net lipid oxidation[212]; inhibits hepatic ketogenesis; and increases the rate of amino acid transport[213] and protein synthesis in muscle, adipose tissue, and liver. The glucagon-to-insulin ratio is the major determinant of the degree of gluconeogenesis. During starvation, the ratio is increased (increased glucagon and decreased insulin levels), and gluconeogenesis is promoted; in the fed state the reverse is true. After most (but not all)[145] types of major surgery[209] there is an increase in the plasma glucagon level, although in some[145] the value peaks later than that of cortisol, some 18–48 hours after injury or surgery.[209] As in starvation, there is an increased glucagon-to-insulin ratio. Insulin levels decrease during surgery,[214] possibly owing to suppression of secretion by elevated levels of catecholamines[214,215] or increased urinary losses.[216] This suppression can be abrogated by α-adrenergic blockade.[217] The hormonal milieu of low insulin with elevated counterregulatory hormones is thought to be a stimulus to gluconeogenesis. In some septic patients this mechanism may fail and cause hypoglycemia, a situation associated with poor survival rates.[218] Postoperatively, the insulin level is increased, and this is thought to be caused by increases in both plasma glucose and epinephrine-induced β-adrenergic stimulation. Unlike during starvation, however, the plasma insulin concentrations are often markedly increased above the basal value, although they are inappropriately low for the prevailing level of glycemia.

Somatostatin is a hormone found in the pancreatic D cells and the hypothalamus that suppresses release of GH, insulin, and glucagon.[218,219] When somatostatin was infused into patients, the rate of glucose production decreased, as did the rate of clearance. If insulin is also infused into patients receiving somatostatin, the rate of glucose clearance returns to basal level, normalizing glucose kinetics. It thus appears that glucagon is a major mediator of gluconeogenesis. The lesser role of the catecholamines in the abnormal glucose metabolism of burn patients was demonstrated when propranolol failed to reduce the rates of glucose production or glucose cycling.[220] It is likely that catecholamines and glucagon work synergistically: Either one, infused alone into normal subjects, causes only transient elevation in gluconeogenesis; when they are infused simultaneously, gluconeogenesis is more prolonged.[221]

Growth Hormone

GH is a polypeptide secreted by the anterior pituitary. Its secretion is stimulated by hypothalamic GH-releasing factor and inhibited by somatostatin.[222] GH is important in the regulation of growth during the prenatal and neonatal periods and childhood. GH stimulates the secretion of insulin growth factor-1 (IGF-1) and -2 (IGF-2). The effects of GH are biphasic. Initial exposure (2–3 hours) may produce insulin-like effects, but after longer exposure counterregulatory and anabolic effects appear.[223] The latter results in increased incorporation of amino acids into structural proteins, glucose intolerance caused by insulin resistance, and increased lipolysis caused by increase sensitivity to the lipolytic effects of catecholamines. IGF-1 mediates the anabolic and skeletal growth-promoting activity effects of GH. IGF-1 also has insulin-like actions. Infusion of IGF-1 for 5 days did not change the rate of glucose oxidation, increased lipid oxidation, raised resting energy expenditure, and reduced protein oxidation. It is thought that IGF-1 facilitates anabolism by directly reducing protein oxidation and enhancing insulin sensitivity so that insulin and GH stimulate protein synthesis.[224] The IGF-binding proteins modify the availability of IGF-1 and its action. Six binding proteins have been identified, with the majority of circulating IGF-1 bound to IGF-binding protein-3 (IGFBP-3). IGFBP-1 plays a major role in regulating unbound free IGF-1.

Immediately after injury, burns, and surgery, concentrations of GH in the blood are elevated,[224,225] the increase being roughly proportional to the degree of trauma. However, after a day they decline to preoperative/preinjury concentrations. In severe trauma the pulsatile nature of GH secretion persists but the bursts occur less frequently.[226] IGF-1, IGF-2, and IGFBP-3 were reduced 40–60% after trauma, whereas IGFBP-1 and IGFBP-4 increased.[227,228]

Thyroid Hormones

In acute illnesses that do not involve the thyroid there are profound alterations in thyroid homeostasis. A decrease in serum T_3 concentrations, low or normal T_4, normal free T_4, increased reverse T_3, and normal thyroid-stimulating hormone (TSH) often accompany nonthyroidal illness. This *sick euthyroid syndrome* is seen during postoperative convalescence, after trauma, after extensive burns, and during sepsis. After emergency surgery among patients older than 70 years, this syndrome was associated with markedly elevated cortisol and norepinephrine concentrations, high Acute Physiologic and Chronic Health Evaluation (APACHE) II scores, and mortality.[229] The mechanism of sick euthyroid syndrome development is still unclear. Some have pointed to the lack of TSH elevation in the face of a low serum T_3 concentration and questioned if the problem is too little stimulation by thyrotropin-releasing hormone (TRH). This view was reinforced by a postmortem study of the paraventricular nuclei of patients with antemortem sick euthyroid syndrome. There was a positive correlation between antemortem serum T_3 and TSH with total postmortem TRH messenger RNA in the nuclei.[230] TSH concentrations are within normal ranges; however, nocturnal secretion resembles the pattern found in central hypothyroidism with lower nocturnal surges.[231,232] Additionally, sialylation (by oligosaccharide) of TSH is decreased, possibly explaining the altered TSH bioactivity.[233]

Elevated serum levels of IL-6 are associated with the low serum T_3 concentrations during illness as are serum concentrations of soluble TNF-α receptors (see the section Tumor Necrosis Factor). However, studies with normal subjects infused with endotoxin indicated that TNF does not play a role in endotoxin-induced thyroid hormone changes.[234] Short- (4-hour) and long-term (42-day) infusion of recombinant IL-6 decreases T_3, but not T_4, concentrations.[235,236] It is unclear whether elevated IL-6 is one of the causes of the sick euthyroid syndrome or is just an associated phenomenon. Dopamine infusion decreases basal TSH concentrations, inhibits the TSH response to TRH, decreases both serum T_4 and T_3 levels, and may aggravate sick euthyroid syndrome.[237] Cessation of dopamine infusion results in an increase in TSH, T_4, and T_3.[238,239] There has been interest in treating sick euthyroid syndrome with thyroid hormone and TRH.[239] In a randomized double-blind, placebo-controlled trial T_3 administration in cardiac surgery patients having cardiopulmonary bypass did not have dramatic effects on hemodynamics.[240,241]

The plasma-free T_4 concentration remains in the normal range despite reduced total T_4 concentration because of a decrease in thyroxine-binding globulin. During stress, the synthesis of thyroxine-binding globulin by the liver is reduced, and there may also be accelerated consumption (protease cleavage).[242]

The most intriguing aspect of thyroid metabolism in the critically ill patient is that, despite low T_3 and T_4 levels, many of these patients are hypermetabolic.

Counterregulatory Hormone Interactions

The hormones glucagon, catecholamines, and cortisol are called *counterregulatory hormones* because they oppose the effects of insulin and act synergistically to increase hepatic glucose production. Shamoon's group[221] explored the short-term effects in healthy subjects of the combined infusion of hydrocortisone, glucagon, and epinephrine designed to simulate the plasma levels found in moderate injury. They observed increased glucose production (gluconeogenesis) and decreased glucose clearance; the effect was more pronounced when all three hormones were administered together than when they were infused individually or in groups of two, suggesting that they act synergistically.[221] A possible reason for this synergism is that glucagon increases intracellular cAMP, especially in the liver, by a non–β-receptor mechanism.[203] This could amplify the actions of epinephrine. Cortisol acts synergistically with epinephrine and other β-agonists (an action used in the treatment of asthma). Proposed mechanisms include cortisol-induced inhibition of catechol-o-methyl transferase and blockade of catecholamine reuptake.[243,244] Glucocorticoids prevent $β_2$-adrenergic receptor down-regulation by increasing $β_2$-receptor production, as evidenced by increased $β_2$-receptor mRNA.[245] Additionally, the glucocorticoids may reduce cytokine levels, which is important because both IL-1 and TNF have been observed to down-regulate β-receptors.[245,246] Simultaneous infusion of the three hormones also caused negative nitrogen and potassium balances, glucose intolerance, hyperinsulinemia, insulin resistance, sodium retention, and peripheral leukocytosis.[247,248] In only one study was significant sustained hypermetabolism observed.[247] The nitrogen losses appear to be mainly caused by the effects of cortisol, because nitrogen balance during cortisol infusion was similar to that seen during infusion of all three hormones. The nitrogen losses were also not of the magnitude observed after accidental injury. With hormone infusions, there were significant alterations in leucine flux and oxidation, but only small increases in 3-methyl histidine excretion, indicating little muscle breakdown.[248] Therefore, other mediators must cause the proteolysis and massive nitrogen loss observed among patients. Also, normal subjects were not febrile and did not have increased acute phase-reactant proteins and decreased serum iron. Treatment protocols in which the pyrogenic (stimulates IL-1 secretion) steroid etiocholanolone[249] was injected into healthy subjects resulted in fever, leukocytosis, and hypoferremia without elevations in the counterregulatory hormones, hyperglycemia, or negative nitrogen balance. Infusion of the counterregulatory hormones plus etiocholanolone simulated more of the features of the response to injury than when they were administered individually.[250] Thus, both endocrine and inflammatory mediators are active in the response to injury and sepsis.

Immune System Connection: Cytokines

There are also nonendocrine factors that figure prominently in the response to stress. The cytokines are major mediators of the stress response that are produced by cells (e.g., lymphocytes, macrophages) of the immune system. Some cytokines (e.g., TNF-α, interferon-γ [IFN-γ], IL-1, IL-6, IL-8) are proinflammatory (type I), whereas others (e.g., IL-4, IL-10, IL-13) are anti-inflammatory (type II). Some (e.g., IL-12) induce cellular immunity by inducing uncommitted helper T-cells toward the TH1 phenotype, whereas others (e.g., IL-10) induce the TH2 phenotype and enhance humoral immunity.[251] The inflammatory response is controlled by the balance between the proinflammatory and anti-inflammatory cytokines.[252] For example, survival from sepsis was correlated with the recurrent secretion of proinflammatory, rather than anti-inflammatory, cytokines,[253] indicating that the inflammatory response is necessary to overcome sepsis. Cytokines interact closely with endocrine hormones,[254] as demonstrated by the marked elevations in ACTH and cortisol observed after IL-6 was administered to cancer patients.[255] Alternately, endocrine hormones affect cytokine secretion (e.g., cortisol suppresses IL-1 and TNF-α secretion).

Cytokines operate via endocrine, paracrine, autocrine, and juxtacrine mechanisms (Table 19-2).[254] Therefore, plasma concentrations may not completely reflect cytokine activity. The cytokines are components

TABLE 19-2
Definitions

Endocrine: transported by the blood, effective at distant tissues
Paracrine: acting locally on adjacent cells
Autocrine: acting back on the cells that produce the substance
Juxtacrine: acting on immediately adjacent cells

of a complex network of receptors, receptor-antagonists, and cytoplasmic-signaling molecules.[256] Soluble receptors are generated by proteolytic cleavage of membrane-bound receptors or by de novo production and release of different receptors. These circulating soluble receptors bind cytokines and may neutralize cytokine actions or act as carrier proteins that protect the cytokine from proteolysis.[257]

Interleukin-1

IL-1, a proinflammatory cytokine secreted by macrophages and endothelial cells, occurs in two physiologically indistinguishable forms, IL-1α and IL-1β. IL-1 often operates in conjunction with other proinflammatory cytokines (e.g., TNF-α and IL-6) to affect almost every body system.[258,259] For example, IL-1 induces the secretion of granulocyte colony-stimulating factor, granulocyte-macrophage colony-stimulating factor, and IL-6 by endothelial cells, helper T cells, bone marrow stroma cells, and fibroblasts.[260-262] Granulocyte colony-stimulating factor and granulocyte-macrophage colony-stimulating factor, in turn, activate marrow progenitor cells, causing leukocytosis.[263] IL-1β is probably the most potent endogenous pyrogen stimulating prostaglandin E_2 production in the hypothalamus.[264,265] In addition to the circulating form of IL-1, there is a membrane-bound form that, via a juxtacrine mechanism, induces IL-8 secretion (another proinflammatory cytokine).[266] Infusion of endotoxin into healthy subjects increased IL-1β concentrations. Peak TNF-α levels were seen before the IL-1β peak levels and were not correlated, indicating that the two cytokines are regulated independently.[267] Similar increases in IL-1 were seen in healthy subjects after intravenous CRH administration.[268] Acute stress, such as coronary angioplasty, but not post–endoscopic retrograde cholangiopancreatography pancreatitis, increased plasma IL-1 concentrations.[268] The IL-1 response to aortic surgery was found to be short-lived.[269] IL-1β was elevated during sepsis and was higher in survivors than patients who succumbed.

The activity of IL-1 is tightly controlled by the naturally occurring IL-1 receptor antagonist (IL-1ra), which is structurally similar to IL-1β, but lacks agonist activity.[259] IL-1ra is secreted by monocytes, macrophages, and neutrophils.[270] Serum IL-1ra concentrations are also increased after injury. Plasma IL-1ra concentrations were increased at the termination of vascular operations,[271] after endotoxin infusions in human volunteers,[272] and in septic patients.[27-273] The concentrations of IL-1ra remained elevated even when IL-1 concentrations were normal.[272,273] Endotoxin infusion increased IL-1 and glucocorticoids in parallel, whereas glucocorticoids inhibited both IL-1 and IL-1ra secretion, indicating that IL-1ra is not part of the glucocorticoid anti-inflammatory mechanism.[274] Yet, when endotoxin was administered to volunteers pretreated with glucocorticoids, IL-1ra secretion was unaffected, indicating that it could act in concert with glucocorticoids to antagonize proinflammatory cytokines.[275] The infusion of IL-1ra in septic patients reduced the activation of the coagulation and fibrinolytic systems.[276] Clinical trials performed to ascertain whether the infusion of IL-1ra into septic shock patients reduced mortality have yielded disappointing results.[277]

In addition to IL-1ra, IL-1β activity is regulated by soluble (circulating) IL-1 receptors. Type I receptors bind IL-1ra and IL-1α with high affinity but IL-1β poorly, and thus indirectly have IL-1 agonist activity.[278,279] In contrast, soluble type II IL-1 receptors bind IL-1β avidly, but bind IL-1α and IL-1ra poorly, so they are anti-inflammatory.[279] After major surgery (e.g., cardiac surgery and thoracoabdominal aneurysm repair,[280] burns,[281] and sepsis) both IL-1ra and soluble type II IL-1 receptors were elevated, whereas less extensive surgery only increased IL-1ra.[282]

Tumor Necrosis Factor

TNF is a polypeptide, pleiotropic cytokine produced by monocytes, macrophages, and other cells.[283] It is a member of a family of homotrimeric membrane-associated proteins with proinflammatory and apoptosis-inducing properties.[284] It, along with IL-1, is a major mediator of septic shock and is also implicated in the pathophysiology of other diseases such as rheumatoid arthritis. It has immunomodulating actions that include activation of T cells, promotion of adhesion molecule expression on endothelial cells and granulocytes, activation of coagulation pathways, and, with IL-1, induction of endothelial nitric oxide production.[283-286] Induction of endothelial nitric oxide production results in venodilation and increased microvascular permeability. Elevated plasma concentrations of TNF-α after a stress are often short-lived, yet it is an initiator of the inflammatory cascade. Additionally, it operates as a local mediator, such as in the joint spaces in rheumatoid arthritis.

After major surgery (e.g., esophagostomy and open cholecystectomy), plasma TNF-α concentrations were elevated immediately on termination of the surgery.[287,288] However, TNF-α concentrations were significantly lower 24 hours after surgery.[288] After distal gastrectomy, concentrations were not elevated.[287,289] No TNF-α elevations were observed after laparoscopic surgery.[290] After major trauma plasma TNF-α, IL-6, and IL-8 concentrations increased in correlation with the level of endotoxemia.[291] TNF-α peaked earlier than the other two cytokines. Ex vivo studies showed that after 2–6 days whole blood from trauma patients was less able to produce TNF coincident with TNF inhibitory activity in the sera.[292] This anti-inflammatory activity includes increased concentrations of soluble TNF receptors p55 and p75.[293] After severe burns, elevation of serum TNF-α concentrations was seen in only approximately one-half of the patients[294] and often not after débridement.[295] Yet, it is important to realize that TNF often operates via apocrine and paracrine mechanisms, and serum concentrations may not be elevated.

TNF-α, along with IL-1, IL-6, and IL-8, is a major mediator of the local and systemic abnormalities that occur during sepsis and septic shock.[296] It is the uncontrolled production of TNF that appears to be a major cause of septic shock and multiple organ dysfunction.[297] TNF activity is modulated by soluble forms of the p55 and p75 kD membrane receptors.[298-300] Septic shock is thought to be caused by TNF-α concentrations greater than soluble TNF receptor concentrations.[298] Peak TNF-α levels were reached earlier (2–4 hours) than those of the two TNF-soluble receptors (4–8 hours). The importance of the TNF and soluble-TNF receptor relationship was shown by the association of a high membrane-associated TNF-α to TNF receptor ratio with the development of multiple organ dysfunction.[301] High ratios were also found when septic burn patients were compared with nonseptic burn patients.[302] During sepsis[303] and after trauma[304] and burn injury[302] the concentration of the soluble-TNF receptors p55 and p75 increases, often in concentrations many times greater than TNF in an attempt to control the outbreak of septic shock and multiple organ dysfunction.[276,303]

TNF is secreted by macrophages upon exposure to endotoxin and *Candida albicans* organisms. Higher plasma concentrations occur with positive bacterial cultures and with gram-negative, as opposed to gram-positive, infections.[305] In septic shock from an abdominal source, high serum TNF was associated with increased survival,[305] although in another study plasma type II phospholipase A$_2$ concentrations, which correlated with TNF concentrations, were associated with reduced survival.[306] In humans the nature of the TNF response may be dependent on genetic factors, as there are polymorphisms of the TNF-α gene.[307]

Administration of TNF to animals results in most of the manifestations of septic shock: hypotension, metabolic acidosis, hemoconcentration, hyperglycemia, hyperkalemia, hemorrhagic lesions of the gastrointestinal tract, and acute tubular necrosis.[308] Waage and colleagues[309] noted a correlation between TNF levels, degree of septic shock, and subsequent death in patients with meningococcemia. Michie and colleagues[310] found that serum levels of TNF peaked 90–180 minutes after normal subjects received infusions of endotoxin. Associated with this peak were increases in plasma ACTH and epinephrine concentrations, body temperature, and heart rate. Pretreatment with ibuprofen did not affect the increase in TNF level, but did suppress the increase in body temperature and ACTH. Ibuprofen administration before endotoxin challenge in healthy subjects demonstrated different kinetics for releasing the p75- and p55-soluble TNF receptors.[311] Dimeric TNF receptors (p80) administered to healthy volunteers infused with endotoxin failed to affect endotoxin-related symptoms and delayed, but did not diminish, the febrile response.[312]

TNF-α acts synergistically with IL-1 to depress myocardial function,[313] with TNF produced in the myocardium being an important contributor.[314] Low TNF-α concentrations induce myocardial depression via a non–TNF-dependent process, whereas higher concentrations may act via a process that includes inducing inducible nitric oxide synthetase (iNOS).[315] There is some evidence that TNF-mediated caspase-3 apoptosis causes extensive lymphocyte apoptosis during sepsis that may contribute to impaired immune responses.[316] Epinephrine, used to support the blood pressure of septic shock patients, inhibits TNF-α production during the infusion of endotoxemia in humans[317] by a β_2-receptor mechanism.[318]

TNF-α and other cytokines (e.g., IL-6, IFN-γ, IL-1) have been implicated as mediators of cachexia.[319] They are among the causes of anorexia and may decrease gastric and intestinal motility.[319,320] TNF can dramatically decrease the synthesis and activity of lipogenic enzymes in cultured adipocytes,[321] which mirrors the decreased lipogenesis observed with whole body measurements in septic and injured patients. TNF-α can induce lipolysis by stimulating Gi proteins and decreasing lipoprotein lipase activity.[322,323] TNF is also one of the stimulators of acute-phase protein synthesis[324] and induces insulin resistance in adipo-

cytes, likely at the level of phosphatidylinositol-3-kinase.[325] In addition, TNF may stimulate peripheral muscle proteolysis.[326–328]

Interleukin-6

IL-6, secreted by immune cells and adipocytes,[329] is a pivotal mediator in the stress response. It influences (via the signal transducer gp130) the growth and differentiation of hematopoietic precursor cells, B lymphocytes, and T lymphocytes; regulates acute phase protein synthesis[330,331]; causes release of immunoglobulins; and stimulates the HPA axis. Along with IL-1 and IL-2, IL-6 increases the synthesis and release of CRH and ACTH.[332] IL-6 is under the tonic negative control of glucocorticoids and up-regulates the number of glucocorticoid receptors.[332] Alternately, glucocorticoids work in coordination with IL-6 and TNF-α to stimulate hepatic amino acid transport, increase IL-6 receptor expression, and prime liver cells to produce acute phase proteins.[333] When administered to healthy volunteers, recombinant IL-6 suppressed testosterone concentrations without changing gonadotropin levels. Therefore, IL-6 must either induce resistance to LH, suppress Leydig's cell steroidogenesis, or both.[334]

IL-6 concentrations are elevated after most major injuries and during sepsis. Concentrations of IL-6 were found to peak 24 hours after major surgery.[335,336] Along with IL-10, but not TNF-α or IL-1β, IL-6 levels were elevated after esophagectomy and pulmonary lobectomy. IL-6 concentrations were not elevated after lesser surgery (e.g., mastectomy and laparoscopic cholecystectomy).[337] Laparoscopic surgery (abdominal hysterectomy and cholecystectomy) resulted in lower concentrations of IL-6 than open procedures.[338,339] Infection is also accompanied by elevations in IL-6, with higher concentrations found in bacteremic compared with nonbacteremic patients.[340] In studies of septic patients, IL-6 concentrations were often higher in nonsurvivors than survivors.[331,341,342] After trauma, IL-6 and IL-8 concentrations became elevated after initial increases in TNF-α and correlated with endotoxemia.[291] Similarly after burns, IL-6 concentrations were elevated and correlated positively with protein turnover and catabolism.[343]

As with IL-1 and TNF-α, there are IL-6–soluble receptors in plasma and wounds[344] that constitute a controlling mechanism for IL-6 activity. The feedback system for IL-6 activity is theorized to involve IL-6 stimulation of the production of C-reactive protein, which, in turn, stimulates IL-6–soluble receptor production.[345]

IL-6 is involved with many of the metabolic responses to injury. One of its major functions is the stimulation of the acute phase protein response. Additionally, IL-6 administered to healthy subjects caused hyperglycemia and increased glucagon concentrations, but did not affect insulin concentrations.[346] IL-6 also increases serum triglycerides by increasing very low-density lipoprotein production. These lipoproteins are reportedly scavengers of endotoxin.[347]

Other Cytokines

Other cytokines are operative during the response to stress. IL-2 is secreted by activated T cells (TH1) in response to stimuli such as IL-1 and causes generation and proliferation of antigen-specific cytotoxic and helper T cells required for cell-mediated immunity. IL-2 production is reduced in injured patients, and the volume of production is inversely correlated with the severity of injury.[348] This decreased IL-2 synthesis is likely caused by excessive prostaglandin E_2 output by inhibitory monocytes.[349] Prostaglandin E_2 is associated with reduced cytokine production,[350] inhibited lymphocyte-mediated cytolysis, and inhibition of lymphocyte mitogenesis.[350] Partial restoration of IL-2 synthesis can occur by blocking the cyclo-oxygenase pathway with indomethacin.[349] After injury there is reduced cellular immunity and more prominence of humoral (TH2) immunity (with a shift to more of the

CD8 suppressor/cytotoxic T-lymphocyte subset). Besides a reduction in IL-2 production, there is increased production of soluble IL-2 receptors and IL-4 by CD8 cells.[351-354] IL-4 is an anti-inflammatory cytokine, also called *B-cell differentiating factor*, that induces T-cell differentiation to TH2 type cells. IL-2 is used in the treatment of malignancies, but when given in large doses cause a response similar to that seen after injury and sepsis—weight gain caused by fluid retention, noncardiogenic pulmonary edema, hyperpyrexia, nephrotoxicity, and hepatotoxicity.[355,356] IL-2 infusions increase plasma levels of ACTH, cortisol, GH, endothelin-1, IFN-γ, and TNF-α.[357,358] Attempts at tempering this stress response have been made using soluble TNF receptor p75:IgG chimera to block TNF.[359]

IFN-γ, a glycoprotein released by stimulated T lymphocytes, is another mediator of the immune stress response.[360] It activates macrophages to release IL-1, TNF,[361] granulocyte colony-stimulating factor and macrophage colony-stimulating factor[262]; increases IL-2 receptors on monocytes; and reduces release of prostaglandin E_2[362] and urokinase-type plasminogen activator.[361] It reduces immune suppressor activity by inhibiting prostaglandin E_2 release as well as inhibiting viral replication.

Other Mediators

Our understanding of the homeostatic changes that occur during sepsis has been revolutionized by the discovery that a gas, nitric oxide, is a potent endogenous vasodilator (Figure 19-2) and neurotransmitter. Nitric oxide, along with carbon monoxide, is an inhibitory regulator of the HPA axis. They both act through guanylcyclase. Carbon monoxide is formed by the catabolism of heme moieties by heme oxygenase,[363] whereas nitric oxide is produced from arginine.

The profound vasodilatation that occurs during septic shock has been ascribed to cytokine (TNF-α, IL-1β, and IFN-γ)-mediated induction of iNOS in vascular endothelial cells and cardiac monocytes, leading to elevated synthesis of nitric oxide from arginine.[364,365] Direct evidence of expression of iNOS in human septic shock has yet to be confirmed,[366] although it has been detected in alveolar macrophages from adult respiratory distress syndrome patients with sepsis.[367] It is likely that in human sepsis endothelial NOS, rather than iNOS, is up-regulated.[368] Inhibition of nitric oxide synthetase with N-nitro-L-arginine methyl ester restored arterial blood pressure and systemic vascular resistance in patients with septic shock. It also decreased the elevated myocardial stroke volume and cardiac index[369] but was

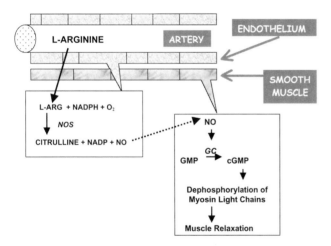

FIGURE 19-2 Nitric oxide (NO) is synthesized in the endothelium of blood vessels and then diffuses to the adjacent smooth muscle cells. This paracrine action results in vasodilation. (L-ARG = L-arginine; cGMP = cyclic guanosine monophosphate; GC = guanylyl cyclase; NADP = nicotinamide-adenine dinucleotide phosphate; NADPH = nicotinamide-adenine dinucleotide phosphate [reduced form]; NOS = nitric oxide synthetase.)

associated with increased mortality.[370] The latter is likely because of nonselective inhibition by N-nitro-L-arginine methyl ester of neuronal, inducible, and endothelial nitric oxide synthetase.[365] The N-nitro-L-arginine methyl ester inhibition of nitric oxide synthetase also unmasks endothelin-1 vasoconstriction.[371] Endothelin-1, a 21-amino-acid peptide, is a powerful endothelium-produced vasoconstrictor. Its production is elevated during shock, low flow states, and ischemia. The degree of vasodilation in septic shock is thought to be caused by a balance between vasodilating nitric oxide and vasoconstricting endothelin-1.[372,373]

Endocrine-Immune System Interaction

There are many close interactions between the endocrine and immune systems. It has long been recognized that pharmacologic doses of glucocorticoids suppress cellular immunity. This may be partially because of steroid-induced reduced responsiveness to IL-12, a cytokine that promotes cellular immunity.[374] Glucocorticoids cause release of neutrophils from the bone marrow, reduce circulating monocytes and macrophages, and sequester T cells in the bone marrow. They also cause lysis of immature T cells; inhibit IFN-γ, IL-1,[375] and IL-2 production; block phospholipase A$_2$ (responsible for prostaglandin and leukotriene production); and inhibit the action of certain proteases involved in inflammation.[376] There are glucocorticoid receptors on leukocytes; peripheral leukocytes have also been observed to secrete ACTH when infected by a virus or exposed to endotoxin.[377]

The neuroendocrine axis was long thought to be mainly concerned with triggering endocrine hormone release and stimulating the sympathetic nervous system. However, it also modulates immunologic function, whereas immunomediators, such as cytokines, also modulate neuroendocrine function.[378] Interestingly, many of the mediators originally thought to be secreted only by the hypothalamus and pituitary are also secreted by other body systems, especially immune-related cells. For example, prolactin is also secreted by activated T cells and thymocytes and binds to receptors of the cytokine superfamily.[379,380] Prolactin receptors are found on up to 80% of thymic lymphoid cells and all peripheral B cell macrophages, and 70% of T cells.[381] Prolactin acts via autocrine and paracrine mechanisms to regulate cellular immunity.[382–384] The role of prolactin in the stress response is unclear, although after prolonged abdominal exploration, but not lesser surgery (cholecystectomy and herniorrhaphy), serum levels were elevated for up to 5 postoperative days.[385–387]

Other neuroendocrine substances also have immune activity. α-MSH is thought to have anti-inflammatory (acting as a TNF-α antagonist), antipyretic, and antimicrobial actions.[378,388–391] The central melanocortin system, along with leptin and insulin, may also be a component of the adipostat (or lipostat), the mechanism that regulates adipose mass.[392,393] Leptin, which is produced by adipocytes, appears to stimulate proopiomelanocortin, and the α-MSH produced binds to the melanocortin receptor MC4-R that decreases appetite and activates lipid metabolism.[394] The exact function of α-MSH during the stress response is still being elucidated. Somatostatin is secreted not only by the hypothalamus and pancreas, but also by immune cells such as thymocytes.[395] There are somatostatin receptors on immune cells and when they are stimulated by low concentrations of somatostatin, they have inhibitory effects, whereas at higher concentrations no effects are seen.[396,397]

In addition to their functions as immune mediators, some of the cytokines and growth factors are active via autocrine and paracrine mechanisms in the hypothalamic-pituitary region.[398,399] Cytokines, including IL-1, IL-2, IL-6, IFN-γ, and TNF, have effects on the HPA axis. The teleologic explanation is that the cytokines transmit stimuli (e.g., the presence of bacteria, viruses, and antigens) that are not recognizable by the central and peripheral nervous systems.[400] IL-1 stimulates intracerebral noradrenaline and dopamine,[401] ACTH, and CRF release. Brown and coworkers demonstrated that IL-1 and IL-2 enhance the expression of the mRNA to proopiomelanocortin.[402] Controversy exists as to whether IL-1 directly stimulates ACTH secretion by pituitary cells or directs the release of CRF from hypothalamic cells.[403] (It is possible that this depends on the type of IL-1, α or β.) It has also been observed that IL-1 and IFN-γ[404] stimulate release of ACTH-like substances (and endorphins) from peripheral white blood cells. Additionally, IL-1 is expressed in the human adrenal gland and may stimulate cortisol secretion by autocrine or paracrine mechanisms.[405] IL-6 can also cause ACTH secretion from pituitary cells via a leukotriene mechanism.[406] IL-10 is produced not only in lymphocytes, but also in pituitary and hypothalamic cells, and regulates CRF and ACTH production.[407] These actions of the proinflammatory cytokines on the hypothalamic-pituitary axis represent an anti-inflammatory and immunosuppressive negative feedback system because the ultimate outcome is the increased secretion of glucocorticoids.[408] Alternately, pretreatment with glucocorticoids can suppress the IL-1α activation of CRF.[409]

IL-6 administered as part of cancer therapy caused secretion of AVP and also release of CRH, again demonstrating the influence of the cytokines on the HPA axis.[410] It also increases brain tryptophan and serotonin metabolism.[411] IL-11, a member of the IL-6 cytokine family, and leukemia inhibitory factor, another cytokine-like mediator, are also involved in HPA activity.[412]

BIOCHEMICAL CHANGES AFTER INJURY AND SEPSIS

Carbohydrate Metabolism

The major fuel source for healthy humans is glucose. It enters the circulation either from endogenous sources (glycogenolysis and gluconeogenesis) or from external ones (via the digestive tract or intravenously). It can then be (1) metabolized to carbon dioxide, water, and energy, (2) converted and stored as glycogen, or (3) converted to fat. Insulin facilitates glucose uptake by cells, promotes glycogen synthesis, and opposes gluconeogenesis. Catecholamines and glucagon stimulate glycogenolysis, renal gluconeogenesis, and hepatic gluconeogenesis; cortisol also stimulates the latter. Although the liver is the site of most gluconeogenesis, some have estimated as much as 25% of gluconeogenesis occurs in the kidney.[413]

A prominent feature of the response to injury or sepsis is hyperglycemia. This hyperglycemia is thought to ensure a ready supply of glucose to predominantly glucose-consuming cells, such as the wound and inflammatory and immune cells.[414] Hyperglycemia is initially caused by the mobilization of liver glycogen; however, the hyperglycemia persists beyond exhaustion of the glycogen supply, owing to a marked increase in hepatic glucose production plus reduced glucose clearance. This increase in glucose production is caused by hepatic gluconeogenesis, which uses amino acids, lactate, pyruvate, and glycerol as substrates. The lactate and pyruvate arise from glycogenolysis and glycolysis in peripheral tissues, especially muscle. The amino acids arise from the breakdown of muscle, the glycerol from the metabolism of triglycerides (fat). The increase in hepatic glucose production is marked. In normal subjects approximately 200 g of glucose is produced daily. Noninfected burn patients may produce 320 g per day and infected ones 400 g per day. The magnitude of the increase in glucose production after abdominal hysterectomy was associated with the duration that the peritoneum was open.[415] In addition to the increase in hepatic glucose production there is reduced clearance of glucose because of resistance to the actions of insulin coupled with insulin levels that are inadequate to maintain normoglycemia. Some investigators[416] have suggested that the insulin levels are inadequate because of the suppression of insulin secretion by high epinephrine concentrations, along with increased insulin turnover causing increased insulin clearance.[417] Epinephrine inhibits insulin secretion by reducing insulin exocytosis; this can be reversed with α-adrenergic blockade.[415] β-Adrenergic activity, on the other hand, is responsible for the increased hepatic glucose production. Other mechanisms also contribute to the hyperglycemia. There is reduced nonoxidative glucose disposal resulting from decreased muscle glycogen synthetase activity.[418–420] This is also a result of insulin resistance.[421] Unlike the response of healthy subjects to hyperglycemia, stress-induced hyperglycemia does not increase glucose disposal nor does it reduce the elevated hepatic glucose production.[422]

Insulin resistance in peripheral tissues hinders cellular glucose uptake and is thought to be caused by a postreceptor defect in extrahepatic tissues. This defect does not appear to be caused by impaired signaling of phosphatidylinositol-3-kinase,[423] but to impaired activity of the intracellular glucose transport system (e.g., glucose transporter-4). Insulin resistance persisted for at least 5 days after both open and laparoscopic cholecystectomies.[424,425] The incremental response to increases in insulin concentration is maintained,[426] but the ability to reduce blood glucose concentrations per insulin concentration is markedly diminished.[427] Despite the resistance to insulin, the overall peripheral uptake of glucose is often nearly *normal* because of increased non–insulin-mediated glucose uptake. Also, the normal amount of peripheral glucose uptake may be fueled by the large amounts of glucose (because of hyperglycemia) being presented to the partially resistant insulin pathway.[428] However, relative to the blood glucose concentration, the uptake is low.[429] The intracellular glucose oxidization pathway is intact so that the *rate* of glucose oxidation is unchanged.[420] Yet, the *relative* (to the prevailing blood glucose concentration) *and even overall amount* of glucose that is oxidized is decreased because of the relatively reduced glucose uptake into the cell.[419]

Glucose can be oxidized to produce ATP, water, and CO_2; converted to glycogen for storage in the liver and muscles; or converted to fat. The latter process is called *lipogenesis* and occurs in both liver and adipose tissue, although the latter appears to be the main site for lipogenesis.[430,431] Under normal circumstances carbohydrate intake inhibits fat oxidation, increases glucose oxidation, and promotes fat storage.[432] Lipogenesis is quantitatively unimportant in humans because the rate of lipogenesis does not exceed the rate of lipid oxidation.[433] Yet, when carbohydrate intake exceeds total energy expenditure lipogenesis becomes a more important pathway[434] and respiratory quotients may exceed 1.0, indicating net lipogenesis. This may be seen among patients receiving glucose infusions of greater than 4 mg per kg per minute.[435] Critically ill patients administered intravenous glucose at a rate of 4 mg per kg per minute as part of glucose-based TPN exhibited some increased hepatic de novo lipogenesis, despite achieving a respiratory quotient of only 0.90.[436] This lipogenesis occurred despite the fact that during surgical or septic stress, lipogenetic capability is reduced. This reduction is possibly secondary to TNF and, maybe, IL-1β, which inhibit lipogenesis in human adipocytes.[437] TNF can also induce apoptosis of preadipocytes and adipocytes.[438]

Fat Metabolism

Fat can be either used as an immediate energy source or stored. Exogenously administered long-chain triglycerides are metabolized into free fatty acids and glycerol. The free fatty acids can be metabolized as fuel or can be re-esterified back to triglycerides. In the fed (high-insulin) state re-esterification predominates and lipolysis is inhibited; in the starved state, with a high glucagon-to-insulin ratio, fat is metabolized to free fatty acids (lipolysis) and then oxidized as fuel, with the associated production of ketone bodies by the liver mitochondria. The ketone bodies are then transported to other organs to be used as fuels. The oxidation of exogenous lipids blocks the lipolysis of endogenous fat. It appears that fat mobilization, with the increase in free fatty acids, impairs muscle glucose uptake and oxidation.[439]

After injury there is a marked increase in lipolysis mainly because of increased β$_2$-adrenergic activity caused by elevated concentrations of circulating catecholamines (Figure 19-3).[440,441] Increased concentrations of cortisol, glucagon, TNF-α, IL-1, β-endorphin, interferon-α, and interferon-γ may also play a role in stimulating lipolysis.[175,204,442,443] β$_2$-Receptor stimulation increases cAMP concentrations, which, in turn, (via protein kinase A–induced phosphorylation) stimulates hormone-sensitive lipase activity.[442,444] This activity is inhibited by insulin, which promotes lipogenesis. The role of the newly discovered β$_3$-adrenergic receptor in human lipolysis is still unclear.[445] The lipolytic response to β$_2$-stimulation is greater in lean, than obese, subjects.[446] There are regional variations in the lipolytic rate, with visceral fat cells having the fastest rate because of increased activity of β$_2$- and β$_3$-receptors and reduced activity of α$_2$-adrenergic receptors. Stimulation of α$_2$-adrenergic receptors inhibits lipolysis by inhibit-

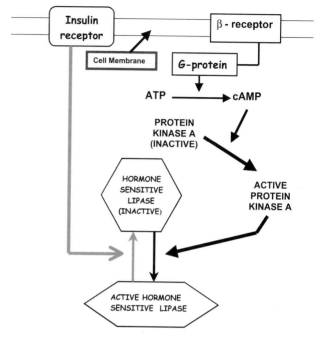

FIGURE 19-3 Lipolysis occurs in adipocytes after stimulation by various mediators, especially β-adrenergic agonists such as epinephrine. This stimulation results in the activation of hormone-sensitive lipase, which breaks up triglycerides into fatty acids and glycerol. The glycerol is then transported to the liver where it enters the gluconeogenic pathway. Insulin inactivates hormone-sensitive lipase, thus inhibiting lipolysis. (ATP = adenosine triphosphate; cAMP = cyclic adenosine monophosphate.)

ing cAMP production.[442] Subcutaneous fat has reduced lipolytic activity because of increased activity of insulin and α$_2$-adrenergic receptors.[447]

Trauma patients exhibit increased lipolysis and use fat as the major fuel source.[218] Plasma glycerol and free fatty acid levels are elevated, fatty acid and glycerol turnover are accelerated,[448–450] and lipid oxidation is increased. Lipoprotein lipase is the capillary endothelium membrane-bound enzyme that hydrolyzes triglycerides (bound to very low-density lipoproteins and chylomicrons) to glycerol and fatty acids. Heparin releases this enzyme into the blood stream,[451] causing an immediate increase in the intravascular hydrolysis of lipids. After trauma, muscle lipoprotein lipase activity is increased, but adipose tissue lipoprotein lipase is decreased.[452] In sepsis, muscle lipoprotein lipase activity is decreased. Thus, there appears to be a difference between trauma and sepsis.[453] Studies with labeled (^{14}C) palmitate and labeled long-chain triglyceride emulsion (Intralipid) have demonstrated increased oxidation and clearance.[453,454] It is also interesting to note that in severely injured and burn patients the ratio of the rate of appearance of free fatty acids to the rate of appearance of glycerol increases, indicating that rate of re-esterification is greater in adipose tissues.[455] This apparently *futile* cycle in adipose tissue may be one of the causes of hypermetabolism in these patients. Treatment with propranolol decreased the rate of appearance of glycerol and free fatty acids in burn patients; this process thus appears to be mediated adrenergically.[220] The increase in lipolysis also increases the amount of glycerol available for gluconeogenesis.

During the period of stress after surgery and trauma and during infection, the plasma levels of ketones remain low, even during calorie deprivation.[456,457] This is surprising given the increased availability of bloodborne free fatty acids caused by lipolysis. Studies of patients after elective surgery have demonstrated a two- to threefold increase in ketones 3 hours after surgery; thereafter levels decreased toward normal.[458] Forearm extraction of β-hydroxybutyrate and acetoacetate decreases immediately after surgery. The cause of this reduced ketone production and use have been ascribed mainly to the elevated plasma insulin concentrations as well as the increased alanine concentrations and the increased uptake and β-oxidation of free fatty acids.[459]

Protein Metabolism

Injury (surgical, traumatic, burn) and sepsis accelerate protein breakdown,[460] which is manifested by increased urinary nitrogen loss, increased peripheral release of amino acids, and inhibition of muscle amino acid uptake.[461] The amino acids originate from both injured tissue and uninjured skeletal muscle and are transported to the liver for conversion to glucose (gluconeogenesis) and for protein synthesis. The negative nitrogen balance (catabolism) observed in such patients represents the net result of breakdown and synthesis: Breakdown is increased and synthesis either increased or diminished.[462] In burned children the volume of protein breakdown was equally elevated during both the acute and convalescent phases but synthesis increased in the latter phase, creating a positive nitrogen balance.[463] Catabolic activity is thought to be mediated partially by cortisol[464] and by TNF-α, IL-1, IL-6, and IFN-γ. It is the balance between these catabolic hormones and anabolic hormones, such as insulin and insulin-like growth factors, that determine the degree of catabolism. Current thinking is that skeletal muscle proteolysis begins with release of myofilaments from myofibrillar proteins by the calpain enzymes followed by their lysis by the lysosomal Ca^{++}-activated, ATP-ubiquitin–dependent proteolytic pathway.[465,466] The amino acids released by proteolysis provide some of the substrate for the concomitant increased hepatic gluconeogenesis. However, reducing the rate of hepatic gluconeogenesis with somatostatin does not decrease the rate of peripheral protein breakdown, demonstrating that the accelerated rate of hepatic glucose production is not linked to the elevated level of peripheral protein breakdown.[428] The liver also contributes to catabolism through the increased clearance of α-amino nitrogen (urea). After surgery the rate of this conversion is doubled.[467]

After injury the hepatic synthesis of selected proteins (acute phase reactants) increases, whereas that of others decreases. These proteins are involved in humoral immunity (e.g., immunoglobulins), inflammation, and coagulation (e.g., fibrinogen). Other acute phase reactants include complement, C-reactive protein, haptoglobin, α₁-acid glycoprotein, α₁-antitrypsin, α₁-antichymotrypsin, ceruloplasmin, ferritin, and serum amyloid A.[468] The degree of acute phase response is proportional to the level of tissue injury.[463] Stimulators of the acute phase reactants include IL-1, IL-6, TNF, and IFN-γ, along with some role for the glucocorticoids.

Proteins whose synthesis decreases include binding proteins (e.g., albumin, transthyretin [prealbumin]), retinols, transferrin, and CBGs. Cytokines such as IL-6, but not the counterregulatory hormones, mediate this decreased protein production.[469] In critically ill patients, hypoalbuminemia may be caused not only by a decreased albumin synthetic rate, but also to a shortened half-life.[470] The plasma albumin concentration is also reduced by transcapillary escape facilitated by increased capillary permeability and extracellular expansion after fluid resuscitation. Therefore, acute changes in plasma albumin concentrations after surgery or trauma are caused by fluid fluxes. Prealbumin has a shorter half-life and is a better postoperative indicator of nutritional status. The reason for the decreased synthesis of binding proteins has been explained by the free hormone hypothesis: The decrease in binding proteins allows for more free retinoid, cortisol, and thyroid hormone.[471]

Energy Metabolism

Most often, stressed patients have elevated resting metabolic rates. After elective surgery, the increase is approximately 10–15% above preoperative values. The peak occurs around the third postoperative day and the period of hypermetabolism has been reported to last at least 21 days in critically ill trauma[472] and burn[473] patients. Patients with sepsis have increases of 20–40%, whereas those with burns experience the greatest increases (up to 120%, essentially the increase is proportional to the extent of the burn).[474] After subarachnoid hemorrhage, resting energy expenditure was 18% above predicted for at least the initial 5 days.[475] Mechanically ventilated trauma patients had lower increases in energy expenditure (17%) than spontaneously breathing patients likely because they were sedated and had no or minimal work of breathing.[476] This increase in energy expenditure appears to be mediated by the altered metabolic milieu.[477] Catecholamines infused into normal subjects increase the metabolic rate,[478] and this increase is even greater when cortisol, glucagon, and catecholamines are infused together.[479] Some have ascribed the increased energy expenditure to increased protein oxidation[429] and synthesis.[480] Yet, this may not always be the case. Lowry et al.[481] noted that after elective surgery there was only modest change in energy expenditure, despite an increase in protein turnover. This implied there was little relation between the two. The other metabolic process that may contribute to the increase in energy expenditure is the substantial increase in carbohydrate and fat futile cycling, a process that causes a major increase in energy expenditure.[481] The teleologic reason for this increase in futile cycling is that it affords these patients the flexibility to adapt quickly to changes in energy substrate demands.[220] Fever also plays a role in hypermetabolism.[482]

Various environmental factors may also affect energy expenditure. Elevated ambient temperature (and humidity) has been shown to reduce the energy expenditure of burn patients by reducing evaporative losses and, in turn, reducing the need to generate increased energy to maintain body temperature.[481,483]

NUTRITIONAL SUPPORT

Understanding the changes wrought on the metabolic milieu by the response to stress is important when planning the nutritional support of an injured or septic patient. Because injured and septic patients do not respond to the intake of exogenous nutrients in the same manner as do postabsorptive or starved subjects, the effectiveness of nutritional support is often limited by an underlying hostile metabolic environment that reduces the use of administered nutrients. This has vastly complicated the design of nutritional regimens and has led to multiple strategies aimed at overcoming these limiting factors.

The administration of exogenous glucose and carbohydrates to injured or septic patients either does not or only minimally diminishes the rate of gluconeogenesis.[436,484] This is in contradistinction to refeeding starved patients in whom carbohydrate administration reduces gluconeogenesis and lipolysis. Despite the reduced use of glucose, it is still important to administer carbohydrates because some body tissues are unable to readily use other substrates. Furthermore, glucose and carbohydrate intakes stimulate the secretion of additional insulin, which promotes protein synthesis[485] and has an antilipolytic affect.[486,487] Yet, the appearance of hyperglycemia limits the amount of glucose and carbohydrate that can be administered. The degree of hyperglycemia induced by total parenteral nutrition is directly proportional to the rate of glucose infusion and the degree of injury. Elderly patients are more predisposed to develop hyperglycemia.[488] Excessive glucose loads should be avoided.[489] Excess glucose is metabolized to carbon dioxide and converted to glycogen, but it is not as readily converted to fat, owing to a block in net lipogenesis.[490] The administration of large glucose loads to such patients results in further increases in energy expenditure because of sympathetic nervous system stimulation.[491] This increase in metabolic rate (oxygen consumption), along with increased carbon dioxide production, requires increased minute ventilation. It is thus recommended that glucose intake for such patients be limited to less than 4 mg/kg per minute.[491,492]

Critically ill, stressed (trauma, sepsis) patients often derive as much as 80% of their energy requirement from fat. Fat emulsions containing polyunsaturated long-chain triglycerides are administered intravenously. Most patients readily clear and oxidize these triglycerides, but a small portion with severe sepsis are unable adequately to clear and to oxidize fat.[490] Stressed patients used fat to provide as much as 50% of nonprotein calories. Jeejeebhoy and colleagues[487] compared nutritional formulations containing carbohydrate (glucose) as their sole nonprotein source to those containing approximately equal amounts of glucose and fat. They found that the two formulations are equally nitrogen sparing.[487]

The provision of protein to stressed patients is an important aspect of nutritional support. Adequate nonprotein calories (from lipid and carbohydrates) must be provided, so that the infused amino acids can be used as substrate for protein synthesis rather than as an energy substrate to alleviate nitrogen losses. Exogenous protein or amino acids are often administered to injured patients in an attempt to attenuate the breakdown of endogenous proteins by providing an alternate source of amino acids for gluconeogenesis and protein synthesis. Unfortunately, in such states proteolysis is relatively unresponsive to the usual negative feedback mechanisms, including the administration of exogenous glucose, protein, or amino acids. Therefore, exogenous amino acids and protein are not well used, and nitrogen balance remains negative well into the convalescent stage. This has piqued interest in using anabolic substances, especially insulin, to improve nitrogen use. Among the major consequences of glucose and carbohydrate administration is the stimulation of insulin secretion. At lower doses insulin decreases protein breakdown by inhibiting the ATP-ubiquitin proteosome proteolytic pathway[493] and may also stimulate protein synthesis when there is adequate availability of intracellular amino acids.[494] At higher doses it is thought to also stimulate protein synthesis. Alternately, suppression of insulin secretion, such as occurred during stress hormone infusion (cortisol, glucagon, epinephrine) in healthy subjects, increased whole body nitrogen losses and the forearm efflux of amino acids.[495] The administration of small doses of insulin to burn patients increased skeletal muscle protein synthesis[496] and improved wound matrix formation.[497] The provision of hypocaloric parenteral nutrition with high-dose insulin improved nitrogen balance in postoperative cancer patients.[498] However, the anabolic effects of insulin on protein metabolism were not evident in enterally fed trauma patients. Therefore, the route of nutrient intake may play a role in insulin's anabolic effects.[499]

Other anabolic substances that have or are being studied include GH, IGF-1, and anabolic steroids.[500] GH administration in critically ill patients receiving nutritional support has been observed to reduce nitrogen loss and improve phosphate retention. However, outcome studies of GH administration in the critically ill demonstrated no improvement in patient outcome.[501,502] Moreover, one study reported excess mortality in critically ill patients, which may be attributable to the diabetogenic and lipolytic properties of GH.[503] Therefore, GH may not be a viable anabolic substance for the acute critically ill and may be more useful in the convalescent period. IGF-1 and its binding protein, IGFBP-3, are both reduced during stress.[504] Like GH, IGF-1 stimulates protein synthesis at lower doses, and at higher doses also reduces proteolysis.[505] It has advantages when compared with GH because it is not diabetogenic (it enhances insulin sensitivity) and is effective when GH resistance is present. The administration of IGF-1 for 3 days decreased protein oxidation and when administered along with its binding protein, IGFBP-3, attenuated catabolism in burn patients.[504,506] More study of

these substances is under way. Another effort was to administer anabolic steroids, which have positive effects on muscle size and strength, but may have detrimental psychological, cardiovascular, and thrombotic effects.[507] These hormones increased amino acid and water uptake and increased fat use in catabolic patients, but failed to promote significant increases in visceral protein synthesis.[508] Anabolic steroids may be more useful in restoring muscle mass in noncritically ill patients.[509, 510]

Glutamine has been the focus of much study because it may be important in the maintenance of gut and immunologic integrity during critical illness. Glutamine is the most abundant amino acid in blood and by itself may be an insulin-independent stimulator of gluconeogenesis.[511] It is a primary fuel for rapidly dividing cells such as enterocytes and immunocytes.[512] It is also involved in the interorgan transport of nitrogen. Evidence from animal studies has indicated that glutamine may be an essential amino acid during critical illness and that parenteral and enteral glutamine-supplemented nutrition may prevent bacterial translocation. The data in humans are less compelling.[513] Glutamine is rather insoluble and thus is difficult to administer. Some success has been achieved infusing it as the L-amino acid, glutamine-dipeptides or alanylglutamate. Initial reports indicate that in some catabolic patients glutamine-containing nutrition may improve gut structure and function, exert an anabolic effect, and reduce morbidity, hospital costs, infection rates, and length of hospital stay.[514,515] More studies are needed to ascertain whether glutamine administration improves outcome.[516]

GENDER AND THE STRESS RESPONSE

Certain aspects of the response to stress differ between male and female subjects. Compared with male subjects, in female subjects activation of the sympathetic system is attenuated or, alternately, sympathoadrenal inhibition is augmented.[517] Similarly, male subjects have greater increases in arginine vasopressin and ACTH in response to physostigmine than female subjects, indicating differential sensitivity of the HPA axis.[518] Traumatized women had increased serum IGF-1 and minimal changes in transthyretin (prealbumin) concentrations, whereas among traumatized men both were decreased.[519] Serum concentrations of IGF-binding protein-3 increased as injury severity increased in traumatized women. The opposite relationship was found among traumatized men.[520] Most interesting was the observation of significantly better prognoses among septic women than septic men. This was associated with high proinflammatory TNF concentrations in the men and high anti-inflammatory IL-10 in the women.[521] Differences in cytokine expression were also found. Monocytes from men produced more soluble IL-1 type II receptors than monocytes from women.[522]

In summary, the response to injury and sepsis results in profound disordering of physiological homeostasis. Major alterations occur in almost every body system mediated by the outpouring of bioactive substances by the CNS and endocrine, immune, and hematopoietic systems. The underlying metabolic milieu is upset and the ability to metabolize endogenous substrates and exogenous nutrients altered. Yet, despite the continued discovery of many of the mediators of this complex response over the past two decades, many aspects of the response are still not understood. Further investigation is needed to unravel the remaining mysteries so that ways to attenuate the detrimental effects of the stress response and accentuate its beneficial aspects may be developed.

REFERENCES

1. Mallory GK, White PD, Saicedo-Salgar J. The speed of healing of the myocardial infarction: a study of the pathologic anatomy in seventy-two cases. Am Heart J 1939;18:47–671.
2. Jetter WW, White PD. Rupture of the heart in patients in mental institutions. Ann Intern Med 1944;21:783–802.
3. Allen C, Glasziou P, Del Mar C. Bed rest: a potentially harmful treatment needing more careful evaluation. Lancet 1999;354:1229–1233.
4. Dietrick JE, Whedon GD, Shorr E. Effects of immobilization upon various metabolic and physiologic functions of normal men. Am J Med 1948;4:3–36.
5. Graveline DE, Barnard GW. Physiological effects of a hypodynamic environment: short-term studies. Aerospace Med 1964;35:1194–1200.
6. Miller PB, Johnson RL, Lamb LE. Effects of four weeks of absolute bed rest on circulatory functions in man. Aerospace Med 1964;35:1194–1200.
7. Vogt FB, Johnson PC. Plasma volume and extracellular fluid volume change associated with 10 days bed recumbency. Aerospace Med 1967;38:21–25.
8. Saltin B, Blomqvist G, Mitchell JH, et al. Response to exercise after bed rest and after training: a longitudinal study of adaptive changes in oxygen transport and body composition. Circulation 1968;38(Suppl 7):1–55.
9. Gaffney FA, Nixon JV, Karlsson ES, et al. Cardiovascular deconditioning produced by 20 hours of bedrest with head-down tilt (–5 degrees) in middle-aged men. Am J Cardiol 1985;56:634–638.
10. Convertino V, Hung J, Goldwater D, et al. Cardiovascular responses to exercise in middle-aged men after 10 days of bedrest. Circulation 1982;65:134–140.
11. Flye MW. Disorders of Veins. In DC Sabiston (ed), Textbook of Surgery. Philadelphia: WB Saunders, 1986;1709–1730.
12. Blomqvist CG, Nixon JV, Johnson RL, et al. Early cardiovascular adaptation to zero gravity stimulated by head-down tilt. Acta Astronaut 1980;7:543–553.
13. Lathers CM, Diamandis PH, Riddle JM, et al. Acute and intermediate cardiovascular responses to zero gravity and to fractional gravity levels induced by head-down or head-up tilt. J Clin Pharmacol 1990;30:494–523.
14. Johnson PC, Driscoll TB, Carpenter WR. Vascular and extravascular fluid changes during six days of bedrest. Aerospace Med 1971;42:875–878.
15. Maillet A, Pavy-Le Traon A, Allevard AM, et al. Hormone changes induced by 37.5-h head-down tilt (-6 degrees) in humans. Eur J Appl Physiol 1994;68(6):497–503.
16. Henricksen L, Sjersen P. Effect of "vein pump" activation upon venous pressure and blood flow in human subcutaneous tissue. Acta Physiol Scand 1977;100:14–21.
17. Thompson FJ, Barnes CD, Wald JR. Interactions between femoral venous afferents and lumbar spinal reflex pathways. J Auton Nerv Syst 1982;6:113–126.
18. Taylor HL, Henschel A, Brozek J, et al. Effects of bedrest on cardiovascular function and work performance. J Appl Physiol 1949;2:223–235.
19. Chobanian AV, Lille RD, Tercyak A, et al. The metabolic and hemodynamic effects of prolonged bed rest in normal subjects. Circulation 1974;49:551–559.
20. Hyatt KH, Kamenetsky LG, Smith WM. Extravascular dehydration as an etiologic factor in post-recumbency orthostatism. Aerospace Med 1969;40:644–650.
21. ten Harkel AD, Baisch F, Karemaker JM. Increased orthostatic blood pressure variability after prolonged head-down tilt. Acta Physiol Scand Suppl 1992;604:89–99.
22. Hung J, Goldwater D, Convertino V, et al. Mechanics for decreased exercise capacity after bedrest in normal middle-aged men. Am J Cardiol 1983;51:344–348.
23. Goldberger AL, Goldwater D, Bhargava V. Atropine unmasks bed-rest effect: a spectral analysis of cardiac interbeat intervals. J Appl Physiol 1986;61:1843–1848.
24. Robinson BF, Epstein SE, Beiser GD, et al. Control of heart rate by the autonomic system. Studies in man on the interrelation between baroreceptor mechanism and exercise. Circ Res 1966;19:400–411.
25. Melada GA, Goldman RH, Luetscher JA, et al. Hemodynamics, renal function, plasma renin and aldosterone in man after 5 to 14 days of bedrest. Aviat Space Environ Med 1975;46:1049–1055.
26. Maass H, Transmontano J, Baisch F. Response of adrenergic receptors to 10 days head-down tilt bed rest. Acta Physiol Scand Suppl 1992;604:61–68.
27. Leftheriotis G, Legrand MS, Abraham P, et al. Calf vein compliance increases following bed rest after aortocoronary bypass surgery. Clin Physiol 1998;18(1):19–25.
28. Gaffney FA, Buckey JC, Lane LD, et al. The effects of a 10-day period of head-down tilt on the cardiovascular responses to intravenous saline loading. Acta Physiol Scand Suppl 1992;604:121–130.
29. Convertino VA, Doerr DF, Ludwig

DA, Vernikos J. Effect of simulated microgravity on cardiopulmonary baroreflex control of forearm vascular resistance. Am J Physiol 1994;266: R1962–R1969.

30. West JB. Ventilation-Blood Flow and Gas Exchange (3rd ed). Philadelphia: JB Lippincott, 1977.

31. Laver MB, Hallowell P, Goldblatt A. Pulmonary dysfunction secondary to heart disease: aspects relevant to anesthesia and surgery. Anesthesiology 1970;33:161–192.

32. Schulz H, Hillebrecht A, Karemaker JM, et al. Cardiopulmonary function during 10 days of head-down tilt bed rest. Acta Physiol Scand Suppl 1992;604:23–32.

33. Macklern PT. Respiratory mechanics. Ann Rev Physiol 1978;40:157–184.

34. Minh VD, Kurihara N, Friedman PJ, et al. Reversal of pleural pressure gradient during electrophrenic stimulation. J Appl Physiol 1974;37:496–504.

35. Tisi GM. Preoperative evaluation of pulmonary function. Am Rev Respir Dis 1979;119:293–310.

36. Lumb PD. Perioperative Pulmonary Physiology. In DC Sabiston, FC Spencer (eds), Surgery of the Chest (5th ed). Philadelphia: WB Saunders, 1990.

37. Craig DB, Wahba WM, Don HE. Airway closure and lung volumes in surgical positions. Can Anaesth Soc J 1971;18:92–99.

38. Marini JJ, Tyler ML, Hudson LD, et al. Influence of head-dependent positions on lung volume and oxygen saturation in chronic airflow obstruction. Am Rev Respir Dis 1984;129:101–105.

39. Beckett WS, Vroman NB, Nigro D, et al. Effect of prolonged bed rest on lung volume in normal individuals. J Appl Physiol 1986;61(3):919–925.

40. Hillebrecht A, Schulz H, Meyer M, et al. Pulmonary responses to lower body negative pressure and fluid loading during head-down tilt bed rest. Acta Physiol Scand Suppl 1992;604:35–42.

41. Cardus D. Oxygen alveolar-arterial tension differences after ten days recumbency in man. J Appl Physiol 1967;23:934–967.

42. Booth FW. Physiologic and biochemical effects of immobilization on muscle. Clin Orthop 1987;219:15–20.

43. MacDougall JI, Ward GR, Sale DG, et al. Bio-chemical adaptation of human skeletal muscle to heavy resistance training and immobilization. J Appl Physiol 1977;43:700–703.

44. Witzmann FA, Kim DH, Fitts RH. Effect of hindlimb immobilization on the fatigability of skeletal muscle. J Appl Physiol 1983;54:1242–1248.

45. Watson PA, Stein JP, Booth FW. Changes in actin synthesis and alpha-actin mRNA content in rat muscle during immobilization. Am J Physiol 1984;247:C39–C44.

46. Booth FW, Seider MJ. Recovery of skeletal muscle after three months of hindlimb immobilization in rats. J Appl Physiol 1979;47:435–439.

47. Goldspink DF. The influence of immobilization and stretch on protein turnover of rat skeletal muscle. J Physiol (Lond) 1977;264:267–282.

48. Ferrando AA, Lane HW, Stuart CA, et al. Prolonged bed rest decreases skeletal muscle and whole body protein synthesis. Am J Physiol 1996;270:E627–E633.

49. Savolainen J, Vaanen K, Vihko V, et al. Effect of immobilization on collagen synthesis in rat skeletal muscles. Am J Physiol 1987;252:R883–R888.

50. Reiser PJ, Kasper CE, Moss RL. Myosin subunits and contractile properties of single fibers from hypokinetic rat muscles. J Appl Physiol 1987;63:2293–2300.

51. Ferrando AA, Stuart CA, Shefield-Moore M, Wolfe RR. Inactivity amplifies the catabolic response of skeletal muscle to cortisol. J Clin Endocrinol Metab 1999;84(10):3515–3521.

52. Rifenberick DH, Max SR. Substrate utilization by disused rat skeletal muscles. Am J Physiol 1974;226:295–297.

53. Holloszy JO, Booth FW. Biochemical adaptations to endurance exercise in muscle. Physiol Rev 1976;38:273–291.

54. Ferrando AA, Tipton KD, Bamman MM, Wolfe RR. Resistance exercise maintains skeletal muscle protein synthesis during bed rest. J Appl Physiol 1997;82(3):807–810.

55. Rubin CT, Lanyon LE. Regulation of bone formation by applied dynamic loads. J Bone Joint Surg 1984;66A:397–402.

56. Wbedon GD. Disuse osteoporosis: physiological aspects. Calcif Tissue Int 1984;36(Suppl 1):S146–S150.

57. Donaldson CL, Hulley SB, Vogel JM, et al. The effect of prolonged bed rest on bone mineral. Metabolism 1970;19:1071–1084.

58. Smith MC, Rambaut PC, Vogel JM, et al. Bone Mineral Measurement—Experiment M078. In RS Johnston, LF Dietlein (eds), Biomedical Results from Skylab. Cited by A LeBlanc, V Schneider, J Krebs, et al. Spinal bone mineral after 5 weeks of bed rest. Calcif Tissue Int 1987;41:259–261.

59. Hulley SB, Vogel JM, Donaldson CL, et al. The effect of supplemental oral phosphate on the bone mineral changes during prolonged bed rest. J Clin Invest 1971;50:2506–2518.

60. Nishimura Y, Fukuoka H, Kiriyama M, et al. Bone turnover and calcium metabolism during 20 days bed rest in young males and females. Acta Physiol Scand Suppl 1994;616:27–35.

61. Zerwekh JE, Ruml LA, Gottschalk F, Pak CY. The effects of twelve weeks of bed rest on bone histology, biochemical markers of bone turnover, and calcium homeostasis in eleven normal subjects. J Bone Miner Res 1998; 13(10):1594–1601.

62. LeBlanc A, Schneider V, Krebs J, et al. Spinal bone mineral after 5 weeks of bed rest. Calcif Tissue Int 1987;41:259–261.

63. Takata S, Yamashita Y, Masaki K, et al. Effects of bed rest on bone metabolism in patients with femoral neck fracture. Ann Physiol Anthropol 1993;12(6):321–325.

64. Nilsson BER. Post-traumatic osteopenia. Acta Orthop Scand 1966;91:1–55.

65. Rose GA. Immobilization osteoporosis. Br J Surg 1966;53:769–774.

66. Minaire P, Meunier P, Edouard C, et al. Quantitative histological data on disuse osteoporosis: comparison with biological data. Calcif Tissue Res 1974;17:57–73.

67. van der Wiel, Lips P, Nauta J, et al. Intranasal calcitonin suppresses increased bone resorption during short-term immobilization: a double-blind study of the effects of intranasal calcitonin on biochemical parameters of bone turnover. J Bone Miner Res 1993;8(12):1459–1465.

68. Ruml LA, Dubois SK, Roberts ML, Pak CY. Prevention of hypercalciuria and stone-forming propensity during prolonged bed rest by alendronate. J Bone Miner Res 1995;10(4):655–662.

69. Moses FM. The effect of exercise on the gastrointestinal tract. Sports Med 1990;9:159–172.

70. Dooley CP, Schlossmacher B, Valenzuela JE. Modulation of esophageal peristalsis by alterations of body position: effect of bolus viscosity. Dig Dis Sci 1989;34:1662–1667.

71. Moore JG, Datz FL, Christian PE, et al. Effect of body posture on radionuclide measurements of gastric emptying. Dig Dis Sci 1988;33:1592–1595.

72. Mojaverian P, Vlasses PH, Kellner PE, et al. Effects of gender, posture, and age on gastric residence time of an indi-

gestible solid: pharmaceutical considerations. Pharm Res 1988;5:639–644.

73. Sjovall H, Forssell H, Haggendal J, et al. Reflex sympathetic activation in humans is accompanied by inhibition of gastric HCO3-secretion. Am J Physiol 1988;255(6 Pt 1):G752–G758.

74. Evans DF, Foster GE, Hareastle JD. Does exercise affect small bowel motility in man. Gut 1989;A1012.

75. Sikirov B-A. Etiology and pathogenesis of diverticulosis coli: a new approach. Med Hypoth 1988;26:17–20.

76. LeBlanc A, Schneider V, Spector E, et al. Calcium absorption, endogenous excretion, and endocrine changes during and after long-term bed rest. Bone 1995;16(Suppl 4):301S–304S.

77. Blotner H. Effect of prolonged physical inactivity on tolerance of sugar. Arch Intern Med 1945;75:39–44.

78. Pawlson LG, Field JB, McCally M, et al. Effects of two weeks of bedrest on glucose, insulin and human growth hormone in response to glucose and arginine stimulation. Aerospace Med Abstr 1968;105.

79. Lipman RL, Schnure JJ, Bradley Em, et al. Impairment of peripheral glucose utilization in normal subjects by prolonged bed rest. J Lab Clin Med 1970;76:221–230.

80. Altman DF, Baker SD, McCally M, et al. Carbohydrate and lipid metabolism in man during prolonged bedrest. Clin Res 1969;17:543.

81. Stuart CA, Shangraw RE, Prince MF, et al. Bed-rest–induced insulin resistance occurs primarily in muscle. Metabolism 1988;37:802–806.

82. Shangraw RE, Stuart CA, Prince MF, et al. Insulin responsiveness of protein metabolism in vivo following bedrest in humans. Am J Physiol 1988;255:E548–E558.

83. Vernikos-Danellis J, Leach CS, Winget CM, et al. Changes in glucose, insulin and growth hormone levels associated with bedrest. Aviat Space Environ Med 1976;47:583–587.

84. Samel A, Wegmann HM, Vejvoda M. Response of the circadian system to 6 degree head-down tilt bed rest. Aviat Space Environ Med 1993;64(1):50–54.

85. Pequinot JM, Guell A, Gauquelin G, et al. Epinephrine, norephedrine and dopamine during a 4-day head-down bed-rest. J Appl Physiol 1985;58:157–163.

86. Stamatakis JD, Kakkar VV, Lawrence D, et al. Failure of aspirin to prevent postoperative deep vein thrombosis in patients undergoing total hip replacement. BMJ 1978;1:1031.

87. Bergqvist D, Efsing HO, Hallbrook T, et al. Thromboembolism after elective and post-traumatic hip surgery—a controlled prophylactic trial with dextran 70 and low-dose heparin. Acta Chir Scand 1979;145:213–218.

88. Schlosser V. Klinik, Prophylaxe und Therapie der Lungenembolie aus chirurgischer Sicht. In D Bergqvist (ed), Postoperative Thromboembolism: Frequency, Etiology, Prophylaxis. New York: Springer-Verlag, 1983.

89. Dalen J, Alpert J. Natural history of pulmonary embolism. Prog Cardiovasc Dis 1975;17:257–270.

90. Havig O. Deep vein thrombosis and pulmonary embolism. An autopsy study with multiple regression analysis of possible risk factors. Acta Chir Scand Suppl 1977;478:1–120.

91. Shull KC, Nicholaides AN, Fernandes e Fernandes J, et al. Significance of popliteal reflux in relation to ambulatory venous pressure and ulceration. Arch Surg 1979;114:1304–1306.

92. Haimovici H. Pathophysiology of Postphlebitic Syndrome with Leg Ulcer. In H Haimovici (ed), Haimovici's Vascular Surgery: Principles and Techniques. Norwalk, CT: Appleton & Lange, 1989;971–978.

93. Hewson W. Experimental Inquiries. In D Bergqvist (ed), Postoperative Thromboembolism: Frequency, Etiology, Prophylaxis. New York: Spring-Verlag, 1983;41.

94. Sevitt S. The structure and growth of valve-pocket thrombi in femoral veins. J Clin Path 1974;27:517–528.

95. Karino, T, Motomiya M. Vortices in the pockets of a venous valve. Microvasc Res 1981;21:247.

96. Malone PC, Hamer JD, Silver IA. Oxygen tension in venous valve pockets. Thromb Haemost 1979;42:230.

97. Hume M, Sevitt S, Thomas LP. Venous Thrombosis and Pulmonary Embolism. Cambridge: Harvard University Press, 1970.

98. Lough J, Moore S. Endothelial cell injury induced by thrombin or thrombi. Lab Invest 1975;33:130–135.

99. Mansfield A. Alterations in fibrinolysis associated with surgery and venous thrombosis. Br J Surg 1972;59:754–757.

100. Clark C, Cotton LT. Blood flow in deep veins of legs. Recording technique and evaluation of methods to increase flow during operation. Br J Surg 1968;55:211–214.

101. Bird AD. Effect of surgery, injury, and prolonged bedrest on calf blood flow. Aust NZ J Surg 1972;41:374–379.

102. Warlow C, Ogston D, Douglas AS. Deep venous thrombosis of the legs after strokes. Part I: Incidence and predisposing factors. BMJ 1976;1:1178–1183.

103. Marik PE, Andrews L, Maini B. The incidence of deep venous thrombosis in ICU patients. Chest 1997;111:661–664.

104. Blattler W. Ambulatory care for ambulant patients with deep vein thrombosis. J Mal Vasc 1991;16(2):137–141.

105. Partsch H, Kechavarz B, Kohn H, Mostbeck A. The effect of mobilization of patients during treatment of thromboembolic disorders with low-molecular-weight heparin. Int Angiol 1997;16(3):189–192.

106. Gmunder FK, Baisch F, Bechler B, et al. Effect of head-down tilt bed rest (10 days) on lymphocyte reactivity. Acta Physiol Scand Suppl 1992;604:131–141.

107. Klokker M, Secher NH, Madsen P, et al. Adrenergic beta 1- and beta 1+2-receptor blockade suppress the natural killer response to head-up tilt in humans. J Appl Physiol 1997;83(5):1492–1498.

108. Buckingham JC. Hypothalamo-pituitary responses to trauma. Br Med Bull 1985;41:203–211.

109. Goschke H, Bar E, Girard J, et al. Glucagon, insulin, cortisol, and growth hormone levels following major surgery: their relationship to human prolactin and growth hormone release during surgery and other conditions of stress. J Clin Endocrinol Metab 1972;35:840–851.

110. Newsome HH, Rose JC. The response of adrenocorticotrophic hormone and growth hormone to surgical stress. Horm Metab Res 1978;10:465–470.

111. Korpassy A, Stoekel H, Vecsec P. Investigations of hydrocortisone secretion and aldosterone excretion in patients with severe prolonged stress. Acta Anaesthesiol Scand 1972;16:161–168.

112. Cochrane JP, Forsling ML, Gow NM, et al. Arginine vasopressin release following surgical operations. Br J Surg 1981;68:209–213.

113. Cuthberson DP. The disturbance of metabolism produced by bony and non-bony injury with notes on certain abnormal conditions of bone. Biochem J 1930;24:1244–1263.

114. Kinney JM (ed), The Application of Indirect Calorimetry to Clinical Studies. Assessment of Energy Metabolism in Health and Disease. Columbus, OH: Ross Laboratories, 1980;42–45.

115. Imamura M, Clowes GHA Jr, Blackburn GL. Liver metabolism and gluconeogenesis in trauma and sepsis. Surgery 1975;77:868–880.

116. Lequesne LP, Cochrane JPS, Feldman NR. Fluid and electrolyte disturbances after trauma: the role of adrenocortical and pituitary hormones. Br Med Bull 1985;41:212–217.

117. Meguid MM, Brennan MF, Aoki TT, et al. Hormone-substrate interrelationships following trauma. Arch Surg 1974;109:776–783.

118. Kuntscher FR, Galletti PM, Hahn C, et al. Alterations of insulin and glucose metabolism during cardiopulmonary bypass under normothermia. J Thorac Cardiovasc Surg 1985;89:97–106.

119. Frayn KN. Substrate turnover after injury. Br Med Bull 1985;4:232–239.

120. Oppenheim WL, Williamson DH, Smith R. Early biochemical changes and severity of injury in man. J Trauma 1980;20:135–140.

121. Rolih CA, Ober KP. The endocrine response to critical illness. Med Clin North Am 1995;79:211–224.

122. Chernow B, Alexander HR, Smallridge RC, et al. Hormonal responses to graded surgical stress. Arch Intern Med 1987;147:1273–1277.

123. Webster EL, Torpy DJ, Elenkou IJ, et al. Corticotropin-releasing hormone and inflammation. Ann N Y Acad Sci 1998;840:21–23.

124. Rivier C, Plotsky P. Mediation by corticotropin-releasing factor (CRP) of adenohypophyseal hormone secretion. Annu Rev Physiol 1986;48:475–498.

125. Crozier TA, Drobnick L, Stafforst D, et al. Opiate modulation of the stress-induced increase of vasoactive intestinal peptide (VIP) in plasma. Horm Metab Res 1988;20:352–356.

126. Ametz BB. Endocrine reactions during standardized surgical stress: the effects of age and methods of anaesthesia. Age Ageing 1985;14:96–101.

127. Noel GL, Suh HK, Stone JG, et al. Human prolactin and growth hormone release during surgery and other conditions of stress. J Clin Endocrinol Metab 1972;35:840–851.

128. McCann SM, Kimura M, Karanth S, et al. Role of nitric oxide in the neuroendocrine responses to cytokines. Ann N Y Acad Sci 1998;840:174–184.

129. Breslow MJ, Jordan DA, Christopherson R, et al. Epidural morphine decreases postoperative hypertension by attenuating sympathetic nervous system hyperactivity. JAMA 1989;261:3577–3581.

130. Chan V, Wang C, Yeung RTY. Pituitary-thyroid response to surgical stress. Acta Endocrinol 1978;88:490–498.

131. Von Bormann B, Weidler B, Dennhardt R, et al. Influence of epidural fentanyl on stress-induced elevation of plasma vasopressin after surgery. Anesth Analg 1983;62:727–732.

132. Dreyfuss D, Leviel F, Paillard M, et al. Acute infectious pneumonia is accompanied by a latent vasopressin-dependent impairment of renal water excretion. Am Rev Respir Dis 1988;138:583–589.

133. McAlpine HM, Cobbe SM. Neuroendocrine changes in myocardial infarction. Am J Med 1988;84(Suppl 3A):61–66.

134. McAlpine HM, Morton JJ, Leckie B, et al. Neuroendocrine activation after acute myocardial infarction. Br Heart J 1988;60:117–124.

135. Widerlov E, Ekman R, Jensen L, et al. Arginine vasopressin, but not corticotropin-releasing factor, is a potent stimulator of adrenocorticotropic hormone following electroconvulsive treatment. J Neural Transm 1989;75:101–109.

136. Moran WH, Mittenberger FW, Shuayl WA, et al. Relationship of anti-diuretic hormone secretion to surgical stress. Surgery 1964;56:99–107.

137. Wu WH, Zbuzek VK. Vasopressin and anesthesia and surgery. Bull N Y Acad Med 1982;58:427–442.

138. Erkut ZA, Pool C, Swaab DF. Glucocorticoids suppress corticotropin-releasing hormone and vasopressin expression in human hypothalamic neurons. J Clin Endocrinol Metab 1998;83:2066–2073.

139. Salata RAM, Jarrett DB, Verablis JG, et al. Vasopressin stimulation of adrenocorticotropin hormone (ACTH) in humans. J Clin Invest 1988;81:66–74.

140. Gaillard RC, Riondel AM, Ling N, et al. Corticotropin releasing factor activity of CRF 41 in normal man is potentiated by angiotensin 11 and vasopressin but not desmopressin. Life Sci 1988;43:1935–1944.

141. Reisine T. Neurohumoral aspects of ACTH release. Hosp Pract 1988;23:77–96.

142. Engquist A, Fog-Moller F, Christiansen C, et al. Influence of epidural analgesia on the catecholamine and cyclic AMP response to surgery. Acta Anaesthesiol Scand 1980;24:17–21.

143. Brandt MR, Olguard K, Kehlet H. Epidural analgesia inhibits renin and aldosterone response to surgery. Acta Anaesthesiol Scand 1979;23:267–272.

144. Engquist A, Brandt MR, Fernandes A, et al. The blocking effects of epidural analgesia on the adrenocortical and hyperglycemia responses to surgery. Acta Anaesthesiol Scand 1977;21:330–335.

145. Kehlet H. Epidural analgesia and the endocrine-metabolism response to surgery: update and perspectives. Acta Anaesthesiol Scand 1984;28:25–127.

146. Segewa H, Mori K, Kasai K, et al. The role of the phrenic nerves in the stress response in upper abdominal surgery. Anesth Analg 1996;82:1215–1224.

147. George JM, Reier CE, Lanese RR, et al. Morphine anaesthesia blocks cortisol and growth hormone response to surgical stress in humans. J Clin Endocrinol Metab 1974;38:736–741.

148. Walsh ES, Paterson JL, O'Riordan JBA, et al. Effect of high dose fentanyl anaesthesia on the metabolic and endocrine response to cardiac surgery. Br J Anaesth 1981;53:1155–1165.

149. Woolf PD, Hamill RW, Lee LA, et al. Free and total catecholamines in critical illness. Am J Physiol 1988;254:E287–E291.

150. Davies CL, Molyneux SG, Newman RJ. HPLC determination of plasma catecholamines in road accident casualties. Br J Clin Pharmacol 1981;13:283P.

151. Frayn KN, Little RA, Maycock PE, et al. The relationship of plasma catecholamines to acute metabolic and hormonal responses to injury in man. Circ Shock 1985;6:229–240.

152. Benedict CR, Grahame-Smith DG. Plasma noradrenaline and adrenaline concentrations and dopamine-beta-hydroxylase activity in patients with shock due to septicemia, trauma, and haemorrhage. QJM 1978;185:1–20.155.

153. Jaattela A, Alho A, Avikainen V, et al. Plasma catecholamines in severely injured patients: a prospective study on 45 patients with multiple injuries. Br J Surg 1975;62:177–181.

154. Sametz W, Metzler H, Greis M, et al. Perioperative catecholamine changes in cardiac risk patients. Eur J Clin Invest 1999;26:582–587.

155. Yoshizumi M, Mikitagawa T, Ozawa Y, et al. Changes in plasma free and sulfoconjugated catecholamines during the perioperative period of cardiac surgery: effect of continuous infusion of dopamine. Biol Pharm Bull 1998;21:787–791.

156. Davies CL, Newman RJ, Molyneux SG, et al. The relationship between plasma catecholamines and severity of injury in man. J Trauma 1984;24:99–105.

157. Nistrup-Madsen S, Fog-Moller F, Christiansen C, et al. Cyclic AMP, adrenaline, and non-adrenaline in plasma during surgery. Br J Surg 1978;65:191–193.

158. Butler MJ, Britton BJ, Wood WG, et al. Plasma catecholamine concentrations during operations. Br J Surg 1977;64:786–790.

159. Stanley TH, Berman L, Green O, et al. Plasma catecholamine and cortisol responses to fentanyl-oxygen anesthesia for coronary-artery operations. Anesthesiology 1980;53:250–253.

160. Halter JB, Pflug AE, Porte D. Mechanism of plasma catecholamine increases during surgical stress in man. J Clin Endocrinol Metab 1977;45:936–940.

161. Ester M. Assessment of sympathetic nervous function in humans from norepinephrine plasma kinetics. Clin Sci 1982;62:247–254.

162. Ester M, Jennings G, Korner P, et al. Measurements of total and organ specific kinetics in humans. Am J Physiol 1984;247:E21–E28.

163. Hilsted J, Christiansen NJ, Madsbad S. Whole body clearance of norepinephrine. J Clin Invest 1983;71:500–505.

164. Christiansen NJ, Hilsted J, Hegedus L, et al. Effects of surgical stress and insulin on cardiovascular function and norepinephrine kinetics. Am J Physiol 1984;247:E29–E34.

165. Leinhardt DJ, Arnold J, Shipley KA, et al. Plasma norepinephrine concentrations do not accurately reflect sympathetic nervous system activity in human sepsis. Am J Physiol 1993;265:E284–E288.

166. Deibert DC, DeFronzo RA. Epinephrine-induced insulin resistance in man. J Clin Invest 1980;65:717–721.

167. Waldhaus WK, Gasic S, Bratusch-Marrain P, et al. Effect of stress hormones on splanchnic substrate and insulin disposal after glucose ingestion in healthy humans. Diabetes 1987;36:127–135.

168. Fryberg DA, Gelfand RA, Jahn LA, et al. Effects of epinephrine on human muscle glucose and protein metabolism. Am J Physiol 1995;268:E55–E59.

169. Hendler RG, Sherwin RS. Epinephrine-stimulated glucose production is not diminished by starvation: evidence for an effect on gluconeogenesis. J Clin Endocrinol Metab 1984;58:1014–1021.

170. Matthews DE, Pesola G, Campbell RG. Effects of epinephrine on amino acid and energy metabolism in humans. Am J Physiol 1990;258:E948–E956.

171. Fong YM, Albert JD, Tracy K, et al. The influence of substrate background on the absolute metabolic response to epinephrine and cortisol. J Trauma 1991;31:1467–1476.

172. Tayek JA, Katz J. Glucose production, recycling, Cori cycle, and gluconeogenesis in humans: relationship to serum cortisol. Am J Physiol 1997;273:E476–E484.

173. Darmaun D, Mathews DE, Beir DM. Physiological hypercortisolemia increases proteolysis, glutamine and alanine production. Am J Physiol 1988;255:E366–E373.

174. Dinneen S, Alzaid A, Miles S, et al. Metabolic effects of nocturnal rise in cortisol on carbohydrate metabolism in normal humans. J Clin Invest 1993;92:2283–2290.

175. Divertie GD, Jensen MD, Miles JM. Stimulation of lipolysis in humans by physiological hypercortisolemia. Diabetes 1991;40:1228–1232.

176. Louard RJ, Bhushan R, Gelfand RA, et al. Glucocorticoids antagonize insulin's antiproteolytic action on skeletal muscle in humans. J Clin Endocrinol Metab 1994;79:278–284.

177. Dahanukar SA, Thatte UM, Deshumukh OD, et al. The influence of stress on the psychoneural-endocrine-immune axis. J Postgrad Med 1996;42:12–14.

178. Munck A, Naray-Fejes-Toth A. Glucocorticoids and stress: permissive and suppressive actions. Ann NY Acad Sci 1994;746:115–131.

179. Ottosson M, Lonnoroth P, Bjontorp P, et al. Effects of cortisol and growth hormone on lipolysis in human adipose tissue. J Clin Endocrinol Metab 2000;85:799–803.

180. Morand EF, Leech M. Glucocorticoid regulation of inflammation: the plot thickens. Inflamm Res 1999;48:557–560.

181. Lendingham IM, Watt I. Influence of sedation on mortality in critically ill multiple trauma patient. Lancet 1983;1:1270.

182. Wagner RL, White PF, Kan PB, et al. Inhibition of adrenal steroidogenesis by the anesthetic etomidate. N Engl J Med 1984;310:1415–1421.

183. Moore RA, Allen MC, Wood PJ, et al. Perioperative endocrine effects of etomidate. Anaesthesia 1985;40:124–130.

184. Ganong WR. The stress response—a dynamic overview. Hosp Pract 1988;23:155–171.

185. Newsome NH, Rose JC. The response of human adrenocorticotrophic hormone and growth hormone to surgical stress. J Clin Endocrinol 1971;33:481–487.

186. Vogeser M, Felbinger TW, Kilger E, et al. Corticosteroid-binding globulin and free cortisol in the early postoperative period after cardiac surgery. Clin Biochem 1999;32:213–216.

187. Perrot D, Bonneton A, Dechaud H, et al. Hypercortisolism in septic shock is not suppressible by dexamethasone infusion. Crit Care Med 1993;21:396–401.

188. Garrel DR. Corticosteroid-binding globulin during inflammation and burn injury: nutritional modulation and clinical implications. Horm Res 1996;45:245–251.

189. Bladon PT, Rowlands TE, Whittaker JA, Oakley RE. Serum cortisol binding capacity measured with Concanavalin-A-Sepharose in patients with a recent inflammation response. Clin Chim Acta 1996;253:9–20.

190. Barton RN, Passingham BJ. Effect of binding to plasma proteins on the integration of plasma cortisol concentrations after accidental injury. Clin Sci 1981;61:399–405.

191. Calogero AE, Norton JA, Shappard BC, et al. Pulsatile activation of the hypothalamic-pituitary-adrenal axis during major surgery. Metabolism 1992;41:839–845.

192. McIntosh TK, Lothrop DA, Lee A, et al. Circadian rhythm of cortisol is altered in postsurgical patients. J Clin Endocrinol Metab 1981;53:117–122.

193. Lanuza DM. Postoperative circadian rhythms and cortisol stress response to two types of cardiac surgery. Am J Crit Care 1995;4:212–220.

194. Doncaster HD, Barton RN, Horan MA, et al. Factors influencing cortisol-adrenocorticotropin relationships in elderly women with upper femur fractures. J Trauma 1993;34:49–55.

195. Jeffries MK, Vance ML. Growth hormone and cortisol secretion in patients with burn injury. J Burn Care Rehabil 1992;13:391–395.

196. Rivier C, Rivest S. Effect of stress on the activity of the hypothalamic-pituitary-gonadal axis: peripheral and central mechanism. Biol Reprod 1991;45:523–528.

197. Chrousos GP, Torpy DJ, Gold PW. Interactions between the hypotha-

lamic-pituitary-adrenal axis and the female reproductive system: clinical implications. Ann Int Med 1998;129:229–240.

198. Spratt DI, Cox P, Orar J, et al. Reproductive axis suppression in acute illness is related to disease severity. J Clin Endocrinol Metab 1993;76:1548–1554.

199. Semple CG, Mitchell R, Hollis S, Robertson WR. An investigation of LH pulsatility in burned men by bioassay and radioimmunoassay. Acta Endocrinol (Copenh) 1992;126:404–409.

200. Lindh A, Carlstrom K, Eklund J, et al. Steroid and prolactin during and after major surgical trauma. Acta Anesthesiol Scand 1992;36:119–124.

201. Batrinos ML, Panitsa-Faflia C, Koutsoumanis C, et al. Surgical stress induces a marked and sustained increase of adrenal androgen secretion in postmenopausal women. In Vivo 1999;13:147–150.

202. Chibber VL, Soriano C, Tayek JA. Effects of low-dose and high-dose glucagon on glucose production and gluconeogenesis in humans. Metabolism 2000 49:39–46.

203. Lyengar R, Schwartz TL, Brinbaumer L. Coupling of glucagon receptors to adenylcyclase. J Biol Chem 1979;254:1119–1123.

204. Perea A, Clemente F, Martinell J, et al. Physiological effect of glucagon in human isolated adipocyte. Horm Metab Res 1995;27:372–375.

205. Carlson MG, Snead WL, Campbell PJ. Regulation of free fatty acid metabolism by glucagon. J Clin Endocrinol Metab 1993;77:11–15.

206. Jensen MD, Heiling VJ, Miles JM. Effects of glucagon on free fatty acid metabolism in humans. J Clin Endocrinol Metab 1991;72:308–315.

207. Wise JK, Hendler R, Felig R. Influence of glucocorticoids on glucagon secretion and plasma amino acid concentrations in man. J Clin Invest 1973;52:2774–2782.

208. Unger RH, Orce L. Glucagon and the delta cell. N Engl J Med 1981;304:4518–4575.

209. Russell RCG, Walker CJ, Bloom SR. Hyperglucagonemia in the surgical patient. BMJ 1985;1:10–12.

210. DelPratto S, Riccio A, Vigili de Kreutzenberg S, et al. Basal plasma insulin levels exert a qualitative but not quantitative effect on glucose-mediated glucose uptake. Am J Physiol 1995;268:E1089–E1095.

211. Jacob S, Hauer B, Becker R, et al. Lipolysis in skeletal muscle is rapidly regulated by low physiological doses of insulin. Diabetologia 1999;42:1171–1174.

212. Groop LC, Bonadonna RC, Shank M, et al. Role of free fatty acids and insulin in determining free fatty acid and lipid oxidation in man. J Clin Invest 1991;87:83–89.

213. Bonadonna RC, Saccomani MP, Cobelli C, et al. Effect of insulin on system amino acid transport in human skeletal muscle. J Clin Invest 1993;91:514–521.

214. Holter JB, Pflug AE. Effects of anesthesia and surgical stress on insulin secretion in man. Metabolism 1980;29:1124–1127.

215. Unger RH. Glucagon and insulin: glucagon ratio in diabetes and other catabolic illnesses. Diabetes 1971;20:834–838.

216. Meguid MM, Aun F, Soeldner JS. The effect of severe trauma on urine loss of insulin. Surgery 1976;79:177–181.

217. Nakoo K, Miyata M. The influence of phentolamine on adrenergic blocking agent on insulin secretion during surgery. Eur J Clin Invest 1977;7:41–45.

218. Giovanni I, Boldrini G, Castagneto M, et al. Respiratory quotient and patterns of substrate utilization in human sepsis and trauma. JPEN J Parenter Enteral Nutr 1983;7:226–231.

219. Wolfe RR, Burk JF. Somatostatin infusion inhibits glucose production in burn patients. Circ Shock 1982;9:521–527.

220. Wolfe RR, Hemdon DN, Jahoor F, et al. Effect of severe burn injury on substrate cycling by glucose and fatty acids. N Engl J Med 1982;317:397–408.

221. Shamoon H, Hendler R, Sherwin RS. Synergistic interactions among anti-insulin hormones in the pathogenesis of stress hyperglycemia in humans. J Clin Endocrinol Metab 1981;52:1235–1241.

222. Thoss VS, Perez J, Probst A, Hoyer D. Expression of five somatostatin receptor mRNAs in the human brain and pituitary. Naunyn Schmiedebergs Arch Pharmacol 1996:354:411–419.

223. Felig P, Marliss EB, Cahill GF. Metabolic response to human growth hormone during prolonged starvation. J Clin Invest 1971;50:411–421.

224. Hussain MA, Schmitz O, Mengel A, et al. Insulin-like grown factor 1 stimulates lipid oxidation, reduces protein oxidation and enhances insulin sensitivity in humans. J Clin Invest 1993;92:2249–2256.

225. Aarimaa A, Gryvalahati E, Viikari J, et al. Insulin, growth hormone, and cate-cholamines as regulators of energy metabolism in the course of surgery. Acta Chir Scand 1978;144:411–422.

226. Melarvie S, Jeevanandam M, Holaday NJ, et al. Pulsatile nature of growth hormone levels in critically trauma victims. Surgery 1995;117:402–408.

227. Jeevanandam M, Holaday NJ, Petersen SR. Plasma levels of insulin-like growth factor binding protein-3 in acute trauma patients. Metabolism 1995;44:1205–1208.

228. Davies SC, Wass JAH, Ross RJM, et al. The induction of a specific protease for insulin-like growth factor binding protein-3 in the circulatory during severe illness. J Endocrinol 1991;130:469–473.

229. Girvent M, Maestro S, Hernandez R, et al. Euthyroid sick syndrome associated endocrine abnormalities and outcome in elderly patients undergoing emergency operations. Surgery 1998;123:560–567.

230. Fliers F, Guldenaar SE, Wiersinger WM, et al. Decreased hypothalamic thyrotropin-releasing hormone gene expression in patients with nonthyroidal illness. J Clin Endocrinol Metab 1997;82:4032–4036.

231. Adriaanse R, Romijn JA, Branbant G, et al. Pulsatile thyrotropin secretion in nonthyroidal illness. J Clin Endocrinol Metab 1993;77:1313–1317.

232. Bartalena L, Martino E, Brandi LS, et al. Lack of nocturnal serum thyrotropin surge after surgery. J Clin Endocrinol Metab 1990;70:293–296.

233. Magner J, Roy P, Fainter L, et al. Transient decreased sialylation of thyrotropin (TSH) in a patient with the thyroid sick syndrome. Thyroid 1997;7:55–61.

234. van der Poll T, Endert E, Coyle SM, et al. Neutralization of TNF does not influence endotoxin induced changes in thyroid hormone metabolism in humans. Am J Physiol 1999;276:R357–R362.

235. Stouthard JM, van der Poll T, Endert E, et al. Effects of acute and chronic interleukin-6 administration on thyroid hormone metabolism in humans. J Clin Endocrinol Metab 1994;79:1342–1346.

236. van der Poll T, Van Zee KJ, Endert E, et al. Interleukin-1 receptor blockade does not effect endotoxin-induced changes in plasma thyroid hormone and thyrotropin concentrations in man. J Clin Endocrinol Metab 1995;80:1341–1346.

237. Kaptein EM, Spencer CA, Kamiel MB, et al. Prolonged dopamine administration and thyroid hormone economy in

normal and critically ill subjects. J Clin Endocrinol Metab 1980;51:387–393.

238. Van den Berghe G, de Zegher F, Lauwers P, et al. Dopamine and the sick euthyroid syndrome in critical illness. Clin Endocrinol (Oxf) 1994;41:731–737.

239. Van den Berghe G, de Zegher F, Vlasselaers D, et al. Thyrotropin-releasing hormone in critical illness: from a dopamine-dependent test to a strategy for increasing low serum tri-iodothyronine, prolactin and growth hormone concentrations. Crit Care Med 1996;24:590–595.

240. Bennett-Guerrero E, Jimenez JL, White WD, et al. Cardiovascular effects of intravenous triiodothyronine in patients undergoing coronary artery bypass graft surgery. A randomized, double-blind, placebo-controlled trial. Duke T3 study group. JAMA 1996;275:687–692.

241. Broderick TJ, Wechsler AS. Triiodothyronine in cardiac surgery. Thyroid 1997;7:133–137.

242. Afandi B, Schussler GC, Arafah AH, et al. Selective consumption of thyroxine-binding globulin during cardiac bypass surgery. Metabolism 2000;49:270–274.

243. Kaisner S. Mechanism of hydrocortisone potentiation of responses to epinephrine and norepinephrine in rabbit aorta. Circ Res 1969;24:383–395.

244. Geddes BA, Jones TR, Dvorsky RJ, et al. Interaction of glucocorticoids and bronchodilators on isolated guinea pig trachea and human bronchial smooth muscle. Am Rev Respir Dis 1974;110:420–427.

245. Chung KF. The complementary role of glucocorticoids and long-acting beta-adrenergic agonists. Allergy 1998;53:7–13.

246. Singh M, Notternan DA, Metakis L. Tumor necrosis factor produces homologous desensitization of lymphocyte beta-2-adrenergic responses. Circ Shock 1993;39:375–378.

247. Bessey PQ, Watters JM, Aoki TT, et al. Combined hormonal infusion stimulates the metabolic response to injury. Ann Surg 1984;200:264–280.

248. Gelfand RA, Matthews DE, Bier DM, et al. Role of counterregulatory hormones in the catabolic response to stress. J Clin Invest 1984;74:2238–2248.

249. Watters JM, Bessey PQ, Dinarello CA, et al. The induction of interleukin-1 in humans and its metabolic effects. Surgery 1985;98:298–305.

250. Watters JM, Bessey PQ, Dinarello CA, et al. Both inflammatory and endo-crine mediators stimulate host responses to sepsis. Arch Surg 1986;121:179–190.

251. Elenkov IJ, Papanicolou DA, Wilder RL, et al. Modulatory effects of glucocorticoids and catecholamines on human interleukin-12 and interleukin-10 production: clinical implications. Proc Assoc Am Physicians 1996;108:374–381.

252. Riche FC, Cholley BP, Panis YH, et al. Inflammatory cytokine response in patients with septic shock secondary to generalized peritonitis. Crit Care Med 2000;28:433–437.

253. Weighardt H, Heidcke CD, Emmanuilidis K, et al. Sepsis after major visceral surgery is associated with sustained and interferon-gamma resistant defects of monocyte cytokine production. Surgery 2000;127:309–315.

254. Cryssikopoulos A. The relationship between the immune and endocrine systems. Ann N Y Acad Sci 1997;816:83–93.

255. Mastrakos G, Chroousos GP, Weber JS. Recombinant interleukin-6 activates the hypothalamic-pituitary-adrenal axis in humans. J Clin Endocrinl Metab 1993;77:1690–1694.

256. Rubinstein M, Dinarello CA, Oppenheim JJ, et al. Recent advances in cytokines, cytokine receptors and signal transduction. Cytokine Growth Factor Rev 1998;9:175–181.

257. Fernandez-Botran R. Soluble cytokine receptors: basic immunology and clinical applications. Crit Rev Clin Lab Sci 1999;36:165–224.

258. Dinarello CA. Interleukin-1. Cytokine Growth Factor Rev 1997;8:253–265.

259. Dinarello CA. The interleukin-1 family: 10 years of discovery. FASEB J 1994;8:1314–1325.

260. Kaushansky K, Lin N, Adamson JW. Interleukin 1 stimulates fibroblasts to synthesize granulocyte macrophage- and granulocyte colony-stimulating factors. J Clin Invest 1988;81:92–97.

261. Clark SC, Kame R. The human hematopoietic colony-stimulating factors. Science 1987;236:1229–1236.

262. Miyajima A, Miyatake S, Schreurs J, et al. Co-ordinate regulation of immune and inflammatory responses by T-cell-derived lymphokines. FASEB J 1988;2:2462–2473.

263. Broudy VC, Kaushansky K, Harlan J, et al. Interleukin 1 stimulates human endothelial cells to produce granulocyte colony stimulating factors. J Immunol 1987;139:464–468.

264. Dinarello CA. Cytokines as endoge-nous pyrogens. J Infect Dis 1999;179(Suppl 2):S294–S304.

265. Dinarello CA, Gatti S, Bartfai T. Fever: links with an ancient receptor. Curr Biol 1999;9:R147–R150.

266. Kaplanski L, Farnarier C, Kaplanski S, et al. Interleukin-1 induces interleukin-8 secretion from endothelial cells by a juxtacrine mechanism. Blood 1994;84:4242–4248.

267. Cannon JG, Tomkins RG, Gelfand JA, et al. Circulating interleukin-1 and tumor necrosis factor in septic shock and experimental endotoxin fever. J Infect Dis 1990;161:79–84.

268. Schulte HM, Bamberger CM, Eisen H, et al. Systemic interleukin alpha and interleukin-2 secretion in response to acute stress and to corticotropin-release hormone in humans. Eur J Clin Invest 1994;24:773–777.

269. Baigrie RJ, Lamount PM, Dallman M, et al. The release of interleukin-1 beta (IL-1) precedes that of interleukin-6 (IL-6) in patients undergoing major surgery. Lymphokine Cytokine Res 1991;10:253–256.

270. Avend WP, Malyak M, Guthridge CJ, et al. Interleukin-1 receptor antagonist: role in biology. Ann Rev Immunol 1998;16:27–55.

271. Kruimel JW, Pesmon GJ, Sweep CG, et al. Depression of plasma levels of cytokines and ex-vivo cytokine production in relation to the activity of the pituitary-adrenal-axis, in patients undergoing major vascular surgery. Cytokine 1999;11:382–388.

272. Fischer E, Van Zeek KJ, Marano MA, et al. Interleukin-1 receptor antagonist circulates in experimental inflammation and in human disease. Blood 1992;79:2196–2200.

273. Rogy MA, Coyle SM, Oldenburg HS, et al. Persistently elevated soluble tumor necrosis factor receptor and interleukin-1 receptor antagonist levels in critically ill patients. J Am Coll Surg 1994;178:132–138.

274. Arzt E, Sauer J, Polmucher T, et al. Glucocorticoids suppress interleukin-1 receptor antagonist synthesis following induction by endotoxin. Endocrinology 1994;134:672–677.

275. Santos AA, Schelting MR, Lynch E, et al. Elaboration of interleukin-1-receptor antagonist is no attenuated by glucocorticoids after endotoxemia. Arch Surg 1993;128:138–144.

276. Boermeester MA, van Leeuwen PA, Coyle SM, et al. Interleukin-1 block-ade attenuates mediator release and dysregulation of the hemostatic mecha-

nism during human sepsis. Arch Surg 1995;130:739–748.

277. Van Zeek KJ, Coyle SM, Calvano SE, et al. Influence of IL-1 receptor block-ade on the human response to endotox-emia. J Immunol 1995;154:1499–1507.

278. Preas HL Jr, Reda D, Tropea M, et al. Effects of recombinant soluble type I interleukin-1 receptor on human inflammatory responses to endotoxin. Blood 1996;88:2465–2472.

279. Vannier E, Karser A, Atkins MB, et al. Elevated circulating levels of soluble interleukin-1 receptor type II during interleukin-2 immunotherapy. Eur Cytokine Netw 1999;10:37–42.

280. O'Noallain EM, Puri P, Mealy K, et al. Induction of interleukin-1 receptor antagonist (IL-1ra) following surgery is associated with major trauma. Clin Immunol Immunopathol 195;76:96–101.

281. Mandrup-Poulsen T, Wogensen LD, Jensen M, et al. Circulating interleu-kin-1 receptor antagonist concentra-tions are increased in adult patients with thermal injury. Crit Care Med 1995;23:26–33.

282. Priutt JH, Welborn MB, Edwards PD, et al. Increased soluble interleukin-1 type II receptor concentrations in post-operative patients and in patients with sepsis syndrome. Blood 1996;87:3282–3288.

283. Tracey KJ, Cerami A. Tumor necrosis factor: a pleiotropic cytokine and ther-apeutic target. Annu Rev Med 1994;45:491–503.

284. Tannahill CL, Fukuzuka K, Marum T, et al. Discordant tumor necrosis factor-alpha superfamily gene expression in bacterial peritonitis and endotoxemic shock. Surgery 1999;126:349–357.

285. Dinarello CA. Role of pro and anti-inflammatory cytokines during inflam-mation: experimental and clinical find-ings. J Biol Homeost Agents 1997;11:91–103.

286. Shanley TP, Warner RL, Ward PA. The role of cytokines and adhesion molecules in the development of inflammatory injury. Mol Med Today 1995;1:40–45.

287. Aosasa S, Ono S, Mochizuki H, et al. Activation of monocytes and endothelial cells depends on the severity of surgical stress. World J Surg 2000;24:10–16.

289. Helmy SA, Wahby MA, El-Nawaway M. The effect of anaesthesia and sur-gery on plasma cytokine production. Anaesthesia 1999;54:733–738.

289. Curtis GE, McAtear CA, Formela L, et al. The effect of nutritional status on

the cytokine and acute phase protein responses to elective surgery. Cytokine 1995;7:380–388.

290. Reith HB, Kaman S, Mittelkotter O, et al. Cytokine activation in patients undergoing open or laparoscopic cholecystectomy. Int Surg 1997;82:389–393.

291. Jiang J, Tian K, Chen H, et al. Kinetics of plasma cytokines and its clinical sig-nificance in patients with severe trauma. Chin Med J (Engl) 1997;110:923–926.

292. Majetschak M, Flach R, Heukamp T, et al. Regulation of whole blood tumor necrosis factor product upon endo-toxin stimulation after severe blunt trauma. J Trauma 1997;43:880–887.

293. Keel M, Ecknauer E, Stocker R, et al. Different pattern of local and systemic release of proinflammatory and anti-inflammatory mediators in severely injured patients with chest trauma. J Trauma 1996;40:907–914.

294. Vindenes HA, Ulvestad E, Bjerkenes R. Concentrations of cytokines in plasma of patients with large burns: their rela-tion to time after injury, burn size, inflammatory variables, infection, and outcome. Eur J Surg 1998;164:647–656.

295. Papini RP, Wilson AP, Steer JA, et al. Plasma concentrations of tumour necrosis factor-alpha and interleukin-6 during burn wound surgery and dress-ing. Br J Plast Surg 1997;50:354–361.

296. Ottaway CA, Fong IW, de Silva B, et al. Integrative aspects of a human model of endotoxemia. Can J Physiol Pharmacol 1998;76:473–478.

297. Strieter RM, Kunkel SL, Bone RC. Role of tumor necrosis factor-alpha in disease stated and inflammation. Crit Care Med 1993;21(Suppl):S447–S463.

298. Neilson D, Kavanaugh JP, Rao PN. Kinetics of circulating TNF-alpha and TNF soluble receptors following sur-gery in a clinical model of sepsis. Cytokine 1996;8:938–943.

299. Ertel W, Scholl FA, Gallati H, et al. Increased release of soluble tumor necrosis factor receptors into blood during clinical sepsis. Arch Surg 1994;129:1330–1337.

300. Aderka D. The potential biological and clinical significance of the tumor necro-sis factor receptors. Cytokine Growth Factor Rev 1996;7:231–240.

301. Pellerini JD, Puyana JC, Lachak PH, et al. A membrane TNF-alpha/TNFR ratio correlates to MODS score and mortality. Circ Shock 1996;6:389–396.

302. Zhang B, Huang YH, Chen Y, et al. Plasma tumor necrosis factor-alpha, its

soluble receptors and interleukin-1 beta levels in critically burned patients. Burns 1998;24:599–603.

303. Goldie AS, Fearon KC, Ross JA, et al. Natural cytokine antagonists and endogenous antiendotoxin core anti-bodies in sepsis syndrome. The Sepsis Intervention Group. JAMA 1995;274:172–177.

304. Cinat ME, Waxman K, Granger GA, et al. Trauma causes sustained elevation of soluble tumor necrosis factor recep-tors. J Am Coll Surg 1994;176:529–537.

305. Riche F, Panis Y, Laishe MJ, et al. High tumor necrosis factor serum level is associated with increased survival in patients with abdominal septic shock: prospective study in 59 patients. Sur-gery 1996;120:801–807.

306. Endo S, Inadak K, Nakoe H, et al. Plasma levels of type III phospholipase A2 and cytokines in patients with sep-sis. Res Commun Mol Pathol Pharma-col 1995;90:413–421.

307. Mira JP, Cariou A, Gral F, et al. Asso-ciation of TNF2, a TNF-alpha pro-moter polymorphism, with septic shock susceptibility and mortality: a multicenter study. JAMA 1999;282:561–568.

308. Tracey KJ, Beutler B, Lowry SP, et al. Shock and tissue injury induced by recombinant human cachectin. Sci-ence 1986;234:470–474.

309. Waage A, Halstensen A, Espevik T. Association between tumor necrosis factor in serum and fatal outcome in patients with meningococcal disease. Lancet 1987;1:355–357.

310. Michie HR, Mangue KR, Spriggs DR, et al. Detection of circulating tumor necrosis factor after endotoxin admin-istration. N Engl J Med 1988;318:1481–1486.

311. Spinas GA, Keller U, Brockhaus M. Release of soluble receptors for tumor necrosis factor (TNF) in relation to cir-culating TNF during experimental endotoxemia. J Clin Invest 1992;90:533–536.

312. Suffredini AF, Reda D, Banks SM, et al. Effects of recombinant dimeric TNF receptor on human inflammatory responses following intravenous endo-toxin administration. J Immunol 1995;155:5038–5045.

313. Cain BS, Meldrum DR, Dinarello CA, et al. Tumor necrosis factor-alpha and interleukin-1 beta synergistically depress human myocardial function. Crit Care Med 1999 27:1309–1318.

314. Meldrum DR, Meng X, Dinarello CA,

et al. Human myocardial tissue TNF alpha expression following acute global ischemia in vivo. J Mol Cell Cardiol 1998;30:1683–1689.

315. Muller-Werdan U, Engelamann H, Werdan K. Cardiodepression by tumor necrosis factor-alpha. Eur Cytokine Netw 1998;9:689–691.

316. Hotchkiss RS, Swanson PE, Freeman BD, et al. Apoptotic cell death in patients with sepsis, shock and multiple organ dysfunction. Crit Care Med 1999;27:1230–1251.

317. Van der Poll T, Coyle SM, Barbosa K, et al. Epinephrine inhibits tumor necrosis factor alpha and potentiates interleukin-10 production during human endotoxemia. J Clin Invest 1996;97:713–719.

318. Guirao X, Kumar A, Katz J, et al. Catecholamines increase monocyte TNF receptors and inhibit TNF through beta-2-adrenoreceptors. Am J Physiol Endocrin Metab 1997;273:E1203–E1208.

319. Yeh SS, Schuster MW. Geriatric cachexia: the role of cytokines. Am J Clin Nutr 1999;70:183–197.

320. Uehara A, Sekiya C, Takasugi Y. Anorexia induced by IL-1 involvement of corticotropin-releasing factor. Am J Physiol 1989;257:R613–R617.

321. Torti FM, Dieckmann B, Beutler B, et al. A macrophage factor inhibits adipocyte gene expression: an in-vitro model of cachexia. Science 1985;229:867–869.

322. Doerrier W, Feingold KR, Grunfeld C. Cytokines induce catabolic effects in cultured adipocytes by multiple mechanisms. Cytokine 1994;6:478–484.

323. Gasic S, Tian B, Green A. Tumor necrosis factor alpha stimulates lipolysis in adipocytes by decreasing Gi protein concentrations. J Biol Chem 1999;274:6770–6775.

324. Moldawer LL, Copeland EM III. Proinflammatory cytokines, nutritional support and the cachexia syndrome: interactions and therapeutic options. Cancer 1997;79:1828–1839.

325. Liu LS, Spelleken M, Rohrig K, et al. Tumor necrosis factor-alpha acutely inhibits insulin signaling in human adipocytes: implication of the p80 tumor necrosis factor receptor. Diabetes 1998;47:515–522.

326. Espat NJ, Copland EM, Moldawer LL. Tumor necrosis factor and cachexia: a current perspective. Surg Oncol 1994;3:255–262.

327. Tisdale MJ. Wasting in cancer. J Nutr 1999;129(Suppl):243S–246S.

328. Paslisso G, Rizza MR, Mazziotti G, et al. Advancing age and insulin resistance: role of plasma factor-alpha. Am J Physiol 1998;275:E294–E299.

329. Mohamed-Ali V, Goodrick S, Rawesh A, et al. Subcutaneous adipose tissue releases interleukin-6, but not tumor necrosis factor-alpha, in vivo. J Clin Endocrinol Metab 1997;82:4196–4200.

330. Bosze S, Kajtar J, Szabo R, et al. Synthesis, solution conformation and interleukin-6 related activities if interleukin-6 peptides. J Ped Res 1998;52:216–228.

331. Torpy DJ, Bornstein SR, Chrousos GP. Leptin and interleukin-6 in sepsis. Horm Metab Res 1998;30:726–729.

332. Angeli A, Maseia RG, Sartori ML, et al. Modulation by cytokines of glucocorticoid action. Ann N Y Acad Sci 1999;876:210–220.

333. Fischer CP, Bode BP, Takahasi K, et al. Glucocorticoid-dependent induction of interleukin-6 receptor expression in human hepatocytes facilitates interleukin-6 stimulation of amino acid transport. Ann Surg 1996;223:610–619.

334. Tsigos C, Papinicolaou DA, Kurou I, et al. Dose-dependent effects of recombinant human interleukin-6 on the pituitary-testicular axis. J Interferon Cytokine Res 1999;19:1271–1276.

335. Akgus S, Ertel NH, Mosenthal A, et al. Postsurgical reduction of serum lipoproteins: interleukin-6 and the acute phase response. J Lab Clin Med 1998;131:103–108.

336. Shito M, Veda M, Wakabayashi G, et al. Pathophysiological response of cytokines and vasoactive agents in patients undergoing total gastrectomy. Eur J Surg. 1998;164:115–118.

337. Yamauchi H, Kobagashi E, Yoshida T, et al. Changes in immune-endocrine response after surgery. Cytokine 1998;10:549–554.

338. Bellon JM, Manzano L, Larrad A, et al. Endocrine and immune response after injury after open and laparoscopic cholecystectomy. Int Surg 1998;83:24–27.

339. Yuen PM, Mak TW, Yim SF, et al. Metabolism and inflammatory responses after laparoscopic and abdominal hysterectomy. Am J Obstet Gynecol 1998;179:1–5.

340. Otto G, Branconier J, Andreasson A, et al. Interleukin-6 and disease severity in patients with bacteremic and non-bacteremic febrile urinary tract infection. J Infect Dis 1999;179:172–179.

341. Wakenfield CH, Barclay GR, Fearon

KC, et al. Proinflammatory mediator activity, endogenous antagonists and the systemic inflammatory response in intraabdominal sepsis. Scottish Sepsis Intervention Group. Br J Surg 1998;85:818–825.

342. Adamik B, Zimecki M, Wlaszczyk A, et al. Immunological status of septic and trauma patients. 1. High tumor necrosis factor alpha serum levels in septic and trauma patients are not responsible for increased mortality: a prognostic value of interleukin-6. Arch Immunol Ther Exp (Warsz) 1997;45:169–175.

343. De Bandt JP, Chollet-Martin S, Hernvann A, et al. Cytokine response to burn injury: relationship with protein metabolism. J Trauma 1994;36:624–628.

344. Hisano S, Sakamoto K, Ishhiko T, et al. IL-6 and soluble IL-6 receptor levels change differently after surgery both in the blood and in the operative field. Cytokine 1997;9:447–452.

345. Jones SA, Novick D, Horiuchi S, et al. C-reactive protein: a physiological activator of interleukin-6 receptor shedding. J Exp Med 1999;189:599–604.

346. Tsigos C, Papinicolaou DA, Kyrou I, et al. Dose-dependent effects of recombinant human interleukin-6 on glucose regulation. J Clin Endocrinol Metab 1997;82:4167–4170.

347. Grunfeld C, Feingold KR. Regulation of lipid metabolism by cytokines during host defense. Nutrition 1996;12:524–526.

348. Abraham E, Regan RE. The effects of hemorrhage and trauma on interleukin 2 production. Arch Surg 1985;120:1341–1344.

349. Faist E, Meures A, Aker CC, et al. Prostaglandin E_2 (PGE_2)-dependent suppression of interleukin alpha (IL-2) production in patients with major trauma. J Trauma 1987;27:837–848.

350. Faist E, Mewes A, Strasser T, et al. Alteration of monocyte function following major injury. Arch Surg 1988;123:287–292.

351. Ziedler S, Bone RC, Baue AE, et al. T-cell reactivity and its protective role in immunosuppression of burns. Crit Care Med 1999;27:66–72.

352. Shirakawa T, Tokunaga A, Onda M. Release of immunosuppressive substances after gastric resection is more prolonged than after mastectomy in humans. Int Surg 1998;83:210–214.

353. Schinkel C, Zimmer S, Durda PJ, et al. Kinetics of soluble interleukin receptor

after mechanical and burn trauma. Burn Care Rehabil 1997;18:210–213.

354. DiPiro JTm, Howdieshell TR, Goddard JK, et al. Association of interleukin-4 plasma levels with traumatic injury and clinical course. Arch Surg 1995;130:1159–1162.

355. Lee RE, Lotze MT, Skibber JM, et al. Cardiovascular effects of immunotherapy with interleukin 2 killer cells. J Clin Oncol 1988;17:51–59.

356. Conant EF, Fox KR, Miller WT. Pulmonary edema as a complication of interleukin-2 therapy. AJR Am J Roentgenol 1989;152: 749–752.

357. Baars JW, de Boer JP, Wagstaff J, et al. Interleukin-2 induces activation of coagulation and fibrinolysis: resemblance to the changes seen during experimental endotoxemia. Br J Haematol 1992;82:295–301.

358. Raab C, Weidmann E, Schmidt A, et al. The effects of interleukin-2 treatment on endothelin and the activation of the hypothalamic-pituitary-adrenal axis. Clin Endocrinol (Oxf) 1999;50: 37–44.

359. Wigmore SJ, Maingay JP, Pearon KC, et al. Effects of interleukin-4 on pro-inflammatory cytokine production and the acute phase response in healthy individuals and in patients with cancer or multiple organ failure. Clin Sci (Colch) 1998;98:347–354.

360. Vilcek J, Gray PW, Rinderknecht E, et al. Interferon gamma: a lymphokine for all seasons. Lymphokine Res 1985;11:1–10.

361. Collort MA, Belin D, Vassalli JD, et al. Gamma interferon enhances macrophage transcription of the tumor necrosis factor/cachectin interleukin 1 and urokinase genes which are controlled by short-lived repressors. J Exp Med 1986;164:2113–2118.

362. Boraschi D, Censini S, Tagliabue A. Interferon reduces macrophage suppressive activity by inhibiting prostaglandin E_2 release and inducing interleukin 1 production. J Immunol 1984;133:764–768.

363. Mancuso C, Preziosi P, Grossman AB, et al. The role of carbon monoxide in the regulation of neuroendocrine function. Neuroimmunomodulation 1997;4:225–229.

364. Duke T, South M, Stewart A. Activation of the L-arginine nitric oxide pathway in severe sepsis. Arch Dis Child 197;76:203–209.

365. Parratt JR. Nitric oxide in sepsis and endotoxemia. J Antimicrob Chemother 1998;41(Suppl A):31–39.

366. Kirkeboen KA, Strand OA. The role of nitric oxide in sepsis: an overview. Acta Anaesthesiol Scand 1999;43:275–288.

367. Kobayacshi A, Hashimoto S, Kooguchi K, et al. Expression of inducible nitric oxide synthetase and inflammatory cytokines in alveolar macrophages of ARDS following sepsis. Chest 1998;113:1632–1639.

368. Bhagat K, Hingorani AD, Palacios M, et al. Cytokine-induced venodilation in humans in vivo: eNOS masquerading as iNOS. Cardiovasc Res 1999;41:754–764.

369. Avontuur JA, Tutein Nolthenius RP, Buijk SL, et al. Effect of L-NAME, an inhibitor of nitric oxide synthesis on cardiopulmonary function in human septic shock. Chest 1998;113:1640–1646.

370. Avontuur JA, Tutein Nolthenius RP, van Badegom JW, et al. Prolonged inhibition of nitric oxide synthesis in severe septic shock: a clinical study. Crit Care Med 1998;26:660–667.

371. Avontuur JA, Boomsma F, van den Meiracker AH, et al. Endothelin-1 and blood pressure after inhibition of nitric oxide synthesis in human septic shock. Circulation 1999;99:271–275.

372. Groeneveld AB, Hartemink KJ, de Groot MC, et al. Circulating endothelin and nitrate-nitrite relate to hemodynamic and metabolic variables in human septic shock. Shock 1999;11:160–166.

373. Sanai L, Haynes WG, Mackenzie A, et al. Endothelin production in sepsis and the adult respiratory distress syndrome. Intensive Care Med 1996;22:52–56.

374. Franchimont D, Galon J, Gadina M, et al. Inhibition of the Th1 immune response by glucocorticoids: dexamethasone selectively inhibits IL-12 induced Stat4 phosphorylation in T lymphocytes. J Immunol 2000;164: 1768–1774.

375. Nathan CE. Secretory products of macrophages. J Clin Invest 1987;79:319–326.

376. Besedovsky H, del Ray A, Sorkin E, et al. Immunoregulatory feedback between interleukin 1 and glucocorticoid hormones. Science 1986;233:652–655.

377. Buckingham JC. A role for leukocytes in the control of adrenal steroid genesis. J Endocrinol 1984;114:1–2.

378. Berczi I, Chalmers IM, Nagy E, et al. The immune effects of neuropeptides. Ballieres Clin Rhematol 1996;10:227–257.

379. Larrea F, Sanchez-Gonzalez S, Mendez I, et al. G protein-coupled receptors as targets for prolactin actions. Arch Med Res 1999;30:523–543.

380. Goffin V, Binart N, Clement-Lacroix P, et. al. From the molecular biology of prolactin and its receptor to the lessons learned from knockout mice models. Genet Anal 1999;15:189–201.

381. Leite De Moraes MC, Touraine P, Gagnerault MC, et al. Prolactin receptors and the immune system. Ann Endocrinol (Paris) 1995;56:567–570.

382. Draca S. Prolactin as an immunoreactive agent. Immunol Cell Biol 195;73:481–483.

383. Matera L. Action of pituitary and lymphocyte prolactin. Neuroimmunomodulation 1997;4:171–180.

384. De Mello-Coelho V, Savino W, Postel-Vinay MC, et al. Role of prolactin and growth hormone on thymus physiology. Dev Immunol 1998;6:317–323.

385. Peter S, Bozorgzadeh A, Lamate H, et al. Prolactin response to the severity of surgical insult. J Natl Med Assoc 1999;91:262–264.

386. Redondo M, Rubio V, de la Pena A, et al. The effects of the degree of surgical trauma and glucose load on concentration of thyrotropin, growth hormone and prolactin under enflurane anaesthesia. Horm Metab Res 1997;29:66–69.

387. Muzii L, Marana R, Marana E, et al. Evaluation of stress-related hormones after surgery by laparoscopy or laparotomy. J Am Assoc Gynecol Laparosc 1996;3:229–234.

388. Coates PJ, Donloch J, Hale AC, et al. The distribution of immuno-reactive α-melanocyte-stimulating hormone cells in the adult human pituitary gland. J Endocrinol 1986;111:335–342.

389. Catania A, Lipton JM. The neuropeptide alpha-melanocyte-stimulating hormone: a key component of neuroimmunomodulation. Neuroimmunomodulation 1994;1:93–99.

390. Taherzadeh S, Sharma S, Chhajlani V, et al. Alpha-MSH and its receptors in regulation of tumor necrosis factor-alpha production by human monocyte/macrophages. Am J Physiol 1999;276:R1289–R1294.

391. Cutuli M, Cristiani S, Lipton JM, et al. Antimicrobial effects of alpha-MSH peptides. J Leukoc Biol 2000;67:233–239.

392. Loftus TM. An adipocyte-central nervous system regulatory loop in the control of adipose homeostasis. Semin Cell Dev Biol 1999;10:11–18.

393. Cone RD. The central melanocortin system and its role in energy homeostasis. Ann Endocrinol (Paris) 1999; 60:3–9.

394. Pankov YA. Adipose tissue as an endocrine organ regulating growth, puberty and other physiological functions. Biochemistry (Moscow) 1999;64:601–602.

395. Savino W, Arzt E, Dardenne M. Immunoneuroendocrine connectivity: the paradigm of the thymus-hypothalamus/pituitary axis. Neuroimmunomodulation 1999;6:126–136.

396. Hofland LJ, van Hagen PM, Lamberts SW. Functional role of somatostatin receptors in neuroendocrine and immune cells. Ann Med 1999;31(Suppl 2):23–27.

397. van Hagen PM. Somatostatin receptor expression in clinical immunology. Metabolism 1996;45(8 Suppl 1):86–87.

398. Arzt E, Pereda MP, Castro CP, et al. Pathophysiological role of the cytokine network in the anterior pituitary gland. Front Neuroendocrinol 1999;20:71–95.

399. Turnbull AV, Rivier CL. Regulation of the hypothalamic-pituitary-adrenal axis by cytokines: actions and mechanisms of action. Physiol Rev 1999;79:1–71.

400. Weigent DA, Blalock JE. Associations between the neuroendocrine and immune systems. J Leukoc Biol 1995;58:137–150.

401. Dunn AJ, Wang J, Ando T. Effects of cytokines on cerebral neurotransmission. Comparison with the effects of stress. Adv Exp Med Biol 1999;461:117–127.

402. Brown SL, Smith LR, Blalock JE. Interleukin 1 and interleukin 2 enhance proopiomelanocortin gene expression in pituitary cells. J Immunol 1987;139:3181–3183.

403. Sapolsky R, Rivier C, Yamamoto G, et al. Interleukin I stimulates the secretion of hypothalamic corticotropin-releasing factor. Science 1987;238:522–524.

404. Smith EM, Blalock JE. Human lymphocyte production of corticotropin and endorphin-like substances: association with leukocyte interferon. Proc Natl Acad Sci U S A 1981;78:7530–7534.

405. Gonzalez-Hernandez JA, Bornstein SR, Eluhart-Bornstein M, et al. Clin Exp Immunol 1995;99:137–141.

406. George DT, Abeles FB, Mapes CA, et al. Effect of leukocyte endogenous mediators on endocrine pancreas secretory responses. Am J Physiol 1977;233:E240–E245.

407. Smith EM, Cadet P, Stefano GB, et al. IL-10 as a mediator in the HPA axis and brain. J Neuroimmunol 1999;100:140–148.

408. Anisman H, Baines MG, Berczi I, et al. Neuroimmune mechanisms in health and disease: 1. Health. CMAJ 1996;155:867–874.

409. Buckingham JC, Loxley HD, Taylor AD, et al. Cytokines, glucocorticoids and neuroendocrine function. Pharmacol Res 1994;30:35–42.

410. Mastorkas G, Weber JS, Magiakou MA, et al. Hypothalamic-pituitary-adrenal axis activation and stimulation of systemic vasopressin secretion by recombinant interleukin-6 in humans: potential implications for the syndrome of inappropriate vasopressin secretion. J Clin Endocrinol Metab 1994;79:934–939.

411. Brakhudaryan N, Dunn AJ. Molecular mechanisms of action of interleukin-6 on the brain, with special reference to serotonin and the hypothalamo-pituitary-adrenocortical axis. Neurochem Res 1999;24:1169–1180.

412. Auernhammer CJ, Melemed S. Interleukin-11 stimulates proopiomelanocortin gene expression and adrenocorticotropin secretion in corticotroph cells: evidence for a redundant cytokine network in the hypothalamo-pituitary-adrenal axis. Endocrinology 1999;140:1559–1566.

413. Stumvoll M, Meyer C, Mitrakou A, et al. Renal glucose production and utilization: new aspects in humans. Diabetologia 1997;40:749–757.

414. Chiolero R, Revelly JP, Tappy L. Energy metabolism in sepsis and injury. Nutrition 1997;13(Suppl 9):45S–51S.

415. Schricker T, Carli F, Schreiber M, et al. Time of peritoneal cavity exposure influences postoperative glucose production. Can J Anaesth 1999;46:352–358.

416. Turinsky J, Saba TM, Scovill WA, et al. Dynamics of insulin secretion and resistance after burns. J Trauma 1977;17:344–350.

417. Dahn MS, Lange P, Mitchell RA, et al. Insulin production following injury and sepsis. J Trauma 1987;27:1031–1038.

418. Thorell A, Nygren J, Hirshman MF, et al. Surgery-induced insulin resistance in human patients: relation to glucose transport and utilization. Am J Physiol 1999;276:E754–E761.

419. Green CJ, Campbell IT, O'Sullivan E, et al. Septic patients in multiple organ failure can oxidize infused glucose, but non-oxidative disposal (storage) is impaired. Clin Sci (Colch) 1995;89:601–609.

420. Saced M, Carslon GL, Little RA, et al. Selective impairment of glucose storage in human sepsis. Br J Surg 1999;86:813–821.

421. Bak JF. Insulin receptor function and glucagon synthase activity in human skeletal muscle: physiology and pathophysiology. Dan Med Bull 1994;41:179–192.

422. Ki Y, Jarviner H. Acute and chronic effects of hyperglycemia on glucose metabolism. Diabetologia 1990;33:579–585.

423. Strommer L, Permert J, Arnelo U, et al. Skeletal muscle insulin resistance after trauma: insulin signaling and glucose transport. Am J Physiol 1998;275:E351–E358.

424. Thorell A, Efendic S, Gutniak M, et al. Insulin resistance after abdominal surgery. Br J Surg 1994;81:59–63.

425. Hawthorne GC, Ashworth L, Albertic KG. The effect of laparoscopic cholecystectomy on insulin sensitivity. Horm Metab Res 1994;26:474–477.

426. Brandi LS, Santoro D, Natali A, et al. Insulin resistance of stress: sites and mechanisms. Clin Sci 1993;85:525–535.

427. Wolfe RR, Durkot MJ, Allsop JR, et al. Glucose metabolism in severely burned patients. Metabolism 1979;28:1031–1039.

428. Wolfe RR. Herman Award Lecture 1996: Relation of metabolic studies to clinical nutrition—the example of burn injury. Am J Clin Nutr 1996;64:800–808.

429. Nelson KM, Long CL, Bailey R, et al. Regulation of glucose kinetics in trauma patients by insulin and glucagon. Metabolism 1992;41:68–75.

430. Aarsland A, Chinkes D, Wolfe RR. Hepatic and whole body fat synthesis in humans during carbohydrate overfeeding. Am J Clin Nutr 1997;65:1774–1782.

431. Vernon RG, Barber MC, Travers MT. Present and future studies on lipogenesis in animals and human subjects. Proc Nutr Soc 1999;58:541–549.

432. Stubbs RJ, Prentice AM, James WP. Carbohydrates and energy balance. Ann N Y Acad Sci 1997;819:44–69.

433. Jequier E. Carbohydrates as a source of energy. Am J Clin Nutr 1994;59(Suppl):682S–685S.

434. Hellerstein MK. De novo lipogenesis in humans: metabolic and regulatory aspects. Eur J Clin Nutr 1999;53(Suppl):S52–S65.

435. Guenst JM, Nelson LD. Predictors of total parenteral nutrition-induced lipogenesis. Chest 1994;105:553–559.

436. Tappy L, Schwarz JM, Schneiter P, et al. Effects of isoenergetic glucose-based or lipid-based parenteral nutrition on glucose metabolism, de novo lipogenesis, and respiratory gas exchanges in critically ill patients. Crit Care Med 1998;26:860–867.

437. Delikat SE, Galvani DW, Zuzel M. The metabolic effects of interleukin 1 beta on human bone marrow adipocytes. Cytokine 1995;7:338–343.

438. Prins JB, Niesler CU, Winterford CM, et al. Tumor necrosis factor-alpha induces apoptosis of human adipose cells. Diabetes 1997;46:1939–1944.

439. Rennie MJ, Holloszy JO. Inhibition of glucose uptake and glycogenolysis by availability of substrate in cell-oxygenated perfused skeletal muscle. Biochem J 1977;168:161–173.

440. Fellander G, Nordenstrom J, Tjader I, et al. Lipolysis during abdominal surgery. J Clin Endocrinol Metab 1994;78:150–155.

441. Herndon DN, Nguyen TT, Wolfe RR, et al. Lipolysis in burned patients is stimulated by the beta-2-receptor for catecholamines. Arch Surg 1994; 129:1301–1305.

442. Miles JM. Lipid fuel metabolism in health and disease. Curr Opin Gen Surg 1993;78–84.

443. Doerrler W, Feingold KR, Grunfeld C. Cytokines induce catabolic effects in cultured adipocytes by multiple mechanisms. Cytokine 1994;6:478–484.

444. Carey GB. Mechanisms regulating adipocyte lipolysis. Adv Exp Med Biol 1998;441:157–170.

445. Granneman JG. Why do adipocytes make the beta 3 adrenergic receptor? Cell Signal 1995;7:9–15.

446. Townsend RR, Klein S, Wolfe RR. Changes in lipolytic sensitivity following repeated epinephrine infusion in humans. Am J Physiol 1994;266:E155–E160.

447. Arner P. Differences in lipolysis between human subcutaneous and omental tissues. Ann Med 1995;27:435–438.

448. Carpentier YA, Askanazi J, Elwyn DH, et al. Effects of hypercaloric glucose infusion on lipid metabolism in injury and sepsis. J Trauma 1979;19:649–654.

449. Nordenstrorn J, Carpentier YA, Askanazi J, et al. Free fatty acid mobilization and oxidation during total parenteral nutrition in trauma and infection. Ann Surg 1983;198:725–735.

450. Galster AD, Bier DM, Cryer P, et al. Plasma palmitate turnover in subjects with thermal injury. J Trauma 1984;24:938–945.

451. Persson E, Nordenstrom J, Vinnars E. Plasma clearance of fat emulsion during continuous heparin infusion. Acta Anaesthesiol Scand 1987;31:189–192.

452. Robin AP, Askanazi J, Greenwood MRC, et al. Lipoprotein lipase activity in surgical patients: influence of trauma and sepsis. Surgery 1981;90:401–408.

453. Nordenstrom J. Utilization of exogenous and endogenous lipid for energy production during parenteral nutrition. Acta Chir Scand Suppl 1982;510:1–42.

454. Robin AP, Nordenstrom J, Askanazi J, et al. Influence of parenteral carbohydrate on fat oxidation in surgical patients. Surgery 1984;195:608–618.

455. Schricker T, Berroth A, Pfeiffer U, et al. Assessment of perioperative glycerol metabolism by stable isotope tracer technique. Nutrition 1997;13:191–195.

456. Smith R, Fuller DJ, Wedghe JH, et al. Initial effect of injury on ketone bodies and other blood metabolites. Lancet 1975;1:1–3.

457. Avary JC, Siegel JH, Nakatani T, et al. A biochemical basis for depressed ketogenesis in sepsis. J Trauma 1986;26:419–425.

458. Schofiel PS, Frent TJ, Sugden MC. Ketone-body metabolism after surgical stress or partial hepatectomy. Biochem J 1987;241:475–481.

459. Hartl WA, Jauch KW, Kimmig R, et al. Minor role of ketone bodies in energy metabolism by skeletal muscle tissue during the postoperative course. Ann Surg 1988;207:95–101.

460. Shaw JF, Wildbore M, Wolfe RR. Whole body protein kinetics in severely septic patients. Ann Surg 1987;205:288–294.

461. Hasselgren PO, James JH, Fischer JE. Inhibited muscle amino acid uptake in sepsis. Ann Surg 1986;203:360–365.

462. Jahoor F, Wolfe RR. Regulation of protein catabolism. Kidney Int 1987;82(Suppl 22):581–593.

463. Jahoor F, Desai M, Hemdon DN, et al. Dynamics of the protein metabolic response to burn injury. Metabolism 1988;37:330–337.

464. Brown JA, Gore DC, Jahoor F. Catabolic hormones alone fail to reproduce the stress-induced efflux of amino acids. Arch Surg 194;129:819–824.

465. Mansoor O, Beaufrere B, Boirie Y, et al. Increased mRNA levels for components of the lysosomal, Ca^+-activated, and ATP-ubiquitin-dependent proteolytic pathways in skeletal muscle from head trauma patients. Proc Natl Acad Sci U S A 1996;493:2714–2718.

466. Williams AB, Decourtens-Myers GM, Fischer JE, et al. Sepsis stimulates release of myofilaments in skeletal muscle by a calcium-dependent mechanism. FASEB J 1999;13:1435–1443.

467. Heindorff HA. The hepatic catabolic stress response: hormonal regulation of urea synthesis after surgery. Dan Med Bull 1993;40:224–234.

468. Stahl WM. Acute phase protein response to tissue injury. Crit Care Med 1987; 15:545–550.

469. Banks RE, Forbes MA, Storr M, et al. The acute phase protein response in patients receiving subcutaneous IL-6. Clin Exp Immunol 1995;102:217–223.

470. Speiss A, Mikalunas V, Carlson S, et al. Albumin kinetics in hypoalbuminemic patients receiving total parenteral nutrition. JPEN J Parenter Enteral Nutr 1996;20:424–428.

471. Ingenbleck Y, Young V. Transthyretin (prealbumin) in health and disease: nutritional implications. Ann Rev Nutr 1994;14:495–533.

472. Monk DN, Plank LD, Franch-Arcas G, et al. Sequential changes in the metabolic response in critically injury patients during the 25 days after blunt trauma. Ann Surg 1996;223:395–405.

473. Khorram-Sefat R, Behrendt W, Heiden A, et al. Long-term measurements of energy expenditure in severe burn injury. World J Surg 1999;23:115–122.

474. Turner WW, Ireton CS, Hunt JL, et al. Predicting energy expenditures in burn patients. J Trauma 1985;25:11–16.

475. Hersio K, Takala J, Kari A, et al. Patterns of energy expenditure in intensive-care patients. Nutrition 1993;9:127–132.

476. Brandi LS, Santini L, Bertolini R, et al. Energy expenditure and severity of injury and illness indicies in multiple trauma patients. Crit Care Med 1999;27:2684–2689.

477. Askanazi J, Forse RA, Weissman C, et al. Ventilatory effects of the stress hormones in normal man. Crit Care Med 1986;14:602–606.

478. Weissman C, Askanazi J, Forse RA, et al. The metabolic and ventilatory response to the infusion of stress hormones. Ann Surg 1986;203:408–412.

479. Gil KM, Forse RA, Askanazi J, et al. Energy Metabolism in Stress. In JS Garrow, D Halliday (eds), Substrate and Energy Metabolism. London: John Libbey, 1985;203–212.

480. Wilmore DW, Aulick LH. Metabolic changes in burned patients. Surg Clin North Am 1978;58:1173–1187.

481. Lowry SF, Leyaspi A, Jeevanandam M, et al. Body protein kinetics during perioperative intravenous nutritional support. Surg Gynecol Obstet 1986; 163:303–309.

482. Frankenfield DC, Smith JS Jr, Cooney RN, et al. Relative association of fever and injury with hypermetabolism in critically ill patients. Injury 1997;28:617–621.

483. Kelemenn JJ III, Cioffi WG Jr, Mason AD Jr, et al. Effect of ambient temperature on metabolic rate after thermal injury. Ann Surg 1996;223:406–412.

484. Tappy L, Berger M, Schwarz JM, et al. Hepatic and peripheral glucose metabolism in intensive care patients receiving continuous high- or low-carbohydrate enteral nutrition. JPEN J Parenter Enteral Nutr 1999;23:260–269.

485. Wolfe RR. Substrate utilization/insulin resistance in sepsis/trauma. Ballieres Clin Endocrinol Metab 1997;11:645–657.

486. Fellander G, Nordenstrom J, Ungerstedt U, et al. Influence of operation on glucose metabolism and lipolysis in human adipose tissue: a microdialysis study. Eur J Surg 1994;160:87–95.

487. Jeejeehoy KN, Anderson GH, Nakhooda AF, et al. Metabolic studies in total parental nutrition. J Clin Invest 1976;52:125–136.

488. Watters JM, Kirkpatrick SM, Hopbach D, et al. Aging exaggerates the blood glucose response to total parenteral nutrition. Can J Surg 1996;39:481–485.

489. Shaw JHF, Wolfe RR. Determinations of glucose turnover and oxidation in normal volunteers and septic patients using stable and radio-isotopes: the response to glucose infusion and total parenteral feeding. Aust NZ J Surg 1986;56:785–791.

490. Lindholm M, Rossner S. Rate of elimination of the intralipid fat emulsion from the circulation in intensive care patients. Crit Care Med 1982;11:740–747.

491. Wolfe RR, O'Donnell TF, Stone MD, et al. Investigation of factors determining the optimal glucose infusion rate in total parenteral nutrition. Metabolism 1980;29:892–900.

492. Burke JF, Wolfe RR, Mullany CJ, et al. Glucose requirements following burn injury. Parameters of optimal glucose infusion and possible hepatic and respiratory abnormalities following excessive glucose intake. Ann Surg 1979;190:274–279.

493. Grizard J, Dardevet D, Balage M, et al. Insulin action on skeletal muscle protein metabolism during catabolic states. Reprod Nutr Dev 1999;39:61–74.

494. Wolfe RR. Effects of insulin on muscle tissue. Curr Opin Clin Nutr Metab Care 2000;3:67–71.

495. Bessey PQ, Lowe KA. Early hormonal changes affect the catabolic response to trauma. Ann Surg 1993;218:476–491.

496. Ferrando AA, Chinkes DL, Wolfe SE, et al. A submaximal dose of insulin promotes net skeletal muscle protein synthesis in patients with severe burns. Ann Surg 1999;229:11–18.

497. Pierre EJ, Barrow RE, Hawkins HK, et al. Effects of insulin on wound healing. J Trauma 1998;44:342–345.

498. Pearlstone DB, Wolf RF, Berman RS, et al. Effect of systemic insulin on protein kinetics in postoperative cancer patients. Ann Surg Oncol 1994;1:321–332.

499. Clements RH, Hayes CA, Gibbs ER, et al. Insulin's anabolic effect is influenced by route of administration of nutrients. Arch Surg 1999;134:274–277.

500. Demling RH, Orgill DP. The anticatabolic and wound healing effects of the testosterone analog oxandrolone after severe burn injury. J Crit Care 2000;15:12–17.

501. Koea JB, Breier BH, Douglas RG, et al. Anabolic and cardiovascular effects of recombinant human growth hormone in surgical patients with sepsis. Br J Surg 1996;83:196–202.

502. Voerman BJ, Srack van Schijndel RJ, de Boer H, et al. Effects of human growth hormone on fuel utilization and mineral balance in critically ill patients on full intravenous nutritional support. J Crit Care 1994; 9:143–150.

503. Takala J, Ruokonene E, Webster NR, et al. Increased mortality associated with growth hormone treatment in critically ill adults. N Engl J Med 1999;341:785–792.

504. Herndon DN, Ramzy PI, DebRoy MA, et al. Muscle protein catabolism after severe burn: effects of IGF-1/IGFBP-3 treatment. Ann Surg 1999;229:713–722.

505. Miers WR, Barrett EJ. The role of insulin and other hormones in the regulation of amino acid and protein metabolism in humans. J Basic Clin Physiol Pharmacol 1998;9:235–253.

506. Cioffi WG, Gore DC, Rue LW III, et al. Insulin-like growth factor-1 lowers protein oxidation in patients with thermal injury. Ann Surg 1994;220:310–319.

507. Wu FC. Endocrine aspects of anabolic steroids. Clin Chem 1997;43:1289–1292.

508. Young GA, Yule AG, Hill GL. Effects of an anabolic steroid on plasma amino acids, proteins and body composition in patients receiving intravenous hyperalimentation. JPEN J Parenter Enteral Nutr 1983;7:221–225.

509. Ferreifa IM, Verreschi IT, Nery LE, et al. The influence of 6 months of oral anabolic steroids on body mass and respiratory muscles in undernourished COPD patients. Chest 1998;114:19–28.

510. Demling RH, DeSanti L. Oxandrolone, an anabolic steroid, significantly increases the rate of weight gain in the recovery phase after major burns. J Trauma 1997;43:47–51.

511. Perriello G, Nurjhan N, Stumvoll M, et al. Regulation of gluconeogenesis by glutamine in normal postabsorptive humans. Am J Physiol 1997;272:E437–E445.

512. Hall JC, Heel K, McCauley R. Glutamine. Br J Surg 1996;83:305–312.

513. Buchman AL. Glutamine: is it a conditionally required nutrient for the human gastrointestinal system? J Am Coll Nutr 1996;15:199–205.

514. Ziegler TR, Szeszycki EE, Estivariz CF, et al. Glutamine: from basic science to clinical applications. Nutrition 1996; 12(Suppl):S68–S70.

515. Jones C, Palmer TE, Griffiths RD. Randomized clinical outcome study of critically ill patients given glutamine-supplemented enteral nutrition. Nutrition 1999;15:108–115.

516. Sacks GS. Glutamine supplementation in catabolic patients. Ann Pharmacother 1999;33:348–354.

517. Hinojosa-Laborde C, Chapa I, Lange D, Haywood JR. Gender differences in sympathetic nervous system regulation. Clin Exp Pharmacol Physiol 1999;26:122–126.

518. Rubin RT, Sekula LK, O'Toole S, et al. Pituitary-adrenal cortical responses to low-dose physostigmine and arginine vasopressin administration in normal women and men. Neuropsychopharmacology 1999;20:434–446.

519. Houston-Bolze MS, Downing MT, Sayed AM, Meserve LA. Gender differences in the responses of insulin-like growth factor-1 and transthyretin (prealbumin) to trauma. Crit Care Med 1996;24:1982–1987.

520. Houston-Bolze MS, Downing MT, Sayed AM, Williford JH. Serum insulin-like growth factor binding protein-3

responds differently to trauma in men and women. Crit Care Med 1996;24:1988–1992.

521. Schroder J, Kahlke V, Staubach KH, et al. Gender differences in human sepsis. Arch Surg 1998;133:1200–1215.

522. Daun JM, Ball RW, Cannon JG. Glucocorticoid sensitivity of interleukin-1 agonist and antagonist secretion: the effects of age and gender. Am J Physiol Regul Integr Comp Physiol 2000;278:R855–R866.

20

Obesity and Weight Control

DANIEL J. HOFFMAN AND DYMPNA GALLAGHER

Being overweight and obese results from a positive energy balance created by excess energy intake, insufficient energy expenditure, or both. Human energy expenditure is composed of three distinct segments, the largest of which is the resting energy expenditure, which accounts for 60–70% of total energy expenditure. The thermic effect of feeding, or diet-induced thermogenesis, accounts for 10% of total energy expenditure and is the energy used to metabolize and digest food. Finally, the most controllable and variable component is physical activity, which accounts for 15–30% of total energy expenditure, but can reach as much as 60% in highly trained athletes.

DEFINITION OF OBESITY

The hallmark of obesity is excess adipose tissue. Body weight adjusted for stature is universally used as an alternative to the measurement of adipose tissue mass in the evaluation of individuals or populations for obesity.[1] Body mass index (BMI; Quetelet's index), which is body weight in kilograms divided by stature in meters squared, was an attempt by the nineteenth century mathematician Lambert-Adolf-Jacques Quetelet to describe the relationship between body weight and stature in humans.[2] The common use of BMI represents an effort to derive a measure of adiposity by adjusting body weight for individual differences in stature.[3] Many studies have shown that BMI is a reasonable measure of adiposity,[1,4–7] given that body weight and stature are simple, inexpensive, safe, and practical measurements to acquire. Current guidelines adopted by national[8] and international committees establish being overweight as BMI greater

than or equal to 25 kg/m^2 and obesity as BMI greater than 30 kg/m^2.

PREVALENCE

The prevalence of being overweight and obese is increasing world-wide. Between the National Health and Nutrition Examination Survey (NHANES) II (1976–1980) and NHANES III, phase I (1988–1991), the incidence of being overweight increased by 8%. Between NHANES III, phase 1 and NHANES III, phase 2 (1991–1994), a further increase of 6% occurred.[9] Despite the fact that obesity is increasing in all parts of society, the prevalence of obesity typically falls along gender, racial, and economic lines such that more women than men, more blacks than whites, and more persons from low than high income sectors are overweight and obese.

However, the epidemic is not confined to the United States alone. The WHO MONICA study[10] has collected data in 48 populations (1983–1988), with the majority from European populations, and reported that between 1983 and 1986, the average prevalence was 15% in men and 22% in women. These data reflect an average increase in the prevalence of obesity of approximately 10–40% over the past 10 years. These data have been corroborated by individual national studies as summarized in Table 20-1.

CLASSIFICATION OF OBESITY

As described earlier, clinicians frequently use the BMI to define who is overweight.[11,12] The normal limits of BMI are 20–25 for men and 19–24 for women. Being

TABLE 20-1
Obesity Trends (Body Mass Index $\geq$ 30) in Five European Countries

Country (Author and Date)	Years	Age (years)	Prevalence (%) in Men	Prevalence (%) in Women
England (London Department of Health, 1995)[146]	1980–1995	16–64	6–16	8.0–16.5
Finland (Seidell, 1998)[147]	1978–1993	20–75	10–14	10–11
Former East Germany (Heinman, personal communication, 1996)	1985–1992	25–65	13.7–20.5	22.2–26.8
Netherlands (Seidell, 1997)[148]	1987–1995	20–59	6.0–8.4	8.5–8.3
Sweden (Kuskowska, 1993)[149]	1980–1989	16–84	4.9–5.3	8.7–9.1

Source: Adapted from Obesity. Preventing and Managing the Global Epidemic. Report of the WHO Consultation on Obesity. Geneva, June 3–5, 1997, Table 3.5. World Health Organization, 1998.

overweight is associated with a BMI between the upper limit of normal and 30, and obesity with a BMI greater than 30.[4,13] BMI is independent of frame size, but there is a direct relationship (i.e., the larger the frame the larger the BMI) among those with equal proportions of body composition components. The main weakness of using the BMI for classifying a person as overweight or obese is that persons who are muscular may be misclassified as overweight, despite the fact that the person is simply overmuscular for his or her respective height.

Researchers have attempted to use skin fold measurements to classify obesity. Seltzer and Mayer[5] did so using the triceps skin fold. They suggested that at age 12 years in boys a triceps skin fold greater than 18 mm indicates obesity and for girls the value is any greater than 22 mm. The critical thickness increases with age until among those 30–50 years, a triceps skin fold of 23 mm for men and 30 mm for women indicates obesity. If one accepts the equivalent fat content calculated from skin fold thicknesses to be acceptable for the classification of obesity, one might accept more than 25% body fat for men and more than 30% for women as the lower limits of obesity. Durnin and Womersley[6] developed a table of equivalent fat content for men and women and demonstrated that skin fold thickness gradually decreases with age. They summed the thicknesses of four skin folds (biceps, triceps, subscapular, suprailiac) and reported the following approximate sums for four age groups of men: 17–29 years, 80 mm; 30–39 years, 70 mm; 40–49 years, 50 mm; and 50 years and older, 45 mm. A similar trend of lower magnitude was reported for women, the values were as follows: 16–29 years, 65 mm; 30–39 years, 60 mm; 40–49 years, 45 mm; and 50 years and older, 40 mm.

A variety of other techniques are now available for assessing body fat; however, what percentage of fat constitutes obesity has differed, depending on the pur-

poses of the study, the population, and other variables. Thus, the selection of criteria has varied and there has been no consensus, although it appears possible to select practical guidelines. Body fat in excess of 25% of body weight for men and 30% for women appears to be a reasonable criterion for excessive body fat, whereas more than 40% body fat for men and 50% for women could define severe or morbid obesity. The relationship between obesity and morbidity has resulted in considerable debate over the years because increased morbidity is associated with both high and low BMI (above 35 or below 15), and some believe that the central question is one of fatness rather than weight. Thus, answers to the question regarding what amount of fat constitutes a health risk have yet to be made.[14-16]

The definition of obesity changes depending on the perspective of the classification scale. For example, if physiological strain (respiratory, cardiovascular, thermal) serves as a criterion, the respective strains brought about by common stresses such as exercise intensity, environmental conditions such as heat and humidity, hypobaria and hyperbaria, and hypoxia could be used for classification purposes. In that case, the 25% body fat criterion for men and 30% for women may be too high. Similarly, these criteria may be too lax in light of current health attitudes and the emphasis on leanness. Thus, obesity criteria should be not only population specific but also meaningful in terms of health or pathologic or physiological strain criteria.

Bray[17] has stressed the multiple causes of obesity and has classified obesity anatomically and etiologically. His anatomic classification focuses on fat storage pattern: localized or generalized. The etiologic classification focuses on the type, postulated mechanism, and treatment of obesity. The types of obesity include hypothalamic, endocrine, nutritional, genetic, drug induced, and sedentary lifestyle induced. Although lack of exercise is involved in only one category, exercise interacts with a variety of regulatory and metabolic mechanisms, such as glucose and insulin metabolism, catecholamine metabolism, lipolysis, and peripheral receptor activity.

Classification by volume of adipose tissue cells requires valid and reliable measurements of cell size and total body fat from which to calculate cell number.[18] Adipocyte size and number both vary among regional fat deposits, both within and between individuals. Those who develop obesity later in life are largely normocellular. Bjorntorp[19] has suggested that these two types of obesity may respond differently to therapy.

A more recent classification based on regional distribution of body fat depends on the ratio of the circumference measurements of the waist and hip, also known as the *waist-to-hip ratio*.[20,21] The waist-to-hip ratio reflects the relative amount of visceral adipose tissue, and high ratios, in both men and women, have been associated with an increased risk of cardiovascular disease, including myocardial infarction, angina pectoris, stroke, and death.[21] This is thought to be because of the rapid release of fats from and a high turnover of fatty acids in the visceral adipose tissue[22-24] and is discussed later in this chapter (see the section Cardiovascular Disease).

PHYSIOLOGICAL RISKS

Obesity has been linked to a variety of conditions that adversely affect physiological function and health status (Table 20-2): cardiovascular, respiratory, temperature regulation, and metabolic disturbances.[25] To begin this section it is helpful to discuss the physiology of adipose tissue because it is the neuroendocrinology that forms the basis from which many of the physiological effects of obesity arise.

Adipose tissue is a special tissue for energy storage, and it is peculiar because specific progenitor cell types have not been clearly described. In addition, adipocytes contain receptors that are responsive to neurogenic and hormonal stimulation. These two aspects of adipose tissue are described briefly in the following sections.

That precursor and preadipocyte cells differentiate is known, but the factors that regulate adipocyte differentiation are not known. It has been suggested that the condensation of mesenchymal cells around blood vessels is responsible for development of primitive fat organs. Adipocytes are observed after tissue vascularization. Thus, the interaction of precursor cells and preadipocytes with capillary endothelial cells may be important, as are constituents in blood such as growth hormone responsible for adipocyte development. In

TABLE 20-2
Conditions Associated with Obesity

Cardiovascular
  Reduced myocardial function: arrhythmias
  Enlarged heart: congestive heart failure
  Arteriosclerosis: coronary heart disease
  Cerebrovascular disease
  Hypertension
  Varicoses
  Hypoxia syndromes: pulmonary hypertension
  Edema
Respiratory
  Reduced pulmonary function: hypoventilation
  Sleep apnea
  Loss of sensitivity to CO_2
  Pneumonia
  Dyspnea on exertion
Metabolic
  Diabetes mellitus type II
  Hyperinsulinemia
  Cirrhosis of the liver
  Gout
  Hyperlipidemia
  Gallbladder disease
  In women, osteoarthritis in weight-bearing joints
Thermoregulatory
  Reduced heat tolerance
Other
  Menstrual and ovarian abnormalities
  Complications of pregnancy
  Appendicitis
  Peptic ulcer
  Endometrial carcinoma, other cancer, leukemia
  Greater risk at surgery
  Poor tolerance for anesthesia
  Compromised mobility: greater risk of accidents
  Greater risk of suicide

Source: Adapted from references 65, 93–95, and 97, with permission.

addition, adipogenic serum activity may also play a role in differentiation; such activity has been demonstrated in serum from last-trimester pregnant women and from umbilical cord blood.[26] The effects of such serum are ascertained by the responsiveness of cell cultures.

Adipose tissue is innervated by the sympathetic nervous system. The concentration of norepinephrine in adipose tissue is on the order of 40 ng/g of tissue. Both β-adrenoreceptors and β-receptors are present. Although the β_1-receptor has been thought to be associated with lipolytic activity, there is the possibility that a new β-adrenoreceptor subtype is responsible. The α_2-

receptors demonstrate antilipolytic action. In addition to stimulating lipolysis through sympathetic activation of adipocytes, lipolysis may also be stimulated by catecholamines released from the adrenals. Denervation of adipose tissue leads to increased lipid mass, whereas electrical stimulation leads to fatty acid release. Blocking of sympathetic activity inhibits lipid mobilization.[27]

Regional differences have been observed in adipose tissue lipolysis: Lipolytic activity is greater in omental than in subcutaneous tissue. Lesser insulin action and α_2-adrenoreceptor antilipolytic activity are thought to be responsible. Catecholamines appear less lipolytic in gluteal and femoral subcutaneous adipose tissue than in similar abdominal tissue. Perhaps there is enhanced α_2-adrenoreceptor responsiveness in the gluteal and femoral tissue. Site variation in receptor distribution, as well as the signals from the receptors, may play a role in regulation. Development of regional forms of obesity, such as the protruding abdominal (android) type or the gluteal-femoral (gynecoid) type, may depend on regional receptor and signal variations. The android type is predominant in men and the gynecoid in women. The android type has been associated with elevated free fatty acids in the portal system and impaired glucose metabolism by the liver.[21,28]

Sex hormones may also be important in influencing fat distribution: Testosterone treatment in women increases the size of upper body adipocytes, and estrogen therapy in men increases fat cell numbers in the thighs.[29] Progesterone appears to increase femoral lipoprotein lipase activity in women, which appears to be inhibited by testosterone. Estradiol and testosterone exhibit lipolytic action in adipocytes from the abdominal region. In addition, long-term exposure to corticosteroids might increase femoral lipoprotein lipase activity and decrease abdominal lipolysis.[30]

In addition to sex hormones influencing fat distribution, growth hormone plays an important role as well. It is believed that growth hormone acts in coordination with the sex hormones to regulate the amount of adipose tissue that is deposited centrally.[31] As may be seen by simple visual observation, men tend to accumulate more adipose tissue centrally and women more peripherally. Although only cross-sectional, several studies have found that the level of testosterone is inversely correlated with the amount of visceral adipose tissue.[32] Likewise, a high waist-to-hip ratio is correlated with low levels of both sex hormones and growth hormone. Some studies have found that replacing growth hormone in growth hormone–deficient subjects reduced the amount of visceral adipose tissue. There was not a decrease in the insulin resistance of these subjects.[33]

Still, it remains unclear whether or not the growth hormone deficiency occurs before the onset of obesity and insulin resistance or vice versa.

Related to the regulation of fat distribution, it was reported that human immunodeficiency virus–positive persons who received protease inhibitors in combination with other drug treatments designed to reverse human immunodeficiency virus–associated weight loss, experienced an increase in weight and an increase in central adiposity.[34] The U.S. Centers for Disease Control and Prevention reported that 62 cases of abnormal fat accumulation occurred in persons receiving protease inhibitors.[35] In addition to an increase in central adiposity, patients reported breast enlargement, thickening of the neck, and the presence of buffalo humps. Subsequent studies have reported that treating such cases with recombinant human growth hormone has been successful in reversing the abnormal deposition of adipose tissue.[36] Although the exact mechanism of why treatment with protease inhibitors is associated with this abnormal fat accumulation is unknown, some have suggested that hypercortisolism may be partly responsible, whereas others suggest that changes in the hormone, metabolic, or both profiles of persons with human immunodeficiency virus positive are partly responsible.[37] Further studies are being conducted on both the cause and treatment of this particular pathology.

Cardiovascular Disease

The association between being excessively overweight or obese and cardiovascular disease has been described for many years as the circulation of obese patients has been studied.[38–43] In two prospective studies of coronary heart disease (CHD) in which skin fold measurements were used to calculate adiposity, it was found that the projected increase in coronary disease risk was related to greater fatness in middle-aged men.[44,45] Nevertheless, controversy exists. Keys et al.[44] presented a discussion of the problem and calculated the probability of CHD-related deaths in relation to BMI for men from the Chicago Gas Company study, the U.S. railroad study, and some European studies. The probability of a CHD-related death was increased at the extremes of the BMI distribution (i.e., very low and very high values). Keys et al. concluded that risk of heart disease increases substantially only at the extremes of underweight and overweight or fatness. Bloom and coworkers[46] also found rates of CHD and cardiovascular disease to be higher in the most obese men than in nonobese ones, no matter whether the men were normotensive or hypertensive. These results were obtained in a prospective epidemiologic study of a cohort of Japanese-American men aged 45–65 years who were followed for 12 years in the Honolulu Heart Program.

Hypertension is of considerable consequence in obesity because of associated atherosclerosis, arterial wall damage, retinopathy, and renal vascular disease. Bloom's group[46] concluded that for obese persons hypertension is associated with increased risk of cardiovascular disease. Messerli and colleagues[47,48] postulated that in obese hypertensive persons, the circulating blood volume is large and the relatively greater venous return adds a load to the left ventricle (LV) already burdened by high afterload caused by arterial hypertension. They suggested that the double burden on the LV may enhance the long-term risk of congestive heart failure. Messerli's group noted disparate effects of obesity and hypertension on total peripheral resistance and intravascular volume (i.e., the former was relatively lower and the latter relatively higher in obese subjects), and the effects partially offset each other. Comparison of obese men with normal blood pressure and with hypertension revealed expansion of extracellular and interstitial fluid in the hypertensive group. The volumes paralleled the degree of obesity.[49]

Obese patients have been found to have greater cardiac output, stroke volume, left ventricular filling pressure, and left ventricular eccentric hypertrophy than nonobese ones. The decrease in arterial pressure with weight loss may well be caused by decreased adrenergic activity leading to decreased cardiac output along with some lowering of vascular resistance. The relatively elevated cardiac output, in hypertensive obese patients, along with relatively restricted arterial capacity, may well be associated with the low vascularity of adipose tissue. Increased blood viscosity may contribute to the elevated arterial pressure in grossly obese persons.[50]

When morbidly obese patients underwent gastric restriction and subsequently achieved substantial weight loss, follow-up echocardiography revealed that the mean LV dimension in diastole and mean blood pressure were significantly decreased. The conclusions were that cardiac chamber enlargement, LV hypertrophy, and LV systolic dysfunction occur in many morbidly obese patients and that these functions may improve after substantial weight loss (Table 20-3).[51] Similar observations were made by Rubal and Elmesallamy,[52] who compared observations on obese women and control subjects. The obese women had greater mean blood pressure, LV wall thickness, LV enddiastolic volume, LV mass, and left atrial and aortic root dimensions. The investigators concluded that significant structural changes in the myocardium occur in obese subjects, even though they are free of cardiovascular symptoms.

TABLE 20-3

Comparison of Cardiac Size, Wall Thickness, and Function of 34 Morbidly Obese Patients before and after Weight Loss

Echocardiographic Variable	Number	Before Weight Loss (Mean ± SD)	After Weight Loss (Mean ± SD)	P Value
LV internal dimension in diastole (cm)				
Normal (3.6–5.5)	21	5.0 ± 0.3	4.8 ± 0.3	NS
Enlarged (>5.5)	13	6.0 ± 0.2	5.1 ± 0.2	<.02
LV internal dimension in systole (cm)				
Normal (3.7)	19	3.2 ± 0.2	3.0 ± 0.2	NS
Enlarged (>3.7)	15	4.7 ± 0.2	3.5 ± 0.2	<.01
LV fractional shortening (%)				
Normal (28–44)	21	35 ± 3	37 ± 3	NS
Low (<28)	13	22 ± 2	31 ± 2	<.01
LV posterior wall thickness (cm)				
Normal (0.6–1.1)	16	0.9 ± 0.1	0.9 ± 0.1	NS
Increased (>1.1)	18	1.3 ± 0.1	1.3 ± 0.1	NS
Right ventricle internal dimension (cm)				
Normal (0.7–2.3)	24	1.8 ± 0.1	1.7 ± 0.1	NS
Enlarged (<2.3)	10	2.5 ± 0.1	2.3 ± 0.2	NS
Body weight (kg)	34	135 ± 8	79 ± 6	<.005

LV = left ventricle; NS = not significant.
Source: Adapted from MA Alpert, BA Terry, DL Kelly. Effect of weight loss on cardiac chamber ventricular function in morbid obesity. Am J Cardiol 1985;55:783–786.

Persons with the obesity-hypoventilation syndrome (Pickwickian syndrome) have a relatively larger pulmonary blood volume (pulmonary circulatory congestion), most likely because of pulmonary arterial vasoconstriction and hypertension secondary to hypoxia and hypercapnic acidemia.[53] The linking of left- and right-sided heart problems with CHD and hypertension, as can occur in grossly obese persons, severely limits functional cardiovascular and respiratory capacity.

Another risk factor for CHD associated with obesity is hyperlipidemia.[54-57] Serum triglyceride concentrations tend to be more elevated than total cholesterol, and the proportion of high-density lipoprotein cholesterol tends to be lower in many obese subjects.[56] Serum lipids have been shown to be elevated after experimental production of obesity via simple overeating of a diet high in carbohydrates.[58]

As discussed earlier, the pattern of body fat distribution is an independent risk factor for developing CHD. It was first noted in the 1950s that the distribution of adipose was more closely related to diabetes, hypertension, and CHD than the amount of adipose tissue.[59] Specifically, CHD is associated with the male or android pattern of distribution,[21,54,60] which consists of a relatively high (>1.0) waist-hip circumference ratio, in contrast to the female or gynecoid pattern, in which body fat is greater around the hips and thighs (ratio <1.0). Relatively higher plasma concentrations of triglycerides and total cholesterol and lower concentrations of high-density lipoproteins have been observed with the male pattern of fat distribution.[60,61] This has been reported to be the result of increased lipolytic activity in visceral adipose cells.[62,63] Because this activity is not well regulated by insulin, there is an increased flux of free fatty acids to the liver, which promotes not only high concentrations of free fatty acids, but also lower insulin sensitivity. These changes may be part of the causal pathway in the association between visceral adipose tissue and the increased risk for insulin resistance, dyslipidemias, diabetes, and CHD.

Investigation of the children who participated in the Bogalusa Heart Study[64] showed that several risk factors for CHD increased with age, including BMI, total serum cholesterol, and diastolic blood pressure. With increased body fat, especially in boys, total serum cholesterol and triglycerides increased also, particularly low-density and very low-density lipoproteins.[65,66]

In a person at rest blood flows through adipose tissue at a rate of approximately 2–3 ml per minute per 100 g of tissue.[67] Alterations in pressure-flow relationships have been observed in the adipose tissue vascular bed in response to changes in oxygen tension, pH, circulating

blood volume, mechanical factors, exercise, temperature, sympathetic nerve activity, and several hormones.[68] Because the vascular beds in adipose tissue also serve as blood volume reservoirs, displacement or augmentation of the contained volume has central cardiovascular effects. In general, adipose tissue blood flow is related inversely to fat cell volume but directly to the number of fat cells.[67] After prolonged fasting and weight loss, which produces a reduction in cardiac output, there is a relatively increased number of fat cells per unit of adipose tissue weight, which is accompanied by a relatively greater blood flow. These changes reduce the total blood flow to the smaller fat cell volume.[69]

Respiration

Deposition of fat over the thoracic cavity and within and over the abdomen increases the likelihood of regressive changes in pulmonary function (e.g., the functional residual volume of the lung is decreased with moderate or gross obesity). The smaller functional residual volume is brought about by thoracic cavity squeeze. Both the mass of overlying adipose tissue and an elevated diaphragm contribute to the squeeze.[70-72] The lesser functional residual volume is to a large extent associated with reduction in the expiratory reserve volume; the residual volume remains relatively unchanged or elevated (Table 20-4).[73] Abnormalities in the ventilation-perfusion distribution of gases and lung mechanics may be associated with the reduction in expiratory reserve volume.

TABLE 20-4

Respiratory Function in Normal and Obese Subjects Categorized by Weight-to-Height Ratios

Variable	Weight-to-Height Ratio ($kg \times cm^{-1}$)	
	Normal (0.60–0.69)	Obesity (1.10–1.19)
Vital capacity (% P)	108 ± 5	69 ± 14
Expiratory reserve volume (L)	1.35 ± 0.14	0.48 ± 0.18
Expiratory reserve volume (% P)	100 ± 8	32 ± 11
Functional residual capacity (% P)	80 ± 4	75 ± 14
Residual volume (% P)	63 ± 6	141 ± 37
Maximal voluntary ventilation (% P)	102 ± 7	61 ± 12

% P = percentage of predicted value.
Source: Adapted from CS Ray, DY Sae, G Bray, et al. Effects of obesity on respiratory function. Am Rev Respir Dis 1983;128:501–506.

The mechanical work of breathing, reflected in a higher oxygen cost of breathing,[74] is increased in obesity. The intercostal muscles being forced to move the large adipose tissue mass overlying the thorax and the contracting diaphragm work against an enlarged and distended abdomen. As the increased work of breathing occurs at reduced lung volume, a feeling of respiratory distress occurs that reduces the desire and ability to exercise.

Obesity-hypoventilation syndrome occurs in approximately 5% of severely obese patients. It is characterized by hypoventilation, periodic respiration, somnolence, cyanosis, polycythemia, right ventricular hypertrophy, and heart failure; this constellation was dubbed the *Pickwickian syndrome* by Burwell and coworkers.[75] The expiratory reserve volume and chest wall compliance are reduced, along with alveolar volume and gas exchange.[67] Shallow breathing at a low lung volume causes small airway closure and regional atelectasis that lead to increased venous admixture, physiological shunting, nonuniformity of pulmonary capillary perfusion, and increased physiological dead space.[76] There is decreased respiratory response to hypoxia and hypercapnia. Pulmonary hypertension in the obesity-hypoventilation syndrome has several causes[77]: pulmonary vasoconstriction secondary to hypoxia and acidosis, biventricular hypertrophy, elevated pulmonary venous pressure, and transpulmonary diastolic pressure gradient.[67] When the syndrome does occur, sleep apnea may lead to sudden death. Fortunately, some of the features of the obesity-hypoventilation syndrome can be reversed by weight reduction such as the hypoventilation and the respiratory response to carbon dioxide, but impaired response to hypoxia may persist.[67,69] In some patients a ketogenic diet caused increased carbon dioxide response independent of changes in body weight or pulmonary mechanics.[78]

Exercise Tolerance

Several respiratory factors have been identified that limit exercise tolerance in obese persons: (1) increased metabolic and associated ventilatory requirements to perform exercise; (2) increased cost of breathing because of the high breathing frequency and the interfering chest wall and abdominal fat; and (3) pulmonary insufficiency related to the heavy work of breathing and lung atelectasis. These changes in pulmonary function exacerbate the ventilatory strain associated with exercise by obese persons, and the high metabolic cost of breathing reduces exercise tolerance and the amount of work accomplished in a given time, thus increasing the imbalance between energy intake and expenditure.

Sleep Apnea

The syndrome of obstructive sleep apnea in obese persons is caused by increased pharyngeal resistance and decreased airway patency, and both are important determinants in airway collapse or occlusion during sleep. White and colleagues[79] found that both weight and weight-to-height ratio were significantly related to pharyngeal resistance ($r = 0.53$ and 0.59, respectively) and indicated that these relationships increase with age. The apnea problem, as it relates to obesity, may also be associated with a markedly reduced total respiratory compliance during recumbency compared with that of healthy subjects.[53]

Temperature Regulation

When exposed to heat or cold, healthy persons maintain relatively constant body temperature by a variety of physiological responses. Exercise causes increased heat production, and when it is performed in a hot and humid environment it can strain the body's heat loss capability. Blood flow through the skin is increased during heat stress, to afford greater heat loss by evaporation. During exercise there is competition between the requirements of the working muscles and circulation through the skin. In obese persons, relatively less blood flow is allocated to the skin, to facilitate heat loss, and this compromises heat balance. Thus, obese persons are less tolerant of exposure to heat or exercise in a warm or hot and humid environment than are nonobese people, often suffering hyperthermia and even shock and collapse. There are several reasons.

First, an obese person is rounder and, so, has a smaller surface-area-to-body-mass ratio. As heat exchange with the environment by convection, radiation, and evaporation is proportional to body surface area exposed, a small ratio is associated with less heat exchange per unit mass. Second, the specific heat of fat stored in adipose tissue is lower than that of water or other tissue. Thus, for a given heat load, persons with excessive adipose tissue exhibit a greater increase in body temperature per kilogram of body weight. Third, the heat-activated sweat gland density of obese persons is lower owing to stretching of the skin to accommodate the fat mass (Table 20-5), which may compromise evaporative capacity.[80] Fourth, the cardiorespiratory system of obese persons may be taxed at a relatively lower exercise intensity in warm or hot environments because of the necessity to supply blood

TABLE 20-5

Average Density and Calculated Total of Heat-Activated Sweat Glands in Obese and Lean Men and Women *

Subjects (No.)	Statistics	Heat-Activated Sweat Gland $\times$ cm^{-2}	Surface Area (Dubois) (m^2)	Total Heat-Activated Sweat Glands (millions)
Obese men (3)	$\bar{X}$	46.7	1.89	1.04
	SD	$\pm$ 17.2	$\pm$ 0.32	$\pm$ 0.33
Lean men (6)	$\bar{X}$	59.2	1.69	1.00
	SD	$\pm$ 12.5	$\pm$ 0.03	$\pm$ 0.22
Obese women (6)	$\bar{X}$	74.5	2.00	1.48
	SD	$\pm$ 9.9	$\pm$ 0.11	$\pm$ 0.19
Lean women (4)	$\bar{X}$	99.8	1.55	1.56
	SD	$\pm$ 11.8	$\pm$ 0.08	$\pm$ 0.25

$\bar{X}$ = mean.
*Subjects sat in 47°C $\pm$ 1°C dry-bulb, 24°C $\pm$ 1.5°C wet bulb environment for 45 minutes before measurements were made. Heat-activated sweat gland data were determined from 46 skin sites, 18 on the trunk and 28 on the limbs, with a starch-iodine–impregnated bond paper technique.
Source: Adapted from O Bar-Or, HM Lundegren, LI Magnusson, et al. Distribution of heat activated sweat glands in obese and lean men and women. Hum Biol 1968;40;235–248.

to working muscle and to the skin for effective heat loss.[81] Last, there is a significantly lower volume of skin blood flow in proportion to central body temperature in obese persons who exercise in the heat. The skin blood flow is important to support heat loss to the environment, and the relatively lower flow reduces heat loss (Table 20-6).[82]

In summary, it seems that obese persons are more susceptible to hyperthermia when exercising in warm or hot environments, particularly if evaporative cooling associated with sweating is compromised.[83-86] Healthy, young, obese subjects engaged in basic military training or late summer or early fall football practice have suf-

TABLE 20-6

Average Slope of the Forearm Blood Flow/Deep Body Temperature (Esophageal Temperature) Relationship in a Thermoneutral[a] and a Warm[b] Environment

Subjects	Statistic	Thermoneutral[a]	Warm[b]
Obese (N = 5)	$\bar{X}$	7.35	8.92
	SEM	$\pm$ 0.69	$\pm$ 1.09
Lean (N = 5)	$\bar{X}$	10.26[c]	12.08[c]
	SEM	$\pm$ 0.78	$\pm$ 0.54

$\bar{X}$ = mean.
[a]Thermoneutral environment: T_{db} = 22°C, T_{wb} = 14°C.
[b]Warm environment: T_{db} = 38°C, T_{wb} = 20°C.
[c]$P < .05$ when comparing data from lean and obese subjects.
Source: Adapted from NB Vroman, ER Buskirk, JL Hodgson. Cardiac output and skin blood flow in lean and obese individuals during exercise in the heat. J Appl Physiol 1983;55:69–74.

fered heat injury and even death, especially before being effectively acclimated to the heat.[81]

In a cold environment, subcutaneous fat provides thermal insulation, which is approximately two to four times as effective as an equivalent amount of lean tissue. In tolerable cold (minimally clothed) an obese person who accomplishes a fixed work task has a lower body surface temperature for a higher deep body temperature than a lean person.[81] The higher deep body temperature in obese persons occurs despite only a modest increase in metabolism brought about by shivering or other means of heat production. In lean persons exposure to cold air, and particularly cold water (e.g., 15°C, 59°F), can elevate metabolism two- to threefold, but similar exposure of obese people produces little if any increase in metabolism.[87,88] Body cooling activates a variety of mechanisms (Table 20-7). In general, obese subjects activate fewer physiological and behavioral mechanisms. Although the perception of thermal comfort among the obese is not much different than among the lean, they tolerate cold considerably better, suffering less physiological strain.

O'Hara and colleagues[89] introduced an interesting idea in their concept of *treatment* of obesity by exercise in the cold. The investigators exposed six obese men for 10 days to a cold environment (–34°C) in which they performed various types of exercise for approximately 3.5 hours per day. The mean daily energy expenditure for the exercise was 1,242 kcal. After early cold-induced diuresis of approximately 1 kg that may also have involved water loss from partially depleted glycogen stores, substantial body fat was also lost, which was well sustained 2 months after completion of the experi-

TABLE 20-7

Mechanisms Activated by Moderate Body Cooling in Lean and Obese Subjects

Mechanism	Lean	Obese
Physiological		
Stimulation of cutaneous thermal receptors	Yes	Yes
Cutaneous vasoconstriction	Yes	Yes
Increased secretion of epinephrine and norepinephrine	More	Less
Thyroid-stimulating hormone secretion	More	Less
Semiconscious increase in motor activity	More	Less
Shivering	More	Less
Piloerection	Yes	Yes
Behavioral		
Body curling and extremity protection	More	Less
Add clothing	More	Less
Seek warmer environment	Frequently	Less so

TABLE 20-8

Mean Daily Heat Debt, Metabolic Heat Production, and Cumulative Caloric Turnover Incurred by Obese Women (N = 7) during 90 Minutes of Exercise in Cool Water*

Statistic	Mean Daily Heat Debt (kcal)	Metabolic Heat Production (kcal)	Cumulative Caloric Turnover (kcal)
$\bar{X}$	186	380	566
SEM	±10	±3	±13
Range	135–215	305–470	496–620

$\bar{X}$ = mean.

*Underwater cycle ergometer in 17–22°C water.

Source: Adapted from LM Sheldahl, ER Buskirk, ER Loomis, et al. Effects of exercise in cool water on body weight loss. Int J Obesity 1982;6:29–42.

mental regimen. O'Hara's group[90] cited additional evidence that substantial body fat loss can occur among soldiers who work hard in an Arctic environment. Sheldahl and colleagues[91] attempted to confirm such results among women who exercised at approximately 36–40% of their aerobic power for approximately 90 minutes per day five times per week for 8 weeks in cool water (17–22°C; 62–68°F). Some women lost a small amount of body weight and fat, but the losses were insignificant. Although the women experienced considerable heat debt and associated calorie turnover (on the order of 500–600 kcal/day; see Table 20-8), their appetite, satiety, and associated kilocalorie intake were apparently unaltered. In contrast to the studies of O'Hara's group, who demonstrated effective loss of body weight and fat, Sheldahl and coworkers could not confirm such results, perhaps because the temperature was not as cold and the exposure shorter lived.

Subsequent to the work on men by O'Hara's group,[89] Murray and coworkers[92] performed a cold exposure experiment on somewhat obese women in a –20°C environment. The women exercised 200 minutes per day at approximately 30% of their aerobic power for 5 days during the winter months. The women lost approximately 0.5 kg of fat, a relatively inconsequential change compared with the losses of men and of the women themselves when they exercised in a warmer environment. The investigators gave several possible reasons why exercising in the cold did not produce greater loss of body fat in the women: (1) lower exercise intensity (the most plausible explanation), (2) greater stability of

fat stores, (3) avoidance of caffeine (a stimulator of lipolysis), and (4) translocation of fat to deep fat depots.

Altered Metabolism

Obese persons are at an increased risk for developing non–insulin-dependent diabetes, which is generally preceded by a change in the insulin resistance of the individual.[93] Typically, obese persons have a higher blood concentration of insulin and a decreased rate of hepatic insulin extraction.[94–96] Glucose uptake and use by skeletal muscle may also be decreased, but by increasing insulin secretion from the pancreas, a more normal blood sugar level is maintained. The primary increase in pancreatic insulin secretion presumably is mediated by the pancreatic nerves, but excessive carbohydrate intake may also provoke increased insulin secretion. Belfiori and coworkers[97] have suggested that insulin resistance in obesity is caused by the failure of key enzyme depression of catabolic pathways.

Several hypotheses exist that may explain the relationship between obesity and the development of insulin resistance and non–insulin-dependent diabetes. First, it has been found that obese patients tend to have a decreased number of glucose transporters, Glut 4, on the plasma membrane of cells, resulting in a decreased ability to remove glucose from the blood.[98] Second, it has been reported that the transport of glucose transporters to the cell surface is reduced during exposure to high concentrations of glucose.[99]

Patients who are hypertensive as well as obese have higher fasting or glucose-stimulated circulating insulin concentrations than those who are normotensive, even though the nonobese hypertensive patients may also have insulin resistance.[100] This observation reveals the

TABLE 20-9
Common Metabolic Alterations with Obesity *

Greater insulin secretion
Insulin resistance
    Skeletal muscle
    Adipocytes after hypertrophy
Hyperlipidemia
Growth hormone insensitivity to hypoglycemia

*In each instance, regular exercise has a counter effect.

possibility of an important relationship between blood pressure and insulin that does not involve obesity. Diet-induced loss of weight and fat in obese persons restores insulin sensitivity before blood pressure becomes more normal. In obese patients with hypertension, diet and exercise decrease insulin concentrations and increase insulin sensitivity while they lower blood pressure.[96] Thus, regular exercise can be regarded as a useful adjunctive therapeutic measure for obese persons, including those who have diabetes or hypertension. Some common metabolic alterations associated with obesity are listed in Table 20-9; for each, exercise produces a counter effect.

It has been postulated that a gain in body fat (body energy stores) is strongly influenced by overall sympathetic tone, the defect in obesity being associated with a deficiency of circulating norepinephrine rather than failure to respond to the neurotransmitter.[101] Abnormal hypotha-

lamic neural output is at least partially responsible for any diminished sympathetically released norepinephrine in obese persons. Obese subjects may have an inadequate ability to elevate sympathetic tone in the presence of food, which suggests the use of ephedrine-methylxanthine mixtures as a metabolic stimulant: The former increases the norepinephrine content of sympathetic nerve terminals and the latter inhibits the breakdown of cyclic adenosine monophosphate in the tissues and antagonizes the inhibitory effects of adenosine on norepinephrine secretion. In obese persons, this drug mixture normalizes the thermogenic response to a meal and increases fasting metabolic rate and 24-hour energy expenditure (Table 20-10).

Thermogenesis

The production of heat by the body, *thermogenesis*, can be induced by a single nutrient (cholesterol, protein, fat), a meal, exercise, or drugs and in summation accounts for the total energy expenditure of the individual. Although some aspects of thermogenesis may be modified by exercise or drugs, some are not so easily changed or are at least more difficult to measure. For example, the thermic effect of food in obese subjects was found reduced in some,[102,103] but not all,[104,105] studies. Thus, it remains equivocal as to whether or not changes in body composition are results or causes of changes in the thermic effect of feeding. Danforth[106] concluded that the decreased heat production is inversely related to the extent of insulin resistance and

TABLE 20-10
Changes in Metabolism with Sympathomimetics[a]

	Percentage Increase in Resting Metabolic Rate over 150 Minutes in Response to Sympathomimetics, a 300-kcal (1.25 MJ) Meal, or Both in Eight Lean and Eight Postobese Subjects	
Treatments[b]	*Lean (%)*	*Postobese (%)*
Ephedrine	4.82 ± 0.97	5.68 ± 0.87
Ephedrine/methylxanthines	10.4 ± 1.4	10.9 ± 1.2
Meal	15.2 ± 1.5	5.65 ± 0.67[c]
Meal plus both drugs	22.6 ± 2.5	16.7 ± 1.2[c]

	Percentage Change in Daily Energy Intake and Expenditure during Treatment with Sympathomimetics		
Group	*Intake (%)*	*Energy Expenditure (%)*	*Balance (%)*
Lean	0 ± 2.6	+0.5 ± 0.6	−0.7 ± 2.5
Formerly obese	−16.2 ± 4.0[c]	+8.1 ± 2.6[c]	−24.3 ± 2.4[c]

[a]Values, mean ± standard error.
[b]Drug doses: ephedrine, 22 mg; methylxanthines, 30 mg caffeine, and 50 mg theophylline.
[c]Significant difference between treatments, $P < .02$.
Source: Adapted from AG Dulloo, DS Miller. Obesity: a disorder of the sympathetic nervous system. World Rev Nutr Diet 1987;50:1–56.

TABLE 20-11

Obese Subjects' Reasons for Decreased Adherence to Conditioning Program Activities after Its Termination, and Frequency of Mention

Stated Reason	Obese Subjects* (%)
Inability to find or make time, job demands, young children and family demands, pressure of university coursework or research, sick relative to care for, and move to new house	61 (11)
Poor self-discipline or motivation, no car for transportation to an exercise program, no parking proximal to exercise facilities, no exercise facilities near home, and hiatus between program termination and availability of other supervised exercise	44 (8)
Loss of social support afforded by the conditioning program group	33 (6)
Another leisure exercise mode with aerobic component pursued	17 (3)
Disappointment with weight loss during program	6 (1)

*Percentage of subjects citing reason, with number of subjects citing reason given in parentheses. Many participants cited multiple reasons and all are included.
Source: Reprinted with permission from PC MacKeen, BA Franklin, WC Nicholas, et al. Body composition, physical work capacity and physical activity habits at 18-month follow-up of middle-aged women participating in an exercise intervention program. Int J Obesity 1983;7:61–71.

can partially be restored by weight loss; the thermogenic defect in obesity may be the consequence of a slower carbohydrate storage rate and greater inhibition of gluconeogenesis. It is well known that overfeeding increases the basal metabolic rate (BMR) and underfeeding decreases it in both lean and obese subjects. The respective changes are not exclusively related to changes in fat-free body mass or the metabolically active tissue mass. Generally, lean people have lower BMRs than obese ones,[107] and after weight loss the BMR of obese individuals is reduced.[108,109]

Exercise increases heat production and energy expenditure, although for most people who are not dedicated athletes, this rarely means more than a 50% increase in BMR over 24 hours. The elevation in energy expenditure with regular exercise is a desirable adjunct to any weight loss regimen, but it is distinctly secondary to restriction of calorie intake. For most people, regulation of food intake appears to be closely related to energy expenditure,[110] except with rather continuous exhausting exercise, when appetite cannot keep up with energy expenditure and body weight is lost.[81] In obese persons the ability to deliver oxygen to working muscle and the rate of its use by these muscles (aerobic power, $\dot{V}O_2$max) may be reduced, depending on age, sex, and history. Thus, their relative fitness to perform hard work is reduced, causing them to limit activity to relatively low exercise intensity and for shorter periods.

It is difficult for obese people to develop the exercise habit, and even if they join a supervised exercise program they generally do not continue to exercise when they leave the program (Table 20-11).[81,111,112] Several reasons for lessening activity were cited, but available time, poor motivation, and loss of social support predominated. A list of beneficial effects is presented in Table 20-12; the most important one is increased energy expenditure.

TABLE 20-12

Beneficial Effects of Regular Exercise for Obese Person

Physiological effects
    Increased daily energy expenditure
    Relatively decreased appetite
    Increased or preserved muscle mass
    Reduced body fatness (aided by dietary restriction)
    Increased functional capacity
    Decreased plasma insulin concentration
    Increased tissue sensitivity to insulin, skeletal muscle
    Decreased serum triglyceride concentration
    Decreased heart rate both at rest and during submaximal exercise
    Decreased systolic blood pressure
    Increased stroke volume
    Decreased peripheral vascular resistance
    Decreased cardiac work, submaximal exercise
    Increased flexibility
    Better motor coordination
Psychological effects
    Reduced fatigue on the job, recreational activities
    Increased self-satisfaction and acceptance
    Improved self-perception, image
    Improved social interactions
    Improved self-esteem and confidence
    More balanced perspective about regular exercise

Source: Adapted from L Landsberg. Insulin and hypertension: lessons from obesity. N Engl J Med 1997;317:378–379; F Belfiori, S Lanello, AM Rabuazzo. Insulin resistance in obesity: a critical analysis at enzyme level. Int J Obesity 1979;3:301–323; and ER Buskirk. Obesity. In JS Skinner (ed), Exercise Testing and Exercise Prescription for Special Cases. Philadelphia: Lea & Febiger, 1987;149–173.

Drugs can stimulate thermogenesis. The sympathomimetic amines have already been mentioned. A special issue of the *International Journal of Obesity* (1987) was devoted to the topic, and in it Munro provides an overview of drug treatment for obesity.[113] The potential for increasing metabolism by use of thermogenic agents such as sympathomimetic amines is encouraging. Pasquali and colleagues[114] report results using ephedrine hydrochloride and etilefrine hydrochloride in different groups of obese patients. They observed approximately a three-point drop in BMI when these drugs were administered for 3 months. They concluded that the drugs may be especially valuable for obese patients who are chronically adapted to low-energy expenditure or who have documented thermogenic defects.

Drug therapy, discussed in greater detail later in this chapter, is recommended when necessary to satisfy a specific need for weight reduction, such as that associated with elective surgery (see Pharmacotherapy). In terms of long-term treatment, it is viewed as unethical to justify such treatment until there is extensive documentation of evidence of both drug efficacy and safety.

TREATMENTS FOR OBESITY

Psychology of Obesity

It would be inappropriate to describe the various treatments for obesity without offering some insight into the psychology of obesity and the effects that being obese may have on a person's mental well-being. Although no study has been able to describe a specific psychological profile that places a person at greater risk for becoming obese, certain characteristics do seem to promote behavior that favors fat deposition. For example, persons who are prone to overeating, lack of awareness of hunger and satiety, and exaggerated misperceptions of body image tend to be overweight or obese. Still, these characteristics tend to be found in persons who are obese already, rather than those who become obese.

Nonetheless, the most important issues related to the psychology of obesity center around the psychological effect and the social costs of being obese. It has been reported that obese persons tend to have low levels of self-esteem, a factor that can inhibit the ability to adhere to treatment plans. In addition, without a healthy sense of self-worth many obese persons may not feel *worthy* of being thin.

Compounding the effects of low self-esteem among the obese is the fact that many studies have reported discrimination against the obese.[115] For example, it is more difficult for an overweight person to be hired for work

in which image is important. Something as simple as the size of seats in movie theatres or on airplanes can limit an obese person's enjoyment of these activities. One study even found that when young children (5–8 years of age) were shown a variety of pictures of people of different ages, races, and body size, the majority of children indicated that the person with whom they would most not like to play was the overweight person.[116]

All of these effects culminate in what is described as a poor quality of life. For example, compared with lean persons, obese women are less likely to marry, obese persons in general attain lower levels of education and earn considerably less during their lifetimes, and tend to remain in a low socioeconomic status.[117] The degree to which an obese person would give up being obese is expressed dramatically by one subject who lost weight after gastric bypass surgery and stated that he or she would rather become an amputee than return to the former morbidly obese state.[118]

Therefore, efforts to reduce the weight of both obese and overweight persons are central to the study of obesity. The various treatments available range from simple caloric restriction to a more radical approach in which the size of the stomach is surgically reduced. Each of these treatments is effective to a degree and almost all of them require proper and full compliance of the subject. Unfortunately, in terms of weight loss programs for the disabled, little information is available. What is known is that the same approaches may be used given the restrictions of each type of disability. For example, persons who are mildly disabled, but can perform certain exercises, are encouraged to maintain lean body mass and restrict calories to lose weight. Persons with more severe disabilities are more restricted in the options they can choose, generally being limited to only caloric restriction. Nonetheless, a thorough knowledge of each type of treatment is beneficial for health practitioners who are attempting to help both healthy and disabled persons either maintain their current weight or lose excess weight.

Dietary Regimens

Body weight and fat loss can be achieved with dietary (calorie) restriction if energy expenditure is maintained or increased. As with exercise, the success of weight loss from dietary restriction is highly dependent on adherence to the prescribed regimen. The types of diets, together with a rough description and general experience using the diet are included in Table 20-13. Care must be taken to ensure that restricted diets contain all essential nutrients. Many who have worked extensively

TABLE 20-13
Categories of Weight Loss Diets

Type of Diet	Description	Characteristics
Unrestricted calories Nutritionally balanced	Liquid homogenate	Monotonous
Restricted calories		
Varied items	Mixed low-calorie diet (800–1,200 kcal)	Carefully controlled calorie intake, palatable (satisfying)?
Formula	Liquid homogenate	Carefully controlled calorie intake, monotonous
Nutritionally unbalanced (may also be calorically restricted), altered proportion of macronutrients	High-protein, or high-carbohydrate, low-fat	Less efficient calorie use, reduced fat deposition, difficult to compensate for excluded foods
	Low-carbohydrate, high-fat or high-protein	Ketosis, decreased appetite, small excretory loss of calories, difficult to compensate for excluded foods
Focus on a specific food item	Grapefruit, kelp, vitamin B_6, and so forth	Promote lipolysis, reduced efficiency of calorie use, monotonous
Calorically dilute	High-fiber, low-fat	Slowed ingestion rate (more chewing required), impaired digestion, absorption of nutrients, satiety inducing
Fasting		
Very few calories	Protein or protein-carbohydrate mixture, 300–600 kcal/day	Reduces body fat, spares body proteins, ketosis
Total fast		Reduces body fat and protein, highly ketogenic

Source: Reprinted with permission from JR Vasselli, MP Cleary, TB Van Itallie. Modern concepts of obesity. Nutr Rev 1983;41:361–373.

with obese patients, even though they may initially use specific starter diets, prefer to wean to a well-balanced diet containing a variety of good foods, with limits on quantity that are compatible with goals for weight loss or maintenance.

The calorie equivalent of stored body fat (triacylglyceride) is between 9.0 and 9.3 kcal/g. Nevertheless, body weight loss is not composed of stored fat alone; although it consists largely of fat, it contains water and protein as well. Thus, the calorie equivalent of 6.5–8.0 kcal/g of weight is lost. Early during weight loss induced by diet restriction, more water is lost and the calorie equivalent might be as low as 2.5 kcal/g. These values translate to approximately 1,200 kcal/lb of weight lost when starting a weight reduction program and increase to approximately 3,500 kcal/lb as weight loss continues.

Exercise Programs

To reduce body weight and fat, exercise must involve reasonably high energy expenditure.[119,120] Movement of the body mass is important. This can be accomplished by walking, hiking, stair climbing, lawn mowing, dancing, jogging, or cross-country skiing, among other activities. Table 20-14 lists the approximate calorie turnover associated with several common activities. Values with respect to individual differences in body weight are included. Weight-supported activities include bicycling (or indoor cycle ergometer riding) and particularly swimming. Significant calorie turnover can be generated if the speed of pedalling or stroking is appreciable and sustained.

Given that physical activity increases energy expenditure, it is important to consider a physically active lifestyle for both prevention and treatment of obesity. A physically active lifestyle can help improve cardiorespiratory fitness; promote flexibility, mobility, and physical self-confidence; modify risk factors associated with the development of cardiovascular disease and maturity-onset diabetes; allow weight loss with larger food intake that still is nutritionally adequate; and preserve a higher RMR than that commonly observed with diet restriction. Development of a regular physical activity regimen can create appreciation of the need for total lifestyle management. Such lifestyle management may well involve choosing foods that help reduce body fat and maintain

TABLE 20-14
Approximate Calorie Expenditure for 1 Hour of Physical Activity[a]

Activity	Body Weight				
	56.8 kg 125 lb	68.2 kg 150 lb	79.5 kg 175 lb	90.9 kg 200 lb	113.6 kg 250 lb
Sitting, writing, or reading	60	72	84	96	120
Domestic housework	204	246	282	318	408
Walking (2 mph)	174	210	240	276	148
Walking (3 mph)[b]	240	300	360	450	510
Jogging (5.0 mph)	300	360	420	510	620
Cycling (6.0 mph)	240	300	360	400	480
Mowing grass (power)	204	246	282	318	402
Mowing grass (manual)	228	270	312	348	444
Bowling (nonstop)	240	300	360	430	510
Dancing (moderate)	210	252	288	330	390
Dancing (vigorous)	288	342	396	450	540
Golf (walking)	198	240	288	330	408
Skiing (cross-country; 5 mph)	312	426	480	530	640
Swimming (moderate crawl)	240	288	336	378	480

[a]Approximate values for activities that can be undertaken by many obese persons. Values vary with rate of exercise and efficiency with which activity is performed. Interpolation and extrapolation can be used for subjects who differ in weight.
[b]3 mph = 80 meters per minute.
Source: Adapted from F Belfiori, S Lanello, AM Rabuazzo. Insulin resistance in obesity: a critical analysis at enzyme level. Int J Obesity 1979;3:301–323; and ER Buskirk. Obesity. In JS Skinner (ed), Exercise Testing and Exercise Prescription for Special Cases. Philadelphia: Lea & Febiger, 1987;149–173.

optimal weight. Thus, the aims of a physically active lifestyle are to increase energy expenditure, preserve muscle and metabolically active tissue mass, provide enjoyment, and emphasize healthy lifestyle awareness. Nevertheless, an obese sedentary person contemplating a more active lifestyle is well advised to proceed slowly, preferably with competent professional assistance.

For obese persons, walking is an effective way to start an exercise program. The pace and distance covered can be regularly increased until an acceptable calorie turnover is achieved. Walking a mile uses essentially as much energy as jogging or running a mile; thus distance covered is important in structuring a simple exercise regimen for an obese person. In addition, a simple lifestyle change is more likely to be continued than a more complex one. A walking regimen can mean less reliance on vehicular transportation, using stairs instead of elevators, parking at a distance from the job, or walking to deliver a message rather than phoning. Walking with a companion or as part of a sightseeing or hiking group provides important social support.

Warnold and coworkers[121] structured slow and rapid walking regimens for obese patients who were approximately 40% body fat. Slow walking ranged from 25–42 m per minute (0.93–1.57 mph) and rapid walking from 45–75

m per minute (1.68–2.80 mph). Each patient started with a slow walk, although even the rapid rate would be regarded as slow by many lean people. We have usually used a similar approach when working with obese subjects (i.e., start with slow walking, then go to faster walking, and then to other activities). Table 20-15 lists the advantages of walking; Table 20-16 lists additional activities undertaken by obese subjects with whom we have worked.

Unfortunately, most obese people cannot swim well enough (although most float quite readily) to use swim-

TABLE 20-15
Advantages of Walking

Avoids musculoskeletal problems associated with running
Avoids traffic hazards of cycling
Avoids inconvenience of trying to find a swimming pool or special recreational facilities
Requires no extraordinary skill
Can be done almost anywhere and at any time
Can produce a training effect
Is inexpensive
Affords socializing with a companion while walking
Affords exercising a pet and sharing the pet's companionship

TABLE 20-16

Simple Physical Activities Recommended for Obese Subjects

Walking
Stair climbing
Walking and jogging
Selected strength and flexibility exercises
Dancing, with or without partner: aerobic, simple steps to
    music
Distance swimming
Walking purposefully in waist-deep water
Cycling, perhaps on tricycle
Cycling in water
Treading in water, with or without flotation device

TABLE 20-17

*Factors That Could Enhance Adherence to an
Exercise Program*

Select appropriate exercise
    Emphasize movement of body mass
    Emphasize all opportunities for walking
    Emphasize that all daily activities are exercise
Provide realistic expectations, no miracles
    Amount of exercise, intensity, and duration
    Time commitment and frequency
    Physiological and psychological changes
Start slowly
Select convenient hours
Select pleasant surroundings
Provide individual attention
Encourage group activity, socialization
Have highly motivated group leader
Record results, use some self-monitoring
Provide positive feedback about changes in weight, fatness,
    exercise capacity, heart rate, blood pressure, serum lip-
    ids, glucose, insulin, uric acid
Use deposit and refund (rewards)
Emphasize education: self, family members, close friends,
    and companions; gain understanding of energy turnover
    brought about by diet and exercise

ming as a means of regular exercise. Nevertheless, alternative activities can be undertaken in the water: using a kickboard with or without kick fins, kicking while grasping the side of a pool, walking or jogging in waist-deep water, cycling an immersed ergometer, or striding in a deeper pool while suspended in a harness or buoyed up by a flotation device. Such exercise in water avoids much weight bearing and reduces strain on joints by using the water to provide buoyancy.[91,122,123] Sheldahl and colleagues[91] showed that women can cycle an ergometer in water for 90 minutes or longer and expend upward of 400 kcal per exercise session while maintaining "near thermal neutrality." This relatively comfortable in-water exercise for obese persons could logically be extended for longer periods, as many of them find it more tolerable than weight-bearing exercise.

Exercise and Safety

Goodman and Kenrick[124] noted that when obese persons participated in a walk-jog program, they had a higher incidence of injury than leaner ones. Pollock and colleagues[125] found that for men who participated in a regular exercise program the incidence of injuries was significantly related to their fatness. Franklin and associates[126] found that among 23 middle-aged obese women, seven sustained foot or leg injuries severe enough to force temporary discontinuation or modification of their activity. Most injuries occurred during the first 8 weeks of the program, despite their exercise of extreme caution in undertaking all physical activity gradually and after adequate warm-up and routine stretching. Nevertheless, in a well-organized and supervised physical activity program, the injury rate is acceptably low and the injuries minor. Injury remains something to plan for, but it should not warrant undue concern.

Table 20-17 lists a variety of factors that contribute to a successful exercise program for obese persons. Personal preparation, selection of appropriate apparel and footwear, and foot care all are important. Orthotic devices that provide heel support or compensatory foot pronation may be necessary so that exercise can be undertaken more safely and more enjoyably. Nevertheless, exercise can give rise to physiological and pathologic hazards (Table 20-18). Careful physical examination and a complete medical history can obviate many of these problems.

Complex behavior modifications are likely to be necessary if a weight reduction regimen is going to result in permanent beneficial lifestyle changes. Table 20-19 lists characteristics of obese persons who are likely to benefit from an exercise program. In an attempt to ascertain the successful strategies employed to maintain desirable weight once weight loss is achieved, Wing and Jeffrey[127] questioned 42 men and 22 women who were originally, on average, 43% overweight and who had sustained a weight loss of 10 kg (22 lb) or more for 1 year (Table 20-20). These *successful* individuals were most concerned about appearance, but more than one-half paid attention to diet and exercise.

TABLE 20-18
Potential Hazards of Exercise for Obese Persons

Precipitation of angina pectoris or myocardial infarction
Excessive increase in blood pressure; isometric exercise
Aggravation of degenerative arthritis and other joint problems
Ligamentous injuries
Injury from falling
Excessive sweating, chafing
Hypoloydration and reduced circulating blood volume to the skin
Heat stroke or heat exhaustion
Lower extremity edema

Source: Adapted from N Grey, DM Kipnis. Effect of diet composition on the hyperinsulinemia of obesity. N Engl J Med 1971;285:827–831; L Landsberg. Insulin and hypertension: lessons from obesity. N Engl J Med 1997;317:378–379; and ER Buskirk. Obesity. In JS Skinner (ed), Exercise Testing and Exercise Prescription for Special Cases. Philadelphia: Lea & Febiger, 1987;149–173.

Pharmacotherapy

In obese individuals for whom dietary and exercise interventions fail to achieve weight loss, pharmacotherapy is yet another technique. Weight loss drugs are recommended as adjuncts to diet and exercise. The NHLBI 1999 guidelines[8] recommend the adjuvant use of drugs in patients with a BMI greater than or equal to 27 kg/m^2, with accompanying risk factors or disease such as hypertension, dyslipidemia, CHD, type II diabetes, and sleep apnea, and in some patients with a BMI greater than or equal to 30 kg/m^2, with no such risk factors or disease.

The most common medications used for the treatment of obesity are phentermine, sibutramine, and orlistat. Phentermine received approval by the Food and Drug Administration as an antiobesity agent in 1959 and is used today as an appetite suppressant. Otherwise known as an anorexiant medication, which suppresses appetite,

TABLE 20-19
Characteristics of Obese Persons Who Are Most Likely to Benefit from an Exercise Program

Slightly or moderately obese
Became obese as an adult
Had not previously tried to lose weight
Sincerely desires weight reduction
Psychologically adjusted to pursuit of weight-reduction goal
Can intelligently follow directions
Has no complicating disease or disability
Is willing to make the commitment
Can find the time and facilities

TABLE 20-20
Most Popular Strategies of Formerly Obese Persons for Maintaining Weight Loss

Strategy	% Using Strategy
Frequent weighing	75
Reduced snacking	60
Reduced meal portions	60
Better food selection	57
Increased exercise	55

Source: Reprinted with permission from ER Buskirk. Obesity. In JS Skinner (ed), Exercise Testing and Exercise Prescription for Special Cases. Philadelphia: Lea & Febiger, 1987;149–173.

phentermine is a sympathomimetic amine that stimulates the release of norepinephrine.[128] The magnitude of weight loss with phentermine is reported to be approximately 4 kg with trials over 20 weeks or less.[129] Reported side effects include palpitations, tachycardia, elevated blood pressure, CNS stimulation (e.g., restlessness), dry mouth, constipation, and sexual dysfunction. Phentermine is contraindicated in persons with advanced arteriosclerosis, symptomatic cardiovascular disease, moderate to severe hypertension, hyperthyroidism, glaucoma, agitated states, or a history of drug abuse. Phentermine is approved for short-term weight loss treatment.

For a brief period, phentermine was coadministered with another class of drugs called *fenfluramines*. The use of this combination therapy, referred to as *fen-phen*, was halted in 1997 when the U.S. Centers for Disease Control reported 24 cases of valvular heart disease in women receiving this combination.[130] After the report, the number of cases of valvular disease in persons taking fen-phen increased because of heightened physician scrutiny. Several research studies were undertaken to both validate and describe this pathology. It was reported that persons taking fen-phen for longer than 6 months were at a higher risk for developing valvulopathy,[131] characterized by irregular thickening and chordal fusion of the mitral valve.[132]

Sibutramine (Meridia) received approval by the Food and Drug Administration as an obesity treatment drug in 1997. A reuptake inhibitor of 5-hydroxytryptamine and noradrenaline, sibutramine prolongs the period of time that serotonin and noradrenalin are active in the brain, resulting in appetite suppression and minimal elevations in energy expenditure.[133] A dosage of 15 mg per day over 6–12 months resulted in 5.5–6.5 kg weight loss.[134] Sibutramine is not advised for use in patients with a history of hypertension, CHD, congestive heart failure, arrhythmias, or stroke[8] and is contraindicated in patients with uncontrolled hypertension who are taking monoamine oxidase inhibitors or other antiobesity drugs. Sibutramine is available for long-term management of obese patients.

Orlistat (Xenical) is the most recent weight loss drug to receive approval by the U.S. Food and Drug Administration (April 1999). This is a new category of drug that selectively inhibits gastrointestinal lipases, which reduces the absorption of dietary fats. The amount of calories absorbed into the body as fat is reduced by 30%. U.S.-[135] and European-[136] based multicenter trials have collectively studied over 4,000 patients followed for 1–2 years. After 1 year of treatment, the average weight loss was 10% of initial body weight compared with 6% in placebo. After 2 years of treatment, orlistat-treated patients maintained 8% of weight loss compared with 5% in placebo. Additional benefits of orlistat, 120 mg, 3 times per day,[137] plus diet included improvements in fasting low-density lipoprotein cholesterol and insulin levels[135,136] and blood glucose levels.[135] Side effects of this drug include gastrointestinal symptoms (flatus with discharge, oily spotting, fecal urgency, fatty or oily stool, oily evacuation, fecal incontinence, and increased defecation), which lessen in severity over time. Supplementation with multivitamins is recommended because of potential loss of fat-soluble micronutrients such as vitamins. Orlistat, therefore, has potential for long-term management of obese patients in conjunction with an appropriate diet.

Surgical Treatment of Obesity

Each of the previously discussed treatments of obesity has been found to be successful or unsuccessful depending on many factors, such as the degree of obesity, a significant history of obesity, the age of the patient, various psychobehavioral factors, and last, the adherence to a particular treatment plan. In considering each of these options it has been found that as the severity of obesity increases and persists, with repeated failures and an increase in the number of comorbidities, the last step in managing obesity is through surgical intervention.[137] Before recommending surgery, the practitioner evaluates the patient's medical history, obesity treatment history, and presence or absence of comorbidities. Surgery is recommended for the patient who has a BMI greater than 35 or is 100% over their ideal body weight, presents with a number of comorbidities, and has attempted dietary, behavioral, or pharmacologic treatments without success.[138,139]

The history of obesity surgery is long and filled with radical approaches that have proven to be both unsuccessful and harmful to the patient. Some early surgeries resulted in chronic ulcers, whereas others had a high rate of mortality.[140] Surgical interventions for obesity have improved greatly in more recent years and are typically designed to reduce the number of calories a person consumes or absorbs by creating either malabsorption, gastric restriction, or both.

Gastric restriction reduces the capacity of the stomach and is accomplished by surgically creating a small pouch in the stomach into which only 15 ml of food may enter and is followed by a 9-mm elastic band through which the food then passes into the remainder of the stomach.[141] This surgery has been found to be beneficial in the short-term; however, with time the banding may relax, allowing the quantity of food ingested to increase. To counter this problem, an adjustable gastric band is attached to a subcutaneous opening through which saline may be injected, thereby inflating the band, creating the pouch when needed. Still, neither of these techniques has been shown to be successful over long-term periods and for some persons a different form of surgery is recommended.

The most successful form of obesity surgery is gastric bypass, also called *intestinal bypass*.[138] The idea behind gastric bypass is that by both reducing the capacity of the stomach and allowing ingested food to enter the small intestine more quickly, the amount of food both ingested and absorbed is reduced. The operation basically creates a 15-ml pouch at the top of the stomach, sealing off the rest of the stomach and attaches the proximal jejunum to the base of the pouch, allowing the food to bypass the duodenum. Patients who have undergone gastric bypass have lost up to 50% of their original weight and weight maintenance is highly dependent on adhering to dietary recommendations (avoiding overeating or eating energy-dense foods) and maintaining a regular exercise routine.[142] This suggests that behavior modification remains an important part of any obesity treatment, including surgery.

The success of surgical approaches to obesity is more than simply weight loss. It has been found that persons who undergo surgery to lose weight often have overall improved quality of life and health. Most long-term studies after surgery have found that patients who lose a significant amount of weight and remain at that weight are less diabetic (83% had normal glucose levels),[143] reduce their hypertension (only 14% of patients were hypertensive postoperatively compared with 58% preoperatively),[144] and improve respiratory insufficiency. Of course, there are some side effects and complications to gastric bypass, such as *dumping* (the rapid emptying of food into the small intestine resulting in palpitations, nausea, and dizziness generally brought about by the ingestion of energy-dense foods), diarrhea, and vitamin deficiencies.[145] Most of the side effects can be controlled through both dietary education, improved patient compliance, and the use of nutritional supplements.

SUMMARY

The prevalence of persons who are overweight or obese is increasing in almost all developed countries and even in some developing countries. Efforts to reduce this prevalence have not succeeded and efforts continue to find noninvasive treatments for obesity, such as pharmacologic or dietary practices. Still, it remains clear that the primary risk factors for obesity are lack of physical activity and diets high in calories and fat. Gross obesity constitutes a disabling condition that compromises physiological function and leads to, or is associated with, considerable morbidity, particularly chronic disease. The development of cardiovascular, respiratory, and neuromotor problems leads to disability, which then promotes a sedentary lifestyle. This lifestyle results in a reduction of lean body mass, further reducing exercise tolerance. The result of this cycle impairs a grossly obese person's ability to participate in exercise programs, but it is important to remember that any exercise is helpful. Moreover, it is important to consider that multiple interventions are most useful, including attention to identifiable medical problems and the patient's psyche, diet, and exercise.

REFERENCES

1. Keys A, Fidanza F, Karvonen MJ, et al. Indices of relative weight and obesity. J Chron Dis 1972;25:329–343.

2. Quetelet LAJ. A Treatise on Man and the Development of his Faculties. In Comparative Statistics in the 19th Century. Farnborough: Gregg International Publishers, 1973.

3. Garrow JS, Webster JD. Quetelets's index (W/H2) as a measure of fatness. Int J Obes 1985;9:147–153.

4. Thomas AE, McKay DA, Cutlip MB. A nomograph method for assessing body weight. Am J Clin Nutr 1976;29:302–304.

5. Seltzer CC, Mayer J. A simple criterion of obesity. Postgrad Med 1965;38:A101–A107.

6. Durnin JVGA, Womersley J. Body fat assessed from total body density and its estimation from skinfold thickness measurements on 481 men and women aged 16 to 72 years. Br J Nutr 1974;32:77–97.

7. Buskirk ER. Obesity: a brief overview with emphasis on exercise. Fed Proc 1974;33:1948–1951.

8. National Heart, Lung, and Blood Institute. Clinical Guidelines on the Identification, Evaluation, and Treatment of Overweight and Obesity: The Evidence Report. Bethesda, MD: National Institutes of Health, 1998.

9. Kuczmarski RJ, Carroll MD, Flegal, KM, Troiano RP. Varying body mass index cutoff points to describe overweight prevalence among U.S. adults: NHANES III. Obesity Research 1997;5(6):542–548.

10. The World Health Organization. WHO MONICA Project. Project: risk factors. Int J Epidemiol 1989;18(Suppl 1):S46–S55.

11. Deurenberg P, Weststrate JA, Seidell JC. Body mass index as a measure of body fatness: age- and sex-specific prediction formulas. Br J Nutr 1991;65:105–114.

12. Gallagher D, Visser M, Sepulveda D, et al. Body mass index as an estimate of fatness across gender, age, and ethnic groups. Am J Epidemiol 1996;143(3):228–239.

13. Bray GA. Obesity in America: an overview of the second Fogarty International Center Conference on Obesity. Int J Obesity 1979;3:363–375.

14. Fitzgerald FT. The problem of obesity. Annu Rev Med 1981;32:221–231.

15. Keys A. Overweight, obesity, coronary heart disease and mortality. Nutr Rev 1980;38:297–307.

16. Allison DB, Zannolli R, Faith MS, et al. Weight loss increases and fat loss decreases all-cause mortality rate: results from two independent cohort studies. Int J Obes Relat Metab Disord 1999;23(6):603–611.

17. Bray GA (ed). Comparative Methods of Weight Control. Westport, CT: Technomic, 1980.

18. Hirsch J, Batchelor B. Adipose tissue cellularity and human obesity. Clin Endocrinol Metab 1976;5:299–311.

19. Bjorntorp P. The Fat Cell. A Clinical View. In GA Bray (ed), Recent Advances in Obesity Research II. London: Newman, 1978.

20. Bjorntorp P. Regional patterns of fat distribution. Ann Intern Med 1985;103:994–995.

21. Buskirk ER, Puhl S. Adipose Tissue Distribution and Metabolic Consequences. In OA Levander (ed), AIN Symposium Proceedings Nutrition 87. Washington, DC: The American Institute of Nutrition, 1987;97–102.

22. Lapidus L, Bengtsson C, Larsson B, et al. Distribution of adipose tissue and risk of cardiovascular disease and death: a 12 year follow-up of participants in the population study of women in Gothenburg, Sweden. BMJ 1984;289:1261–1263.

23. Larsson L, Svardsudd K, Welin L, et al. Abdominal adipose tissue distribution, obesity and risk of cardiovascular disease and death: 13 year follow-up of participants in the study of men born in 1913. BMJ 1984;288:1401–1404.

24. Ducimetiere P, Richard J, Cambien F. The pattern of subcutaneous fat distribution in middle-aged men and the risk of coronary heart disease: the Paris Prospective Study. Int J Obes Relat Metab Disord 1986;10:229–240.

25. Van Itallie TB. Health implications of overweight and obesity in the United States. Ann Intern Med 1985;103:983–988.

26. Kuri-Harcuch W, Carrera-DeLaTorre B, Arkuch-Kuri S, et al. Human adipogenic serum activity increases during pregnancy. Int J Obes 1985:9:299–306.

27. Trayhurn P, Ashwell P. Control of white and brown adipose tissues by the autonomic nervous system. Proc Nutr Soc 1987;46:135–142.

28. Arner P. Role of antilipolytic mechanisms in adipose tissue distribution and function in man. Acta Med Scand Suppl 1988;723:144–152.

29. Kissebah AH, Peiris AN, Evans DJ. Mechanisms associating body fat distribution to glucose intolerance and diabetes mellitus: window with a view. Acta Med Scand Suppl 1988; 723:78–89.

30. Rebuffe-Scrive M. Steroid hormones and distribution of adipose tissue. Acta Med Scand Suppl 1988;723:121–134.

31. Bjorntorp P. Endocrine abnormalities of obesity. Metab Clin Exp 1995; 44(Suppl 3):21–23.

32. Cowell CT, Briody J, Loyd-Jones S, et al. Fat distribution in children and adolescents—the influence of sex and hormones. Horm Res 1997;48(Suppl 5): 93–100.

33. Alford FP, Hew FL, Christopher MC, Rantzau C. Insulin sensitivity in growth hormone (GH)-deficient adults and effect of GH replacement therapy. J Endocrinol Invest 1999;22(Suppl 5):28–32.

34. Miller KD, Jones E, Yanovski JA, et al. Visceral abdominal-fat accumulation associated with use of indinavir. Lancet 1998;351(9106):871–875.

35. Mann M, Piazza-Hepp T, Koller E, et al. Unusual distribution of body fat in AIDS patients: a review of adverse events reported to the Food and Drug Administration. Aids Patient Care STDS 1999;13(5):287–295.

36. Wanke C, Gerrior J, Kantaros J, et al. Recombinant human growth hormone improves the fat redistribution syndrome (lipodystrophy) in patients with HIV. AIDS 1999;13(15):2099–2103.

37. Lo JC, Mulligan K, Tai VW, et al. "Buffalo hump" in men with HIV-1 infection. Lancet 1998;351(9106):867–870.

38. Alexander JK. Obesity and the circulation. Mod Concepts Cardiovasc Dis 1963;32:799–803.

39. Amad KH, Brennan JC, Alexander JK. The cardiac pathology of chronic exogenous obesity. Circulation 1965; 32:740–749.

40. Prodger SH, Dennig H. A study of the circulation in obesity. J Clin Invest 1932;11:789–806.

41. Robinson SC, Brucer M. Hypertension, body build and obesity. Am J Med Sci 1940;199:819–829.

42. Terry AH. Obesity and hypertension. JAMA 1923;81:1283–1284.

43. Eckel RH, Krauss RM. American Heart Association call to action: obesity as a major risk factor for coronary heart disease. AHA Nutrition Committee. Circulation 1998;97:2099–2100.

44. Keys A, Aravanis C, Blackburn H, et al. Coronary heart disease: overweight and obesity as risk factors. Ann Intern Med 1972;77:15–27.

45. Paul O. A longitudinal study of coronary heart disease. Circulation 1963; 28:20–31.

46. Bloom E, Reed D, Katsuhiko Y, et al. Does obesity protect hypertensives against cardiovascular disease? JAMA 1986;256:2972–2975.

47. Messerli FH, Christie B, DeCarvalho JGR, et al. Obesity and essential hypertension, hemodynamics, intravascular volume, sodium excretion and plasma renin activity. Arch Intern Med 1981;141:81–85.

48. Messerli FH, Sundgaard-Rise K, Resin E, et al. Disparate cardiovascular effects of obesity and arterial hypertension. Am J Med 1983;74:802–812.

49. Raison J, Achmastos A, Asmar R, et al. Extracellular and interstitial fluid volume in obesity with and without associated systemic hypertension. Am J Cardiol 1986;57:223–226.

50. Messerli FH. Cardiovascular effects of obesity and hypertension. Lancet 1982; 1:1165–1168.

51. Alpert MA, Terry BA, Kelly DL. Effect of weight loss on cardiac chamber size, wall thickness and left ventricular function in morbid obesity. Am J Cardiol 1985;55:783–786.

52. Rubal BJ, Elmesallamy FH. Cardiac adaptations in a group of obese women. J Obes Weight Reg 1984;3:236–247.

53. Luce JN. Respiratory complications of obesity. Chest 1980;78:626–631.

54. Barakat HA, Burton DS, Carpenter JW, et al. Body fat distribution, plasma lipoproteins and the risk of coronary heart disease of male subjects. Int J Obesity 1987;12:473–480.

55. Garn SM, Bailey SM, Block WD. Relationships between fatness and lipid level in adults. Am J Clin Nutr 1979;32:733–735.

56. Kannel WB, Gordon T, Castelli WP. Obesity, lipids and glucose intolerance. The Framingham Study. Am J Clin Nutr 1979;32:1238–1245.

57. Miettinen TA. Cholesterol production in obesity. Circulation 1971;44:842–850.

58. Anderson JT, Lawler A, Keys A. Weight gain from simple overeating. II. Serum lipids and blood volume. J Clin Invest 1957;36:81–88.

59. Vague J. La differenciation sexuelle, facteur determinant des formes de l'obesite. Presse Med 1947;30:339–340.

60. Larson B, Svardsudd K, Wein L, et al. Abdominal adipose tissue distribution, obesity and risk of cardiovascular disease and death: 13-year follow-up of participants in the study of men born in 1913. BMJ 1984;288:1401–1404.

61. Lemieux I, Pascot A, Tchernof A, et al. Visceral adipose tissue and low-density lipoprotein particle size in middle-aged versus young men. Metab Clin Exp 1999;48(10):1322–1327.

62. Fujioka S, Matsuzawa Y, Tokunaga K, et al. Contribution of intraabdominal fat accumulation to the impairment of glucose and lipid metabolism in human obesity. Metabolism 1987;36:54–59.

63. Bjorntorp P. Abdominal obesity and the development of non-insulin dependent diabetes mellitus. Diabetes Metab Rev 1988;4:615–662.

64. Frericks RR, Webber LS, Srinivasan SR, et al. Relation of serum lipids and lipoproteins to obesity and sexual maturity in white and black children. Am J Epidemiol 1978;108:486–496.

65. Freedman DS, Burke GL, Harska DW, et al. Relationship of changes in obesity to serum lipid and lipoprotein changes in childhood and adolescence. JAMA 1985;254:515–520.

66. Berenson GS, McMahan CA, Voors AW, et al. Occurrence of Multiple Risk-Factor Variables for Cardiovascular Disease in Children. In GS Berenson, CA McMahan (eds), Cardiovascular Risk Factors in Children. New York: Oxford University Press, 1980;311–320.

67. Alexander JK. The Heart and Obesity. In JW Hurst (ed), The Heart, Arteries and Veins (5th ed). New York: McGraw-Hill, 1982;1584–1590.

68. Rosell S, Belfrage E. Blood circulation in adipose tissue. Physiol Rev 1979;59:1078–1104.

69. Alexander JK, Peterson KL. Cardiovascular effects of weight reduction. Circulation 1972;45:310–318.

70. Bedell GN, Wilson WR, Seebohm PM. Pulmonary function in obese persons. J Clin Invest 1958;37:1049–1060.

71. Buskirk ER, Bartlett HL. Pulmonary Function and Obesity. In RB Tobin, MA Mehlman (eds), Advances in Modern Human Nutrition. Vol I. Park Forest South, IL: Pathotox, 1980;211–224.

72. Bartlett HL, Buskirk ER. Body composition and the expiratory reserve volume in lean and obese men and women. Int J Obesity 1983;7:339–343.

73. Ray CS, Sae DY, Bray G, et al. Effects of obesity on respiratory function. Am Rev Respir Dis 1983;128:501–506.

74. Cherniak RM, Guenter CA. The effi-

ciency of the respiratory muscles in obesity. Can J Biochem Physiol 1961; 39:1215–1222.

75. Burwell CS, Robin ED, Whaley RD, et al. Extreme obesity associated with alveolar hypoventilation—a pickwickian syndrome. Am J Med 1956;21:811–818.

76. Said SI. Abnormalities of pulmonary gas exchange in obesity. Ann Intern Med 1960;53:1121–1124.

77. Rochester DF, Enson Y. Current concepts in the pathogenesis of the obesity-hypoventilation syndrome: mechanical and circulatory factors. Am J Med 1974;57:402–420.

78. Fried PI, McClean PA, Phillipson EA, et al. Effect of ketosis on respiratory sensitivity to carbon dioxide in obesity. N Engl J Med 1976;294:1081–1086.

79. White DP, Lombard RM, Cadieux RJ, et al. Pharyngeal resistance in normal humans: influence of gender, age and obesity. J Appl Physiol 1985;58:365–371.

80. Bar-Or O, Lundegren HM, Magnusson LI, et al. Distribution of heat activated sweat glands in obese and lean men and women. Hum Biol 1968;40:235–248.

81. Buskirk ER, Bar-Or O, Kollias J. Physiological Effects of Heat and Cold. In N Wilson (ed), Obesity. Philadelphia: FA Davis, 1969;119–139.

82. Vroman NB, Buskirk ER, Hodgson JL. Cardiac output and skin blood flow in lean and obese individuals during exercise in the heat. J Appl Physiol 1983;55:69–74.

83. Bar-Or O, Lundegren HM, Buskirk ER. Heat tolerance of exercising obese and lean women. J Appl Physiol 1969;26:403–409.

84. Schvartz E, Saar E, Benar D. Physique and heat tolerance in hot-dry and hot-humid environments. J Appl Physiol 1973;34:799–803.

85. Wyndham CH. The physiology of exercise under heat stress. Annu Rev Physiol 1973;35:193–220.

86. Epstein Y, Shapiro Y, Brill S. Role of surface area-to-mass ratio and work efficiency in heat intolerance. J Appl Physiol 1983;54:831–836.

87. Buskirk ER, Kollias J. Total body metabolism in the cold. Bull N J Acad Sci 1969;17–25.

88. Buskirk ER. Cold Stress: A Selective Review. In LJ Folinsbee, et al. (eds), Environmental Stress. New York: Academic Press, 1978;249–266.

89. O'Hara WJ, Allen C, Shephard RJ. Treatment of obesity by exercise in the cold. Can Med Assoc J 1977;8:773–785.

90. O'Hara WJ, Allen C, Shephard RJ. Loss of body weight and fat during exercise in a cold chamber. Eur J Appl Physiol 1977;37:205–218.

91. Sheldahl LM, Buskirk ER, Loomis JL, et al. Effects of exercise in cool water on body weight loss. Int J Obesity 1982;6:29–42.

92. Murray SJ, Shephard RJ, Greaves S, et al. Effects of cold stress and exercise on fat loss in females. Eur J Appl Physiol 1986;55:610–618.

93. Pi-Sunyer F. Weight and non-insulin-dependent diabetes mellitus. Am J Clin Nutr 1996;63(Suppl):423S–425S.

94. Peiris AN, Mueller RA, Smith GA, et al. Splanchnic insulin metabolism in obesity: Influence of body fat distribution. J Clin Invest 1986;78:1648–1657.

95. Grey N, Kipnis DM. Effect of diet composition on the hyperinsulinemia of obesity. N Engl J Med 1971;285:827–831.

96. Landsberg L. Insulin and hypertension: lessons from obesity. N Engl J Med 1997;317:378–379.

97. Belfiori F, Lanello S, Rabuazzo AM. Insulin resistance in obesity: a critical analysis at enzyme level. Int J Obesity 1979;3:301–323.

98. Simkin V. Urinary 17-ketosteroid and 17-ketogenic steroid excretion in obese patients. N Engl J Med 1961;264:974–977.

99. Kurtz BR, Givens JR, Kominder S, et al. Maintenance of normal circulating levels of delta-androstenedione and dehydroepiandrosterone in simple obesity despite increased metabolic clearance rates: evidence for a serve-controlled mechanism. J Clin Endocrinol Metab 1987;64:1261–1267.

100. Ferrannini E, Buzzigola G, Bonadonna R, et al. Insulin resistance in essential hypertension. N Engl J Med 1987;317:350–357.

101. Dulloo AG, Miller DS. Obesity: a disorder of the sympathetic nervous system. World Rev Nutr Diet 1987;50:1–56.

102. Pitlet PL, Chappius PL, Aecheson K, et al. Thermic effect of glucose in obese subjects studied by direct and indirect calorimetry. Br J Nutr 1976;35:282–292.

103. Swaminathan R, King RFGJ, Holmfield J, et al. Thermic effect of feeding carbohydrate, fat, protein and mixed meal in lean and obese subjects. Am J Clin Nutr 1985;42:177–181.

104. Felig P, Cunningham I, Levitt M, et al. Energy expenditure in obesity in fasting and postprandial state. Am J Physiol 1983;244:E45–E51.

105. Segal KR, Gutin B. Thermic effects of food and exercise in lean and obese women. Metabolism 1983;32:581–589.

106. Danforth E. Diet and obesity. Am J Clin Nutr 1985;42:1132–1145.

107. James WPT. Elevated metabolic rates in obesity. Lancet 1978;1:1122–1125.

108. Welle SL, Armatruda JM, Forbes GB, et al. Resting metabolic rate of obese women after rapid weight loss. J Clin Endocrinol Metab 1984;59:41–74.

109. den Besten C, Vansant G, Weststrate JA, Deurenberg P. Resting metabolic rate and diet-induced thermogenesis in abdominal and gluteal-femoral obese women before and after weight reduction. Am J Clin Nutr 1988;47:840–847.

110. Mayer J, Roy P, Mitra KP. Relation between caloric intake, body weight and physical work: studies in an industrial male population in West Bengal. Am J Clin Nutr 1956;4:169–175.

111. Franklin BA, MacKeen PC, Buskirk ER. Body composition effects of a 12-week physical conditioning program for normal and obese middle-aged women, and status at 18-month follow-up. Int J Obes 1978;2:394.

112. MacKeen PC, Franklin BA, Nicholas WC, et al. Body composition, physical work capacity and physical activity habits at 18-month follow-up of middle-aged women participating in an exercise intervention program. Int J Obes 1983;7:61–71.

113. Munro JF. Drug treatment of obesity: an overview. Int J Obes 1987;(Suppl 3):13–15.

114. Pasquali R, Cesari MP, Besteghi L, et al. Thermogenic agents in the treatment of human obesity: preliminary results. Int J Obes 1987;11(Suppl 3):23–26.

115. Kolotkin RL, Head S, Hamilton M, Tse KJ. Assessing impact of weight on quality of life. Obes Res 1995;3:49–56.

116. Allon N. The Stigma of Overweight in Everyday Life. In BB Wolman (ed), Psychological Aspects of Obesity: A Handbook. New York: Van Nostrand Reinhold, 1982.

117. Kral JG, Sjostrom LV, Sullivan MEE. Assessment of quality of life before and after surgery for severe obesity. Am J Clin Nutr 1992;55:611S–614S.

118. Rand CSW, MacGregor AMC. Successful weight loss following obesity surgery and the perceived liability of morbid obesity. Int J Obes Relat Metab Disord 1991;15:577–579.

119. Buskirk ER. Obesity. In JS Skinner (ed), Exercise Testing and Exercise Prescription for Special Cases. Philadelphia: Lea & Febiger, 1987;149–173.

120. Oscai LB. The Role of Exercise in Weight Control. In J Wilmore (ed), Exercise and Sports Sciences Review. Vol I. New York: Academic Press, 1973;103–123.

121. Warnold I, Carlgren G, Krotkiewski M. Energy expenditure and body composition during weight reduction in hyperplastic obese women. Am J Clin Nutr 1978;31:750–763.

122. Castronic M. Jog in the pool—no pain. J Phys Ed 1976;74:8–18.

123. Evans BW, Cureton KJ, Purvis JW. Metabolic and circulatory responses to walking and jogging in water. Res Q 1867;49:442–449.

124. Goodman CE, Kenrick MM. Physical fitness in relation to obesity. Obesity Bariatric Med 1975:4:12–15.

125. Pollock ML, Gettman LR, Milesis CA, et al. Effects of frequency and duration of training on attrition and incidence of injury. Med Sci Sports 1977;9:31–36.

126. Franklin B, Buskirk ER, Hodgson J, et al. Effects of physical conditioning on cardiorespiratory function, body composition and serum lipids in relatively normal-weight and obese middle-aged women. Int J Obes 1979;3:97–109.

127. Wing RR, Jeffrey RW. Successful losers: a descriptive analysis of the process of weight reduction. Obesity Bariatric Med 1978;7:190–191.

128. Kordik CP, Reitz AB. Pharmacological treatment of obesity: therapeutic strategies. J Med Chem 1999;42:181–201.

129. Weintraub M. A double blind clinical trial in weight control. Arch Intern Med 1984;144:1143–1148.

130. US Department of Health and Human Services. Cardiac valvuopathy associated with exposure to fenfluramine or dexfenfluramine: interim public health recommendations. MMWR Morb Mortal Wkly Rep 1997;46(45):1061–1066.

131. Ryan DH, Bray GA, Helmcke F, et al. Serial echocardiographic and clinical evaluation of valvular regurgitation before, during, and after treatment with fenfluramine or dexfenfluramine and mazindol or phentermine. Obes Res 1999;7(4):414–416.

132. Steffee CH, Singh HK, Chitwood WR. Histologic changes in three explained native cardiac valves following use of fenfluramine. Cardiovasc Pathol 1999;8(5):245–253.

133. Connoley IP, Heal DH, Stock MJ. A study in rats of the effects of sibutramine on food intake and thermogenesis. Br J Pharmacol 1995;114:387P.

134. Meridia Monograph. Mt Olive, NJ: Knoll Pharmaceuticals, 1997.

135. Davidson MH, Hauptman J, DiGirolamo M, et al. Weight control and risk factor reduction in obese subjects treated for 2 years with orlistat. JAMA 1999;281:235–242.

136. Sjostrom L, Rissanen A, Andersen T, et al. Randomized placebo-controlled trial of orlistat for weight loss and prevention of weight regain in obese patients. European Multicentre Orlistat Study Group. Lancet 1998; 352:167–173.

137. Stunkard AJ. Current views on obesity. Am J Med 1996;100(2):230–236.

138. Kalfarentzos F, Dimakopoulos A, Kehagias L, et al. Vertical banded gastroplasty versus standard or distal Roux-en-Y gastric bypass based on specific selection criteria in the morbidly obese: preliminary results. Obes Surg 1999;9(5):433–442.

139. Crampton NA, Izvornikov V, Stubbs RS. Silastic ring gastric bypass: results in 64 patients. Obes Surg 197;7(6):489–494.

140. Kremen AJ, Linner JH, Nelson CH. An experimental evaluation of the nutritional importance of proximal and distal small intestine. Ann Surg 1954;140:439.

141. Fielding GA, Rhodes M, Nathanson LK. Laparoscopic gastric banding for morbid obesity. Surgical outcome in 335 cases. Surg Endosc 1999;13(6):550–554.

142. Freeman JB, Kotlarewsky M, Phoenix C. Weight loss after extended gastric bypass. Obes Surg 1997;7(4):337–344.

143. Pories WJ, Swanson MS, MacDonald KG, et al. Who would have thought it? An operation proves to be the most effective therapy for adult-onset diabetes mellitus. Ann Surg 1995;222:339–352.

144. Kral JG. Surgical Treatment of Obesity. In GA Bray, C Bouchard, WPT James (eds), Handbook of Obesity. New York: Marcel Dekker, 1998.

145. Bray GA, Bouchard C, James WPT (eds). Handbook of Obesity. New York: Marcel Dekker, 1998;986.

146. London Department of Health. Obesity: Reversing the Increasing Problem of Obesity in England. A Report from the Nutrition and Physical Activity Task Forces. London: London Department of Health, 1995.

147. Seidell JS, Rissanen AM. Time trends in the worldwide prevalence of obesity. In: Bray GA, Bouchard C, James WPT (eds). Handbook of Obesity. New York: Marcel Dekker, 1998;79–91.

148. Seidell JC. Time trends in obesity: an epidemiological perspective. Horm Metab Res 1997;29(4):155–158.

149. Kuskowska-Wolk A, Bergstrom R. Trends in body mass index and prevalence of obesity in Swedish women. 1980–1989. J Epidemiol Community Health 1993;47:195–199.

21

Thermoregulation and the Effects of Thermomodalities

Daniel E. Lemons, Georgia Riedel, and John A. Downey

"La fixité du milieu intérieur est la condition de la vie libre."* Thus Claude Bernard emphasized the biological significance of the constancy of internal conditions in the body, and he clearly recognized that temperature control was a factor in this constancy. Fever, or elevated body temperature, had been recognized since biblical times as an indication of illness, but not until the development of the thermometer in the eighteenth century could accurate temperature measurements be made. This led to a more definitive understanding of its significance and control. It is now clear that, in humans and other warm-blooded animals, deep body temperature is regulated to a fine degree most of the time, despite exposure to wide extremes of environmental temperature. This phenomenon is labeled *homeothermy*, in contrast to *poikilothermy*, variation of body temperature with the environmental temperature. Humans with certain neurologic and other medical conditions may lose the regulation of body temperature and become effectively poikilotherms. We now recognize that constancy itself is not the critical result of many regulated systems including thermoregulation, but rather adjustment of the regulated variable to the appropriate level for the existing conditions. Thus, under nonpathologic conditions, the regulated central body temperature changes from night to day, during exercise, and over the monthly female menstrual cycle.

BODY TEMPERATURE

The temperature in different body regions may vary significantly from each other at any given time. When discussing body temperature it is important to distinguish both the temperatures of different body regions, and the thermoregulatory consequences of the differences. The skin is exposed to wide variations of ambient temperature (T_a) and skin temperature (T_s) changes as a consequence, initiating some thermoregulatory responses. Central body temperature (T_b) is much less variable, but when T_b changes, more powerful corrective responses are initiated. This is not to deny that skin temperature influences the thermoregulatory response; it does, but core temperature changes of equal size produce far greater effector responses.

Skin temperature varies because of exposure to the environment and change in the circulation of the blood to the skin caused primarily by thermoregulatory adjustment. The temperatures of the fingers and toes vary most (up to 30°C) and that of the proximal part of the limbs and the trunk less (3–4°C). Humans are often most aware of their skin temperature and may misconstrue the meaning of what they sense. Cold fingers on a cool day, for instance, may be interpreted as a failure to thermoregulate when, in fact, they are the result of appropriate thermoregulatory conservation of deep body heat. Mean skin temperature is a derived value that is useful for characterizing thermoregulatory responses. It is usually the weighted average of the skin temperature of six to eight sites on the limbs and trunk.

Central or deep body temperature would ideally be found by measuring the temperature of the mixed venous blood as it returns to the heart or of specific sites in the body (particularly the anterior hypothalamus) where evidence suggests the principal central regulators of temperature are located. Because it is rarely possible to measure temperature in these locations, less ideal sites must be used. Traditionally, temperature measured rectally has

---

*Independent life depends upon the constancy of the internal environment.

been the most reliable and constant. This is true when the body is in thermal balance, whether at rest, during exercise, or with a fever, but rectal temperature does not accurately reflect rapid changes in body heat. When, for example, hot saline is injected into a vein to cause an increase in oral temperature, a compensatory vasomotor reaction occurs in the skin even though rectal temperature is unchanged (Figure 21-1). The rectal temperature is usually approximately 0.3°C higher than the temperature of the aortic blood.[1] Vaginal temperature and bladder temperature (the latter is measured by thermistor within an indwelling catheter, as during surgery) also accurately reflect the body temperature when it is constant or slowly changing, but they do not reflect rapid changes in central temperature. Oral temperature more accurately reflects the temperature of the blood, owing to the dense vascular supply to the undersurface of the tongue. It is easy to obtain but it is also easily distorted, particularly if the patient has eaten or drunk recently or breathes through the mouth while the thermometer is in place. Probably the best approximation of the deep body temperature and its changes is in the lower end of the esophagus, where the heart lies close to the esophagus. Taking a temperature there, however, is unpleasant for most patients, who will tolerate it only under exceptional circumstances. In experimental situations and in the clinic, temperature is also frequently measured at the eardrum using infrared sensors.

Normal Body Temperature

Body temperature is remarkably similar across individuals when measurements are taken under standard circumstances. Ivy[2] measured the oral temperatures of 276 medical students in class between 8:00 and 9:00 AM and found mean body temperature to be 36.7±0.2°C.

Diurnal (Circadian) Changes

Body temperature varies throughout the day, being minimal (approximately 36.1°C) in the early morning (4:00–6:00 AM) and maximal (37.4°C) in the late afternoon (Figure 21-2).[3] This variation is one manifestation of the circadian rhythms that are recognized in many areas of physiology, which are affected by sleeping, eating, and light and are regulated by a complex of hormonal changes.[4] The cycle changes with travel (e.g., when a person flies east to west for 8–10 hours the cycle readjusts slowly over 3–4 days to the new time). Similarly, when people change shifts from day to night or work very long hours, as medical students and residents do, their diurnal rhythms are disrupted.

Age

Regulation of body temperature is different in newborns than in adults, owing in part to the immaturity of the

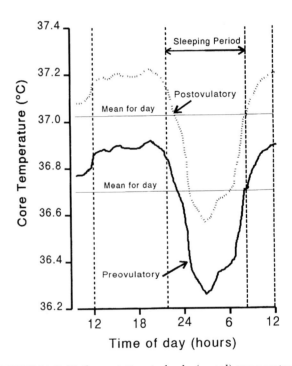

FIGURE 21-2 Daily variation in body (rectal) temperature. The lower curve was obtained in the first (preovulatory) half of the menstrual cycle, the upper curve in the second (postovulatory) half (values represent mean of eight subjects). Shaded area is the sleeping period. (Reprinted with permission from K Brück. Human Physiology. Berlin: Springer Verlag, 1989.)

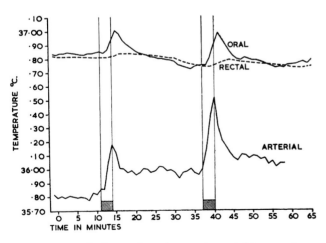

FIGURE 21-1 Oral, rectal, and central arterial temperatures before and after two intravenous injections of hot saline. Vertical bars mark the injection periods.

infant's nervous system. The difference is more pronounced in premature infants. Babies have a relatively higher ratio of surface area to mass than adults and consequently a more rapid heat exchange with the environment. Consequently, they have difficulty thermoregulating, in both hot and cold environments. Babies rarely shiver; rather they use their highly calorigenic brown fat to produce large amounts of heat. Brown fat cells have this capability partly because they are rich in mitochondria. Babies' sweat glands are immature and largely localized on the face and head. Premature babies, especially those born more than 8 weeks before term, do not sweat at all at birth.

At the time of delivery many babies are washed in cool water and exposed to (for them) cool environments, putting them in danger of developing hypothermia. The ideal room temperature for a baby that is well wrapped is somewhere between 25° and 27°C, and it is even warmer for very small infants. Conversely, if children are kept wrapped in too heavy blankets and exposed to heat they can suffer heat stroke.[5]

There is increasing evidence that thermoregulatory control is less effective in elders because of both changes in the neural control system and in behavior. Elderly persons seem less able to sense changes in skin temperature[6] and then may not respond appropriately to them. There is evidence, too, that elders have abnormal autonomic nervous system responses that are manifested in control of blood pressure and circulation in general, as well as in thermoregulation. This is evidenced by reduced shivering[7] and sweating,[6] which may be explained in part by reduced acclimatization during seasonal change. In addition, older people may take any of several medications for hypertension, gastrointestinal complaints, anxiety, or insomnia, among other conditions. Such medications can seriously affect the sensitivity of the thermoregulatory system. Because elders frequently have abnormal thermoregulation, they account for a large proportion of persons who develop hypothermia and heat stroke. In the context of associated medical conditions, either can prove lethal.

Gender

Preovulatory women have the same oral temperature as men, but at ovulation their body temperatures tend to rise 0.2–0.5°C and remain at that level through the remainder of the cycle (see Figure 21-2). Several hormones, including pregnenolone and pregnanediol, are involved in this increase in temperature. The special circumstances of abnormal thermoregulation in women during menopause (hot flashes) are discussed in Chapter 25. Men and women respond to thermal stresses in somewhat different ways. In the heat, sweating begins in women at a higher skin temperature than in men and women sweat less profusely. In the cold, women have a lower skin temperature than men and lose heat approximately 10% more slowly.

This phenomenon is caused in part by more effective vasoconstriction in women and to thicker subcutaneous tissues.[8] Some of these differences in thermoregulation between men and women, especially in the heat, may be caused by different states of acclimatization and can be abolished by appropriate training and exposure.[9]

Geography and Race

Geography and race may each play a role in human thermoregulatory responses. Three possible processes are involved in the differences seen between groups. The process of *acclimatization* is the physiological adjustments over days and longer to climate. *Habituation* is the blunting of physiological responses to environmental temperature. *Adaptation* is the process of genetic change in populations caused by natural selection. All humans respond to cold with vasoconstriction, a rise in the metabolic rate and shivering. However, circumpolar residents often have a blunted shivering response and a greater fall in T_b, thus, they exhibit habituation.[10] They also appear to allow greater heat transfer to the body shell in the cold than inhabitants of temperate climates. This altered response would serve to keep peripheral regions warmer and possibly prevent cold damage at the expense of allowing the core to cool. People living in temperate climates but with primitive technology may also experience significant cold exposure at night. Australian aborigines experience nighttime temperatures near 0°C with little or no protection and do not raise their metabolic rates in response. Consequently, their body temperature fell more than nonacclimatized controls, although their body thermal conductance was lower.[11] It is important to note that extreme environments are not always experienced as extreme because humans have always had the ability to alter their microenvironment. Eskimos, for instance, are able to maintain a comfortable microenvironment through clothing and shelter, which reduces their need to acclimatize to the cold.

MECHANISMS FOR THE REGULATION OF BODY TEMPERATURE

Body temperature is the result of a dynamic balance between heat production and heat loss, both of which are adjusted by the central hypothalamic thermoregulatory controller. As with any control system, the one for thermoregulation can be characterized as having five elements:

1. Regulated, variable, body temperature
2. Sensory system to report the value of the regulated variable
3. Set point value for the desired level of the regulated variable
4. Effectors whose activity can alter the value of the regulated variable
5. Controller that integrates afferent sensory information, compares it to the set point, and activates the effectors

A great deal is known about the input and output characteristics of this control system, whereas less is known about the hypothalamic controller itself.

Sensory Component: Temperature Receptors

Cutaneous Temperature Sensors
The sensory component of the thermoregulatory feedback system must provide an accurate assessment of the state of the body temperature. Sensory information

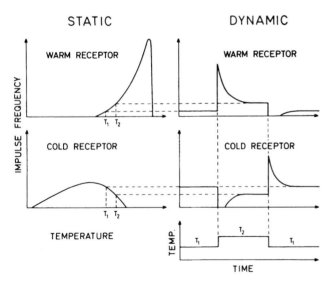

FIGURE 21-3 Diagram of the firing response of the cold and warm receptors of the skin. The left side shows the static response to steady temperature changes. The right side shows the dynamic response to rapid increases and decreases in temperature. (Reprinted with permission from H Hensel. Handbook of Sensory Physiology II, The Somatosensory System. Berlin: Springer Verlag, 1973.)

reaches the controller from temperature-sensitive structures in both superficial and deeper, central regions of the body. Two types of undifferentiated nerve endings in the skin respond specifically to changes in temperature.[12] These thermal receptors, which appear to be morphologically similar, respond differently to heating and cooling (Figure 21-3). One receptor type responds to heating with a transient rapid burst of action potentials that is followed by a reduced frequency of action potentials that is still greater than the rate before heating. These receptors have a tonic discharge between 15° and 20°C. The warm receptor afferents are predominantly of the C-fiber type. The warm receptor response is seen on the top right of Figure 21-3. The upper left of Figure 21-3 shows the static action potential rate of these neurons after their initial dynamic overshoot in response to temperature increases. Over a wide temperature range, the steady-state action potential frequency is proportional to the temperature. The second receptor type responds to cooling also with a transient burst of activity followed by an elevated static action potential rate. The steady-state discharge rate is roughly inversely proportional to the temperatures from 25° to 33°C, but at low temperatures the static rate diminishes. It appears that the temperature receptors in the skin provide information to the CNS that reflects (1) the absolute temperature of the skin of various areas of the body, (2) the direction of temperature change, and (3) the rate of change of the temperature. By integrating this information, the CNS gains an indication of the overall thermal state of the body shell.

Temperature receptors are present throughout the skin and superficial areas of the body, but they vary in density. There are more in the fingers, face, and genitalia, and fewer in the proximal part of the extremities and in the trunk, particularly on the back. In total, the neural activity from skin receptors gives an indication of the overall thermal state of the periphery and serves as an early warning to the CNS of potential changes in body heat so that appropriate, though short-term, physiological responses can be initiated to minimize any perturbation.

Central and Deep Body Temperature Sensors
Research on homeothermic animals employing ablation techniques and the warming or cooling of selected areas of the brain have clearly indicated that there are also temperature-sensitive structures in the anterior preoptic region of the hypothalamus and that temperature changes of as little as 0.1°C can initiate appropriate peripheral thermoregulatory responses.[13,14] Microelectrode recording techniques from single nerve cells in the

hypothalamus have demonstrated both cells that respond selectively to cooling or heating with changes in electrical firing activity and cells that do not change their activity with temperature.[15,16] These populations of hypothalamic cells, working together, may be the central thermostat that senses and integrates body temperature information and coordinates the responses that hold body temperature at the desired level.[17]

Direct studies of hypothalamic function are not possible in humans, but there is good evidence that central thermoregulatory structures are present and that they respond in a manner similar to those in other mammals. The return of warm or cool blood from an extremity to the central regions of the body causes peripheral vasomotor responses.[18] Intravenous infusion of measured amounts of hot or cold saline produced the appropriate vasomotor response in the hand of normal humans and showed a sensitivity in the central receptors to changes of as little as 0.1°C. Extensive studies of patients with spinal cord transection confirmed the responses to central temperature change (Figure 21-4). For example, when central temperature was caused to fall to approximately 35.6°C, shivering occurred in the innervated muscles above the level of spinal cord transection, even when the sentient skin of the body was not cooled (and, therefore, there was no peripheral sensory input of cooling). In like manner, warming of the central regions of the body induced sweating above the level of 37.4°C, even when the sentient skin was cool. There was a synergistic relationship between the temperature of the skin and the central temperature: When both central and peripheral cooling took place, the responses occurred earlier and appeared more vigorous than with cooling of either skin or central temperature alone. The same thing happened on the warm side of the response. The most likely location for the temperature-sensitive structures in the CNS is in the anterior preoptic hypothalamus; injuries in this region can cause disorders of temperature regulation.

There is also convincing evidence in animals and humans of temperature-sensitive sites in structures in other regions of the deep body, including the proximal great veins, pulmonary vessels,[19] heart,[20] and abdominal viscera.[21] In particular, there is evidence in both nonhuman mammals[22] and humans[23] of thermosensitive structures in the spinal cord, although these tend to be rather less sensitive than those in other areas of the CNS and the responses they induce are sluggish. They may contribute to the amount of residual thermoregulatory ability of spinal cord–injured patients, as discussed later in this chapter. Studies indicate that spinal thermosensors are primarily of the warm type.[24] The deep body

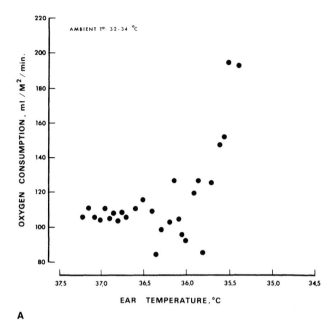

A

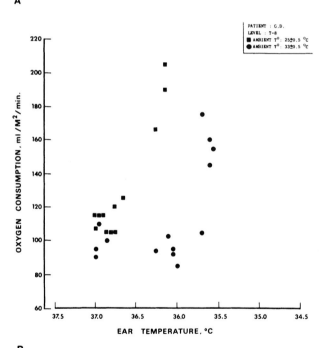

B

FIGURE 21-4 A. Metabolic response of patients with spinal cord transection to a decrease in core temperature. Shivering increases oxygen consumption and causes additional heat production. **B.** Metabolic response of patients with spinal cord transection to a decrease in core temperature. The lower ambient temperature causes shivering to begin at a significantly higher core temperature; the threshold for the response is altered by the skin temperature.

temperature receptors may turn out to provide the most important sensory information for the controller because it is the core body temperature that is defended rather than the temperature of the superficial regions.

Thermoregulatory Effectors

Two classes of thermoregulatory effector mechanisms are available to homeotherms: (1) behavioral, including postural adjustments, selection of a thermal environment, and addition or removal of insulating clothing, and (2) physiological, including vasomotor adjustments, piloerection, sweating, panting, and shivering and nonshivering thermogenesis. These effectors are not used equally, but are a hierarchy of responses that can be sequentially activated as the thermal stress increases.

Behavioral Responses

In all animals, including humans, the most basic response to externally applied heating or cooling is to seek a better thermal environment or a more advantageous posture. In fact, most human thermoregulation is behavioral.[25] This behavior is seen in all vertebrates,

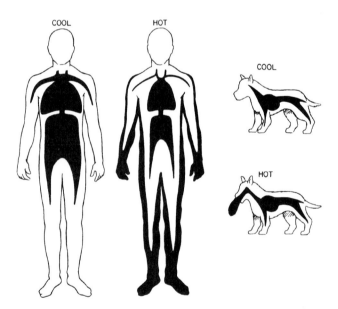

FIGURE 21-5 Schematic illustration of altered distribution of blood volume in heat-stressed humans and dogs. In the human, heat is most efficiently dissipated from the skin of the extremities, but in a furred animal such as a dog heat release occurs most efficiently from the tongue, where panting produces a high rate of evaporation from the surface. (Reprinted with permission from LB Rowell. Thermal Stress. In JT Shepherd, FM Abboud [eds], The Handbook of Physiology. American Physiological Society, Washington, DC, 1983.)

including fish, amphibians, and reptiles, whose major mechanism of body temperature control is selection of an appropriate thermal environment.[26,27]

Modern humans attempt to avoid extremes of temperature by modifying either their dress or their environment, the environment being modified by such means as room heating or air conditioning. These modifications are so effective that even people living in extremely cold climates may experience only short-term and limited cold stress. Postural changes (e.g., curling up in a ball when cool or extending arms and legs when warm) may significantly alter heat exchange with the environment, and they occur even during sleep. Regular participants in winter outdoor sports are aware of the evolution of significant technological solutions for minimizing cold exposure, even in extremely cold environments.

Physiological Responses

Vasomotor Responses   Control of blood flow to the skin regulates the flow of heat from the core to the periphery of the body. At rest almost all heat production occurs in the core regions, and without vascular convection, which transports heat to the surface, death by hyperthermia would result within 2–3 hours, even in a cool environment. Increased skin circulation raises skin temperature, increasing the thermal gradient between the skin and environment, thus augmenting heat loss from the skin by radiation and convection. Both radiative (electromagnetic) and convective heat losses from the body are directly proportional to the thermal gradient between the skin and environment.

In the heat, blood flow to the skin may increase dramatically. This is made possible by both redistribution of blood flow from other regions to the skin (Figures 21-5 and 21-6) and increased cardiac output (see Figure 21-6).

If the ambient temperature is greater than the skin temperature, increased skin circulation actually hastens the onset of hyperthermia by carrying additional heat into the body core. In these conditions, decreased skin circulation reduces heat loss or gain in the periphery.

The peripheral circulation is controlled by the autonomic nervous system, and not all peripheral vascular beds respond in the same way to thermal stress. The circulation of the skin of the fingers and toes, for example, is under much greater thermoregulatory control than that of the trunk, and only the skin circulation takes part in thermoreflexes. The blood flow to the muscles remains relatively constant unless the muscles are actually heated or cooled. The primary means of fine adjustment of body temperature is variation of blood flow to the skin, and in an ambient temperature of approximately 24–32°C, most, if not all, of the heat balance of a naked human at rest is achieved through small adjustments in skin perfusion.

When the body is exposed to temperatures above 30°C, there is progressive cutaneous vasodilatation, which enhances heat loss to the environment. When this loss is not effective and body temperature begins to rise, panting or sweating begins.

Sweating The high heat of evaporation of water (approximately 0.5–0.6 kcal/g) affords a potent method of eliminating heat from the body when regulation demands much heat loss. The avenues of evaporative heat loss are the lungs and respiratory passages and sweating onto skin surfaces. The air expired from the lungs is saturated with water vapor taken up by evaporation from the respiratory passages. In many vertebrates, increased ventilation (panting) serves as an effective way to increase heat loss. (This is why the dog in the heat in Figure 21-5 increases blood flow to the tongue and nasal area instead of to the skin.) In humans this mechanism is relatively less important, even though respiratory rate is significantly increased by fever or by body heating.

In humans, heat loss by evaporation occurs mostly through sweat excreted on the skin. There are two types of sweat glands. Eccrine sweat glands secrete a dilute solution containing sodium chloride, urea, lactic acid, and several trace elements. They are distributed over the whole body and are under the control of the sympathetic cholinergic nerves. Their production of sweat is abolished by atropine.[2] Apocrine glands, which are found in association with hair follicles, particularly in the axillae, nipples, and pubic region, secrete a creamy substance that gives rise to body odor. The apocrine glands respond to adrenergic transmitters, and their activity is not abolished by atropine.

The eccrine glands are stimulated by heating and may produce as much as 15 kg of sweat per day; thus, the body can lose large amounts of heat.[28] Central body temperature, mean skin temperature, and local skin temperature all can influence the rate of sweating.[29] Humans who lack sweat glands (anhydrosis) are unable to tolerate heat stress.

Piloerection The raising of hair follicles on the skin by contraction of piloerector muscles (*goose* or *duck bumps*) results in trapping of air on the skin and increases surface insulation. This is effective for hairy animals but not for humans.

Thermogenesis The body's basal metabolic activity (basic metabolic rate) is the minimum level of heat production and occurs at rest when the ambient temperature is between 26° and 30°C. This temperature range is called the *thermoneutral zone*. In the thermoneutral

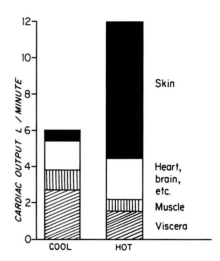

FIGURE 21-6 (*Left*) Estimated distribution of cardiac output between skin and other major organs at rest in normothermia. (*Right*) Expected distribution during hyperthermia $T_b > 39°C$. (Reprinted with permission from LB Rowell. Thermal Stress. In JT Shepherd, FM Abboud [eds], The Handbook of Physiology. American Physiological Society, Washington, DC, 1983.)

zone, the fine regulation of body temperature is largely accomplished by small vasomotor adjustments, which alter heat loss from the skin. When the ambient temperature is below the thermoneutral temperature, vasoconstriction occurs. If this is not enough to prevent a decrease in body temperature, increased heat production is initiated through shivering.

Shivering is the involuntary, rhythmic contraction of muscles. Initially invisible, it may take the form of muscle tensing. With colder temperatures the muscle contractions are visible. Often, they start in the patient's shoulders, and ultimately they extend to all muscles of the body. Shivering is a potent source of increased heat production by which oxygen consumption can be increased as much as 500% for short periods and as much as 200–300% for longer periods. It is mediated by the somatic nerves and requires an intact spinal cord and posterior hypothalamus. No shivering occurs below the level of a spinal cord transection or in limbs paralyzed by poliomyelitis.

Body heat production can also be increased by eating, or exercising, or by the secretion of calorigenic hormones such as norepinephrine. In acclimatized animals there is evidence of nonshivering thermogenesis, particularly in association with an increased amount of adrenergic and thyroid hormones, but nonshivering thermogenesis has not been demonstrated as clearly in adult humans. In fact, in the cold, totally paralyzed humans exhibited no increased heat production over at least several hours.[30] The human β₃-adrenergic receptor seems to be specifically involved in activating cellular thermogenesis.[31]

THERMOREGULATORY CONTROLLER(S)

Activation of Thermoregulatory Responses

Appropriate thermoregulatory reflexes can be activated by heating or cooling only the skin, well before any changes in central deep body temperature take place. Warming[32] or cooling[18] the skin in one part of the body causes vasodilatation or vasoconstriction elsewhere so quickly that these reactions can be mediated only by neurologic reflex. These reflex human responses are transient unless there is a decrease or increase in central temperature, at which time the vasomotor changes continue and are enhanced (Figure 21-7).[18]

Sudden, extreme cooling of the whole body can initiate shivering, which often produces an increase in central temperature, owing to the concomitant vasoconstriction and increased heat production. Skin cooling alone produces shivering for only a few minutes that does not resume until the central temperature falls below the basal level. If central temperature continues to fall, the intensity of the shivering progressively increases.

Between approximately 24° and 32°C, the thermoneutral zone neither increased heat loss by sweating nor increased heat production; the adjustment of cutaneous blood flow is sufficient to maintain thermal homeostasis. Below this range, intense cutaneous vasoconstriction and increased metabolism increase conservation and production of heat. Above the thermoneutral zone, skin blood flow increases dramatically and sweating increases to enhance heat loss at the surface. Heat production also increases slightly because of the increased cardiac work required to sustain the increased blood flow to the skin. These dynamics are shown in Figure 21-7.

Heating of an area of the skin can cause sweating elsewhere in the body, also before central temperature increases.[33] When the central body temperature increases, the sweating induced by skin heating is enhanced and continues as long as the central rise continues.

Central heating or cooling without changes in skin temperature, as occurs in laboratory studies and some clinical situations, causes the appropriate peripheral response, but often only after a significant decrease or increase in central temperature. When both peripheral and central heating or cooling occur there is a synergistic response with an earlier and more vigorous reaction.[23,34,35] In summary, it appears that there is a high degree of control of central body temperature, whereas skin temperature varies greatly.

A number of models have been developed to describe and predict thermoregulatory responses. The most widely used general model[13] assumes a single controller in the hypothalamus. Other types of regulatory schemes may also be consistent with experimental studies, including a model with a separate controller for each effector.[36] Each of these models is able to accurately account for and predict many of the responses of the thermoregulatory system. Sophisticated mathematical models have also been developed to account for the input and output relationships of the thermoregulatory system and predict the body's thermal state. The most advanced whole body thermoregulatory models to date are multielement, distributed parameter models that can determine dynamic radial temperature profiles through the body, based on experimentally determined sensory inputs and effector outputs, and knowledge of the mechanisms of heat transfer within and out of the body.[37-39]

A more complete understanding of normal thermoregulatory control will give greater insight into abnormal conditions, particularly those seen in rehabilitation medicine, when, for example, there is disruption of the nervous system, absence of effector organs (e.g., congenital absence of sweat glands), or a change in the skin (e.g., burns), or when drugs render the body incapable of mobilizing the normal mechanisms. In addi-

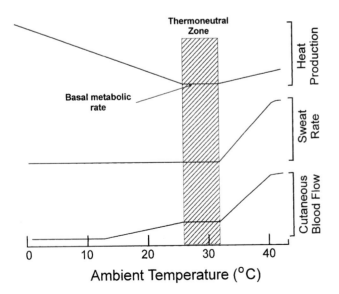

FIGURE 21-7 Schematic of physiological responses to ambient temperature changes.

tion, it is important in all aspects of medicine, particularly rehabilitation medicine, to recognize that the competing regulatory systems in the body can diminish the efficiency of any one system. For example, exercise, which increases heat production and changes the distribution of cardiac output to the exercising muscle and away from many organs including the skin, can significantly load the body with excess heat to be lost, leading to thermal collapse (hyperthermia), especially in a hot environment. The perfusion demands of the exercising muscle take precedence over the need for skin perfusion for heat loss, resulting in a reduction in heat loss at the same time that heat production is increased by the exercising muscle. Regulation of blood pressure by adjustment of the circulatory system to ensure adequate perfusion of the brain and the vital body organs can likewise be compromised by exposure to heat. An enormous amount of blood must be shifted to the skin to speed heat loss. Sweating can also significantly deplete the circulating blood volume, interfering with the regulation of body fluid volume.

ALTERATIONS IN BODY TEMPERATURE AND THERMOREGULATION

Regulation of Body Temperature during Exercise

Exercise causes an increase in body temperature that is proportional to the metabolic work performed and to the independent ambient temperatures over wide extremes.[40] This increase in body temperature with exercise may be caused by an adjustment of the set point of body temperature and not simply by overload of the body's heat loss mechanisms. However, in extremes of temperature, activities such as marathon running in the heat or in cold, wet climates, may cause the system to be overloaded, and hyperthermia or hypothermia can occur.

When exercise is terminated, the temperature returns toward normal, but it takes as long as 45–60 minutes to return to the basal level. Consequently, temperature measurements taken shortly after exercise do not accurately reflect basal body temperature. The increase in temperature during exercise cannot be abolished with antipyretic drugs such as aspirin.[41]

Fever

The most commonly recognized abnormality of human body temperature is fever resulting from infections or

inflammation. The increase in body temperature during fever is caused by setting of the thermoregulatory system to a new set point and not to a breakdown of thermoregulation or overload of the system. At the onset of fever, after an infection or injection of a pyrogen, the body acts as if it were too cool and behavioral changes and intense cutaneous vasoconstriction occur, increasing conservation of heat followed by shivering (chill), which increases heat production. These continue until a new higher level of body temperature, equal to the elevated set point, is reached. When the body temperature reaches the higher level it remains constant, and the thermoregulatory system responds to heating or cooling quantitatively in the same fashion as before the fever. This indicates that the sensitivity of the regulation of body temperature is as precise in fever as at normal levels.[42] When the cause of the fever is removed or the fever is abolished by antipyretics that act on the CNS, the body mobilizes heat loss mechanisms: behavioral (casting off covers or clothing; Figure 21-8), vasodilatation, and sweating, and temperature is reduced to its prefever levels.

Fever occurs under a great variety of clinical circumstances, but it appears that the pathophysiology of the fever is common to all. The entrance of a bacterial pyrogen into the body causes phagocytic cells of the body to synthesize and release cytokines such as interleukin-1 and interleukin-6 among others.[43] The cytokines initiate

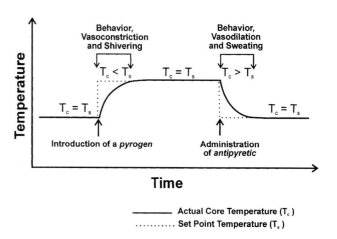

FIGURE 21-8 Schematic diagram of the change in body temperature before, during, and after the onset of fever. Note that during the time when there is a difference between the set point of body temperature (*dotted line*) and the actual body temperature (*solid line*), the appropriate thermoregulatory effectors are activated to bring the actual body temperature to the set point temperature.

the febrile response by an as yet unknown mechanism that appears to involve at least two intermediaries, which in turn act on the CNS. One of these intermediaries is a prostanoid derived from arachidonic acid released from the brain, metabolized to the prostaglandin endoperoxide, and then converted to prostaglandin, prostacyclin, and thromboxane. These products appear to act directly on the thermoregulatory control center in the hypothalamus. This effect can be blocked by use of a nonsteroidal, anti-inflammatory drug such as aspirin. The production of interleukin-1, interleukin-6, and other cytokines can be initiated by bacteria, fungi, viruses, or immune reactions, and each pyrogen may activate a different cytokine.[43] Much is yet unknown about the central generation of fever, and new hypotheses continue to be developed for how pyrogens, cytokines, and hypothalamic intermediaries produce the response.[44,45]

Cortisone is also antipyretic, but its action is to prevent arachidonic acid release from the brain membrane phospholipids.[46,47] When a patient is febrile, it is important to recognize that body temperature is regulated at the new, higher, level. If it is desirable to reduce the temperature, it is important to use antipyretic agents to reset the body's thermostat and then to use physical means to enhance heat loss. Attempting to lower a fever with ice baths or ice blankets alone produces the same rather violent reaction in the body as an attempt to reduce a normal body temperature from 37° to 36°C, and the increased physiological stress could well be detrimental.

Whether fever is beneficial during infection or should be abolished is not clear. In some ectotherms infected with pathogens, survival is enhanced by allowing fever to persist, but this is not so in others.[48] In rabbits infected with *Pasteurella multocida*, survival was greatest in those that had a febrile response of 1.50–2.25°C,[49] and death rates were high when fever was abolished.[50] Other studies were inconsistent. In humans no studies have shown a clear benefit for abolishing fever. Hyperpyrexia can cause complications such as febrile convulsion in children, and the increased metabolism and hyperpnea can be harmful to patients with cardiopulmonary disease. Until more conclusive studies are performed, it would seem to be logical to reduce fever to a comfortable level (approximately 38.0–38.5°C) with antipyretics but not to strive to abolish it altogether.

Surgery

Patients are deliberately cooled for a number of surgical procedures including open heart surgery,[51] but hypo-thermia is frequently an unintended by-product of anesthesia.[52] Violent shivering during recovery is common and attempts have been made to either prevent hypothermia[53] or to facilitate rewarming.[54] A dramatic and life-threatening increase in body temperature occurs rarely during anesthesia in what is termed *malignant hyperthermia*. In this condition there is a disruption of normal calcium regulation in skeletal muscle brought on by the anesthetic agent, which causes hyperactivity of the muscle, large increases in heat production, and rapid elevation of body temperature. The reaction has been associated with a mutation of the ryanodine receptor as well as a mutation in the gene encoding the dihydropyridine receptor.[55]

Spinal Cord–Injured Patients

Spinal cord–injured patients may have abnormal body temperature regulation or may be less able to respond effectively to changes in ambient temperature, particularly during other physiological stresses. The amount of impairment depends on the level and completeness of the lesion. With high spinal injury, when a large portion of the skin is insentient, the patient may be especially insensitive to changes in heat or cold, particularly if the sentient skin is clothed. For example, in a cold environment a patient wearing a warm jacket and mittens may become seriously hypothermic if the lower part of the body is inadequately clothed and yet may not be aware of hypothermia until the warm sentient skin is cooled by the cool recirculating blood.[35] In like fashion, a patient may be in a very warm bath and not be aware of the changes in the central body temperature, particularly if the sentient skin is relatively cool until core temperature has risen significantly.

On the output side of the thermoregulatory system, some of the effector mechanisms are lost. Patients do not shiver below the level of their lesion, so the heat increase so produced is limited. With a high spinal injury, heat production may increase by only 10–15% over resting levels, placing the patient at risk of hypothermia in a cold environment.

Vasomotor control of the lower body may also be seriously impaired when sympathetic outflow is damaged. Because of this, heat would be neither conserved nor lost in response to central temperature changes. Some slow, sluggish, and relatively ineffectual vasomotor control appears to occur at the spinal cord level, and sweating is equally ineffectual below the level of the spinal lesion.[56]

In spinal cord–injured patients it is relative thermal stability, not relative poikilothermy, that is remarkable, and many questions remain as to how this is accomplished. In managing or guiding patients, particularly those with a high spinal lesion, the physician should recommend appropriate adjustment of the environment with air conditioning and heating to help regulate body temperature. Laboratory studies are needed to determine what extremes of temperature are tolerated well. In addition, thermoregulation should be studied in fully rehabilitated spinal-injured patients, particularly those who are in the workforce or who engage in strenuous physical activity such as Olympic-style athletics. Appropriate guidelines and adjustments should then be made based on these studies.

Conditions such as skin disease, burns, and amputations may well compromise the ability either to sense temperature changes or to alter blood flow to the skin or sweating rate.

Drugs can modify thermoregulatory effectiveness, too. Any anesthetic agent can reduce the sensitivity of the CNS, inducing a state of poikilothermia. This effect can last for some time after consciousness begins to return, leaving patients hyperthermic or hypothermic, depending on the environment and how well clothed they are.

Alcohol is a CNS depressant that reduces the sensitivity of the thermoregulatory system and a direct peripheral vasodilator that increases heat loss. The two effects together can be particularly dangerous in the cold, but they also impair regulation in the heat. Drugs such as tranquilizers, sleeping pills, and antihypertensives also affect the CNS and thus may be particularly damaging to elders.

Narcotics, especially street drugs, can either be sedatives (e.g., heroin, morphine) and make the user susceptible to hypothermia in the cold or stimulants (e.g., cocaine, a metabolic stimulant). A massive cocaine overdose can cause serious, sometimes life-threatening, hyperthermia.

PHYSIOLOGICAL EFFECTS OF PHYSICAL THERAPEUTIC THERMOMODALITIES

Vasomotor effects after the therapeutic use of heat or cold vary, depending on the location, intensity, and duration of the application. Local heating directly causes vasodilation in heated skin. Local heating or cooling of a sufficiently large area of the skin may also cause reflex vasodilation or vasoconstriction elsewhere in the body, although this effect may be transitory if the central body temperature remains unchanged. Thus, heating the skin of the trunk causes vasodilation of the skin of the extremities. In the case of diabetes or arteriosclerotic peripheral vascular disease, using this reflex response may be a safe and useful way to augment peripheral blood flow. It can increase peripheral blood flow without causing the tissue damage that could result from a direct increase in the peripheral tissue temperature, which would raise metabolism and potentially result in ischemia.

Heat applied to the surface may eventually raise the temperature of tissues beneath the skin. Diathermy and ultrasound are able to deposit energy into deeper tissues. Heating muscle may produce increased perfusion, although it is unclear how large the increase in blood flow is. Roemer et al.[57] found four different patterns of temperature change in the muscle of dogs subjected to microwave heating. Low rates of energy deposition produced an increase in muscle temperature to a steady state several degrees higher than the baseline. High rates of energy deposition produced a 10°C increase in muscle temperature that was followed by large oscillations in muscle temperature. They ascribed the temperature oscillations to alternating cycles of hyperemia followed by reduced muscle blood flow. They suggested that the thermally induced hyperemia caused tissue cooling that was followed by renewed tissue warming when the blood flow rate was reduced. Their results suggest that with deep heating, the tissue may need to be warmed substantially before significant increases in blood flow occur. Sekins et al.[58] found that in humans, diathermy applications that produced an increase in muscle temperature of approximately 42°C or greater resulted in an increase in muscle blood flow. Hogan et al.[59] found that muscle arterioles of the rat actually constricted during heating of 3–4°C. In one study in which ultrasound was applied to human subjects according to common clinical protocols, no increase in blood flow could be detected.[60] Thus, although deep heating may have therapeutic effects, these effects may not be mediated by increased blood flow unless the temperatures achieved exceed 42°C.

Application of heat to joints produces variable, and on occasion, paradoxical effects. When heat or cold is applied over a knee joint, the overall blood flow of the area is increased or decreased as expected.[61] However, the temperature within the joint may actually decrease secondary to application of heat (hot packs) or increase with cold (cold packs).[62] When the joint is exposed to diathermy or ultrasound, the temperature is increased and blood flow is increased.[63]

Raising the central body temperature such as with diathermy or a hot bath causes a sustained increase in blood flow to all the peripheral tissues and can be an effective means of getting heat and its effects into deep body tissues such as the spine and paraspinal tissues, as well as muscle. There are, however, other effects of temperature change. Nerve conduction rate is increased by warming and slowed by cooling. The stretch receptor sensitivity in muscle and tendons is reduced with cooling,[64] and when the central body temperature is raised, the gamma efferent activity (that activity that tends to increase the sensitivity of stretch receptors in muscles) is reduced.[65] In addition, the general sympathetic activity is increased with cooling of the body, and this may affect the responses of the stretch receptors in a beneficial way.

Another effect of the thermal application is that the competitive bombardment of the CNS by the thermal sensation may reduce the perception of the noxious sensations.[66-68] Thus, heating an area may decrease the perception of pain elsewhere. The effects of heat, cold, and stretch on connective tissue have been reviewed[69] and in general, heating increases and cooling diminishes the elasticity of connective tissue. This effect may modify the responses to exercise and stretch.

Despite the understanding of the vasomotor and other effects of heating and cooling, the evidence for therapeutic benefit is less well established. Subjectively, pain reduction is commonly reported with either heating or cooling; however, controlled trials have revealed little benefit in some postsurgical rehabilitation programs.[70] Reviews of thermotherapy[71-74] confirm its usefulness in general to decrease inflammation.[75] However, prostaglandin-mediated inflammation can be aggravated by cold, whereas acute exudative inflammations are helped with cold, and chronic proliferative inflammations are helped by heat.

SUMMARY

Body temperature is a tightly regulated physiological variable whose set point changes depending on the conditions. Regulatory adjustments result in a balance between heat production and heat loss, a balance brought about by an intricate system of thermosensitive structures in skin, brain, and many other regions of the body, that causes appropriate adjustments in the peripheral regions of the body. The response of humans to activity, environment, stress, and illness can be understood and predicted with knowledge of the basic systems of physiological controls.

REFERENCES

1. Cooper KE, Kenyon JR. A comparison of temperature measured in the rectum oesophagus, and on the surface of the aorta during hypothermia in man. Br J Surg 1957;44:616–619.

2. Ivy AC. What is normal or normality? Q Bull Northwestern Univ Med Sch 1944;18:22–32.

3. Pembry MS. Animal Heat. In Schafer (ed), Textbook of Physiology. Edinburgh: Pentland, 1898.

4. Arendt J. Melatonin. Clin Endocrinol (Oxf) 1988;29:205–229.

5. Goodyear JE. Heat hyperpyrexia in an infant. Med Sci Law 1979;19:208–209.

6. Robertshaw D. Man in Extreme Environments, Problems of the Newborn and Elderly. In K Cena, JA Clark (eds), Bioengineering, Thermal Physiology and Comfort. Amsterdam: Elsevier, 1981.

7. Paton BC. Accidental hypothermia. Pharmacol Ther 1983;22:331–377.

8. Hardy JD, Du Bois EF. Differences between men and women in their response to heat and cold. Proc Natl Acad Sci U S A 1940;26:389–398.

9. Fox RH, Lofstedt BE, Woodward PM. Comparison of thermoregulatory function in men and women. J Appl Physiol 1969;26:444–453.

10. Young JL. Homeostatic Responses to Prolonged Cold Exposure: Human Cold Acclimatization. In MJ Fregly, CM Blatteis (eds), Handbook of Physiology. New York: Oxford University Press, 1996;419–438.

11. Hammel HT, Elsner RW, LeMesssurier DH, et al. Thermal and metabolic responses of Australian Aborigine exposed to moderate cold in summer. J Appl Physiol 1959;14:605–615.

12. Pierau FK. Peripheral Thermosensors. In MJ Fregly, CM Blatteis (eds), Handbook of Physiology. New York: Oxford University Press, 1996;85–104.

13. Hammel HT. Regulation of internal body temperature. Annu Rev Physiol 1968;30:641–710.

14. Jessen C. Independent clamps of peripheral and central temperatures and their effects on heat production in the goat. Annu Rev Physiol 1981;11–22.

15. Boulant JA. Hypothalamic Control of Thermoregulation: Neurophysiological Basis. In PJ Morgane, J Panksepp (eds), Handbook of the Hypothalamus: Behavioral Studies of the Hypothalamus. New York: Marcel Dekker, 1980;1–82.

16. Heller HC. Hypothalamic Thermosensitivity in Mammals. In L Giradier, J Seydoux (eds), Effectors of Thermogenesis. Basel: Experientia, 1978.

17. Boulant JA. Hypothalamic Neurons Regulating Body Temperature. In MJ Fregly, CM Blatteis (eds), Handbook of Physiology. New York: Oxford University Press, 1996;105–126.

18. Pickering GW. The vasomotor regulation of heat loss from the human skin in relation to external temperature. Heart 1932;16:115–135.

19. Bligh J. The receptors concerned in the respiratory response to humidity in sheep at high ambient temperature. J Physiol 1963;168:747–763.

20. Downey JA, Mottram RF, Pickering GW. The location by regional cooling of central temperature receptors in the conscious rabbit. J Physiol (Lond) 1964;170:415–441.

21. Rawson RO, Wuick KP. Evidence of deep body thermoreceptor response to intraabdominal heating of the ewe. J Appl Physiol 1970;28:813.

22. Simon E, Rautenberg W, Jessen C. Initiation of shivering in unanesthetized dogs by local cooling within the vertebral canal. Experieutia 1965;21:476–477.

23. Downey JA, Chiodi HP, Darling RC. Central temperature regulation in the spinal man. J Appl Physiol 1967;22:91–94.

24. Simon E, Schmid HA, Pehl U. Spinal neuronal thermosensitivity in vivo and in vitro in relation to hypothalamic neuronal thermosensitivity. Prog Brain Res 1998;115:25–47.

25. Satinoff E. Behavioral Thermoregulation in the Cold. In MJ Fregly, CM Blatteis (eds), Handbook of Physiology. New York: Oxford University Press, 1996;481–505.

26. Heller HC, Crawshaw LI, Hammel HT. The thermostat of vertebrate animals. Sci Am 1978;239(2):102–113.

27. Crawshaw LI, Moffitt BP, Lemons DE, Downey JA. The evolutionary development of vertebrate thermoregulation. Am Scientist 1981;69:543–550.

28. Kuno Y. Human Perspiration. Springfield, IL: Charles Thomas, 1956.

29. Nadel ER, Mitchell JW, Saltin B. Peripheral modifications to the central drive for sweating. J Appl Physiol 1971;31:828–833.

30. Johnson RH, Smith AC. Oxygen consumption of paralyzed men exposed to cold. J Physiol (Lond) 1963;169:584–591.

31. Emorine LJ, Marullo S, Briend-Sutren MM, et al. Molecular characterization of the human beta 3-adrenergic receptor. Science 1989;245:1118–1121.

32. Kerslake DM, Cooper KE. Vasodilation in the hand in response to heating the skin elsewhere. Clin Sci 1950;9:31–47.

33. Randall WC, Rawson RO, McCook RD. Central and peripheral factors in dynamic thermoregulation. J Appl Physiol 1963;18:61–64.

34. Benzinger TH. Heat regulation: homeostasis of central temperature in man. Physiol Rev 1969;49(4):671–759.

35. Downey JA, Miller JM, Darling RC. Thermoregulatory responses to deep and superficial cooling in spinal man. J Appl Physiol 1969;27:209–212.

36. Satinoff E. Neural organization and evolution of thermal regulation in mammals. Science 1978;201:16–22.

37. Werner J. Do black-box models of thermoregulation still have any research value? Contribution of system-theoretical models to the analysis of thermoregulation. Yale J Biol Med 1986;59:335–373.

38. Wissler EH. Mathematical Simulation of Human Thermal Behavior Using Whole Body Models. In A Shitzer, RC Eberhart (eds), Heat and Mass Transfer in Medicine and Biology. New York: Plenum, 1985;325–373.

39. Werner J. Modeling Homeostatic Responses to Heat and Cold. In MJ Fregly, CM Blatteis (eds), Handbook of Physiology. New York: Oxford University Press, 1996;613–626.

40. Nielsen M. Regulation der Korpertemperatur bei muskalarbeit. Scand Arch Physiol 1938;79:193–230.

41. Downey JA, Darling RC. Effect of salicylates on elevation of body temperature during exercise. J Appl Physiol 1962;17:323–325.

42. Cooper KE, Cranston WI, Snell ES. Temperature regulation during fever in man. Clin Sci 1964;27:345–356.

43. Blatteis CM, Sehic E. Cytokines and fever. Ann N Y Acad Sci 1998;840:608–618.

44. Netea MG, Kullberg BJ, Van Der Meer JW. Do only circulating pyrogenic cytokines act as mediators in the febrile response? A hypothesis. Eur J Clin Invest 1999;29:351–356.

45. Saper CB. Neurobiological basis of fever. Ann N Y Acad Sci 1998;856:90–94.

46. Cranston WI, Hellon RF, Mitchell D. Intraventricular injections of drugs which inhibit phospholipase A2 suppress fever in rabbits. J Physiol (Lond) 1983;339:97–105.

47. Gill W, Wilson S, Long WBI. Steroid hypothermia. Surg Gynecol Obstet 1978;146:944–946.

48. Berman HJ, Kluger MJ. Fever and antipyresis in the lizard Dipsosaurus dorsalis. Am J Physiol 1976;321:198–203.

49. Kluger MJ, Vaughn LK. Fever and survival in rabbits infected with Pasteurella multocida. J Physiol (Lond) 1978;282:243–251.

50. Vaughn LK, Veale WL, Cooper KE. Antipyresis effect on mortality rate of bacterially infected rabbits. Brain Res Bull 1980;7:175–180.

51. Murphy DA, Armour JA. Influences of cardiopulmonary bypass, temperature, cardioplegia, and topical hypothermia on cardiac innervation. J Thorac Cardiovasc Surg 1992;103:1192–1199.

52. Sessler DI. Central thermoregulatory inhibition by general anesthesia. Anesthesiology 1991;75:557–559.

53. Sessler DI, McGuire J, Hynson J, et al. Thermoregulatory vasoconstriction during isoflurane anesthesia minimally decreases cutaneous heat loss. Anesthesiology 1992;76:670–675.

54. Hynson JM, Sessler DI. Intraoperative warming therapies: a comparison of three devices. J Clin Anesth 1992;4:194–199.

55. Jurkat-Rott K, McCarthy T, Lehmann-Horn F. Genetics and pathogenesis of malignant hyperthermia. Muscle Nerve 2000;23:4–17.

56. Secendorf R, Randall WC. Thermal reflex sweating in normal and paraplegic man. J Appl Physiol 1961;16:796–800.

57. Roemer RB, Oleson JR, Cetas TC. Oscillatory temperature response to constant power applied to canine muscle. Am J Physiol 1985;249:R153–R158.

58. Sekins KM, Lehmann JF, Esselman P, et al. Local muscle blood flow and temperature responses to 915MHz diathermy as simultaneously measured and numerically predicted. Arch Phys Med Rehabil 1984;65:1–7.

59. Hogan RD, Franklin TD, Avery KS, Burke KM. Arteriolar vasoconstriction in rat cremaster muscle induced by local heat stress. Am J Physiol 1982;242:H996–H999.

60. Snortum AL. Blood flow responses to ultrasound dosage and direct surface cooling as measured by venous occlusion plethysmography [Thesis]. New York: Columbia University, 1989.

61. Bonney GLW, Hughes RA, Janus O. Blood flow through the normal human knee segment. Clin Sci 1951;11:167.

62. Horvath SM, Hollander JL. The influence of physical therapy procedures on the intra-articularly temperature of normal and arthritic subjects. Am J Med Sci 1949;218:543.

63. Harris R, Millard JG. Clearance of radioactive sodium from the knee. Clin Sci 1956;15:9.

64. Eldred E, Schnitzlein HN, Buckwald SJ. Response of muscle spindles to stimulation of sympathetic trunk. Exp Neurol 1960;2:13.

65. Euler C, Von Soderberg U. Co-ordinated changes in temperature thresholds for thermoregulatory reflexes. Acta Physiol Scand 1958;42:112–129.

66. Fischer F, Solomon S. Therapeutic Heat. New Haven, CT: Elizabeth Licht, 1958.

67. Parsons CM, Goetzl FR. Effect of induced pain on pain threshold. Proc Soc Exp Biol Med 1945;60:3327.

68. Ernst E, Fialka V. Ice freezes pain? A review of the clinical effectiveness of analgesic cold therapy. J Pain Symptom Manage 1994;9(1):56–59.

69. Hardy M, Woodall W. Therapeutic effects of heat, cold, and stretch on connective tissue. J Hand Ther 1998;11(2):148–156.

70. Konrath GA, Lock T, Goitz HT, Scheidler J. The use of cold therapy

after anterior cruciate ligament reconstruction. A prospective, randomized study and literature review. Am J Sports Med 1966;24(5):629–633.

71. Downey JA. Physiological effects of heat and cold. Am J Phys Ther Assoc 1964;44:713–717.

72. Nanneman D. Thermal modalities: heat and cold. A review of physiologic effects with clinical applications. AAOHN J 1991;39(2):70–75.

73. Tepperman PS, Devlin M. Therapeutic heat and cold. A practitioner's guide. Postgrad Med 1983;73(1):69–76.

74. Oosterveld FG, Rasker JJ. Treating arthritis with locally applied heat or cold. Semin Arthritis Rheum 1994;24(2):82–90.

75. Schmidt KL, Ott VR, Rocher G, Schaller H. Heat, cold and inflammation. Z Rheumatol 1979;38(11–12):391–404.

22

Peripheral Vascular Function

DANIEL E. LEMONS AND JOHN A. DOWNEY

The peripheral circulation is a mass transport system that moves gases, such as oxygen and carbon dioxide, and other molecules, such as glucose and hormones, throughout the body, serving each tissue's needs. To understand the control of the limb circulation it is also important to consider aspects that serve systemic rather than local needs. First, the peripheral vascular system is a primary effector in the regulation of systemic blood pressure through its ability to alter the distribution of blood flow and to change total peripheral resistance, thereby buffering systemic pressure fluctuations. Second, it is the most important pathway for the transport of heat from the central body to the surface where it can be lost. Without this latter pathway, humans, along with the other mammals and birds, would be unable to sustain their high rate of metabolism without rapidly overheating. As discussed later, the local metabolic needs and the systemic baroregulatory and thermoregulatory demands on blood flow cannot always be met simultaneously and compromises must often be made.

Blood flow to the limbs varies over a wide range, depending on the need for its three primary functions: mass transfer in support of limb metabolism, regulation of systemic blood pressure, and heat transfer for systemic thermoregulation. At rest, in a neutral temperature environment, the circulation to the forearm may be 2–4 ml $\cong$ 100 ml^{-1} tissue $\cong$ min^{-1}, but in the heat this may increase to 15 ml $\cong$ 100 ml^{-1} $\cong$ min^{-1}. The major portion of this increase occurs in the skin, where up to 50% of the cardiac output (CO) may be directed during heat stress. During exercise the muscle blood flow may increase from the resting value of 2–3 to nearly 250 ml $\cong$ 100 ml^{-1} tissue $\cong$ min^{-1}. The arterial, venular, and neural elements that permit this range of flows and the

circumstances under which they occur are covered in this chapter.

HEMODYNAMIC FUNDAMENTALS OF BLOOD FLOW

Pressure and Other Physical Factors Affecting Blood Flow in Vessels: Simple Circuits

To understand limb circulatory control it is necessary to consider the relationship between pressure, viscosity, geometry, and flow in the vessels. The name for this area of study is *rheology*, the study of the flow and deformation of matter. The Poiseuille-Hagen equation describes the role of the critical physical factors influencing blood flow through a single vessel:

$$\forall = (P_1 - P_2)\frac{\pi r^4}{8Ln} \qquad [1]$$

In this equation, $\forall$ is the volumetric blood flow and it is determined directly by the pressure difference from one end of the vessel to the other ($P_1 - P_2$), and the radius of the vessel raised to the fourth power. As the radius, pressure difference, or both increase, so does the flow. $\forall$ is inversely related to the vessel length (L) and the viscosity of the blood, n, so that increases in these parameters decrease the flow through the vessel. The single most important determinant of blood flow is the radius of the vessel. When the radius of a vessel doubles while all other parameters remain the same, the flow through the vessel increases 16-fold, because the flow depends on the fourth power of the radius. When the vessels of a vascular bed dilate together, as happens during exercise, the blood flow through the bed can increase enormously.

The last term in equation 1, which includes the variables of vessel radius and length and the blood viscosity, can be thought of as the conductance of the vessel to blood flow. The greater the conductance, the more readily blood flows through the vessel. Equation 1 may then be simplified as follows:

$$\forall = (P_1 - P_2) \times K \qquad [2]$$

where K is the conductance. As in electrical circuits, the inverse of the conductance (K) is the resistance (R). The greater the R, the less blood will flow at the same perfusing pressure. The product of $1 \div R$ or K and the pressure difference yields the same result:

$$\forall = (P_1 - P_2) \div R \qquad [3]$$

This of course is directly analogous to Ohm's law of electrical current flow, which states that current flow equals the voltage drop across an element divided by the electrical resistance.

Even though R is partially determined by vessel length and blood viscosity, it is generally assumed the changes in R are caused mostly by changes in vessel radius. This is because vessel length does not usually vary over short time frames, and viscosity, although somewhat flow dependent, does not change a great deal for a given vessel. As discussed later, the vascular resistance of a tissue or of the entire peripheral circulation is a useful index of the functioning of the intact autonomic nervous system. However, R is not measured directly, but rather is calculated according to the rearrangement of equation 3:

$$R = (P_a - P_v) \div \forall \qquad [4]$$

In this equation, P_a and P_v are, respectively, the arteriolar inlet and the venular outlet pressures for a vascular bed. In humans, when the entire peripheral circulation is considered, the inlet pressure is usually the systemic pressure, P_a, and $\forall$ may be measured invasively or noninvasively. The outlet pressure of the peripheral circulation is usually taken to be close to central venous pressure, which may be either measured or more likely assumed to be a value from 0–5 mm Hg. R for the entire circulation is usually calculated with P_v

ignored because it is small, and thus, equation 4 simplifies to the following equation:

$$R = P_a \div \forall \qquad [5a]$$

or

$$\forall = P_a \div R \qquad [5b]$$

Often studies on humans report only limb blood flow measurements and then ascribe blood flow changes to alterations in vascular diameters or tone. As can be seen in equation 5b, P_a also determines flow, and if changes in this driving pressure are not accounted for, then changes in blood flow cannot be accurately interpreted; limb blood flow may change because the systemic pressure has changed and not because vascular tone has been altered. The most useful way to report changes in vascular control is in terms of vascular conductance, which is specific to the actual responses of vascular smooth muscle and its effect on vessel diameter.

Blood Flow in Vascular Beds Arranged in Series and in Parallel

The entire circulatory system can be thought of as two primary circulations, the systemic, which is sustained by the left side of the heart, and the pulmonary, which is sustained by the right side of the heart; each includes many vessels connected in parallel. Figure 22-1 shows this generalized view. This entire circulation, or components of it, can be analyzed in the same way that electrical circuits can, with resistive-, capacitive-, and pressure-producing components. Figure 22-2 shows the circulation diagrammed according to this analogy. The batteries represent the right and left sides of the heart, producing a potential difference around the circuit that produces the flow.

As with resistors in an electrical circuit, the total resistance of vessels connected in series equals the sum of the resistances of each of the vessels. Thus, the total resistance down the arterial tree from the aorta to a given precapillary arteriole equals the sum of the resistance to flow at each vessel generation. The small radii of the terminal arterioles of the microcirculation produce the highest resistance to flow, and consequently, they are the principal vessels controlling total peripheral resistance.

Because the circulation mostly consists of many vessels in parallel, it is necessary to understand how total resistance is determined by the resistance in parallel ele-

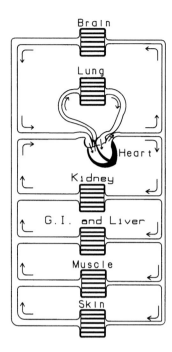

FIGURE 22-1 Schematic view of the human circulatory system. The total circulation passes through the right side of the heart and lung, then returns to the left side of the heart where it is distributed by the arterial system to the organs. The blood passes through many parallel pathways to the various regions and through many more parallel pathways within each organ. (G.I. = gastrointestinal tract.)

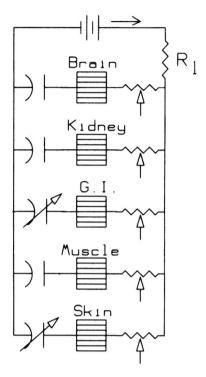

FIGURE 22-2 Electrical equivalent of the human circulatory system. The heart is represented by the battery at the top. Resistor R_1 represents the resistance of the distributing arterial system, whereas the variable resistors before each vascular bed represent the arteriolar resistances, which are the main components of peripheral resistance. The capillaries are parallel conductance pathways of low resistance. All venous beds are represented as capacitors because they can expand to store blood, but the cutaneous and splanchnic beds are represented as variable capacitors because they have the greatest range of capacity and can pool large amounts of blood under certain conditions. (G.I. = gastrointestinal tract.)

ments. For vascular beds arranged in parallel, the reciprocal of the total vascular resistance equals the sum of the reciprocal of the resistances of the parallel vascular beds as shown in the following equation:

$$1 \div R_t = 1 \div R_{hrt} + 1 \div R_{br} + 1 \div R_{kid} + 1 \div R_{spl} + 1 \div R_1 \quad [6]$$

where R_t, R_{hrt}, R_{br}, R_{kid}, R_{spl}, and R_1 are the total, heart, brain, kidney, splanchnic, and limb circulation resistances.

When resistances are in series, the total resistance of the circuit changes by the same amount as the resistance change in any of the series elements. Thus, if the resistance in one element increased by 10 arbitrary resistance units (RU), the total resistance would also increase by 10 RU. In a parallel circuit an increase in 10 RU of one parallel element would increase the reciprocal of total resistance by $1 \div 10$ RU or $1 \div R_t + 1 \div 10$. In this case the total resistance is much less affected by the resistance change in a single parallel element. Table 22-1 illustrates this point by showing the result of increasing limb resistance from 40–140 RU. If these circulations

were connected in series, the result would be a 100 RU increase in R_t, or a 100% change. In a parallel arrangement, the 100 RU increase in limb resistance results in only a 5% increase in total resistance.

When the CO, which produces the driving pressure, remains the same, and one of the parallel vascular beds dilates so that its resistance to flow decreases, such as the skin during heat stress, then the entire vascular resistance falls, thereby reducing systemic pressure. This is more easily seen when equation 5a is applied to the entire circulation and rearranged as below:

$$P_a = CO \cong R_t \quad [7]$$

When R_t falls, then P_a must also fall unless there is an increase in CO.

TABLE 22-1
Series and Parallel Vascular Resistances

Vascular Bed	Series Resistance (R)	Parallel (1/R)	Series Resistance (R)	Parallel (1/R)
Heart	10	0.100	10	0.100
Brain	10	0.100	10	0.100
Kidney	20	0.050	20	0.050
Splanchnic	20	0.050	20	0.050
Limbs	40	0.025	140	0.007
Sum	100	0.33	200	0.31
Total resistance	100	3.08	200	3.26
% increase	—	—	100	5.8

R = resistance.

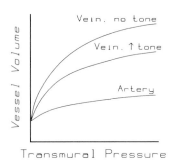

FIGURE 22-3 Relationship between transmural pressure and volume for arteries and veins. Arteries have little change in volume with pressure because their walls are muscular and stiff. Veins have relatively little smooth muscle and expand easily as the transmural pressure is increased. Veins that are innervated become stiffer and have a reduced volume-pressure curve when there is sympathetic activity as shown by the middle curve.

To maintain systemic pressure when one vascular bed is dilated, it is necessary to increase the resistance to flow in one of the parallel vascular beds, to increase CO, or both, thus preventing a change in P_a. This is what occurs during heat stress when the splanchnic bed may constrict as the cutaneous beds dilate so that P_a remains unchanged.

FEATURES OF ARTERIES AND VEINS

Compliance of the Vessel Wall

The adjustment of peripheral vascular resistance depends on the ability of individual vessels to change their diameters, which is determined by the internal pressure and the distensibility of the vessel wall, or its compliance. Arteries and veins differ significantly in their compliance. Figure 22-3 shows compliance curves for an artery and a vein, revealing the relationship between their internal pressure and their diameter. Veins increase their volume to a much greater degree than arteries as the internal pressure increases, and thus have much greater compliance than arteries. For this reason veins are often called the capacitance vessels of the circulation.

Compliance is not a static property of a vessel. In Figure 22-3 the middle compliance curve is for the same vein at a higher level of sympathetic tone. As sympathetic activity increases, the smooth muscle in the vessels contracts and the walls become less compliant; hence, the relationship between pressure and diameter is altered.

Compliance is a consequence of an active component, the smooth muscle, which contracts and relaxes, and a passive connective tissue component, which stretches as external forces are applied to it. Vessels have varying proportions of smooth muscle, connective tissue collagen, and elastin. Elastin is more distensible than collagen and vessels such as the aorta and its major branches have a large amount of elastin, giving them highly elastic, distensible properties. Small arteries consist mostly of smooth muscle and are consequently highly inelastic. Veins have little smooth muscle, hence their greater compliance.

The small arteries and arterioles (vessels smaller than 1 mm) are responsible for the greatest pressure decrease along the arterial tree because of their high resistance. The plot in Figure 22-4 of the intravascular pressure from the left ventricle to the right atrium reveals that the greatest pressure change occurs in the arteriolar resistance vessels. For this reason, these vessels are called the *resistance vessels*. Because of the great resistance of the terminal arterioles, the pressure at the entrance of the capillary circulation is typically only 15–30 mm Hg. Arterioles are inelastic but well endowed with smooth muscle, with their diameters determined almost entirely by the contractile state of their smooth muscle. Consequently, their resistance can vary over a wide range as the smooth muscle relaxes and contracts in response to local and systemic factors.

Passive and Active Changes in Vessel Size

Because each vessel segment and vascular bed has different intrinsic properties, a nomenclature has developed to distinguish the mechanisms producing diameter changes. At a fixed perfusion pressure, in the absence of

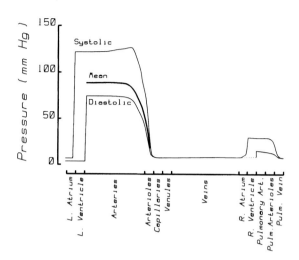

FIGURE 22-4 Systolic, diastolic, and mean pressure distribution in the heart and vascular system. The major decrease in pressure occurs in the small distributing arterioles of the systemic and pulmonary circulation that are referred to as the *resistance vessels*. Venous pressures are low.

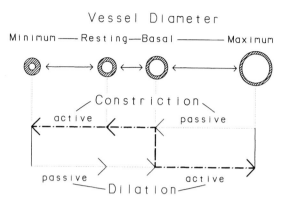

FIGURE 22-5 Resting and basal vascular tone. At a given perfusing pressure, and in the absence of neural, hormonal, and local influences, a vessel has a *basal* diameter. Increases or decreases from this diameter (*heavy lines, – · –*) require *active* processes such as sympathetic nerve activity, hormones, or local metabolites, whereas the return to the basal diameter (*dotted lines*) requires only the removal of these influences, and is thus called *passive vasoconstriction or vasodilation*. Under normal circumstances most arteries have some tonic sympathetic tone maintaining their *resting* diameter. Further increases in constrictor influence diminish the diameter until the vessel either is closed or at its minimum diameter. This constriction is termed *active vasoconstriction*. The return from the maximally constricted to the resting or basal state is called *passive vasodilation* because it requires only the removal of constrictor influences. To increase beyond the basal diameter either dilator nerves, hormones, or local factors are required, and such increases are termed *active vasodilation*. The return from the maximum diameter requires only the removal of the active vasodilator influences and is termed *passive vasoconstriction*.

sympathetic and hormonal input, each vessel has an intrinsic diameter called its *basal* or *intrinsic* diameter. This diameter is the result of the passive, or connective tissue, and active, or smooth muscle, properties of the vessel. Increases or decreases from this intrinsic or basal diameter are caused by active processes that modify the contractile state of the smooth muscle. Figure 22-5 shows changes from the basal diameter (dashed line) as dash-dot lines. When sympathetic nerves are present and when they are tonically active, the vessel diameter is smaller than its basal diameter; this diameter, which is called the *resting* diameter, is achieved by *active vasoconstriction* via the sympathetic nerves. Constriction of the vessel beyond its resting diameter is also an active process requiring increased sympathetic activity or hormonal factors. Dilation of the vessel from the constricted state to resting or basal levels is called *passive vasodilation* because it only requires the withdrawal of sympathetic vasoconstrictor tone or constrictor hormones. In Figure 22-5 this process is indicated by horizontal dotted lines.

Dilation of arterioles beyond their basal level is possible when substances such as epinephrine, acetylcholine, or bradykinin are released, or local metabolites such as lactate or CO_2 are present. In some tissues such as skeletal muscle there are also sympathetic vasodilator nerves. As indicated in Figure 22-5, dilation beyond the basal diameter is called *active vasodilation* because it is caused by added extrinsic stimulation, whereas the return to the basal diameter is a passive process called

passive vasoconstriction, which requires only the withdrawal of the dilator nerve activity or hormone. Active dilation of the veins has not yet been demonstrated.

CELLULAR ASPECTS OF VESSEL FUNCTION

Mediators of Vascular Smooth Muscle Contractile State

Because vascular resistance is determined almost entirely by the diameter of the resistance vessels, and the diameter changes from the resting diameter in all vessels depend on the contractile state of the smooth muscle, it is important to briefly review the factors that influence smooth muscle contractile function. The role of the sympathetic nerves has already been mentioned and the release of norepinephrine (NE), and in some cases acetylcholine, by these nerves is for most limb vessels the most important means of controlling vascular tone. The sympathetic nerve terminal and smooth muscle cell are diagrammatically represented in Figure 22-6.

Sympathetic Nerves

Nerve-Muscle Synapse In contrast to the junction between somatic nerves and striated muscle, where the axons end in a terminal button with a narrow cleft separating it from the muscle, the sympathetic nerve has enlargements called *varicosities* along its length where neurotransmitter is released. These are not always closely apposed to each smooth muscle cell. The cleft between nerve and muscle is typically 5–50 nm wide, so considerable diffusion time is often required for NE to reach the smooth muscle cell after it is released from the nerve. Because not all the cells in the muscle are close to the nerve varicosities, either the transmitter must diffuse to the distant cells, or the depolarization induced in the nearby cells must spread electronically to the other cells via gap junctions.

The time course of smooth muscle activation is slower than that found in the somatic nerve-striated

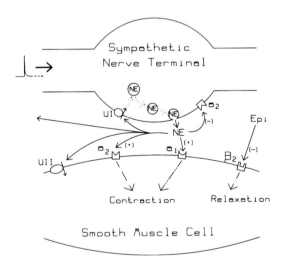

FIGURE 22-6 Synapse between the sympathetic nerve terminal and the smooth muscle cell. Action potentials traveling down the nerve initiate the release of norepinephrine (NE) from synaptic vesicles into the cleft. NE may traverse the synaptic cleft and bind to α_1-, α_2-, or β_2-receptors, causing either contraction or relaxation. Ultimately, NE may be taken back into the nerve or muscle via active uptake, reuptake I (UI), or reuptake II (UII), respectively, or it may be degraded or diffuse away from the synapse. Presynaptic α_2-receptors mediate negative feedback to the release of NE from the nerve. A (+) indicates that the pathway shown increases vascular tone and a (–) the opposite. β_2-receptors are usually extrajunctional and respond mostly to circulating epinephrine (Epi).

muscle synapse. Inactivation of the response is also slower, and is caused by (1) enzymatic breakdown of the NE by catechol-O-methyl transferase in the cleft, (2) Na^+-K^+-ATPase dependent reuptake into the sympathetic nerve (reuptake I), or into the smooth muscle cell (reuptake II), and (3) diffusion into the interstitial space and ultimately into the capillaries. Because some NE released from the nerve finds its way into the blood stream, plasma NE gives an indication of the level of sympathetic activity. An increase in sympathetic activity results in an increase in plasma NE, which lags behind the onset of activity by 2–3 minutes.

The NE that is released from the sympathetic nerves is synthesized by the nerve from tyrosine, which is first converted to dopamine in the nerve's cytoplasm. The dopamine is then packaged in 40- to 60-nm synaptic vesicles, which also contain the enzyme dopamine-β-hydroxylase, which converts dopamine to NE. When action potentials traveling down the nerve arrive at the nerve varicosity, an inward Ca^{++} current raises the intraneuronal Ca^{++} concentration initiating the fusion of vesicles with the membrane. After fusion with the membrane, the vesicles rupture, releasing their contents into the junctional cleft.

The synaptic vesicles of the nerve contain vasoactive substances besides NE, including adenosine triphosphate (ATP) and an assortment of peptides, depending on where the nerve is located.[1] These substances are coreleased along with NE into the cleft and also affect the contractile state of the smooth muscle cell. The precise role in the regulation of vascular tone is not clear.

Receptors for Vasoactive Agents Found on the Nerve and Smooth Muscle Cells The concept of cellular receptors was postulated long before it was known what the cellular components were. Receptors have been traditionally defined by pharmacologic means using various drugs found to be either agonists (initiators) or antagonists (inhibitors) of a given effect. Using such techniques it has been possible to establish the existence of several major categories of receptor (adrenergic, muscarinic, dopaminergic, histaminergic), each of which has two to many subtypes. Many of these membrane receptors have now been isolated, sequenced, and cloned.[2] Occupancy of these receptors by the appropriate agent or ligand activates a many-stepped intracellular pathway leading to constriction or dilation of vessels. Vessels usually have receptors for more than one type of substance, some which cause constriction and others dilation.

Figure 22-6 shows that sympathetic nerves have α_2-receptors, usually referred to as *presynaptic receptors*. These receptors bind NE that the nerve releases and mediate feedback inhibition of the release of neurotransmitter, regulating the amount of neurotransmitter released into the cleft. Sympathetic nerves may have muscarinic, purinergic, neuropeptide Y, and other receptors that also are involved in inhibition of NE release.

Adrenergic Pathways and the G Proteins

The adrenergic receptors, designated AR, have been divided into two major subclasses, αAR and βAR, based on the ability of drugs such as isoproterenol (βAR) or phenylephrine (αAR) to activate or propranolol (βAR) or phentolamine (αAR) to block them. There are at least two to three distinct forms of each of these receptor subclasses, α_1AR, α_2AR, β_1AR, β_2AR, and β_3AR, three of which (α_1AR, α_2AR, β_2AR) are found in the vessels of the limb. Both of the α_1ARs cause constriction when activated, and the β_2AR causes dilation. Table 22-2 lists these receptors, their location in the various vascular beds of the limbs, their agonist and antagonist ligand, their actions when activated, and the intracellular second messenger systems they activate.

When an agonist binds an adrenergic receptor, the receptor interacts with a membrane resident G protein, so called because of its GTPase activity, which in turn mobilizes one or more multistepped intracellular effector pathways.[3-5] There are many forms of the G protein involved in the transmembrane signaling of receptor systems. The G protein that is coupled to the β_2AR, G_s, activates the membrane-bound enzyme adenylate cyclase. Adenylate cyclase catalyzes the production of cyclic adenosine monophosphate (cAMP), which initiates other cytosolic processes, leading ultimately to smooth muscle relaxation.

The α_1AR and the α_2AR both cause vasoconstriction, but use different intracellular pathways to do so. The α_2ARs interact with a G protein called G_i which inhibits adenylate cyclase causing a reduction in cAMP levels in the cell. This leads to vasoconstriction via the removal of some tonic cAMP-mediated smooth muscle cell relaxation. Some workers have suggested that other effector pathways might also be activated by G_i which could also lead to smooth muscle cell contraction.[6] G_i may, for instance, directly affect ion channels in the membrane.

The α_1AR appears to act through a G protein that has been designated G_p[7] to initiate the phospholipase C–mediated hydrolysis of membrane phosphatidylinositol 4,5-bisphosphate into two components. The first, inositol, 1,4,5-trisphosphate, releases calcium from intracellular stores (the sarcolemma), and the second, diacylglycerol, directly activates protein kinase C,

which may affect contractile state through a separate mechanism.

Activation of the Contractile Proteins

The mechanism of smooth muscle contraction is similar to the sliding filament cross-bridge model of skeletal muscle, but the regulation of cross-bridge formation is more complex in smooth muscle. As in skeletal muscle, intracellular calcium is one of the most important initiators of smooth muscle contractile activity, but only a transient increase in cytosolic calcium is required to initiate a sustained contraction of the muscle. The calcium that activates the muscle comes predominantly from the sarcoplasmic reticulum, and it is rapidly taken back up after its release. Calcium-dependent calmodulin catalyzes the phosphorylation of myosin light chain kinase, which in turn phosphorylates the myosin light chain that forms the cross-bridge with actin-producing contraction. All pathways that increase cytosolic free calcium increase smooth muscle tone, and conversely most pathways that cause smooth muscle relaxation do so at least in part by reducing cytosolic free calcium. There are, however, other pathways that may sensitize or desensitize the contractile proteins to calcium and thereby cause an increase or a decrease in cross-bridge formation with no change in intracellular calcium. The βAR vasodilatory pathway may both decrease intracellular calcium and also phosphorylate myosin light chain kinase at a site that reduces its activity, thus causing relaxation by two mechanisms.[8]

Hormones and Other Vasoactive Influences on Smooth Muscle Tone

Many substances and physical factors modify vascular tone. Some are tonic influences that are usually present at some level, whereas others occur only under certain conditions such as exercise, stress, or hemorrhage. Table 22-2 lists the membrane receptors for a number of important vasoactive substances along with their actions in the cardiovascular system and the mechanisms, if known, by which they modify tone.

Acetylcholine

Acetylcholine causes vasodilation of most vascular smooth muscle via activation of muscarinic receptors. The cholinergic vasodilator system of the limbs, particularly the limb muscle, is controlled by the higher brain centers that increase their activity during fight or flight responses or psychological stress.[9,10] Before the discovery of endothelium-derived relaxing factor (EDRF), acetylcholine was thought to directly relax smooth muscle,

TABLE 22-2
*Vascular Endothelial and Smooth Muscle Cell Membrane Receptors Mediating Vascular Tone**

Receptor Type	Tissues	Agonists	Antagonist	Action	Coupling System	Intermediate Enzyme	Second Messengers	References
Adrenergic								
α_1	Most VSM	NE>Epi>>Iso	Prazosin	Vasoconstriction	G_p	PLC	IP_3, DAG	3,4
α_2	Peripheral vein VSM, small arterioles VSM, sympathetic nerves	NE>Epi>>Iso	Yohimbine	Vasoconstriction, decreased NE release	G_i, G_k (?)	Decreased AC, increased g_k	Decreased cAMP	3,4,6
β_1	SA node, ventricles	Iso>Epi>NE	Propranolol	Increased rate, increased contractility	G_s	AC	cAMP	3,4
β_2	Skeletal muscle VSM	Iso>Epi>NE	Atenolol	Vasodilation	G_s	AC	cAMP	3,4
Cholinergic								
M_1 (?)	VSM, endothelium, sympathetic nerves	ACh, carbachol	Pirenzepine, atropine, PTX?	Vasoconstriction, vasodilation, decreased NE release	G_p (?), EDRF	PLC, GC	IP_3, cGMP	11,78
M_2 (?)	VSM, endothelium, sympathetic nerves	ACh, carbachol	AF-DX116	Vasoconstriction, vasodilation, decreased NE release	G_i (?), EDRF	Decreased AC, GC	cAMP, cGMP	11,78,79
	SA node, AV node	—	PTX, atropine	Decreased rate; decreased conduction	G_k (?)	$I_{k.ACH}$	—	11
M_3 (?)	VSM, endothelium, sympathetic nerves	ACh, carbachol	P-fluorohexahydroisol	Vasoconstriction, vasodilation, decreased NE release	G_p (?), EDRF	PLC, GC	IP_3, cGMP	11,78,79
Purinergic								
P_2x	VSM	ATP>AMP>adenosine	$ANAPP_3$	Vasoconstriction	ROC-(Ca^+)	—	—	14
P_2y	Endothelium	ATP>AMP>adenosine	$ANAPP_3$	Vasodilation	EDRF	—	—	14
Adenosine								
A_1	VSM	Adenosine, ATP(?)	—	Vasodilation	G_i	AC	cAMP	15
A_2	VSM	Adenosine, ATP(?)	—	Vasodilation	G_s	AC	cAMP	15

Receptor	Location	Agonist	Antagonist	Response	Coupling system	Intermediate enzyme	Second messenger	References
Histaminergic								
H_1	Postcapillary venule endothelium, endothelium	2-Methylhistamine, histamine	Pyrilamine	Increased capillary permeability	G_p	PLC	IP_3	80,81
H_2	VSM	4-Methylhistamine, histamine	Burimamide	Vasodilation	—	—	—	80,81
Serotonergic								
$5\text{-}HT_{1c}$ (?)	VSM	α-methyl-5-HT	—	Vasoconstriction	G_p (?)	PLC	IP_3	18–20,86
$5\text{-}HT_{1b}$ (?)	Endothelium	α-methyl-5-HT	Methysergide	Vasodilation	EDRF (NO)	GC	cGMP	18–20
$5\text{-}HT_{1a}$ (?)	VSM	5-Carboxyamidotryptamine	—	Vasodilation	G_s (?)	AC	cAMP	19
$5\text{-}HT_2$	VSM	—	Ritanserin	Vasoconstriction	G_p (?)	PLC	IP_3	18–20,86
$5\text{-}HT_3$	Sensory nerve	—	ICS205930	—	ROC	—	—	18,86
Peptidergic								
Substance P (SP)	Endothelium	—	—	Vasodilation	EDRF	GC	cGMP	82,83
Neuropeptide Y (NPY)	VSM	—	—	Vasoconstriction	—	—	—	84
Vasoactive intestinal polypeptide (VIP)	VSM	—	—	Vasodilation	—	AC	cAMP	85
Antidiuretic hormone (vasopressin) V_{1A}	VSM	—	—	Vasoconstriction	—	PLC	IP_3/DAG	86
Atrial natriuretic protein (ANP)								
A	VSM (0.5%)	α-ANP	—	Vasodilation	—	GC	cGMP	84
B	VSM (95%)	α-ANP	—	Na^+ clearance	—	GC	cGMP	86

ACh = acetylcholine; AMP = adenosine monophosphate; ATP = adenosine triphosphate; AV = atrioventricular; Epi = epinephrine; 5-HT = serotonin; NE = norepinephrine; PTX = pertussis toxin; SA = sinoatrial; VSM = vascular smooth muscle.

*Known membrane receptors of vascular endothelium or smooth muscle that mediate vascular tone. Coupling systems are G protein (G_x), receptor-operated ion channel (ROC), or endothelium dependent (EDRF). Intermediate enzymes are phospholipase C (PLC), adenylate cyclase (AC), or guanylate cyclase (GC). Second messengers are inositol trisphosphate (IP_3), cyclic adenosine monophosphate (cAMP), cyclic guanosine monophosphate (cGMP), or diacylglycerol (DAG). Not all receptor types are known, and uncertainty about the specific type is indicated by a question mark. Intracellular pathways are known only for some receptor systems, and those that are as yet undetermined are indicated by "—".

but now it is known that the vascular endothelium must be present, and that if it is not, acetylcholine is a vasoconstrictor. There are five known subtypes of muscarinic receptors, designated M_{1-5}, but only the first three are pharmacologically identified; M_4 and M_5 are so far only known because of cloning studies,[11] whose amino acid sequences are highly homologous with the adrenergic receptor family.[12] It is not clear which receptors are found in the peripheral vessels. Like the adrenergic receptors, the muscarinic receptors are coupled to G proteins as listed in Table 22-2. There are also muscarinic receptors on the sympathetic nerves and when occupied they inhibit the release of NE by the nerve.

Purines

ATP causes vasoconstriction when applied to smooth muscle, but when the endothelium is present and it is applied inside the vessel lumen, it causes vasodilation.[13] The vasodilation occurs via EDRF. ATP is a cotransmitter with NE in many sympathetic nerves, and the sympathetic nerves of some small arterioles seem to release mostly or only ATP and thus are sympathetic-purinergic.[14] Adenosine receptors are treated as a separate receptor group with two subtypes, A_1 and A_2. Although adenosine is a purine, it is far more potent at these receptors than is ATP, adenosine diphosphate, or AMP. Both subtypes are found in the heart,[15] but the A_2 receptors appear to be the receptors mediating vasodilation in blood vessels.

Histamine

Histamine is a potent vasodilator found in the walls of mammalian arteries and veins[16] and in mast cells from which it is released during the inflammatory process. NE appears to exert a tonic inhibitory influence on histamine release from either neuronal or nonneuronal stores; a decrease in NE results in an increase in histamine release. The importance of histamine in circulatory control is not clear.[17] The vasodilation to histamine in some tissues is dependent on an intact endothelium, but receptors on the smooth muscle also mediate vasodilation.

Serotonin

Serotonin, which is named for the serum from which it was originally isolated and its vasoconstrictor action, has both vasodilator and vasoconstrictor activity. There are thought to be at least five receptor subtypes (see Table 22-2), some of which are structurally related to the adrenergic receptors.[18] Most circulating serotonin is contained in platelets, and its action on smooth muscle depends on whether there is an intact endothelium. If the endothelium is present, serotonin binds to receptors on the luminal side and causes the formation of EDRF, which then causes vasodilation. If there are no endothelial cells present, serotonin binds to smooth muscle and, depending on the tissue and vessel type, may cause either vasodilation or vasoconstriction.[19] Serotonergic nerve fibers have been found in some vascular beds, but none is reported in the vessels of the limbs.[20]

Angiotensin II

Angiotensin II is a much more potent vasoconstrictor on a molar basis than NE. Angiotensin II is produced in the circulation from the parent molecule, α_2-globulin or renin substrate, a protein circulating in the plasma. The juxtaglomerular cells release the enzyme renin into the circulation when sympathetic activity to the juxtaglomerular cells of the kidney is increased, plasma sodium is decreased, arterial pressure of the renal artery is diminished, or all three. Renin catalyzes the conversion of α_2-globulin to angiotensin I. When angiotensin I passes through the lung and some other organs, it is converted by converting enzyme of the endothelial cells into angiotensin II. Angiotensin II then binds to specific receptors in the arterioles, causing vasoconstriction. So far angiotensin II has not been shown to cause venoconstriction.

Vasopressin (Antidiuretic Hormone)

Vasopressin or antidiuretic hormone is released by the posterior pituitary in response to reductions in plasma osmolality or volume. Perhaps its primary function is the stimulation of the distal and collecting tubules of the kidney to increase their permeability to water, resulting in increased reabsorption, but it is also a potent vasoconstrictor of arterioles. Antidiuretic hormone may be important during hemorrhage in augmenting the vasoconstriction in muscle and other peripheral beds to preserve central blood volume.[21]

Neuropeptides (Coreleased with Norepinephrine by Sympathetic Nerves)

A variety of vasoactive peptides may be coreleased with NE from the sympathetic nerves, including neuropeptide Y, vasoactive intestinal protein, somatostatin, dynorphin, and galanan.[1] The significance of these peptides for normal blood flow regulation is not known, but they may be modulator substances producing effects that persist for some time (30 minutes) after their release. They are usually only released at high rates of sympathetic nerve activity and may be important during times of high stress or in pathologic states.

Endothelium-Derived Relaxing Factor

Acetylcholine, ATP, histamine, serotonin, substance P, and some other substances normally cause vasodilation, but have the opposite effect when the endothelium has been removed. These substances cause vasodilation by first binding to the endothelial cells, which then release a diffusible factor, endothelium-derived relaxing factor (EDRF), which then causes the smooth muscle cells to relax. There is a tonic release of EDRF by most vessels that partially dilates the vessels, and if EDRF production is pharmacologically inhibited, systemic blood pressure increases. Chronic exercise augments the release of EDRF during the first few weeks.[22,23] Physical factors such as stretch and flow velocity (shear stress) cause EDRF to be released, and platelets are able to cause EDRF release.[24,25] Thus, an intact endothelium prevents the constriction caused by platelets and the factors such as serotonin that they release, whereas the absence of endothelium favors vasoconstriction in the presence of platelets. EDRF also inhibits platelet aggregation and adhesion to the vessels.

EDRF dilates the smooth muscle cells by elevating cyclic guanosine monophosphate, which then causes smooth muscle cell relaxation through an unknown mechanism. It is now thought that nitric oxide is an EDRF because it is able to reproduce the effects of EDRF and is inhibited by the same agents that inhibit EDRF. L-Arginine appears to be the source of nitric oxide in the endothelial cell.[26] However, in some vascular beds, prostacyclin is the EDRF and inhibition of cyclo-oxygenase blocks the vasodilation.[27]

Endothelium-Derived Contracting Factor and Endothelin

Endothelial cells also may produce a constricting factor or factors in response to stretch (endothelium-derived contracting factor) that seems to involve a prostanoid, and some endothelia produce a 21-amino acid peptide vasoconstrictor called *endothelin*. The role of endothelium-derived contracting factor and endothelin is even less well characterized than that of EDRF.

Atrial Natriuretic Factor

Atrial natriuretic factor is released from the atrium in response to stretch and is a vasodilator peptide at high doses in vitro. In humans its major physiological role appears to be the elevation of renal blood flow and stimulation of greater fluid reabsorption by the kidney tubules. Atrial natriuretic factor does not appear to be important in the regulation of limb blood flow in humans.

Local Metabolic and Thermal Influences

During muscular exercise local pH decreases, and local metabolites increase, directly dilating the arterioles. Microcirculatory studies have shown that the smallest

arterioles, those that regulate the level of capillary perfusion, are the most sensitive to pH.[28]

The microvessels as well as some of the large superficial veins have an enhanced response to NE at temperatures lower than 37°C, and these same vessels have many adrenergic receptors of the α_2AR subtype. The response of the α_2AR pathway is inversely related to temperature such that cooling enhances the vasoconstriction caused by NE or epinephrine, but this is not true of the α_1AR pathway, whose response is directly related to temperature. The inverse thermal response of the α_2AR pathway may be an important local mechanism helping to adjust the level of blood flow to the appropriate level. During exercise, the constrictor effect of sympathetically released NE would be diminished in the terminal arterioles of muscle because high temperature along with local metabolite accumulation and low pH would dilate arterioles, helping to increase muscle perfusion. The cutaneous vessels with many α_2ARs would have an enhanced response in the cold to the sympathetically released NE, thus further reducing skin blood flow and consequently heat loss from the body.

SYSTEMIC ELEMENTS OF CIRCULATORY CONTROL

Blood Pressure Regulation

Baroreflex System

Systemic blood pressure is regulated within limits by an effective negative feedback baroreflex system that monitors pressure in the great vessels and attempts to minimize change by adjusting CO and vascular resistance via the autonomic nervous system. The role of the arterial, or high pressure, baroreceptors in the baroreflex system was first investigated in 1836,[29] and nearly 100 years later, Cramer[30] showed that there are also baroreceptors in the great veins, atrium, and pulmonary vessels. Both sets of baroreceptors respond to stretch with an increase in firing rate that increases their tonic inhibition of the medullary sympathetic outflow and their excitation of vagal outflow.

The high- and low-pressure baroreceptors appear to have distinct roles in the regulation of blood pressure. The high-pressure baroreceptor nerves, located in the carotid sinus and the aortic arch, enter the *medulla oblongata* via the IXth and Xth cranial nerves (see Chapter 4, Figure 4-1), and mediate the rapid responses to fluctuations of systemic arterial pressure. When systemic pressure increases by a few millimeters of mercury, there is increased stretch in the walls of the aortic arch and carotid body, which causes the baroreceptor nerves to increase their firing rate. Because these nerves have an inhibitory effect on the medullary sympathetic center, the result of increased arterial pressure is a decrease in sympathetic outflow to the blood vessels and the heart, causing a decrease in peripheral resistance and CO and a lowering of systemic arterial pressure.

The low pressure, cardiopulmonary baroreceptors located in the atrial and ventricular walls and in the lung also increase their rate of firing as pressure increases. These nerves also inhibit the medullary sympathetic center, but their pattern of activity during stretch and relaxation is different from that of the arterial baroreceptors. These receptors do not sense the beat-to-beat variation in systemic arterial pressure and do not respond as rapidly as the high-pressure baroreceptors to pressure change. It seems that their role is not the rapid correction of blood pressure, but rather in its long-term regulation. They also are important in mediating the adjustments to orthostatic stress via vasoconstriction of some vascular beds.

The difference between these two pressure-sensing pathways has been revealed by studies that eliminate just one or both of them. When the high-pressure baroreceptor nerves are cut, systemic pressure initially increases but then returns to the same average value, with wide fluctuations about that value. When the low-pressure baroreceptors are also denervated, the average blood pressure increases.[31,32] This indicates that the low-pressure sensors are necessary for maintaining the absolute level of average blood pressure. The high-pressure baroreceptor pathway does not operate around an absolute pressure set point, but rather operates around a set point established by some other system, perhaps the cardiopulmonary receptor pathway. The arterial baroreceptor set point appears to be changed in conditions such as some forms of hypertension in which the regulated pressure is much higher than normal or during exercise when the regulated pressure is temporarily increased.

Chemosensors

The arterial chemosensors located in the carotid and aortic bodies serve as sensory elements for both cardiovascular and pulmonary feedback control. They increase their firing rate when Po_2 and pH decrease and when Pco_2 increases. Stimulation of these receptors during hypoxia may result in increased CO, heart rate, vasoconstriction, and venoconstriction, as well as increased ventilation. In contrast to the baroreflex system, however, the chemoreceptor influence on blood flow is not entirely clear and may be far less important under normoxic conditions than during hypoxemia.[33]

Thermoregulation

The circulation probably first evolved to transport gases and important biological molecules and cells, but in birds and mammals, it is also important for the regulation of heat dissipation. The mechanisms by which the blood transports heat have been poorly understood. For many years it was thought that heat entered and left the circulation much as oxygen does, and that the primary exchange site was the capillaries.[34] It is now clear that heat, being much more diffusible than oxygen, is not carried by vessels as small as capillaries, because their rate of flow is slower than the radial diffusion of heat through the tissue. Experimental and theoretical studies have shown that most heat enters and leaves the circulation in vessels that are 40 μm or larger.[35,36] This means that by the time arterial blood from the warm core reaches small arterioles in the limb it is thermally equilibrated with the surrounding tissue and no longer carries any heat. Blood velocity is so high in the large arteries and veins (>1 mm) that little heat is lost or gained from them, so they function mainly as conduit vessels, just as they do for oxygen.

Later, the precise way in which the circulatory patterns are altered to facilitate heat loss are discussed. It is sufficient for now to point out that blood flow to the skin may be high, up to 8 liters min^{-1}, and only a small fraction of that flow serves a nutritive function. The large capacity for blood flow to the skin is entirely for the purpose of regulating body temperature by increasing heat dissipation at the surface.

DISTRIBUTION OF THE LIMB CIRCULATION

The four principal types of limb tissue receiving blood flow are skin, adipose tissue, muscle, and bone. Blood flow to the adipose tissue and bone is the least variable and least important for the systemic functions already mentioned.

Bone

Bone blood flow serves to both sustain the bone cells and facilitate ion exchange, particularly calcium.[37] The main vessels run in the cavity of the bone and branches feed the marrow and the intricate system of channels in the bone. The difficulty in measuring bone blood flow noninvasively has limited the data available for humans, but radioactive microsphere measurements in dogs revealed that cortical and cancellous bone received 2.5 and 38.3 ml $\cong$ 100 ml^{-1} tissue $\cong$ min^{-1}, respectively, or over 9% of CO.[38]

Adipose Tissue

The adipose tissue, which in the limb is mostly distributed subcutaneously, requires an adequate circulatory supply for gas exchange and nutritive exchange plus the transport of free fatty acids released from fat cells. The vessels in adipose tissue are innervated by sympathetic fibers and they constrict when sympathetic nerves are stimulated. These vessels do not appear to participate in the systemic baroreflex or thermoregulation, but they do dilate during prolonged exercise, suggesting that they facilitate free fatty acid delivery under such conditions.[39]

Skin

Anatomy

The skin is organized into two layers, the epidermis, a layer of keratinized squamous epithelial cells, and the dermis, which contains the blood vessels as well as the glands of the skin, the nerves, and the hair follicles. A review of the skin circulation can be found elsewhere.[40] Figure 22-7 shows the vascular organization. The main supply vessels to the skin are feeder arteries and veins that branch from the major vessels of the subcutaneous tissue. After they enter the dermal layer these vessels connect to the deep cutaneous plexus, a plexus of larger countercurrent arteries and veins. From this deep cutaneous plexus arise perpendicular riser vessels that feed the more superficial and much smaller arteriolar plexus. Arterioles rising from this plexus feed the capillary loops near the upper layer of the dermis. After the blood passes through the capillary loops it enters the superficial venous plexus, which has a high capacity to pool blood and has mistakenly been assumed to be an important site of heat transfer from the blood that passes through the capillaries.[41] The capillary loops of the human nailfold can be visualized noninvasively,[42] and most of the information on human capillary function is derived from such studies.

In some skin areas of the extremities, there are special vascular elements called *arteriovenous anastomoses*, which connect the rising precapillary arterioles to the venous plexus, bypassing the capillaries. These highly muscular and highly innervated vessels provide an alternate route for blood from the arteriole to the venular side of the circulation. The greatest density of arterio-

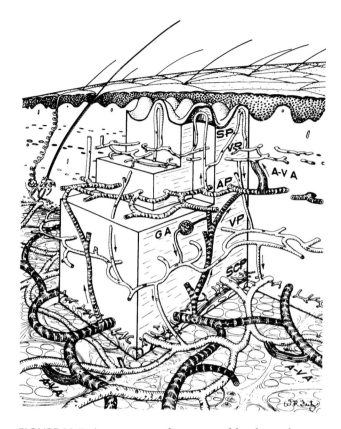

FIGURE 22-7 Arrangement of cutaneous blood vessels combining features normally characteristic of specific regions. (AP = arteriolar plexus; A-VA = arteriovenous anastomosis; GA = arteriovenous glomus; SCP = cutaneous plexus; SP = subpapillary plexus layer; VP = venous plexus.) (Reprinted with permission from HV Sparks. Skin and Muscle. In PC Johnson [ed], Peripheral Circulation. New York: Wiley, 1978.)

venous anastomoses is in the tips of the digits, and there are few in forearm skin.[43] When they are opened as they are during heat stress, a much higher volume of blood can pass through the skin than would be possible if the blood had to pass through the capillary circulation. Even though the skin accounts for only approximately 5% of the body's volume, blood flow through the arteriovenous anastomoses may be so great that the skin receives 50% of the CO. Blood that passes through the arteriovenous anastomosis into the superficial venous plexus may transfer its heat in the later vessels, although no experiments have yet demonstrated this to be true.

Nerve Supply

The control of the skin blood flow in the hand and foot is different from that of the forearm, upper arm, calf, and thigh, hereafter designated the *proximal limb regions.* In the hand and foot there is a high resting level of sympathetically maintained vascular tone, whereas in the proximal limb skin resting sympathetic tone is slight. Figure 22-8 compares the blood flow responses of the hand and the forearm with nerve block and deep body cooling and heating. Virtually all of the dilation and constriction in the hand is caused by decreases or increases in sympathetic constrictor nerve activity, but as seen in Figure 22-8, the forearm skin vessels contain both vasoconstrictor and vasodilator nerves. The active dilator nerves are important in heat-induced thermoregulatory vasodila-

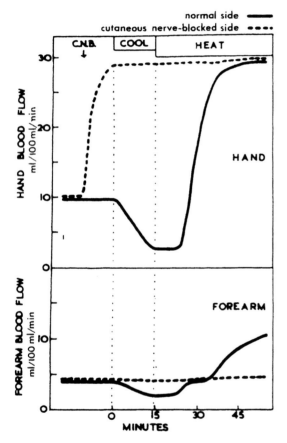

FIGURE 22-8 Schematic representation of changes in blood flow in normal and nerve-blocked hand and forearm during body cooling and heating. At cutaneous nerve block, on one side vasomotor nerves to the hand and forearm skin were blocked with local anesthetic solution. (CNB = cutaneous nerve-blocked.) (Reprinted with permission from IC Roddie. Circulation to Skin and Adipose Tissue. In JT Shepherd, FM Abboud [eds], Handbook of Physiology. Section 2: The Cardiovascular System, Vol. III. Peripheral Circulation and Organ Blood Flow, Part 1. Bethesda: American Physiological Society, 1983.)

tion of proximal limb skin, and these can be blocked by atropine, suggesting that these are cholinergic nerves. When sweating begins, there is a further increase in blood flow that is mostly caused by the local release with the sweat of vasoactive substances such as bradykinin.

The proximal limb vasodilator nerves do not seem to play a role in the baroreflex, but the vasoconstrictor nerves to the extremities and proximal limb do.

Muscle

The skeletal muscle of the limbs is 40% of the total body mass and can receive a large percentage of the CO during exercise. The blood vessels in skeletal muscle of the limbs have a large range of tone, and the basal flow rate of $2-5 \text{ ml} \cong 100 \text{ ml}^{-1} \cong \text{min}^{-1}$ can increase to $240 \text{ ml} \cong 100 \text{ ml}^{-1} \cong \text{min}^{-1}$ during heavy exercise. The large increase from the basal level is possible partially because the capillaries are not all perfused at rest and are recruited as the work intensity increases the demand for oxygen.

Anatomy

Figure 22-9 shows the microvasculature (vessels < 60–80 μm in diameter) of the cat tenuissimus and biceps femoris muscles.[44] The arteries and veins travel through the tissue as countercurrent pairs from the main limb vessels to the final branching of the terminal arterioles that feed the capillaries. The secondary vessels run parallel to the muscle fibers as do the capillaries. Terminal vessels that are perpendicular to the muscle fibers connect the capillaries to the secondary vessels. Myrhage and Eriksson suggest that the arrangement of these vessels forms a fundamental unit in skeletal muscle, shown in Figure 22-9 as a cylinder.[44]

Nerve Supply

The muscle vessels contain sympathetic vasoconstrictor nerves and possibly sympathetic vasodilator nerves, the latter being difficult to directly demonstrate. The αAR receptors on the smooth muscle are innervated but the β_2AR are not, suggesting that they respond mostly to circulating epinephrine that is released from the adrenals. When the sympathetic nerves to muscle are cut, there is a two- to threefold increase in blood flow, indicating that in comparison with the skin, there is less sympathetically mediated resting tone. The increase flow of up to 100-fold is not caused by sympathetic withdrawal, but rather active vasodilation of the muscle vascular bed by either neuronal, hormonal, or local pathways.

FUNCTIONAL REGULATION OF BLOOD FLOW

Now that the fundamental cellular and systemic elements involved in blood flow regulation have been discussed, it is possible to consider how these work in commonly encountered situations of postural change, exercise, thermal stress, and psychological stress.

Orthostatic Adjustment

The basic cardiovascular challenge is the maintenance of adequate perfusion to the organs of the body. The brain is the preeminent organ with regard to perfusion and given its inability to function without a constant supply of oxygenated blood and its position above heart level in many vertebrates, rapid adjustments must be made to maintain adequate perfusion pressure during postural change.

Figure 22-10 summarizes the cardiovascular events during movement from prone to upright posture. The normal sequence is as follows:

1. Pooling of blood in the organs below heart level caused by gravity

2. Reduction of central venous return and a fall in central venous pressure (panel 5, central blood volume)

3. Reduction of cardiac filling because of reduced venous return to the right side of the heart (panel 2, right atrial pressure falls; panel 4, stroke volume declines), and consequent fall in CO_2, via the Frank-Starling mechanism (panel 3, CO)

4. Sensing of the fall in central venous pressure or right atrial pressure by the low-pressure cardiopulmonary baroreceptors that reduce their firing rate and thereby:

   a. Disinhibit the medullary sympathetic centers causing sympathetic activity to increase with ensuing peripheral vasoconstriction (panels 7 and 8, decreases in forearm, splanchnic and renal blood flow) and

   b. Reduce input to the vagal nucleus decreasing vagal outflow and thereby allowing heart rate to increase (panel 6, heart rate)

5. Reduction of arterial systolic blood pressure because of the reduced CO (panel 1, arterial pressure)

6. Sensing of the fall in systolic blood pressure by the carotid body and aortic arch baroreceptors that also reduce their rate of firing and disinhibit the sympathetic centers and stimulate the vagal centers of the medulla

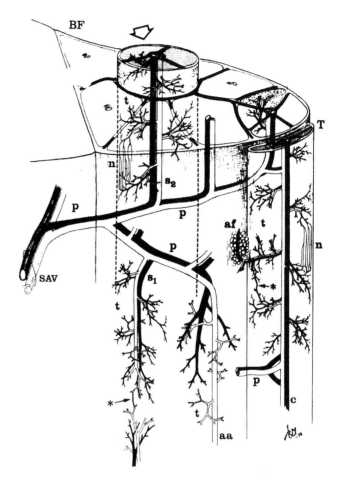

FIGURE 22-9 The vascular arrangement in the thin cat tenuissimus muscle (T) and in the thicker biceps femoris muscle (BF). The terminal arterioles and venules (t) branch in a two-dimensional pattern in the thin muscle and three-dimensionally within a cylinder (basic unit, *large arrow*) of muscle fibers in the thick muscle. (aa = arterial anastomosis connecting ends of primary arteries; af = fascia containing adipose tissue adjacent to the tenuissimus muscle; c = central vessel; n = capillary network; p = primary vessel; SAV = supplying artery and vein; s_1 and s_2 = secondary vessels; * = arterial anastomosis.) (Reprinted with permission from R Myrhage, E Eriksson. Arrangement of the Vascular Bed in Different Types of Skeletal Muscles. In F Hammersen, K Messmer [eds], Skeletal Muscle Microcirculation. Basel: Karger. Boston: Cambridge University Press, 1984.)

As the right side of Figure 22-10 shows, walking activates the venous pump, *second heart*, which facilitates the return of venous blood and the return of central venous pressure to its supine value. As a result, all of the parameters return to their original supine values.

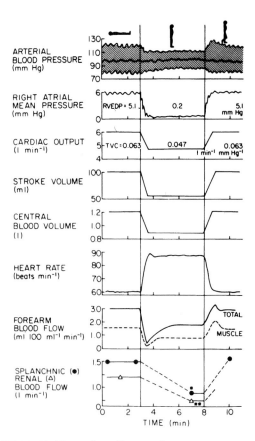

FIGURE 22-10 Normal cardiovascular responses to upright posture (*middle panel*) and activation of muscle pumping by gently contracting the leg muscles without movement (*right panel*). Numbers in panel 2 (right atrial pressure) show right ventricular end-diastolic pressure (RVEDP). Numbers in panel 3 (cardiac output) show total vascular conductance (TVC). Time courses for changes in cardiac output and derived variables and for splanchnic and renal flows are approximate. (Reprinted with permission from LB Rowell. Human Circulation. New York: Oxford University Press, 1986.)

Exercise

As with most of the previous discussion, it is not possible to discuss the limb circulation in isolation from circulation to other parts of the body or the functioning of the heart. This is particularly true in the case of exercise when much of the increase in blood flow occurs in the muscles of the working limbs, but at the expense of blood flow to other organs. Exercise, therefore, is discussed within a systemic fashion, as is circulatory adjustments to thermal stress in the following section. For in-depth reviews of exercise physiology the reader is referred elsewhere[45-48] and to Chapter 16.

Pattern of Cardiovascular Responses to Exercise

There is a predictable cardiovascular response to exercise depending on the fitness of the individual and the intensity of the exercise, as well as the state of hydration, ambient temperature, age, and disease.

Cardiac Function Figure 22-11 shows the response of three classes of individuals of differing fitness to graded increases in oxygen uptake resulting from increasing work load. The three classes of individuals represent a range of work capacity as measured by their maximal oxygen uptake capacity, $\dot{V}O_2$max, from very low in the patients with mitral stenosis to very high in the elite endurance athletes. CO increases more or less in a linear fashion almost up to the point that $\dot{V}O_2$max is reached. The resting CO of approximately 6 liters min^{-1} is similar in all three groups, but the maximum attainable value is much greater in the athletes who can reach a CO greater than 40 liters min^{-1}. Maximum heart rate is similar for all groups, although the most fit have a much lower resting rate because of both lower sympathetic activity and higher resting vagal tone. The initial increase in heart rate is thought to be primarily via withdrawal of vagal tone, whereas increases above 100 beats min^{-1} are the result of increased sympathetic activity to the heart.[49]

Interestingly, stroke volume does not change significantly as $\dot{V}O_2$ increases, partly because of the decreased filling time that results from the increase in heart rate. Stroke volume is much greater in the fit individuals, and for this reason athletes are able to maintain the same level of CO as untrained individuals at a much lower heart rate. The reasons for the increased stroke volume in athletes is not well understood, but it appears that their end-diastolic volume is increased,[50] and ventricular dimensions are increased.[51] It has also been suggested that there is an increase in cardiac contractility with conditioning, but most reviewers do not support this hypothesis.[45,52,53]

Sympathetic Nerve Activity The horizontal dashed line in the heart rate panel of Figure 22-11, which intersects the ordinate at 100 beats per minute, is to indicate that at this heart rate there is an increase in sympathetic nerve activity that both serves to increase heart rate and to increase vasoconstriction in nonexercising vascular beds such as the renal and splanchnic. The bottom panel of the figure shows the decrease in splanchnic and renal blood flow as a percentage change from control. At the same time that vasoconstriction begins, there is an increase in circulating NE because of the overflow of sympathetically released NE into the circulation.

Systemic Blood Pressure In the section on hemodynamics of blood flow it was pointed out that increases in vascular conductance of a vascular bed must be matched by either a similar reduction in conductance of another bed, by an increase in CO, or both, if systemic blood pressure is not to fall. From the previous discussion, it is clear that both of these mechanisms are used to maintain blood pressure during exercise. The reduction in blood flow to renal, splanchnic, and other nonexercising beds contributes to the maintenance of systemic blood pressure while the vascular conductance is increasing dramatically in the working muscles. These regional flow reductions alone are not sufficient, however, to maintain blood pressure, and an increase in CO is essential. Actually, the increase in CO and vascular resistance in some vascular beds more than compensates for the decreased vascular resistance in the exercising muscle, and blood pressure may actually increase.

The observed increase in blood pressure with exercise suggests that there is a resetting of the baroreceptor set point during exercise. Rowell[45] has reviewed the arguments for and against baroreflex resetting and concluded that blood pressure is unquestionably as tightly regulated during exercise as at rest and appears to be regulated at a higher level, but the sensitivity of the response to systemic pressure changes is unaltered.

Increases in Muscle Perfusion and the Redistribution of Regional Blood Flow during Exercise

As muscular contractions begin, the demand for oxygen and for metabolite removal increases rapidly, and there is a need for increased blood flow. Muscle has a remarkable ability to increase its blood flow from the resting value of 3–5 ml $\cong$ 100 ml^{-1} $\cong$ min^{-1} to greater than 240 ml $\cong$ 100 ml^{-1} $\cong$ min^{-1}.[54] Blood flow in exercising muscle of rats may exceed 340 ml $\cong$ 100 ml^{-1} $\cong$ min^{-1}, and it is not clear what is the actual limit to vascular conductance in humans. How is muscle blood flow increased by such a dramatically large amount? First, there is a large increase in the number of capillaries that are perfused. During rest, microcirculatory studies show that only a part of the available capillaries are perfused at any given time; the precapillary arterioles open and shut periodically. The control of this microcirculatory behavior is not clear, but evidence points to local metabolic factors, including pH, PO_2, PCO_2, K$^+$, ATP, adenosine, osmolarity, and temperature.[17] These factors may cause the precapillary arterioles to dilate or constrict as their concentrations or levels wax and wane.[55] As exercise becomes intense and capillarity has reached its maximum, O_2 delivery may not be adequate to sustain aerobic metabolism. At such a point there is a constant maximal local vasodilatory stimulus at the precapillary arterioles and a strong sys-

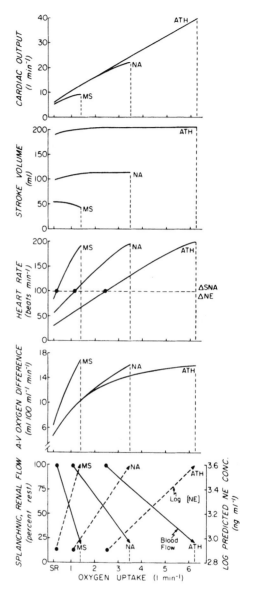

FIGURE 22-11 Representative cardiovascular responses to graded dynamic exercise in three groups of individuals whose levels of maximum oxygen consumption ($\dot{V}O_2$max) are low (patients with *pure* mitral stenosis [MS]), normal (normally active subjects [NA]), or high (elite endurance athletes [ATH]). The dashed vertical line shows the $\dot{V}O_2$max for each group. The horizontal dashed line in the third panel shows the heart rate where plasma NE (ΔNE) and sympathetic nerve activity (ΔSNA) increases. These solid circles are transferred to the splanchnic and renal blood flow and the NE-oxygen uptake axes in the bottom panel. They show that in each group splanchnic and renal flows begin to decrease when heart rate reaches 100 beats min^{-1}, and that plasma NE concentration also begins to increase rapidly at this heart rate. (Reprinted with permission from LB Rowell. Human Circulation. New York: Oxford University Press, 1986.)

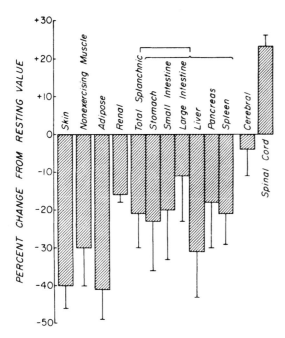

FIGURE 22-12 Human-like redistribution of blood flow during mild dynamic exercise (cycling) in conscious baboons as measured from the distribution of radioactive microspheres. (Reprinted with permission from LB Rowell. Human Circulation. New York: Oxford University Press, 1986.)

temic cardiovascular response that results in both increased CO and a redistribution of blood flow to exercising muscle and away from nonexercising tissues.

In humans there is vasoconstriction in the visceral organs and nonexercising muscle, and initially in the skin, to help meet increasing demand for blood flow in working muscle. Although it is difficult to measure regional blood flow changes in humans, a study in baboons, where radiolabeled microspheres were used to quantify blood flow changes, revealed that all regions measured except the spinal cord had reduced blood flows[56] (Figure 22-12). The largest decreases were in the skin, nonexercising muscle, adipose tissue, and liver. To gain a better quantitative sense of how flow reductions in these beds increase the blood flow available to the exercising muscle, Rowell[45] compared the blood flow distribution at rest and maximal exercise in the same three groups of subjects shown in Figure 22-11. Figure 22-13 demonstrates that although blood flow reductions in renal, hepatic, gastrointestinal tract, and other organs are significant, they account for only a small part of the total increase in flow to the working muscle, and that the additional blood flow must come from an increase in CO.

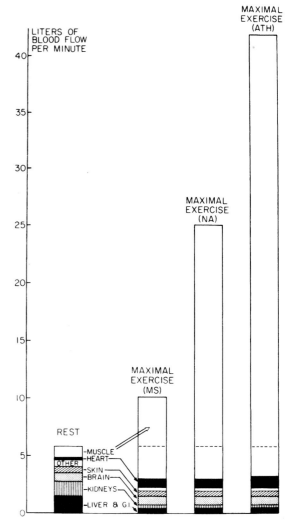

FIGURE 22-13 Total cardiac output and its distribution during rest and brief exercise requiring maximum oxygen consumption in three groups depicted in Figure 22-11. During exercise blood flow to nonexercising regions, except the heart, was almost the same in all three groups. The higher coronary flow in athletes reflected the greater tissue mass; the volumetric blood flow should have been the same. (ATH = elite endurance athletes; MS = patients with *pure* mitral stenosis; NA = normally active subjects.) (Reprinted with permission from LB Rowell. Human Circulation. New York: Oxford University Press, 1986.)

Despite the relatively small contribution of flow redistribution to the increase in blood flow to exercising muscle, it is not negligible, particularly in the mitral stenosis group, which has a limited ability to increase CO and where the redistributed flow represents approximately 30–40% of the total increase in flow to the exercising muscle. In the untrained normal subject and the athlete the redistribution of flow accounts for only 12–17% and 6–10% of the total increase in flow to exercising muscle.

Increased Oxygen Extraction during Exercise

In addition to an increased flow to exercising muscle, there is a greater ability of muscle to extract oxygen, increasing the arteriovenous oxygen gradient. The efficiency of O_2 extraction is expressed as the arterial-venous O_2 difference. During rest the arterial-venous O_2 difference of muscle is approximately 4.5 ml 100 ml^{-1}, or approximately 23% extraction (see the fourth panel of Figure 22-11). As $\dot{V}O_2$max is approached, this value reaches 17–18 ml 100 ml^{-1}, or approximately 85% extraction. The greater extraction of O_2 from the blood is caused by several factors. First, the perfusion of more capillaries both shortens the average O_2 diffusion distance and increases the diffusion area from the capillary to the muscle fiber.[55] Transit time of the blood through the capillary may also increase somewhat.

The geometry of the capillaries is also changed during muscle contraction from a relatively straight tube when the muscle is relaxed, to a highly curved, serpentine configuration that may increase the capillary to muscle fiber surface area ratio.

The O_2 extraction of nonexercising tissues is also increased because of the decreased flow velocity through them. At rest, when their flow is higher, these tissues have a low oxygen extraction efficiency, and during exercise they can extract the same amount of oxygen from a much lower blood flow because the blood transit time is reduced.

Effects of Chronic Exercise on Muscle Blood Flow

Figure 22-13 shows the physiological result of long-term training. The maximum heart rate is not increased, but stroke volume is, and consequently, CO is greatly improved. In the limbs one of the principal changes in the vascular system is the increase in muscle capillarity. This increase is not the dynamic increase seen in all individuals as muscular work begins, but rather, is an increase in the maximum number of capillaries available for exchange. One study found that sedentary individuals had 329 capillaries per square millimeter and that after 8 weeks of training they had 395 capillaries per square millimeter.[57] In the same study the number of capillaries per muscle fiber increased from 1.36 to 2.00.

Competition for Blood Flow between Thermoregulation and Muscle Metabolism

In the next section the limb vascular responses to heat stress are discussed in detail; for now it is sufficient to say that blood flow to the skin is a critical mechanism by which mammals lose the excess heat they continually produce. Even in a cool environment extended muscular exercise generates a great deal of excess heat that must be lost to the environment if overheating is not to occur. As we have seen previously, exercising muscle increases its blood flow up to 100-fold and can create a demand for blood flow that exceeds the maximum CO of the heart. At the same time, the skin, which is at first vasoconstricted during exercise, must soon begin to dilate to allow the blood to carry heat to the surface where it can be lost. Thus, the competing drives for thermoregulation, blood pressure maintenance, and maintenance of muscle metabolism, which together exceed CO, cannot all be fully satisfied.

When the skin begins to dilate after prolonged exercise in a cool environment, there is a pooling of blood in the cutaneous veins that ultimately reduces central venous volume, cardiac filling pressure, and stroke volume. This is a gradual change that has been called *cardiovascular drift*. To compensate for the decrease in stroke volume and to maintain CO, heart rate increases.[58] After a time of exercise, especially in the heat, the renal, hepatic, and splanchnic beds are further constricted.

Heat and Cold Stress

In endotherms the vascular system facilitates the necessary removal of the large excess of centrally produced heat in neutral and warm environmental conditions. In this section the precise nature of the circulatory responses to heat and cold are discussed; a complete discussion of thermoregulation can be found in the chapter on human thermoregulation (see Chapter 21).

In thermoneutral conditions (26–28°C in nude humans), the only active thermoregulatory mechanism is the regulation of skin blood flow, and thermoneutrality is called the *zone of maximum vasomotor instability*. Waxing and waning of skin blood flow of the extremities provide for the minute-to-minute variation in heat loss and conservation in this state in which metabolic heat production is lowest. The importance of vascular heat transfer during the resting state is illustrated in Figure 22-14 in which a simulation of the human thermal state without any heat transfer in the blood is shown. At rest approximately 70% of body heat production occurs in the viscera, heart, and brain, centrally located areas. If the heat produced in these areas could escape only by molecular diffusion through the tissues the simulation shows that the body core temperature would not reach a steady-state temperature until it was approximately 80°C. A lethal temperature would be reached in only 3 hours.

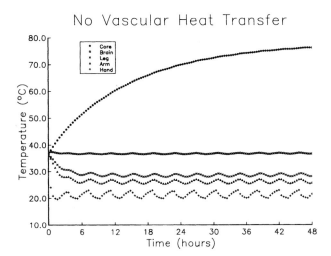

No Vascular Heat Transfer

FIGURE 22-14 Simulation of human body temperature change at rest in a thermoneutral environment. The model assumed that the circulation functioned normally except that it did not carry any heat. It also assumed that metabolic heat production was constant. The core body temperature (*open circles*) rose slowly, reaching a lethal temperature of 42°C by approximately 3 hours. It did not reach a steady-state temperature until 48 hours. Leg, arm, and hand temperatures decreased because their resting heat production is low and their heat loss is high. Under normal conditions their temperatures are maintained because they receive warm blood from the body core.

Centrally Mediated Response to Skin or Body Cooling

When the skin is cooled there is rapid vasoconstriction that is partly central in origin. Cutaneous thermal sensors relay information to the spinal cord and hypothalamus where all thermosensory information is integrated, and an increase in sympathetic drive to the cutaneous vessels causes the vasoconstriction. This initial response is transient, and blood flow returns to resting values unless the recirculating blood from the limb produces some central body cooling that activates a more persistent thermoregulatory response. During intense cutaneous vasoconstriction the minimally perfused skin, along with the underlying subcutaneous fat, provide a layer of insulation, and the temperature gradient from the skin surface into the muscle becomes almost linear,[59] yielding the lowest possible heat transfer from the body.

Local Vascular Response to Cooling

Temperature also has a direct effect on the vascular smooth muscle and the sympathetic nerves. Falling temperature directly enhances the response of the $\alpha_2 AR$ pathway, and in the skin veins and terminal muscle arterioles, where there are many $\alpha_2 ARs$, moderate local cooling (to 25°C) causes further constriction when some sympathetic tone is present.[60-62]

Cold-Induced Vasodilation   Long ago Sir Thomas Lewis observed a curious response to low temperature in the blood flow to human fingers[63] (Figure 22-15). He found that when the hand is immersed in ice water, there is an initial intense vasoconstriction that reduces blood flow to a minimum. However, after 30–40 minutes of continued immersion, blood flow increases, raising the finger temperature, and then again decreases. This oscillating blood flow to the fingers then continues with a frequency of one cycle of constriction and dilation every 30–40 minutes or less. This *Lewis* or *hunting* reaction is hypothesized to be a tissue-protective feature of hand blood flow, which minimizes the loss of body heat to the cold water by vasoconstricting and allowing the hand to become very cold, and then periodically warming the hand to prevent freezing and tissue damage. Such an explanation is appealing and may or may not be correct, but the mechanism behind this behavior is now understood.

During the initial rapid cooling of the hand, the central and local response is to constrict the blood vessels via increased sympathetic outflow and a cooling-induced increase in $\alpha_2 AR$ responsiveness, respectively. This greatly diminishes blood flow and thereby reduces heat transfer to the hand from the central body, causing hand temperature to quickly fall. After 10–20 minutes, the hand temperature becomes so low that sympathetic neurotransmission and the αAR receptor pathway are blocked,[64] and NE concentration eventually decreases because of the circulation and reuptake and metabolism. The smooth muscle contractile mechanisms are probably also partially paralyzed. The vascular smooth muscle then begins to relax and the flow of warm blood from the central body increases, warming the surrounding tissue including the sympathetic nerves. When the sympathetic nerves have warmed sufficiently, they begin to release NE again, which causes renewed vasoconstriction. This cycle is then repeated until cooling of the hand ceases. Animal experiments[65] have confirmed that this is the mechanism by which cold-induced vasodilation occurs.

Centrally Mediated Vascular Response to Heat

When humans enter a hot environment, thermal sensors in the skin relay the information to the hypothalamus and spinal cord, and the first response is the dilation of cutaneous vessels. If exposure to heat is prolonged and intense enough to increase the temperature of the body, then skin blood flow eventually reaches its maximum level of 7–8 liters min^{-1}. Sweating greatly increases the

FIGURE 22-15 Cold-induced vasodilation. Skin temperature of the index finger cooled in crushed ice. The periodic increases in skin temperature were also called the *hunting* or *Lewis reaction*. (Reprinted with permission from T Lewis. Observations on the reactions of the vessels of the human skin to cold. Heart Clin Sci 1930;15:177–208.)

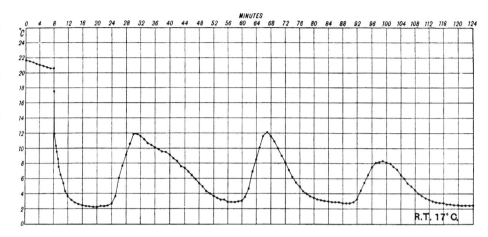

ability of the skin to dissipate heat, and without it, the large blood flow to the skin would be insufficient for effective body cooling. The increase in skin blood flow is achieved through both a redistribution of blood flow away from splanchnic regions and muscle and an increase in CO.[45]

During whole body heating in humans, forearm blood flow immediately begins to increase, followed by an increase in blood flow to the feet and legs.[41] This increased blood flow is largely in the skin because even though much of the muscle mass is near the surface, there is no evidence that its blood flow increases during heat stress. At about the time forearm blood flow begins to increase, sweating also begins. With a sustained increase in body temperature, there is a persistent increase in forearm blood flow, and to support such a large flow increase, CO increases by 6.6 liter min^{-1}. There is a simultaneous decrease in splanchnic, renal, and muscle blood flow, contributing another 1.2 liter min^{-1} to skin blood flow, and allowing an increase in skin blood flow of 7.8 liter min^{-1}. The increased vascular resistance of the splanchnic, renal, and muscle beds and the increase in CO together do not completely compensate for the large increase in vascular conductance of the skin so that arterial pressure decreases for the first 30–40 minutes, after which it slowly returns to normal. Increased pooling of blood in the cutaneous veins causes right arterial mean pressure to slowly decrease throughout the period of heat exposure, until it approaches 0.5 mm Hg. Stroke volume increases, as does heart rate, to increase CO.

The vasoconstriction in viscera and muscle and the increase in CO are sympathetically mediated, but are not initiated by the baroreflex system. The response seems to be solely driven by the thermoregulatory centers, because raising arterial pressure back to normal by elevating and then occluding the legs does not alter

either the vasoconstriction or the heart rate response, which continues to increase.

Local Vascular Responses to Heating   Directly applied heat dilates cutaneous vessels that have some vasoconstrictor tone, and this has often been interpreted as an important local mechanism of thermoregulation and heat loss. Cutaneous veins contract less well to applied NE when they have been warmed to 39°C from 34°C, and if they have been partially constricted with NE, they dilate when warmed.[66] Heating reduces the α_2AR response to NE, and in vessels such as terminal arterioles and cutaneous veins, in which such receptors predominate, heat has a major effect on blood flow. The effect of heat on other receptor-mediated constrictor and dilator pathways is not known.

Heating with diathermy, ultrasound, or hot packs is a common practice in physical medicine and rehabilitation, and one of the therapeutic goals of these treatments is to increase blood flow (see reference 67 for an extensive review of the use of the heat therapeutically). In animals, in which intense local heating is possible, there is a critical temperature between 41° and 44°C beyond which a pronounced vasodilation may occur. The physiological basis of this dilation is not known. One study showed that temperature oscillation of the heated dog thigh occurred after 30–40 minutes with a pattern similar to cold-induced vasodilation.[68] The temperature oscillations appeared to be caused by the primary effect of heat on the vessels, which caused them to dilate, followed by the cooling effect of the increased blood flow, which caused them to return somewhat to their original diameters. If heating was intense enough, there was sometimes a long lasting period of oscillation in temperature.

Heating does not always cause vessels to dilate, and one study demonstrated that moderate heating constricts the small arterioles of skeletal muscle.[69] This is of interest because a study in humans[70] found that ultrasound applied to the calf at the maximal allowed clinical dosage of 3 W/cm^2 slightly increased vascular resistance. It is quite likely that heating of soft tissues to less than the critical temperature for vasodilation either has no effect on blood flow or slightly diminishes it. However, increasing temperature, like decreasing temperature, has a complex effect on limb blood flow that depends on intensity and duration of the heating.

Psychological Stress

Subjects exposed to psychological stress have increased blood flow to forearm skeletal muscle via a cortical pathway mediated by sympathetic cholinergic nerves.[71] Neither the skin nor the calf muscles appear to respond to stress with vasodilation.[10] Severe stress does not have much effect on the cutaneous vessels. Mild stress such as a taxing intellectual task or unexpected loud sounds causes transient vasoconstriction of the skin vessels via the sympathetic nerves. Such stimuli are used to test the integrity of the autonomic nervous system and the cutaneous vascular sympathetic responses.

Diving

The diving reflex is present in many species and, from an evolutionary viewpoint, is retained in humans. The response includes parasympathetic bradycardia and sympathetic vasoconstriction of some vascular beds, including renal, splanchnic, and muscular. Water and cold on the face, which are sensed by trigeminal afferents, initiate the response. In diving mammals and birds, in which diving is an important part of day-to-day survival, the diving reflex is similar to that in humans, but may be more dramatic, with a nearly complete cessation of blood flow to muscle.[72] Diving bradycardia is a useful test of vagal integrity, and it is reduced or absent in patients with some degree of parasympathetic failure.

TISSUE FLUID BALANCE: TRANSCAPILLARY FLUID EXCHANGE AND THE LYMPHATIC CIRCULATION

Dynamics of Fluid Balance: Starling Forces and Their Current Reinterpretation

An important consequence of vascular regulation in the limbs and of certain pathologic states is the alteration of limb fluid balance. In 1896 Starling proposed that plasma proteins, which are largely retained within the capillary lumen, counteract the hydrostatic pressure inside capillaries (P_C), minimizing the loss of fluid from the vascular to the interstitial space.[73] Although this may seem obvious now, it was a remarkable insight considering the small osmotic pressure exerted by plasma proteins relative to the total osmotic pressure of the plasma and interstitial fluid (ISF). Starling suggested that capillaries might produce a net fluid filtration at their arteriolar end because the hydrostatic pressure is relatively high there, exceeding plasma oncotic pressure (A_C), but have a net reabsorption at their venular end where the hydrostatic pressure is considerably lower than A_C. He assumed that A_C remained constant along the capillary. Thirty years later Landis measured the filtration and reabsorption of single capillaries in the frog mesentery exposed to a range of hydrostatic pressures and found that there was a linear correlation between fluid flux and P_C as would have been predicted by Starling's hypothesis. He calculated the flux across the capillary wall per unit surface area, J_v/A, and proposed an equation to describe the factors governing fluid flux:

$$J_V \div A = L_P \left[(P_C - P_I) - \phi (A_C - A_I) \right] \qquad [8]$$

where L_p is the hydraulic permeability of the capillary endothelium, $P_C - P_I$ is the net hydrostatic pressure gradient, ϕ is the reflection coefficient, or the degree of impermeability of the endothelium to proteins, and $A_C - A_I$ is the net oncotic pressure gradient. If $\phi = 1$, then the endothelium is totally impermeable to proteins, which would result in A_I, the interstitial oncotic pressure, being zero. The usual value for ϕ is approximately 0.9.

The Starling-Landis model was universally adopted and has been presented in all physiology texts for the past 60 years. Since the late 1980s it has become clear that while equation 8 is fundamentally correct for any capillary region, it is rarely true that capillaries reabsorb at their venular ends.[74,75] When better methods were developed to measure interstitial hydrostatic pressure, P_I, it was found to be usually below atmospheric, in the range of –2 to –6 mm Hg. When P_I, A_I, and A_C were measured and P_C calculated, it rarely matched the measured value. Usually, measured P_C was significantly higher than its predicted value. Using the Landis experimental preparation, Michel[74] found that he could replicate Landis's findings if he measured the transient filtration (J_V/A) after a change in P_C, but if he measured net fluid flux in the steady state, the transient and steady-state responses were the same if P_C exceeded A_C, but were different when P_C was less than A_C. In the later case, reabsorption occurs when P_C transiently falls, but if it remains low, net filtration becomes zero.

These findings necessitated a rethinking of the way the Starling-Landis model is applied. It is clear now that their model may serve as a lumped model for the entire peripheral circulation, but that it is unlikely to be true for most individual capillaries. The only capillaries that maintain sustained reabsorption are those of the renal medulla, the gastrointestinal tract, and the lymph nodes.[76,77] It has been estimated that one-half the lymphatic flow is reabsorbed by the capillaries of the lymph nodes; thus, lymph flow measured at the thoracic duct is one-half the total lymphatic reabsorption from the ISF. In the limbs, there is likely to be only filtration from the capillaries, which produces a steady, low-level flow into the ISF, which flows at the same rate into the lymphatics. When the ISF volume changes, both P_I and A_I change in ways that tend to minimize further changes in filtration. For instance, when ISF increases, P_I increases and A_I decreases, reducing the rate of filtration. This buffering effect can be overwhelmed when lymphatic flow is blocked, or when endothelial permeability is increased, and the increase in ISF exceeds the lymphatic flow causing edema results.

Lymphatics

The lymphatic circulation completes the necessary circuit from the ISF back to the systemic circulation.

Lymphatic capillaries have leaky endothelial junctions that permit protein and fluid to enter from the interstitium and eventually flow back to the central venous circulation. Flow proceeds from the lymphatic capillaries to larger and larger vessels that enter lymph glands. From the glands, lymph flows through still larger vessels and enters the thoracic or right lymphatic duct, which is connected to the innominate vein. The total flow through the thoracic duct is only 2–4 liters per day. As previously mentioned, the capillaries in the lymph nodes are one of the few examples of capillaries that regularly reabsorb fluid, returning lymphatic fluid to the circulation and reducing the apparent lymph flow as measured at the innominate vein. The pressures in the lymphatic circulation are low (0–2 mm Hg). Small increases in ISF hydrostatic pressure may collapse the lymphatic vessels and reduce or prevent the flow of lymph. These increases in P_I also reduce filtration, however, and limit further edema. Pathologic states in which L_p is increased or ϕ falls below 0.9 may lead to large increases in ISF volume, large increases in P_I, and blockage of the lymphatics. Edema resolves slowly in such cases, depending on reabsorption by the capillaries to reduce the ISF volume, producing a decrease in P_I sufficient to allow the restoration of lymphatic flow.

REFERENCES

1. Gibbons IL. Morphological evidence for regional diversification of autonomic cotransmission in different parts of the cardiovascular system. Proc XVII IUPS Cong 1989;1:28.

2. Kobilka BK, Matsui J, Kobilka TS, et al. Cloning, sequencing, and expression of the gene coding for the human platelet alpha-2-adrenergic receptor. Science 1987;238:650–656.

3. Levitzki A. Beta-adrenergic receptors and their mode of coupling to adenylate cyclase. Physiol Rev 1986; 66(3):819–854.

4. Weiss ER, Kelleher DJ, Woon CW, et al. Receptor activation of G proteins. FASEB J 1988;2:2841–2848.

5. Robishaw JD, Foster KA. Role of G proteins in the regulation of the cardiovascular system. Annu Rev Physiol 1989;51:229–244.

6. Limbird LE. Receptors linked to inhibition of adenylate cyclase: additional signaling mechanisms. FASEB J 1988;2:2686–2695.

7. Fain JN, Wallace MA, Wojcikiewicz RJH. Evidence for involvement of guanine nucleotide-binding regulatory proteins in the activation of phospholipases by hormones. FASEB J 1989;2:2569–2574.

8. Kamm KE, Stull JT. Regulation of smooth muscle contractile elements by second messengers. Annu Rev Physiol 1989;51:299–313.

9. Abrahams VC, Hilton SM, Zbrozyna AW. The role of active muscle vasodilation in the alerting stage of the defense reaction. J Physiol (Lond) 1964;171:189–202.

10. Rusch NJ, Shepherd JT, Webb RC, Vanhoutte PM. Different behavior of the resistance vessels of the human calf and forearm during contralateral isometric exercise, mental stress and abdominal respiratory movements. Circ Res 1981;48(Pt 2):I118–I130.

11. Lechleiter J, Peralta E, Clapham D. Diverse functions of muscarinic acetylcholine receptor subtypes. Trends Pharmacol Sci 1989;(Suppl):34–38.

12. Dohlman HG, Caron MG, Lefkowitz RJ. A family of receptors coupled to guanine nucleotide regulatory proteins. Biochemistry 1987;26:2657–2664.

13. Kennedy C. Possible Roles for Purine Nucleotides in Perivascular Neurotransmission. In G Burnstock, SG Griffith (eds), Nonadrenergic Innervation of Blood Vessels. Vol I, Putative Neurotransmitters. Boca Raton, FL: CRC Press, 1988;65–76.

14. Burnstock G. Sympathetic purinergic transmission in small blood vessels. Trends Pharmacol Sci 1989;9:116–117.

15. Romano F, MacDonald SG, Dobson JG Jr. Adenosine receptor coupling to adenylate cyclase on rat ventricular myocyte membranes. Am J Physiol 1989;257:H1088–H1095.

16. Howland RD, Spector S. Disposition of histamine in mammalian blood vessels. J Pharm Exp Ther 1972;182:239–245.

17. Shepherd JT. Circulation to Skeletal Muscle. In JT Shepherd, FM Abboud (eds), Handbook of Physiology, Sec 2:

The Cardiovascular System. Vol III, Peripheral Circulation and Organ Blood Flow, Part 1. Bethesda, MD: American Physiological Society, 1983;319–370.

18. Hartig PR. Molecular biology of 5-HT receptors. Trends Pharmacol Sci 1989;10:64–69.

19. Angus JA. 5-HT receptors in the coronary circulation. Trends Pharmacol Sci 1989;10:89–90.

20. Griffith SG. Serotonin (5-HT) as a Neurotransmitter in Blood Vessels. In G Burnstock, SG Griffith (eds), Non-adrenergic Innervation of Blood Vessels. Vol I, Putative Neurotransmitters. Boca Raton, FL: CRC Press, 1988;27–40.

21. Cowley AW Jr. Vasopressin and Cardiovascular Regulation. In AC Guyton, JE Hall (eds), Cardiovascular Physiology IV. International Review of Physiology, Vol 26. Baltimore: University Park Press, 1982;189–242.

22. Johnson LR, Parker JL, Laughlin MH. Chronic exercise training improves Ach-induced vasorelaxation in pulmonary arteries of pigs. J Appl Physiol 2000;88:443–451.

23. Lash JM, Bohlen HG. Time- and order-dependent changes in functional and NO-mediated dilation during exercise training. J Appl Physiol 1997;82(2):460–468.

24. Davies PF. Flow-mediated endothelial mechanotransduction. Physiol Rev 1995;75:519–560.

25. Butler PB, Weinbaum S, Chien S, Lemons DE. Endothelium-dependent, shear-induced vasodilation is rate-sensitive. Microcirculation 2000;7:53–65.

26. Moncada S. Biosynthesis of nitric oxide from L-arginine: a path for the regulation of cell function and communication. Biochem Pharmacol 1989;38:1709–1715.

27. Koller A, Sun D, Kaley G. Role of shear stress and endothelial prostaglandins in flow- and viscosity-induced dilation of arterioles in vitro. Circ Res 1993;72:1276–1284.

28. McGillivray KM, Faber JM. Selective effect of metabolic control on beta 2-adrenergic mediated contraction of microvascular smooth muscle. FASEB J 1988;2(6):A1873.

29. Cooper A. Some experiments and observations on tying the carotid and vertebral arteries, and the pneumogastric phrenic and sympathetic nerves. Guy's Hosp Rep 1836;1:457–472.

30. Cramer W. On the action of veratrum viride with some remarks on the inter-relationship of the medullary centres. J Pharmacol 1915;7:63–82.

31. Persson PB, Ehmke H, Kirchheim H. Cardiopulmonary-arterial baroreceptor interaction in control of blood pressure. News Physiol Sci 1989;4:56–59.

32. Persson PB. Cardiopulmonary receptors in "neurogenic hypertension." Acta Physiol Scand Suppl 1988;570:1–54.

33. Eyzaguirre C, Fitzgerald RS, Lahiri S, Zapata P. Arterial Chemoreceptors. In JT Shepherd, FM Abboud, SR Geiger (eds), Handbook of Physiology, Sec 2: The Cardiovascular System. Vol III, Peripheral Circulation and Organ Blood Flow, Part 2. Bethesda, MD: American Physiological Society, 1983;557–622.

34. Pennes HH. Analysis of tissue and arterial blood temperatures in the resting human forearm. J Appl Physiol 1948;1:93–122.

35. Lemons DE, Chien S, Crawshaw LI, et al. The significance of vessel size and type in vascular heat transfer. Am J Physiol 1987;253:R128–R135.

36. Weinbaum S, Jiji LM, Lemons DE. Theory and experiment for the effect of vascular microstructure on surface tissue heat transfer—Part I: anatomical foundation and model conceptualization. ASME J Biomech Eng 1984;106:321–330.

37. Kelley PJ. Pathways of Transport in Bone. In JT Shepherd, FM Abboud (eds), Handbook of Physiology, Sec 2: The Cardiovascular System. Vol III, Peripheral Circulation and Organ Flow, Part 1. Bethesda, MD: American Physiological Society, 1983;371–396.

38. Morris MA, Kelly PJ. Use of tracer microspheres to measure bone blood flow in conscious dogs. Calcif Tissue Int 1980;32:69–76.

39. Bulow J, Madsen J. Adipose tissue blood flow during prolonged heavy exercise. Pflugers Arch 1976;363:231–234.

40. Sparks HV. Skin and Muscle. In PC Johnson (ed), Peripheral Circulation. New York: John Wiley & Sons, 1978;193–230.

41. Roddie IC. Circulation to Skin and Adipose Tissue. In JT Shepherd, FM Abboud (eds), Handbook of Physiology, Sec 2: The Cardiovascular System. Vol III, Peripheral Circulation and Organ Blood Flow, Part 1. Bethesda, MD: American Physiological Society, 1983;285–318.

42. Fagrell B. Microcirculation of the Skin. In NA Mortillaro (ed), The Physiology and Pharmacology of the Microcircu-lation. New York: Academic Press, Inc, 1984;133–180.

43. Clark ER. Arterio-venous anastomoses. Physiol Rev 1938;18:229–247.

44. Myrhage R, Eriksson E. Arrangement of the Vascular Bed in Different Types of Skeletal Muscles. In F Hammersen, K Messmer (eds), Skeletal Muscle Microcirculation. Basel: Karger, 1984;1–14.

45. Rowell LB. Human Circulation. New York: Oxford, 1986.

46. Astrand P-O, Rodahl K. Textbook of Work Physiology. New York: McGraw-Hill, 1977.

47. Marshall RJ, Shepherd JT. Cardiac Function in Health and Disease. Philadelphia: WB Saunders, 1968.

48. Wade OL, Bishop JM. Cardiac Output and Regional Blood Flow. Oxford: Blackwell, 1989.

49. Christensen NJ, Brandsborg O. The relationship between plasma catecholamine concentration and pulse rate during exercise and standing. Eur J Clin Invest 1973;3:299–306.

50. Rerych SK, Scholz PM, Sabiston DC, Jones RH. Effects of exercise training on left ventricular function in normal subjects: a longitudinal study by radionuclide angiography. Am J Cardiol 1980;45:244–252.

51. Morganroth J, Maron BJ, Henry WL, Epstein SE. Comparative left ventricular dimensions in trained athletes. Ann Intern Med 1975;82:521–524.

52. Sjostrand T. The regulation of the blood distribution in man. Acta Physiol Scand 1952;26:312–327.

53. Blomqvist CG, Saltin B. Cardiovascular adaptations to physical training. Annu Rev Physiol 1983;45:169–189.

54. Andersen P, Saltin B. Maximal perfusion of skeletal muscle in man. J Physiol (Lond) 1985;366:233–249.

55. Granger HJ, Borders JL, Meininger GA, et al. Microcirculatory Control Systems. In NA Mortillaro (ed), The Physiology and Pharmacology of the Microcirculation. New York: Academic Press, 1983;209–236.

56. Hohimer AR, Hales JR, Rowell LB, Smith OA. Regional distribution of blood flow during mild dynamic leg exercise in the baboon. J Appl Physiol 1983;55:1173–1177.

57. Andersen P, Henriksson J. Capillary supply of the quadriceps femoris muscle of man: adaptive response to exercise. J Physiol (Lond) 1977;270:677–691.

58. Ekelund L-G. Circulatory and respiratory adaptation during prolonged exer-

cise. Acta Physiol Scand Suppl 1967;292:1–38.

59. Bazett HC. Temperature Sense in Man. Temperature: Its Measurement and Control in Science and Industry. New York: Reinhold, 1941;489–501.

60. Faber JE. Effect of local tissue cooling on microvascular smooth muscle and postjunctional alpha-2 adrenoceptors. Am J Physiol 1988;255:H121–H130.

61. Flavahan NA, Vanhoutte PM. Effect of cooling on alpha-1 and alpha-2 adrenergic responses in canine saphenous and femoral veins. J Pharm Exp Ther 1986;238(1):139–147.

62. Vanhoutte PM, Flavahan NA. Effects of temperature on alpha adrenoceptors in limb veins: role of receptor reserve. Fed Proc 1986;45:2347–2354.

63. Lewis T. Observations upon the reactions of the vessels of the human skin to cold. Heart 1930;15:177–208.

64. Rusch NJ, Shepherd JT, Vanhoutte PM. The effect of profound cooling on adrenergic neurotransmission in canine cutaneous veins. J Physiol (Lond) 1981;311:57–65.

65. Gardner CA, Webb RC. Cold-induced vasodilation in isolated, perfused rat tail artery. Am J Physiol 1986;251:H176–H181.

66. Cooke JP, Shepherd JT, Vanhoutte PM. The effect of warming on adrenergic neurotransmission in canine cutaneous vein. Circ Res 1984;54:547–553.

67. Lehmann JF, DeLateur BJ. Therapeutic Heat. In JF Lehmann (ed), Therapeutic Heat and Cold. Baltimore: Williams & Wilkins, 1982;404–562.

68. Roemer RB, Oleson JR, Cetas TC. Oscillatory temperature response to constant power applied to canine muscle. Am J Physiol 1985;249:R153–R158.

69. Hogan RD, Franklin TD, Avery KS, Burke KM. Arteriolar vasoconstriction in rat cremaster muscle induced by local heat stress. Am J Physiol 1982; 242:H996–H999.

70. Snortum A. Application of ultrasound through a cold coupling medium permits increased treatment duration and intensity but fails to improve muscle blood flow [Thesis]. New York: Columbia University, 1989.

71. Blair DA, Glover WE, Greenfield ADM, Roddie IC. Excitation of cholinergic vasodilator nerves to human skeletal muscles during emotional stress. J Physiol (Lond) 1959;148:633–647.

72. Blix AS, Folkow B. Cardiovascular Adjustments to Diving in Mammals and Birds. In JT Shepherd, FM Abboud, SR Geiger (eds), Handbook of Physiology, Sec 2: The Cardiovascular System. Vol III, Peripheral Circulation and Organ Blood Flow, Part 2. Bethesda, MD: American Physiological Society, 1983;917–946.

73. Michel CC. Starling: the formulation of his hypothesis of microvascular fluid exchange and its significance after 100 years. Exp Physiol 1997;82:1–30.

74. Michel CC. Capillary permeability and how it may change. J Physiol (Lond) 1988;404:1–29.

75. Renkin EM. Cellular aspects of transvascular exchange: a 40-year perspective. Microcirculation 1994;1(3):157–167.

76. Curry FE. Regulation of water and solute exchange in microvessel endothelium: studies in single perfused capillaries. Microcirculation 1994;1(1):11–26.

77. Hu X, Weinbaum S. A new view of Starling's hypothesis at the microstructure level. Microvasc Res 1999;58:281–304.

78. Ashkenazi A, Peralta EG, Winslow JW, et al. Functional diversity of muscarinic receptor subtypes in cellular signal transduction and growth. Trends Pharmacol Sci 1989;(Suppl):16–22.

79. Duckles SP. Acetylcholine. In G Burnstock, SG Griffith (eds), Nonadrenergic Innervation of Blood Vessels. Vol. I, Putative Neurotransmitters. Boca Raton, FL: CRC Press, 1988;15–26.

80. Carson MR, Shasby SS, Shasby MD. Histamine and inositol phosphate accumulation in endothelium: cAMP and G protein. Am J Physiol 1989;257:L259–L264.

81. Tsuru H. Histamine Receptors in the Cardiovascular System. In PM Vanhoutte, SF Vatner (eds), Vasodilator Mechanisms. New York: Karger, 1983;70–80.

82. Burnstock G. Nonadrenergic Innervation of Blood Vessels—Some Historical Perspectives. In G Burnstock, SG Griffith (eds), Nonadrenergic Innervation of Blood Vessels. Vol I, Putative Neurotransmitters. Boca Raton, FL: CRC Press, 1988;1–14.

83. Owman C. Role of Neural Substance P and Coexisting Calcitonin Gene-Related Peptide (CGRP) in Cardiovascular Function. In G Burnstock, SG Griffith (eds), Nonadrenergic Innervation of Blood Vessels. Vol I, Putative Neurotransmitters. Boca Raton, FL: CRC Press, 1988;77–100.

84. Polak JM, Bloom SR. Atrial Natriuretic Peptide (ANP), Neuropeptide Y (NPY) and Calcitonin Gene-Related Peptide (CGRP) in the Cardiovascular System of Man and Animals. In G Burnstock, SG Griffith (eds), Nonadrenergic Innervation of Blood Vessels. Vol I, Putative Neurotransmitters. Boca Raton, FL: CRC Press, 1988;127–144.

85. Edvinsson L, Uddman R. Vasoactive Intestinal Polypeptide (VIP): A Putative Neurotransmitter in the Cardiovascular System. In G Burnstock, SG Griffith (eds), Nonadrenergic Innervation of Blood Vessels. Vol I, Putative Neurotransmitters. Boca Raton, FL: CRC Press, 1988;101–126.

86. Receptor Nomenclature Supplement. TIPS January, 1991.

23

Growth and Development

KERSTIN ML. SOBUS AND JERIE BETH KARKOS

Central nervous system (CNS) impairment often presents with growth and/or developmental delays beyond accepted norms. Indeed, the most common presentation of a developmental disability is failure to achieve age appropriate developmental skills.[1] Early identification of deviation is thought to be important because of the potential for improvement of outcome through educational and rehabilitative services for children with, or at risk for, developmental disability. Additionally, treatment goals for an identified child are incomplete unless the maturational effect of growth and development has been considered. Lastly, as the parent is primarily responsible for child care and stimulation, the pediatric specialist must not only understand normal and abnormal growth and development, but normal and abnormal parent–child interaction.

GROWTH

Normal growth is an increase in physical size and dimensions relative to age and maturity. Growth occurs at predictable, maturity-related rates, more rapidly in infancy and pubescence than in middle childhood. Body proportions also change during age-specific growth. In the newborn, the head is relatively large, the face is round, and the abdomen is prominent, and compared with adults, the trunk and extremities are short. Specific body parts grow at selective rates during certain ages: Head growth is fastest in infancy; trunk in infancy and adolescence; extremities from 1 year through puberty.[2,3] With changing body proportion there is a shift in the center of gravity from the xiphoid process in the newborn to the sacral promontory in late childhood.[4] Body posture also changes over time with growth in skeletal

height and muscle mass increase. The typical 2- to 3-year-old child has a mild lumbar lordosis with protuberant abdomen. By early school age, increased strength, particularly of the abdominal muscles, leads to a more mature pelvic alignment and decreased lordosis. Changing body size and proportions in a child or adolescent with physical disability may alter orthotic needs or ambulatory potential.[5]

The rate of growth of an individual over time is a more sensitive indicator of health or disease than the absolute size at any single measurement. All parameters of growth, height, weight, and head circumference should be serially measured in a consistent manner and recorded on the standard growth chart for immediate comparison. Values outside the plus or minus 2 standard deviation range on the normal distribution curve or a continued and unexplained shift in growth trend indicate a need for evaluation. Transient shifts in growth parameters may occur in the first 4–18 months of life, but should reach a stable rate by 1.5 years of age. Genetic factors begin to influence ultimate height and weight, generally after 6 months of age.[5,6]

Monitoring Growth

Growth aberration, if present at birth, may indicate genetic, metabolic, or congenital conditions that are associated with developmental disability. Some endocrinologic, systemic, and skeletal disorders may lead to growth retardation, failure to thrive, or both.[7,8] Infants with neurologic impairment and oral motor dysfunction are at significant risk for acquired failure to thrive and must be monitored. They may feed too slowly, be limited in texture tolerance, or have metabolic requirements that make it difficult to meet caloric needs for adequate organ growth by mouth. They may require feeding adaptations, nutritional supplementation, both, or possibly enteral feeding tubes, along with close monitoring, to ensure adequate appropriate nutritional and fluid intake. Normative charts for diagnostic groups thought to be at risk for growth problems are being developed to monitor more effectively. An accepted normative growth chart is available for children with Down syndrome.[9,10] A normative growth curve has been developed for children with quadriplegic cerebral palsy, noting the mean in height and weight is at approximately the tenth percentile of the normal population. However, controversy remains, with the recommendations for clinical use of this specific tool still being debated.[11]

Some neurologic lesions affect growth, resulting in asymmetry. Limb shortening or atrophy may be seen with brachial plexus palsy sustained at birth, congenital varicella syndrome, or myelodysplasia.[12,13] Less commonly, upper motor neuron lesions present from birth or acquired in early childhood may also be associated with underdevelopment of an extremity.[5] Hemihypertrophy may be seen with neurocutaneous syndromes, most commonly neurofibromatosis; soft tissue abnormalities or vascular abnormalities as seen in Klippel-Trenaunay-Weber syndrome; inflammatory disorders such as juvenile rheumatoid arthritis; and dysmorphogenic syndromes such as Beckwith-Wiedemann syndrome, Langer-Giedion syndrome, Russell-Silver syndrome, and epidermal nevus syndrome.[14] With an awareness of growth trends, the clinician can anticipate and plan for changes needed in orthotics, wheelchairs, and other adaptive devices. Clinical awareness of adolescent growth trends is necessary in timing of definitive surgical treatment for leg length discrepancy and scoliosis.[5]

Head Circumference

Head circumference measurement is a useful indication of brain growth in infancy and early childhood because the fontanels can normally be open until 12–18 months and the calvarial sutures do not unite firmly until approximately puberty. The average head circumference is 34–35 cm at birth and increases by approximately 12 cm during the first year, representing more than half of the total growth until maturity.[2,15] Head circumference is measured with a tape placed firmly over the glabella and supraorbital ridges anteriorly and on the maximal protuberance of the occiput posteriorly. Head circumference should be obtained routinely up to 3 years of age and thereafter if CNS pathology is suspected. Concern for possible CNS abnormality should always arise and be investigated when head circumference falls outside plus or minus 2 standard deviations

from the mean or *crosses percentiles* because of deceleration or acceleration of head growth.[2,5,16,17]

Head size increases rapidly during the first year of life to reflect the growth and maturation of the brain. Excessive enlargement of head circumference may be benign (familial) or pathologic, most commonly caused by hydrocephalus with elevated intracranial pressure, a space-occupying lesion, or metabolic storage disease. Excessively enlarging head caused by hydrocephalus is a common presentation seen after intraventricular hemorrhage in the premature infant. Hydrocephalus can also be congenital, secondary to structural abnormalities such as aqueductal stenosis or with the Chiari's malformation associated with myelodysplasia. Microcephaly can also be congenital (commonly secondary to anomaly, perinatal viral infection, genetic, or metabolic disorder) or acquired (commonly secondary to severe anoxic encephalopathy or cerebral atrophy associated with a degenerative or genetic disorder of the CNS).[5]

Height

The full-term newborn is 50 cm in length at birth, normally increasing by 50% in the first 12 months.[2] Adult height can be estimated by doubling body length at 2 years. Girls attain maximal growth velocity before menarche and cessation 2 years thereafter. Boys, on the other hand, grow fastest in the late puberty concurrent with the appearance of facial hair on the cheeks and chin.[18] Accurate serial measurements are important when monitoring for aberrance in growth. Recumbent length is much more precise than standing height in children under 5 years of age and for those who have difficulties with standing. For children with marked deformity of the spine or lower extremities, height prediction can be approximated, if the child is over age 6, by obtaining a measure of arm span. When there is significant bilateral lower extremity atrophy because of a lower motor neuron lesion or malformations of the legs, sitting height may be a better indicator of general growth than total height. When significant asymmetry is noted of lower extremities, one should always compare measurements from the same side of the body.

Weight

The average full-term neonate weighs approximately 3,400 g, with a range of 2,500–4,600 g in 95% of the cases. Newborns below 2,500 g are categorized as low-birth-weight infants. This includes those who are born at term, but are small for gestational age, and those infants delivered prematurely, at less than 37 weeks of gestation. A full-term infant usually doubles his or her birth weight by 5 months and triples by 1 year.[5] Weight should be measured consistently, to detect early the child who may be aberrantly changing percentiles on his or her growth chart.[2] Infants and young children should be weighed while only wearing underwear, to avoid guesswork from seasonal changes in clothing.

NEUROMATURATION

The neurophysiological basis for achieving new development is an ascending process of CNS maturation.[16,19,20] In neonates and young infants, motor behavior is influenced by primitive reflexes at the spinal cord and brain stem level (Table 23-1). These reflex patterns generate predictable and stereotypic movements and postures. During the first 6–8 months of life as neurologic maturation of the cortical pathways progresses, these reflexes gradually become integrated. Movement progress from obligatory primitive, mass movement reflex patterns to allow voluntary control of limbs and trunk. More sophisticated postural responses emerge between 2 and 14 months of age (see Table 23-1). Obligatory or persistent primitive reflexes are the earliest markers of abnormal neurologic maturation.[20-27] The neurodevelopmental evaluation is performed to detect abnormalities of tone and reflexive and protective responses and can be performed in the neonate. An abnormal examination result indicates *risk* for later disability and can be used to flag a high-risk group for careful monitoring. Appearance of postural responses is a useful indicator of readiness for specific motor milestones (e.g., rolling, sitting, or standing).[5,20,26]

DEVELOPMENT

Development is typically subdivided into various categories, such as gross motor, fine-motor, adaptive, visual motor, speech, language, cognitive, and emotional. Under normal circumstances, the acquisition and refinement of advancing new skills proceed along a predictable sequence and timetable commonly measured in *milestones*. Development of motor skills, for example, progresses in a cephalocaudal direction and proximal-distal fashion. The sequence and rate of motor development is consistent among infants.[26] The understanding of normal progression of development translates into therapy emphasis on ensuring proximal stability and control before emphasis on distal control. Oral motor feeding skills are gained in sequence parallel to gain of voluntary head and trunk stability. Individual variations may occur within certain limits, more likely in the

TABLE 23-1

Developmental Markers of Central Nervous System Maturation

Primitive Reflex	Postural Responses
Moro	Head righting
Startle	Body righting
Rooting	Parachute reactions
Galant	Protective reactions
Positive supporting	Equilibrium reactions
Asymmetric tonic neck	—
Palmar grasp	—
Plantar grasp	—
Automatic neonatal walking	—
Placing	—
Neck righting	—
Tonic labyrinthine	—

timing than in the sequence of obtaining specific milestones.[27] CNS abnormalities are manifested by developmental delays beyond the accepted normal deviations. The type and degree of developmental delay provide fruitful information to guide diagnostic evaluation or management. Psychosocial factors and parenting practices may also influence development, particularly in adaptive developmental tasks.[5] Multiple developmental models exist that form the basis for evaluation, none of which is all encompassing. Developmental assessment properly includes multiple perspectives to provide a comprehensive view of factors that may affect global development.

Developmental evaluation is a comparison of the child's behavior relative to age-specific normative data. Thorough assessment depends on a process that allows medical, behavioral, and developmental history-taking, physical and neurodevelopmental examination, and formal measurement of developmental milestones. The young child should be examined in a nonthreatening environment, which may be difficult in a doctor's office. It is best performed with the child wearing regular clothing and before formal physical examination that requires undressing and therefore might make the child upset, cry, or uncooperative (Figure 23-1).[5] Developmental evaluation is complementary to a standard neurologic examination, designed to identify and localize indications of specific CNS lesions. In infants and children with physical disabilities it is important to note not only the accomplishment of a task, but also the quality of motor performance.[5] Behaviors observed should be noted and compared with those seen in the home and community. A child's style of coping with

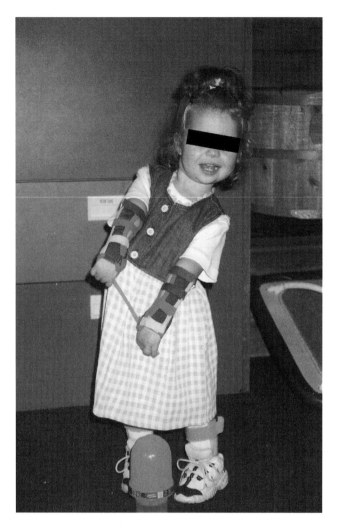

FIGURE 23-1. Developmental evaluations are best done in a nonthreatening environment.

difficult tasks gives insight into his or her personality and temperament.

Cognitive Development

Cognitive development refers to the increasing ability of the child to interpret sensory events; register and retrieve information from memory; and manipulate schemata, images, symbols, and concepts in thinking, reasoning, problem solving, and the acquisition of knowledge and beliefs about the environment.[5,28] Piaget was a psychologist who saw cognitive development as the result of neurophysiological maturation, environmental stimulation, experience, and cognitive reorganization. He described the child as transitioning through four major stages of cognitive development as the child learns to process, adapt, and manage increasingly complex problems: sensorimotor, preoperational, concrete operations, and formal operations.[5,29]

During the sensorimotor stage from birth to 2 years, learning comes from the senses, with visual, auditory, tactile, proprioceptive, and olfactory images forming *thought* until formal language develops. During this stage the infant's response transitions from immature reflex and sensorimotor responses to purposeful and increasing complex motor abilities. The infant develops skills to organize and exercise control over the environment and interpret more complex sensory data. The preoperational stage (2–7 years) begins as speech and language are acquired. During this period, the child develops the tools for representative schemes symbolically through language, imitation, imagery, symbolic play, and drawing. Although the child learns through imaginative play, the child has difficulty discerning reality from fantasy.[5,29,30] In this stage, the child is prelogical. He or she learns to compare and contrast physical characteristics, but can only consider one dimension at a time. The child is unable to reverse or generalize perception. A child at this age is egocentric. Between 7 and 11 years the child enters the stage of concrete operational thought. The child learns that some actions are reversible and learns to take more than one dimension into consideration. The child develops logical problem solving and can manipulate groups of categories, classification systems, and hypothetical theories.[5,29,30] The formal operational stage usually occurs around age 11–15 years, although not all attain it. Abstract comprehension is now possible. The child is able to consider multiple factors in problem solving using internal language to analyze multiple general concepts. He or she is now able to use both inductive and deductive reasoning.[29,30]

Intelligence level is one measure of cognitive function. Evaluations of cognitive skills may be hampered in the child with motor impairment because of reliance of standardized tests on motor expression, particularly in the younger child, who normally has relatively limited verbal expression compared with the older child. The ability to reliably assess the intelligence of an infant and provide an IQ score for school age is controversial. The variation in prediction at different ages at least in part reflects age-related test items, care taking, environment, and the marked resilience of the young CNS. Nevertheless, early cognitive assessment is useful in assessment of risk for mental impairment.

Mild mental impairment cannot be reliably diagnosed in infancy. Similarly, mental superiority cannot be reliably diagnosed in early infancy. Great parental apprehension is raised when the former is considered. The mentally impaired infant is delayed in all aspects of development, although often less so in gross motor tasks, unless cerebral palsy is present. The term *mental retardation* is properly used to refer to cognitive function that is below average intellectual functioning as measured by a standard test of intelligence. Intelligence is a composite of both cognitive functioning or thinking ability and adaptive behavior or ability to adapt to one's environment.

Mental retardation is divided into four levels of function. Mild mental retardation (85% of individuals with mental retardation) is defined by an IQ between 55 to 69. Moderate mental retardation (10%) is defined by an IQ between 40 and 54. Severe mental retardation (5%) is defined by an IQ between 25 and 38, and profound mental retardation (1–2%) by an IQ below 25.[31]

Mental retardation is a result of a variety of etiologies, often multifactorial in origin. These factors may include chromosome errors, genetic endowment, maternal infection (rubella, syphilis, acquired immunodeficiency syndrome, toxoplasmosis), maternal use of alcohol or narcotics, prenatal and postnatal infection, brain injury, and heavy metal exposure.[26,31]

Individuals with mild mental retardation are often able to live independently. Eighty percent can be employed and more than 80% marry. Individuals with severe or profound mental retardation need life-long supervision for safety and judgment. Those with moderate mental retardation can, with repetitive training, accomplish a job. They can, with time, learn self-help tasks and attend to personal hygiene.[31]

Developmental Models and Personality Development

Theories of personality development are numerous. Advice given to parents over the years is reflective not only of evolving theory, but cultural influences. The psychoanalytic theory from the nineteenth century incorporates Sigmund Freud's work on human motivation and sexual development, which was extrapolated from the study of adults. Erikson later modified Freud's theory into eight stages that describe emotional development across the lifespan, conceptualizing personality development as a progressive resolution of conflict between personal needs and social demands.[32] According to Erikson's theory, personality evolves according to steps predetermined by the individual's readiness to react with a widening social world.[5] During the first 18 months (trust/mistrust), infants develop a relationship with their caregivers, usually their mothers, as their basic needs are met. They attain feelings of comfort and confidence that demands will be consistently fulfilled. This general state of trust allows the toddler to constantly *test* behaviors, such as that seen in the typical *terrible twos*. These behaviors reflect an important milestone in the child's life, offering the parent an opportunity to teach the child early coping skills and self-discipline. Behavior that does not endanger the child or encroach on the rights of others is allowed, whereas distraction and temporary time out are used for behavior that cannot be ignored. If the child does not perceive his or her needs to be consistently met, the frustrated infant is at risk to develop a sense of mistrust, or insecure attachment behavior, which manifests as maladaptive behavior such as tantrums, emotional distance, and withdrawal. Withdrawal, in turn, may not give positive feedback to the parent, who then may feel inadequate to meet the infant's needs. Sick or very low-birth-weight infants who require long hospitalizations, painful procedures, or feeding interventions are common populations at risk to develop maladaptive behaviors. Professional assistance is often required to provide the parents with basic skills regarding their infant's special needs and to facilitate positive activities for the parent and the infant. During the toddler stage, the child enters the phase of autonomy versus shame and doubt. The now ambulatory child exercises some self-direction and control, "holding on and letting go." The all too common phrase "Me do it" is proclaimed. The child learns mastery over basic bodily functions (potty training), which can be reassuring to him or her. For those with physical disabilities the issue of autonomy is critical and the child needs to be given opportunities for control and mobility. Professionals working with the child and family should assist with the promotion of independence rather than inadvertently encouraging a passive role by the child. During the third stage, at 3–5 years, the child masters initiative versus guilt. The child demonstrates an increased understanding of task and plan strategies for play. He or she becomes aware of sharing, obligation, and reward. During this period, the child becomes aware of his or her own sex and experiences a sexual attraction to the parent of the opposite sex. With resolution of this crisis, the child identifies with the same sex parent. In the next stage, industry versus inferiority, the child enters school and seeks his place among peers. Parents of children with special needs may experience an increased awareness of their child's limitations intellectually, physically, or both, arousing concerns about school entry. For children with limitations in their ability to learn or to compete in recreational activities, stress may occur from adjusting to school.[5]

Robert Havighurst, in the mid-twentieth century, proposed human development as a continuum of life skills gained throughout the lifespan by progressive achievement of developmental tasks at specific stages (Table 23-2). He proposed the idea of the "teachable" moment, a time when a person is most sensitive to learning as related to a particular developmental task, maturational readiness so to speak.[33]

Temperament describes a child's particular style of behavior, as it affects interaction with his or her environment and bond with parent figure. Temperament, as a concept developed by Thomas and Chess in 1986 from their study of 133 children throughout childhood, is a composite of nine dimensions that can be grouped into three *clusters* to describe risk for future emotional and behavioral problems: the easy, difficult, or slow-to-warm-up child. The crucial factor to the child's outcome is the parent–child match. The easy child requires low-intensity parent interventions, and thus is considered to be a "good child," easy to parent, with a relatively low risk of behavioral or emotional problems. The difficult child is considered to be at highest risk (70%) of developing behavioral difficulties. These are the children who often require significant parenting skill, energy, and sensitive intervention, without which undesirable characteristics may be fostered.[34]

TABLE 23-2
Developmental Tasks

Development tasks for early childhood
  Walk, talk, take solid foods, dress
  Learn sexual differences and modesty
  Develop physiological stability, control waste
  Develop simple concepts of social, physical reality
  Relate emotionally to others
  Distinguish right, wrong; conscience
Developmental tasks for middle childhood
  Develop physical skills for games
  Build wholesome attitude toward self
  Get along with peers, groups, institutions
  Learn *three R's*
  Learn skills and concepts for daily life
  Learn appropriate male or female social role
Developmental tasks for adolescence
  Develop emotional independence of parents and adults
  Develop socially and civically responsible behavior
  Develop sexual identity, more mature relationships, accept physique, and use body effectively
  Prepare for economic independence, job

Source: RJ Havighurst. Developmental Tasks and Education. David McKay Co. 1952;5.

DEVELOPMENTAL MILESTONES

First Two Years

Gross Motor

During the newborn period muscle tone is predominantly with semiflexion of the extremities.[35] When positioned prone, the infant turns his or her head from side to side with neck hyperextension, causing the mouth to sweep against the surface. In supported sitting, full support is required, the back is rounded, and the head drops forward. With supported standing and tilted forward, automatic reflex stepping may be elicited for 3–4 weeks. Several primitive reflexes can be seen or elicited, but should not be obligating in nature.[20]

With progression of CNS maturation, the 4-month-old infant develops increasing motor control with balance flexion and extension tone. As the primitive reflexes are becoming integrated, the postural righting responses are emerging. In supine, the infant's head is usually in midline. With a pull-to-sit maneuver, the infant tucks the chin holding his or her head in midline; some abdominal muscle activity and flexing of the upper and lower extremities may be noted.[36] In supportive sitting, the cervical and thoracic spine is straight. In prone, the infant raises the head to 90 degrees and may lift the chest slightly. The infant may roll from prone to supine.[5]

At 7 months, the primitive reflexes should be well integrated, and the postural responses should be emerging in all positions, allowing the infant an increased freedom of movement and higher transitional skills.[37,38] The infant can now roll both supine to prone and vice versa, transition from prone to quadruped on hands and knees.[38,39] In quadruped the legs are abducted, externally rotated, and the abdomen is sagging. The infant may rock in quadruped. From quadruped, the infant may transition to sitting, and the infant can maintain sitting if placed. During sitting, there is active rotation of the upper trunk and reaching with hands in a limited range. The infant may begin to pull to stand and begin to cruise sideways with lateral leg abduction movements.[5]

At 10 months, mobility and exploration of the environment expand quickly.[39,40] In sitting, the infant can reach up to 10 in. forward without losing balance.[5] The infant can creep on hands and knees with reciprocal movements. Transition to standing continues to improve through half kneeling. Momentary independent standing begins.

As the infant becomes more autonomous at 14 months, the gait pattern advances with independent walking descriptive of a *toddler*.[40] The infant's arms are in a high-guard position, with wide base of support and excessive hip and knee flexion in swing phase. There is slight valgus of the knees and ankle, and with foot strike the full sole contacts the floor. The infant may start to creep up stairs. By 18 months the gait pattern matures with a narrower base of support, heel strike, and arms in low-guard position.[41–43] The toddler can walk backward and sit in a small chair. The toddler imitates the parents' routines such as sweeping, dusting, and carrying or hugging a doll.

Fine Motor: Visual Development

The newborn infant can visually fix and follow a bright object for a limited time and extent. During the first month of life the infant's visual ability increases, with the baby able to follow objects to the side to 45 degrees. By 2 months, visual tracking across midline develops to 180 degrees. At 4–6 months the infant can coordinate hand and eye function.

Hand function and grasp are dynamic transitions during the first 18 months that continues to mature during childhood. The newborn's grasp is reflexive, with the fingers clutching on contact without thumb activity. Release of the object is involuntary. At 2 months the infant develops a pronated grasp of an object placed in the hand and can begin to move a rattle. At 3 months the infant pulls on clothing while being dressed and grasps objects that touch his or her hand. By 4 months of age, the infant voluntarily grasps a rattle or cube with a flexion pattern. At 5 months the cube is grasped with all flexed fingers and adducted thumb pressing the cube against the ulnar side of the palm. The radial palmar grasp emerges at 6 months, with the cube held on the radial side of the palm with flexed fingers and adducted thumb. Objects are released only reflexively unless simultaneously held by the mouth or the other hand, allowing transfer of the object. The 4- to 6-month-old infant enjoys randomly activating toys that produce sound. At 7 months, the radial palmar grasp matures with thumb opposition emerging with some wrist extension. The radial digital grasp develops at 8 months with fingertip and opposed thumb, with space noted between object and palm. Objects are now easily transferred from one hand to another. Small objects may be picked up by grasping between thumb and the side of the partly flexed finger in a scissors grip. At 9 months the inferior pincer grasp emerges, enhancing the child's ability to finger feed (small dry cereal or crackers). The index finger is used independent for pinch while keeping other fingers bent. The 9-month-old child can now point, poke, and grasp with the pads of the index finger and thumb. The infant finds joy in banging toys or a spoon on a table and dropping toys

over the edge of a table. At 12 months, the infant has a fine pincer grasp, with small objects picked up using only the tips of the index finger and thumb. He or she can release an object into a small container. The 14-month-old now can stack two cubes and enjoys scribbling with a marker or crayon. The child holds the marker in the full length of the palm. He or she picks up a small pellet and places it in a bottle. Self-feeding skills advance with the ability to use a spoon. However, frequent spilling occurs with the toddler holding the spoon in overpronation.[44]

At 18 months, hand dominance emerges and is established by 2 years. At 18 months the toddler can build a three-cube tower and at 2 years has mastered the eight-cube tower or aligning the cubes horizontally. The 18-month-old child enjoys turning pages in a book, usually turning two to three at a time, but by 2 years has mastered turning one at a time and listens to stories with pictures.

Feeding Skill Development

As in motor skills, there is maturation in feeding skills over the first several months of life. The newborn infant is reflex bound and automatically makes certain oral motor movements. Ordinarily, feeding and swallowing reflexes are refined into voluntary control of the oral-preparation and oral phase of swallow, resulting in normal growth and progression of the child's ability to handle textures and boluses. Knowing the normal sequence and time frames of feeding skill development is necessary in evaluation and monitoring the child with developmental disability who is at risk for dysphagia, failure to thrive, or both.

In the neonate, anatomic structure dictates an obligate pattern of suckling in an extension-retraction pattern. This is because of restricted room in the oropharynx compared with the older child and adult. The tongue is relatively more prominent in the mouth, lying entirely within the oral cavity. Furthermore, lateral movement is restricted by fatty tissue in the cheeks, which functions as a *sucking pad*. Respiration is coordinated with swallow, with longer sequencing between inspiration, suck, swallow, and respiration. The neonate is an obligate nose breather anatomically, unable to efficiently breathe through the mouth. Particularly with any respiratory compromise, the neonate may be forced to choose between adequate oxygen and food, placing him or her at risk for failure to thrive.[45]

By 6 months, the infant is able to perform a true suck, whereby the posterior tongue moves up and down with the mandible to pull liquid from the nipple. At this age "infant cereal" or "baby food" is most commonly begun for infants in the United States. The infant begins by sucking from the spoon, with the infant unable to move the upper lip to clean the spoon of its contents. By 9 months, he or she is able to do so and also coordinate tongue movements in an attempt at materializing food to the gums. The child can now shift food to the cutting edge of the teeth and begin a more mature rotatory jaw movement in chewing. It is not until this rotatory component is present that the child can grind meat.[45]

By 1 year, lip closure during swallow from a spoon appears. Until 18–24 months, however, the child is unable to close the lips fully around a cup because of a lack of jaw stability. It is not until 2 years of age that the child is able to maturely use the lateral corners of the lips to move food, lateralize the tongue, and achieve fully controlled rotatory jaw movement instead of more immature up and down biting movements of the infant.[45]

The maturation of feeding skills is more directly influenced by developmental changes in the nervous system, rather than anatomic changes related to growth. Teeth may be important for sensory feedback in the development of feeding. Anatomic relationships of the head and neck change with growth. The oral cavity enlarges around the tongue, the fat pads disappear, the neck grows longer, and the larynx gradually descends from the C-4 level to the C-6 level in later childhood. The tip of the epiglottis no longer extends to the soft palate, as it reaches only to the lower portion of the tongue. Because of neurodevelopment, growth, and anticipated changes in tone with age, the infant with developmental disability must be monitored for declines in feeding success.[45]

Speech and Language Development

The newborn infant may initially appear to only communicate with one cry; however, with time, that cry changes to indicate different needs such as hunger or fatigue. The young infant becomes quiet when he or she hears a voice or rattle and turns the head to the sound source. Over the next 16 weeks, the infant starts to coo and makes *laughing* noises.[46] The mother and infant may engage in vocal play with the infant producing vowels and some consonant sounds involving tongue and lip activity. At 4–5 months the infant may make *raspberries*, blow bubbles, and vocalize when content. Some nasal sounds (*m, n*) and lip sounds may be noted. Vowel-like cooing with consonants modifying the vowel are noted with babbling. At 7 months double consonant and vowel combinations develop including *ma, da,* and *do,* and some single words may emerge. At 10 months, the infant shouts for attention and imitates speech sounds and words. The infant waves bye-bye, uses *mama* and *dada* with understanding, and stops behaviors when told "no." With play activities the infant

retrieves an object hidden from view. At 1 year the child starts using labeling words. At 14 months the toddler can understand simple commands and by 18 months can point to named body part or single pictures. The 18-month-old child has 3–50 words and uses two-word utterances with 25% intelligibility.[46] Although normal toddlers may vary greatly in their rate and style of language acquisition, a hearing test and a language assessment should be obtained if an 18-month old uses no words or just *mama* and *dada* and does not point to what he or she wants.

Developmental Task: Sleep

Development of a physiological sleep habit is one of the first active tasks of the infant. Conversely, it is the rare child who does not experience sleep disturbance at some point. Sleep needs differ among people, but ordinarily seem to be fairly constant per individual, although dependent on age. In the first few months of life, infants sleep as many as 16–20 hours per day. By 2 years, the average is approximately 12 hours and by 13 years approximately 8. Seventy percent of babies sleep through the night or easily settle by 3 months of age, another 13% settle by 6 months of age, and 10% never sleep through the night. After age 6 months, however, one-half of all infants wake in the night again.[47] As basic fears manifest in the second year of life and the child becomes more aware of and frightened of separation from the parent, reluctance to go to sleep and nightmares become major issues, only partially abated through the use of a *transitional* object such as a pacifier or special blanket. By age 3, when a strong sense of object permanence appears, sleep disturbance shifts to more complex nightmares caused by the child's difficulty in discerning fantasy from reality. Early encouragement of a consistent bedtime ritual that may include a bath, book reading, falling asleep in a consistent bed, and insistence that a child stay in bed when he or she attempts to get up in the middle of the night encourages a healthy sleep hygiene behavior, so inappropriate patterns will be easy to extinguish if they develop.[48]

Two- to Three-Year-Old Children

Gross Motor

The 2-year-old child's postural stability and balance improve to allow advanced motor skills. The child delights in running everywhere and can start to jump with feet in place. Stairs can be ascended and descended without help in marked time (one step at a time). By 3 years the child can run well, pedal a tricycle, and broad jump. Stairs can now be ascended by alternating feet.[5]

Fine Motor

The 2-year-old child's grasp advances to holding the marker by securing its shaft between thumb and fingers. The child can fold a paper imitatively and copy a vertical line. By age 3 the toddler is able to copy a circle and imitate building a three-cube bridge. The 3-year-old child enjoys playing ball and catches a tossed ball with arms extended and hugging the ball against the body. The 3-year-old child can *parallel* play and may begin to take turns. With self-help, the 3-year-old child may achieve toilet training day and night. He or she can assist with washing and drying the hands and face and unbutton or unzip his or her clothing.[5,39,46]

Speech and Language Development

The average 2-year-old child has a 300-word vocabulary and uses phrases and two-word sentences. The 2-year-old child refers to him- or herself by name and using "me" and "mine." The child can follow simple directions. The 3-year-old child talks in three-word sentences, and frequent questions include "what," "who," and "where." The child uses future tense and can follow directions with prepositional commands, such as "put it under." The 3-year-old child can give his or her full name, identify him- or herself as a girl or boy, and identify three colors.[5,46,48]

A hearing test and language assessment are also indicated if a child is 2 years old and is not putting two words together, has a vocabulary less than 20 words, has speech that is unintelligible to the parents, or does not understand commands or questions without gestures.[31]

Developmental Task: Toilet Training

Shortly after a child learns to walk, parents turn their attention to toilet training, with the common belief being that ambulation is a necessary prerequisite for potty training. Toileting behavior emerges from physiological maturation of bowel and bladder control combined with behavioral toilet readiness, described at length in many writings of T. Berry Brazelton.[49] Signs of fully developed bowel and bladder continence are not recognized by the child until 2–3 years of age. Potty training should be presented at a time when the individual child brings readiness and understanding of conforming to the expectation of continence. This occurs, in the average child, at approximately 2 years of age when the following prerequisites are met: the child is ready to sit down; has receptive speech; can demonstrate independence to communicate "no"; is capable of understanding a process with steps and cause and effect; has both a desire and an ability to imitate and please important adults around him or her; has play that demonstrates a capacity and a desire to put things where they belong; and can indicate both *need to go* and when he or she is *going*.[50] The natural desire to please allows an intrinsic reward system that reinforces the *pleasantness* of continence over incontinence. If the child has a consistent emptying pattern, then he or she may be timed to go to the potty shortly before the physiological need. Because potty-training readiness generally coincides with the initiative versus guilt stage and the toddler's need to control his or her body, a cooperative approach is most successful with *reward for success*. Pressure in the form of frequent *pottying* or scolding often backfires by prolonging the process or resulting in stool holding and constipation.

Four to Five Years

Gross Motor

The 4-year-old child shows advanced motor skills with increased skills at the park and playgrounds. The 4-year-old child is able to ride a tricycle well, climb on playground equipment, and throw a ball overhand. Stairs are managed easily by alternating feet up and down, and hopping on one foot is mastered. The plantar arch of the foot has matured, giving a more adult appearance to the feet. The 4-year-old child can sit up directly from supine without rolling to the side, as the abdominal muscle strength has improved.[5,39,46] At 5 years of age the child can enjoy skipping, walking on tiptoes and heels, and even balance on one foot for 10 seconds. The 5-year-old child has advanced to throwing a ball with a diagonal arm and body rotation. He or she now catches the ball in the hands rather than hugging it with full arms against body.[5]

Fine Motor

The 4-year-old child has developed more mature fine motor skills. Mature manipulation of the pencil is noted, with moving the pencil with finger and wrist movement. Drawing skills have advanced from copying a circle (3 years) to copying a cross and drawing a circle person with head, eyes, and extremities. Paper can be cut with a scissors. The 4-year-old child can also button and lace, feed him- or herself neatly, and pour from a pitcher. The child can wash and dress. At 5 years the child can comb his or her hair and brush the teeth. Some 5-year-old children still need assistance with tying shoelaces. The 5-year-old child can copy a square and triangle and draw a person with all base body parts, including body, and may elaborate with complex scenes or backgrounds.[5,39,46]

Language Development

Articulation of the 4-year-old child may still be somewhat immature, but is largely intelligible in context. Complex parts of speech develop including adverbs, past tense, and adjectives. Cognitive linguistic skills advance with the ability to give accounts of recent experiences, storytelling, and frequent questions including "why," "when," and "how." The 4-year-old child can repeat four-digit series and understand the opposites of analogies. By 5 years speech is fluent and articulation is clear, with responses to questions more succinct and relevant. The 5-year-old child can follow three-part commands, count to 10, and recite address, age, and phone number.[5,48] Concern should be raised if word endings are consistently missed after age 5 years.

Developmental Task: Social Development

As the 4-year-old child develops the concepts of sharing, play with peers becomes more interactive than parallel. One-fifth of 3- to 6-year-old children have an imaginary friend, generally an animal or human-like figure with a described name, character, and appearance. The imaginary friend is seen most often in creative children with above average intelligence. This imaginary friend may be real to the child until 10 years of age.

Self-care skills improve with the ability of the 4-year-old child to distinguish the front and back of a garment and thus can dress and undress with supervision. The 5-year-old child can dress with limited adult supervision and brush teeth and comb hair, but may still need assistance with shoelaces. The 4-year-old child can start assisting with tasks at home and run simple errands nearby the home.

Six to Twelve Years

By age 8 years, the child has complete basic gross motor skills and high-level balance development and is independent in basic personal self-care skills such as hygiene, bathing, toileting, dressing, mobility, functional communication, and safety. The child's focus now transitions from care-free play activities to structured learning.[51] A 6-year-old child enters full-day school and is expected to work on academic tasks while sitting quietly at a desk. Motor skills and eye-hand coordination continue to develop with skills such as riding a bicycle without training wheels, roller skating, mature catching, and throwing a ball. Self-help skills include appropriate use of a fork, spreading with a knife, and in most cases tying shoelaces.[5] The ability to read with the mastery of decoding the written words

and understanding the content of a passage occur during the first grade. The child also learns basic addition and subtraction. By 7 years, most children have learned the days of the week, can tell time, and are beginning to reason in concrete terms. Handwriting is becoming better organized, although written letters may occasionally be reversed, but this error generally disappears by 8 years.[5,29]

With advancing grades, the child must apply reading comprehension and follow written directions and use mathematic principles. Cognitive development has reached the concrete operational stage.[29] By age 9, the typical child can demonstrate true sequencing such as day, month, and year. Simple multiplication and division concepts are performed by this age. In middle childhood, children share well with peers, understand play "by the rules," listen to authority, and take responsibility for their own acts. Lasting friendships are formed, most commonly of the same gender. Preadolescents can reason through problems and situations and begin to understand social and political issues.[48]

As cognitive-linguistic demands increase, the middle school child must process more abstract, more complex, and *decontextualized* information. Subtle difficulties in auditory processing, receptive or expressive language skill acquisition, cognitive maturation, specific learning disability, or shortened attention span may become more obvious as cognitive-linguistic demands increase, but are difficult to classify.[52] Many children with physical disabilities have motor limitations that further complicate formal cognitive and learning skill assessment. Because of the paucity of standardized tools available for this population, informal tools must be used, and the index of suspicion must be high. Creative ways of assessing learning, which do not rely on motor response, should be stressed. Assistive technology can be used to facilitate motor response, both for evaluation and to maximize performance. Children with fine motor incoordination precluding legible and efficient handwriting, for example, may find success with computer access. The rehabilitation professional is in an excellent position to closely monitor and advocate for appropriate evaluation to amplify the child's potential and to minimize negative outcomes.

Thirteen to Eighteen Years

The adolescent or teenage years are those of physical and sexual maturity and crucial intellectual and social expansion.[5,53] Physical growth and sexual maturation occur at an explosive pace in early adolescence, emphasizing normal and pathologic individual differences.[54]

The adolescent with a physical disability may lose mobility when a sudden change in size outstrips available strength and range of motion to support weight. With diminished freedom of movement, obesity may become part of a vicious cycle of physical inactivity. Diminished mobility may impair appropriate peer contact, which results in social isolation.

Children with physical, cognitive, or emotional disabilities may experience social failure, particularly if several areas of disability are involved. Those with inattention are likely to be impulsive, have difficulty with self-modulation, and fail to focus on social nuances. Those with cognitive-linguistic impairments are likely to experience difficulties in peer communication and, therefore, social skill acquisition. Difficulties may include delayed ability to perform a social task secondary to impairment in verbal pragmatics (use of language in a situationally appropriate context), social prediction and social memory (ability to predict consequences of actions and words based on previous experiences), and affective matching (ability to communicate and interpret nonverbal social expression).[55] The stage of formal operational thought emerges, with the adolescent now achieving abstract thought and problem solving. He or she is now able to make complex plans based on hypothetical ideas. He or she is able to develop insight into his or her own and other's feelings and behaviors. An individualized moral code and social judgment develop. Prevocational and vocational planning begins, requiring accurate self-assessment for successful choice making. Development of an accurate and healthy self-image is perhaps the most vital developmental task of the adolescent age group (see Table 23-2). The normal adolescent's struggle to achieve a healthy, mature self-image and social interaction may be aggravated by medical issues, school absences, and need for physical assistance in activities of daily living. Coping strategies change as a child matures. Hospitalization or unnatural situations may reinforce undesired coping strategies (passive-aggression, rationalizing, avoidance, quitting, clowning, regression) that are maladaptive in preparation for adult life. Perpetuation of dependency and unresolved issues of identity may hinder development of a mature personality. The transition from complete dependence on the family to the self may not occur without transitional planning.[55] For the adolescent with chronic disability, individual counseling may be beneficial to assist with transition to college or vocational training. Additional therapy for physical disabilities may be necessary at this age in order to adapt to changes in body size and dimensions that occur with the growth spurt during this age. Also, direct therapy can assist with transition to

independent living, in learning how to organize and plan for personal care assistance and manage daily living tasks such as meal preparation and homemaking activities.[5] Role playing and teaching of social skill strategies can prepare the adolescent for comfort in both routine and novel social interactions.

Evaluation Tools

Over the years, many developmental assessment instruments have been developed for infants and children (Figure 23-2). Some of them examined all areas of development, whereas others concentrated on selective aspects of function. A number of assessment instru-

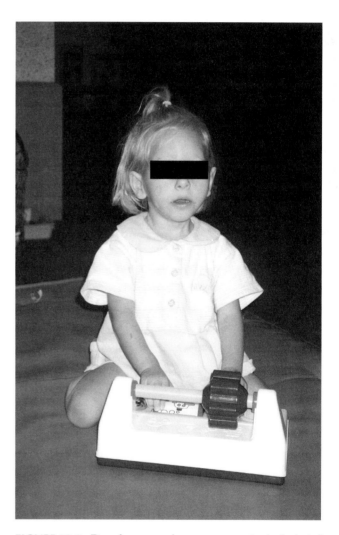

FIGURE 23-2. Developmental assessments include brief screens or in-depth diagnostic evaluations based on educational or clinical need.

ments have also been established for children with certain physical disabilities, which include testing of tone and reflexes, functional independence, hand function, or activities of daily living. Some assessments can be used at all ages in childhood, whereas others are age specific.[5] Developmental screens are properly used to test whole populations of children, identifying those at risk for unsuspected aberration and referral for more in-depth diagnostic assessment. Screening tools must be brief, inexpensive, valid, reliable, and broad, allowing for frequent administration. These tools are useful in identifying infants who are showing signs of possible delays or neurologic risk. These screens also are used by agencies to identify children who may benefit from early intervention services. A commonly taught screen for children 0–6 years old is the Denver Developmental Screening Test.[56-58] The Bayley Infant Neurodevelopmental Screen, based on the Early Neuropsychologic Optimality Rating Scales, enables screening of neurologic functions (reflexes, tone), neurodevelopment (movement, symmetry), and development (object permanence, imitation, language, movement, posture) in the child 0–2 years in less than 10–15 minutes.[59] The Bayley Scales of Infant Development, a more detailed assessment instrument, is considered by many to be the best instrument to assess global development from age 2–30 months, giving a *developmental index*, with fair correlation with IQ scores obtained after age 24 months. It can be used with older, developmentally delayed children, giving *age-equivalent* scores. This test requires trained examiners and takes approximately 30–45 minutes to administer.[60] For comprehensive developmental screening, parent training, and home programs, the Hawaii Early Learning Profile and Batelle Developmental Inventory are commonly used.[61] Although the Batelle Developmental Inventory takes approximately 1–2 hours to administer, its major strength is that standardized adaptations for testing handicapped children are provided.[58] The Peabody Motor Scales and the Bruininks-Oseretsky Test of Motor Proficiency are examples of tools to assess for gross or fine motor delays.[62,63] The Gross Motor Functional Measure is a standardized and validated observational test designed to demonstrate changes over time in children with cerebral palsy. *Functional*, in the test, is defined as the child's degree of achievement of motor behavior when instructed to perform or placed in a particular position. The test dimensions include activities in prone and supine positions, progressing to lying, rolling, sitting, crawling, kneeling, standing, walking, running, and jumping. All items are achievable by 5-year-old children with normal motor development.[64,65] Speech and language delays must be assessed early as communication is the basis for more advanced learning. The Peabody Picture Vocabulary test is a useful screening task that assesses one-word vocabulary between age 2.5 years and adulthood.[66] The preschool Language Scale-3 measures auditory comprehension and verbal expression separately, which is helpful in isolating specific areas of language deficit between the ages of 1 and 6 years. A discrepancy between the scores may reflect the need for further language evaluation, particularly in the school-aged child. In any child with suspected speech or language delays, a hearing test must be performed as well.[67]

Test instruments aimed at assessment of functional capabilities, independent task performance, and need for caregiver assistance or modification include the Functional Independence Measure for Children, The Pediatric Evaluation of Disability Inventory, and The Tufts Assessment of Motor Performance.[68-70] The Functional Independence Measure for Children, which takes approximately 15 minutes to administer, is a discipline-free test of disability developed to assess functional mobility, locomotion, self-care, sphincter control, communication, and social cognition using developmental norms. In addition to measuring functional skills, the Functional Independence Measure for Children assesses the overall cost of caregiver assistance needed to accomplish daily tasks so that a certain quality of life is achieved and sustained. Its brevity lends itself to frequent reassessment and is therefore useful in tracking outcomes after interventions over time and across health, developmental, and community settings. Because it has two national pediatric databases, the measure can be used to compare program outcomes with national norms.[68] The Pediatric Evaluation of Disability Inventory, a standardized evaluation that takes approximately 30–45 minutes to administer, assesses activities of daily living normally performed independently by young children up to age 7.5 years and can be scored by raw score or normative standard score.[71] Although lengthy, this test combines test elements used in special education and rehabilitation medicine, which allows it to be a particularly useful tool for monitoring progress, goal-setting, and evaluating program elements. The test includes three content domains (i.e., self-care, mobility, and social function) and evaluates functional skill level, caregiver's assistance, and use of mechanical modifications or devices within a domain. Tests that evaluate children with specific physical disabilities are: The Functional Activities Score, Spina Bifida Neurologic Scale, The Child Amputee Prosthetic Project Functional Status Inventory, and the Prosthetic Upper Extremity Functional Index.[72-77]

REFERENCES

1. Levy SE, Hyman SL. Pediatric assessment of the child with developmental delay. Pediatr Clin North Am 1993;40(3):465.
2. Behrman RE, Vaughan VC III (eds). Nelson Textbook of Pediatrics (13th ed). Philadelphia: WB Saunders, 1987;6–112.
3. Dipchand AI (ed). The HSC Handbook of Pediatrics (9th ed). St Louis: Mosby-Year Book, 1997.
4. Palmer CD. Study of the center of gravity in the human body. Child Dev 1944;15:99.
5. Molnar G, Alexander M. Pediatric Rehabilitation (3rd ed). Philadelphia: Hanley & Belfus, 1999;13–28.
6. Hay W, Groothuis J (eds). Current Pediatric. Diagnosis and Treatment. Stamford CT: Appleton & Lange, 1995.
7. Smith DW. Growth and its disorders: basics and standards, approach and classifications, growth deficiency disorders, growth excess disorders, obesity. Major Prog Pediatr 1977;15:1.
8. Tachdjian M. Pediatric Orthopedics. Philadelphia: WB Saunders, 1990.
9. Cronk C, Crocker AC, Pueshal SM, et al. Growth charts of children with Down Syndrome: 1 month to 18 years of age. Pediatrics 1998;81:102–110.
10. Cooley WC, Graham JM. Down syndrome: an update and review for the primary pediatrician. Clin Pediatr 1991;30:233.
11. Krick J, Murphy-Miller P, Zeger S, Wright E. Pattern of growth in children with cerebral palsy. J Am Diet Assoc 1996;96(7):680.
12. Eng GD, Koch B, Smokvinda MD. Brachial plexus palsy in neonates and children. Arch Phys Med Rehabil 1980;59:458.
13. Paryani SG, Arvin AM. Intrauterine infection with varicella-zoster virus after maternal varicella. N Engl J Med 1986;314:1542.
14. Green M. Pediatric Diagnosis: Interpretation of Symptoms and Signs in Different Age Periods (4th ed). Philadelphia: WB Saunders, 1986.
15. Nellhaus G. Head circumference from birth to eighteen years. Practical composite international and interracial graphs. Pediatrics 1968;41:106.
16. Swaiman KF, Wright FS (eds). Pediatric Neurology. 2nd ed. St Louis: CV Mosby, 1994.
17. Volpe JJ, Hill A. Neurologic Disorders. In GB Avery (ed), Neonatology: Pathophysiology and Management of the Newborn. Philadelphia: JB Lippincott, 1987.
18. Finkelstein JW. The endocrinology of adolescence. Pediatr Clin North Am 1980;27:53.
19. Egan DF. Developmental Examination of Infants and Preschool Children. Clinics in Developmental Medicine, Number 112. Philadelphia: JB Lippincott, 1990.
20. Fiorentino M. A Basis for Sensorimotor Development—Normal and Abnormal: The Influence of Primitive, Postural Reflexes on the Development and Distribution of Tone. Springfield, IL: Charles C Thomas, 1981;10–167.
21. Bobath K. A neurophysiologic basis for the treatment of cerebral palsy. Clin Dev Med 1980;75.
22. Taft LT, Cohen HJ. Neonatal and Infant Reflexology. In J Hellmuth (ed), Exceptional Infant. Seattle: Special Child Publications, 1967.
23. Twitchell TE. Attitudinal reflexes. Phys Ther 1965;45:411.
24. Twitchell TE. Normal motor development. Phys Ther 1965;45:419.
25. Menkes JH. Textbook of Child Neurology (5th ed). Baltimore: Williams & Wilkins, 1995.
26. Capute A, Accardo P. Developmental Disabilities in Infancy and Childhood. Baltimore: Paul H Brookes, 1991;335–348.
27. Scherzer A, Tscharnuter I. Early Diagnosis and Therapy in Cerebral Palsy: A Primer on Infant Developmental Problems. New York: Marcel Dekker, 1990.
28. Mussen PH, Conger JJ, Kagan J. Child Development and Personality. New York: Harper & Row, 1974.
29. Piaget J, Inhelder B. The Psychology of the Child. New York: Basic Books, 1969.
30. Newman BM, Newman PR. Development Through Life: A Psychosocial Approach. Pacific Grove, CA: Brooks/Cole, 1991.
31. Stoudemire A. Human Behavior: An Introduction for Medical Students (3rd ed). Philadelphia: Lippincott-Raven, 1998;261–315.
32. Hoffman L, Paris S, Hall E, Shell R. Developmental Psychology Today. New York: McGraw-Hill, 1988.
33. Havighurst RJ. Developmental Tasks and Education. David McKay Co. 1952;5.
34. Thomas A, Chess S. Temperament in Clinical Practice. New York: Guilford Press, 1986.
35. Dubowitz V, Dubowitz L. The neurologic assessment of the preterm and full-term infant. Clin Dev Med 1981;79.
36. Paine SR, Brazelton TB, Donovan DE, et al. Evolution of postural reflexes in normal infants and the presence of chronic brain syndromes. Neurology 1964;14:1036.
37. Brazelton TB. Behavioral Competence of the Newborn Infant. In GB Avery (ed), Neonatology: Pathophysiology and Management of the Newborn. Philadelphia: JB Lippincott, 1987.
38. Gesell AL, Amatruda CS. Developmental Diagnosis. In H Knobloch, B Pasamanick (eds), The Infancy and Early Childhood. New York: Harper & Row, 1974.
39. Knobloch H, Stevens F, Malone AF. Manual of Developmental Diagnosis: The Administration and Interpretation of the Revised Gesell and Amatruda Developmental and Neurological Examination. Hagerstown, MD: Harper & Row, 1980.
40. Illingsworth RS. The Development of the Infant and Young Child: Normal and Abnormal. Edinburgh: Churchill Livingstone, 1987.
41. Statham L, Murray MP. Early walking pattern of normal children. Clin Orthop 1971;79:8.
42. Burnett CN, Johnson EW. Development of gait in childhood. Dev Med Child Neurol 1971;13:196.
43. Sutherland DH, Olshen R, Cooper L, Woo-Sam J. The development of mature gait. J Bone Joint Surg 1980;62A;336.
44. Illingworth RS. Basic Developmental Screening 0-4 Years. Boston: Blackwell Scientific Publications, 1990;18.
45. Stevenson R, Allaire J. The development of normal feeding and swallowing. Pediatr Clin North Am 1991;38:439.
46. McMillan J, Oski F, Stockman J, Niebrug P. The Best of the Whole Pediatrician Catalogs I-III. Philadelphia: WB Saunders, 1984;69.
47. Moore T, Ucko LE. Night waking in early infancy, part 1. Arch Dis Child 1957;32:333.
48. Chamberlin R. Anticipatory Guidance. In RA Hoekelman (ed), Primary Pediatric Care. St Louis: Mosby, 1987;149.
49. Brazelton TB. A child-oriented approach

to toilet training. Pediatrics 1962;29: 278–281.

50. Brozelton TB, et al. Physiological and clinical considerations regarding toilet training: an updated review. Pediatrics 1999;103(Suppl 6, pt 2):1345.

51. Gesell A, Ilg FL. The Child from Five to Ten. New York: Harper & Row, 1946.

52. Montgomery JW. Easily overlooked language disabilities during childhood and adolescence. Pediatr Clin North Am 1992;39(3):513–524.

53. Bax M, Hart H, Jenkins S. Assessment of speech and language in the young child. Pediatrics 1988;66:350.

54. Gesell A, Ilg FL, Ames LB. Youth, the Years from Ten to Fifteen. New York: Harper & Row, 1956.

55. Brooks RB. Self-esteem during the school years: its normal development and hazardous decline. Pediatr Clin North Am 1992;39(3):537–550.

56. Frankenburg WK, Dodds JB. The Denver Developmental Screening Test. J Pediatr 1967;71:181.

57. Frankenburg WK, Dodds JB, Fandal AW. Denver Developmental Screening Test Revised Manual. Denver: University of Colorado Medical Center, 1970.

58. Aylward G. Practitioner's Guide to Developmental and Psychological Testing. New York: Plenum Medical Book Co, 1994;17.

59. Bayley Infant Neurodevelopmental Screener Standardization Manual. The Psychological Corporation, San Antonio, 1996.

60. Bayley N. Manual for the Bayley Scales of Infant Development. New York: Psychology Corp, 1969.

61. Parks S, Furuno S, O'Reilly KA, et al. HELP . . . at Home. Palo Alto, CA: VORT Corporation, 1988.

62. Folio R, Fewll RR. Peabody Developmental Motor Scales and Activity Cards. Hingham, MA: Teaching Resources Corporation, 1983.

63. Bruininks RH. Bruininks-Oseretsky Test of Motor Proficiency. Examiner's Manual. Circle Pines, MN: American Guidance Services, 1978.

64. Gross Motor Measure Group. Gross Motor Function Measures. Hamilton, Ontario: Chedoke-McMaster Hospital, 1990.

65. Russell DJ, Rosenbaum PL, Cadman DT, et al. The gross motor function measure: a means to evaluate the effects of physical therapy. Dev Med Child Neurol 1989;31:341.

66. Aylward G. Practitioner's Guide to Developmental Psychological Testing. New York: Plenum Book Co, 1994;54.

67. Perkins WH. Speech Pathology: An Applied Behavioral Science. St Louis: CV Mosby, 1971.

68. Granger C, Braun S, et al. Guide for Use of the Uniform Data Set for Medical Rehabilitation. Functional Independence Measure for Children (WEEFIM), Version 1.5. New York: SUNY Research Foundation, 1991.

69. Haley S, Coster W, et al. Pediatric Evaluation of Disability Inventory (PEDI): Development, Standardization and Administration Manual, Version

1.0. Boston: New England Medical Center Hospital, 1992.

70. Haley SM, Inacio C, Gans BM. Tufts Assessment of Motor Performance, Pediatric Clinical Version. Boston: New England Medical Center Hospital, 1991.

71. PEDI Research Group, Department of Rehabilitation Medicine. Pediatric Evaluation of Disability Inventory. Boston: New England Medical Center Hospital, 1992.

72. Sousa JC, Gordon LH, Shurtleff DB. Assessing the development of daily living skills in patients with spina bifida. Dev Med Child Neurol 1976;17(Suppl 37):134.

73. Sousa JC, Telzrow RW, Holm RA, et al. Developmental guidelines for children with myelodysplasia. Phys Ther 1983;63:21.

74. Oi S, Matsumoto S. Purposed grading scoring system for spina bifida: SPINA BIFIDA, Neurologic scale (SBNS). Child Nerv Syst 1992;8:337.

75. Pruitt S, Varni J, Setogughi Y. Functional status of children with limb deficiency: development and initial validation of an outcome measure. Arch Phys Med Rehabil 1996;77:1233.

76. Pruitt S, Varni JW. Functional status in limb deficiency: development of outcome measure for preschool children. Arch Phys Med Rehabil 1998;79:405.

77. Huggins M, Wright S, et al. The Prosthetic Upper Extremity Functional Index (PUFI): Presentation of an approach to measurement of a child's use of an upper extremity prosthesis. Grand Rapids, MI: ACPOC, 1998.

24

Aging of Organ Systems

GERALD FELSENTHAL, TAMAR S. FERENCE,
AND MARK ALLEN YOUNG

AGING, A DEFINITION

Aging represents a maturational process that includes a series of genetically programmed events that are influenced by external factors such as nutrition, activity, environment, and illness. The aging of human organ systems has implications for affecting function and a human's ability to maximize quality of life.

Contemporary medicine's ability to fight disease and manage chronic illness has resulted in a substantial improvement in longevity in the general population. As we move swiftly ahead in the new millennium, mean life expectancy continues to increase dramatically, defying lifespan trends observed earlier in the twentieth century when normal life projections averaged only 49 years.[1] The segment of the population older than 85 years is projected to grow the most by the year 2020.[2] With the advancement of modern medical knowledge and the widespread availability of new life-sustaining procedures, technology, and therapies, it is estimated that the average age of survival now is rapidly approaching 80 years. This phenomenon has been shaped by a variety of external factors as well, including growing recognition of the importance of proper nutrition, diet, and exercise. There is accumulating scientific evidence regarding the essential antiaging physiological role of vitamins, nutrients, and supplements.[3,4]

REHABILITATION'S ROLE

Physical medicine and rehabilitation continue to play vital roles in the maintenance or restoration of function of the aged patient by systematically evaluating and rehabilitating the musculoskeletal and neuromuscular systems as well as determining and modifying the functional implications of the aging process. As older people survive life-threatening illnesses and disability, the effects of normal aging on the integrity of organ systems continue to be exerted in a dramatic way, and the physiatrist and other clinicians are in a unique position to conduct a functional assessment and modify the functional consequences.

CHAPTER OVERVIEW

This chapter provides an overview of the effects of the normal aging process on individual organ systems. This is followed by a specific discussion of functional issues that are affected by the aging human organ system. In reviewing the effects of age on specific organ systems, it is important to draw a distinction between the normal aging process and the *modified aging process.* Often the normal aging process is modified by the coexistence of disease and concurrent illness, which exert their effects on the organ systems, thus affecting the *normal* aging and maturational process. An appropriate example of this is the 60-year-old man whose aging process has been significantly accelerated because of the effects of advanced insulin-dependent diabetes. The normal aging and maturational process is frequently blurred by pathophysiological illnesses such as diabetes and atherosclerosis.

The *rule of thirds* is a convenient way to categorize the aging process. This rule of thumb conveniently attributes the aging process to three influences: normal aging, pathophysiology, and disuse.

NERVOUS SYSTEM

Anatomic and Physiological Changes with Aging

With aging, gross parenchymal changes have been reported within the brain.[5] Brain weight has been estimated to decrease by 15–20% by age 80 and protein content by 25–30%.[6] Gender differences have been reported with the male brain showing greater volume loss in the whole brain and in the frontal and temporal lobes, whereas the female brain shows greater loss in the hippocampus and parietal lobes.[7] The cerebral cortex shows loss of neurons and dendritic arborization with a concomitant increase in neuroglial density with advancing age.[8,9] The genesis of new neuronal cells in the adult human brain has not been demonstrated except for the hippocampus.[10] The greatest changes are noted in the precentral gyrus, the superior temple gyrus, and the area striatum, with the postcentral gyrus being relatively unaffected.[8] An age-related decrease in the neuronal density occurs within the primary and secondary somatosensory cortex, within area 3, lamina IV, where the thalamocortical fibers are thought to terminate.[11] With the exception of the locum ceruleus, nuclei of the brain stem are thought to show little age-related neuronal loss, although an 18% reduction of thalamic neurons has been reported.[11]

Intraneuronal organelles such as neurofibrillary tangles, lipofuscin, and granulovacuoles accumulate. Senile plaques containing amyloid deposits, degenerating hypertrophic neuritic processes, and intracellular organelles form and may be a precursor of Alzheimer's disease. Degenerative changes evidenced by increased lipofuscin granules are found in most sensory spinal cord neurons by 60 years of age.[12]

A loss of myelin and evidence of axonal involution in the ascending pathways of the dorsal column (medial lemniscal pathways) have been noted.[12] There is a loss of large myelinated fibers proportional to the decreasing number of posterior spinal nerve roots.[13,14]

Anatomic cranial nerve changes with aging have been reported. The olfactory receptor cells, bulb, and tract exhibit a loss of neurons and nerve fibers and an increased amount of astroglia and corpora amylacea. There is a smaller response to odors and less ability to allocate attentional resources and slowing in olfactory cognitive processing.[15] Similarly, there is a reported decrease in taste with aging.[16] There are changes in the

components of the acoustic nerve including sensory, neural, vascular, supporting, synaptic, mechanical, or all of these structures within the peripheral, central, or both auditory systems.[17] The optic nerve displays similar changes for both peripheral and central projections.[18]

Electrophysiological studies indicate that aging is associated with a general slowing of alpha frequency in the electroencephalogram.[5] Numerous neurochemical changes have been reported within the aging brain (catecholamines, serotonin, γ-aminobutyric acid, acetylcholine). The functional significance of these changes has yet to be established.[5,14] Morphologic manifestations of aging within the peripheral nervous[19] and autonomic nervous systems[20] are noted in sensory ganglion cells, nerve and dorsal root, peripheral receptors, dorsal columns, anterior horn cell, motor nerve and ventral root, motor nerve endings, and striated muscle. Myelin changes include bubbling, demyelination and remyelination of axons, and onion bulb formation.[19] Encapsulated receptors (pacinian and Meissner's) show changes in morphology and decreases in number.[14] The loss of Meissner's corpuscles is greater in the foot than the finger.[21] These encapsulated receptors subserve the sensory functions of touch, vibration sensation, and two-point discrimination, and these aging changes may account for the decrease in these sensory functions with aging.[22-26] Quantitative vibratory sensation testing indicates a decrease in sensitivity of 97% in the legs of healthy patients between 20 and 80 years of age.[27] Table 24-1 lists the relative decrement of various functions between ages 25 and 75.[5] Proprioceptive threshold in the toes increases approximately 50% after age 60[28] and may affect joint position sensation as far as the knee.[29] Whether there are aging changes in the density or structure of free nerve endings of myelinated fibers that mediate pain is contradictory in different studies.[14,19] An increase in threshold to some kinds of painful stimuli in the aged has been reported[19,30] as has age-related changes in temperature[31] and light touch sensation.[22]

Age-related decrease in density of myelinated fibers has been demonstrated in peripheral nerves as well as somatic nerves.[14] For the sural nerve, the maximum fiber density is achieved by the third decade, with a decline to 54% of this maximum by 90 years of age.[32] With aging and remyelination and demyelination of the peripheral nerves, nerve fibers demonstrate an increase in segmental demyelination, wallerian degeneration, decrease in mean internodal length, presence of regeneration clusters, and accumulation of endoneurial collagen.[33,34]

Electrophysiological studies have demonstrated a decrease in the amplitude of evoked action potentials and conduction velocities and an increase in distal

TABLE 24-1
Relative Decrement of Various Functions, Ages 25–75ª

Function	Little or No Change	<20%	20–40%	40–60%	>60%
Vocabulary	X				
Information	X				
Comprehension	X				
Digits forward	X				
Touch sensation, fingers and toes[b]	X				
Two-point discrimination, finger[b]	X				
Raven progressive matrices:					
Tying bow		X			
Manipulating safety pin		X			
Simple reaction time		X			
Hand tapping		X			
Finger dexterity		X			
Foot tapping		X			
Tandem stepping		X			
Rising from chair with support			X		
Putting on shirt			X		
Managing large button			X		
Zipping garment			X		
Cutting with knife			X		
Speed of handwriting			X		
Digit symbol substitution			X		
Foot dorsiflexion			X		
One leg standing, eyes open			X		
Vibration sense, upper extremities				X	
Leg flexion				X	
Vibration sense, lower extremities					X
One leg standing, eyes closed					X

ªCross-sectional study.
[b]Longitudinal studies.
Source: Reprinted with permission from R Katzman, R Terry. Normal Aging of the Nervous System. In R Katzman, JW Rowe (eds), Principles of Geriatric Neurology. Philadelphia, F.A. Davis, 1992;18–58, with modified additions from AR Potvin, K Syndulko, WN Tourtellotte, et al. Human neurologic function and the aging process. J Am Geriatr Soc 1980;28:1–9.

latencies with aging. Sensory and motor peripheral and central nerve conduction demonstrates a decline of 1–2 m per second per decade.[35] In the 70- to 88-year-old subject group, the amplitude of the sensory-evoked action potential is one-third of 18- to 25-year-old subjects.[36] A combination of large fiber loss and segmental demyelination has been suggested as the cause of these observations. Clinically, in the elderly, there may be difficulty in distinguishing between the normal changes of aging and the pathologic changes of a peripheral neuropathy.[37]

Histochemical studies of striated muscle from normal elderly subjects show evidence of fiber size variation, hyaline or granular degeneration, loss of striations, clumps of pyknotic nuclei, increased fat and connective tissue, and fiber type grouping.[34,38] There are aging changes in the sarcolemma, sarcoplasmic reticulum, Z lines, T system, and mitochondria.[39,40] Muscle spindles undergo capsular thickening, lamellar fibrosis, and a mild degree of intrafusal fiber loss.[41]

There is a one-third to one-half reduction in total muscle mass between ages 30 and 80,[42,43] with a loss of 1% per year after age 70.[44] Between ages 50 and 80 there is a 30% decrease in cross-sectional area of muscles.[45] Existing motor units of elderly persons contain a larger number of muscle fibers than those of younger persons.[46] This suggests that the number of motor units and anterior horn cells decreases with aging[47] and is estimated to be approximately 200 cells per spinal segment per decade.[48] This is substantiated by histopathologic analysis showing fiber type grouping.[44,49,50] Electromyographic data show an age-related decrease of greater than 50% in the number of motor units between ages 20 and 80 years[51,52] occurring particularly in the largest and fastest conducting motor units.[53] Absence of weakness is ascribed to collateral reinnervation by surviving motor units.

Loss of muscle fibers begins at approximately age 25 and by age 80 there is a decrease of approximately 39%.[43,51,54,55] There is a relative stability of type I fibers with aging[39,51,55] and a loss of type II,[56] especially type IIB, fibers.[44] Biopsy studies show a 15–25% reduction in type IIA and IIB cross-sectional areas.[57] The decrease in cross-sectional area of type II fibers is greater in the lower than the upper extremities.[49] This may reflect decreased weight-bearing activities in the elderly, with continuation of upper extremity activities (non–weight-bearing sedentary activities).[39] Metabolically, capacity for aerobic and anaerobic metabolism shows little change with age after adjusting for change in area of fiber type.[44,49,58,59] Speed of muscle contraction time lengthening with age, an increased time to peak tension of muscle twitch, a lower force cross-sectional area, and easier fatigability in the elderly have been noted.[60–62]

Neurologic Examination Changes with Aging

Cognition

The Baltimore Longitudinal Study of Aging has demonstrated age-related declines in some of the measures testing cognition (Benton Visual Retention test, Concept Problem Solving, Paired Associate Learning), but other measures remained stable or increased over time (Wechsler Adult Intelligence Scale [WAIS] Vocabulary, Digit Span Forward, Memory for Text).[63] The Baltimore Longitudinal Study of Aging demonstrated that declines of cognitive function are a part of the normal aging process but start later in life and are of smaller magnitude than previously assumed. Little change in functioning was found as a result of these cognitive aging changes. In a study of subjects aged 70–102 years interviewed at baseline and then again 3–6 years later, cognitive performance decreased in tests of episodic memory and cognitive speed and the Mini-Mental State Examination, but not in the National Adult Reading Test.[64] In a cross-sectional versus longitudinal study, a small decline in scores on the Mini-Mental State Examination was demonstrated with increasing population age in the cross-sectional analysis, but was masked by a learning effect in the longitudinal study.[65]

Tone

Mild axial or limb tone increase (gegenhalten or rigidity) may occur with aging. The etiology may be basal ganglia or extrapyramidal dysfunction.[66] This is noted more in the lower extremities than in the upper extremities.[67] Pyramidal signs are always pathologic as are asymmetric motor findings.

Reflexes

With aging the ankle jerk is frequently absent.[68] The knee jerk may also be absent.[69] The clinical use of the blink and the release reflexes (palmomental, glabellar, grasp, and snout) has been reviewed. These reflexes are frequently seen as an incidental abnormality in old age. An asymmetric grasp reflex is sensitive but not specific for abnormal brain function. Lack of inhibition is more important than the presence or absence of the blink or release reflexes.[70] Multiple primitive reflexes are rare in healthy old age. Single primitive reflexes can be found in an increasing proportion of healthy aging subjects.[71]

Muscle Strength and Endurance

There is an age-related decrease in muscle strength that is of the same order of magnitude as the noted decrease in muscle mass.[72] Muscle strength peaks in the third decade with minimum decline until age 50 after which there is a more rapid decline in strength.[19,66] The age-related decline appears to be greater in the back and lower extremity muscles than in the upper extremity muscles and greater in the proximal than in the distal muscles.[49,73] Between ages 30 and 80, strength is reduced approximately 40% in the leg and back muscles and 30% in the arm muscles.[74] Another investigator reports that the mean strength of back, arm, and leg muscles decreases as much as 60%, largely reflecting a progressive loss of muscle mass at an average of 4% per decade from 25 to 50 years of age and 10% per decade after age 50.[75] Specific studies indicate decreased strength with aging in grip and pinch strength,[76] elbow flexors,[62,77] knee extension,[78] and plantar flexors.[62,77] Reduction of strength reflects the reduction in the number of functional motor units.[52]

Aerobic capacity or endurance as determined by maximal oxygen uptake during exercise declines an average of approximately 1% per year after the third decade.[79] Relative muscle endurance does not appear to decrease with age as long as older people work at the same relative intensity (as a percentage of their maximum strength) as younger people.[39,80]

Aging is not synonymous with disuse; disuse exacerbates the changes that occur with aging.[81] As activities of daily living represent an increasing percentage of a person's maximum aerobic capacity, an elderly person may become disinclined to perform the activities of daily living.[82] Aging muscles are more easily injured by their own contractions.[83] With training of sufficient intensity, elderly subjects can increase strength as effectively as younger subjects.[82] Increase in strength can also lead to functional improvement in activities such as stair climbing and gait velocity.[84] Table 24-2[85] gives a summary of muscle adaptations to aging and training by the elderly.

Range of Motion

Cross-sectional studies report decreases in flexibility of the shoulder, elbow, wrist, hip, knee, ankle, and spine with aging.[86] The flexibility of a typical sedentary 70-year-old subject may show a 20–30% decrease.[87,88] Decreased range of motion may be secondary to changes in connective tissue in tendons, joint capsules, muscles, and ligaments.[89] Range of motion and aerobic exercises have been reported to improve range of motion.[90] Poor flexibility at the ankles, knees, hips, and shoulders affects adversely on posture, balance, and gait.

Posture

Kaufman[91] has reviewed the common postural changes seen with aging. Typical postural changes of the spine are the head-forward position, accentuated kyphosis of the thoracic spine, and loss of the normal lumbar lordosis, either increased or decreased. The arms may be extended to counterbalance the anterior thrust position of the head. In the upper extremities, there may be scapular protraction (rounding of the shoulders), increased flexion at the elbows, ulnar deviation at the wrist, and flexion of the fingers. In the lower extremities, there may be increased hip and knee flexion and decreased ankle dorsiflexion. The base of support is often widened. These postural adjustments are the result of a combination of neuromusculoskeletal influences as well as lifestyle.

Balance

Walking is a balance-displacement activity. Decreased balance has been noted in 13% of 65- to 69-year-old community-living persons and in more than 46% of people 85 or more years old.[92,93] To maintain static balance, the body's center of gravity, located over the second sacral vertebra, should remain over its base of support. Activities displacing the center of gravity, such as leaning, require dynamic balance, which returns the center of gravity to S_2 over the base of support. This

TABLE 24-2

Summary of Muscle Adaptations to Aging and Training by the Elderly

Variable	Aging	Training
Muscle mass	Decrease	Increase or no change
Type I %	Increase	No change
Type II %	Decrease	No change
Type I area	No change	Increase
Type II area	Decrease	Increase
Oxidative capacity	Decrease	Increase
Glycolytic capacity	No change	No change
Capillary density	Decrease	Increase
Contraction time	Increase	Decrease or no change
Relaxation time	Increase	Decrease or no change
Shortening velocity	No change	Increase

Source: Reprinted with permission from DT Kirkendall, WE Garrett. The effects of aging and training on skeletal muscle. Am J Sports Med 1998;26:598–602.

requires coordinated efforts of afferent mechanisms or sensory systems (visual, vestibular, and proprioceptive) and efferent mechanisms or motor systems (upper and lower extremity muscle strength and joint flexibility). Components of visual function contributing to balance include static and dynamic acuity, contrast sensitivity, depth perception, and peripheral vision. Proprioceptive sensory input comes from muscle and tendon receptors, articular mechanoreceptors, and deep pressure receptors on the plantar aspect of the feet. The vestibular system includes the peripheral sensory component (inner ear semicircular canals and the otolithic organs, utricle and saccule), central processing component including the pons and cerebellum (combines visual, vestibular, and proprioceptive information), and motor control component (ocular muscles and spinal cord). Reflexes used by the body to regulate postural control are the vestibulo-ocular reflex and the vestibulospinal reflex. The vestibulo-ocular reflex ensures ocular stability and orientation of the head in space. The vestibulospinal reflex influences skeletal muscles in the neck, trunk, and limbs and generates compensatory body movement that maintains head and postural control (righting reflex).[94] All components are affected by aging.[95,96]

There is increased postural sway with aging under both static and dynamic conditions.[97] The initiation of postural muscular responses or latency to balance displacement is delayed 20–30 msec in healthy aged individuals.[98,99] Older subjects take multiple small steps in response to a large displacement of balance (stepping strategy), whereas younger subjects take a single corrective step as a compensatory mechanism to maintain balance.[100] In younger people, sway compensation is mainly through the ankle joint (so-called ankle strategy), but older people tend to use muscle responses at the hip, possibly because of a lack of muscle strength, proprioceptive inputs, or both.[101] With aging, there is an increase in reaction time.[102] There is a decreased ability to stand on one leg, particularly with the eyes closed.[103] Activities performed at least part of the time on one foot include ambulation as the center of gravity falls outside of the base of support of the body for 80% of the stride length[104] as well as stepping activities such as ascending and descending stairs.

Gait

With aging there is a reported increase in difficulty in walking, with 15% reporting difficulty between ages 65 and 69 and 49% after age 85.[105] Comfortable walking speed declines at a rate of 2.5–4.5% per decade up to age 62 and at a rate of 16% for men and 12% for women thereafter.[106] Controlling for leg length, height,

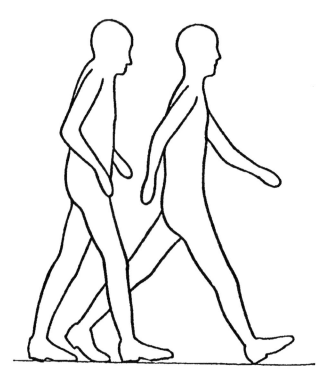

FIGURE 24-1 Diagram illustrates the differences in the sagittal positions of the body of older (*left*) and younger (*right*) men at the instant of heel strike. (Reprinted with permission from MP Murray, RC Kory, BH Clarkson. Walking patterns in healthy old men. J Gerontol 1969;24:176.)

or both may eliminate gender differences.[107] Cadence remains the same, but there is a shorter step length, an increased double-support stance period, decreased push-off power, and a more flat-footed landing.[104] Older men compared with younger men show shorter step length and a wider based gait, flexed posture, decreased pelvic rotation, decreased excursions of hip flexion-extension, decreased extension of the ankle and decreased elevation of the heel of the rear limb, decreased heel-floor angle and decreased elevation of the toe of the forward limb, decreased shoulder flexion on the forward arc of the arm swing, and decreased elbow extension on the backward arc. There is less vertical and more lateral oscillation of the head[108] (Figure 24-1). Women develop a narrow-based, short-step-length, waddling gait.[109] They tended to have valgus deformities of the knee[110] and decreased foot placement and clearance during stair descent.[111]

Vision

With aging, there are multiple changes in the eye and with vision. The importance of vision as one of the modalities affecting balance has been previously discussed. Visual acuity declines substantially between ages 60 and 80.[112] The aging pupil is smaller with, not uncommonly, minor differences between sides.[113] The speed of pupillary constriction is slower, the latency is prolonged,[114] and the reaction to light is diminished.[112] Dark adaptation decreases because of a combination of optical and retinal changes.[115] There is age-related contraction of the visual fields[116,117] and decreased range of eye movement, especially elevation.[118] There is ptosis of the upper eyelid (blepharoptosis), which may give a symptomatic visual field restriction during down-gaze activities such as reading.[119] The velocity of saccadic movements diminishes with age.[120] Accommodation of the lens declines (presbyopia). Color perception deteriorates, particularly for short wavelength colors.[121] The lens tends to become less uniform in its refractive index, scattering light and causing glare.[122]

Hearing

The prevalence of hearing loss among persons 65 years of age or older is 40%.[123] There are four patterns of presbycusis: sensory, neural, mechanical, and metabolic.[124] In men, there is a progressive loss of hearing starting in the third decade, particularly and initially involving the higher sound frequencies. This is caused by a peripheral presbycusis and may cause an impairment in speech understanding.[125] Central presbycusis is caused by changes in auditory pathways in the brain stem and cortex and occurs in 23–35% of elderly persons.[126] Central presbycusis causes low-frequency hearing loss[127] and affects sentence recognition and word understanding. As mentioned previously, there are age-related anatomic and physiological changes effecting the components of the hearing system including the sensory, neural, vascular, supporting, synaptic, and mechanical structures within the peripheral and central auditory systems.[17]

Cardiovascular

Age-related changes in cardiovascular structure and function increase the probability of disease, modify the threshold at which symptoms and signs arise, and affect the clinical course and prognosis. Evidence is mounting that life-style and diet can modify age-associated increases in arterial stiffness and pressure.[128,129] For example, dietary sodium has a greater effect on arterial pressure with age. More recent studies indicate that the effect of lifestyle on cardiovascular function may be far greater than that of aging.

Heart
A modest increase in left ventricular wall thickness with age is normal in normotensive persons, and an exaggerated increase occurs in hypertensive patients. Left atrial dimension increases with age, even in otherwise healthy persons. An increase in myocyte size underlies heart wall thickening.[128]

Vasculature
Atrial walls stiffen with age, and the aorta becomes dilated and elongated. This appears to result not from atherosclerosis but from changes in the amount and nature of elastin and collagen, as well as from calcium deposition. Changes in the cross-linking of collagen may render it less elastic. With aging, glycoprotein eventually disappears from elastin fibrils, elastin becomes frayed, and its calcium content increases.[128]

Cardiovascular Function
The early diastolic filling rate progressively slows after the age of 20, so that by 80 years of age, the rate is reduced up to 50%. Despite the slowing of left ventricular filling early in diastole, end-diastolic volume is not usually reduced in healthy elderly persons. The at-rest filling volume during each cardiac cycle is roughly the same regardless of age. Thus, in healthy persons, more filling occurs later in diastole to compensate for the slowed early filling. This latter filling response is caused

by atrial enlargement and a more vigorous atrial contraction and is manifested on auscultation as a fourth heart sound (atrial gallop). Atrial stiffening and the associated increase in pulse wave velocity appear to cause the increase in systolic blood pressure associated with aging.[130]

The increase in systolic pressure affects left ventricular afterload. The left ventricle may empty incompletely during each cardiac cycle, leading to a reduced ejection fraction and ventricular dilatation. Left ventricular wall thickness may increase sufficiently to normalize wall stress, thus maintaining normal cavity size and ejection fraction; this occurs in healthy older persons whose increase in systolic blood pressure is clinically normal.[131] Epidemiologic studies show that these untreated elderly persons with increased systolic blood pressure are at higher risk for cardiovascular events.

The resting ejection fraction is not reduced in older men and women whose resting end-diastolic and end-systolic volumes are comparable with those of younger persons. Stroke volume also remains constant with age. In healthy men, the supine basal heart rate does not change with aging; in the sitting position, the heart rate decreases slightly.[131]

Effects of Exercise

The maximum exercise capacity and maximal oxygen consumption decline with age, but to a variable extent among individuals. Elderly persons in good physical condition can match or exceed the aerobic capacity of unconditioned younger persons. This indicates either that physical deconditioning causes the decline in some older persons or that physical conditioning can retard aging's effect on cardiorespiratory function.[132]

In summary, the aerobic capacity of both middle-aged and older men can increase with endurance training and is mediated by adaptions in peripheral and cardiac mechanisms. Compared with younger persons, healthy elderly persons have a substantially lower heart rate during high levels of physical exertion. During vigorous exercise, the left ventricular stroke volume is not reduced in healthy elderly persons.

Pulmonary

When assessing age-related changes in the respiratory system, it is difficult to distinguish between disease effects and aging effects. Age-related changes in structure and function are more greatly affected by disease than by the process of aging itself. For example, smoking increases the levels of oxidants in the lung[133] and negatively affects the preservation of respiratory function with aging. Other causes of decline of respiratory function with age include previous respiratory infection, nutritional status, environmental pollution, and increased bronchial responsiveness to irritants. Because no other internal organ is so intimately exposed to external environmental influences as the lung, it is difficult even in the absence of disease to differentiate clearly between physical and physiological changes of aging itself and those brought about by a lifetime sum of diverse inspired *environmental* insults.

The most important age-related change in the large airways is a reduction in the number of glandular epithelial cells. This results in reduced production of protective mucus and thus impaired defense against respiratory infection. There are few changes in the bronchi, but the area of the alveoli falls, and the alveoli and alveoli ducts enlarge. Functional residual capacity, residual volume, and compliance increase. There is deposition of amyloid in lung vasculature and alveolar septa.[134]

Small airways suffer qualitative and quantitative changes in the supportive elastin and collagen, with coiling and rupture of fibers and consequent dilatation of alveolar ducts and air spaces[135] and increased tendency for small airways to collapse during expiration. This results in hypoventilation and failure to clear dependent sputum and thus further risk of lower respiratory infection.

The major age-related change in the respiratory muscles is a reduction in the proportion of type IIA fibers (fast-fatigue resistant) with consequent impairment of strength and endurance.[136] Such changes lead to impaired reserve to combat respiratory challenges consequent on acute respiratory disease. Ossification of costal cartilages and loss of disk spaces combined with muscle changes produce impaired mobility of the thoracic cage.

Lung volumes decrease gradually with age. Forced expiratory volume in 1 second and forced vital capacity as well as the ratio of forced expiratory volume in 1 second to forced vital capacity all decrease in the elderly.[137] Flow in the small airways also declines with age. There is an increased tendency for small airways to collapse sooner during expiration.

A variety of age-related changes produce relative inefficiency in control and monitoring of ventilation. Kronenberg and Drage[138] suggested impaired ventilatory responses to both hypoxia and hypercapnia at rest in old age. Elderly people are less able to perceive acute bronchoconstriction (cause still unclear), resulting in decreased awareness of respiratory symptoms, and

increased mortality from acute respiratory problems.[139] Mucociliary clearance is reduced in old age.[140] Maximal oxygen uptake also declines with age.

Overall lack of fitness (deconditioning) exacerbates all the age-related changes detailed previously, leading to further compromise in the elderly.

Gastrointestinal

For the most part, the digestive system maintains normal functioning in the elderly. Up to 40% of healthy elderly people complain of a dry mouth. Although baseline salivary flow decreases with aging, stimulated salivation is unchanged in both healthy and edentulous geriatric patients.[141] Chewing power is diminished, probably because of decreased bulk of the muscles of mastication.[142] Nilsson et al. demonstrated a weakening of the orolabial pump when the system was stressed by forced repetitive swallows, but not during single swallows (baseline function). The higher prevalence of multiple swallows to clear the oral cavity observed in the elderly reflects an age-related change in the pattern of swallowing rather than an alternation in morphodynamics.[143] There is delay in the initiation of the pharyngeal swallow, decrease in the duration of the pharyngeal swallow, and decrease in the opening duration of the cricopharyngeus. Thus, a large portion of the bolus may enter the valleculae before laryngeal elevation, increasing the risk of aspiration. In general, the coupling between oral and pharyngeal phases of swallowing was diminished with aging.[144] Despite early data to the contrary, the physiological function of the esophagus in otherwise healthy individuals is well-preserved with increasing age, with the exception of very old patients.[145]

Most studies on gastric histology have found evidence of an increased prevalence of atrophic gastritis in people older than 60 years.[146] Aging results in an overall decline in gastric acid output.[147] Gastric emptying of solids remains intact in the elderly, although liquid emptying is prolonged.[148]

Small bowel histology and transit time do not appear to change with age in humans. Small bowel absorptive capacity for most nutrients remains intact. Several histologic changes have been demonstrated in the colon,[147] and colonic transit time decreases with aging. Anorectal physiological changes in the elderly include decreased resting anal sphincter pressure and decreased rectal wall elasticity.

Anatomic studies on the liver reveal an age-related decrease in weight, number, and size of hepatocytes.[149] The major functional changes in older patients are

TABLE 24-3

Effects of Age on Serum Hormone Levels

Increased Levels	Normal Levels	Decreased Levels
Atrial natriuretic peptide	Calcitonin	Corticotropin[b]
Insulin	Cortisol[a]	Thyroid-stimulating hormone[c]
Norepinephrine	Epinephrine	Growth hormone
Parathormone	Prolactin	Insulin-like growth factor-1 (somatomedin C)
Vasopressin	Thyroxine (T_4)	Renin
		Aldosterone
		Triiodothyronine (T_3)

[a]Mildly increased in some studies.
[b]May be normal.
[c]May be normal; in approximately 15% of persons older than age 65, thyroid-stimulating hormone is increased because of autoimmune thyroiditis, not because of age.
Source: Reprinted with permission from WB Abrams, MH Beers, R Berkow, et al. (eds), Metabolic and Endocrine Disorders. In The Merck Manual of Geriatrics (2nd ed). Whitehouse Station, NJ: Merck Research Laboratories, 1995;981–984.

TABLE 24-4

Effects of Age on Serum Levels of Steroids and Related Hormones

Increased Levels	Normal Levels	Decreased Levels
Elderly women		
Follicle-stimulating hormone	Total testosterone	Androsterone
		Dehydroepiandrosterone
Luteinizing hormone	—	Dehydroepiandrosterone sulfate
Ovarian testosterone[a]	—	Estradiol
		Estrone
		Progesterone
Elderly men		
Dihydrotesterone[b]	—	Androstenedione
		Androsterone
Follicle-stimulating hormone	—	Dehydroepiandrosterone
		Dehydroepiandrosterone sulfate
Luteinizing hormone	—	—
Free estradiol	—	Testosterone
Free esterone	—	Bioavailable testosterone

[a]May be normal.
[b]High in men with benign prostatic hyperplasia, but tends to be normal in men without benign prostatic hyperplasia.
Source: Reprinted with permission from WB Abrams, MH Beers, R Berkow, et al. (eds), Metabolic and Endocrine Disorders. In The Merck Manual of Geriatrics (2nd ed). Whitehouse Station, NJ: Merck Research Laboratories, 1995;981–984.

reduction in hepatic blood flow, altered clearance of certain drugs, and delayed hepatic regeneration after injury.

Several alterations of adult gastrointestinal disease occur in the elderly. Acute abdominal pain appears to mute with age. Pain localization is often atypical in elderly patients. The causes of acute abdominal pain differ as well. A multicenter review found that 25% of emergency room patients older than 70 years had cancer as the etiology of pain, whereas below age 50 they had malignancy as the explanation in less than 1% of cases.[150] Acute appendicitis may have few overt abdominal signs and may therefore progress more frequently to gangrene and perforation.[151]

Gastroesophageal reflux disease has a higher prevalence rate and a greater number of associated complications in the elderly.[146] Gastroduodenal ulcer disease has a several-fold greater incidence, hospitalization rate, and mortality in the elderly because of an increase in injurious agents (such as *Helicobacter pylori*, medications) and impaired defense mechanisms.

In conclusion, normal physiological changes in the aged gastrointestinal tract are few. Therefore, one must weed out and actively treat gastrointestinal tract disorders of the elderly and not ascribe these symptoms to the aging process.[141] Elderly patients have diminished reserve capacity to accommodate illness and should be thoughtfully evaluated and treated early in the course of the disease to prevent irreversible deterioration.[152]

Endocrine

With aging, many aspects of the endocrine system change. Some endocrine organs and axes become hypoactive, either from diseases or physiological down-regulation; some change little or not at all; and a few become hyperactive. These diverse and at times striking changes result from changes in hormone production and secretion rates, metabolic clearance rates, and tissue responsiveness or sensitivity. Serum hormone levels reflect the sum of all these changes (Tables 24-3 and 24-4).[153]

Clinical Significance of Changes

Knowledge of expected hormonal changes may be clinically useful. For example, the increase in serum insulin caused by insulin resistance requires weight loss and exercise to protect the patient from the adverse effects of hyperinsulinemia. The increase in parathormone leads to accelerated bone resorption and, in women, requires calcium supplements and estrogen replacement therapy, both of which suppress bone resorption and parathormone secretion. The increase in vasopressin predisposes the elderly to hyponatremia (hypo-osmolarity, water intoxication). Drug-induced hyponatremia is seen almost exclusively in persons older than 60 years. The high serum level of atrial natriuretic peptide, a potent diuretic, may contribute to nocturia in older people. Growth hormone secretion decreases markedly with aging, and the response to all stimuli is then blunted.[154]

Skin

Aging of the skin is a highly complex process. The epidermis that serves a barrier function to skin is still able to do so in elderly, but its moisture content and cohesiveness are reduced, coupled with an increase in renewal time of damaged cells.[155] These changes are manifest clinically as dry, rough skin. Epidermal thickness decreases only slightly with age.[156] Another hallmark of aged skin is flattening of the dermal-epidermal junction, which manifests as an enhanced susceptibility to simple trauma and shearing forces. The number of epidermal Langerhans' cells, involved in immune surveillance, is reduced in aging skin, causing increased risk of skin cancer. The physiological changes in the dermis with aging include decrease in number and size of fibroblasts; decreased ability of fibroblasts to produce extracellular matrix components such as collagen and elastin, causing decreased rate of healing and increased susceptibility to shearing force trauma; and decreased vascularity, causing pale skin and impaired thermoregulation. In addition, sweat glands are reduced in number and function in aged skin, further reducing the ability to thermoregulate. Aging reduces and disorganizes the nerve supply of the skin, therefore causing an increased threshold to pain. Graying of the scalp and beard hair is caused by reduction (gray hair) or loss (white hair) of melanin from hair follicles. Nails grow more slowly in the elderly and are brittle and longitudinal. There is evidence that topical retinoids, a metabolite of vitamin A, may improve clinical features of aged skin.[157]

Bone and Joints

There are three principal functions of the musculoskeletal system: provide mechanical support and protection to the soft tissue structures; permit movement of the limbs; and enable calcium homeostasis by acting as a mineral reservoir. It is notable that the first two of these functions are frequently compromised in the aged patient and are the root cause of pain and disability in people older than age 65.[158]

The process of senescence affects articular cartilage and skeletal structures as well as soft tissues. As aging occurs, osteoarthritis, osteoporosis, reduced range of motion, and stiffness set in. The alterations in the body that occur with age happen because of a variety of mechanisms: accumulation of degradation products such as proteoglycan in tissue matrix; decrease in mesenchymal stem cell production; and decreased synthetic ability of differentiated cells (osteoblast and chondrocyte) and reduction in matrix.[159]

As aging sets in there, the amount of calcium in the skeleton declines. This process is accelerated in women for 5 years after menopause.[160] Changes in skeletal structure cause bone to become weaker and more vulnerable to fractures.[161] It is thought that with age, the bony cortex becomes thinner because of inner medullary cavity expansion leading to microfractures.[162]

Bone remodeling is a process of bone formation and resorption that deploys special types of cells known as *osteoblasts* and *osteoclasts*. Age-related bone loss is attributable to excessive osteoclastic activity. Increased osteoclastic activity is linked to menopausal decline in ovarian function.[163] Another reason for elevated osteoclastic activity in the elderly is dietary vitamin D deficiency along with reduced sun exposure.

Articular Cartilage

Articular cartilage serves an important role in the human skeleton by cushioning the subchondral bone and providing a low friction surface for unrestricted movement. Articular cartilage is an avascular, aneural tissue that withstands the challenge of biomechanical stress. Mechanical features of cartilage that are altered with age include a decrease in tensile stiffness, fatigue resistance, and strength but no change in compressive properties. Many of these changes are attributable to age-related decrement in tissue water content. Another important change occurring in the aged patient is an alteration in the two main matrix constituents of the chondrocyte: proteoglycan (aggrecan) and type II collagen. With age, there is a reduction in proteoglycan aggregation, and collagen increases in fiber diameter and cross-linking.[158] These changes lead to cartilage fibrillation and loss.

The normal aging process causes cartilage to wear down, which leads to osteoarthritis. This is associated with alterations in other joint tissues. There is irregular thickening and remodeling of the subchondral bone with associated sclerosis and cysts. The joint capsule may show thickening, distortion, and fibrosis. Chronic synovitis and osteophytosis may occur.[158] Joints typically involved in order of frequency are knees, first metatarsal phalangeal, distal interphalangeal, carpal metacarpal, hips, cervical spine, and lumbar spine. Large weight-bearing joints usually show the greatest clinical disability secondary to pain and limitation of functional activities.[164]

Soft Tissue Structure

With age, there are significant changes in ligaments, intervertebral disks, tendons, and joint capsules. As water content of tissue declines with age, tissues become more susceptible to external damage. Changes in tensile strength of tendons and ligaments and joint capsule integrity also occur.[158]

Genitourinary System

Reduced kidney function, often seen in the older adult patient as a consequence of illness and chronic disease, adversely affects optimal regulation of composition and volume of extracellular fluid. The effect of atherosclerosis, infection, diabetes, and age-related alterations may have a substantial effect on kidney function.

The normal aging process can bring about significant changes in the anatomic appearance of the nephron. A decrease in parenchymal mass and a net reduction in kidney weight occur.[165] A significant reduction in the size and quantity of nephrons is also common. On a microscopic level, parenchymal mass reduction results in changes in the architecture of the interstitial spaces between the tubule structures. As the weight of the kidneys experience an age-related decline, a net reduction in glomeruli occurs.[166] It is estimated that the amount of sclerotic glomeruli increase to 12% after age 50 from 1–2% during the third to fifth decades. Many of the alterations in kidney function observed in old age, independent of coexisting illness and disease, are attributable to alterations in intrarenal blood supply. Pathophysiological changes can be imposed by various disease processes, including hypertension, diabetes, atherosclerosis, and pyelonephritis.

Functional Changes

As a direct consequence of the normal aging process, there is a well-recognized reduction in plasma flow from 600 ml in young adults to 300 ml during the octogenarian years.[167] There is also a significant decline in glomerular filtration rate, as determined by inulin or creatinine clearance values. Creatinine clearance is generally thought to be stable until age 45 when a linear decrease is noted.[167]

Despite declining glomerular filtration rates in advancing age among relatively healthy patients, there is not generally an observed elevation in serum creatinine. The reason for this is that muscle mass (containing creatinine) also is known to decrease with age at virtually the same rate as the glomerular filtration rate declines.

Tubular structures, responsible for excretory and resorptive functions, change with age. The aged kidney is able to sustain normal homeostatic mechanisms including optimization of acid–base balance and electrolyte concentrations. During abnormal stress situations, however, water and salt processing is adversely affected in the geriatric patient, resulting in a malfunctioning of the normal sodium excretory and conservational mechanism. Maintenance of normal potassium balance is another challenge of the aged kidney.

Sexuality

Sexuality, an essential part of human existence, is undoubtedly affected by the normal and pathologic aging process. *Sexuality* is defined as the expression of a person's femaleness or maleness through personality, body dress, and behavior.[168] The primary obstacles to sexuality in the older individual are medical, social, and psychological barriers.

Old age confers a gradual change in sexual function. Advancing age and falling testosterone levels can result in multiple organ consequences and have been linked to heightened risk for myocardial infarction and bone fracture.[169,170] Although no specific definable menopause transition occurs for men, a gradual decline in testosterone levels occurs after the third decade. This decline does not go below a baseline threshold, leaving most men in their seventh decade with testosterone levels in the same range as their younger counterparts.

Physiological changes that interfere with the sexual experience of older men include testicular crenation (gradual atrophy) and the onset of penile flaccidity, requiring a greater degree of tactile stimulation to achieve erection and engorgement. A truncation of orgasmic time and an increase in *down time* is not uncommon. Ejaculatory force and volume are also decreased.

Disease states also contribute to impotence in older men. These include arthritis, emphysema, prostatitis, diabetes, heart disease, heart failure, hypertension, pelvic steal syndrome, stroke, stress incontinence, and Peyronie's disease. Medications can also have a dramatic effect on potency.

Women, too, undergo changes accompanied by the normal aging process. Hormonal adjustments are obviously far more pronounced in woman patients. Reduced estrogen production ascribable to menopause is universally seen. Physical issues include a change in shape and configuration of the vaginal wall. Increased vaginal dryness and thinning may also occur, which can result in bleeding and pain during coitus. A heightened increase in vaginal infection can occur in response to less acidic vaginal secretions.

Hematology and Immunology

With age, hematopoietic inactive adipose tissue replaces red hematopoietic active tissue[171] and cellularity is reduced to 30% of its original baseline.[172] Peripheral blood lymphocyte concentrations decline with age. This results in alteration in quantity of CD4 T-helper cells. CD8 T-suppressor cells, B lymphocytes, and granulocyte effector cells are also affected by age. Although anemia is common in old age, several studies of healthy seniors failed to reveal abnormalities in hemoglobin.[173] Several secondary factors in older patients can contribute to anemia such as infection, diet, disease, and medications. The role of antioxidant vitamins such as vitamin E have been described in preventing normal aging.

Homeostatic Changes

The ability of the elderly to regulate their internal body temperature and to adjust to different thermal environments deteriorates with aging.[174] In response to hot environments, there is a reduction in ability to increase cutaneous blood flow.[175] Sweating decreases in the elderly.[176] The response to a cold environment is also impaired with decreased cutaneous vasoconstrictor response and a less effective shivering response.[177] Fever response in the presence of infection is blunted.[178] There is a diminished sense of thirst in the elderly, and few older people take any fluids between meals.[179] These facts coupled with orthostatic hypotension, which occurs in 11–30% of older persons,[180] indicate the need to advise patients and modify activity and exercise prescriptions to recommend appropriate environmental temperature restrictions with avoidance of rapid movements and encouragement of fluid replacement.

The elderly have altered pain perception and tend to minimize pain reporting. They may attribute pain to normal aging and expectations of aging in a form of age-

ism: "What do you expect? I am old." They may require higher levels of stimulation before reporting pain. Underlying this change in pain perception and reporting is a loss of peripheral sensory fibers, an apparent decline in the functional response of nociceptive primary afferent Aδ and C fibers, alterations in central nervous system biochemistry, and diminished central nervous system electrophysiological activity to incoming noxious stimuli. These changes may be counterbalanced to some extent by a parallel loss of endogenous pain inhibitory systems.[14]

EXERCISE IN THE ELDERLY

As more individuals live longer, it is imperative to determine the extent and mechanisms by which exercise and physical activity can improve health, functional capacity, quality of life, and independence in this population.[181]

Participation in a regular exercise program is an effective intervention modality to reduce or prevent a number of functional declines associated with aging (see the section Muscle Strength and Endurance and Range of Motion). Furthermore, the trainability of older individuals is evidenced by their ability to adapt and respond to both endurance and strength training.

Endurance training can help maintain and improve various aspects of cardiovascular function (as measured by maximal $\dot{V}o_2$, output, and arteriovenous O_2 difference) as well as enhance submaximal performance.[132] Importantly, reductions in risk factors associated with disease states (heart disease, diabetes, and so forth) improve health status and contribute to an increase in life expectancy.[182–184]

Strength training helps offset the loss in muscle mass and strength typically associated with normal aging.[185,186] Additional benefits from regular exercise include improved bone health and, thus, reduction in risk of osteoporosis; improved postural stability, thereby reducing the risk of falling and associated injuries and fractures[187,188]; and increased flexibility and range of motion. Evidence also suggests that regular exercise provides some psychological benefits related to preserved cognitive function,[189] alleviation of depression symptoms and behavior, and improved concept of personal control and self-efficacy.

REFERENCES

1. National Center for Health Statistics. Vital Statistics of the United States, Life Tables. Vol II, Sec 6. Washington, DC: US Government Printing Office, 1985;88–104.

2. Stein B, Felsenthal G. Geriatric Rehabilitation. In BJ O'Young, MA Young, SA Stiens (eds), Physical Medicine and Rehabilitation Secrets.

Philadelphia: Hanley & Belfus, 1996; 428–435.

3. Gaby SK, Machlin LJ. Vitamin Intake and Health: A Scientific

Review. New York: Marcel Dekker, 1991.

4. Rimm EB. Vitamin E consumption and the risk of coronary heart disease in men. N Engl J Med 1993;328:1450–1455.

5. Katzman R, Terry R. Normal aging of the nervous system. In R Katzman, JW Rowe (eds), Principles of Geriatric Neurology. Philadelphia: FA Davis, 1992;18–58.

6. Goldman J, Cote LJ. Aging of the Brain: Dementia of the Alzheimer's Type. In E Kandel, J Schwartz, TM Tessell (eds), Principles of Neural Science (3rd ed). Norwalk, CT: Appleton & Lange, 1991;974–983.

7. Murphy DG, DeCarli C, McIntosh AR, et al. Sex differences in human brain morphometry and metabolism: an in vivo quantitative magnetic resonance imaging and positron emission tomography study on the effect of aging. Arch Gen Psychiatry 1996;53:585–594.

8. Brody H. Organization of the cerebral cortex: III. A study of aging in the human cerebral cortex. J Comp Neurol 1955;102:511–556.

9. Anderson B, Rutledge V. Age and hemisphere effects on dendritic structure. Brain 1996;119:1983–1990.

10. Eriksson PS, Perfilieva E, Bjork-Eriksson T, et al. Neurogenesis in the adult human hippocampus. Nature Med 1998;4:1313–1317.

11. Brizzee KR. Gross Morphometric Analyses and Quantitative Histology of the Aging Brain. In JM Ordy, KR Brizzee (eds), Neurobiology of Aging. London: Plenum Press, 1975;401–424.

12. Prineas JW, Spencer PS. Pathology of the Nerve Cell Body in Disorders of the Peripheral Nervous System. In PJ Dyck, PK Thomas, EH Lambert (eds), Peripheral Neuropathy. Philadelphia: WB Saunders, 1975;253–295.

13. Corbin KB, Gardner ED. Decrease in number of myelinated fibers in human spinal roots with age. Anat Rec 1937;68:63–74.

14. Gibson SJ, Helme RD. Age differences pain perception and report: a review of physiological, psychological, laboratory and clinical studies. Pain Rev 1995;2:111–137.

15. Murphy C, Wetter S, Morgan CD, et al. Age effects on central nervous system activity reflected in the olfactory event-related potential: evidence for decline in middle age. Ann N Y Acad Sci 1998;855:598–607.

16. Matsuda T, Doty RL. Regional taste sensitivity to NaCl: relationship to subject age, tongue locus and areas of stimulation. Chem Senses 1995;20:283–290.

17. Weinstein BE. Disorders of Hearing. In R Tallis, H Fillit, JC Brocklehurst (eds), Brocklehurst's Textbook of Geriatric Medicine and Gerontology (5th ed). Edinburgh: Churchill Livingstone, 1998;673–684.

18. Dolman CL, McCormick AQ, Drance SM. Aging of the optic nerve. Arch Ophthalmol 1980;98:2053–2058.

19. Schaumberg HH, Spencer PS, Ochoa J. The Aging Human Peripheral Nervous System. In R Katzman, R Terry (eds), The Neurology of Aging. Philadelphia: FA Davis, 1983;111–122.

20. Brizzee KR, Ordy JM. Effects of Age on Visceral Afferent Components of the Autonomic Nervous System. In JM Ordy, KR Brizzee (eds), Sensory Systems and Communication in the Elderly. New York: Raven Press, 1979;283–296.

21. Winkelmann RK. Nerve changes in the aging skin. Adv Biol Skin 1965;6:51–61.

22. Thornbury JM, Mistretta CM. Tactile sensitivity as a function of age. J Gerontol 1981;36:34–39.

23. Dyck PJ, Schultz PW, O'Brien PC. Quantitation of touch-pressure sensation. Arch Neurol 1972;26:465–473.

24. Stevens JC. Aging and spatial acuity of touch. J Gerontol (Psych Sci) 1992;47:35–40.

25. Verillo RT. Age related changes in sensitivity to vibration. J Gerontol 1980;35:185–193.

26. Frisena RD, Gescheider GA. Comparison of child and adult vibrotactile thresholds as a function of frequency and duration. Percept Psychophysiol 1977;22:100–103.

27. Potvin AR, Syndulko K, Tourtellotte WN, et al. Human neurologic function and the aging process. J Am Geriatr Soc 1980;28:1–9.

28. Kokmen E, Bossemeyer RW, Williams WJ. Quantitative evaluation of joint motion sensation in an aging population. J Gerontol 1978;1:62–67.

29. Skinner HB, Barrack RL, Cook SD. Age-related decline in proprioception. Clin Orthop 1984;184:208–211.

30. Procacci P, Bozza G, Buzzelli G, et al. The cutaneous pricking pain sensation in old age. Gerontol Clin 1970;12:213–218.

31. Jamal GA, Hansen S, Weir AI, et al. An improved automated method for the measurement of thermal threshold. I. Normal subjects. J Neurol Neurosurg Psychiatry 1985;48:354–360.

32. Tohgi H, Tsukagoshi H, Toyokura Y. Quantitative changes with age in normal sural nerves. Acta Neuropath (Berl) 1977;38:213–220.

33. Drac H, Babiuch M, Wisniewska W. Morphological and biochemical changes in peripheral nerve with aging. Neuropathol Pol 1991;29:49–67.

34. Jennekens FGI, Tomlinson BE, Walton JN. Histochemical aspects of five limb muscles in old age: an autopsy study. J Neurol Sci 1971;14:259–276.

35. Dorfman LJ, Bosley TM. Age-related changes in peripheral and central nerve conduction in man. Neurology 1979;29:38–44.

36. Buchthal F, Rosenfalck A. Evoked action potentials and conduction velocity in human sensory nerves. Brain Res 1966;3:1–122.

37. Munoz M, Boutros-Toni F, Preux PM, et al. Prevalence of neurological disorders in Haute-Vienne department (Limousin region-France). Neuroepidemiology 1995;14:193–198.

38. O' Sullivan DJ, Swallow M. The fibre size and content of the radial and sural nerves. J Neurol Neurosurg Psychiatry 1968;31:464–470.

39. Cress ME, Schultz E. Aging muscle: functional, morphologic, biochemical and regenerative capacity. Topics Geriatr Rehabil 1985;1(1):11–19.

40. Cummings WJK. Aging in Neuromuscular Disease. In R Tallis, H Fillit, JC Brocklehurst (eds), Brocklehurst's Textbook of Geriatric Medicine and Gerontology (5th ed). Edinburgh: Churchill Livingstone, 1998;1115–1129.

41. Swash M, Fox KP. The effect of age on human skeletal muscle: studies of the morphology and innervation of muscle spindles. J Neurol Sci 1972;16:417–432.

42. Tzankoff SP, Norris AH. Effect of muscle mass decrease on age-related BMR changes. J Appl Physiol 1977;43:1001–1006.

43. Lexell J, Taylor CC, Sjostrom M. What is the cause of ageing atrophy? Total number, size and proportion of different fiber types studied in whole vastus lateralis muscle from 15- to 83-year-old men. J Neurol Sci 1988;84:275–294.

44. Aniansson A, Hedberg M, Henning GB, et al. Muscle morphology, enzymatic activity and muscle strength in elderly men: a follow-up study. Muscle Nerve 1986;9:585–591.

45. Booth FW, Weeden SH, Tseng BS. Effect of ageing on human skeletal muscle and motor function. Med Sci Sports Exerc 1994;26:556–560.

46. Stalberg E, Borges O, Ericsson M, et al.

The quadriceps femoris muscle in 20–70 year old subjects: relationship between knee extension torque, electrophysiological parameters and muscle fibre characteristics. Muscle Nerve 1989;12:382–389.

47. Tomlinsson BE, Irving D. The number of limb motor neurons in the human lumbosacral cord throughout life. J Neurol Sci 1977;34:382–389.

48. Kawamura Y, O'Brien P, Okazaki H, et al. Lumbar motoneurons of man II: the number and diameter distribution of large- and intermediate- diameter cytons in motoneuron columns of spinal cord of man. J Neuropathol Exp Neurol 1977;36:861–870.

49. Grimby G, Danneskiold-Samsoe B, Hvid K, et al. Morphology and enzymatic capacity in arm and leg muscles in 78–81 year old men and women. Acta Physiol Scand 1982;115:123–134.

50. Lexell J, Downham D, Sjostrom M. Distribution of different fibre types in human skeletal muscles: fiber type arrangement in m. vastus lateralis from three groups of healthy men between 15 and 83 years. J Neurol Sci 1986;72:211–222.

51. Brown WF. A method for estimating the number of motor units in thenar muscles and the changes in motor unit control with ageing. J Neurol Neurosurg Psychiatry 1972;35:845–852.

52. Campbell MJ, McComas AJ, Petito F. Physiological changes in ageing muscles. J Neurol Neurosurg Psychiatry 1973;36:174–182.

53. Wang F-C, de Pasquia V, Delwaide PJ. Age-related changes in fastest and slowest conducting axons of thenar motor units. Muscle Nerve 1999;22:1022–1029.

54. Lexell J, Downham D. What is the effect of ageing on type 2 muscle fibres? J Neurol Sci 1992;107:250–251.

55. Lexell J, Henriksson-Larsen K, Winblad B, et al. Distribution of different fiber types in human skeletal muscles: effects of aging studied in whole muscle cross sections. Muscle Nerve 1983;6:588–595.

56. Grimby G, Saltin B. The ageing muscle. Clin Physiol 1983;3:209–218.

57. Coggan AR, Spina RJ, Rogers MA, et al. Histochemical and enzymatic characteristics of skeletal muscle in master athletes. J Appl Physiol 1990;68:1896–1901.

58. Larsson L. Morphological and functional characteristics of aging skeletal muscle in man. A cross sectional study. Acta Physiol Scand Suppl 1978;457:1–36.

59. Essen-Gustavsson B, Borges O. Histochemical and metabolic characteristics of human skeletal muscle in relation to age. Acta Physiol Scand 1986;126:107–114.

60. Florini JR, Ewton DZ. Skeletal muscle fiber types and myosin ATPase activity do not change with age or growth hormone administration. J Gerontol 1989;44:B110–B117.

61. Vandervoort AA, Hayes KC, Belanger AY. Strength and endurance of skeletal muscle in the elderly. Physiother Can 1986;38:167–173.

62. Davies CTM, Thamos DO, White MJ. Mechanical properties of young and elderly human muscle. Acta Med Scand Suppl 1986;711:219–226.

63. Shock NW, Greulich RC, Costa PT, et al. Normal Human Aging. Baltimore: US Department of Health and Human Services, 1984.

64. Korten AE, Henderson AS, Christensen H, et al. A prospective study of cognitive function in the elderly. Psychol Med 1997;27:919–930.

65. Unger JM, van Belle G, Heyman A. Cross-sectional versus longitudinal estimates of cognitive change in nondemented older people: a CERAD study. J Am Geriatr Soc 1999;47:559–563.

66. Barclay L, Wolfaon L. Normal Aging: Pathophysiologic and Clinical Changes. In L Barclay (ed), Clinical Geriatric Neurology. Philadelphia: Lea & Febiger, 1993;13–20.

67. Odenheimer G, Funkenstein HH, Beckett L, et al. Comparison of neurologic changes in successfully aging persons vs the total aging population. Arch Neurol 1994;51:573–580.

68. Klawans HL, Tufo HM, Ostefield AN, et al. Neurological examinations in an elderly population. Div Nerv Syst 1971;32:274–279.

69. Hobson W, Pemberton J. The health of the elderly at home. BMJ 1958;I:587–593.

70. Thomas RJ. Blinking and the release reflexes: are they clinically useful. J Am Geriatr Soc 1994;42:609–613.

71. Jenkyn LR, Reeves AG, Warren T, et al. Neurologic signs in senescence. Arch Neurol 1985;42:1154–1157.

72. Evans WJ. What is sarcopenia? J Gerontol 1995;50A:5–8.

73. Knortz KA. Muscle physiology applied to geriatric rehabilitation. Topics Geriatr Rehabil 1987;2:1–12.

74. Asmusson E. Aging and Exercise. In SM Horvath, M Yousef (eds), Environmental Physiology: Aging, Heat and Altitude. Amsterdam: Elsevier, 1980.

75. Faulkner JA, Brooks SV. Age-Related Immobility: The Roles of Weakness, Fatigue, Injury and Repair. In JA Buckwalter, VM Goldberg, SL Woo (eds), Musculoskeletal Soft-Tissue Aging: Impact on Mobility. Rosemont, IL: American Academy of Orthopaedic Surgeons, 1993;187–194.

76. Mathiowetz V, Kashman N, Volland G, et al. Grip and pinch strength: normative data for adults. Arch Phys Med Rehabil 1985;66:69–74.

77. Pearson MB, Bassey EJ, Bendall MJ. The effects of age on muscle strength and anthropometric indices within a group of elderly men and women. Age Ageing 1985;14:230–234.

78. Danneskiold-Samsoe B, Kofod V, Munter J, et al. Muscle strength and functional capacity in 78–81-year-old men and women. Eur J Appl Physiol 1984;52:310–314.

79. Morey MC, Cowper PA, Feussner JR, et al. Two-year trends in physical performance following supervised exercise among community-dwelling older veterans. J Am Geriatr Soc 1991;39:549–554.

80. Brown M. Selected physical performance changes with aging. Topics Geriatr Rehabil 1987;2(4):68–76.

81. Buckwalter JA. Decreased mobility in the elderly. Phys Sports Med 1997;25(9):127–136.

82. Evans WJ. Exercise, nutrition, and aging. Clin Geriatr Med 1995;11(4):725–734.

83. Faulkner JA, Brooks SV, Zerba E. Skeletal muscle weakness and fatigue in old age: underlying mechanisms. Ann Rev Gerontol Geriatr 1990;10:147–166.

84. Fiatarone MA, O'Neill EF, Ryan ND, et al. Exercise training and nutritional supplementation for physical frailty in very elderly people. N Engl J Med 1994;330:1769–1775.

85. Kirkendall DT, Garrett WE. The effects of aging and training on skeletal muscle. Am J Sports Med 1998;26:598–602.

86. Smith EL, Gilligan C. Fitness Declines and Assessment in Older Adults. In TF Drury (ed), Assessing Physical Fitness and Physical Activity in Population Based Surveys. Washington, DC: Government Printing Office, 1989.

87. Adrian MJ. Flexibility in the Aging Adult. In EL Smith, RC Serfass (eds), Exercise and Aging: The Scientific Basis. Hillside, NJ: Enslow Publishing, 1981;45–58.

88. Canada Fitness Survey: Fitness and Lifestyle in Canada. Ottawa: Canadian

Fitness and Lifestyle Research Institute, 1983.

89. Johns RJ, Wright V. Relative importance various tissues in joint stiffness. J Appl Physiol 1962;117:824–828.

90. Munns K. Effect of Exercise on Range of Joint Motion in Elderly Subjects. In EL Smith, RC Serfass (eds), Exercise and Aging: The Scientific Basis. Hillside, NJ: Enslow Publishing, 1981;167–178.

91. Kaufman T. Posture and age. Top Geriatr Rehabil 1987;2(4):13–28.

92. Sixt E, Landahl S. Postural disturbances in a 75-year old population. I. Prevalence and functional consequences. Age Ageing 1987;16:393–398.

93. Gerson LW, Jarjoura D, McCord G. Risk of imbalance in elderly people with impaired hearing and vision. Age Ageing 1989;18:31–34.

94. Tideiksaar R. Disturbances of Gail, Balance, and the Vestibular System. In R Tallia, H Fillit, JC Brocklehurst (eds), Brocklehurst's Textbook of Geriatric Medicine and Gerontology (5th ed). Edinburgh: Churchill Livingstone, 1998;595–609.

95. Ring C, Nayok USL, Isaacs B. The effect of visual deprivation and proprioceptive change on postural sway in healthy adults. J Am Geriatr Soc 1989;37:745–749.

96. Rosenhall U, Rubin W. Degenerative changes in the human vestibular sensory epithelial. Acta Otolaryngol 1975;79:67–81.

97. Baloh RW, Fife TD, Zwerling L, et al. Comparison of static and dynamic posturography in young and older normal people. J Am Geriatr Soc 1994;42:405–412.

98. Stelmach GE, Teasdale N, DiFabio RP, et al. Age-related decline in postural control mechanisms. Int J Aging Hum Dev 1989;29:205–223.

99. Woollacott MH. Changes in posture and voluntary control in the elderly: research findings and rehabilitation. Top Geriatr Rehabil 1990;5:1–11.

100. Luchies CW, Alexander NB, Schultz AB, et al. Stepping responses of young and old adults to postural disturbances: kinematics. J Am Geriatr Soc 1994;42:506–512.

101. Manchester D, Woollacott M, Zederbauer-Hylton N, et al. Vestibular and somatosensory contributions to balance control in the older adult. J Gerontol 1989;44:M118–M127.

102. Sherwood DE, Selder DJ. Cardiorespiratory health, reaction time and aging. Med Sci Sports 1979;11:186–189.

103. Bohannon RW, Larkin PA, Cook AC. Decrease in timed balance test scores with aging. Phys Ther 1984;64:1067–1070.

104. Winter DA, Patla AE, Frank JS, et al. Biomechanical walking pattern changes in the fit and healthy elderly. Phys Ther 1990;70:340–347.

105. Dawson D, Hendershot G, Fulton J. Aging in the Eighties: Functional Limitations of Individuals Age 65 and Over. Advance Data from Vital and Health Statistics, Number 113. Hyatteville, MD: Public Health Service, 1987.

106. Himann JE, Cunningham DA, Rechnitzer PA. Age related changes in speed of walking. Med Sci Sports Exerc 1988;20:161–166.

107. Alexander NB. Gait disorders in older adults. J Am Geriatr Soc 1996;44:434–451.

108. Murray MP, Kory RC, Clarkson BH. Walking patterns in healthy old men. J Gerontol 1969;24:169–178.

109. Murray MP, Kory RC, Sepic SB. Walking patterns of normal women. Arch Phys Med Rehabil 1970;51:637–650.

110. Azar GJ, Lawton AH. Gail and stepping as factors in the frequent falls of elderly women. Gerontologist 1964;4:83–84,103.

111. Simoneau CG, Cavanagh PR, Ulbrecht JS, et al. The influence of visual factors in fall-related kinematic variables during stair descent by older women. J Gerontol 1991;46:M188–M195.

112. Pitts DG. Effects of Aging on Selected Visual Functions: Dark Adaptation, Visual Acuity Stereognosis and Brightness Contrast. In R Sekuler, D Kline, K Dismutes (eds), Aging and Human Visual Function. New York: Alan R Liss, 1982;131–159.

113. Lowenfeld IE. Pupillary Changes Related to Age. In HS Thompson (ed), Topics in Neuro-ophthalmology. Baltimore: Williams & Wilkins, 1979;1214–1250.

114. Bowine PR, Smith SA, Smith SE. Dynamics of the light reflex and the influence of age on the human pupil measured by television pupillometry. J Physiol (Lond) 1979;293:1–10.

115. Coile DC, Baker HD. Foveal dark adaptation, photopigment regeneration and aging. Vis Neurosci 1991;9:27–39.

116. Jaffe GJ, Alvarado JA, Juster RP. Age-related changes of the normal visual field. Arch Ophthalmol 1986;104:1021–1025.

117. Owsley C, Ball K, McGwin G, et al. Visual processing impairment and risk of motor vehicle crash among older adults. JAMA 1998;279:1083–1088.

118. Chamberlain W. Restriction in upward gaze with advancing age. Trans Am Ophthalmol Soc 1970;68:235–244.

119. Sridharan GV, Talis RC, Leatherbarrow B, et al. A community survey of ptosis of the eyelid and pupil size of elderly people. Age Ageing 1995;24:21–24.

120. Pitts MC, Rawles JM. The effect of age on saccadic latency and velocity. Neuroophthalmology 1988;8:123–129.

121. Roy MS, Podgor MJ, Collier B, et al. Color vision and age in a normal North American population. Graefes Arch Clin Exp Ophthalmol 1991;229:139–144.

122. Butler RN, Faye EE, Guazzo E, et al. Keeping an eye on vision: primary eye care of age-related ocular disease. Geriatrics 1997;52:30–41.

123. Strom K. An analysis of 1995 haring instrument sales. Hearing Rev 1996;3:8–36.

124. Goins MA. Geriatric Hearing Loss. In G Felsenthal, SJ Garrison, FU Steinberg (eds), Rehabilitation of the Aging and Elderly Patient. Baltimore: Williams & Wilkins, 1994;339–350.

125. Pathy MSJ. Neurologic Signs in Old Age. In R Tallis, H Fillit, JC Brocklehurst (eds), Brocklehurst's Textbook of Geriatric Medicine and Gerontology (5th ed). Edinburgh: Churchill Livingstone, 1998;423–434.

126. Cooper JC, Gates GA. Hearing in the elderly—the Framingham cohort, 1983–1985: Part II. Prevalence of central auditory processing disorders. Ear Hear 1991;12:304–311.

127. Hansen CG, Reske-Nielsen E. Pathological studies in presbycusis. Arch Otolaryngol 1965;82:115–132.

128. Abrams WB, Beers MH, Berkow R, et al. (eds). Cardiovascular Disorders. In The Merck Manual of Geriatrics (2nd ed). Whitehouse Station, NJ: Merck Research Laboratories, 1995;425–481.

129. Lakatta EG. Cardiovascular aging research: The next horizons. J Am Geriatr Soc 1999;47:613–625.

130. Pearson JD, Morrell CH, Brant LJ, et al. Age-associated changes in blood pressure in a longitudinal study of healthy men and women. J Gerontol 1997;52A:M177–M183.

131. Yamakado T, Takagi E, Okubo S, et al. Effects of aging on left ventricular relaxation in humans. Analysis of left ventricular isovolumic pressure decay. Circulation 1997;95:917–923.

132. Ades PA. Cardiac rehabilitation in older coronary patients. J Am Geriatr Soc 199;47:98–105.

133. Richards GA, Theron AJ, Van der Merwe CA, et al. Spirometric abnormalities in young smokers correlate with increased chemiluminescence response of activated blood phagocytes. Am Rev Resp Dis 1989;139:181–187.

134. Connolly MJ. Age-Related Changes in the Respiratory System. In R Tallis, H Fillit, JC Brocklehurst (eds), Brocklehurst's Textbook of Geriatric Medicine and Gerontology (5th ed). Edinburgh: Churchill Livingstone, 1998;1073–1078.

135. Verbeken EK, Cauberghs M, Mertens I, et al. The senile lung. Comparison with normal and emphysematous lungs. 1. Structural aspects. Chest 1992;101:793–799.

136. Brook MH, Kaiser KK. Muscle fibertypes: how many and what kind. Arch Neurol 1970;23:369–379.

137. Tager IB, Segal MR, Speizer FE, Weiss ST. The natural history of forced expiratory volumes. Effect of cigarette smoking and respiratory symptoms. Am Rev Respir Dis 1988;138:837–849.

138. Kronenberg RS, Drage CW. Attenuation of the ventilatory and heart responses to hypoxia and hypercopria with aging in normal men. J Clin Invest 1973;52:1812–1819.

139. Connolly MJ, Crowley JJ, Charan NB, et al. Reduced subjective awareness of bronchoconstriction provoked by methacholine in elderly asthmatic and normal subjects as measured on a simple awareness scale. Thorax 1992;47:410–413.

140. Goodman RM, Yergin BM, Landa JF, et al. Relationship of smoking history and pulmonary function tests to tracheal mucous velocity in non-smokers, young smokers, ex-smokers and patients with chronic bronchitis. Am Rev Respir Dis 1978;117:205–214.

141. Lovat LB. Age related changes in gut physiology and nutritional status. Gut 1996;38:306–309.

142. Karlsson S, Persson M, Carlsson GE. Mandibular movement and velocity in relation to state of dentition and age. J Oral Rehabil 1991;18:1–8.

143. Nilsson H, Ekberg O, Olsson R, Hindfelt B. Quantitative aspects of swallowing in an elderly nondysphagic population. Dysphagia 1996;11:180–184.

144. Tracey JF, Logeman JA, Kahrilas PJ, et al. Preliminary observations on the effects of age on oropharyngeal deglutition. Dysphagia 1989;4:90–94.

145. Brandt LJ. Upper gastrointestinal diseases and the elderly: an interview. Intern Med World Rep 1995; 10(Suppl):1–2.

146. Bird T, Hall MR, Schade RO. Gastric histology and its relation to anaemia in the elderly. Gerontology 1977;23:309–321.

147. Baime MJ, Nelson JB, Castell DO. Aging of the Gastrointestinal System. In WR Hazzard, EL Bierman, JP Blass, et al. (eds), Principles of Geriatric Medicine and Gerontology (3rd ed). New York: McGraw-Hill, 1994;665–681.

148. Kao CH, Lai TL, Wang SJ, et al. Influence of age on gastric emptying in healthy Chinese. Clin Nucl Med 1994;19:401–404.

149. Keefe EB. Abnormal liver tests and liver disease in the elderly. Practical Gastroenterol 1993;17:16A–17A.

150. Telfer S, Fenyo G, Holt PR, et al. Acute abdominal pain in patients over 50 years of age. Scand J Gastroenterol 1988;23:47–50.

151. Arnbjornsson E, Adren-Sandberg A, Bengmark S. Appendicectomy in the elderly: incidence and operative findings. Ann Chir Gynaecol 1983;72:223–228.

152. Snape WJ Jr. Gastrointestinal disorders in the elderly. II. Bowel dysfunction in the elderly: a growing problem. Intern Med World Rep 1995;10(13):14–24.

153. Abrams WB, Beers MH, Berkow R, et al. (eds). Metabolic and Endocrine Disorders. In The Merck Manual of Geriatrics (2nd ed). Whitehouse Station, NJ: Merck Research Laboratories, 1995;981–984.

154. Winger JM, Hornick T. Age-associated changes in the endocrine system. Nurs Clin North Am 1996;31:827–844.

155. Balin AK, Pratt LA. Physiological consequences of human skin aging. Cutis 1989;43:431–436.

156. Lavker RM. Structural alterations in exposed and unexposed aged skin. J Invest Dermatol 1979;73:59–66.

157. Griffiths CEM. Aging of the Skin. In R Tallis, H Fillit, JC Brocklehurst (eds), Brocklehurst's Textbook of Geriatric Medicine and Gerontology (5th ed). Edinburgh: Churchill Livingstone, 1998;1293–1297.

158. Dieppe P, Tobias J. Bone and Joint Aging. In R Tallis, H Fillit, JC Brocklehurst (eds), Brocklehurst's Textbook of Geriatric Medicine and Gerontology (5th ed). Edinburgh: Churchill Livingstone, 1998;1131–1135.

159. Buckwalter JA, Woo SLY, Goldberg VM, et al. Soft tissue aging and musculoskeletal function. J Bone Joint 1993;75A:1533–1548.

160. Pouilles JM. Effect of menopause on femoral and vertebral loss. J Bone Miner Res 1995;10:1531–1536.

161. Bellantoni M, Madoff D. Osteoporosis and Back Pain: Diagnosis, Treatment and Prevention. In MA Young (ed), Spinal Rehabilitation. Philadelphia: Hanley Belfus, 1995;641–656.

162. Todd RC, Freeman MAR. Isolated trabecular fatigue fractures in the femoral neck. J Bone Joint Surg 1972;54B:723–728.

163. Garnero P, Sornay-Rendu E, Chapuy MC, et al. Increased bone turnover in late postmenopausal woman is a major determinant of osteoporosis. J Bone Miner Res 1996;11:337–349.

164. Hicks JE, Shah JP. Medical and Rehabilitative Management of Rheumatic Diseases. In B O'Young, MA Young, SA Stiens (eds), PM&R Secrets. Philadelphia: Hanley & Belfus, 1997;386–398.

165. Jassal V, Fillit H, Oreopoulos DG. Aging of the Urinary Tract. In R Tallis, H Fillit, JC Brocklehurst (eds), Brocklehurst's Textbook of Geriatric Medicine and Gerontology (5th ed). Edinburgh: Churchill Livingstone, 1998;919–924.

166. McLachlan MSF. The ageing kidney. Lancet 1978;2:143–145.

167. Holtenberg NK. Senescence and the renal vasculature in normal man. Circ Res 1974;34:309–316.

168. Stiens SA, Westheimer RK, Young MA. Satisfying Sexuality Despite Disability. In BJ O'Young, MA Young, SA Stiens (eds), Physical Medicine and Rehabilitation Secrets. Philadelphia: Hanley & Belfus, 1996;62–67.

169. Swartz CM, Young MA. Male hypogonadism: risks for myocardial infarction and bone fracture. Comp Ther 1988;14:421–424.

170. Swartz CM, Young MA. Low serum testosterone and myocardial infarction in geriatric male in-patients. J Am Geriatr Soc 1987;35:39–44.

171. Kricun ME. Red yellow marrow conversion. Skeletal Radiol 1985;14:10–19.

172. Liu PI, Takanarai H, Yatani R, et al. Comparative studies of bone marrow from the United States and Japan. Ann Clin Lab Sci 1989;19:345–351.

173. Garry PJ, Goodwin JS, Hunt WC. Iron status and anemia in the elderly: new findings and a review of previous studies. J Am Geriatr Soc 1983;31:389–399.

174. Collins KJ, Exton-Smith AN. Thermal homeostasis in old age. J Am Geriatr Soc 1983;31:519–524.

175. Kenney WL. Control of heat-induced cutaneous vasodilation in relation to age. Eur Appl Physiol 1988;57:120–125.

176. Inoue Y, Nakao M, Araki T, et al. Regional differences in the sweating responses of older and younger men. J Appl Physiol 1991;71:2453–2459.

177. McCarter RJM. Energy Utilization. In EJ Masoro (ed), Handbook of Physiology. Sec 11: Aging. New York: Oxford University Press, 1995.

178. Norman DC, Grahn D, Yoshikawa TT. Fever and aging. J Am Geriatr Soc 1985;33:859–863.

179. Hunt TE. Homeostatic malfunctions in the aged. BC Med J 1980;22:379–381.

180. Moder SC, Josephson KR, Rubenstein LZ. Low prevalence of postural hypotension among community-dwelling elderly. JAMA 1987;258:1511–1514.

181. Mazzeo R, Cavanagh P, Evans W, et al. Exercise and physical activity for older adults. Med Sci Sports Exerc 1988;30(6):992–1008.

182. Seals D, Hagberg J, Hurley BF, et al. Endurance training in older men and women. I. Cardiovascular responses to exercise. J Appl Physiol 1984;57:1024–1029.

183. Kohrt W, Malley M, Coggan A, et al. Effects of gender, age, and fitness level on response of Vo_2 max to training in 60–71 year olds. J Appl Physiol 1991;71:2004–2011.

184. Forman D, Manning R, Hauser E, et al. Enhanced left ventricular diastolic filling associated with long-term endurance training. J Gerontol 1992;47:M56–M58.

185. Frontera WR, Meredith CN, O'Reilly KP, et al. Strength training and determinants of Vo_2 max in older men. J Appl Physiol 1990;68:329–333.

186. Frontera WR, Meredith CN, O'Reilly KP, et al. Strength conditioning in older men: skeletal muscle hypertrophy and improved function. J Appl Physiol 1988;64:1038–1044.

187. Wolf SL, Barhart HX, Kutner NG, et al. Reducing frailty and falls in older persons: an investigation of Tai Chi and computerized balance training. Atlanta FICSIT Group. Frailty and Injuries: Cooperative Studies of Intervention Techniques. J Am Geriatr Soc 1996;44:489–497.

188. Judge JO, Lindsey C, Underwood M, et al. Balance improvements in older women: effects of exercise training. Phys Ther 1993;73:254–265.

189. Chodzko-Zajko WJ, Moore KA. Physical fitness and cognitive functioning in aging. Exerc Sport Sci Rev 1994;22:195–220.

25

Women's Health Issues

FREDI KRONENBERG, SHARON E. ROBINSON, DAVID A. ROHE, JAN WEINGRAD SMITH, AND JOAN E. EDELSTEIN

Women's physiological development centers on the preparation for, occurrence of, and aftermath of motherhood. Hormonal changes related to childbearing affect every system throughout the life-span. This chapter describes the bodily responses to puberty, menstruation, pregnancy, postpartum period, and menopause.

CHILDHOOD

In the first trimester of pregnancy, the association between the hypothalamus and the anterior pituitary is established in the fetus and is stimulated by gonadotropins produced by the fetus in the second and third trimesters.[1] At birth the ovary contains 1–2 million oocytes.[2] By puberty the germ cell mass is reduced to approximately 300,000–500,000. Reduction results from cycling changes in the ovary during childhood.[3] During early childhood, levels of gonadotropins are low, there is negligible response of the pituitary gland to gonadotropin-releasing hormone (GnRH), and the hypothalamus is suppressed.

PUBERTY

Puberty, often referred to as an individual event, is a combination of physiological and chemical changes that occurs as children grow into adulthood. During adolescence, girls move through the process of physiological maturity, which may or may not coincide with emotional maturity.[4] The general progression of events begins with the initiation of rapid growth and continues with thelarche (breast development), pubarche (growth of pubic and axillary hair in response to increased production of adrenal androgens), and menarche.[1]

Although the exact triggers of puberty are not known, authorities agree that elevated levels of luteinizing hormone (LH), particularly at night, precede the appearance of secondary sex characteristics. As the time of puberty approaches, neurons in the hypothalamus increase their pulsatile secretions of GnRH. This heightens the response of the pituitary gland, which increases production of gonadotropins. These substances stimulate follicular growth, development in the ovary, and increased production of steroid hormones. Increasing levels of estrogen, produced by the ovaries, provide a feedback loop to the hypothalamus. This structure responds by increasing its pulsatile secretions of GnRH, which, in turn, stimulate the secretion of LH and follicle-stimulating hormone (FSH). LH and FSH stimulate the development of the ovarian follicles, which, in turn, produce additional estrogen and increasing levels of progesterone.[1,5]

MENSTRUATION

Menarche

Menarche is the initiation of menstruation. The first menstrual cycle occurring at menarche signals the beginning of reproductive capability for young women. The occurrence of menarche is a visible signal that a continuum of neurologic, chemical, structural, and behavior changes are on schedule. It represents a stage in the development of the relationship between the anterior pituitary gland, the hypothalamus, and the ovary, referred to as the *hypothalamic-pituitary axis*. The cumulative effects of the changing levels of hormones result in the cycling responses of the uterus and menstruation.

In response to GnRH secreted by the hypothalamus, the anterior pituitary secretes the gonadotropic hormones FSH and LH, which cause follicular growth, maturation, and subsequent extrusion of a mature ovum. Production of the ovarian estrogen β-estradiol occurs as the follicle matures. Once the mature ovum is ruptured from its follicle, the theca cells lining the follicle's cavity accelerate the production of progesterone. The theca cell–lined cavity of the extruded ovum is called the *corpus luteum*. Varying levels of estradiol and progesterone are the feedback to the hypothalamus and pituitary that causes a cycle increase and decrease in their production of the gonadotropic hormones. The result of the recurring change in hormonal secretion is a pattern of follicular stimulation and maturing.[1]

Progesterone secreted from the corpus luteum maintains the thickened lining of the uterus while the egg traverses the fallopian tube and, if not fertilized, until it disintegrates. As the corpus luteum ceases its production of progesterone, the levels of FSH and LH begin to pulse upward. These hormones stimulate yet another follicle to begin its process of maturation and lead to spasms of the arterioles in the uterine lining, causing necrosis and shedding of the endometrium.[1]

Figure 25-1 is a classic visual description of the interrelationships between the hypothalamus, pituitary gland, ovaries, and uterus.[5] The figure shows the changing levels of estrogen and progesterone and their effects on the uterine lining. Note that in describing the menstrual cycle, the first day of bleeding or shedding of the necrosed endometrium is day 1 and that ovulation occurs approximately 14 days before the first day of bleeding. The ovarian cycle and the menstrual cycle begin together with the shedding of the endometrial lining and the increase in FSH. The follicular phase of the ovarian cycle occurs as the menstrual and proliferative phase of the menstrual cycle affects the endometrium.

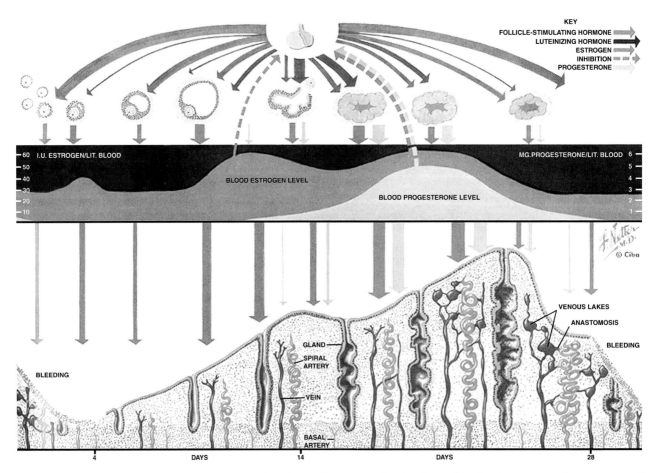

FIGURE 25-1 Pituitary-ovary-endometrium relationships during the menstrual cycle. (Reproduced with permission from F Netter. The Ciba Collection of Medical Illustrations. Vol 2. The Reproductive Tract. Plate 26. Summit, NJ: Ciba Pharmaceutical Products, 1997;115.)

The luteal phase of the ovarian cycle corresponds to the secretory phase of the endometrium.[5]

The most common cycle length is 28 days, but many women experience variations during their lives. Cycles from 24 to 35 days are not unusual.[6] Variations occur in the number of the days of bleeding (menstrual phase; 1–5) or in the number of days of proliferation (10–17), although the secretory phase does not vary. The day of ovulation can be calculated by counting back from the first day of bleeding.[1]

Age of Onset

Changes associated with puberty usually begin between 8 and 14 years of age and occur over a 2- to 4-year span.[1] Young girls can be categorized as early maturing and late maturing according to the chronologic age at which these developmental changes start. Those who begin the process at a younger age tend to be smaller, with broader hips and narrower shoulders than those who begin later. At menarche, most young women are at 96% of their adult height and 80% of their adult weight.[7]

The age of puberty and menarche has become increasingly younger over the past centuries as the interrelationship between endocrine, skeletal, chemical, and physical factors have come to the trigger point for menarche at increasingly younger ages.[8,9] A 10-year prospective study found the average age of menarche to be 12.83, with the range of individual events from 9.14 to 17.70 years.[10] Data collected in a more recent cross-sectional study of clinicians in 225 pediatric practices suggest differences in the timing of the onset of puberty across racial groups with secondary sex characteristics appearing earlier and in a different sequence in black adolescents as compared with whites.[9] Reasons for this trend include improved living conditions, other socioeconomic factors, reduction of life-threatening illnesses, and improved nutrition, as well as genetics.[11]

The timing of the onset of menarche is influenced by body composition. Frisch and McArthur have described a trigger point that is achieved when the ratio of lean body mass to fat reaches approximately 17% of body weight as fat. Their reference for normal weight was a woman who weighed approximately 103 lb; therefore, the absolute percent of body fat may vary somewhat for girls who weigh more than 103 lb.[12] Those who mature earlier have a higher body fat ratio, lower total body water content, and less lean body mass, and these relationships appear to persist when compared after menarche with later maturing girls.[13] Estrogen is stored in fat tissue, and the amount of body fat has an influence on estrogen metabolism. Girls with body fat levels at the extremes of overweight and underweight may experience abnormal ovulatory or bleeding cycles.

Skeletal Effects

The timing of menarche influences skeletal maturity.[14] Immediately before the onset of menarche, growth in height accelerates maximally.[15] Changes in bone mass and pelvic breadth occur during the years immediately preceding and after menarche. Moerman has compared the time relationship in the attainment of adult body dimensions and pelvic diameters between girls maturing early and those maturing late.[7] Late maturing girls have completed more growth in height and pelvic diameters at menarche and therefore have less to complete afterward than early maturing girls. At early menarche, the pelvis is smaller, but more time is available to complete its growth.[7,16]

Estrogen is essential to the development of the genetically determined amounts of bone.[17,18] The critical level of estrogen is achieved just before menarche and must be maintained to participate in the dynamic nature of bone development and resorption. Low estrogen conditions, such as amenorrhea and delayed puberty, can lead to decreased bone mass.[19] Trabecular bone is more sensitive to the metabolic conditions that influence bony growth and loss and show changes sooner than cortical bone.[20]

Athletic Effects

Adolescent athletes who engage in intense physical training and who undergo a weight loss of 10–15% may experience endocrine changes that result in amenorrhea or anovulation. The physiological alternations are caused both by a decreased production of estrogen by the ovaries and a deficit of estrogen from fat storage. Bone health is affected by low estrogen levels, leading to accelerated demineralization, rapid bone resorption, and delay in epiphyseal closure. Calcium intake should be closely monitored and supplemented for young women with habitually low body fat.[21,22]

PREGNANCY

The normal maternal physiological adaptation to pregnancy represents a series of systematic changes that provide the foundation for the growth, development, birth, and nourishment of the developing fetus and new infant. Although fetal growth and development are compartmentalized from the changes in the mother, they are linked by the effects of hormones produced by fetal tissues.

Adolescent Pregnancy

Gynecologic maturity is reached within several years of the onset of menarche. Reproductive maturity can be described in several ages, including chronologic, skeletal, chemical, and gynecologic.[14] The pattern of pelvic growth affects the outcomes of adolescent pregnancy with greater incidence of pelvic inlet contraction and cephalopelvic disproportion, leading to increased rates of operative deliveries for chronologically younger pregnant adolescents who have matured early.[23,24] Although younger teens may not be emotionally ready for pregnancy, those who have achieved menarche early and are gynecologically mature have no greater risks for the obstetric outcomes of pregnancy caused by reproductive system function than their young adult counterparts.

Ovulation, Fertilization, and Uterine Preparation

After ovulation, when the theca cells of the corpus luteum are secreting progesterone, the endometrium becomes secretory, as glycogen collects in the endometrial cells. The glands have a jagged, saw-toothed appearance. Arterioles proliferate and are tortuous, and capillaries are prominent. The endometrium, now termed *decidua*, is rich with protein-secreting glands and arteriole blood supply and is primed for implantation of the fertilized ovum.[5]

The maturing ovum, containing 23 chromosomes, is swept into the fallopian tube by its fimbriae and is transported toward the cornu of the uterus by ciliary action in conjunction with peristalsis of the tubular smooth muscle. After being fertilized by the sperm, which contributes 23 chromosomes during that journey, the cell with its full complement of 46 chromosomes, is termed the *zygote*. Within hours, the cell divides many times to become a mass named the *morula*. Some cells divide more rapidly than others, developing a membrane over the more slowly dividing cells, except at one end. At the same time, the cells secrete a semifluid substance that transforms the mass into a spherical structure termed the *blastocyst*. Ectodermal cells with small tentacle-like projections termed *trophoblasts* cover this vesicle. The cells at the end of the sphere not covered by the membrane differentiate into the beginning cells of the embryo. During this process, the cell mass is traveling the length of the fallopian tube.[5]

A fertilized egg that implants in the fallopian tubes is defined as an *ectopic pregnancy*. Because there is limited room for expansion of the circumference of the tube, ectopic pregnancy represents an obstetric emergency. The tube ruptures, and life-threatening hemorrhage can occur. Symptoms include sudden lower quadrant pain, usually without bleeding, in a woman who has experienced 6–8 weeks of amenorrhea. Often women have not yet confirmed pregnancy at this point. Consequently, any woman of reproductive age who presents with this picture should have a rapid pregnancy test and be treated emergently until ectopic pregnancy is ruled out.[25]

Role of the Placenta

The placenta serves as the site of respiration, excretion, nutrient absorption, and endocrine hormone production. It also shields the fetus from foreign proteins, most bacteria, and maternal blood cells. It develops in the second week after ovulation.[26]

The blastocyst adheres to a spot on the endometrial wall and begins the process of penetrating the epithelium and the mother's circulatory system 2–3 days after entering the uterus. Implantation involves the invasion of the endometrium by the trophoblast cells surrounding the blastocyst. Once it is burrowed into the decidua, the surface layer of endometrial cells closes over the developing mass within the endometrium.[1,27] From this point the trophoblast cells invade the endometrium, opening the arterioles, venules, and glands, and hollowing the intervillous lakes in which the chorionic villi, which are the structural and functional units of the placenta, will rest.[28] The villi are the bridge across which materials pass between the fetal and maternal compartments. Throughout pregnancy, the syncytiotrophoblast serves as the place for gas and nutrient exchange and is an active endocrine unit synthesizing steroid and polypeptide hormones, such as estrogen, progesterone, and human placental lactogen. These substances are necessary for the development and maintenance of pregnancy. Hormones, in concert with others produced by the fetus, enter the maternal circulation, influencing maternal physiological adaptations and stimulating systemic changes in the mother that support gestation.[1,28]

Cardiovascular and Hematologic Changes

Beginning in the first trimester, significant cardiovascular and hematologic changes occur in the mother that ensure an adequate oxygen-carrying capacity for the fetoplacental unit, as well as the mother's own needs.

Although these changes are normal in pregnancy, they would represent cardiac pathology in a nonpregnant person.[29] They include changes in anatomy, blood volume, cardiac output, and systemic vascular resistance that can result in cardiac enlargement, sinus tachycardia, cardiac murmurs, and peripheral edema.[29,30]

Table 25-1 summarizes the alternations that are necessary to ensure an oxygen and nourishment supply system to the fetus without putting the mother's needs at risk.

Common discomforts of pregnancy that result from cardiovascular changes include a maternal perception of the increase in heart rate as palpitations, and, in later pregnancy, supine hypotension, termed *vena cavae syndrome*. This is caused by pressure on the inferior vena cavae by the enlarging uterus when the women remains supine for any length of time. The mother's heart sounds may not be appreciated in the usual locations as the diaphragm pushes the heart slightly upward and dextrorotates it.[30]

Respiratory Changes

The cardiovascular and hematologic adaptations ensure that increased red blood cells, hemoglobin, and plasma volume increase in the oxygen-carrying capacity of the maternal system. Changes occur in the respiratory system, which ensures there will be additional oxygen present. Early in pregnancy, the diaphragm rises approximately 4 cm, which causes the anatomic displacement of the heart described above. The subcostal angle widens as the transverse diameter of the thoracic cage increases by 2 cm. The circumference of the thoracic cavity increases approximately 6 cm. Progesterone causes a reduction in the total pulmonary resistance, which allows the airways to conduct more air.[31] Progesterone may also be responsible for stimulating a physiologic dyspnea, resulting in a slightly lowered P_{CO_2} level. The mild respiratory alkalosis causes the woman to have an increased desire to breathe.[32] These changes result in the movement of increased amounts of oxygen into the lungs and into the circulation. Although the normal adaptations of the respiratory system to pregnancy do not impair respiratory function, any pre-existing or coincident condition that impacts mechanical or chemical respiration may be more serious during gestation.

Nutritional Considerations

In normal pregnancy, changes in digestive peristalsis, appetite, absorption, and metabolism of nutrients; sensitivity of maternal cells to insulin; and decreased gluco-

TABLE 25-1

Cardiovascular and Hematologic Changes in Normal Pregnancy

Parameter	Normal Pregnancy
Blood volume	Increases to 30–50% above nonpregnant level
Red cell mass	Increases to 20–30% above nonpregnant level
Hematocrit	Decreases to an average of 37%
Cardiac output	Increases 30–40% above nonpregnant level
Heart rate	Increases to maximum of 15–20 bpm by 32 weeks
Peripheral resistance	Decreases
Blood pressure	Small decreases in second trimester may return to prepregnant levels in third trimester

Source: Data from JA Pritchard. Changes in the blood volume during pregnancy and delivery. Anesthesiology 1965;26:393; JA Pritchard, RH Adams. Erythrocyte production and destruction during pregnancy. Am J Obstet Gynecol 1960;79:750; and SC Robson, S Hunter, RJ Boys, W Dunlop. Serial study of factors influencing changes in cardiac output during human pregnancy. Am J Physiol 1989;256:H1060.

neogenesis all ensure a constant supply of growth substrate to the fetal compartment, while meeting the mother's metabolic needs.

During the first trimester, there is a drain of glucose and amino acids from the maternal to the fetal compartment without any changes in the role of insulin. This often leads to hypoglycemia in the mother, as well as decreased gluconeogenesis, hypoinsulinemia, and elevated levels of maternal plasma human somatomammotropin.[22] As pregnancy progresses, the fetus and placenta increase in size. The hormones produced by the placenta, namely human placental lactogen, estrogen, cortisol, and progesterone, cause an antagonistic effect in the response of maternal cells to insulin. This effect increases as the surface area of the placenta enlarges. Glucose provides the major fuel for fetal growth. The altered response of maternal cells to the effects of insulin ensures that the maternal cells do not use all available glucose, leaving none in the plasma to cross the placenta. As a result, maternal lipolysis occurs with an increase in circulating free fatty acids that can be used as fuel for maternal cells.[33] This phenomenon is referred to as the *diabetogenic effect of pregnancy*. To compensate for the peripheral insulin resistance, the maternal pancreas increases production of insulin to meet the fuel requirements of maternal cells. Under normal circumstances, the maternal system responds to the challenges of the placental hormones.[22]

Inability of the maternal-fetal-placental compartments to maintain the balance between placental hormone production, insulin resistance, and insulin production leads to pregnancy- or gestationally induced diabetes.[22] At approximately 28 weeks' gestation, most women will be screened for gestational diabetes with a 1-hour, nonfasting, 50-g glucose challenge test. A woman with an elevation in the results of the test should then have the 3-hour glucose tolerance test with preparatory diet. Women with risk factors, such as a first-degree relative with diabetes or obesity, should be screened earlier and more frequently.[34]

Pregnancy requires between 75,000 and 84,000 kcal in total, approximately 300 kcal per day for a woman of normal weight.[35] The prenatal period has been termed an *anabolic state* because of the increase in maternal food intake, the 3.5 kg of fat deposition, and the synthesis of approximately 900 g of new protein distributed among the mother, fetus, and placenta.[35,36]

The body mass index, the relationship of weight to height, is the current standard for evaluating prepregnancy weight status and guiding prenatal weight gain. Table 25-2 shows the current recommendations of the Institute of Medicine for weight gain in pregnancy.[37]

Digestive Changes

To provide the building blocks for maternal needs, as well as fetal growth and development, several changes occur in the digestive system. These include increased appetite; slower peristalsis from the esophagus through the intestinal tract in response to progesterone, estrogen, and relaxin hormones produced by the placenta;

TABLE 25-2
Recommended Total Weight Gain Ranges for Pregnant Women by Prepregnancy Body Mass Index

	Recommended Total Gain[a]	
Weight-for-Height Category	*kg*	*lb*
Low (body mass index <19.8)[b]	12.5–18.0	28–40
Normal (body mass index of 19.8–26.0)	11.5–16.0	25–35
High (body mass index >26.0–29.0)[c]	7.0–11.5	15–25

[a]Young adolescent and black women should strive for gains at the upper end of the recommended range. Short women (<157 cm, or 62 in.) should strive for gains at the lower end of the range.
[b]Body mass index is calculated using metric units.
[c]The recommended target weight gain for obese women (body mass index >29.0) is at least 6.0 kg (15 lb).
Source: Reprinted with permission from Institute of Medicine. Nutrition During Pregnancy, Part I, Weight Gain. Part II, Nutrient Supplements. Washington, DC: National Academy Press, 1990.

and an increase in the absorptive capability of the villous surface of the intestinal tract. Additionally, the muscle tone and motility of the gallbladder decrease, the enlarging uterus displaces the liver, and liver production of plasma proteins, serum enzymes, and serum lipids is altered.[30]

These changes are the causes of some of the common discomforts of pregnancy. Constipation, flatulence, and heartburn may result from decreased peristalsis and relaxation of the pyloric sphincter. Some women experience symptoms of cholestasis as a result of decreased tone and production in the gallbladder. In later pregnancy, as the growing uterus exerts pressure on the stomach and intestines, intake at a single meal may diminish and appetite may decrease.

Renal Changes

Changes in the renal system also contribute to the expansion of blood volume and peripheral vascular relaxation. Outside of pregnancy these alterations, too, would be diagnostic of pathology.[29,30] The structural and functional changes allow the body to cope with increased maternal intravascular volume and metabolic waste. The increased excretion of waste includes fetal waste, which crosses the placenta into the maternal circulation for disposal. Because the expanding uterus presses on the vena cavae, venous return and kidney perfusion are best at night when the woman is recumbent, frequently on her left side. The uterus enlarges with a dextrorotated position, causing greater pressure on the right ureter and kidney than on the left. As a result of pressure on the bladder from the uterus, a woman may experience frequency and stress incontinence.[30] Table 25-3 summarizes changes in the renal system.

Musculoskeletal Changes

Changes in physiology associated with pregnancy change a woman's weight distribution and joint stability. Biomechanical changes may result in some of the discomforts associated with pregnancy. Altered body conformation, which includes enlargement of the breasts and abdomen, can contribute to changes in posture, movement, and the ability to perform activities of daily living.

The center of gravity or center of mass (COM) is the point at which the force of gravity is concentrated on an object. In a nonpregnant woman, the center of gravity is just anterior to the second sacral vertebra. During pregnancy, the larger breasts and abdomen raise the composite COM. In addition, the distended abdomen displaces the COM anteriorly.[38]

TABLE 25-3
Summary of Changes in the Renal System during Pregnancy

Parameter	Alteration	Significance
Bladder	Renal calyces, pelvis, and ureters; elongation, decreased mobility, and hypertonicity of ureters	Dilation (more prominent on right) increased risk of urinary tract infection in pregnancy and postpartum; alter accuracy of 24-hour urine collections
	May last up to 3 months postpartum; decreased tone, increased capacity	Risk of infection; urinary frequency; alteration in accuracy of 24-hour urine collections
	Displaced in late pregnancy; mucosa edematous and hyperemic; incompetence of vesicoureteral valve	Urinary frequency; risk of trauma and infection; risk of reflux and infection; alteration in accuracy of 24-hour urine collections
Renal blood flow	Increases 35–60%	Increased glomerular filtration rate; increased solutes delivered to kidney
Glomerular filtration rate	Increases 40–50%	Increased filtration and excretion of water and solutes; increased urine flow and volume; decreased serum blood urea nitrogen, creatinine, uric acid; altered renal excretion of drugs with risk of subtherapeutic blood and tissue levels
Renal tubular function	Increased reabsorption of solutes (may not always match increase in filtered load)	Maintenance of homeostasis; avoid pathologic solute or fluid loss
	Increased renal excretion of glucose, protein, amino acids, urea, uric acid, water-soluble vitamins, calcium, H_1 ions, phosphorus	Tendency for glycosuria, proteinuria; compensation for respiratory alkalosis; increased nutritional needs (i.e., calcium, water-soluble vitamins)
	Net retention of sodium and water	Accumulation of Na and water to meet maternal and fetal needs
Renin-angiotensin-aldosterone system	Increase in all components; resistance to pressor effects of angiotensin 11	Maintain homeostasis with expanded extracellular volume; retention of water and sodium; balance forces favoring sodium excretion; maintain normal blood pressure
Arginine vasopressin and regulation of osmolarity	Osmostat reset	Retention of water; expansion of plasma volume and other extracellular volume; maintenance of volume homeostasis in spite of reduction in plasma osmolarity

Source: Adapted from S Blackburn, D Loper. Maternal, fetal and neonatal physiology: A clinical perspective. Philadelphia: Saunders, 1992.

The higher center of gravity increases the risk of a loss of standing balance. This is caused by the increased likelihood that the line of gravity, the vertical line from the COM to the supporting surface, will fall outside the base of support, namely the feet. To compensate, the pregnant woman widens her base of support. The augmented stance can be the result of weight gain and heavier thighs.[39] Although the wider base increases gait stability, it may be fatiguing. Walking requires transferring the line of gravity over the stance foot; consequently, the wider stance also increases the amount of lateral weight shift of the COM. Postural changes contribute to the characteristic *waddling* gait of late pregnancy. Any increase in the amount of weight shift during gait increases the energy expenditure. A pregnant woman with significant breast and abdominal enlargement is likely to become more tired than a woman without those anatomic changes.

In addition to the accommodations in the COM, the pregnant woman tends to show postural changes.[40] The anterior abdominal displacement causes a reactive posterior shift of the upper body to bring the line of gravity back over the feet. This shift in trunk posture typically results in an increased lumbar lordotic curve. Abdominal distention tilts the pelvis forward, thereby shifting the center of gravity. In combination with the decreased tone of the abdominal muscles, a significant lordosis can develop. Approximately 15% of women experience severe back pain localized in the sacroiliac region and most intense at night.[30] Because of postural changes and mechanical stress, there is an increased incidence of prolapsed intervertebral disk, most frequently in the fifth lumbar and first sacral nerve root areas.[41]

Strain on muscles and ligaments in compensating for the lordosis causes significant lower back discomfort that can persist postpartum.[30,42] Beginning after the fifth month, backache is caused by exaggeration of the lumbar lordotic curve, weight gain, and relaxation of ligaments, as well as from muscle spasm caused by pressure on nerve roots. The exaggerated curve is associated with a compensatory increase in the thoracic and cervical curves. Change in the spinal alignment can decrease the biomechanical advantage and relationship of the muscles and other supporting structures.[43]

Some consequences of these postural changes, if not addressed, are

1. Further stretching of the abdominal muscles, which are already elongated over the enlarged uterus

2. Shortening of the lumbar paraspinal muscles, making them less efficient for contraction

3. Lengthening of the thoracic paraspinal muscles with the same effect

4. Stretching of the pain-sensitive lumbar anterior longitudinal ligament

5. Rounded shoulders with tipped scapulae

6. Forward head

The composite effect of these postural changes is the frequent musculoskeletal complaints of pain in the low back, thorax, neck, and shoulder, and symptoms of thoracic outlet syndrome. Between 50% and 60% of pregnant women complain of low back pain during their pregnancy.[44] The exaggerated lumbar lordosis is a likely cause of low back pain with the stress on the sensitive anterior longitudinal ligament, on the facet joints, and from the unusual load bearing required of the facet joints and spinous processes.

The increased lumbar lordosis is often associated with an increase in anterior pelvic tilt. Maintenance of the altered pelvic posture accompanied by an increase in upper body mass leads to more vertebral shearing forces, particularly between L-5 and S-1 and between L-4 and L-5. A woman with a spondylolysis can develop a spondylolisthesis, a shift of the vertebral body away from the posterior components of the vertebra. Women who participate in activities requiring extreme spinal extension, such as gymnastics, are particularly prone toward a spondylolysis, which can be aggravated during pregnancy.

The compensatory increased thoracic curve with rounded shoulders and forward head produces tightness in the middle and anterior scalene muscles. The position also tends to depress the clavicles onto the first ribs. Both conditions tend to produce symptoms of thoracic outlet syndrome that mimic the symptoms of carpal tunnel syndrome. The forward head posture produces increased flexion at the cervicothoracic junction and extension at the occipitoatlantoid joints. In addition to contributing to the symptoms of thoracic outlet syndrome, this posture is also associated with the tendency to compromise blood flow in the vertebral arteries, resulting in dizziness, especially when the head is fully extended as in looking up.

In addition to biomechanical changes, pregnant women are vulnerable to hypermobility. Progesterone and relaxin, two placental hormones, are responsible for the characteristic changes that affect ligaments, connective tissue, and the skeleton. Decreased tone in the ligaments and connective tissue increases the mobility of the sacroiliac joints and pubic symphysis. In pregnancy there is a production of the hormone relaxin by the placenta, which results in a softening and relaxing of connective tissue, especially ligaments. In the pelvis this has a significant effect on the integrity of the pelvic ring, particularly the pubic symphysis and the sacroiliac joints.[39] The increased strain on the ligaments stabilizing the sacroiliac joints, in combination with the altered body structure and posture, may be the cause for the lower back pain of pregnancy termed *posterior pelvic pain*. The widening and destabilizing of the pubic symphysis secondary to increases in relaxin may be involved in the pubic pain frequently reported by pregnant women. The decreased sacroiliac stability is translated directly to the pubic symphysis through the closed chain hemipelvic ring. When both joints are unstable, as they begin to be in the first trimester, the result can be significant pain on weight bearing, turning while standing, and rolling in bed.

Ligamentous laxity also affects the ankles and knees. During pregnancy, when the supporting ligaments are not as stiff, the joints are particularly susceptible to trauma. The risk is aggravated by decreased balance and decreased visual field for foot placement. Should a sprain occur, the joint will likely require increased healing time. Ligamentous laxity caused by pregnancy can take up to 2 years to return to the prepregnancy state.

Lower quadrant abdominal pain may result from relaxation of the round ligaments that support the uterus coincident with lax abdominal musculature and the weight of the growing uterus. Characteristically this *round ligament pain* is felt as a pulling, stretching, or pinching pain extending into the vagina. It is important to distinguish these common discomforts of pregnancy from complications of pregnancy such as preterm labor.[30]

Anterior flexion of the head secondary to lordosis and slumping of the shoulder girdle exerts traction on the ulnar and median nerves, which causes aching and numbness in the upper extremities.[45] Breast changes secondary to the influence of estrogen, progesterone, human placental lactogen, increased blood volume, and venous stasis contribute to upper backache. Table 25-4 summarizes the most common peripheral neuropathies encountered in pregnancy, postpartum, and during lactation.

In light of the musculoskeletal changes of pregnancy, women should be cautious and minimize the most likely postural changes and avoid initiating, high-impact exercise on unstable joints. Women who have been actively engaged in regular physical exercise before pregnancy are the most likely to tolerate similar strenuous exercise during pregnancy.[46] To decrease the stress on joints that are biomechanically compromised or unstable because of hormonal influence, the pregnant woman needs education concerning posture[44] and exercise alternatives.

TABLE 25-4
Peripheral Neuropathies during Pregnancy and Lactation

Disorder	Description	Implications
Neuropathies associated with pregnancy		
Bell's palsy	Acute unilateral neuropathy of the seventh cranial nerve leading to facial paralysis with weakness of the forehead and lower face	Three times more frequent during pregnancy; most often occurs in the third trimester or first 2 weeks' postpartum; onset late in pregnancy is usually associated with full recovery and generally requires no treatment if partial or mild
Transient carpal tunnel syndrome	Entrapment and compression of the medial nerve at the wrist, more prominent in dominant hand	May develop in pregnancy because of excessive fluid retention; nocturnal hand pain reported by 20–40% of pregnant women; evidence of this syndrome in approximately 5%; supportive treatment (splinting of wrist at night); few may require surgery; most resolve by 3 months' postpartum; may recur with later pregnancies
Meralgia paresthesia	Unilateral or bilateral entrapment and compression of lateral femoral cutaneous nerve as it passes beneath the inguinal ligament	Associated with obesity and rapid weight gain in pregnancy; also related to trauma and stretch injury; lumbar lordosis in pregnancy may make nerve more vulnerable to compression; develops in third trimester, resolves spontaneously over first 3 months' postpartum
Neuropathies occurring in the intrapartum and postpartum periods		
Postpartum foot drop	Compression of the lumbosacral trunk against the sacral ala by the fetal head or of the common peroneal nerve between leg braces and the fibular head	Most common intrapartum nerve injury; seen most often in women of short stature with large infants; clinical manifestations may not appear until 24–48 hours' postpartum; prognosis is good if only the myelin sheath has been distorted, with improvement in 2–3 months
Other traumatic neuropathies	Compression of the lumbosacral plexus or obturator, femoral, or peroneal nerves against the weakness and palsy	Associated with obstetric practices, including use of lithotomy position, application of forceps, prolonged pressure from the fetal head, or from cesarean delivery; prognosis is good if only the myelin sheath has been distorted, with improvement in 2–3 months
Neuropathies associated with breast-feeding	Pressure on the nerves of the axilla	Occurs during engorgement with numbness and tingling of flexor surface of arms to ulnar distribution of hands that abates as the infant sucks; disappears as engorgement resolves
	Pain and tingling with flexion of the elbow	Seen in women using hand pump
	Transient carpal tunnel syndrome	Develops approximately 1 month after delivery and revolves within a month of weaning

Source: Reprinted with permission from S Blackburn, D Loper. Maternal, Fetal, and Neonatal Physiology; a Clinical Perspective. Philadelphia: Saunders, 1992.

Postpartum Period and Lactation

During the immediate postpartum period, maternal physiological adjustment occurs rapidly. Adaptations, which occurred over the 9 months of pregnancy, are no longer necessary after the infant is delivered. Cardiac output and respiration revert to prepregnancy status. There continues to be a challenge to the renal system, as it must clear the accumulated fluid load of pregnancy.[30]

Women who formula feed return to the nonpregnant functioning of the gastrointestinal tract fairly quickly.[47] For those who breast-feed, gastrointestinal changes that occurred during pregnancy persist to some degree to provide the substrate for milk production. Nursing mothers may experience upper back pain because of the persistence of enlarged breasts heavy with milk. Supportive undergarments are essential. Incorrect positioning of the infant, in which the woman leans over to bring the breast closer to the baby rather than bringing the infant to the breast, may contribute to persistent backache. Correcting the posture during breast-feeding helps relieve these symptoms.[30,42]

After delivery, the abdominal wall and peritoneum remain stretched and lax. This is partially because of rupture of elastic tissue and the prolonged distention of pregnancy. Separation of the rectus muscles leaves the abdomen susceptible to injury and without the normal responses to abdominal pain (e.g., rigidity). Separation, measured in finger breadths, is termed *diastasis recti*, and is a normal sequel to pregnancy that can be resolved with abdominal strengthening exercises.[34,48]

Separation of the pubic symphysis is a relatively rare, but significant, cause of maternal morbidity and possibly long-term disability. During pregnancy, the cartilage that connects the pubic rami, as well as other joints in the pelvis, relaxes so the pelvic girdle can enlarge its diameter at birth. In susceptible women, the normal adjustment weakens the pubic symphysis, causing symptoms of suprapubic pressure or pain, difficulty in walking, or pain when turning in bed. During labor there may be separation of the symphysis or one of the sacroiliac synchondroses. Separation may be palpable and often the woman is unable to walk without assistance. Most women have diminishing symptoms over a period of weeks or months after birth, but for some, symptoms may persist, necessitating the use of pelvic belts and occasionally the use of a wheelchair and, in the extreme cases, surgical correction.[34]

AGING OF THE REPRODUCTIVE SYSTEM IN WOMEN: MENOPAUSE

Aging of the reproductive system in women is integrally interwoven with the inexorable aging process. As a result, it is difficult to separate the consequences of aging from those of menopause. The passage of time causes changes in skin, bone, muscle, blood vessels, and other tissues, and these changes can be modulated by hormones such as estrogen.

Menopause has been the focus of some controversy in medicine. At one extreme are physicians who view menopause as a natural process that requires minimal intervention, if any. At the other extreme are those who view menopause as an estrogen-deficiency disease or an endocrinopathy that requires aggressive treatment.

In this section we focus on the biology of menopause: the changes in biological structure and function that occur in the years during and subsequent to the transition from reproductive cyclicity to nonreproductive acyclicity. The rate and magnitude of these changes vary considerably, as do individual responses to them. Many women have a relatively smooth transition; others, a more difficult one. Thus, physiological change does not necessarily imply major clinical problems. And, in fact, today more women are living longer and are remaining active and healthier than ever before.

Definitions

The word *menopause* is derived from the Greek *mene* (month) and *pausis* (stop). Strictly speaking, menopause is the occurrence of the last menstrual period, but in popular usage it is the period of years during which menstrual cycles become increasingly irregular, culminating in the cessation of menses and followed by a variable number of years during which the body continues to adjust to its new, noncycling state. To facilitate comparisons among research studies we have attempted to standardize definitions and to distinguish discrete stages of reproductive function within what is really a continuum. Definitions are based principally on the degree of regularity of the menstrual cycle. *Perimenopause* generally refers to the transition period before menopause and shortly after the last menstrual period. It typically lasts several years and is characterized by changes in menstrual cycle length or bleeding pattern interspersed with periods of amenorrhea, presumably reflecting hormone fluctuations. *Menopause* is the permanent cessation of menstruation, marking the decrease of ovarian activity. *Natural menopause*, which usually occurs as part of the normal maturation process, is most commonly defined as the absence of menses for 12 consecutive months. Menopause can also be prematurely induced by medical interventions such as surgical removal of both ovaries (surgical menopause) or after radiation, chemotherapy, or other drug administration that suppresses ovarian function (artificial menopause). *Postmenopause* is generally considered to be the period beginning at, or 12 months after, the cessation of menses and continuing indefinitely thereafter. The term *menopause*, or the *menopausal period*, is commonly used to mean the time from menopause onward, or even more broadly, to encompass the perimenopausal period as well. Here, the latter, broader, sense of the word is used.

Age at Natural Menopause

Estimates of the median age at menopause are fairly consistent, ranging from age 49 to 51 years[49-56] using different population samples and despite inconsistent definitions of menopause and various methods of analysis. In some countries of the southern hemisphere, reports of an earlier age at menopause were likely caused by methodologic differences.[57] Figure 25-2 illustrates the range of ages at which cessation of menses occurs.[56]

A variety of physiological, environmental, and sociodemographic factors have been examined to determine their influence on age at menopause. The data are sparse and contradictory. The most compelling data are for cigarette smoking, which is associated with 1–2 years earlier onset of menopause in most studies,[58-62] although not in all.[62] A woman's reproductive history may influence her age at menopause. Menstrual irregularity before age 25 seems to predict earlier menopause.[62] Data on parity are conflicting. Some investigators have reported that nulliparous women experience earlier menopause than parous women,[55,56,58-62] but others found no association.[49,61,63] Also, a lack of agreement exists in reports of relationships between age at natural menopause and age at menarche, age at first birth, number of live births, oral contraceptive use, race, income, and education.[51,55,62] Medical interventions such as chemotherapy[64] or trauma to the blood supply of the ovary[65] may also influence age at menopause.

Transition to Menopause

The transition from regular menstrual cyclicity to menopausal acyclicity is usually a gradual process that lasts several years. The World Health Organization

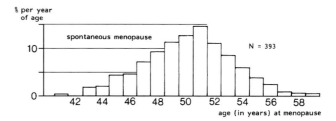

FIGURE 25-2 Age at menopause. (Reprinted with permission from AE Treloar. Menstrual cyclicity and the premenopause. Maturitas 1981;3:255.)

considers the 2–8 years before and 1 year after the final menses to be the perimenopausal period.[66] Women's levels of circulating estradiol reach a peak in the fourth decade of life and then decrease gradually. Thus, the perimenopausal period typically begins in a woman's 40s when clinical changes are noted. Yet subtle endocrine changes can begin in one's 30s. Although the end result is the same (i.e., cessation of menses), the time course, pattern, and magnitude of physical and endocrine changes vary between women, and within women from month to month.

Menstrual Cycle

During the reproductive years, cyclic production of sex steroids and gonadotropins characterizes the menstrual cycle. The ovary is responsible for the cyclic synthesis and secretion of steroid hormones and the release of oocytes. Ovary, hypothalamus, and anterior pituitary act in concert to regulate the endocrine and gametogenic events of the menstrual cycle. The principal ovarian steroids are estradiol produced primarily by the granulosa cells, androstenedione produced primarily by the stroma and thecal cells, and progesterone produced by the corpus luteum. Ovarian function is regulated by the gonadotropins FSH and LH, which are peptides secreted by the anterior pituitary in response to stimulation by GnRH from hypothalamic neurons. The ovarian steroids feed back to the hypothalamus and pituitary and modulate secretion of gonadotropin. GnRH is secreted in pulses, and this episodic secretion is critical to stimulating the pulsatile secretion of LH and FSH. LH pulses vary in frequency and amplitude across the menstrual cycle, being more frequent but lower in amplitude in the follicular than in the luteal phase. These changes in pulsatility are modulated by feedback of steroid hormones, especially progesterone, on the hypothalamus and pituitary.[67]

Endogenous opioid peptides also play a role in the steroid-gonadotropin interrelationships. Endogenous opiates are modulated by ovarian steroids. From a nadir in the early follicular phase, circulating β-endorphin levels increase to peak at midcycle.[68] β-Endorphin exerts inhibitory control on gonadotropin secretion.[69,70]

At the start of a menstrual cycle, when estrogen and progesterone levels are low, the FSH level begins to increase, stimulating follicular growth. Inhibin, a peptide produced by granulosa cells in response to FSH, facilitates the development of one primary follicle through suppression of FSH.[71] LH also increases (negative feedback). Soon, one follicle dominates and others become atretic. The maturing dominant follicle produces an increasing amount of estradiol, which by negative feedback leads to a decline in FSH level and by positive feedback culminates in a peak of estradiol. The high level of estrogen exerts a stimulatory (positive feedback) effect on LH release, whereas LH release is suppressed at low estrogen levels.[72] This high estrogen level just before midcycle triggers the pituitary to release a burst of LH and a concomitant surge of FSH. The follicle ruptures, and ovulation occurs. The high midcycle LH peak is closely followed by a decrease in the estradiol level.

The ovulatory follicle undergoes changes, including vascularization and incorporation of lipids and lutein, a yellow pigment. This luteinization begins before ovulation, resulting in an increase in progesterone. The progesterone facilitates the surge of LH and FSH.[73] After ovulation, the ruptured follicle is converted into a corpus luteum (yellow body), which secretes large amounts of progesterone and some estrogen. These hormone levels increase, reach a peak in the midluteal phase, and via negative feedback inhibit secretion by the pituitary of LH and FSH and thus reduce the stimulus for follicular development. If the oocyte is not fertilized, the corpus luteum deteriorates as lipid levels decline and vascularity decreases. Progesterone and estradiol levels return to the lower follicular phase levels. This decline in the levels of these steroids results in spasm of the spiral arteries of the endometrium, and menses occurs. LH and FSH levels increase owing to release of negative feedback inhibition, permitting the development of a new cohort of follicles and the start of a new menstrual cycle.

This repetitive menstrual cycle pattern becomes irregular during the transition into menopause, principally owing to changes in the structure and function of the ovary.

Changes in the Ovary

The ovaries of older women differ structurally and functionally from those of younger women. With aging, the ovaries become smaller, stromal tissue increases,

and fewer oocytes are present.[74] The decline in the number of oocytes begins before birth. The number of oocytes is greatest (approximately 7 million) in the ovaries of a fetus of approximately 20 weeks. By birth, the number has fallen to approximately 2 million, and by puberty, to less than 300,000.[75] The oocytes are largely lost to atresia, plus a small number to ovulation. Oocyte depletion is accelerated during the perimenopause.[3] Some primordial follicles and corpora lutea have been found in ovaries several years after menopause,[76,77] with some follicular growth and hormone secretion, but fewer and fewer follicles reach maturity, ovulation, and luteinization.[77]

Changes in Menstrual Cyclicity

At approximately age 40 years, although regular menstrual bleeding may continue, hormone patterns may become increasingly variable, apparently owing to aging of the ovary. During this perimenopausal period, changes in menstrual cycle length begin. The patterns of these changes have been documented in two major longitudinal, prospective studies: Treloar and colleagues' in the United States[78] and Vollman's in Switzerland.[79] Records of women's menstrual histories from menarche to menopause establish that the years just preceding menopause are characterized by menstrual cycle irregularity reminiscent of that in the years just after menarche (Figure 25-3). The mean duration of this perimenopausal menstrual cycle irregularity was 5.0 years (Figure 25-4).[56]

Vollman's subjects recorded their daily basal body temperature and reported no midcycle increase in basal body temperature. This suggested that perimenopausal menstrual cycle irregularity was characterized by an increasing number of anovulatory cycles and that shorter cycles resulted from a shorter follicular phase.[79] The menstrual irregularity may be manifested clinically as oligomenorrhea, polymenorrhea, or amenorrhea, but changes in the menstrual pattern do not predict when menses will occur.[80,81]

Endocrine Changes

During the perimenopause, the general trend is one of increasing levels of circulating FSH, while changes in the LH pattern lag somewhat, usually just before menopause, when marked increases in LH are noted (Figure 25-5).[82–84] Estrogen level generally is not markedly decreased in this period.[85] Within these general trends, individual patterns of gonadotropins vary, not only between women, but in one woman over time. The range of hormone levels during this period is from normal premenopausal levels to

FIGURE 25-3 Menstrual cycle lengths: puberty to menopause. (Reprinted with permission from AE Treloar, RE Boynton, BG Behn, et al. Variation of the human menstrual cycle through reproductive life. Int J Fertil 1967;12:93.)

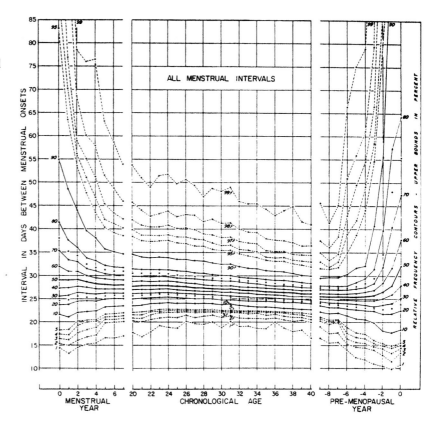

levels characteristics of postmenopausal women. Although menstrual cycles continue, there may be increases in circulating FSH and decreases in peak levels of estradiol at midcycle and during the luteal phase; LH concentrations remain relatively unchanged. Other observed endocrine patterns include (1) high levels of estrogen, FSH, and LH and (2) high LH but low FSH levels.[86] The various patterns of change in FSH and LH levels limit their use as predictors of menopause and may reflect decreased sensitivity to estrogen or altered regulation by the hypothalamus or pituitary, or they may be the result of decreasing levels of inhibin, an ovarian hormone that contributes to the regulation of FSH.[71,72,82,87,88] Circulating FSH and LH levels may continue to increase for 2–3 years after menopause. Thereafter, FSH and LH concentrations begin to decrease (Figure 25-6).[89-91] Postmenopausally, a pulsatile pattern of release still characterizes both LH and FSH secretion.[92]

During reproductive life the principal ovarian steroid is 17-β-estradiol, produced by developing follicles. The ovary also secretes estrone, progesterone, androstenedione, and testosterone.[93] Smaller amounts of estrone, a biologically weaker estrogen than estradiol, are produced by peripheral conversion of androstenedione.[94-96]

In the perimenopausal period, estrogen levels may fluctuate widely and occasionally may even increase before menopause.[97]

During the menopausal period, with the continuing reduction in the number of follicles, cyclic ovarian produc-

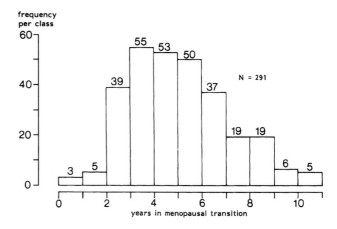

FIGURE 25-4 Duration of the menopausal transition. (Reprinted with permission from AE Treloar. Menstrual cyclicity and the premenopause. Maturitas 1981;3:260.)

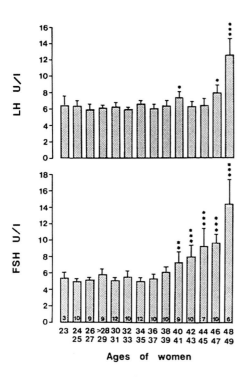

FIGURE 25-5 Age distribution of geometric mean (± error of the mean) of luteinizing hormone and follicle-stimulating hormone plasma concentrations in 127 women aged 23–49 years. The number of women in each age group is given at the base of each column. (*P < .05; **P < .01; ***P < .001.) (FSH = follicle-stimulating hormone; LH = luteinizing hormone.) (Reprinted with permission from EA Lenton, L Sexton, S Lee, ID Cooke. Progressive changes in LH and FSH and LH:FSH ratio in women throughout reproductive life. Maturitas 1988;10:39.)

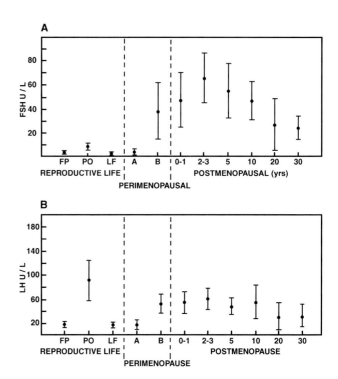

FIGURE 25-6 Plasma follicle-stimulating hormone (FSH) **(A)** and luteinizing hormone (LH) **(B)** values (mean ± SD) at different ages. The normal values in the reproductive phase are given as follicular phase (FP), peak ovulatory phase (PO), and luteal phase (LF). Groups A and B refer to women who are still menstruating who attended the menopausal clinic with apparent climacteric symptoms. Patients in group A had no hot flushes. Group B represents the patients who complained of hot flush symptoms. Follicle-stimulating hormone and luteinizing hormone values at various years after the menopause are also shown. (Reprinted with permission from J Studd, S Chakravarti, D Oran. The climacteric. Clin Obstet Gynaecol 1977;4:6.)

tion of estradiol and progesterone eventually stops, although for several years postmenopausally the ovary is capable of some small degree of estrogen production.[98–131] In postmenopausal women, estrone, produced largely by conversion of adrenal androstenedione, becomes the primary circulating estrogen.[102] This conversion to estrone takes place largely in adipose tissue,[99,103] but also in bone, muscle, and other tissue.[104] With age, conversion of androstenedione to estrone becomes more efficient.[105] Estrogen level in postmenopausal women is correlated with body weight and is particularly high in obese women.[96,99,100,103,106] Circulating estradiol is derived primarily from peripheral conversion of estrone.[107] The progesterone level does not change substantially with age.[106]

Most of the androgen circulating postmenopausally is produced by the adrenal gland. The level of circulating androstenedione is approximately one-half of what it was before menopause: The postmenopausal ovary produces approximately 20% of the circulating androstene-

dione.[85,92,99,101,106,108] Ovarian testosterone secretion drops only slightly, if at all, and the total circulating testosterone level is only slightly lower postmenopausally than it was premenopausally.[85,92,108,109] The decrease in ovarian estrogen production relative to the amount of ovarian testosterone being produced may account for the increased hirsutism some women experience after menopause.[109] Thus, the postmenopausal endocrine environment is quite different from that of the premenopausal period (Figure 25-7).

Fertility in the Perimenopause

Between age 40 and 50 years, when menstrual cycles may become increasingly irregular with long periods of

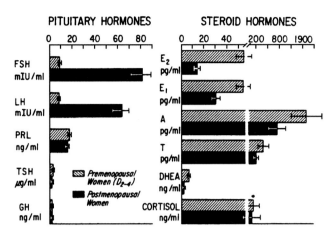

FIGURE 25-7 Circulating levels of pituitary and steroid hormones in postmenopausal women as contrasted with premenopausal women (days 2–4 of menstrual cycle). (A = androstenedione; DHEA = dehydroepiandrosterone; E_1 = estrone; E_2 = 17-β-estradiol; FSH = follicle-stimulating hormone; GH = growth hormone; LH = luteinizing hormone; PRL = prolactin; T = testosterone; TSH = thyroid-stimulating hormone.) (Reprinted with permission from SSC Yen. The biology of menopause. J Reprod Med 1977;18:290.)

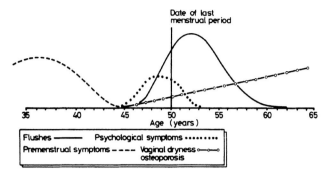

FIGURE 25-8 Occurrence of common problems with respect to the date of the last menstrual period. (Reprinted with permission from J Coope. Menopause: Diagnosis and treatment. BMJ 1984;289:888.)

amenorrhea interspersed between occasional menses, women may not know whether they are still ovulating, and thus fertile. Ovulation has been documented in women throughout the menopausal transition, even when menstrual cycles are irregular and gonadotropin levels are elevated, and as long as 3 years after the last menstrual period.[76,82,110] The incidence of pregnancy is low after age 45 and rare after age 50.[76] Although there is histologic evidence of corpus luteum formation in women after age 50,[76] biochemically, the corpus luteum may be incapable of supporting a pregnancy and the ova may be inadequate for fertilization or implantation.[76,111] However, given the variety of transitional menstrual patterns, sexually active women should be informed of the possibility of pregnancy.

Stress and Menstrual Cyclicity

Midlife may be a time of changes in various aspects of one's life; spouses may become ill, die, or leave. Changes in one's own body, although gradual, normal, and typical, in our culture are a source of stress and distress for many women. This may result in an interest in exercising that did not previously exist (although the question is often, "How little do I have to do?" rather than how much) or that may now be intensified. If working, there may be changes in work environment, both positive (bringing greater responsibilities and chal-

lenges), and negative (loss of job or activities) that are beyond one's control.

We are only just learning how various stressors may influence neuroendocrine and reproductive function.[132] There may be individual differences in responsiveness of the hypothalamic-pituitary-gonadal axis to particular challenges.[133] Although anecdotal reports of the effect of stress on menstrual cyclicity, for example, have been reported for a long time,[134] substantive data supporting this contention in women are scant. In animals, effects of physical stress, emotional stress, or both on the hypothalamic-pituitary-adrenal axis have been shown.[135,136] In women, reproductive cycle disorders may involve weight loss, eating disorders, or excessive exercise.[137–139] It is not known, but worth considering, whether any of these patterns and problems that occur in reproductive years and may result in changes in reproductive hormones and menstrual cyclicity affect the menopausal transition or the physiological experience of menopause.

Signs, Symptoms, and Sequelae of Menopause

The nature and severity of symptoms women experience during the menopausal years vary greatly. Some women cease to menstruate and have no associated symptoms, whereas others experience many problems. When symptoms do appear, they may begin in the perimenopausal period and continue long after menstrual cycles stop, or they may first be manifested after cessation of menses (Figure 25-8).

Hot flashes (hot flushes) are most clearly associated with menopause and a low estrogen level; atrophic vaginitis is also consistently associated with a decline in estrogen level. Many other symptoms have been attributed to menopause, although inconsistently. These include fatigue, headache, memory loss, irritability, poor concentration, crying spells, and dizziness. There is no consensus among physicians, social scientists, and women themselves about which symptoms are attributable to physiological changes underlying menopause, which are caused by general physiological aging, and which are the result of simultaneous psychological or social factors that may beset women at midlife.

To resolve these issues, it must be kept in mind that menopause is a biological process and a sociocultural phenomenon. Women in different cultures have different experiences of menopause and different expectations of symptoms. Both depend in part on their culture's attitudes toward and stereotypes of menopausal women. Whether a woman reports any symptoms, or which symptoms a woman relates to menopause, is influenced by her culture's definition of menopause.[57,112-114] In western societies, hot flashes are the concomitant of menopause most widely accepted as having a biological basis. In Japan and Indonesia, the reported frequency of hot flashes is far less than in the United States.[115,116] Mayan women in Yucatan, Mexico, do not report any symptoms at menopause other than menstrual cycle irregularity.[117] In cultures in which hot flashes are not frequently reported, it is not known whether the physiological changes such as increased heart rate, sweating, and skin temperature, measured in association with hot flashes, are absent, or are present but not attributed to menopause. In Africa, the sweating of hot flashes is sometimes misdiagnosed as malaria.[118] Physiological processes may be affected by factors such as diet, exercise, climate, and the reproductive practices of a culture. It is, therefore, not surprising that the reported prevalence of hot flashes varies widely from culture to culture.

Multiple Effects of Decreased Estrogen Level

Estrogen has multiple effects on the body, especially on the reproductive and urinary systems. Estrogen receptors are present in the ovaries, vagina, cervix, fallopian tubes, distal urethra, and bladder.[119] The rate and magnitude of the change in circulating estrogen level vary among women, as does the rate and extent of the resultant target tissue changes. For some women, physical and physiological changes occur slowly and are barely noticeable; for others, changes are marked and occur rather rapidly. This may be caused by the rate of decrease of hormones, because sudden changes are particularly evident in women whose ovaries have been surgically removed or rendered nonfunctional by radiation or chemotherapy. Drugs or diseases that alter the estrogen level may also affect the extent of the estrogen-related changes. Whether clinical problems are caused by the decline in estrogen level depends on a complex interplay of factors. A synergistic interaction between aging and estrogen depletion causes urogenital atrophy, but the relative contributions of the two components have not been determined.

Vulva

The external genitalia, which are highly vascular during reproductive years, become less vascular as estrogen levels decline.[120] The labia become less sensitive, and less responsive to sexual stimulation.[121] The lower estrogen level leads to a decrease in vulvar skin elasticity and other atrophic changes. Skin conditions such as lichen sclerosis become more prevalent.[122,123] Pubic hair thins and the labia majora, which previously contained much subcutaneous fat, become smaller and more wrinkled as this fat layer is reduced.[122]

Vagina

With a decline in ovarian estrogen production, the vaginal epithelium becomes thin and more susceptible to irritation (atrophic vaginitis). The vagina becomes shorter, narrower, and less flexible and distensible. Vaginal blood flow decreases and vaginal secretions diminish, reducing the protective layer of moisture on the cells lining the vagina and decreasing sexually stimulated fluid production.[124,125] Inadequate lubrication and dryness of the vagina, in conjunction with the structural changes, can result in discomfort during intercourse (dyspareunia), and even bleeding.[122] Women who are sexually active tend to have less vaginal atrophy than women of similar age and estrogen level who are not.[126] These atrophic changes are responsive to estrogen treatment (topical or oral), which increases the thickness of the vaginal mucosa, increases vaginal perfusion, restores vaginal fluid production, and results in lowered pH.[127,128]

The population of micro-organisms in the vagina is also affected by estrogen. Döderlein's lactobacilli and other acidophilic bacteria normally present in the vagina metabolize glycogen, which is plentiful in well-estrogenized cells. The organic acids produced by this metabolism help keep the vaginal pH acidic, thus favoring the lactobacilli over pathogenic bacteria and minimizing vaginal infections.[128] As estrogen levels decline, there are fewer layers of epithelial cells lining the vagina, and cell glycogen content is reduced. There is a reduction in the number of lactobacilli, and a resulting change in pH from acidic to alkaline. This alkaline environment increases the risk of vaginal infection by bacteria such as staphylococci and streptococci.[124,128] Estrogen treatment helps reduce vaginal pH and restore a more favorable balance to the bacterial population.

The range and severity of these problems are great. Some women have minor discomfort, which is remedied by short-term, local estrogen treatment. Others experience significant pain and vaginal dryness so extreme as to make even walking uncomfortable.[129] Few statistics are available on the incidence of these symptoms.

Cervix and Uterus

As estrogen levels decline, atrophic changes occur in the epithelium of the cervix and less mucus is produced by the endocervical glands. The cervix, which once protruded into the vagina, may retract and become flush with the wall of the vagina.[121,130] The uterus decreases in size, the endometrial lining becomes thin, and there is decreased vascularization. Epithelial cells flatten and the glands become inactive. Myometrial fibers change in structure and become atrophic. If fibroids are present, they tend to shrink.[119,122]

Relaxation of the pelvic muscles and other structures supporting the uterus and urinary tract organs may result in a descensus of these organs and consequent discomfort,[121,131] although pelvic relaxation may also be related to parity, birth trauma, and obesity.[104]

Breasts

The breast is also a target organ for estrogen. In the postmenopausal years as a result of a decrease in glandular and subcutaneous fatty tissue, the breasts tend to shrink and become less elastic.[122] Some women's breasts retain their normal appearance, even at an advanced age, and a small number of women report increased breast size, although the explanation for this is not clear.[140]

Skin and Hair

Skin changes with age. It becomes less elastic and more pigmented; sweat and sebaceous gland activity is reduced,[141] and the skin becomes drier. The epidermis thins and subcutaneous fat is reduced, resulting in wrinkling of the skin. Skin contains estrogen receptors and is thus a target tissue for estrogen,[142,143] and it has been demonstrated that estrogen therapy increases epidermal thickness in surgically menopausal women.[144] Hair loss may be noted at sites that are influenced by loss of estrogen (e.g., pubic, axillary, scalp), whereas hair growth may increase on sites presumably affected by the greater relative amount of androgen (e.g., chin, upper lip).

Urinary System

The lower portion of the urinary tract and the lower reproductive tract tissues have a common embryonic origin. Thus, urinary tract tissues are also estrogen sensitive and undergo atrophic changes similar to those in the vaginal epithelium. As estrogen levels decline, the urethral mucosa becomes thin and friable, and vascularity diminishes.[145] These changes may manifest as reduced ability to control urine. Urethral closure pressure, important in the maintenance of continence, may diminish in the years after menopause.[121] Cystitis, urinary frequency, urgency, suprapubic pain, and dysuria may increase after menopause (atrophic urethritis).[104,121,131,140,146] Some of these symptoms respond favorably to estrogen treatment.[140,147] Estrogen loss may also be one cause of a reduction in the support of pelvic organs provided by pelvic muscles, ligaments, and fascia. This may facilitate the occurrence of cystocele, cystourethrocele, and rectocele.[104,121,148] Reduction in the support of the bladder and urethra contributes to diminished urinary control, because periurethral muscles contract less effectively.

Although urinary problems are a troubling complaint of menopausal women, the incidence or seriousness of these problems in the general population is not known. Hagstad and Janson[149] found no significant differences in the percentage of urinary incontinence between menstruating (8.1%) and postmenopausal (11.1%) women; others have observed a significantly higher rate of incontinence in older women.[150,151] Notelovitz[140] reported that 30% of women aged 45–65 years reported nocturia. Rekers[152] reported that among a random sample of postmenopausal women in Holland, the frequency of urinary symptoms were approximately these: incontinence, 26%; urgency, 15%; frequency, 20%; nocturia, 18%; and dysuria, 11%.

Lipoproteins and Coronary Heart Disease

Between puberty and menopause women have a much lower incidence of coronary heart disease (CHD) than men.[153] After menopause, CHD becomes a leading cause of death in women.[154,155] Menopause, not age per se, is the critical factor, as postmenopausal women have a higher risk of CHD than age-matched, menstruating women.[154,156] Clinical and epidemiologic studies have demonstrated that a low level of low-density lipoprotein cholesterol and an elevated level of high-density lipoprotein cholesterol are predictors of reduced risk of CHD in both men and women.[157,158] Throughout adult life, high-density lipoprotein cholesterol levels in women exceed those of men, whereas low-density lipoprotein cholesterol levels in women are lower than those of men until age 50, when they increase and surpass those of men.[159]

Substantial evidence exists that sex steroids play a significant role in the regulation of these serum lipids and lipoproteins. The increase in the female to male ratio of deaths from CHD that occurs at menopause, and the fact that CHD is rare in younger women but high in men younger than 50 years, suggests that estrogen is a critical factor in women's favorable lipoprotein profile and lower risk of CHD before menopause. Studies of the effects of estrogens on lipoproteins, including exogenous estrogen administration to postmenopausal women, have consistently, over many years, demonstrated that estrogens increase high-density lipoprotein cholesterol and decrease low-density lipoprotein cholesterol.[160-163]

Thus, estrogen's role in producing a lipid profile that is correlated with reduced CHD is compelling, despite continued controversy about the effect of postmenopausal estrogen treatment on CHD. Although some studies show no statistically significant effect of estrogen on CHD[155,164] or elevated risk,[165] most demonstrate a beneficial effect.[160,166-170]

Skeletal System

Estrogen's role in bone metabolism becomes extremely significant in postmenopausal women. Chapter 7, Skeletal Physiology and Osteoporosis, is devoted to osteoporosis and bone metabolism.

Hot Flashes

Hot flashes, which affect many women in the menopausal years, are recurrent, transient periods of heat sensation, flushing, sweating, palpitations, and a sense of anxiety, often followed by shivering or chills. The terms *hot flash*, *hot flush*, *night sweat*, and *vasomotor instability* are used interchangeably. More women seek medical treatment for hot flashes than any other menopausal complaint; yet the specific cause and physiology of hot flashes, the most characteristic manifestation of the menopausal period, are still unknown.

Epidemiology and Natural History of Hot Flashes

Information on the prevalence of hot flashes is based principally on studies of menopausal symptoms conducted in several western countries (Great Britain, the Netherlands, Scotland, Sweden, the United States). The prevalence of hot flashes ranges from 24% to 92%, being highest in the first 2 years after menopause

and gradually declining after that.[171-178] Hot flash prevalence rates tend to be higher with surgical menopause than with natural menopause, at least for the first year after ovariectomy.[177-181] Hot flashes have been reported in many different cultures and ethnic groups, including Japanese, Indian, African, American Indian, Mexican American, and Mayan.[115,117,182-186] In Asian countries, several studies report a low frequency of hot flashes.[115,187-189] However, other studies found hot flash frequencies in Asian countries similar to levels in European countries[190,191]; and relatively high rates are reported from Turkey,[192] Tanzania,[193] and other countries.

Findings of studies to identify characteristics that might predispose women to hot flashes have been contradictory. A study of premenopausal and perimenopausal women found hot flash prevalence to be significantly greater among black American women as compared with white American women (53% versus 29%).[194] Although confirming another study that found black American women to be more likely than white women to have hot flashes,[195] the results contrasted with those of Schwingl et al. (1994),[196] who found no increased association between being a black American woman and having hot flashes.

Premenopausal and perimenopausal women also report hot flashes; reported prevalences range from 6% to 61%.[53,149,171-174,178,183] In a study of women who reported hot flashes, 50% of participants reported onset of hot flashes before menopause (sometimes 5, 10, or 15 years before), when menstrual cycles were still regular or were becoming irregular (Figure 25-9).[178] Some women do not begin having hot flashes until a number of years after menstruation has stopped. Hot flashes typically subside within 6 months to 2 years, although they can continue many years, even as long as 40 years after cessation of menstrual cycles (Figure 25-10).[178]

Within and among individuals, the frequency, intensity, and duration of hot flashes vary. For the majority of women experiencing them, frequency and severity peak during the first 2–5 years after menopause. Hot flashes may occur monthly, weekly, or hourly. For approximately 15% of affected women, hot flashes occur many times a day. In the perimenopausal period hot flashes may come and go as menstrual cycles stop and start again. The intensity of hot flashes can vary from mild to severe, and the duration of each episode, although typically lasting 3–5 minutes, occasionally can last 30 minutes or more (Figure 25-11).[197]

Many women experience an aura when a hot flash is about to begin. It is described as a sense of anxiety, a

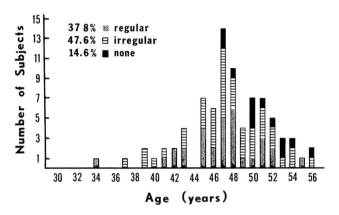

FIGURE 25-9 Age at which hot flashes begin with respect to menstrual cycle status at that time.

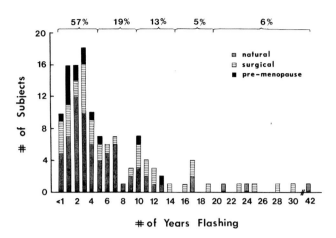

FIGURE 25-10 Number of years women experience hot flashes.

change in heart rate, or a sense of *dis-ease*. The hot flash itself, in addition to the sweating, sensation of heat, and flushing, may include a feeling of panic, suffocation, or frustration.[178]

Hot flashes occur spontaneously; however, some women report specific triggers for their hot flashes, including a warm or confined environment, coffee, alcohol, sex, or stress.[178] Hot flashes are particularly distressing at night, when a woman's sleep often is disrupted several times because she awakens drenched in sweat and must change her nightclothes and sheets. This pattern of sleep, punctuated by awakenings associated with hot flashes, is illustrated in Figure 25-12. The concomitant decreases in chest skin temperature reflect evaporative cooling with each sudden, transient outpouring of sweat. Rapid, marked increases in heart rate accompany the hot flashes. The disrupted sleep leads to fatigue and irritability and can adversely affect spousal and other family and work relationships.

Thermoregulatory Physiology
Hot flashes are marked by a characteristic pattern of thermoregulatory responses and hormone changes that are well documented (Figure 25-13).[178,197-204]

Immediately before the onset of the hot flash, women often report a brief aura that alerts them to an impending hot flash. Increases in heart rate (up to 38%)[178,205,206] and skin blood flow (4–30 times)[175,178] occur during this aura, slightly before the hot flash is sensed. Most women report that the sensation of heat and sweating is predominantly in and on the upper body, and in particular, the chest, neck, face, and scalp. The wave of heat typically is described as spreading upward. Sweat on

the chest and forehead evaporates, resulting in cooling of the skin; it can be measured indirectly as a decrease in skin temperature (see Figure 25-12). The rapid increase in finger temperature (1–7°C) that follows the vasodilatation,[178,207,208] in combination with sweating and the resulting evaporative cooling (thermoregulatory heat loss responses), result in a decrease in internal body temperature (0.1–0.9°C).[178,198,200,203]

Hot flashes may be the body's response to sudden, transient downward resetting of the body's thermostat (temperature set point), which is located in the hypothalamus.[178,200] This set-point resetting would cause the sensation of intense heat and activation of heat loss responses, including behavioral adjustments, cutaneous vasodilation, and sweating, causing a decrease in core temperature. When subsequently the temperature set point returns to normal, the sensation becomes one of chilliness, as body temperature has fallen below nor-

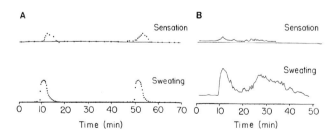

FIGURE 25-11 A, B. Subjective sensation and sweating patterns in discrete and prolonged hot flashes. (Reprinted with permission from F Kronenberg, JA Downey. Thermoregulatory physiology of menopausal hot flashes: a review. Can J Physiol Pharmacol 1987;65:1315.)

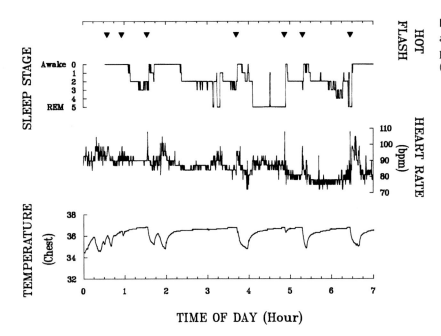

FIGURE 25-12 Association of nocturnal awakenings with hot flashes in a postmenopausal woman (temperatures in Celsius scale). (REM = rapid eye movement.)

mal, and heat conservation (vasoconstriction), heat production (shivering), and behavioral adjustments are activated to bring body temperature back to normal.[207] This constellation of physiological and behavioral changes that characterizes a hot flash suggests an integrated thermoregulatory event whose pattern is the inverse of that during a fever.[204]

Studies by Freedman and colleagues over the past decade have led them to postulate that there is a narrowing of the zone of thermoneutrality (where there is no major thermoregulatory activity) in women who have hot flashes, and that small elevations in core temperature precede most hot flashes.[209,210] They also propose an activation of a central noradrenergic mechanism driving the physiological changes that make up a hot flash.[211] Work remains to be done to fully understand the physiological mechanisms of hot flashes.

Endocrinology

Observation of an abrupt onset of hot flashes after bilateral ovariectomy and the relief of hot flashes with estrogen therapy suggested a relationship between low plasma estrogen levels and hot flashes.[181,212] Reports that levels of circulating estrone and estradiol are lower in women with hot flashes than in women with no hot flashes provide further support for this relationship[213-215]; however, a low estrogen level is not the complete explanation for hot flashes. All postmenopausal women have a low estrogen level, but some never have hot flashes and oth-

ers have them only sporadically or only for a short while.

Hot flashes are not triggered by the high or pulsatile gonadotropin patterns characteristic of menopause, because, despite continued high gonadotropin levels, hot flashes often decline or stop after menopause. Although LH pulses may be temporally correlated with hot flashes,[178,207,208,216] hot flashes occur in women who have no episodic LH release, such as those who have undergone hypophysectomy,[217] in premenopausal or postmenopausal women whose pulsatile LH release has been suppressed by treatment with a GnRH analogue,[218-220] and in women with pituitary insufficiency and hypoestrogenism.[221]

A variety of substances have been found to increase in the peripheral blood in association with hot flashes, including epinephrine,[197,222] neurotensin,[203] β-endorphin, β-lipotropin, adrenocorticotropin,[202] cortisol, androstenedione, dehydroepiandrosterone,[202,216] and growth hormone.[201] Norepinephrine decreases during hot flash episodes[197]; levels of estradiol, estrone,[216] FSH,[207,223] prolactin,[201,208,223] dopamine,[208] and TSH remain the same.[201] Thus, although there is a relationship between low estrogen level and hot flashes, other factors clearly are involved in triggering individual hot flash episodes.

In more recent years there has been increased study of noradrenergic pathways and the possible role in hot flash physiology. 3-Methoxy-4-hydroxyphenylglycol,

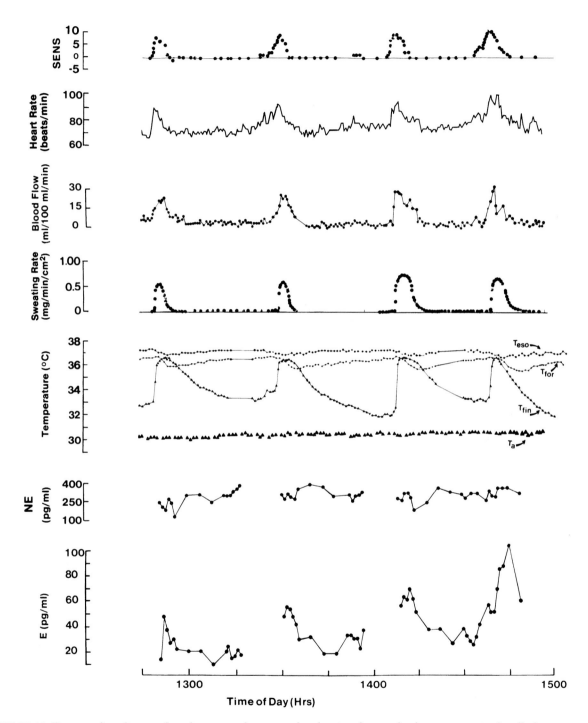

FIGURE 25-13 Pattern of cardiovascular, thermoregulatory, and endocrine changes for four consecutive hot flashes over a 2-hour period. Changes in sensation (SENS), heart rate, blood flow (finger), sweating rate, temperatures (esophageal, forehead, finger, ambient), norepinephrine (NE), and epinephrine (E) are depicted. (Reprinted with permission from F Kronenberg, JA Downey. Thermoregulatory physiology of menopausal hot flashes: a review. Can J Physiol Pharmacol 1987;65:1314.)

a primary metabolite of brain norepinephrine, is elevated in women with hot flashes (compared with asymptomatic women) and during heat-induced hot flashes,[211] suggesting increased brain norepinephrine levels during hot flashes. It is hypothesized that declining estrogen levels affect hypothalamic β_2-adrenergic receptors, and that this would affect central levels of norepinephrine.

Modulating Factors

Environmental temperature influences the frequency and intensity of hot flashes: Cool ambient temperatures reduce the frequency and intensity of hot flashes, and warmer temperatures increase them.[224] Thus, sleeping in a cool room generally may be expected to decrease the prevalence of hot flashes and resultant awakenings.

Sleep Patterns at Menopause

Several survey studies of menopausal symptoms have reported increased complaints of insomnia after menopause as compared with menstruating women.[52,53,172,174] Nighttime awakenings in menopausal women are often associated with hot flashes.[225] Sometimes women awaken 30–60 seconds before feeling the hot flash; at other times they awaken already drenched in sweat. Figure 25-13 illustrates the abrupt change in sleep state associated with the reported hot flashes. If the hot flash is mild, the woman may quickly fall asleep again. If the sweating is profuse she may have to further disrupt her sleep by getting up to change clothes and bedding. Sometimes, the changes in heart rate, sweating, and skin temperature characteristic of hot flashes continue throughout the night and are associated with transient electroencephalographically documented arousals that do not cause conscious awakening (Kronenberg, unpublished observations). These brief arousals may also contribute to poorer quality sleep and diminished functioning the next day.[226] Treatment with estrogen has been shown to decrease nocturnal hot flashes, reduce the frequency of awakenings,[225,227] and decrease the amount of wake time.[228]

Many other complaints of menopausal women (e.g., depression, poor concentration, irritability, anxiety) can negatively affect sleep.[229] Ravnikar et al.[230] suggested that these problems, and the insomnia and hot flashes, may all be interrelated and related to the hormone changes at menopause. Schiff and colleagues[228] reported that estrogen administration improved clinically rated psychological adjustment and reduced hot flashes and improved the quality of sleep. In a survey of women aged 40–55 years, Ballinger[231] found the highest

incidence of psychiatric problems in women 45–49 years old, but observed no clear relationship between psychiatric problems and hot flashes. Ballinger[232] found no correlation between sleep disturbance and menopausal status and reported that sleep disturbances occurred in women both with and without psychiatric disorders. She concluded that although it seems that relationships may exist between hormone levels and hot flashes and hormone levels and psychological function, they may not be the same relationships.

Scharf et al.[233] demonstrated that estrogen therapy reduced the frequency of hot flashes associated with waking from sleep and improved sleep quality. Further verification and elucidation of the relationship between estrogen therapy, sleep improvement, and menopausal symptoms are provided by Polo-Kantola et al.[234] In a prospective, randomized, double-blind, crossover study, symptomatic and asymptomatic menopausal women were given estrogen replacement therapy and questionnaires assessing sleep, menopausal symptoms, and depression. In both symptomatic and asymptomatic women, there was a significant improvement in sleep on estrogen therapy as compared with placebo. Neither estrogen nor FSH level was predictive of improved sleep. However, the women with lowest serum estradiol levels did not have better sleep. Reduction in hot flashes was the strongest predictor of sleep improvement, supporting other reports that hot flashes can cause sleep problems. However, the beneficial effects of estrogen replacement therapy on sleep in asymptomatic women suggest a direct effect of estrogen on brain regions involved in sleep physiology. Beck Depression Scale scores were not improved with estrogen replacement therapy, but memory problems were reduced.

Estrogen's influence on sleep and mood has yet to be fully defined. Estrogen does affect enzymes that control biogenic amines involved in regulating both sleep and mood state,[159] but further research is needed to understand more fully the interrelationships between the many central and peripheral actions of estrogen.

Sexual Functioning during the Menopausal Transition and Beyond

Much of the early research on human sexuality has focused on sexual functioning as it relates to intercourse and orgasm. Now, a broader definition of sexuality and the meaning of a satisfying sexual and sensual life for people of all ages is becoming widely accepted.[235-237] Sexuality, sensuality, love, and affection are important to healthy living for people of all ages. Information reported over the past 15 years on the sex lives of middle-aged and older people[238] supports earlier reports,[239,240] indicating that healthy women can retain interest in and enjoyment of sex throughout life. This information has called into question stereotyped notions of menopausal women as uninterested in or incapable of enjoying sex. Certainly, postmenopausal changes in anatomy and physiology consequent to a decline in estrogen level can affect some aspects of sexual functioning,[241-243] but existing research suggests that although hormone changes may impinge on sexual physiology and function, the degree to which the hormone-induced changes actually disrupt this functioning depends on social, psychological, general health, and other factors.

Anatomic and Physiological Changes

Most of what is known about changes in sexual functioning associated with menopause involves changes in sexual anatomy and physiology that are principally caused by diminished estrogen levels and the resultant decrease in blood flow to the genitourinary area. A change in sexual responsiveness is manifested in a slightly slower time to arousal, lubrication, and clitoral response; and in less lubrication, less vasocongestion, and a shorter lived and less intense orgasm.[120,244] The breast continues to respond to sexual arousal, but with diminished vasocongestive response. Yet not all women exhibit these changes. Some postmenopausal women retain an increase in vaginal blood flow on stimulation comparable with that of premenopausal women.[242] Painful uterine contractions may occur with orgasm.[120,240] The reduction in vaginal lubrication and the dryness and irritation of the vaginal wall predispose to vaginitis. Increase in vaginal pH increases susceptibility to infection. These changes, in combination with a narrower, less flexible vagina, can lead to discomfort, or even pain, during intercourse or any form of genital stimulation. Postcoital bleeding may occur as a result of the thinning of vaginal epithelium. This certainly can lead to the avoidance of sexual activity.

Maintaining sexual activity reduces vaginal atrophy and helps preserve the functional capacity for lubrication.[104,126,148,240,245] Self-stimulation also helps maintain sexual responsiveness and contributes to reducing atrophic changes.[245] Administration of oral or local estrogen can help increase vaginal blood flow, mucosal wall thickness, and vaginal lubrication.[127]

Modification of Sexual Function

Despite the age-related reduction in estrogen level and physiological changes in the urogenital system, women can remain sexually interested and responsive throughout life. A change in function does not imply dysfunc-

tion. Some women experience no change in libido[246]; some report an increase in sexual desire that possibly is caused in part by the relative increase in circulating androgens,[247-249] but also to feeling relief from the fear of pregnancy and the annoyance of birth control. Yet physical discomfort, such as dyspareunia and hot flashes, may cause anxiety and tension, which can negatively affect the desire for sex, and therefore, sexual responsiveness.[126]

Little research has been done on the physiology of the sexual response in postmenopausal women. Masters and Johnson[240] documented that the capacity for orgasm remains intact, although the intensity and duration of the orgasm may be reduced and the overall sexual response is decreased and requires more stimulation. Morrell and coworkers[244] reported that postmenopausal women demonstrate lower estrogen levels and less sexual responsiveness to erotic films than younger (mean age, 31) normally cycling women and older (mean age, 51) cycling women, as measured by vaginal pulse amplitude. Thus, it seems that menopausal status, not age per se, is the critical factor.

Many women are concerned about maintaining a satisfying sexual relationship as they enter their postmenopausal years. An individual's sexual behavior after menopause depends to a great extent on her satisfaction with her sex life before menopause and on the responsiveness and sensitivity of her partner.[239] Genital tract changes do not necessarily affect a woman's capacity as a lover. The problems a woman faces also can be caused by physical changes in her partner, a partner ignorant of the changes that both may be experiencing, or, more likely, the lack of a partner.[250] Demographics indicate that there are far more older women than available men. Masturbation and homosexuality are not practiced by many older women today; thus, many have no sexual outlet. If they do have a partner of the same age or older, his sexual responsiveness is likely to have declined, a phenomenon manifested as increased time to achieve erection and decreased ability to maintain it. Surgery or medication may also affect men's sexual functioning.

But a changing body does not have to mean a reduction in the quality of sexual interaction. Sex is, of course, more than just intercourse, orgasm, and the anatomy and physiology of sex organs. Sensual and sexual arousal can involve the whole body. The slower arousal time that both men and women experience as they grow older can provide an opportunity to explore new ways to heighten sexual enjoyment.

In the 1990s, menopause has emerged as a significant area of clinical and basic research. In this chapter we have presented current information about menopause, including an indication of the range of symptom patterns that may be seen in clinical practice. Although we have focused on symptoms that have been described extensively in western populations, physicians in North America may see patients from a variety of cultural and ethnic backgrounds. It is helpful, therefore, to be aware that women of different cultures may have different perceptions and definitions of whether or how their problems, both psychological and physiological, relate to menopause.

Currently, approximately one-third of American women are 45 years of age or older.[251] Health issues of concern to them, such as osteoporosis and cardiovascular disease, and the relationship of these diseases to the hormonal changes of menopause, have made their way into the media. Today, physicians are treating women who have more medical information than ever before, who ask many questions, and who deserve informed and considered responses.

In concentrating on the physiology of menopause, one risks giving the impression that the changes described are solely caused by menopause, and that all women experience them as problems. Although the biological changes that occur with menopause can cause serious problems for some women, for many others they pose few, if any. Changes associated with menopause are complexly interrelated with concomitant aging processes. The ability and capacity to adapt to these changes vary with each person. We do well to keep in mind Margaret Mead, who spoke of her menopausal years as an energetic and creative time and reported that women in most societies exhibit a postmenopausal zest.[252]

REFERENCES

1. Speroff L, Glass R, Kase N. Clinical Gynecologic Endocrinology and Infertility (6th ed). Baltimore: Lippincott Williams & Wilkins, 1999.

2. Himelstein-Braw R, Byskov AG, Peters H, Faber M. Follicular atresia in the infant human ovary. J Report Fertil 1976;46:55–59.

3. Richardson SJ, Senikas V, Nelson JF. Follicular depletion during the menopausal transition—evidence for accelerated loss and ultimate exhaustion. J Clin Endocrinol Metab 1987;65:1231.

4. Crockett L, Peterson A. Adolescent Development Health Risks and Opportunities for Health Promotion. In S Millstein, A Petersen, E Mightengale (eds), Promoting the Health of Adolescents: New Directions for the Twenty-First Century. New York: Oxford University Press, 1993.

5. Netter F. The Ciba Collection of Medical Illustrations. Vol 2: The Reproductive Tract. Summit, NJ: Ciba Pharmaceutical Products, 1977.

6. Munster K, Schmidt L, Helm P. Length and variation in the menstrual cycle—a cross sectional study from Danish country. Br J Obstetr Gynecol 1992;99:422.

7. Moerman ML. Growth of the birth canal in adolescent girls. Am J Obstetr Gynecol 1982;143:528–532.

8. Wyshak G, Frisch RE. Evidence for a secular trend in menarche. N Engl J Med 1982;306:1033–1035.

9. Herman-Giddens ME, Slora EJ, Wasserman RC, et al. Secondary sexual characteristics and menses in young girls seen in office practice: a study from the Pediatric Research in Office Settings network. Pediatrics 1997;99(4):505–512.

10. Zacharias L, Rand WM, Wurtman RJ. A prospective study of sexual development and growth in American girls: the statistics of menarche. Obstetr Gynecol Surv 1976;31:325.

11. Marshall WA, Tanner JM. Variations in pattern of pubertal changes in girls. Arch Dis Child 1969;44:291–303.

12. Frisch RE, McArthur JW. Menstrual cycles: fatness as a determinant of minimum weight for height necessary for their maintenance or onset. Science 1974;185:949–951.

13. Frisch RE, Revelle R, Cook S. Components of weight at menarche and the initiation of the adolescent growth spurt in girls: estimated total water, lean body weight and fat. Hum Biol 1973;45:469–483.

14. Bayley N. Size and body build of adolescents in relation to rate of skeletal maturing. Child Dev 1943;14:47–90.

15. Tanner JM. Growth at Adolescence (2nd ed). London: Blackwell Scientific, 1962.

16. Stevens-Simon C, Forbes GB, Kreipe RE, McArney ER. A comparison of chronologic age and gynecologic age as indices of biologic maturity. Am J Dis Child 1986;140:702–705.

17. Whitelaw MJ. Experiences in treating excessive height in girls with cyclic oestradiol valerate. Acta Endocrinol 1967;54:473–484.

18. Manolagas SC, Jilka RL. Bone marrow: cytokines and bone remodeling. N Engl J Med 1995;332:305–311.

19. Krokor A. Endocrine, Iatrogenic and Nutritional Cause of Osteopenia. In P Foa (ed), Humoral Factors in the Regulation of Tissue Growth. New York: Springer-Verlag, 1993;194–210.

20. Lyles KW. Osteoporosis Textbook of Internal Medicine (2nd ed). Philadelphia: JB Lippincott, 1991.

21. Tresolini CP, Gold D, Lee L. Osteoporosis: A Curriculum Guide for the Health Professions (2nd ed). San Francisco: National Fund for Medical Education, 1998.

22. Luke B, Johnson T, Petrie R. Clinical Maternal-Fetal Nutrition. Boston: Little, Brown, 1993.

23. Duenhoelter JH, Jimenez JM, Bauman G. Pregnancy performance of patients under fifteen years of age. Obstetr Gynecol 1975;46:49–52.

24. Graham D. The Obstetric and Neonatal Consequences of Adolescent Pregnancy. In ER McAnarney, G Stickle (eds), Birth Defects: Original Article Series. Vol 17(3): Pregnancy and Childbearing during Adolescence. New York: AR Liss, 1981;49–67.

25. Maymon R, Shulman A. Controversies and problems in the current management of tubal pregnancy. Hum Reprod Update 1996;2:541–551.

26. Burrows TD, King A, Loke YW. Trophoblast migration during human placental implantation. Hum Reprod Update 1996;2:307.

27. Navot RW, Scott RT, Doresch K, et al. The window of embryo transfer and the efficiency of human conception in vitro. Fertil Steril 1991;55:114.

28. Alsat E, Guibourdenche J, Luton D, et al. Human placental growth hormone. Am J Obstetr Gynecol 1997;177(6):1526–1534.

29. Creasy R, Resnik R (eds). Maternal Fetal Medicine (4th ed). Philadelphia: WB Saunders, 1999.

30. Blackburn S, Loper D. Maternal, Fetal and Neonatal Physiology: A Clinical Perspective. Philadelphia: WB Saunders, 1992.

31. De Swiet M. Maternal Pulmonary Disorders. In R Creasy, R Resnik (eds), Maternal-Fetal Medicine. Philadelphia: WB Saunders, 1999.

32. Milne JA, Howie AD, Pack AI. Dyspnoea during normal pregnancy. Br J Obstetr Gynaecol 1978;85;260–263.

33. Cousins L, Rigg L, Hollingsworth D, et al. The 24-Hour excursion and diurnal rhythm of glucose, insulin and C-peptide in normal pregnancy. Am J Obstetr Gynecol 1980;153:824–828.

34. Cunningham G, MacDonald P, Gant N, et al. Williams Obstetrics (20th ed). Norwalk, CT: Appleton & Lange, 1997.

35. Baird JD. Some aspects of the metabolic and hormonal adaptation to pregnancy. Acta Endocrinol 1986;112(Suppl 277):11.

36. Kretchmer N, Schumacher LB, Stillman K. Biological factors affecting intrauterine growth. Semin Perinatol 1989;13:169.

37. Institute of Medicine. Nutrition During Pregnancy. Part I: Weight Gain, Part II: Nutrient Supplements. Washington, DC: National Academy Press, 1990.

38. Fries EC, Hellenbrandt FA. The influence of pregnancy on the location of center of gravity: postural stability and body alignment. Am J Obstet Gynecol 1943;46:374.

39. Perkins J, Hamer RL, Loubert PV. Identification and management of pregnancy-related low back pain. J Nurs Mid 1998;43:331–340.

40. Kisner C, Colby LA. Therapeutic Exercises: Foundations and Techniques. Philadelphia: FA Davis, 1996.

41. Aminoff M. Neurologic Disorders. In RK Creasy, R Resnick (eds), Maternal-Fetal Medicine: Principles and Practice (3rd ed). Philadelphia: WB Saunders, 1999.

42. Mantle MJ, Greenwood RM, Currey HLF. Backache in pregnancy. Rheumatol Rehab 1997;16:95.

43. Bullock JE, Jull GA, Bullock MI. The relationship of low back pain to postural changes during pregnancy. Aust J Physiol 1987;15:22–27.

44. Orvieto R, Achiron A, Ben-Rafael Z, et al. Low-back pain of pregnancy. Acta Obstet Gynecol Scand 1994;73:209–214.

45. Crisp WE, DeFrancesco A. The hand syndrome of pregnancy. Obstetr Gynecol 1964;23:433.

46. Clapp JF III, Rokey R, Treadway JL, et al. Exercise in pregnancy. Med Sci Sports Exerc 1992;24:S294–S300.

47. Sandhar BK, Elliott RH, Windram I, Rowbotham DJ. Peripartum changes in gastric emptying. Anesthesia 1992;47(3);196–198.

48. Gilleard W, Brown J. Structure and function of the abdominal muscles in primigravid subjects during pregnancy and the immediate post birth period. Phys Ther 1996;76(7):750–762.

49. Jaszmann L, Van Lith ND, Zaat JCA. The age at menopause in the Netherlands: the statistical analysis of a survey. Med Gynaecol Androl Sociol 1969;4:256–262.

50. Frere G. Mean age at menopause and menarche in South Africa. S Afr J Med Sci 1971;36:21–24.

51. McKinlay S, Jefferys M, Thompson B. An investigation of the age at menopause. J Biosoc Sci 1972;4:161–173.

52. Jaszmann L. Epidemiology of climacteric and post climacteric complaints. Front Horm Res 1973;2:22–34.

53. Thompson B, Hart SA, Durno D. Menopausal age and symptomatology in a general practice. J Biosoc Sci 1973;5:71–82.

54. Treloar AE. Menarche, menopause, and intervening fecundability. Hum Biol 1974;46(1):89–107.

55. van Keep PA, Brand PC, Lehert P. Factors affecting the age at menopause. J Biosoc Sci 1979;6(Suppl):37–55.

56. Treloar AE. Menstrual cyclicity and the premenopause. Maturitas 1981;3:249–264.

57. Obermeyer CM. Menopause across cultures: a review of the evidence. Menopause 2000;7:184–192.

58. Jick H, Porter J, Morrison AS. Relation between smoking and natural menopause. Lancet 1977;1:1354–1355.

59. Kaufman DW, Slone D, Rosenburg L, et al. Cigarette smoking and age at natural menopause. Am J Public Health 1980;70:420–422.

60. Willett W, Stampfer MJ, Bain C, et al. Cigarette smoking, relative weight, and menopause. Am J Epidemiol 1983;117:651–658.

61. McKinlay SM, Bifano N, McKinlay JB. Smoking and age at menopause in women. Ann Intern Med 1985;103:350–356.

62. Stanford JL, Hartge P, Brinton LA, et al. Factors influencing the age at natural menopause. J Chron Dis 1987;40:995–1002.

63. Brand PC, Lehert PH. A new way of looking at environmental variables that may affect the age at menopause. Maturitas 1978;1:121–132.

64. Richards MA, O'Reilly SM, Howell A, et al. Adjuvant cyclophosphamide, methotrexate and fluorouracil in patients with axillary node-positive breast cancer: an update of the Guy's/Manchester trial. J Clin Oncol 1990;8:2032–2039.

65. Ravn P, Lind C, Nilas L. Lack of influence of simple premenopausal hysterectomy on bone mass and bone metabolism. Am J Obstet Gynecol 1995;172:891–895.

66. World Health Organization. Research on the Menopause in the 1990s: Report of a WHO Scientific Group. Geneva: WHO Technical Report Series, 1996;866.

67. Veldhuis JD, Christiansen E, Evans WS, et al. Physiological profiles of episodic progesterone release during the midluteal phase of the human menstrual cycle: analysis of circadian and ultradian rhythms, discrete pulse properties, and correlations with simultaneous luteinizing hormone release. J Clin Endocrinol Metab 1988;66:414–421.

68. Wehrenberg WB, Wardlaw SL, Frantz AG, et al. Beta-endorphin in hypophyseal portal blood: variations throughout the menstrual cycle. Endocrinology 1982;111:879–881.

69. Reid RL, Hoff JD, Yen SSC, et al. Effect of exogenous Beta-endorphin on pituitary hormone secretion and its disappearance rate in normal human subjects. J Clin Endocrinol Metab 1981;52:1179–1183.

70. Ferin M, Van Vugt D, Wardlaw S. The hypothalamic control of the menstrual cycle and the role of endogenous opioid peptides. Recent Prog Horm Res 1984;40:441–485.

71. McLachlan RI, Robertson DM, Healy DL, et al. Circulating immunoreactive inhibin levels during the normal human menstrual cycle. J Clin Endocrinol Metab 1987;65:954.

72. Speroff L, Glass RH, Kase NG. Clinical Gynecologic Endocrinology & Infertility. Baltimore: Williams & Wilkins, 1989.

73. March CM, Marrs RP, Goebelsmarm U, et al. Feedback effects of estradiol and progesterone upon gonadotropin and prolactin release. Obstet Gynecol 1981;58:10–16.

74. Nicosia SV. The aging ovary. Med Clin North Am 1987;71:1–10.

75. Baker TG. A quantitative and cytological study of germ cells in human ovaries. Proc R Soc Lond Biol 1963;158:417–433.

76. Novak ER. Ovulation after fifty. Obstet Gynecol 1970;36:903–910.

77. Costoff A, Mahesh VB. Primordial follicles with normal oocytes in the ovaries of postmenopausal women. J Am Geriatr Soc 1975;23:193–195.

78. Treloar AE, Boynton RE, Behn BG, et al. Variation of the human menstrual cycle through reproductive life. Int J Fertil 1967;12:77–126.

79. Vollman RF. The Menstrual Cycle. Philadelphia: WB Saunders, 1977.

80. Kaufert PA, Gilbert P, Tate R. Defining menopausal status: the impact of longitudinal data. Maturitas 1987;9:217–226.

81. McKinlay SM, Brambilla PJ, Posner JG. The normal menopausal transition. Maturitas 1992;14:103–115.

82. Sherman BM, West JH, Korenman SG. The menopausal transition: analysis of LH, FSH, estradiol, and progesterone concentrations during menstrual cycles of older women. J Clin Endocrinol Metab 1976;42:629–636.

83. Reyes FI, Winter JSD, Faiman C. Pituitary–ovarian relationships preceding the menopause. Am J Obstet Gynecol 1977;129:557–563.

84. Lenton EA, Sexton L, Lee S, et al. Progressive changes in LH and FSH and LH:FSH ratio in women throughout reproductive life. Maturitas 1988;10:35–43.

85. Chang RJ, Judd HL. The ovary after menopause. Clin Obstet Gynecol 1981;24:181–191.

86. Metcalf MG, Donald RA, Livesey JH. Pituitary–ovarian function in normal women during the menopausal transition. Clin Endocrinol 1981;14:245–255.

87. Marrs RP, Lobo R, Campeau JD, et al. Correlation of human follicular fluid inhibin activity with spontaneous induced follicular maturation. J Clin Endocrinol Metab 1984;58:704–709.

88. Sherman BM. Endocrinologic and Menstrual Alterations. In DR Mishell Jr (ed), Menopause: Physiology and Pharmacology. Chicago: Year Book Medical Publishers, 1987;41–51.

89. Wide L, Nillius SJ, Gensell C, et al. Radioimmunosorbent assay of follicle-stimulating hormone and luteinizing hormone in serum and urine from men and women. Acta Endocrinol (Copenhagen) 1973;174:1–58.

90. Chakravarti S, Collins WP, Forecast JD, et al. Hormonal profiles after the menopause. BMJ 1976;2:784–786.

91. Studd J, Chakravarti S, Oram D. The climacteric. Clin Obstet Gynaecol 1977;4:3–29.

92. Judd HL. Reproductive Hormone Metabolism in Postmenopausal Women. In BA Eskin (ed), The Menopause. Comprehensive Management. New York: Masson, 1980;55–71.

93. Somma M, Sandor T, Lanthier A. Site of origin of androgenic and estrogenic steroids in the normal human ovary. J Clin Endocrinol 1969;29:457–466.

94. Baird DT, Horton R, Longcope C. Steroid dynamics under steady-state conditions. Recent Prog Horm Res 1969;25:611–664.

95. Baird DT, Fraser IS. Blood production and ovarian secretion rates of estradiol-17 and estrone in women throughout the menstrual cycle. J Clin Endocrinol Metab 1974;38:1009–1017.

96. Casey ML, MacDonald PC. Origin of Estrogen and Regulation of Its Formation in Postmenopausal Women. In HJ Buschman (ed), The Menopause. New York: Springer-Verlag, 1983;1–8.

97. Santoro N, Brown JR, Adel T, Skurnick JH. Characterization of reproductive hormone dynamics in the perimenopause. J Clin Endocrinol Metab 1996;81:1495–1501.

98. Poliak A, Jones GES, Goldberg B, et al. Effect of human chorionic gonadotropin on postmenopausal women. Am J Obstet Gynecol 1968;101:731–739.

99. Vermeulen A, Verdonck L. Factors affecting sex hormone levels in postmenopausal women. J Steroid Biochem 1979;11:899–904.

100. Vermeulen A. Sex hormone status of the postmenopausal woman. Maturitas 1980;2:81–89.

101. Longcope C, Hunter R, Franz C. Steroid secretion by the postmenopausal ovary. Am J Obstet Gynecol 1980;138:564–568.

102. Grodin JM, Siiteri PK, MacDonald PC. Source of estrogen production in post-menopausal women. J Clin Endocrinol Metab 1973;36:207–214.

103. MacDonald PC, Edman CD, Hemsell DL, et al. Effect of obesity on conversion of plasma androstenedione to estrone in postmenopausal women with and without endometrial cancer. Am J Obstet Gynecol 1978;130:448–455.

104. Edman CD. The Climacteric. In HJ Buchsbaum (ed), The Menopause. New York: Springer-Verlag, 1983;23–33.

105. Hemsell DL, Grodin JM, Brenner PF, et al. Plasma precursors of estrogen-II. Correlation of the extent of conversion of plasma androstenedione to estrone with age. J Clin Endocrinol Metab 1974;38:476–479.

106. Meldrum DR, Davidson BJ, Tataryn IV, et al. Changes in circulating steroids with aging in postmenopausal women. Obstet Gynecol 1981;57:624–628.

107. Judd HL, Shamonki IM, Frumar AM, et al. Origin of serum estradiol in post-menopausal women. Obstet Gynecol 1982;59:680–686.

108. Vermeulen A. The hormonal activity of the post-menopausal ovary. J Clin Endocrinol Metab 1976;42:247–253.

109. Judd HL, Judd GE, Lucas WE, et al. Endocrine function of the postmenopausal ovary: concentration of androgens and estrogens in ovarian and peripheral blood. J Clin Endocrinol Metab 1974;39:1020–1024.

110. Sherman BM, Korenman SG. Hormonal characteristics of the human menstrual cycle throughout reproductive life. J Clin Invest 1975;55:699–706.

111. Kaufman SA. The Menopause. In TW McElin, JJ Sciarra (eds), Gynecology and Obstetrics. New York: Harper & Row, 1981;1–11.

112. Flint M. The menopause: reward or punishment. Psychosomatics 1975;16:161–163.

113. Kaufert P, Syrotuik J. Symptom reporting at the menopause. Soc Sci Med 1981;15E:173–184.

114. Kaufert PA, Gilbert P, Hassard T. Researching the symptoms of menopause: an exercise in methodology. Maturitas 1988;10:117–131.

115. Lock M, Kaufert P, Gilbert P. Cultural construction of the menopausal syndrome: the Japanese case. Maturitas 1988;10:317–332.

116. Agoestina T, van Keep PA. The climacteric in Bandung, West Java province, Indonesia: a survey of 1025 women between 40–55 years of age. Maturitas 1984;6:327–333.

117. Beyene Y. Cultural significance and physiological manifestations of menopause: a biocultural analysis. Cult Med Psychiatry 1986;10:47–71.

118. Thornton JG. Menopausal hot flushes: personal experience in Africa. Trop Doct 1984;140:135.

119. Brown KH, Hammond CB. Urogenital atrophy. Obstet Gynecol Clin North Am 1987;15:13–32.

120. Sarrel PM. Sexuality in the middle years. Obstet Gynecol Clin North Am 1987;4:49–62.

121. Bergman A, Brenner PF. Alterations in the Urogenital System. In DR Mishell Jr (ed), Menopause: Physiology and Pharmacology. Chicago: Year Book Medical Publishers, 1987;67–75.

122. Voet RL. End Organ Response to Estrogen Deprivation. In HJ Buchsbaum (ed), The Menopause. New York: Springer-Verlag, 1983;9–22.

123. Barber HRK. Perimenopausal and Geriatric Gynecology. New York: Macmillan, 1988.

124. Semmens JP, Wagner G. Estrogen deprivation and vaginal function in postmenopausal women. JAMA 1982; 248:445–448.

125. Tsai CC, Semmens JP, Semmens EC, et al. Vaginal physiology in postmenopausal women: pH value, transvaginal electropotential difference, and estimated blood flow. South Med J 1987;80:987–990.

126. Bachmann GA, Lieblum SR, Kermmann E, et al. Sexual expression and its determinants in the post-menopausal woman. Maturitas 1984;6:19–29.

127. Semmens JP, Tsai CC, Semmens EC, et al. Effects of estrogen therapy on vaginal physiology during menopause. Obstet Gynecol 1985;66:15–18.

128. Bergh PA. Vaginal Changes with Aging. In JL Breen (ed), The Gynecologist and the Older Patient. Rockville, MD: Aspen, 1988;299–311.

129. Cobb JO. Understanding Menopause. Toronto: Key Porter Books, 1988.

130. Singer A. The uterine cervix from adolescence to the menopause. Br J Obstet Gynaecol 1975;82:81–99.

131. Karafin LJ, Coll ME. Lower urinary tract disorders in the postmenopausal woman. Med Clin North Am 1987;71:111–122.

132. Ferin M. Clinical review 105: stress and the reproductive cycle. J Clin Endocrinol Metab 1999;84:1768–1774.

133. Berga SL. Functional Hypothalamic Chronic Anovulation. In EY Adashi, JA Rock, Z Rosenwaks (eds), Reproductive Endocrinology, Surgery and Technology. Vol 1. Philadelphia: Lippincott-Raven, 1996;1061–1076.

134. Reifenstein EC. Psychogenic or "hypothalamic" amenorrhea. Med Clin North Am 1946;30:1103–1114.

135. Chrousos GP, Gold PW. The concepts of stress and stress system disorders. Overview of physical and behavioral homeostasis. JAMA 1992;267:1244–1252.

136. Dunn AJ, Berridge CW. Physiological and behavioral responses to corticotropin-releasing factor administration: Is CRF a mediator of anxiety or stress responses? Brain Res Rev 1990;15:71–100.

137. Luger A, Deuster PA, Kyle SB, et al. Acute hypothalamic-pituitary-adrenal responses to the stress of treadmill exercise. Physiologic adaptations to training. N Engl J Med 1987;316:1309–1315.

138. Warren MP. Eating Disorders and the Reproductive Axis. In EY Adashi, JA Rock, Z Rosenwaks (eds), Reproductive Endocrinology, Surgery and Technology. Vol 1. Philadelphia: Lippincott-Raven, 1996;1039–1060.

139. Prior CJ. Exercise-Associated Menstrual Disturbances. In EY Adashi, JA Rock, Z Rosenwaks (eds), Reproductive Endocrinology, Surgery and Technology. Philadelphia: Lippincott-Raven, 1996;1077–1092.

140. Notelovitz M. Gynecologic problems of menopausal women: part 3. Changes in extragenital tissues and sexuality. Geriatrics 1978;33:51–58.

141. Kligman AM, Grove GL, Balin AK. Aging of Human Skin. In CE Finch, EL Schneider (eds), The Biology of Aging. New York: Van Nostrand Reinhold, 1985;820–841.

142. Stumpf WE, Sar M, Joshi SG. Estrogen target cells in the skin. Experientia 1974;30:196–198.

143. Hasslequist MB, Goldberg N, Schroeter A, et al. Isolation and characterization of the estrogen receptor in human skin. J Clin Endocrinol Metab 1980;50:76–82.

144. Brincat M, Studd J. Skin and Menopause. In DR Mishell Jr (ed), Menopause: Physiology and Pharmacology. Chicago: Year Book Medical Publishers, 1987;103–114.

145. Corlett RC. Urinary Tract Disorders. In HJ Buchsbaum (ed), The Menopause. New York: Springer-Verlag, 1983;131–138.

146. Smith P. Age changes in the female urethra. Br J Urol 1972;44:667–676.

147. Brown ADG. Postmenopausal urinary problems. Clin Obstet Gynecol 1977;4:181–206.

148. Notelovitz M. Gynecologic problems of menopausal women: part 1. Changes in genital tissues. Geriatrics 1978;33:24–30.

149. Hagstad A, Janson PO. The epidemiology of climacteric symptoms. Acta Obstet Gynecol Scand Suppl 1986;134:59–65.

150. Thomas TM, Plymat KR, Blannin J, et al. Prevalence of urinary incontinence. BMJ 1980;281:1243–1245.

151. Brocklehurst JC, Fry J, Griffiths LL, et al. Urinary infection and symptoms of dysuria in women aged 45–64 years, their relevance to similar findings in the elderly. Age Ageing 1972;1:41–47.

152. Rekers H. Urogenital Problems. In L Zichella, M Whitehead, PA van Keep (eds), The Climacteric and Beyond. Park Ridge, NJ: Parthenon, 1988;145–146.

153. Tsang R, Gleuck CJ. Atherosclerosis, a pediatric perspective. Curr Probl Pediatr 1979;9:3–37.

154. Gordon T, Kannel WB, Hjortland MC, et al. Menopause and coronary heart disease: the Framingham Study. Ann Intern Med 1978;89:157–161.

155. Pfeffer RI, Whipple GA, Kurosak TT, Chapman JM. Coronary risk and estrogen use in postmenopausal women. Am J Epidemiol 1978;107:479–487.

156. Kannel WB, Hjortland MC, McNamara PM, et al. Menopause and risk of cardiovascular disease. The Framingham Study. Ann Intern Med 1976;85:447–452.

157. Castelli WB, Doyle IT, Gordon T, et al. HDL cholesterol and other lipids in coronary heart disease. The Cooperative Lipoprotein Phenotyping study. Circulation 1977;55:767–772.

158. Gordon T, Castelli WP, Hjortland MP, et al. The Framingham Study. High lipoprotein as a protective factor against coronary heart disease. Am J Med 1977;62:707–714.

159. Heiss G, Tamir I, Davis CE, et al. Lipoprotein-cholesterol distributions in selected North American populations: the Lipid Research Program prevalence study. Circulation 1980;61:302–315.

160. Bush TL, Barrett-Connor E. Noncontraceptive estrogen use and cardiovascular disease. Epidemiol Rev 1985;7:80–104.

161. Wallace RB, Hoover J, Barrett-Connor E, et al. Altered plasma lipid and lipoprotein levels associated with oral contraceptive and oestrogen use. Lancet 1979;2:111–115.

162. Cauley JA, LaPorte RE, Kuller LH, et al. Menopausal estrogen use, high density lipoprotein cholesterol subfractions and liver function. Arteriosclerosis 1983;49:31–39.

163. Wahl P, Walden C, Knopp R, et al. Effect of estrogen/progestin potency on lipid/lipoprotein cholesterol. N Engl J Med 1983;308:862–867.

164. Rosenberg L, Armstrong B, Jick H. Myocardial infarction and estrogen therapy in post-menopausal women. N Engl J Med 1976;294:1256–1259.

165. Wilson PWF, Garrison RJ, Castelli WP. Postmenopausal estrogen use, cigarette smoking, and cardiovascular morbidity in women over 50. N Engl J Med 1985;313:1038–1043.

166. Ross RK, Paganini-Hill A, Mack TM, et al. Menopausal oestrogen therapy and protection from death from ischemic heart disease. Lancet 1981;1:858–860.

167. Bush TL, Miller VT. Effects of Pharmacologic Agents Used During Menopause: Impact on Lipids and Lipoproteins. In DR Mishell Jr (ed), Menopause: Physiology and Pharmacology. Chicago: Year Book Medical Publishers, 1987;187–208.

168. Bain C, Willett W, Hennekens CH, et al. Use of postmenopausal hormones and risk of myocardial infarction. Circulation 1981;64:42–46.

169. Stampfer MJ, Colditz GA, Willett WC, et al. Postmenopausal estrogen therapy and cardiovascular disease. N Engl J Med 1991;325:756–762.

170. Kennedy DL, Baum C, Forbes MB. Noncontraceptive estrogens and progestins: use patterns overtime. Obstet Gynecol 1985;65:441–446.

171. Goodman MJ, Stewart CJ, Gilbert F Jr. Patterns of menopause. A study of certain medical and physiological variables among Caucasian and Japanese women living in Hawaii. J Gerontol 1977;32:291–298.

172. McKinlay SM, Jefferys M. The menopausal syndrome. Br J Prev Soc Med 1974;28:108–115.

173. Jaszmann L, Van Lith ND, Zaat JAC. The perimenopausal symptoms: the statistical analysis of a survey. Parts A & B. Med Gynaecol Androl Sociol 1969;4:268–277.

174. Neugarten BL, Kraines RJ. "Menopausal symptoms" in women of various ages. Psychosomat Med 1965;27:266–273.

175. Smith G, Waters WE. An epidemiological study of factors associated with perimenopausal hot flushes. Public Health 1983;97:347–351.

176. James CE, Breeson AJ, Kovacs G, et al, The symptomatology of the climacteric in relation to hormonal and cytological factors. Br J Obstet Gynaecol 1984;91:56–62.

177. Feldman BM, Voda AM, Gronseth E. The prevalence of hot flash and associated variables among perimenopausal women. Res Nurs Health 1985;8:261–268.

178. Kronenberg F. Hot flashes: epidemiology and physiology. Ann N Y Acad Sci 1990;592:52–86.

179. Sherman BM, Wallace RB, Bean JA, et al. The relationship of menopausal hot flushes to medical and reproductive experience. J Gerontol 1981;36:306–309.

180. Chakravarti S, Collins LAT, Newton JR, et al. Endocrine changes and symptomatology after oophorectomy in premenopausal women. Br J Obstet Gynaecol 1977;84:769–775.

181. Utian WH. The true clinical features of postmenopause and oophorectomy, and their response to oestrogen therapy. S Afr Med J 1972;46:732–737.

182. Lock M. Ambiguities of aging: Japanese experience and perceptions of menopause. Cult Med Psychiatry 1986;10:23–46.

183. Sharma VK, Saxena MSL. Climacteric symptoms: a study in the Indian context. Maturitas 1981;3:11–20.

184. Moore B. Climacteric symptoms in an African community. Maturitas 1981;3:25–29.

185. Wright AL. On the calculation of climacteric symptoms. Maturitas 1981;3:55–63.

186. Kay M, Voda AM, Olivas G, et al. Ethnography of the menopause-related hot flash. Maturitas 1982;4:217–227.

187. Boulet MJ, Oddens BJ, Lehert P, et al. Climacteric and menopause in seven south-east Asian countries. Maturitas 1994;19:157–176.

188. Chompootweep S, Tankeyoon M, Yamarat K, et al. The menopausal age and climacteric complaints in Thai women in Bangkok. Maturitas 1993;17:63–71.

189. Tang G. The climacteric of Chinese factory workers. Maturitas 1994;19:177–182.

190. Punyahotra S, Dennerstein L, Lehert P. Menopausal experiences of Thai women. Part 1: Symptoms and their correlates. Maturitas 1997;26:1–7.

191. Wasti S, Robinson SC, Akhtar Y, et al. Characteristics of menopause in three socioeconomic urban groups in Karachi, Pakistan. Maturitas 1993;16:61–69.

192. Neslihan CS, Bilge SA, Ozturk TN, et al. The menopausal age, related factors and climacteric symptoms in Turkish women. Maturitas 1998;30:37–40.

193. Moore B, Kombe H. Climacteric symptoms in a Tanzanian community. Maturitas 1991;3:229–234.

194. Grisso JA, Freeman EW, Maurin E, et al. Racial differences in menopausal information and the experience of hot flashes. J Gen Intern Med 1999;14:98–103.

195. Langenberg P, Kjerulff KH, Stolley PD. Hormone replacement and menopausal symptoms following hysterectomy. Am J Epidemiol 1997;146:870–880.

196. Schwingl PJ, Hulka BS, Harlow SD. Risk factor for postmenopausal hot flashes. Obstet Gynecol 1994;84:29–32.

197. Kronenberg F, Cote LJ, Linkie DM, et al. Menopausal hot flashes: thermoregulatory, cardiovascular, and circulating catecholamine and LH changes. Maturitas 1984;6:31–43.

198. Molnar GW. Body temperatures during menopausal hot flashes. J Appl Physiol 1975;38:499–503.

199. Sturdee DW, Wilson KA, Pipili E, et al. Physiological aspects of menopausal hot flash. BMJ 1978;2:79–80.

200. Tataryn IV, Lomax P, Bajorek JG, et al. Postmenopausal hot flushes: a disorder of thermoregulation. Maturitas 1980;2:101–107.

201. Meldrum DR, DeFazio JD, Erlik Y, et al. Pituitary hormones during the menopausal hot flash. Obstet Gynecol 1984;64:752–756.

202. Genazzani AR, Petraglia F, Facchinetti F, et al. Increase of proopiomelanocortin-related peptides during subjective menopausal flushes. Am J Obstet Gynecol 1984;149:775–779.

203. Kronenberg F, Carraway RE. Changes in neurotensin-like immunoreactivity during menopausal hot flashes. J Clin Endocrinol Metab 1985;60:1081–1086.

204. Kronenberg F, Downey JA. Thermoregulatory physiology of menopausal hot flashes: a review. Can J Physiol Pharmacol 1987;65:1312–1324.

205. Ginsberg J, Swinhoe J, O'Reilly B. Cardiovascular responses during the menopausal hot flush. Br J Obstet Gynaecol 1981;88:925–930.

206. Nesheim BI, Saetre T. Changes in skin blood flow and body temperatures during climacteric hot flashes. Maturitas 1982;4:49–55.

207. Tataryn IV, Meldrum DR, Lu KH, et al. FSH and skin temperature during menopausal hot flush. Clin Endocrinol Metab 1979;49:152–154.

208. Casper RF, Yen SSC, Wilkes MM. Menopausal flushes: a neuroendocrine link with pulsatile luteinizing hormone secretion. Science 1979;205:823–825.

209. Freedman RR, Woodward S. Core body temperature during menopausal

hot flushes. Fertil Steril 1996;65:1141–1144.

210. Freedman RR, Krell W. Reduced thermoregulatory null zone in post-menopausal women with hot flashes. Am J Obstet Gynecol 1999;181:66–70.

211. Freedman RR. Biochemical, metabolic, and vascular mechanisms in menopausal hot flashes. Fertil Steril 1998;70:332–337.

212. Aksel S, Schomberg DW, Iyrey L, et al. Vasomotor symptoms, serum estrogens and gonadotropin levels in surgical menopause. Am J Obstet Gynecol 1976;12:165–169.

213. Erlik Y, Meldrum DR, Judd HL. Estrogen levels in postmenopausal women with hot flashes. Obstet Gynecol 1982;59:403–407.

214. Abe T, Furvhashi N, Yamaya Y, et al. Correlation between climacteric symptoms and serum levels of estradiol, progesterone, follicle-stimulating hormone, and luteinizing hormone. Am J Obstet Gynecol 1977;129:65–67.

215. Chakravarti S, Collins WP, Thom MH, et al. Relation between plasma hormone profiles, symptoms, and responses to oestrogen treatment in women approaching the menopause. BMJ 1979;1:983–985.

216. Meldrum DR, Tataryn IV, Frurnar AM, et al. Gonadotropins, estrogens, and adrenal steroids during the menopausal hot flash. J Clin Endocrinol Metab 1980;50:685–689.

217. Mulley G, Mitchell JRA, Tattersall RB. Hot flushes after hypophysectomy. BMJ 1977;2:1062.

218. Casper RF, Yen SSC. Menopausal flushes: effect of pituitary gonadotropin desensitization by a potent luteinizing hormone releasing factor agonist. J Clin Endocrinol Metab 1981;53:1056–1058.

219. Lightman SL, Jacobs SJ, Maguire AK. Downregulation of gonadotropin secretion in postmenopausal women by superactive LHRH analogue: lack of effect on menopausal flushing. Br J Obstet Gynaecol 1982;89:977–980.

220. DeFazio J, Meldrum DR, Laufer L, et al. Induction of hot flashes in premenopausal women treated with a long-acting GnRH agonist. J Clin Endocrinol Metab 1983;56:445–448.

221. Meldrurn DR, Erlik Y, Lu JKH, et al. Objectively recorded hot flushes in patients with pituitary insufficiency. J Clin Endocrinol Metab 1981;52:684–687.

222. Mashchak CA, Kletzky OA, Artal R, et al. The relation of physiological changes to subjective symptoms in postmenopausal women with and without hot flushes. Maturitas 1984;6:301–308.

223. Lightman SL, Jacobs HS, Maguire AK, et al. Climacteric flushing: clinical and endocrine response to infusion of naloxone. Br J Obstet Gynaecol 1981;88:919–924.

224. Kronenberg F, Barnard RM. Modulation of menopausal hot flashes by ambient temperature. J Therm Biol 1992;17:43–49.

225. Erlik Y, Tataryn IV, Meldrurn DR, et al. Association of waking episodes with menopausal hot flushes. JAMA 1981;245:1741–1744.

226. Carskadon MA, Dement WC. Nocturnal determinants of daytime sleepiness. Sleep 1982;5:573–581.

227. Thomson J, Oswald L. Effects of oestrogen on the sleep, mood, and anxiety of menopausal women. BMJ 1977;2:1317–1319.

228. Schiff I, Regestein Q, Tulchinsky D, et al. Effects of estrogens on sleep and psychological states of hypogonadal women. JAMA 1979;242:2405–2407.

229. Fry JM. Sleep disorders. Med Clin North Am 1987;71:95–111.

230. Ravnikar VA, Schiff I, Regestein QR. Menopause and Sleep. In HJ Buchsbaum (ed), The Menopause. New York: Springer-Verlag, 1983;161–171.

231. Ballinger CB. Psychiatric morbidity and the menopause: screening of general population sample. BMJ 1975;3:344–346.

232. Ballinger CB. Subjective sleep disturbance at the menopause. J Psychosomat Res 1976;20:509–513.

233. Scharf MB, McDannold MD, Stover R, et al. Effects of estrogen replacement therapy on rates of cyclic alternating patterns and hot-flush events during sleep in postmenopausal women: a pilot study. Clinical Therapeutics 1997;19:304–311.

234. Polo-Kantola P, Erkkola R, Helenius H, et al. When does estrogen replacement therapy improve sleep quality? Am J Obstet Gynecol 1998;178:1002–1009.

235. Davidson JM. The Psychobiology of Sexual Experience. In JM Davidson, RJ Davidson (eds), The Psychobiology of Consciousness. New York: Plenum, 1980;271–332.

236. Weg RB. Sexuality in the Menopause. In DR Mishell Jr (ed), Menopause: Physiology and Pharmacology. Chicago: Year Book Medical Publishers, 1987;127–138.

237. Phillips NA, Rosen RC. Menopause and Sexuality. In RA Lobo (ed), Treatment of the Postmenopausal Woman: Basic and Clinical Aspects. Philadelphia: Lippincott Williams & Wilkins, 1999;437–443.

238. Brecher EM. Love, Sex, and Aging: A Summary. In EM Brecher (ed), Love, Sex, and Aging. A Consumers Union Report. Boston: Little, Brown, 1984;403–408.

239. Kinsey A, Pomeroy W, Clyde M. Sexual Behavior in the Human Female. Philadelphia: WB Saunders, 1953.

240. Masters WH, Johnson VE. Human Sexual Responses. Boston: Little, Brown, 1966.

241. Cawood EH, Bancroft J. Steroid hormones, the menopause, sexuality and well-being of women. Psychol Med 1996;26:925–936.

242. Laan E, van Lunsen RH. Hormones and sexuality in postmenopausal women: a psychophysiological study. J Psychosom Obstet Gynaecol 1997;18:126–133.

243. Dennerstein L, Smith AMA, Morse CA, Burger HG. Sexuality and the menopause. J Psychosom Obstet Gynaecol 1994;15:59–66.

244. Morrell MJ, Dixen JM, Carter CS, et al. The influence of age and cycling status on sexual arousability in women. Am J Obstet Gynecol 1984;148:66–71.

245. Leiblurn S, Bachmann G, Kemmann E, et al. Vaginal atrophy in the postmenopausal woman. JAMA 1983;249:2195–2198.

246. Cutler WB, Garcia CR, McCoy N. Perimenopausal sexuality. Arch Sex Behav 1987;16:225–234.

247. Persky H, Dreisbach L, Miller W, et al. The relation of plasma androgen levels to sexual behaviors and attitudes of women. Psychosomat Med 1982;44:305–319.

248. Sherwin BB, Gelfand MM, Brender W. Androgen enhances sexual motivation in females: a prospective, crossover study of sex steroid administration in the surgical menopause. Psychosomat Med 1985;47:339–351.

249. Bachmann GA, Leilblum SR, Sandler B, et al. Correlates of sexual desire in postmenopausal women. Maturitas 1985;7:211–216.

250. Weg RB. The Physiological Perspective. In RB Weg (ed), Sexuality in The Later Years. New York: Academic Press, 1983;39–80.

251. U.S. Department of Commerce Bureau of Census. Current Population Reports. Series P-25, Numbers 512, 917, 1022. Washington, DC: US Bureau of the Census, 1980.

252. Mead M. PMZ at work. Behav Today 1975;498.

26

Principles of Neuroplasticity: Implications for Neurorehabilitation and Learning

NANCY N. BYL AND MICHAEL MERZENICH

INTEGRATION OF RESEARCH IN NEURAL PLASTICITY INTO THE PRACTICE OF REHABILITATION

Forebrain neurons have the capability of undergoing long-lasting alterations in their responses to hormonal, pharmacologic, and environmental stimulation. The natural processes of development generate profound changes in the central nervous system (CNS). We drive neuronal response changes with specific goal-directed repetitive activities throughout life, and those changes collectively account for new skill development and for skill refinement with practice. Such goal-oriented repetitive behaviors driving positive changes in neuronal *representations* can be particularly useful for remediating the consequences of injury, disease, and aging. Numerous studies have provided insight into behavioral, molecular, and cellular mechanisms operating in adaptive brain plasticity processes.[1-3]

The findings from research in the neuroscience of plasticity have yielded novel strategies for the diagnosis and treatment of neurologic, neuropsychiatric, and neuromuscular disorders. This research has provided a foundation for understanding important neurologic effects of hormones, growth factors, and modulatory neurotransmitters, including their receptors, in development and aging. Research is also enabling the use of tissue transplantations for regeneration, aggressive interventions for neuroprotection and prevention of cell death, and rehabilitation strategies to maximize restoration of function.[4-9] Researchers and clinicians in the twenty-first century will undoubtedly expand our understanding of neuroplasticity and its applications to patient care.

Rehabilitation is the process of maximizing learning. The integration of basic neuroscience findings into clinical practice is a critical dimension of *best practice*. Neuroscientists have documented that the CNS is adaptable during development and throughout life. The nervous system can also recover from serious disease and injury through spontaneous adaptation and healing. We know that the appropriate rate and extent of recovery can be enhanced with environmental enrichment, intensive behavioral training, and drugs that positively enable or facilitate brain plasticity processes. Even the physiological effects of aging appear to be slowed if neurons remain actively engaged and rewarded.[10,11] Despite this revolutionary growth of knowledge, implementation of these findings into clinical practice has been limited. The lack of integration of basic science and clinical practice can be attributed to the researcher, clinician, patient, and third-party payer.

All too often the researcher is focused on the narrow perspective of a fundamental neuroscience subdiscipline. Researchers actively communicate with others in their field through scientific publications and formal meetings. However, most basic science researchers have little, if any, contact with clinicians. Many are primarily interested in pursuing their line of scientific inquiry. Chapter 27 exemplifies an excellent integration of basic science research and clinical application.

Practicing clinicians in neurorehabilitation may create a barrier to integrating basic science in clinical practice. For example, familiar treatment approaches dominate practice, even when the neuroscientific premises underlying these approaches are uncertain, and even though there is often no quantitative validation of their success. Many practitioners are unfamiliar with the current basic neuroscience literature. Others are familiar with recent research findings, but do not understand how to translate those findings into practice. Still others are unwilling to accept an even high probability that new research findings provide clear evidence that should support a change in practice. Failure to integrate basic science understanding into clinical practice significantly limits the potential for effective treatment of patients with disabling neurologic problems.

In some situations, the patient is the obstacle to applying current research findings into practice. To achieve maximum plasticity, patients must be committed to their recovery. They must be willing to engage in repetitive, attended, goal-directed behaviors. There is limited measurable neural adaptation generated by passive movements or passive stimuli. To achieve enduring positive changes in neural processing, the patient has to attend to stimuli, make decisions about them, and receive feedback. There are many instances in which patients are not convinced that their efforts will make a difference. In some cases, patients are not motivated to be compliant. They would prefer a drug or a surgical procedure to solve the problem. In still other situations, the neural insult itself alters patient motivation, cognition, or both, creating emotional instability or problems of neglect that forestall any meaningful commitment to recovery.

Another barrier to bringing new scientific evidence into practice is the current health care system. We live in a society in which economics largely drive the health care system. When a physician or a therapist recommends a new approach to intervention, the third-party payer usually denies payment for services considered *experimental*. Further, the third-party payer may refute claims that findings from animal studies should or can be applied to the care of human subjects. For example, animal studies confirm that the greatest spontaneous recovery occurs 30 days after a cerebrovascular accident. More recently, it has been shown that we can drive further neural adaptation and improve outcomes beyond that 30-day period with repetitive, goal-directed, fine-motor tasks.[12] Still, when physicians refer patients for continued therapy after 30 days, most third-party payers are likely to deny reimbursement.

As we continue to expand the science of learning-based brain plasticity, it is critical that we find ways to improve the interface between the scientist, practitioner, patient, and third-party payer. We must develop interdisciplinary research that makes partners of neuroscience researchers and regularly informed rehabilitation practitioners. In addition, the consumers and the third-party payers must be kept up to date on the current research findings in neuroplasticity and its realistic applications to practice.

INTEGRATION OF SENSORY INFORMATION AND MOTOR CONTROL

In all higher order perceptual processes, the brain must correlate sensory inputs with motor outputs to accurately assess and control the body's interaction with the environment. A problem in the somatic sensory system affects the motor output system. Both systems are adaptive; functional adaptation involves the interaction between both systems. Although the operation of these two systems is often studied separately, the systems are interrelated in complex ways and at multiple levels in the healthy nervous system.

Sensory systems provide an internal representation of the outside world that guides the movements that make up our behavioral repertoires. These movements are controlled by the motor systems of the brain and the spinal cord. Our perceptual skills are a reflection of the capabilities of sensory systems to detect, analyze, and estimate the significance of physical stimuli. Our agility and dexterity are a reflection of the capabilities of the motor systems to plan, coordinate, and execute movements. The task of the motor systems in controlling movement is the reverse of the task of sensory systems in generating an internal representation. Perception is the end product of sensory processing, whereas the internal representation (images of the desired movement and its goals) is the beginning of motor processing.

In sensory psychophysics, we look at the attributes of a stimulus: its quality, intensity, location, movement, and duration. In motor psychophysics we look at the organization of action: the intensity of the contraction, the recruitment of distinct populations of motor neurons, the accuracy of the movement, the coordination of the movements, and movement speed. In both sensory and motor systems, the complexity of our behaviors depends, in part, on the multiplicity of modalities that we have available to us. In somatic sensation, we have the distinct modalities and submodalities for pain, temperature, light touch, deep touch, vibration, proprioception, kinesthesia, and stretch, whereas in the motor system we have submodalities of reflex responses, rhythmic motor patterns, and voluntary movements.[13] Although all motor movements require integration of sensory information, the relationship is particularly complex in voluntary motor movements. Voluntary motor movements require contraction and relaxation of muscles, recruitment of appropriate muscles, appropriate timing and sequencing of muscle contraction and relaxation, and balanced distribution of body mass to enable appropriate postural adjustments.

The control systems for voluntary movement include

1. Continuous flow of sensory information about the environment, position, and orientation of the body and limbs as well as the degree of contraction of the muscles
2. Spinal cord
3. Descending systems of the brain stem
4. Pathways of the motor areas of the cerebral cortex

Each level of control is provided with sensory information that is relevant for the functions it controls. This information is provided by feedback, feed-forward, and adaptive mechanisms. These control systems are organized both hierarchically and in parallel. The hierarchical organization permits lower levels to generate reflexes without substantially involving higher centers, whereas parallel systems allow the brain to process the flow of discrete types of sensory information to produce discrete types of motor movements.[14,15]

The control of movement is ultimately substantially shaped from (1) the sensory organs innervating muscles (i.e., muscle spindles, which contain the specialized elements that sense muscle length as well as the velocity of changes in length) and (2) Golgi tendon organs that sense muscle tension while the muscle spindles provide the CNS with continuous information about the mechanical state of the muscle. Ultimately, the firing of the muscle spindles depends on both muscle length, the level of gamma activation of the intrafusal fibers, and the interpretation of the signals from the muscle spindles by the nervous system. Inputs from the sensory systems (touch, vision, audition, balance) also play an important role in guiding refined movements. This integral relationship between sensory and motor processing must be kept in mind when discussing neuroplasticity.[16]

ANATOMIC FOUNDATION FOR THE STUDY OF NEUROPLASTICITY

Our principal models for studying cortical plasticity have been based on the representations of hand skin and hand movements in New World owl monkeys (*Aotus*) and squirrel monkeys (*Saimiri*). These primate models were chosen because their central sulci do not usually extend into the hand representational zone in the anterior parietal (S_1) or posterior frontal (M_1) cortical fields.

In other primates, the sulci are deeper and impede precise mapping. Although there are differences in hand use among primates, the hand has the largest topographic representation for the actual size of the extremity in all primates, the detail of this representation is orderly and relatively easily reconstructed, and in the somatosensory domain, the hand has the greatest potential for skilled movements and sensory discrimination. The richness of the neuronal representation in the hand and the access to its cortical representation explain why it has been studied most extensively in neuroplasticity studies. It is critical to remember that the findings from these studies are not limited to the hand, but have general application to other cortical areas.[9,17,18]

Basic Cortical Representations of the Hand Contributing to the Study of Neuroplasticity: Primate Research

Cortical Maps of Cutaneous Afferents

The early maps of the cortical representations of the skin surfaces of the hand were made from surface recordings of evoked responses with response sampling at sites separated by a millimeter or more[19,20] or by mapping sensations evoked by surface stimulation in awake human subjects.[21] Contemporary maps are derived by much more discrete intracortical microelectrode response recordings, commonly with response sampling at densities of approximately 20–50 samples per square meter.[22] These differences in recording precision and recording methods from response mapping studies conducted in different individual animals contributed to the early erroneous conclusion that there was a single representation of the body surface within the four cytoarchitectonic fields of the S_1 cortex.[19,21,23-27]

It is clear that there are at least four different cortical areas within the classic S_1 zone in monkeys. Each map is distinguished by field-specific sources and destinations of anatomic connections. Each of these areas (3b, 1, 2) contains a relatively complete representation of the body.[28-30] Area 3a contains a relatively complete map of muscle and joint afferents, usually partially or nearly completely masking anatomically convergent cutaneous inputs to this site.[31-34] The S_1 area contains a mix of cutaneous and proprioceptive inputs.[35,36] In these cortical areas, representations of the hands have a roughly mirror-image topographic relationship with one another, with representational reversals occurring along the lines of representation of the fingertips between areas 3a and 3b and 1 and 2, or along a line separating duplicative palmar representations between areas 3b and 1.[29,30,37] Macaque monkeys have even further subdivisions in cortical area 2, with sharply segregated zones of exclusively *deep* or predominantly cutaneous afferent zones. These zones may be regarded as more than one functional cortical area.[35]

Cortical representations of the surfaces of the hand have been described for S_1 in humans,[21,38,39] as well as other nonhuman species.[17,19,20,23,25,26,28–30,35,37,40–50] The representations of the hands have a similar general pattern. In addition, the representations of digits are relatively discrete in area 3b in most primates, less so in cortical areas 1 and 2, and rarely so in area 3a. The representation of the thumb of humans and great apes is proportionally large in comparison with other species. The radial margin of the hand is represented lateralward and is discontinuous with the face representation. The wrist and forearm are represented medial to the hand representation. The digits and palmar pads are represented in order proceeding medialward in the cortex, progressing in a radial to ulnar sequence across the hand.

Idiosyncratic variability in representational detail has been described in S_1 in the same species. Documentation of this variability has been most compelling in studies using higher response sampling densities.[17,43,51] Studies suggest that representational differences between individuals of a given species can be as great or greater than are the differences recorded for individuals of different primate species.[17,51] In 3b, this variability has been reported in terms of the size of the entire hand representation, the size of territorial representation of the digits, the size of the dorsal representation, and the relationships of the skin surfaces of the hand bordering the face representation. These idiosyncratic differences are even greater in cortical areas 3a, 1, 2, and 5 than in 3b.[17] In cortical area 3a, some monkeys have large representations of palmar movements and proportionally small digital-movement muscle afferent representations, whereas other individual monkeys have almost no palm-muscle afferent representations. Monkeys have also been described with over half of the field of 3a dominated by cutaneous inputs, contrasted with other monkeys in which few or no cutaneous responses were recorded in the hand zone. Representational feature differences have also been described in a limited number of maps derived in cortical area S_2[52–54] and cortical area 6b.[55]

Movement Maps in Motor Cortical Area 4

Using surface-stimulation mapping, cortical representations of evoked movements of the hand have been defined in nonhuman and human primate species in *primary motor cortex* for area 4 in humans,[21,38] great

apes,[40–42,56] baboons,[32,57–59] macaque monkeys,[40,41,60–65] and New World owl monkeys[66] and squirrel monkeys.[12,67–69] Humans and apes have more refined digital and hand movements than do monkeys.[39,70] Movements evoked by low-level intracortical microstimulation in New World monkeys appear to be less differentiated than are those evoked in macaques or baboons. Representational differentiation appears to parallel the differences in hand dexterity. In New World monkeys, evoked movements of area 4 representations of the four fingers broadly overlap.

As in the sensory cortex, maps derived in M_1 (area 4) in different species also differ in evoked-movement sampling densities. Commonalities and differences are therefore incompletely determined.[67,68] More recently, maps constructed with a sampling density of 20 or more samples per square millimeter have shown that movement representations are internally more complex than was formerly believed, with any given wrist or hand or finger movement represented in a series of discrete islands or patches, and with a variety of neighborhood relationships for different zones of movement representations.[12,66,69,71] Area 4 and a number of surrounding cortical fields from which movements can be evoked have now been identified. These experiments indicate that area 6, supplementary motor cortex, and other zones bordering cortical area 4 are subdivisible into a number of input- and output-specific functional cortical motor areas.[72–74]

Again, maps derived in different individuals in the same species by the use of surface-stimulation methods are highly variable in detail. Sherrington and colleagues[61] provided early information showing that evoked movements could be altered by surface electrical stimulation conditioning or by stimulating a nerve innervating a specific related muscle.[75] This variability and change in response generated by stimulation have been reconfirmed in more contemporary intracortical microstimulation mapping studies.[76,77] Variability in movement maps between individuals and between hemispheres in the same species (macaques) has also been recorded in cortical area 4 surface-mapping experiments by Franz[62] and Lashley.[78] This led to the conclusion that the variability in area 4 movement representations probably reflected differences in motor experiences and abilities of different studied monkeys and led Lashley to conclude that movement representations might be continually changing constructs, altered in their representational details by intervening experiences. Given these continuing dynamics, any point in the motor cortex has *equipotentiality* for representing a broad range of movements.[78]

Documentation of substantial idiosyncratic variability in movement maps was also a main outcome of the human motor cortex studies of Penfield and colleagues.[21,38] Penfield and colleagues mapped the cortex before surgery to provide a more accurate prediction of location and extent of movement representation in each individual patient. In New World monkeys, marked variability between movement representations in different animals and different hands in the same animal has been reported.[12,66,69] M_1 representation of specific movements of the hand preferred for use in small-object retrieval is often more complex, more elaborate, has more complex relationships with the representations of other movements, and is represented over larger total areas than those same movements for the nonpreferred hand. This finding confirmed a prediction of Hughlings Jackson in the midnineteenth century,[79] who argued that the cortex represents specific movement products, with specific muscles and simple component movements represented in combination with other movements that contribute to movement products. Those combinations are much more varied and richly expressed in the representation of a preferred than a nonpreferred hand.

Remodeling of Cortical Hand Representation

It was hypothesized that motor skill learning was associated with changes in representation at the cortical level. This led to many experiments conducted using pavlovian or operant conditioning behaviors and unit recording in the cerebral cortex, which support this conclusion. Ultimately with advances in technology, changes in motor[12,80] and sensory[77,81–97] cortices were documented following specific conditioned behaviors. Changes in representation can be reversed when the associative conditioning is extinguished,[82,83,98] or when the operant conditioned behavior is long unpracticed.[12,87]

Changes in cortical hand representations have also been induced by engaging an adult mammal in a new experience or in an instrumental conditioning regime.[12,22,99] Such studies continue a long history of experiments in which physical changes in the cortex (i.e., in its thickness, layers, compartments, neurons, dendritic branching, spines, synapses) have also been measured following new or *enriched* experiences.[100] Functional changes in response representations are recorded as progressive increases in the representational area, with more specificity, greater sensitivity, more coherent neuronal responses, decreased response thresholds, and higher response strengths. The opposite is reported for repetitive unconditioned inputs or behaviors.[31,34,86,87,89,91–93,95,96,101,102] In one class of

important experiments, primates were challenged with progressively more difficult tasks, and poorly differentiated movements were ultimately replaced with adept movements. These behavioral experiments targeted the primary sensory cortex and the motor cortex.

Repetitive behaviors inducing cortical change do not improve indefinitely. The creation and maintenance of the representation are apparent functions of the level of attention of the subject. Skill acquisition and critical representational plasticity are self-limiting, in the sense that as the behavior becomes more automatic, it become less closely attended. Representational changes induced in the cortex begin to fade and can ultimately disappear, but now the well-learned movement can be replayed from memory.[103] If a movement behavior destined to evolve into a stereotypic form is practiced, an effective, highly statistically, predictable movement sequence is adopted. That enables the storage of the learned behavior in a permanent form that requires only minimal or no behavioral attention. The brain creates a kind of behavioral homeostasis for a well-learned behavior. When behavioral performance declines or brain conditions change and a task becomes difficult, attention to the behavior must again be engaged to produce an invigorated cortical response and to renew a capacity for change.

How is sensorimotor learning sustained when the adaptive representations of the learned behavior have faded? This important issue has not been completely resolved. One potential answer is that the *habit* is represented extracortically in an enduring form. This potential answer has been supported by the finding that learning a new manual skill requires the motor cortex. During learning, a lesion in area 4 significantly impairs the skill. However, overlearned motor skills (e.g., walking) may not be significantly impaired by the occurrence of a lesion in area 4.

Another possible explanation for the generation of long-enduring automatic behaviors is that behaviorally induced changes in the cortex endure in an efficient representational form that sustains key dimensions of representation in a long-enduring form in the cortex itself. This may require engaging only limited distributed populations of cortical neurons to represent the behavior. This proposed explanation is supported by the finding that cortical neuron responses in heavily practiced, overlearned behaviors are commonly strongly correlated with a monkey's discriminative or movement performance abilities. At the same time, there are other highly skilled behaviors that require constant cognitive attention and reinforcement to continue high-level performance. These highly attended behaviors would be expected to continuously engage the cortical plasticity mandatory to change.

Why are skin surface representations consistently orderly, even when great individual variability has been demonstrated?[85,88,92,96,97,104] It has been shown that cortical plasticity mechanisms are coincident input dependent. Connection strengths are increased for behaviorally important inputs that are delivered coincidentally into the cortical network. They are strengthened together to achieve coselection. In Hebb-like mechanisms, one axon excites a second axon repeatedly and persistently until there is an increase in efficiency of the two firing together. These mechanisms create new representational maps of input time continua.[105] The temporal input structure is, by its nature, topographic. Inputs from adjacent skin surfaces are excited with high probability nearly coincidentally in time, with Hebb-like synapses similarly represented in adjacent cortical locations. This coincident input–based plasticity is applicable to other neocortical areas. When movements coconcur in behaviors that are produced together, coincident input–based changes within area 4 are the result.[12]

Cortical Area 3b

Neuroplasticity studies have included training monkeys to pick up small food pellets using the finger tip pads. The behavioral training occurred over a period of less than 1 hour each day (only 100 pellets per day). It took days to weeks to train monkeys at this task. Initial efforts were mostly unsuccessful, but progressive improvements were recorded. It took usually several weeks to train different monkeys under difficult context conditions. Change in the critical cortical representations of the hand was mapped after the task was consistently performed. This differential training was associated with almost a doubling in size of the engaged digit skin representation[22,29] with the engaged skin surfaces represented in correspondingly finer detail.

Cortical Area 4

Similar basic experiments conducted in New World squirrel monkeys documented training-induced changes in area 4. Changes in evoked-movement representations in cortical area 4 were measured by deriving intracortical microstimulation maps of evoked movements on a grain of 15–20 samples per square millimeter. Maps were determined in monkeys under sterile surgical conditions before the small object retrieval task was initiated.[12] After the monkey had perfected the task, as in the somatosensory studies described previously, the same cortical zone was mapped again, in equal detail.

These intracortical microstimulation maps derived before and after such behavioral training showed that major changes in evoked movement representations in cortical area 4 were induced by this practiced motor behavior. Changes in motor cortex were specific to the movements involved in the skill learning. Overall, the representations of digital movements expanded approximately 1.5 times in the motor cortex and approximately two times in the anterior half of cortical area 4. The representation of specific movements employed in the learned movement sequence (e.g., of digit extension) increased severalfold in extent. Movements that coconcurred in the behavior were evoked with higher probability at equal electrical stimulation thresholds in area 4. Movements that were produced in sequence in the learned behavior were *mapped* in neighboring topographic locations in area 4 movement representations. In a repeatedly mapped monkey, changes in cortical maps directly paralleled the studied monkey's task performances.

Changes Induced in Other Sensory and Motor Areas

Plasticity has been induced by similar behaviors in two other S$_1$ areas, areas 1 and 3a. Plastic changes in a cued retrieval task have produced behaviorally specific neuronal response changes on a major scale in different sectors of the premotor area 6,[106] and the supplementary motor area bordering the motor cortex.[107]

Cortical area 3a is normally dominated by inputs from muscle spindles and other deep inputs. It is thought to provide inputs to area 4, contributing to the initiation of movements. Using a reaction time–limited hand movement from a resting position, dramatic representational remodeling was seen with exaggeration of the representation of the specific sensory inputs that cued movement initiation.[31,34,89] In this pellet retrieval behavior, the movement was initiated from the hand or wrist. As the behavior was perfected, movement initiation came to involve all of the joints of the arm, wrist, hand, and fingers (i.e., was initiated fluidly from the entire limb). One major change in cortical area 4 was a progressive increase in cortical territory over which extension of the fingers, hand, wrist, and elbow were evoked together as the behavior was perfected. Such movement combinations were relatively infrequently recorded in monkeys that are naive to this behavior, whereas they were common, and increased progressively, in trained monkeys.

The hand representational zone of cortical area 1 may not be activated during behavioral periods in which the digits are in motion.[85,88,108] This may occur because inputs are inhibited by gating inputs originating from cortical area 4. However, maps derived in monkeys trained to retrieve pellets showed representations of behaviorally engaged digits that were significantly larger in representation than were other digits. Digits that the monkeys never used to pick up pellets, like digits 1 and 5, appeared to be decidedly underrepresented when compared with control hand representations. We hypothesize that when a monkey introduced its fingers into the food well and shifted from extension to flexion and withdrawal, afferent inputs might be momentarily effective in engaging cortical area 1. In any event, area 1 also appears to be remodeled by this behavior, and induced changes in this field presumably contribute to it.

BASIC PRINCIPLES OF NEUROPLASTICITY

As we learn, how does the brain change its representations of inputs and actions? What is the nature of the processes that control the progressive elaboration of performance abilities? In different individuals, what are the sources of variance for emergent performance abilities? These principles are summarized in Table 26-1 and discussed in more detail in the following paragraphs.

The most informative studies on neuroplasticity are those that have been specifically directed toward defining changes induced by learning. One approach has been to document the patterns of distributed neural response representation of specific inputs before and after learning. In particular, neuronal responses have been measured in the primary auditory, somatosensory, and motor cortices in animals. These animal studies have commonly been paired with behavioral studies in humans. Especially when considered together, these animal and human studies provide strong inferences about the ability of the brain to functionally self-organize, not only during development, but also in adulthood, as well as after injury. Based on some basic neuroscience studies, one can identify the basic cortical plasticity processes that contribute to learning.

I. With learning, the distributed cortical representations of inputs and brain actions *specialize* in their representations of behaviorally important inputs and actions in skill learning.

This specialization develops in response to selective cortical neuronal responses that meet the demands of perceptual, cognitive, and motor skill learning.[18,90,92,109,110] This adaptation has been clearly documented in animal studies. For example, if an animal is trained to make progressively finer distinctions about specific sensory stimuli,

TABLE 26-1

Summary: Principles of Neural Adaptivity (Neuroplasticity)

With learning, the distributed cortical representations of inputs and brain actions *specialize* in their representations of behaviorally important inputs and actions for skill learning.

There are important behavioral conditions that must be met in the learning phase of plasticity that enable growth in the number of neuron populations excited, progressively greater specificity in the neuronal representations, and progressively stronger temporal coordination.

With learning, selection of behaviorally important inputs is a product of strengthening input coincidence–based connections (synapses).

The scale of plasticity in progressive skill learning is massive.

Enduring cortical plasticity changes appear to be accounted for by local changes in neural anatomy.

Cortical plasticity processes in child development represent progressive, multiple-staged skill learning.

Cortical field-specific differences in input sources, distributions, and time-structured inputs create different representational structures.

Temporal dimensions of behaviorally important inputs influence representational *specialization*.

The integration time (*processing time*) in the cortex is itself subject to powerful learning-based plasticity.

Learning is modulated as a function of behavioral state.

There are constraints that limit the magnitude of plasticity changes that can occur, such as

  Competition

  Anatomic sources and convergent-divergent spreads of inputs

  Time constants governing coincident input coselection

  Achievable coherences of extrinsic and intrinsic cortical input sources

  Top-down organizational influences

then cortical neurons come to represent those stimuli in a progressively more selective manner.

II. There are important behavioral conditions that must be met in the learning phase of plasticity:

A. If behaviorally important stimuli repeatedly excite cortical neuron populations in a competitively dominant manner in a closely attended behavior, neuron populations selectively responding to these inputs progressively grow in number.

B. Repetitive, behaviorally important stimuli processed in skill learning lead to progressively greater specificity in representations of spectral (spatial) and temporal stimulus dimensions.

C. A growing number of selectively responding neurons discharge with progressively stronger temporal coordination (distributed response synchronicity).

Thus, through the course of progressive skill learning, a more refined basis for processing stimuli and generating the actions critical to the skilled tasks is manifested by these multidimensional changes in cortical responses. Specific aspects of these changes in distributed neuronal response are highly correlated with learning-based improvements in perception, motor control, or cognition.[12,18,22,31,95] In these processes, the brain is not simply changing to record and store content. Instead, the cerebral cortex is selectively refining its processing capacities to fit each task at hand by adjusting its spectral and spatial and temporal filters. Ultimately, it establishes its own general individually specialized processing capabilities. This *learning to learn* determines the facility with which specific classes of information can be stored, associated, and manipulated. These powerful self-shaping processes of the forebrain machinery are not only operating on a large scale during development, but also during adult learning and during the experienced-based management of externally and internally generated information in adults. This self-shaping with experience underlies the development of hierarchically organized perceptual, cognitive, motor, and executive skills.

III. In learning, selection of behaviorally important inputs is a product of strengthening input coincidence–based connections (synapses).

The process of coincident-based input coselection leads to changes in cortical representation. Inputs that nearly simultaneously excite neurons are strengthened together. In skill learning, this principle of concurrent input coselection results inexorably with repetitive practice in:

A. A progressive amplification of cell numbers engaged by repetitive inputs.[18,22,31,87,95]

B. An increase in the temporal coordination of distributed neuronal discharges evoked by successive events that mark features of behaviorally important inputs as a consequence of a progressive increase in positive coupling between nearly simultaneously engaged neurons within cortical networks.[31,97]

C. A progressively more specific *selection* of all of those input features that collectively repre-

sent behaviorally important inputs, expressed moment by moment in time.[87,97]

D. The remapping of temporal neighbors in representational networks at adjacent spatial locations and into continuous representational topographics.[5,104,111]

The basis of the functional creation of the detailed, representational cortical *maps* converting temporal to spatial representations is related to the Hebbian change principle.[105] The operation of coincidence-based synaptic plasticity in cortical networks results in the formation, strengthening, and continuous recruitment of neurons within neuronal *assemblies* that cooperatively represent those behaviorally important stimuli.

IV. Plasticity is constrained by anatomic sources and convergent-divergent spreads of inputs. Every cortical field has

A. Area-specific extrinsic input sources.

B. Specific dimensions of anatomic divergences and convergences (overlaps) of its inputs, limiting dynamically selectable combinative repertoires on the basis of Hebbian input coselection mechanisms.[18,88,91]

C. Anatomic input sources and the overlaps that enable change by establishing input coselection repertoires and limits for the induction of change.

There are relatively strict anatomic constraints at *lower* system levels, where only spatially (spectrally) limited input coincidence-based combinatorial outcomes are possible (e.g., at the spinal cord or brain stem level). At *higher* system levels (cortical), anatomic projection topographies develop with more powerful divergent neurons and neuronal assembly that can respond to complex combinations of features of real-world objects, events, and actions.

V. Plasticity is constrained by the time constants (e.g., how quickly neurons can respond to two stimuli occurring close in time) governing coincident input coselection and by the time structures that allow achievable coherence and integration of extrinsic and intrinsic cortical input sources.

To effectively drive representational changes with coincident input–dependent Hebbian mechanisms, temporally coordinated inputs are a prerequisite, given the short durations (milliseconds to tens of milliseconds) of the time constants that govern synaptic plasticity in the adaptive cortical machinery.[2,112] Consistently noncorrelated or low-discharge-rate inputs induce negative changes in synaptic effectiveness. In addition, repetitive stimuli occurring simultaneously in time can also degrade the representation.[31,34,77,89,93] These negative changes contribute importantly to the learning-driven *election* of behaviorally important inputs.

VI. Cortical field-specific differences in input sources, distributions, and time structured inputs create different representational structures.

For example, there are significant differences in the activity from afferent inputs from the retina, skin, or cochlea generated in a relatively strictly topographically wired V_1 (area 17), S_1 proper (area 3b), or A_1 compared with the inferior, temporal visual, insular somatosensory, dorsotemporal auditory, or prefrontal cortical areas that receive highly diffused inputs. In the former cases, heavy schedules of repetitive, temporally coherent inputs are delivered from powerful, redundant projections from relatively strictly topographically organized thalamic nuclei and lower level associated cortical areas. In the latter cases, while neighboring neurons can share some response properties, neurons or clusters of neurons that respond selectively to learned inputs are distributed widely across cortical areas and share less information with neighboring neurons. Afferent input projections from any given source are greatly dispersed; highly repetitive inputs are common; inputs from multiple, diffuse cortical sources are the rule; and far more varied and complex input combinations are in play. These differences in input schedules, spreads, and combinations presumably largely account for the dramatic differences in the patterns of representation of behaviorally important stimuli at lower versus higher levels.[18,91]

There is a serial progression of differentiation in the central system, resulting in the multilevel functional processing that allows an individual to progressively master more and more elaborate and differentiated perceptual, cognitive, motor, and executive skills. The sources of inputs and their field-specific boundary limit the distributions of modulatory inputs differentiated by cortical layer in different cortical regions and the basic elements and their basic interconnections in the cortical-processing machine, and crucial aspects of input combination and processing at subcortical levels are potentially inherited.[113] Although these inherited aspects of sensory, motor, and cortical processing circuit development constrain the potential learning-based modification of processing within each cortical area, powerful representational changes occur in different forms as a result of environmental interaction and purposeful behavioral practice to refine and specialize our cortical processing machinery at every control level.

VII. Temporal dimensions of behaviorally important inputs also contribute to representational specialization. The cortex refines its representations of the temporal aspects of behaviorally important inputs during learning in at least four ways:

A. The cortex generates more synchronous representations of sequenced input perturbations or events, not only thereby recording their identities but also marking their occurrences.[18,31,93,97,114] This appears to be primarily achieved through increases in positive coupling strengths between interconnected neurons participating in stimulus- or action-specific neuronal cell assemblies.[93,110,115] The progressive, learning-induced generation of synchronously responding neuronal populations results in the following effects:

1. An increase in representational salience because downstream neurons are excited as a direct function of the degree of temporal synchronization of their inputs.

2. An increase in the power of the outputs of a cortical area to drive downstream plasticity because Hebbian plasticity mechanisms operating within downstream cortical (or other) targets also have relatively short time constants, and the greater the synchronicity of their inputs, the more powerfully their change mechanisms are engaged.

3. An increased immunity to noise because simple information abstraction and coding, the distributed neuronal representations of the signal, are converted into a form that is not as easily degraded or altered by *noise*.

4. An increased robustness of complex signal representation for spatially or spectrally incomplete or degraded inputs.

B. For example, in the auditory domain, this information abstraction principle quantitatively explains how the distributed neuronal response representations of speech substantially survive spectral degradation or spectral simplification or reduction up to remarkably high distortion levels at which signal intelligibility actually breaks down in human perception (e.g., why complex information can be delivered in strikingly different spectral forms, such as whispering versus phonated speech, and be equally and interchangeably intelligible).[116]

C. Second, the cortex can select specific inputs through learning to exaggerate the representation of specific input time structures.[18] Conditioning a monkey or a rat with stimuli that have a consistent, specific temporal modulation rate or interstimulus time, for example, results in a selective exaggeration of the responses of neurons at that rate or time separation. In effect, the cortex specializes for expected relatively higher speed or relatively lower speed signal event reception. Both electrophysiological recording studies and theoretical studies suggest that cortical networks richly encode temporal interval as a simple consequence of cortical network dynamics.[117,118] It is hypothesized that the cortex accomplishes time intervals and duration selectivity in learning by positively changing synaptic connection strengths for input circuits that can respond with recovery times and circuit delays that match behavioral important modulation frequency periods, intervals, or durations. Note that studies that also show excessive, rapid, repetitive fine motor movements can sometimes lead to serious degradation in representation if the adjacent digits are driven near simultaneously in time. This may be associated with negative learning and a progressive loss of motor control.[119]

D. Third, the cortex links representations of immediately successive inputs that are presented in a learning context. As a result of Hebbian plasticity, it establishes overlapping and neighborhood relationships between immediately successive parts of rapidly changing inputs, yet retains these individual, distinct cortical representations.[5,120]

E. Fourth, the cortex can generate stimulus sequence-specific (*combination-sensitive*) responses, with neuronal responses selectively modulated by the prior application of stimuli in the learned sequence of temporally separated events.[18]

VIII. The integration time (processing time) in the cortex is itself subject to powerful learning-based plasticity.

Cortical networks engage both excitatory and inhibitory neurons by strong input perturbations. Within a given processing *channel*, cortical pyramidal cells cannot be effectively re-excited by a following perturbation for tens to hundreds of milliseconds. These *integration times* are primarily dictated by the time for recovery from inhibition, which ordinarily dominates poststimulus excitability. This integration time, processing time, or recovery time is commonly measured by deriving a *modulation transfer function*, which defines the ability of cortical neurons to respond to identical successive stimuli within cortical processing channels. These integration times normally range from approximately 15–200 msec in the primary auditory receiving areas.[121-123] Progressively longer processing times are recorded at higher system levels (e.g., in the auditory cortex, they are approximately syllable-length, 200–500 msec in duration in the *belt cortex* surrounding the primary auditory cortex,[124] and roughly a second in duration for dorsolateral temporal cortex [Wernicke's area]).

These time constants govern, and limit, the cortex's ability to chunk (i.e., to separately represent by distributed, coordinated discharge) successive events within its processing channels. Both neurophysiological studies in animals and behavioral training studies in human adults and children have shown that the time constants governing event-by-event complex signal representation are highly plastic. With intensive training in the right form, cortical processing times reflected by the ability to accurately and separately process events occurring at different input rates can be dramatically shortened or lengthened.[18,96,114,125-127]

IX. Plasticity processes are competitive.

If two spatially or spectrally different inputs are consistently delivered nonsimultaneously to the cortex, cortical networks generate input-selective cell assemblies for each input and actively segregate them from one another.[97,104,127-131] Boundaries between such inputs grow to be sharp and are substantially intensity independent. Computational models of Hebbian network behaviors indicate that this sharp segregation of nonidentical, consistently temporally separated inputs is accomplished as a result of a wider distribution of inhibitory versus excitatory responses in the emerging, competing cortical cell assemblies that represent them.

This Hebbian network cell assembly formation and competition appear to account for how the cortex creates sharply sorted representations of the fingers in primary somatosensory cortex,[96,104] and almost certainly accounts for how the cortex creates sharply sorted representations of native aural-language–specific phonemes in lower level auditory cortical areas in the auditory and speech processing system in humans. If inputs are delivered in a constant and stereotyped way from a limited region of the skin or cochlea in a learning context, that skin surface or cochlear sector is an evident competitive winner.[18,31,76] By Hebbian plasticity, cortical networks coselect that specific combination of inputs and represent it within a competitively growing Hebbian cell assembly. The competitive strength of that cooperative cell assembly grows progressively because more and more neurons are excited by behaviorally important stimuli with increasingly coordinated discharges. That means that neurons outside of this cooperative group have greater numbers of more coordinated outputs contributing to their later competitive recruitment. Through progressive functional remodeling, the cortex clusters and competitively sorts information across sharp boundaries dictated by the spectrotemporal statistics of its inputs. It is obviously highly flexible in what can be achieved by that sorting. On the one hand, if it receives information on a heavy schedule that sets up competition for a limited input set, it sorts competitive inputs into a correspondingly small or longer number of largely discontinuous response regions.[132,133]

Competitive outcomes are, again, cortical level dependent. The cortex links events that occur in different competitive groups if they are consistently excited synchronously in time. At the same time, competitively formed groups of neurons come to be synchronously linked in their representations of different parts of the complex stimulus and collectively represent successive complex features of the vocalization, somatosensory sequence, or movements through the coordinated activities of many groups.

Neurons within the two levels of the cortex surrounding A_1 have greater spectral input convergences and longer integration times that enable their facile combination of information representing different spectrotemporal details (i.e., have the combinational capacity to represent different vowels and consonants). Their information extraction is greatly facilitated by the learning-based linkages of cooperative groups that deliver behaviorally important inputs in a highly salient, temporally coordinated form to these fields. With their progressively greater space and time constants, still higher level areas organize competitive cell assemblies that represent still more complex spectral and serial-event combinations.[18] Note that these organizational changes apply over a large cortical scale. In skill learning over a limited period of training, participant neuronal members of such assemblies can easily be increased by many hundredfold, even within a primary sensory area such as S_1 area 3b or A_1.[31,34,97,119,127] In extensive training in complex signal recognition, more than 10% of neurons within temporal cortical areas can come to respond highly selectively to a specific, normally rare, complex training stimulus. The distributed cell assemblies representing those specific complex inputs involve tens or hundreds of millions of neurons and are achieved through repetitive training by enduring effectiveness changes in many billions of synapses.

X. Learning is modulated as a function of behavioral state. At lower levels of cortex, changes are generated only in attended behaviors.[34,87,89,95,98,102] Trial-by-trial change magnitudes are a function of the importance of the input to the animal as signaled by the following factors:

A. The level of attention

B. The cognitive values of behavioral rewards or punishments

C. Internal judgments of practice trial precision or error, based on the relative success or failure of achieving a target goal or expectation

   Little or no enduring change is induced when a well-learned automatic behavior is performed from memory without attention. It is also interesting to note that at some levels of cortex, activity changes can be induced even in nonattending subjects under conditions in which *priming* effects of nonattended reception of information can be demonstrated. For example, if a word is presented and the subject is totally unaware of the word stimulus, yet selects that word out of a random series of words that follows, it is called a *priming effect*.

The modulation of progressive learning is achieved by the activation of powerful reward systems releasing the neurotransmitters acetylcholine, norepinephrine, and dopamine (among others) through widespread projections to the cerebral cortex. Acetylcholine plays a particularly important role in modulating learning-induced change in the cortex.[102,114,127]

Note that the cortex is a *learning machine*, in the sense that during the learning of a new skill, acetylcholine, norepinephrine, dopamine, and others are all released trial by trial with application of the behaviorally important stimulus, behavioral rewards, or both. If the skill can be mastered and thereafter replayed from memory, its performance can be generated without attention. That results in a profound attenuation of the modulation signals from these neurotransmitter sources; plasticity is no longer positively enabled by their release in cortical networks.

XI. Top-down influences constrain cortical representational plasticity. Attentional control flexibly defines an enabling *window* for change in learning.[126] Moreover, progressive learning generates progressively more strongly represented goals and expectations,[134,135] which feed back (1) all across representational systems that are undergoing change, and (2) to modulatory control systems that weigh performance success and error. Strong intermodal behavioral and representational effects have also been recorded in experiments that might be interpreted as shaping expectations in monkeys[136,137] and almost certainly, by analogy, in a human subject who employs, for example, auditory, visual, and somesthetic information to create integrated phonologic representations or to create the movement trajectory patterns that underlie precise hand control or vocal production.

XII. The scale of plasticity in progressive skill learning is massive. Cortical representational plasticity must be viewed as arising from multiple-level systems that are broadly engaged in learning, perceiving, remembering, thinking, and acting. Any behaviorally important input (or consistent internally generated activity) engages many cortical areas, and with repetitive training, drives all of them to change.[18,90-92] Different aspects of any acquired skill are contributed from field-specific changes in the multiple cortical areas that are remodeled in its learning.

It should be noted that in this kind of continuously evolving representational machine, perceptual constancy cannot be accounted for by locationally constant brain representations: Relational representational principles must be invoked to account for it.[92,138] Moreover, representational changes must obviously be coordinated level to level. It should also be understood that plastic changes are also induced extracortically. Although we believe that learning at the cortical level is usually predominant, plasticity induced by learning within many extracortical structures significantly contributes to learning-induced changes that are expressed within the cortex.

XIII. Enduring cortical plasticity changes appear to be accounted for by local changes in neural anatomy. Changes in synapse turnover, synapse number, synaptic active zones, dendritic spines, and the elaboration of terminal dendrites have all been demonstrated to occur in a behaviorally engaged cortical zone.[100,139-142] Through myriad changes in local structural detail, the learning brain is continuously physically remodeling its processing machinery throughout life.

XIV. Cortical plasticity processes in child development represent progressive, multiple-staged skill learning. There are two remarkable achievements of brain plasticity in child development. The first is the progressive shaping of processing to handle the accurate, high-speed reception of the rapidly changing streams of information that flow into the brain. In the cerebral cortex, that shaping appears to begin most powerfully within the primary receiving areas of the cortex. With their early myelination, these main gateways for information into the cortex are receiving strongly coherent inputs from subcortical nuclei, and they can quickly organize their local networks on the basis of coincident input coselection (Hebbian) plasticity mechanisms. The self-organization of the cortical processing machinery spreads outward from these primary receiving areas over time to ultimately refine the basic processing machinery of all of the cortex. The second great achievement, which is strongly dependent on the first, is the efficient storage of massive content compendia in richly associated forms.

During development, the brain accomplishes its functional self-organization through a long parallel series of small steps. At each step, the brain masters a series of elementary processing skills and establishes reliable information repertoires that enable the accomplishment of subsequent skills. Second- and higher order skills can be viewed as both elaborations of more basic mastered skills and creations of new skills dependent on second- and higher order combinatorial processing. That hierarchical processing is allowed by greater cortical anatomic spreads, more complexly convergent anatomic sources of inputs, and longer integration (processing, recovery) times at progressively higher cortical system levels, which allow for progressively more complex combinations of information integrated over progressively longer time epochs as one ascends across cortical processing hierarchies.

As the cortical machinery functionally evolves and consequently physically matures through childhood developmental stages, information repertoires are represented in progressively more salient forms (i.e., with more powerful distributed response coordination). That growing agreement directly controls the power of emerging information repertoires for driving the next level of elaborative and combinatorial changes.[18]

As each elaboration of skill is practiced, in a learning phase, neuromodulatory transmitters allow change in the cortical machinery. The cortex functionally and physically adapts to generate the neurologic representations of the skill in progressively more selective, predictable, and statistically reliable forms. Ultimately, the performance of the skill concurs with the brain's own accumulated, learning-derived *expectations*. The skill can now be performed from memory, without attention (e.g., habit, or automatic). With this consolidation of the remembered skill and information repertoire, the modulatory nuclei enable no further change in the cortical machinery. The learning machine (the cerebral cortex) moves on to the next task or elaboration. In this way, the cortex constructs highly specialized processing machinery that can progressively produce (1) great towers of automatically performed behaviors, and (2) great progressively maturing hierarchies of information-processing machinery that can achieve progressively more powerful complex signal representations, retrievals, and associations. With this machinery in a mature and efficiently operating form, a remarkable capacity for reception, storage, and analysis of diverse and complex associated information is developed.[18]

The flexible, self-adjusting, refined capacity for processing capabilities of the nervous system confers the ability of our species to represent complex language structures. It confers the ability to develop high-speed reading abilities; develop a remarkably wide variety of complex modern-era motor abilities; develop the abstract logic structures of the mathematician, software engineer, or philosopher; and create elaborate, idiosyncratic, experience-based behavioral abilities in all of us.

HOW ARE LEARNING SEQUENCES CONTROLLED? WHAT CONSTRAINS LEARNING PROGRESSIONS?

Perhaps the most important basis of control of learning progressions is representational consolidation. The trained cortex creates progressively more specific and more salient (synchronized) distributed representations of behaviorally important inputs through learning. The power of a cortical area to effectively drive changes wherever its outputs are distributed increases with this growing representational salience.

Progressive myelination is another potentially powerful basis for sequenced learning. Myelination controls the conduction times and therefore the temporal dispersions of input sources to and within cortical areas. At the time of birth, only the core primary extrinsic information entry zones (A_1, S_1, V_1) in the cortex are heavily myelinated.[143,144] Connections to and interconnections between cortical areas are progressively myelinated across the childhood years, proceeding from these core areas out to progressively higher system levels. Myelination in the posterior parietal, anterior, and inferior temporal and prefrontal cortical areas is not mature in the human forebrain until 8–20 years of age. Even in the mature state, it is far less developed at the highest processing levels. Poor myelination at higher levels in the young brain is associated with temporally diffuse inputs. These cortical cells cannot generate reliable representational constructs of an adult quality because they do not as effectively engage input coincidence–based Hebbian plasticity mechanisms. Plasticity is not enabled for complex combinatorial processing until lower level input repertoires are consolidated (i.e., become stable, statistically reliable forms, and highly temporally coordinated).

Another constraint in the development of neural adaptation may be related to development of mature sleeping patterns, especially within the first year of life.[145] Sleep both strengthens the learning-based plastic changes and resets the learning machinery by *erasing* temporary nonreinforced and nonrewarded input-generated changes over the preceding waking period.[146-148] The dramatic shift in the percentage of time spent in rapid eye movement sleep is consistent with a strong early bias toward noise removal in an immature and poorly functioning, unorganized brain. Sleep patterns change dramatically in the older child, in parallel with a strong increase in its daily schedule of closely attended, rewarded, and goal-oriented behaviors.

Top-down modulation controlling attentional windows and learned predictions (expectations and behavioral goals) must be constructed by learning, and the slow development of the effective control of learning must constrain its progression.[18] In the young brain, prediction and error-estimation processes must necessarily be weaker because the stored higher level information repertoires are ill formed and statistically unreliable. As the brain matures, stored information more strongly, progressively, and reliably allows top-down attentional and predictive controls. It also progressively provides a stronger basis for success and error signaling for modulatory control nuclei and progressively enables top-down syntactic feedback to increase representational reliability for accurate reception of high-speed complex-signal input streams such as speech.

The modulatory control systems that enable learning are also plastic, with their processes of maturation constituting an important constraint for progressive learning. These subcortical nuclei are signaled by complex information feedback from the cortex itself. The salience and specificity of that feedback information grow over time. The ability to provide accurate error judging or goal-achievement signaling must grow progressively. The nucleus basalis, nucleus accumbens, ventral tegmentum, and locus ceruleus must undergo their own functional self-organization based on Hebbian plasticity principles to achieve mature modulatory selectivity and power.

INTEGRATING THE PRINCIPLES OF NEUROPLASTICITY INTO PRACTICE

Table 26-1 summarizes the principles of neuroplasticity. Table 26-2 provides a summary of applying the principles of neuroplasticity in rehabilitation and the possible structural changes that could be achieved. Table 26-3 summarizes the possible functional outcomes that could be evaluated as a way of documenting effective treatment. As clinicians, it is most difficult to measure the structural changes. These are more likely measured in basic science studies. However, these changes in structure should be associated with improvement in function. The clinician must apply objective methods of measurement to document changes in clinical function.

SUMMARY

Over the years, learning has been tied to critical periods of development. Particularly in terms of language, it was concluded that if a particular skill or behavior was not accomplished during the critical period, then the opportunity to acquire that skill was lost. Currently, we know that although learning progression is heightened during certain periods, learning is not limited to that period alone.

Development actually refers to a process of neural and behavioral self-organization resulting from a physiological and developmental maturation of the nervous system. However, with increasing interaction with the environment, the brain changes its capacity from a simple to an incredibly specialized representational machine that is adapted to meet the specific inputs that engage it. Language is probably one of the most sophisticated examples of a specialized process affecting brain self-organization at multiple levels. First, the brain has to learn to put meaning to words. Over time one is exposed to millions of English words even though one may not consciously understand all of them. Yet, as we grow, attend school, and continue to have more sophisticated interactions, our brain adapts and we develop massive, language-specific specialization.

The beauty of the brain is that as it self-organizes, it also stores the contents of its learning, creating a foundation that increases in depth and breadth until it can begin to make predictions on even novel inputs to facilitate accurate and efficient operations. The earlier the exposure occurs, the easier it is for the competitive neuronal processes to adapt and to make extensive selective connections. With growing neuronal specificity and representation salience, more powerful predictions are continued until there is greater learning and mastery.

The aging process can take a toll on the ability of the brain to store information. It may reduce both the complexity of the information that we can process and reduce our ability to remember. However, we now know that if we regularly engage in goal-directed activities that include intimate interactions with our environment and with people, we cannot only preserve pathways of representation and prediction, but can continue to adapt and slow down part of the aging process that is experientially practice dependent. Thus, although the critical period can be viewed as developing more powerful specialization in the cortex, cortical plasticity does not shut down after this period. Instead, throughout life, the nervous system adapts to practice-based impairments in skills and abilities in all of us,

TABLE 26-2
Summary of Principles of Neuroplasticity as Applied to Rehabilitation

Requisites for Learning: Guidelines for Applying the Principles of Neuroplasticity in Treatment	*Evidence of Measurable Neuroplastic Changes* after Intervention: Anatomic/Physiological*
Activities must be attended, goal directed	Increase in the area of representation
Behavior must be motivating/fun	Smaller receptive fields
Behaviors must be repeated (and variable)	Improved organization
Behaviors should be linked temporally and spatially, but not simultaneously in time	Improved order of representation
Behaviors must be rewarded	Increased myelination
Give feedback on performance accuracy	Increased complexity of dendrites
Make stimulus strength adequate for detection	Increased strength (amplitude) of evoked responses
Stimulation and behavioral expectations must be progressive in difficulty	Decreased latency of response
Stimulus-induced behaviors need to be integrated into meaningful function	Increased consistency of response (e.g., density of neuronal response)
Behaviors should be age appropriate	Improved selective excitation
Behaviors should be integrated across sensory modalities	Improved autogenic and surround inhibition
Make sensory relevant to desired outputs	Improved neurochemical transmission
Repeat behaviors over time	Normalized location/translocation
Match training behaviors with recovery/developmental periods	Normalized pattern of response
Strengthen responses with multisensory modalities	Increased interconnectedness
Begin stimulation by using the most mature or capable sensory receptors	Spread of healthy neurons to take over function in areas where damage occurred
Behaviors should be performed in different environmental contexts	Early achievement of developmental milestones
Do training in the gravitational positions that facilitate task achievement	Increased specificity of neuronal firing
Preferred behaviors should be rewarded; negative behaviors punished	Improved synchrony of neuronal firing
Accurate behaviors should be repeated	Spatial representational mapping consistent with coincident temporal events
	Increased salience of neuronal responses
	Increased interrelatedness of temporally related neuronal firing
	Change in number and complexity of synapses
	Improved resistance to representational degradation

*Measurements made with a variety of techniques, including neurophysiological mapping after craniotomies, electroencephalography, magnetic source imaging, functional magnetic resonance imaging, electromyography, cortical response mapping with positron emission tomography, and neurochemical analysis of neurotransmitters, growth hormones, inhibitors, corticosteroids, and so forth.

including individuals who have abnormalities in development or impairments from injury or disease.

It was thought that development was the end product of accumulated learning during programmed critical periods. However, we now know that learning does not have to be specifically staged. Rather, complex abilities develop more from systems interactions and integration. We must develop the ability to determine what inputs are reliable and salient and which most effectively create functional and physical brain maturation and adaptation. As we continue to gather information, the nervous system adapts its processing machinery,

and thereby, the complexity of its achievable behaviors. In the face of different types of challenges, we must develop more effective strategies to facilitate neural adaptation, learning, substitution, and representational changes that will allow individuals to have meaningful function despite anatomical or physiological changes in structure.

It should be clear that to meet the conditions of neural adaptivity, behaviors must be attended, repetitive, goal directed, integrated into functional activities and carried out over time with an increasing number of coincident events. Although strong behavioral events can be associ-

TABLE 26-3
Functional Outcomes of Successful Neural Adaptation after Rehabilitation

Improved fine and gross motor coordination
Improved sensory discrimination
Improved balance and postural control
Faster reaction time
Improved accuracy of movements
Improved rhythm and timing of movements
Improved memory storage, organization, and retrieval
Improved alertness and attention
Improved sequencing
Improved logic, complexity, and sophistication of problem solving
Enhanced language skills (verbal and nonverbal)
Improved interpersonal communication
Increased sense of well-being
Increased insight
Increased self-confidence
Improved self-image
Enhanced sign/noise detection; able to make finer distinctions
Increased ability to *chunk* information for memory and use
Enhanced learning skills including faster learning
Early achievement of developmental milestones
Decreased hyperactivity and sensory defensiveness
Expanded ability to perform a skill from memory
Flexible behaviors; variability in task performance
Expanded flexibility for experience-based learning

ated with measurable neural adaptation, new neural connections and synapses must be strengthened with repetition, feedback, and increased complexity. Thus, practical rehabilitation programs must include strong, carefully outlined home programs where family members can assist. Individuals should be coming back periodically to see the therapist to discuss ways to continue to progress in learning. Each patient must become his or her own best therapist. The individual must be motivated to continue to challenge one's self with progressive, attended behavioral activities that get integrated into functional activities. One must work hard to avoid learning negative patterns of movement and behaviors that degrade the neuronal response as opposed to enriching the neuronal response. Maximum opportunities for recovery and neuroplasticity rest with the individual patient with guidance and mentoring from professionals and significant others.

Therapists need to invest significant time in educating patients and their families about the principles of neuroplasticity. The maximum attainment of skill performance cannot necessarily be determined. The original injury can only be used as an estimate of the damage with some indication of prognosis and recovery. The rest of the success of rehabilitation and restoration of function will rest with the motivation and commitment of the individual guided by a knowledgeable rehabilitation practitioner.

REFERENCES

1. Anderson P, Kandel E, Thompson RF, Tonegawa S. Learning and Memory. Cold Spring Harbor, NY: Cold Spring Harbor Laboratory, l996.

2. Buomomano DV, Merzenich MM. Cortical plasticity: from synapses to maps. Annu Rev Neurosci 1998a; 21:149–186.

3. Carew TJ, LeDoux J, Ungerleider LG. Learning and Memory. Cold Spring Harbor, NY: Cold Spring Laboratory, 1999.

4. Wolpaw JR, Schmidt JT, Vaughan TM. Activity-Driven CNS Changes in Learning and Development. New York: New York Academy of Sciences, 1991.

5. Merzenich MM, Recanzone GH, Jenkins WM. How the Brain Functionally Rewires Itself. In M Arbib, JA Robinson (eds), Natural and Artificial Parallel Computations. New York: MIT Press, 1991.

6. Baudry M, Lynch G. Long-Term Potentiation: Biochemical Mechanisms. In B Michel, RF Thompson, JL Davis (eds), Synaptic Plasticity:

Molecular, Cellular and Functional Aspects. Cambridge, MA: MIT Press, 1993;87–115.

7. Filogamo G, Vernadakis A, Gremo F, et al. (eds). Brain Plasticity: Development and Aging. Advances in Experimental Medicine and Biology. New York: Plenum Press, 1997.

8. Erlich YH (ed). Molecular and Cellular Mechanisms of Neuronal Plasticity: Basic and Clinical Implications. Advances in Experimental Medicine and Biology. New York: Pleanum Press, 1998.

9. Merzenich MM, Wright B, Jenkins WM, et al. Cortical plasticity underlying perceptual, motor and cognitive skill development. Implications for neurorehabilitation. Cold Spring Harb Symp Quant Biol 1996;61:1–8.

10. Bennett EL, Rosenzweig MR, Diamond MC. Rat brain: Effects of environmental enrichment on wet and dry weights. Science 1969;146:610–619.

11. Spengler F, Roberts TP, Poeppei D, et al. Realigning transfer and neuronal plasticity in humans trained in tactile

discrimination. Neurosci Lett 1997;232(3):151–154.

12. Nudo RJ, Milliken GW, Jenkins WM, Merzenich MM. Use-dependent alterations of movement representations in primary motor cortex of adult squirrel monkeys. J Neurosci 1995;16:785–807.

13. Prochazka A, Hullinger M. Muscle Afferent Function and Its Significance for Motor Control Mechanisms during Voluntary Movements in Cat, Monkey and Man. In JE Desmedt (ed), Advances in Neurology. Vol 39: Motor Control Mechanisms in Health and Disease. New York: Raven Press, 1983;93–132.

14. Bizzi E, Abend W. Posture Control and Trajectory Formation in Single and Multi-Joint Arm Movements. In JE Desmedt (ed), Advances in Neurology. Vol 39: Motor Control Mechanisms in Health and Disease. New York: Raven Press, 1983;31–45.

15. Desmedt JE. Patterns and Motor Commands During Various Types of Voluntary Movement in Man. In EV Evars, SP Wise, D Bousfield (eds), The

Motor System in Neurobiology. New York: Elsevier, 1985;133–139.

16. Houk JC, Rymer WZ. Neural Control of Muscle Length and Tension. In VB Brooks (ed), Handbook of Physiology, Sec I: The Nervous System. Vol II: Motor Control, Part 1. Bethesda, MD: American Physiological Society, 1981;257–323.

17. Merzenich MM, Nelson RJ, Kaas MP, et al. Variability in hand surface representations in areas 3b and 1 in adult owl and squirrel monkeys. J Comp Neurol 1987;258:281–296.

18. Merzenich MM. Cortical Plasticity Contributing to Child Development; Chapter submitted to Carnegie-Mellon, 2000 (in press).

19. Woolsey CN, Marshall WH, Bard P. Representation of cutaneous tract sensibility in the cerebral cortex of the monkey as indicated by evoked potentials. Bull Johns Hopkins Hosp 1943;60:399–441.

20. Pubols BH, Pubols LM. Somatotopic organization of spider monkey somatic sensory cerebral cortex. J Comp Neurol 1971;141:63–76.

21. Penfield W, Boldrey E. Somatic motor and sensory representations in the cerebral cortex of man as studied by electrical stimulation. Brain 1937; 60:389–443.

22. Xerri C, Merzenich MM, Jenkins W, Santucci S. Representational plasticity in cortical area 3b paralleling tactual-motor skill acquisition in adult monkeys. Cereb Cortex 1999;9:264–276.

23. Powell TPS, Mountcastle VB. Some aspects of the functional organization of the cortex of the postcentral gyrus of the monkey: a correlation of findings obtained in a single unit analysis with cytoarchitecture. Bull Johns Hopkins Hosp 1968;105:301–334.

24. Werner G, Whitsel BC. The Functional Organization of the Somatosensory Cortex. In A Iggo (ed), Handbook of Sensory Physiology. New York: Springer-Verlag, 1971;612–700.

25. Dreyer DA, Schneider RJ, Metz CB, Whitsel BL. Differential contributions of spinal pathways to body representation in postcentral gyrus of Macaca mulatta. J Neurophysiol 1977;36:119–145.

26. McKenna TM, Whitsel BL, Dreyer DA. Anterior parietal cortical topographic organization in macaque monkey: a reevaluation. J Neurophysiol 1982;48:389–417.

27. Iwamura Y, Tanaka M, Sakamoto M, Hikosaka O. Functional subdivisions representing different finger regions in area 3 of the first somatosensory cortex of the conscious monkey. Exp Brain Res 1983;51:315–326.

28. Paul RL, Merzenich MM, Goodman H. Representation of slowly and rapidly adapting cutaneous mechanoreceptors of the hand in Brodmann's areas 3 and 1 of Macaca mulatta. Brain Res 1972;36:229–249.

29. Nelson RJ, Sur M, Felleman DJ, Kaas JH. Representations of the body surface in postcentral parietal cortex of Macaca fascicularis. J Comp Neurol 1980;192:611–643.

30. Sur M, Nelson RJ, Kaas JH. Representations of the body surface in cortical areas 3b and 1 of squirrel monkeys: comparisons with other primates. J Comp Neurol 1982;211:177–192.

31. Recanzone GH, Merzenich MM, Schreiner CS. Changes in the distributed temporal response properties of SI cortical neurons reflect improvements in performance on a temporally-based tactile discrimination task. J Neurophysiol 1992;67:1071–1091.

32. Phillips CG, Powell TPS, Wiesendanger M. Projection from low-threshold muscle afferents of hand and forearm to area 3a of baboon's cortex. J Physiol 1971;217:419.

33. Zarzecki P, Herman D. Convergence of sensory inputs upon projection neurons of somatosensory cortex: vestibular, neck, head, and forelimb inputs. Exp Brain Res 1983;50:408.

34. Recanzone GH, Merzenich MM, Jenkins WM, et al. Topographic reorganization of the hand representational zone in cortical area 3b paralleling improvements in frequency discrimination performance. J Neurophysiol 1992;67:1031–1056.

35. Pons TP, Garraghty PE, Cusick CG, Kaas JH. The somatotopic organization of area 2 in macaque monkeys. J Comp Neurol 1985;241:445–466.

36. Iwamura Y, Tanaka M, Hikosaka O. Overlapping representation of fingers in area 2 of the somatosensory cortex of the conscious monkey. Brain Res 1990;197:516–520.

37. Merzenich MM, Kaas JH, Sur M, Lin C-S. Double representation of the body surface within cytoarchitectonic areas 3b and 1 in "SI" in the owl monkey (Aotus trivirgatus). J Comp Neurol 1978;181:41–73.

38. Penfield W, Rasmussen T. The Cerebral Cortex of Man: A Clinical Study of Localization of Function. New York: Macmillan, 1950.

39. Yang TT, Gallen CC, Schwartz BJ, Bloom FE. Noninvasive somatosensory homunculus mapping in humans by using a large-array biomagnetometer. Proc Natl Acad Sci U S A 1993; 90:3098–3102.

40. Woolsey CN. Patterns of Localization in Sensory and Motor Areas of the Cerebral Cortex. In Biology of Mental Health and Disease. New York: Hoeber, 1951;193–206.

41. Woolsey CN. Organization of Somatic Sensory and Motor Areas in the Cerebral Cortex. In HF Harlow, CN Woolsey (eds), Biological and Biochemical Bases of Behavior. Madison, WI: University of Wisconsin Press, 1958;63–81.

42. Welt C. Topographical Organization of the Somatic Sensory and Motor Areas of the Cerebral Cortex of The Gibbon (Hylobates) and Chimpanzee (Pan) [Dissertation]. Chicago: University of Chicago, 1963.

43. Pons TP, Wall JH, Garraghty PE, et al. Consistent features of the representation of the hand in area 3b of macaque monkeys. Somat Motor Res 1987;4:309–331.

44. Felleman DJ, Nelson RJ, Sur M, Kaas JH. Representations of the body surface in areas 3b and 1 of postcentral parietal cortex of cebus monkeys. Brain Res 1989;268:15–26.

45. Carlson M, Heuerta MF, Cusick CG, Kaas JH. Studies on the evolution of multiple somatosensory representations in primates: the organization of anterior parietal cortex in the New World callitrichid, Saguinus. J Comp Neurol 1986;246:409–426.

46. Krubitzer LA, Kaas JH. The organization of connections of somatosensory cortex in marmosets. J Neurosci 1990;10:952–974.

47. Krishnamurti A, Sanides F, Welker WI. Microelectrode mapping of modality-specific somatic sensory cerebral neocortex in slow loris. Brain Behav Evol 1976;13:267–283.

48. Carlson M, Fitzpatrick KA. Organization of the hand area in the primary somatic sensory area (SmI) of the prosimian primate, Nycticebus cougang. J Comp Neurol 1982;209:280–295.

49. Fitzpatrick KM, Carlson M, Charlton J. Topography, cytoarchitecture and sulcal patterns in primary somatic sensory cortex (SmI) of the prosimian primate, Perodicticus potto. J Comp Neurol 1982;204:196–210.

50. Benjamin RM, Welker WI. Somatic receiving areas of cerebral cortex in the

squirrel monkey (Saimiri sciureus). J Neurophysiol 1957;20:286–299.

51. Merzenich MM. Sources of Intraspecies and Interspecies Cortical Map Variability in Mammals: Conclusions and Hypotheses. In MJ Cohen, F Strumwasser (eds), Comparative Neurobiology: Modes of Communication in the Nervous System. New York: Wiley, 1986;105–116.

52. Robinson CJ, Burton H. Somatotopographic organization in the second somatosensory area of M. fascicularis. J Comp Neurol 1980;192:43–67.

53. Burton H, Robinson CJ. Organization of the S2 Parietal Cortex. Multiple Sensory Representations Within and Near the Second Somatic Area of Cynomolgus Monkeys. In CN Woolsey (ed), Cortical Sensory Organization: Multiple Somatic Areas. Clifton, NJ: Humana, 1981;1–27.

54. Friedman DP. Body Topography in Second Somatic Sensory Area. Monkey S2 Somatotopy. In CN Woolsey (ed), Cortical Sensory Organization: Multiple Somatic Areas. Clifton, NJ: Humana, 1981;121–165.

55. Robinson CJ, Burton H. Organization of somatosensory receptive fields in cortical areas 6b, retroinsular, postauditory and granular insula of M. fascicularis. J Comp Neurol 1980; 192:265–292.

56. Leyton ASF, Sherrington CS. Observations on the excitable cortex of the chimpanzee, orangutan, and gorilla. Q J Exp Physiol 1917;11:135.

57. Hern J, Landgren S, Phillips C, Porter R. Selective excitation of corticofugal neurones by surface-anodal stimulation of the baboon's motor cortex. J Physiol 1962;161:73–90.

58. Phillips CG. Corticomotorneuronal organization. Projections from the arm area of the baboon's motor cortex. Arch Neurol 1967;17:188–195.

59. Waters RS, Samlack DD, Dykes RW, McKinley PA. Topographic organization of baboon primary motor cortex: face, hand, forelimb, and shoulder representation. Somat Motor Res 1990;7:485–514.

60. Ferrier D. Experiments in the brain of monkeys. Proc R Soc Lond B Biol Sci 1975;23:409–430.

61. Sherrington CS. The Integrative Action of the Nervous System. New Haven, CT: Yale University Press, 1906.

62. Franz SC II. Variations in the distribution of motor centers. Psychol Monographs 1915;19:80–161.

63. Chung H-T, Ruch TC, Ward AA. Topographic representation of muscles in the motor cortex of monkeys. J Neurophysiol 1947;10:39–56.

64. Asanuma H, Rosen I. Topographic organization of cortical efferent zones projecting to distal forelimb muscles in the monkey. Exp Brain Res 1972;14:243–256.

65. Humprey DR. Representation of movements and muscles within the primate precentral motor cortex: historical and current perspectives. Fed Proc 1986;45:2687–2699.

66. Gould HJ, Cusick CG, Pons TP, Kaas JH. The relationship of corpus callosum connections to electrical stimulation maps of motor, supplementary motor, and frontal eye fields in owl monkeys. J Comp Neurol 1986; 247:297.

67. Kwan HC, MacKay WA, Murphy JT, Wong YC. Spatial organization of precentral cortex in awake primates. II. Motor outputs. J Neurophysiol 1978;41:1120–1131.

68. Strick PL, Preston JB. Two representations of the hand in area 4 of a primate. I. Motor output organization. J Neurophysiol 1982;48:139–149.

69. Nudo RJ, Jenkins WM, Merzenich MM, et al. Neurophysiological correlates of hand preference in primary motor cortex of adult squirrel monkeys. J Neurosci 1992;12:1918–1947.

70. Levy WJ, Amassian VE, Schmid UD, Jungreis C. Mapping of motor cortex gyral sites non-invasively by transcranial magnetic stimulation in normal subjects and patients. EEG Clin Enceph 1991;43:51–75.

71. Wise SP. Monkey motor cortex: movements, muscles, motoneurons and metrics. Trends Neurosci 1993;16:46–49.

72. Nudo RJ, Masterton RB. Descending pathways to the spinal cord. III. Sites of origin of the corticospinal tract. J Comp Neurol 1990;286:559–583.

73. Dum RP, Strick PL. Medial wall motor areas and skeletomotor control. Curr Opin Neurobiol 1992;2:836–839.

74. He SQ, Dum RP, Strick PC. Topographic organization of corticospinal projections from the frontal lobe: motor areas on the lateral surface of the hemisphere. J Neurosci 1993; 13:952–980.

75. Graham Brown T, Sherrington CS. On the instability of a cortical point. Proc R Soc Lond B Biol Sci 1912;85:249–250.

76. Nudo RJ, Jenkins WM, Merzenich MM. Repetitive microstimulation alters the cortical representation of movements in adult rats. Somat Motor Res 1990;7:463–483.

77. Recanzone GH, Dinse HA, Merzenich MM. Expansion of the cortical representation of a specific skin field in primary somatosensory cortex by intracortical microstimulation. Cereb Cortex 1991;2:181–196.

78. Lashley K. Temporal variation in the function of the gyrus precentralis in primates. Am J Physiol 1923;65:585.

79. Taylor J (ed). Selected Writings of John Hughlings Jackson. New York: Basic Books, 1958.

80. Aou S, Woody CD, Birt D. Increases in excitability of neurons of the motor cortex of cats after rapid acquisition of eye blink conditioning. J Neurosci 1992;12:560–569.

81. Olds J, Disterhoft JF, Segal M, et al. Learning centers of rat brain mapped by measuring latencies of conditioned unit responses. J Neurophysiol 1972;35:202.

82. Disterhoft JF, Stuart DK. Trial sequence of changed unit activity in auditory system of alert rat during conditioned response acquisition and extinction. J Neurophysiol 1976;39:266.

83. Diamond DM, Weinberger NM. Classical-conditioning rapidly induces specific changes in frequency receptive fields of single neurons in secondary and ventral ectosylvian auditory cortical fields. Brain Res 1986;372:357.

84. Weinberger NM, Diamond DM. Dynamic Modulation of the Auditory System by Associative Learning. In GM Edelman, WE Gall, WM Cowan (eds), Auditory Function: Neurobiological Bases of Hearing. New York: Wiley, 1988;485.

85. Merzenich MM, Recanzone GH, Jenkin WM, et al. Cortical Representational Plasticity. In P Rakic, W Singer (eds), Neurobiology of Neocortex. New York: Wiley, 1988;41–67.

86. Weinberger NM, Ashe JH, Metherate R, et al. Retuning auditory cortex by learning: a preliminary model of receptive field plasticity. Concept Neurosci 1990;1:91.

87. Jenkins WM, Merzenich MM, Ochs M, et al. Functional reorganization of primary somatosensory cortex in adult owl monkeys after behaviorally controlled tactile stimulation. J Neurophysiol 1990;63:82–104.

88. Merzenich MM. Development and Maintenance of Cortical Somatosensory Representations: Functional "Maps" and Neuroanatomical Repertoires. In KE Barnard, TB Brazelton (eds), Touch: The Foundation of Experience. Madison, WI: International University Press, 1990;47–71.

89. Recanzone GH, Merzenich MM, Jenkins WM. Frequency discrimination training engaging a restricted skin surface results in an emergence of a cutaneous response zone in cortical area 3a. J Neurophysiol 1991;67:1057–1070.

90. Merzenich MM, Jenkins WM. Cortical Representation of Learned Behaviors. In P Andersen (ed), Memory Concepts. Amsterdam: Elsevier, 1993;437–453.

91. Merzenich MM, Sameshima K. Cortical plasticity and memory. Curr Opin Neurobiol 1993;3:187–196.

92. Merzenich MM, deCharms RC. Neural Representations, Experience and Change. In R Llinas, P Churchland (eds), The Mind-Brain Continuum. Boston: MIT Press, 1996;61–81.

93. Wang X, Merzenich MM, Beitel R, Schreiner C. Representation of species-specific vocalizations in the primary auditory cortex of the marmoset monkey. Spectral and temporal features. J Neurophysiol 1995;74:1685–1706.

94. Xerri C, Cog JO, Merzenich MM, Jenkins WM. Experience induced plasticity of cutaneous maps in the primary somatosensory cortex of adult monkeys and rats. J Physiol Paris 1999;90(3–9):277–287.

95. Recanzone GH, Schreiner CE, Merzenich MM. Plasticity in the frequency representation of primary auditory cortex following discrimination training in adult owl monkeys. J Neurosci 1993;13:87–103.

96. Merzenich MM, Jenkins WM. Reorganization of cortical representations of the hand following alterations of skin inputs induced by nerve injury, skin island transfers, and experience. J Hand Ther 1993;6:89–104.

97. Wang X, Merzenich MM, Sameshima K, Jenkins WM. Remodeling of hand representation in adult cortex determined by timing of tactile stimulation. Nature 1995;378:71–75.

98. Ahissar E, Vaadia E, Ahissar M, et al. Dependence of cortical plasticity on correlated activity of single neurons and on behavioral context. Science 1992;257:1412–1415.

99. Xerri C, Stern J, Merzenich MM. Alterations of the cortical representation of the rat ventrum induced by nursing behavior. J Neurosci 1994;14:1710–1721.

100. Sejnowski TJ. Synapses get smarter. Nature 1996;382:759–760.

101. Woody CD. Understanding the cellular basis of memory and learning. Ann Rev Psychol 1986;37:433.

102. Weinberger NM. Learning-induced changes of auditory receptive fields. Curr Opin Neurobiol 1993;3:570–577.

103. Haier RJJ, Siegel BV Jr, MacLachlan E, et al. Regional glucose metabolic changes after learning a complex visuospatial/motor task: a positron emission tomographic study. Brain Res 1992;570:134–143.

104. Allard TA, Clark SA, Jenkins WM, Merzenich MM. Reorganization of somatosensory area 3b representation in adult owl monkeys following digital syndactyly. J Neurophysiol 1991; 66:1048–1058.

105. Hebb DO. The Organization of Behavior. New York: Wiley, 1949.

106. Mitz AR, Godschalk M, Wise SP. Learning-dependent neuronal activity in the premotor cortex: activity during acquisition of conditioned motor associations. J Neurosci 1992;11:1855–1872.

107. Aizawa H, Inase M, Mushiake H, et al. Reorganization of activity in the supplementary motor area associated with motor learning and functional recovery. Exp Brain Res 1991;84:668–671.

108. Nelson RJ, Smith BN, Douglas VD. Relationships between sensory responsiveness and premovement activity of quickly adapting neurons in areas 3b and 1 of monkey primary somatosensory cortex. Exp Brain Res 1991;84:75–90.

109. Merzenich MM, Allard T, Jenkins WM. Neural Ontogeny of Higher Brain Function: Implications of Some Recent Neurophysiological Findings. In O FranzÈn, P Westman (eds), Information Processing in the Somatosensory System. London: Macmillan, 1991;211–293.

110. Merzenich MM, Tallal P, Peterson B, et al. Some Neurological Principles Relevant to the Origins of—and the Cortical Plasticity Based Remediation of—Language Learning Impairments. In J Grafman, Y Cristen (eds), Neuroplasticity: Building a Bridge from the Laboratory to the Clinic. New York: Springer-Verlag, 1998;169–187.

111. Clark SA, Allard T, Jenkins WM, Merzenich MM. Receptive fields in the body-surface map in adult cortex defined by temporally correlated inputs. Nature 1988;332:444–445.

112. Buonomano DV, Merzenich MM. Net interaction between different forms of short-term synaptic plasticity and slow-IPSPs in the hippocampus and auditory cortex. J Neurophysiol 1998b; 80:1765–1774.

113. Rubenstein JLR, Rakic P. Special issue: genetic control of cortical development. Cereb Cortex 1999;9:521–654.

114. Kilgard MP, Merzenich MM. Plasticity of temporal information processing in the primary auditory cortex. Nature Neurosci 1999;1:727–731.

115. Nagarajan S, Mahncke H, Salz T, et al. Cortical auditory signal processing in poor readers. Proc Natl Acad Sci U S A 1999;96:6483–6488.

116. Nagarajan SS, Blake D, Wright BA, et al. Practice-related improvements in somatosensory discrimination are temporary specific but generalize across skin location, hemisphere, and modality. J Neurosci 1999;18(11):1559–1663.

117. Buonomano DV, Merzenich MM. Temporal information transformed into a spatial code by a network with realistic properties. Science 1995;267:1028–1030.

118. Buonomano TV, Hickmott PW, Merzenich MM. Context-sensitive synaptic plasticity and temporal-to-spatial transformations in hippocampal slices. Proc Natl Acad Sci U S A 1997;94:10403–10408.

119. Byl NN, Merzenich MM, Jenkins WM. A primate genesis model of focal dystonia and repetitive strain injury. Neurology 1996;47:508–520.

120. Merzenich MM, Grajski KA, Jenkins WM, et al. Functional cortical plasticity. Cortical network origins of representational changes. Cold Spring Harb Symp Quant Biol 1991;55:873–887.

121. Schreiner CE, Urbas JV. Representation of amplitude modulation in the auditory cortex of the cat. II. Comparison between cortical fields. Hear Res 1988;32:49–63.

122. Eggermont JJ. Temporal modulation transfer functions for AM and FM stimuli in cat auditory cortex. Effects of carrier type, modulating waveform and intensity. Hear Res 1994;74:51–66.

123. Bieser A, Muller-Preuss P. Auditory responsive cortex in the squirrel monkey: neural responses to amplitude-modulated sounds. Exp Brain Res 1996;108:273–284.

124. Kaas JH, Hacket TA, Tamo MJ. Auditory processing in primate cerebral cortex. Curr Opin Neurobiol 1999;9:164–170.

125. Karni A, Sagi D. Where practice makes perfect in texture discrimination: evidence for primary visual cortex plasticity. Proc Natl Acad Sci U S A 1991;88:4966–4970.

126. Ahissar M, Hochstein S. Attentional control of early perceptual learning. Proc Natl Acad Sci U S A 1993; 90:5718–5722.

127. Kilgard MP, Merzenich MM. Cortical

map reorganization enabled by nucleus basalis activity. Science 1998; 279:1714–1718.

128. Grajski KA, Merzenich MM. Hebb-type dynamics is sufficient to account for the inverse magnification rule in cortical somatotopy. Neural Computation 1990a;2:74–81.

129. Grajski KS, Merzenich MM. Neuronal Network Simulation of Somatosensory Representational Plasticity. In DL Touretzky (ed), Neural Information Processing Systems, Vol 2. San Mateo, CA: Morgan Kaufman, 1990.

130. Somers DC, Todorov EV, Siapas AG, et al. A local circuit approach to understanding integration of long-range inputs in primary visual cortex. Cereb Cortex 1998;8:204–217.

131. Hockfield S, Kalb RG. Activity-dependent structural change during neuronal development. Curr Opin Neurobiol 1993;3:87–92.

132. Kuhl PK. Human adults and human infants show a "perceptual magnet effect" for the prototypes of speech categories, monkeys do not. Percept Psychophys 1991;50:93–107.

133. Kuhl PK. Learning and representation in speech and language. Curr Opin Neurobiol 1994;4:812–822.

134. Kaster S, Pinsk MA, deWeerd P, et al. Increased activity in human visual cortex during directed attention in the absence of visual stimulation. Neuron 1999;22:751–761.

135. Chelazzi L, Duncan J, Miller EK, Desimone R. Responses of neurons in inferior temporal cortex during memory-guided visual search. J Neurophysiol 1998;80:2918–2940.

136. Haenny PE, Maunsell JH, Schiller PH. State dependent activity in monkey cortex. II. Retinal and extraretinal factors in V4. Exp Brain Res 1988;69:245–259.

137. Hsiao SS, O'Shaughnessy DM, Johnson KO. Effects of selective attention on spatial form processing in monkey primary and secondary somatosensory cortex. J Neurophysiol 1993;70:444–457.

138. Phillips WA, Singer W. In search of common foundation for cortical computation. Behav Brain Sci 1997; 20:657–722.

139. Keller A, Arissian K, Asanuma H. Synaptic proliferation in the motor cortex of adult cats after long-term thalamic stimulation. J Neurophysiol 1992;68:295–308.

140. Geinisman Y, deToledo-Morrell L, Morrell F, et al. Structural synaptic correlate of long-term potentiation: formation of axospinous synapses with multiple, completely partitioned transmission zones. Hippocampus 1993; 3:435–445.

141. Kleim JA, Swain RA, Czerlanis CM, et al. Learning-dependent dendritic hypertrophy of cerebellar stellate cells: plasticity of local circuit neurons. Neurobiol Learn Mem 1997;67:29–33.

142. Engert F, Bonhoeffer T. Dendritic spine changes associated with hippocampal long-term synaptic plasticity. Nature 1999;399:66–70.

143. Fleschig P. Anatomie des menschlichen Gehirns und Ruckenmarks auf myelogenetischen Grundlage. Leipzig: Georg Thieme, 1920.

144. Yakolev PI, Lecours AR. The Myelogenetic Cycles of Regional Maturation of the Brain. In A Minkowski (ed), Regional Development of the Brain in Early Life. Oxford: Blackwell, 1967;3–70.

145. Hopson JA. The Dreaming Brain. New York: Basic Books, 1989.

146. Karni A. When practice makes perfect. Lancet 1995;345:395.

147. Qin YL, McNaughton BL, Skaggs WE, Barnes CA. Memory reprocessing in corticocortical and hippocampocortical neuronal ensembles. Philos Trans R Soc Lond B Biol Sci 1997;352:1525–1533.

148. Buzaski G. Memory consolidation during sleep a neurophysiological perspective. J Sleep Res 1998;1:17–23.

27

Plasticity and Regeneration in the Injured Spinal Cord

Michael E. Selzer and Alan R. Tessler

PATTERNS OF SPINAL CORD INJURY

The human spinal cord is injured by one or a combination of mechanisms that include contusion, stretch, compression, and laceration. At the site of impact these forces produce swelling and hemorrhagic necrosis of the gray matter and adjacent white matter, but may leave a rim of spared axons in the peripheral white matter beneath the pia. Over time the edema and hemorrhage disappear, reactive astrocytes establish a scar, and the necrotic areas are eventually replaced by cysts. If the injury has breached the pia, the scar is further thickened by acellular collagenous tissue arising from the meninges.[1] In the spinal cord rostral and caudal to the injury site and in the brain, axons separated from their perikarya undergo wallerian degeneration,[2] and some axotomized neurons isolated from their targets die by retrograde degeneration.[3] Failure of recovery after spinal cord injury is in large part caused by the death of neurons that are not replaced and by the inability of interrupted axons to regenerate.

The American Spinal Cord Injury Association (ASIA) classification of spinal cord injuries is based on a standardized neurologic examination that establishes the segmental level of injury (the most caudal segment with intact sensory and motor function) and the severity of impairment (ASIA).[4] The completeness of spinal cord injury is graded on a five-point ASIA Impairment Scale, which ranges from complete (A) to normal (E) (Figure 27-1). Functional completeness determined by the absence of sensory and motor function on a neurologic examination does not require anatomic discontinuity across the injury.[5] Bunge and his colleagues, for example, observed central nervous system (CNS) nerve fibers crossing the lesion in 50% (8 of 16) of the cases that were complete by clinical criteria.[6] If performed when the injury has stabilized so as to eliminate cases of transient impairment caused by concussion, the neurologic examination assists in predicting motor recovery both at and below the site of injury.[7,8] The amount of initial motor function correlates well with measures of functional recovery. In a multicenter study of quadriplegic patients who were motor complete at C-4, C-5, and C-6, for example, 70–80% of those with some strength in the spinal segment caudal to the intact level (1–2 of 5) recovered to the next caudal level by 4–6 months, whereas only 30–40% of those with no strength (0 of 5) showed recovery.[4] Few (0–9%) patients with complete injuries recover useful motor function compared with those with even a muscle flicker (86%) or those who are motor complete but with spared pin sensation (66–88%).[9]

Incomplete spinal cord injuries have also been classified into five distinct syndromes based on the neuroanatomic localization of the area of damage.[9] The syndromes are associated with selective injury to the anterior or posterior portions of the cord, one side of the cord (Brown-Séquard), and a mixed syndrome. Selective posterior cord damage is rare.[10] The pathophysiological basis of the most common of these syndromes, the central cord syndrome, in which a cervical cord injury causes greater weakness in the upper than the lower extremities, was originally thought to be a hematomyelic cavity in the gray matter that involved the most medial fibers of the corticospinal tract.[11] This was consistent with the traditional view of the corticospinal tract as a somatotopically organized structure with fibers responsible for hand and arm function located medially. In four more recently described

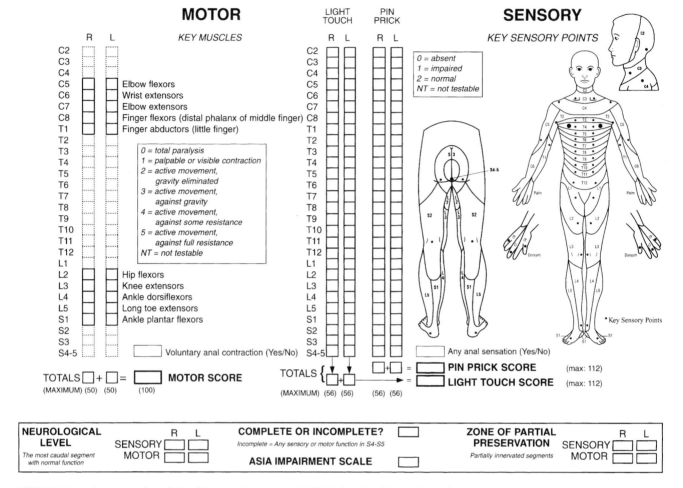

FIGURE 27-1 American Spinal Cord Injury Association (ASIA) Standard Neurological Classification of Spinal Cord Injury. This scale is widely used to document the level and degree of impairment after spinal cord injury and to document progress during recovery. (Reprinted with permission from the American Spinal Cord Injury Association. International Standards for Neurological and Functional Classification of Spinal Cord Injury, revised, 1996.)

cases, however, the gray matter was normal, and axonal damage uniformly distributed throughout the lateral corticospinal tracts.[6] Because the available evidence demonstrates that the corticospinal tract is not somatotopically organized, the disproportionate weakness in the upper extremities is now attributed to the greater importance of the corticospinal tract for upper extremity function than for lower extremity function.[12] Incomplete syndromes have different prognoses that are in part influenced by the patient's age. All patients with lateral hemisection and 80% of patients with central cord syndrome were able to walk at their last follow-up, whereas no patient with the anterior cord syndrome could do so.[10] Virtually all

patients with central cord syndrome younger than 50 years but less than one-half of those older than 50 years were ambulatory.[13]

PATHOPHYSIOLOGY OF SPINAL CORD INJURY

Difference between Effects of Trauma on Brain versus Cord

The spinal cord differs from the brain in its extreme sensitivity to trauma, particularly to concussive injury. Blunt head injuries are commonly followed by a brief loss of consciousness (concussion) without long-lasting sequelae. More severe impacts result in progressively graver neurologic dysfunction. A post-concussion syndrome consisting of headache, dizziness, or other relatively minor symptoms may last up to 4 months and then resolve completely.[14] Greater degrees of head trauma result in diffuse axonal injury,[15] leading to cognitive impairments of varying extent and less frequently to motor or sensory impairments. With even greater forces of impact, brain contusions occur and these lead to more severe focal neurologic deficits, depending on their location. Even penetrating wounds of the brain often lead to relatively isolated neurologic deficits. By contrast, non-penetrating injuries of the spinal cord are much less predictable in gradation. Seemingly mild spinal concussions, seen most frequently in cervical hyperextension, may lead to complete quadriplegia, even in the absence of penetration of the spinal canal or even vertebral fracture.[5] For this reason, it has been difficult for basic researchers to develop a gradeable model of concussive spinal cord injury. Most workers have used variations on the model of Allen,[16] who dropped a weight from varying distances onto the exposed spinal cords of dogs. He and subsequent workers noted that the injured cord initially appeared normal, but after a few hours, a central hemorrhagic necrosis developed that expanded over a period of 1–2 days until the entire cross-section of the cord was destroyed. For years, varying the height or weight of the dropped object did not produce predictable variation in the ultimate degree of functional deficit. However, careful morphologic observations in cats have suggested a correlation between the numbers of surviving axons and the impact intensity, derived from the calculated momentum of a dropped weight at impact divided by the cross-sectional area of the cord.[17] In addition, more sensitive functional scales have been developed[18] that revealed better correlations among magnitude of impact, extent of axon loss, and functional deficit.[19] Nevertheless, it remains true that spinal cord injury has a peculiarly cascading quality such that the range of injury resulting in graded functional loss is small.

The reasons for this peculiar all-or-none character of spinal cord injury are not well understood. A peculiar susceptibility of the spinal cord vasculature to hemorrhage or subsequent spasm and ischemia has been postulated, but this has not been proven. Some experts have pointed to the small diameter of the spinal canal, which would limit the degree of edema that can be tolerated before the cord is compressed. However, the spinal

ASIA IMPAIRMENT SCALE

☐ **A = Complete:** No motor or sensory function is preserved in the sacral segments S4-S5.

☐ **B = Incomplete:** Sensory but not motor function is preserved below the neurological level and includes the sacral segments S4-S5.

☐ **C = Incomplete:** Motor function is preserved below the neurological level, and more than half of key muscles below the neurological level have a muscle grade less than 3.

☐ **D = Incomplete:** Motor function is preserved below the neurological level, and at least half of key muscles below the neurological level have a muscle grade of 3 or more.

☐ **E = Normal:** Motor and sensory function is normal

CLINICAL SYNDROMES

☐ Central Cord
☐ Brown-Séquard
☐ Anterior Cord
☐ Conus Medullaris
☐ Cauda Equina

FIGURE 27-1 *(continued)*

canal is not more restrictive relative to the diameter of the spinal cord than is the cranial cavity relative to the size of the brain. The high concentration of long axon pathways through a small cross-sectional area might confer on the spinal cord an apparent vulnerability because of the exaggerated functional loss that could follow a partial injury. Yet animal studies using surgical transection and contusion models of spinal cord injury have suggested that even if only 10% of axons are spared, it can be difficult to detect a functional deficit.[20-24] Moreover, in their chronic phase, spinal cord injuries result in the development of large cavities that occupy most of the spinal cord cross-section and are surrounded by dense connective tissue through which no axons pass. Although cavitary lesions can be seen in traumatic brain injury, they do not occupy nearly the same proportion of tissue space. The vertebral joints that permit flexion and rotational mobility of the spine and the potential for disk herniations and facet joint dislocations, especially in the cervical spine, appear to account for some of the added vulnerability of the spinal cord, even in the absence of penetrating wounds. Nevertheless, there is a common experience that the spinal cord is unusually susceptible to injury and that this is caused in part by a special tendency for secondary neuronal and oligodendroglial injury to progress in cascade fashion.

Mechanisms of Secondary Neuronal Damage

Necrosis

The initial mechanical spinal cord injury sets in motion a complicated sequence of secondary processes that expand the area of damage over a period of hours to weeks, with the maximum tissue destruction occurring by 12 hours after experimental injury.[25] Evolution of the injury provides an opportunity for treatment, but the mechanisms responsible for the expansion of the lesion are not well understood. Examination of human injuries at autopsy indicates that sustained compression by bone fragments or hematomas is unlikely to play a role.[2] Studies of experimental injuries, however, have identified several interrelated mechanisms that could contribute, including the presence within the cord of hemorrhage, blood breakdown products, and edema.[26] The importance of the accumulation of large concentrations of excitatory amino acids, especially glutamate, has received increasing attention as a critical contributor to cell death.[27-30] Excessive glutamate is thought to act primarily through the *N*-methyl-D-aspartate (NMDA) receptor to cause an increase in intracellular calcium, which in

turn activates calcium-dependent phospholipases, kinases, and proteases that degrade cellular membranes. Activation of phospholipases C and A_2 also produces arachidonate, which is metabolized to thromboxanes, leukotrienes, and free radicals. All of these compounds contribute to tissue destruction.[26,28] Treatments designed to counteract these processes, such as administration of the NMDA receptor antagonist MK-801, have reduced the amount of cellular destruction observed in experimental spinal injuries.[31] High-dose methylprednisolone, which has become part of the standard treatment of acute spinal cord injury in the clinic, is thought to act primarily by suppressing lipid peroxidation and opposing the effects of free radicals.[32] A recent study has raised serious questions regarding the use of high-dose methylprednisolone.[33]

Vascular Changes

Much of the secondary damage may be the result of spinal cord ischemia. Various mechanisms have been proposed to account for the decline in spinal cord blood flow that has been a consistent finding in experimental injuries.[28] Autopsy studies have generally found the major vessels of the spinal cord to be patent.[34] Occlusion of small intramedullary arteries and veins and the anterior sulcal arteries may contribute, however, as may systemic hypotension that is a consequence of cervical cord injuries, and vasospasm caused by the accumulation of substances such as thromboxanes and endogenous opioids released by the injury.[34] Whether the leukocytes, activated microglia, and macrophages that infiltrate and scavenge the injury site contribute to the cellular destruction is controversial, but detailed study of the cellular reaction to a discrete injury of the rat spinal cord suggests that the bulk of the tissue damage precedes the cellular infiltration.[25] The end result of these cellular and biochemical reactions is the death of all cell types present at the injury site and adjacent segments, including neurons, macroglia, microglia, and vascular elements.[25,35] Most of this cell death is necrotic and characterized morphologically by swelling of mitochondria and endoplasmic reticulum, membrane rupture, and phagocytosis by invading scavengers.[36]

Apoptosis

Retrograde death of axotomized neurons, in contrast, occurs by apoptosis.[3,37] Apoptosis results from the activation of an intrinsic cell suicide program and is characterized morphologically by condensation of the nucleus and cytoplasm, intranucleosomal cleavage, and rapid removal of the afflicted cell by resident phagocytes or adjacent cells.[36] Retrograde death of axotomized neurons is difficult to document after spinal cord injury in humans because carefully controlled cell count studies cannot be performed. Information is accumulating from experimental models. Corticospinal tract neurons atrophy slightly but do not die after cervical spinal cord injury in adult rats, but neurons are lost from the red nucleus,[38-40] and several populations of intraspinal neurons both atrophy and disappear.[41,42] In general, immature neurons are more vulnerable to axotomy than mature neurons; axotomy close to the perikaryon is more likely to be lethal than distant injury; and neurons with limited collaterals are more vulnerable than neurons that are richly collateralized. These observations are consistent with the idea that loss of neurotrophic support normally derived from the target plays a critical role in the death of axotomized neurons. Most importantly, the administration of exogenous neurotrophic factors keeps alive diverse groups of neurons that otherwise would have been lost after axotomy, including retinal ganglion cells and neurons of the red nucleus, medial septal nucleus, and Clarke's nucleus.[3] Neurotrophic factors are peptides that cannot reach specific sites within the CNS parenchyma after systemic or intracerebroventricular administration. A promising strategy for providing therapeutic concentrations of these factors is to administer them via transplants of cells genetically modified to express neurotrophic factors (ex vivo gene therapy) or by the injection of a genetically modified virus (in vivo gene therapy).[43]

Increased understanding of the mechanisms of the cell suicide program has generated new approaches to treatment.[44-46] Cell death is often mediated by the activation of a family of at least 10 cytoplasmic cysteine proteases, the caspases, which function both to initiate and to carry out the execution phase of apoptosis by cleaving crucial proteins in the nucleus and cytoplasm.[47,48] Caspases are constitutively expressed as inactive precursors that are proteolytically processed to an active form in response to a proapoptotic signal and then cleave other caspases that are downstream in a rapid cascade. One strategy for preventing neuron death has been to block the execution phase of apoptosis with agents that specifically inhibit a single caspase or that function as general inhibitors of caspases. For example, intraocular injections of a wide-range protease inhibitor (ZVAD-fmd) or of a specific caspase inhibitor (ADEVD-cmk) increased the survival of retinal ganglion cell neurons that otherwise would have died 14 days after optic nerve section.[49] The family of peptides related to the proto-oncogene *Bcl-2*, which is thought to function just proximal to caspase activation,[50] offers another potentially useful point of intervention. Some members of this family, such as *Bcl-2* and

Bcl-xL, have antiapoptotic functions, and others, such as *Bax*, *Bak*, and *Bok*, are proapoptotic. The mechanisms by which these peptides integrate extracellular signals, mitochondrial physiology, and caspase and protease activity are not fully known, but human *Bcl-2* delivered by intraspinal injection of a DNA and lipid plasmid to axotomized Clarke's nucleus neurons prevented retrograde neuron death and significantly attenuated atrophy of the surviving neurons.[51] The interval for effective treatment between the onset of an apoptotic stimulus and the time when cell death becomes inevitable may vary for different types of neurons and has been defined only in a few cases. For example, fetal spinal cord transplants, which are thought to act as a source of neurotrophic factors, can keep axotomized Clarke's nucleus neurons alive if provided at the time of injury,[52] but are completely ineffective if transplantation is delayed for more than 1 week.[53] Caspase inhibitors also increased short-term retinal ganglion cell survival if administered 3 days after injury, but not if administration was delayed until 7 days.[54]

Delayed Oligodendrocyte Apoptosis

Studies of contusion injuries of rat and monkey spinal cord have shown that oligodendrocytes also die by apoptosis in degenerating fiber tracts remote from the area of impact.[55-57] Loss of trophic factors derived from axons that are undergoing wallerian degeneration or secretion of toxic cytokines by infiltrating cells may be responsible. Paradoxically, death may also be induced by neurotrophins through an action on the low-affinity neurotrophin receptor (p75) that is expressed by injured oligodendrocytes.[57] Because oligodendrocytes are responsible for ensheathing multiple CNS axons with myelin, their deaths can amplify the functional deficits that follow spinal cord injury by impairing conduction. Autopsy studies have shown that demyelination is a conspicuous feature of chronic spinal cord injuries in humans.[6] The observation that oligodendrocytes die by apoptosis raises the possibility that they can be kept alive by the same strategies that are being used to rescue axotomized neurons.

REQUIREMENTS FOR FUNCTIONAL RECOVERY

Mechanisms of Spontaneous Recovery

Immediately after spinal cord injury, functional deficits are either maximal, or they may worsen over the next

2–4 days. Thereafter, recovery occurs to variable degrees, and this can be predicted to some extent by the initial neurologic examination[8] and magnetic resonance imaging.[58,59] The mechanisms by which the recovery occurs are not completely known, but they include resolution of edema, various modes of physiological plasticity, collateral sprouting, and dendritic pruning (Figure 27-2). Although each of these mechanisms is known to exist in the mammalian CNS, the degree to which they contribute to recovery or indeed, whether they even occur in human spinal cord injury, is not known.

Resolution of Edema

After spinal cord injury, edema and hemorrhage develop over a period of approximately 24 hours and then slowly resolve. The mechanism of the edema is not completely known, but inflammation,[60] loss of Ca^{2+} from the extracellular space,[61] loss of K^+ and Mg^{2+} from the intracellular space,[62] pressure generated by compression of the swollen cord against the meninges, and ischemia all interact with edema formation in a complex web of events to produce transient dysfunction.[63] The increased pressure in the cord and the alterations in ionic concentrations of the extracellular space result in loss of conduction in some neurons and axons that have not been permanently injured. Over the next several days, as the edema resolves, electrical conduction is restored and physiological function is recovered. However, it has been pointed out that the edema fluid itself is not a predictor of tissue injury severity or progression.[61,64]

Physiological Plasticity

Several phenomena traditionally have been assumed to be based on molecular mechanisms without gross morphologic correlates. Although this is now not strictly true, because ultrastructural or immunohistologic alterations do accompany some of these phenomena, they are largely invisible at the light microscopic level. A term in common use among rehabilitation professionals is *neural plasticity*. *Neural plasticity* refers to the altered physiological responses seen in patients after injury to the nervous system, and after rehabilitative training, that may contribute to recovery. One example is the improvement in locomotion with partial body-weight-supported treadmill training in patients with stroke[65,66] and spinal cord injury[67] (see the series of Special Feature Reviews and Commentaries on this topic in *Neurorehabilitation and Neural Repair*, November 1999). This rapidly developing form of therapy has its basis in two fundamental observations. First, the spinal cord of all vertebrates, including humans, contains neuronal cir-

cuitry that encodes the locomotor pattern, which can be activated by stimulation at supraspinal, suprasegmental, or segmental levels or even by intrathecal drug administration.[68–73] Thus, the activation of locomotor circuitry does not require moment by moment control of individual muscles by the brain. The second key observation was that repeated activation of the central pattern generating circuit by treadmill training could result in long-lasting enhancement of the locomotor output.[68,69,74] In human trials, this resulted in improved locomotion months and even years after training was discontinued.[66,67]

Another well-known example of neural plasticity is the rearrangement of hand representation in the somatosensory cortex after injury to a peripheral nerve[75] or amputation of a digit.[76] The earliest such examples indicated expansion of the cortical representation of adjacent spared body parts for distances of approximately 1.5 mm over the surface of the cortex. Because this amount of remapping was shown to occur almost instantaneously[77] and also represents the distribution of terminals of thalamocortical relay neurons,[78,79] it could be concluded that no synaptic or morphologic plastic changes were required to explain it, but that it might be caused by unmasking of latent synaptic circuitry by removal of ongoing inhibition from the lost afferent pathway. However, at longer recovery times, the territory that could be bridged by shifting sensory maps increased 10-fold.[80] Moreover, even without deafferentation, the area of primary somatosensory cortex activated by stimulating a digit could be increased by repeated sensory overstimulation.[81] Thus, the expansions of sensory receptive fields produced by long-term alterations in afferent input are probably caused by physiological, anatomic, or both physiological and anatomic plastic changes.[82] Changes in central representation of the body have also been demonstrated in cases of CNS injury. When the area of central sensory projections of fingertips was microlesioned in monkeys, previously learned skillful behaviors with the affected hand that depended on finger tip sensation at first deteriorated but then improved. Concomitantly, the central projection for those fingertips shifted to neighboring regions of cortex.[83]

The primary motor cortex also shows plasticity. Training a monkey to perform a skilled task with the digits resulted in an enlargement of the area within the primary motor cortex in which microstimulation elicits movements in the digits. At the same time, the primary motor cortex area representing the wrist and forearm contracted. The reverse occurred with training to perform a movement with the wrist and fore-

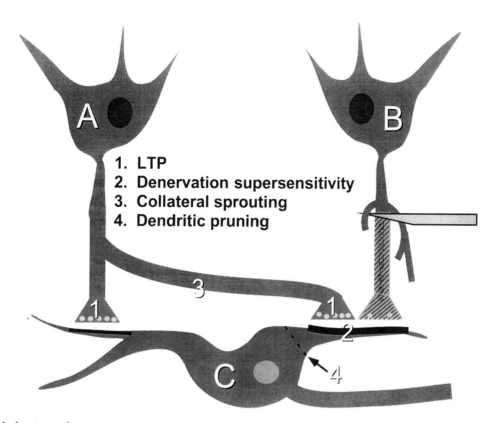

1. LTP
2. Denervation supersensitivity
3. Collateral sprouting
4. Dendritic pruning

FIGURE 27-2 Mechanisms of spontaneous recovery. Neurons A and B represent neighboring pathways afferent to a nucleus in the central nervous system, represented by neuron C. Partial injury to one pathway, represented by cutting of axon B is partially compensated for by plastic changes in the rest of the circuit. The organism may compensate by using pathway A more intensively, giving rise to long-term potentiation (LTP), diagrammed here by an increase in the number of releasable synaptic vesicles (1). Degeneration of pathway B may give rise to an increase in the density of receptors in denuded postsynaptic membranes, which results in denervation supersensitivity (2), diagrammed here as a black thickening of the postsynaptic membrane. Denervated postsynaptic membranes induce collateral sprouting (3) by nearby spared axons, to fill in for lost synaptic terminals. If collateral sprouting is not able to reinnervate denervated dendrites, they undergo pruning (4) (i.e., they wither), permitting the neuron to focus its metabolic activity on those dendrites that are still functional. Finally, injured axons attempt to regenerate, but in mammals this is ordinarily not successful.

arm.[84] A similar phenomenon has been demonstrated on a coarser level with transcranial magnetic stimulation in human subjects. Focal stimulation of the motor cortex was used to evoke thumb movements in one direction. Thumb movements then were practiced in a different direction. Subsequently, transcranial magnetic stimulation evoked movements in or near the recently practiced direction for several minutes before returning to the original direction.[85] Profound and permanent enlargements of motor representation occurred for muscles proximal to an amputation or just rostral to the level of a spinal cord injury.[86] The mechanisms for this are not known. However, pharmacologic studies with lorazepam suggested that the rapid onset temporary changes in motor representa-

tion after ischemic nerve block involve reduction of GABAergic inhibition.[87]

Many other examples have been published of shifts in cortical maps in human patients with peripheral nervous system or CNS lesions and healthy subjects, using transcranial magnetic stimulation, functional imaging, magnetoencephalography, and high-resolution electroencephalography. The mechanisms are not known but the term commonly used to refer to all of them is *neuronal plasticity*. Studies in the aplysia nervous system and in transgenic mice suggest that common molecular mechanisms may be involved in the long-lasting changes included in this terminology.

The word *plasticity* was used by neuroscientists early in connection with the study of the cellular mechanisms underlying memory and learning. The term was applied to a large number of physiological phenomena by which patterns of use and disuse modified the strength of synaptic pathways (e.g., facilitation, potentiation, long-term potentiation [LTP], sensitization, classical and operant conditioning; also synaptic depression, long-term depression [LTD], habituation) and to anatomic rearrangements within a nervous system that had been perturbed by injury (e.g., sprouting, pruning, regeneration). Eventually, the terms *neural plasticity* and *synaptic plasticity* were dismissed by many as trite because they were overused and imprecise. However, the term *neural plasticity* has been resurrected by the community of scientists whose work is relevant to mechanisms of recovery after neural injury because they needed a way to refer in general to a wide assortment of phenomena whose precise mechanisms were not known. In fact, the opprobrium attached to use of the term *neural plasticity* is less warranted now because molecular mechanisms that underlie many of the previously mentioned physiological changes in synaptic efficacy are turning out to be similar and to share common intracellular signaling elements with anatomic rearrangements and other responses to physical and metabolic injury.

The responses of cells to the extracellular environment are mediated by intracellular signal transduction pathways through a large variety of interdigitating cascades of cytoplasmic protein kinases. In these pathways enzymes become activated when they are phosphorylated by a kinase and, in turn, themselves act as kinases to phosphorylate the next kinase in the cascade. Often the phosphorylation cascade is initiated by the binding of a biologically active molecule (e.g., a neurotrophic factor) to a transmembrane receptor whose intracellular portion functions as a kinase (e.g., a tyrosine kinase). In other cases, the cascade is triggered by the entry of calcium through a ligand-activated ion channel, such as occurs when glutamate binds to the NMDA receptor-ion channel complex. The calcium then activates a calcium-dependent kinase, such as protein kinase C. In still other cases, a neurotransmitter (e.g., norepinephrine) or hormone (e.g., insulin) binds to a receptor that is linked by a guanosine triphosphate–binding protein to adenylyl cyclase. The cyclic adenosine monophosphate (AMP) thus generated activates a protein kinase (cAMP-PK). Some kinase cascades are short (i.e., they contain only one or two kinases). Other cascades are much longer. The downstream end of the line for these kinase cascades is the phosphorylation of a transcription factor that binds to DNA and regulates the expression of one or more genes. A great deal of work is directed at identifying all the molecular signals in the pathway between the binding of a ligand to its receptor and the altered expression of one or more genes that trigger such diverse responses of the cell as programmed cell death (apoptosis), increased synthesis and release of synaptic transmitter, or the sprouting of extra branches by spared axons after injury of their neighbors. An example of the molecular convergence of physiological and structural plasticity is the evidence adduced by Kandel and others that increases in the synthesis of neurotransmitter seen in several models of learning in both *Aplysia* and mice involve activation of genes containing cAMP response elements through the phosphorylation of the transcription factors' cAMP response element–binding proteins.[88] What is especially interesting is that the long-term synaptic changes that accompany learning in *Aplysia* include an increase in the number of synaptic contacts, which also appears to be dependent on cAMP response element–binding protein activation.[89] The phenomena studied by some rehabilitation scientists in humans and intact animals are assumed to incorporate many of the transcription-mediated cellular responses that have been studied in more reduced experimental preparations, but these relationships remain to be established.

Denervation Supersensitivity

Neurons that lose a synaptic input become more sensitive to the application of the involved transmitter. At the neuromuscular junction, this *denervation supersensitivity* results from an increase in the number of extrajunctional acetylcholine receptors caused by a loss of electrical activity in the muscle.[90,91] In the rat, depletion of dopamine in the substantia nigra results in supersensitivity to dopamine in the basal ganglia. This supersensitivity can be demonstrated after intraventricular injection of specific dopamine receptor agonists by behavioral responses, by D_1 and D_2 receptor assays, or by ^{14}C-2-deoxyglucose autoradiography.[92,93] Up-regulation of dopamine D_2 receptors has been seen with single photon emission computed tomography in patients with Parkinson's disease,[94] and denervation supersensitivity to dopamine has been postulated to underlie the dyskinetic toxic reactions to L-dopa in patients with Parkinson's disease.[93] Expression of muscarinic acetylcholine receptors[95] and noradrenergic receptors is also up-regulated after denervation in both the CNS and peripheral nervous system, and α-adrenergic supersensitivity by peripheral nociceptors has been proposed as a mechanism for the causalgic pain that follows partial nerve injuries.[96] The phenomenon of up-regulation of receptors on deprivation of the ligand is not restricted to conventional neurotransmitters. Up-regulation of opioid receptors has been demonstrated in enkephalin knockout mice.[97] Thus, denervation supersensitivity appears to be a widespread phenomenon that may characterize most neurotransmitter and neuromodulator systems. By mediating a compensatory enhancement of responsiveness of neurons that have been partially deafferented by spinal cord injury, denervation supersensitivity could account for part of the hyperreflexia or even functional recovery in patients with partial spinal cord injury, but this has not been demonstrated.

Long-Term Potentiation

Changed patterns of use of spared synaptic pathways can alter their strength, and this could contribute to functional recovery after spinal cord injury. Repeated high-frequency stimulation of excitatory glutamatergic pathways to the pyramidal cells of the CA1 region of hippocampus results in a large increase in synaptic efficacy of those pathways that may last hours or even days.[98] This phenomenon, called long-term potentiation (LTP), is seen in several locations in the brain, and the cellular mechanism may vary from location to location.[99-101] In the CA1 region, LTP appears to result from the synchronous occurrence of NMDA receptor activation and a large depolarization of the postsynaptic membrane. This permits a large influx of calcium into the postsynaptic cell, resulting in activation of a retrograde chemical signal directed back to the presynaptic terminal. The nature of the retrograde signal is not known, but both nitric oxide and carbon monoxide have been implicated.[102-104] The retrograde signal causes an increase in the release of glutamate during subsequent synaptic activations. Some investigators have suggested that LTP involves an increased postsynaptic sensitivity to glutamate as well. An important aspect of LTP is that it can be activated either via homosynaptic or heterosynaptic mechanisms. Homosynaptic activation of LTP involves stimulation of the potentiated pathway strong enough so that, in addition to binding to the requisite number of NMDA receptors, a large postsynaptic depolarization is produced via the non-NMDA glutamate receptors. Such a mechanism could be relevant to the type of motor learning that occurs when a new skill is practiced. Heterosynaptic LTP occurs when the potentiated pathway serves as the source of glutamate for NMDA receptor activation, while another pathway synapsing on the same postsynaptic neuron serves to depolarize the postsynaptic membrane. This mechanism could be relevant to associative types of learn-

ing, such as classical and operant (trial and error) conditioning.

Long-Term Depression and Habituation

Stimulation of some synaptic pathways may lead to long-term depression (LTD) of those synapses.[105] As with LTP, there are several different mechanisms involved, depending on the location and type of synapse and the pattern of stimulation, and LTD may be either homosynaptic or heterosynaptic. Homosynaptic LTD results from low-frequency stimulation of the depressed pathway and activation of NMDA receptors. This type of depression could be involved in habituation, a simple form of learning in which monotonously repeated stimuli eventually fail to elicit a response. Heterosynaptic LTD occurs when high-frequency activation of one pathway produces a reduction in response of the postsynaptic neuron to stimulation of the second pathway. This type of LTD is caused by an influx of calcium through voltage-gated calcium channels and subsequent release of calcium from intracellular stores.[106]

Collateral Sprouting

Partial denervation of muscle is followed by sprouting of neurites from neighboring spared axons and reinnervation of the denervated muscle fibers by the sprouts.[107,108] Evidence suggests that when a nerve undergoes partial injury, the Schwann's cells that cap degenerated nerve terminals send out processes to adjacent neuromuscular junctions. Spared axon terminals send out sprouts that follow the Schwann cell processes back to the denervated muscle and there establish a new neuromuscular junction.[109,110] The molecular mechanisms underlying the Schwann's cell–mediated terminal sprouting are not known.

Collateral sprouting in the spinal cord was first demonstrated by Liu and Chambers.[111] They outlined the territory of the central projection of spared dorsal root axons after cutting neighboring dorsal roots in the cat. These results were initially disputed because they were based on degeneration stains, which can give conflicting results. However, sprouting of dorsal root axons and corticospinal tract axons was also demonstrated autoradiographically in cats and monkeys.[112,113] Sprouting of dorsal root axons has also been demonstrated with anterograde tracing methods and immunohistochemically.[114] Although the distance that sprouting neurites grew turned out to be less than originally suggested by Liu and Chambers, the existence of the phenomenon has now been accepted.

In the brain, collateral sprouting has been demonstrated in the septal nucleus,[115] dentate gyrus,[116-118] and CA3 region[119] of the hippocampus. Regardless of location in the CNS, collateral sprouts generally grow no more than 250 μm. An exception is the enlargement of the contralateral projection to the dentate gyrus after ipsilateral entorhinal lesions. In this case, the sprouting fibers may grow as much as 2–3 mm.[118] The mechanisms of sprouting in the CNS are not known, but as at the neuromuscular junction, they appear to involve interactions between cells in the region of axon terminal degeneration and the neighboring spared axons. Microglial or astrocytic proliferation, or other elements of an inflammatory response, do not seem to be required.[120]

The functional significance of sprouting is not clear. It has been suggested that sprouting, also called *reactive synaptogenesis*, contributes to posttraumatic epileptogenesis in the hippocampus.[119] However, because the time course of sprouting in the spinal cord correlates with the development of hyperreflexia and increased muscle tone after spinal transection, it has been suggested that sprouting might be of functional benefit in spinal cord–injured animals by enhancing their ability to support their weight.[112,113]

Dendritic Pruning

Loss of innervation can result in altered postsynaptic neuronal morphology. Dendritic spines that have lost their innervation are lost.[121] Dendritic arbors may be simplified and if insufficient afferent inputs remain, the postsynaptic neuron may atrophy. When different inputs to a neuron are segregated on different parts of the dendritic tree, loss of one afferent pathway results in selective reduction in the size of its territory of the dendritic arbor.[122] This is termed *dendritic pruning*. The mechanisms underlying this dendritic plasticity are unknown, but clusters of polyribosomes have been demonstrated associated with cisternae at the base of dendritic spines. Denervation results in loss of these polyribosomes, whereas reinnervation is associated with their return.[123] Thus, synaptic activity localized to one spine could rapidly influence protein synthesis in that portion of dendrite[124] and thereby affect the size and shape of the dendritic tree.

Required Interventions

From the previously mentioned considerations, it is clear that spinal cord injury results in both immediate and delayed neuronal death. It is also true that in models of CNS injury, axonal rupture is not always immediate, but that some injured axons undergo a process of delayed interruption, probably caused by influx of calcium at the site of tension and subsequent disruption of the cytoskeleton. Despite the plastic properties of the CNS described previously, spinal cord injury is followed by incomplete functional recovery. Optimal recovery would require first that neurons be rescued from cell death to the greatest degree possible. Second, axons must be rescued from rupture to the greatest degree possible. Third, if neurons do die, they must be replaced. Fourth, if axons are severed, they must be encouraged to regenerate. Fifth, regenerated axons must remake their lost synaptic contacts. Sixth, the restored synaptic circuitry must be translated into useful function. The remainder of this chapter focuses on neuronal replacement and axonal regeneration, but clearly, the last requirement (i.e., that restored connections be translated into useful function) links the other requirements directly to traditional rehabilitation strategies and clinical expertise.

REGENERATION IN THE CENTRAL NERVOUS SYSTEM OF VERTEBRATES

Influence of Phylogeny

It is generally accepted that axonal regeneration in the CNS of postnatal animals is more effective among lower species in the phylogenetic tree. Transection of the spinal cord is followed by functional axonal regeneration in lampreys,[125] fishes,[126] and urodele amphibians (newts and salamanders),[127] but not in anuran amphibians (frogs and toads), reptiles, birds, or mammals (see extensive discussions in the classic monograph edited by Windle[128]). The precise reasons for this phylogenetic hierarchy in regenerative ability are not known. Most workers assume that inhibitory molecules in the environment of the injured axons are lacking in lower vertebrates. However, this has not been proven. Some of these molecules are associated with myelin (see following discussion), and because lamprey spinal cord axons lack myelin, this may be one reason for their regenerative ability. However, axons in fish and urodele amphibians are myelinated and yet regeneration is seen in these species. Whether the myelin of species that show regeneration contains mammalian-like neurite growth inhibitors has been disputed.[129,130]

Influence of Glial Phenotype

In higher vertebrates, glial cells have intermediate filaments composed of glial fibrillary acidic protein (GFAP). At the site of a lesion, glial cells proliferate and up-regulate expression of GFAP. This produces a hard gliotic scar, which is thought to form a mechanical barrier that inhibits axonal regeneration. GFAP is also up-regulated in glial cells downstream in the path of axonal regeneration, although it does not proliferate. One of the features that distinguishes nervous systems that show axonal regeneration from those that do not is the special type of glial cells that is present in systems that regenerate. These glial cells are interconnected by desmosomes and contain intermediate filaments that are heteropolymers of keratin subunits rather than GFAP. This type of glial cell has been found particularly in parts of the CNS that show axonal regeneration.[131-136] The reason for this correlation is not clear. It has been speculated that the desmosomes might serve to stabilize the glial architecture at the site of injury, thus preserving correctly *labeled* pathways for axons to grow along.[137] In the lamprey, glial cells may be important in determining the ease and correctness of regeneration, because 80% of the growth cone surfaces of regenerating spinal axons are in contact with glial processes, and processes belonging to glial cells of the rostral and caudal ends of the transected spinal cord precede the axons in bridging the lesion.[137]

Influence of Age

Another commonly accepted generalization is that, within a species, the ability of axons to regenerate decreases with age. Thus, spinal axons regenerate in tadpoles, but not in postmetamorphic frogs.[138-140] Transplants of fetal spinal cord are more successful in bridging a spinal cord transection when performed in neonatal mammals than in adults.[141-143] The reasons for this developmental change are not known, but both extracellular environmental changes and neuron intrinsic changes have been implicated and are discussed here. However, the importance of environmental causes for failure of regeneration may have been overemphasized as a result of the striking observations that some axons of mature CNS can regenerate into peripheral nerve grafts.[144,145] However, in these and subsequent experiments on retinal ganglion cells, it became clear that only a minority of injured axons regenerate into these grafts.[146] This issue has been investigated further in cocultures of retina and optic tectum in rat.[147] When embryonic retinas were cocultured with adult optic tecta, retinal cells sent axons that penetrated into the tectum. However, when postnatal retinas were cocultured with embryonic tecta, retinal cells were unable to regenerate

axons into the tectum. This suggested that the age of the neuron rather than that of its host environment most influences the regenerative ability of axons. Similar conclusions were drawn from experiments in which cocultures of entorhinal cortex and hippocampus were used to test the influence of postnatal age on regeneration of the entorhinodentate pathway of rats.[148]

Specificity

In both invertebrates and vertebrates, the highly specific development of connections between neurons involves four basic types of attractive and repulsive molecular interactions: contact-mediated attraction, chemoattraction mediated by gradients of diffusible molecules, contact-mediated repulsion, and chemorepulsion.[149] Although we have made substantial progress in understanding how developing axons choose their paths, we have little understanding of how these axons decide which cells to form synapses with. Two of the most important questions concerning regeneration are (1) whether regenerating axons are guided in their correct paths and make synapses with their correct target neurons, and if so, (2) whether the same molecular cues are employed as guide developing axons. Chaotic regeneration might produce effects that are even worse than no regeneration at all. For example, it might result in constant pain, but no sensory information that localizes stimuli or gives clues to their modality. Thus, it is critical to know whether any axonal regeneration achieved in the CNS would be specific with regard to pathways taken and synaptic partners selected. The characteristics of regeneration in the CNS of several lower vertebrates have suggested that this is so. After section of the optic nerves of fish and frogs, axons regenerate to the optic tectum in a retinotopically correct way and accurate vision is restored.[150,151] In the frog spinal cord, cut or crushed dorsal roots can regenerate, and muscle sensory neurons form synaptic contacts selectively with appropriate agonist motoneurons.[152] After spinal cord transection in the lamprey, axons regenerate selectively in their original paths.[153-155] Observations on the paths taken by the cut axons early during regeneration and the effects of surgical manipulations on the paths taken by these axons suggested that they may be following guidance cues in their local environment.[156] Regenerating axons form functioning synapses selectively with correct neurons distal to the lesion.[157,158] Much less is known about the specificity of axonal regeneration in mammalian CNS, because this generally requires experimental manipulation, and even then, the amount of regeneration is limited. However, retinal ganglion cell axons that regenerate through peripheral nerve grafts linking the optic nerve with the optic tectum form synapses selectively with neurons in the correct layers of the superior colliculus that are ultrastructurally similar to normal retinotectal synapses.[159]

The molecular mechanisms underlying the specificity shown by regenerating axons in the CNS of lower vertebrates are still unknown. It would seem from work in these lower vertebrate models that some recognition molecules must persist or be re-expressed after injury in the mature nervous system. Indeed, several developmental guidance molecules are expressed in postembryonic spinal cords of lower vertebrates and mammals.[160-162] These guidance molecules act to either attract or repel a growing axon tip that bears receptors for them. It is not yet known whether these molecules affect regenerating axons, but initial reports suggest that expression of some guidance molecules is up-regulated in the spinal cord or supraspinal projecting neurons after spinal cord injury. These include Eph B3,[162] a member of the Eph family of protein tyrosine kinase receptors for the chemorepellent molecules of the ephrin family; netrins,[163,164] molecules that can act as either chemorepellents or chemoattractants, depending on the receptor with which they interact; and the netrin receptor UNC-5.[165] Distribution gradients of ephrin A ligands in the optic tectum of chick and superior colliculus of rodents underlie the specificity of retinotopic innervation of these regions in the anterior-posterior direction. By expressing ephrin A ligands on their surfaces, caudal tectal or superior colliculus cells selectively prevent extension of Eph A type receptor-bearing axons into temporal regions of the retina.[166-168] It is also likely that interactions between ephrin B1–expressing cells in the dorsal tectum repel axons of ventral retinal ganglion cells, which express receptors of the Eph B family.[168] It is not known whether these gradients persist in the mature animal or whether they guide the successful regeneration of retinotopic innervation of the tectum in frogs and fish after optic nerve section.

The correlative data described previously suggest that some of the molecules that guide embryonic axons to their correct targets during development may also influence the ability of axons to elongate during regeneration. Even if injured mature axons are sensitive to the effects of these ligands, however, until much more is known about the precise time course of expression and distribution of the guidance molecules after injury, it is

not possible to determine whether they actually serve to guide growing axon tips in their correct paths.

FACTORS LIMITING REGENERATION IN MAMMALIAN SPINAL CORD

Environmental Factors

Growth Cone Collapsing Factors
Myelin-Associated Growth Inhibitors   Cellular elements of the mature CNS express several molecules that have been shown to inhibit axon growth in tissue culture by causing collapse of the growth cone. When embryonic neurons are grown on adhesive substrates, such as poly-L-lysine or laminin, the leading edge of the growing axon consists of a specialized structure called the *growth cone*. The proximal portion of the growth cone is a flattened expanse called the *lamellipodium*. Along the leading edge of the lamellipodium, fine projections called *filopodia* extend along the substrate. The filopodia contain bundles of 1–12 actin microfilaments composed of fibrous actin (F-actin) and elongate on the extracellular matrix by a process that involves the polymerization of the actin filaments at their distal end.[169] Microtubules concentrate in the region of actively elongating filopodia, and the lamellipodium spreads forward between adjacent elongating filopodia.[170] This mechanism results in the rapid (1–3 mm/day) growth that characterizes early embryonic development. It is not known whether this mechanism also underlies growth cone advance during regeneration, but work in the lamprey suggests that it does not.[171] In this species, the growth cones of cut spinal cord axons lack filopodia, have little actin, and regenerate more slowly than other vertebrate and invertebrate embryonic axons (see discussion on cytoskeletal elements in this section). Because no test of this issue has been performed in mammals, and long-term cultures of lamprey neurons have not been achieved, it is not known whether the differences are caused by species' differences or differences between axon development and regeneration.

Despite the possible differences between embryonic and regenerating growth cones, most work on the molecular mechanisms involved in growth inhibition has employed tissue culture assays, and, therefore, most of our knowledge concerning axon elongation has been derived from these preparations. One growth-inhibiting effect was described by Caroni and Schwab,[172,173] who observed that cultured neurons can grow long processes on peripheral myelin fractions but not on fractions of CNS myelin. They identified two molecules with molecular weights of 35,000 and 250,000 on the surfaces of oligodendrocytes (the cells that make CNS myelin) that cause growth cones to collapse on contact.[172] Both molecules were bound by a single mAb (IN-1), so they are probably structurally related.[173] Purification and microsequencing of a bovine molecule (bNI-220) similar to NI-250 have been reported, and it appears to be unrelated to any previously identified molecular species.[174] The antibody IN-1 neutralized the growth inhibitory activities of NI-35/NI-250 and bNI-220. The mechanism by which these molecules cause growth cone collapse seems to include activation of a G protein[175] and release of calcium from intracellular stores.[176] The excess calcium can activate disaggregation of cytoskeletal elements such as microtubules and actin microfilaments that are important in growth cone motility. One of the most abundant myelin surface proteins, myelin-associated glycoprotein, has also been shown to have growth cone–collapsing activity in vitro.[177-179] The significance of this for regeneration has been questioned because axon outgrowth was not better on CNS myelin of myelin-associated glycoprotein–deficient mice than on myelin of wild type mice.[180] Two chondroitin sulfate proteoglycans, each having neurite growth-inhibiting properties, have been demonstrated on the surfaces of bovine spinal cord oligodendrocytes.[181] These molecules appear to account for some of the growth-inhibiting activity of oligodendrocytes in vitro because treatment with the proteoglycan synthesis inhibitors β-xylosides reduced the synthesis of both of the proteoglycans and reversed the growth cone collapse seen during encounters of neurites with oligodendrocytes. It is not clear how universal the growth-inhibitory effect of oligodendrocytes is. Kobayashi and colleagues[182] found that contact with oligodendrocytes in vitro inhibited the growth of dorsal root ganglion (DRG) cell axons, but not those of retinal cells.

Neuron-Associated Growth Inhibitors Growth cone-collapsing activity is also associated with neuronal membranes. Axons from the nasal side of the developing retina grow selectively to the posterior part of the optic tectum, whereas temporal retinal axons grow to the anterior tectum. When neurons from the nasal and temporal retina of the chick were grown on strips of posterior and anterior optic tectum, the posterior tectal membranes caused collapse of temporal but not nasal retinal growth cones.[183] This growth cone–collapsing activity was ultimately shown to be mediated by ephrins on the surfaces of posterior tectal membranes acting on Eph receptors on the surfaces of

growth cones of temporal retinal neurons[184] and is believed to underlie the specificity of retinotopic innervation of the superior colliculus during development. Evidence suggests a role for ephrin signaling in spinal cord development as well.[185] As we have seen, the re-expression of Eph B3 after spinal cord injury[162] suggests that ephrin signaling may inhibit regeneration of some spinal cord axons.

A similar series of growth cone–collapsing activities were found on neurites of cultured chick CNS and peripheral nervous system.[186] Growth cones collapsed on encountering neurites from alien parts of the nervous system, but continued to advance when they encountered neurites from the same part of the nervous system or a normal target. Unlike NI-35, the neurite-associated collapsing activity did not involve an increase in calcium concentration within the growth cone.[187] Raper and Kapfhammer[188] extracted a protein from chick brain that caused collapse of dorsal root ganglia growth cones.[188] This factor was called *collapsin* and shown to be an 88-kD transmembrane protein belonging to the immunoglobulin superfamily.[189] Collapsin is a member of the semaphorin family of transmembrane and secreted proteins, which have been cloned from several species, including humans.[190-193] The semaphorins are expressed during early development and appear to be important in guiding developing axons to their correct targets. Whether they play a role in inhibiting regeneration in the more mature nervous system has not been determined, but semaphorin expression does persist in the mature CNS, including spinal motor neurons.[161] Another embryonic guidance molecule, netrin[194,195], is expressed by both glial cells and neurons[163-165,196,197] and acts as a secreted chemoattractant when it binds to receptors of the deleted in colorectal cancer (DCC) family.[198-200] However, netrins also act as chemorepellents when they target growth cones bearing receptors of the UNC-5 family.[201-203] It appears that when UNC-5 is complexed with DCC in the growth cone membrane, it converts the chemoattractant effect to chemorepulsion.[200,204] It has not yet been documented that the repulsion involves actual growth cone–collapsing activity, but the persistence of netrins and UNC-5 in the CNS of postembryonic animals suggests that netrin may act as a chemorepellent to some growth cones during regeneration.[164,165,205]

It is important to recognize that these growth cone-collapsing activities require not only the inhibitory molecule, but also the presence of receptors on the surfaces of susceptible neurons. For example, it is assumed that the embryonic growth of axons is not inhibited by myelin-associated growth cone–collapsing factors because of the late development of myelin. However, embryonic neurons from hippocampus, neocortex, and superior colliculus were able to grow long axons when transplanted by atraumatic microinjection into various white matter tracts in the adult mouse.[206,207] This may reflect an absence in these immature neurons of receptors for myelin-associated inhibitory molecules. However, it may also mean that myelin-associated growth inhibitors are less potent when encountered by growing axons in vivo than in vitro and that other molecules expressed at the site of injury are more important.[208]

Astrocyte-Derived Extracellular Matrix Molecules

At the site of CNS injury, a scar is formed by proliferating astrocytes, which also undergo a complex reaction that includes increased synthesis of glial filaments. Axons were long assumed not to regenerate through the astrocytic scar because of the scar's hard consistency and other mechanical features. More recently, however, specific molecular mechanisms have been suggested. Although membrane fractions from gray matter support axon growth in vitro, membrane fractions from astrocytic scars do not.[209] This growth-inhibiting activity appears to be associated with one or more cell surface sulfated glycoproteins, especially chondroitin sulfate proteoglycans.[210-212] The secretion of proteoglycans by reactive astrocytes at the site of injury has been proposed as a mechanism by which the glial scar inhibits axonal regeneration in the CNS (Figure 27-3).[213] In support of this hypothesis, it has been shown that even adult DRG cells could grow long processes when microinjected into spinal cord white matter, unless the procedure was traumatic enough to result in the accumulation of immunohistochemically detectable proteoglycans at the injection site.[208] Thus, one school of thought maintains that in the three-dimensional context of the injured brain and spinal cord, CNS myelin is not the source of significant growth inhibitory activity, but rather it is the proteoglycans secreted at the site of injury that inhibit regeneration. However, DRG cells may not be representative of neurons of the CNS, because they give rise to peripheral processes and adult DRG cells are much easier to grow in culture than mature CNS neurons. The microinjection experiments have not been repeated using adult CNS neurons.

Intraneuronal Factors

Ever since the pioneering studies of Aguayo and his colleagues, showing that CNS axons can regenerate into peripheral nerve grafts,[144,145,214] most explanations for the failure of regeneration in CNS have focused on the role of the extracellular environment. The findings of Schwab and others that CNS myelin contains molecules that inhibit axon elongation in vitro[172,173,215] reinforced this notion and provided an explanation for the influence of age on regeneration, because myelination occurs relatively late in development. However, it has long been apparent that environmental influences cannot explain the decline in regenerative ability in postembryonic mammals. Adult CNS neurons are notoriously difficult to grow in culture on the same substrates that support extensive survival and neurite outgrowth in embryonic neurons. The retinotectal and entorhinal-hippocampal coculture experiments described previously also indicate the importance of intraneuronal factors in limiting regeneration in the mature CNS. Perhaps the most convincing evidence for this concept is the great heterogeneity in intrinsic regenerative ability of neurons in the same animal. After spinal cord transection in the lamprey, identified reticulospinal neurons vary greatly in their ability to regenerate through the same spinal cord environment.[216-218] Moreover, the same axons regenerated better after spinal cord lesioning close to the perikaryon than more distally.[216] Similar results were obtained by Richardson and colleagues,[144] who found that axons belonging to supraspinal projecting neurons in the brain did not regenerate well into peripheral nerve grafts inserted into the spinal cord far from their cell bodies (i.e., at thoracic or lumbar as opposed to cervical levels).[219] Thus, neuron intrinsic factors must contribute greatly to the limitations on regeneration in the CNS. This concept is implicitly recognized in therapeutic approaches aimed at enhancing the intrinsic regenerative abilities of neurons through the use of supplemental trophic factors (see the section Peripheral Nerve Bridges).[143,220-230] In the next few sections, several examples of neuron intrinsic influences on regeneration are reviewed.

Conditioning Lesion Effects

Studies over many years have established that a preceding, or conditioning, lesion can enhance regeneration after a second, or test, lesion.[231] Although changes in the environment at the injury site may contribute, much of the effect has been attributed to changes in the growth properties of the injured neurons themselves. Experimental studies in the rat have taken advantage of special anatomic features of sensory ganglion neurons to show that enhancing an inherently poor regenerative response can increase intraspinal regeneration. DRG neurons have two asymmetric processes originating

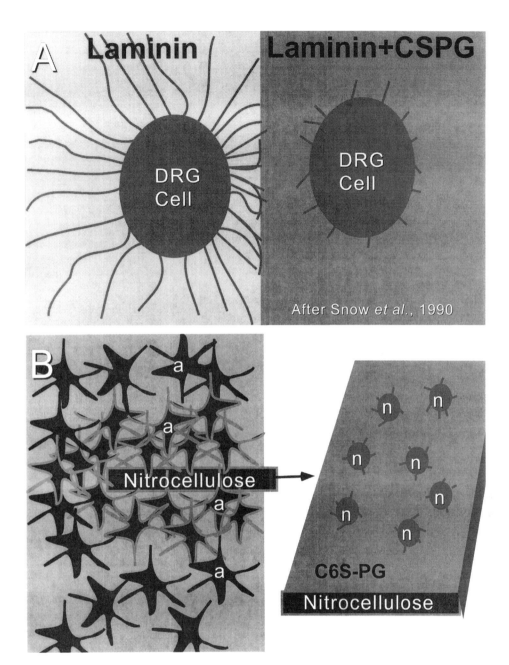

FIGURE 27-3 Astrocytes secrete axon growth inhibitors. Reactive glia in an injured central nervous system produce several molecules that may contribute to inhibition of axon regeneration, including chondroitin-6-sulfate proteoglycan (CSPG). **A.** Dorsal root ganglion (DRG) cells send out long neurites when grown on a substrate of laminin. However, the neurites will not cross onto a lane of substrate in which CSPG is added to the laminin. Neurons grown on the substrate containing CSPG do not send out long neurites. (Diagrammatic representation of work by DM Snow, V Lemmon, DA Carrino, AI Caplan, J Silver. Sulfated proteoglycans in astroglial barriers inhibit neurite outgrowth in vitro. Exp Neurol 1990;109:111–130.) **B.** Astrocytes (a) surrounding an injury to the brain produced by insertion of a nitrocellulose filter become *reactive*. In addition to proliferating and up-regulating glial fibrillary acidic protein, they appear to secrete CSPG. When the nitrocellulose filter is removed, it is coated with cellular elements from brain and with CSPG. Neurons (n) cultured on these nitrocellulose filters do not send out long neurites, as they would if they were grown on a permissive substrate such as laminin. (Diagrammatic representation of work by RJ McKeon, RC Schreiber, JS Rudge, J Silver. Reduction of neurite outgrowth in a model of glial scarring following CNS injury is correlated with the expression of inhibitory molecules on reactive astrocytes. J Neurosci 1991;11:3398–3411.)

from a unipolar axon. Normal maintenance and regeneration of these processes depend on proteins synthesized in perikarya within the sensory ganglia and transported down the axons by fast and slow axonal transport. Injury of the peripheral process within the sciatic nerve initiates a robust metabolic response that leads to regeneration. The growth-related response to injury of the central process is less vigorous[232-234] and, although the axons regenerate within the dorsal root, they fail to penetrate the astrocytic barrier at the dorsal root entry zone and do not regenerate into the spinal cord.[235-237] The central processes that ascend within the dorsal columns also fail to regenerate after spinal cord injury. Several studies have demonstrated that regeneration of the central processes can be enhanced by a peripheral nerve injury that boosts the growth-associated metabolic response within the neuronal perikarya. For example, Richardson and his colleagues found that a conditioning sciatic nerve transection increased by more than 100-fold the number of lumbar DRG neurons whose axons regenerated into a peripheral nerve graft placed in the dorsal columns at the cervical level.[238] Subsequent studies have shown that transecting the sciatic nerve 1–2 weeks before cutting the dorsal columns at the midthoracic level can stimulate sensory axons to grow into the gray matter at the lesion site and up to 4 mm beyond the rostral end of the injury.[239] Concomitant sciatic nerve crush has also allowed limited intraspinal regeneration of cut dorsal roots that had entered the spinal cord by growing along blood vessels.[240] Among the metabolic changes that could enhance regenerative capacity are increased synthesis of growth-associated genes and decreased synthesis of receptors that respond to inhibitory cues within the spinal cord.[240]

Growth-Associated Protein of 43 kD

Growth-associated protein of 43 kD (GAP-43) was discovered in 1981 by Skene and Willard as one of three proteins whose levels increased in the toad retina during regeneration of optic nerve.[241] In the intervening years, GAP-43 has been shown to be transported to the growth cone, where it is preferentially concentrated during development and synaptic remodeling.[242] The function of GAP-43 is still not known, but its molecular structure, biochemical activity, and immunohistochemical localization suggest that its amino end is inserted into the growth cone membrane,[243-245] where it is phosphorylated by protein kinase C,[246] binds calmodulin,[247] and activates a G protein.[248] All of these activities are correlated with axonal development, sprouting, regeneration, or synaptic plasticity in various in vitro and in vivo models.[248,249] The resulting view is that GAP-43 may act in a unique fashion to mediate signal transduction for the reorganization of the cytoskeleton in growth cones and synaptic terminals in response to extrinsic stimuli that activate axon growth and synaptic plasticity, such as LTP.[250-253] In neuroblastoma cells, introduction of anti–GAP-43 antibodies also interfered with the rapid early onset of neurite outgrowth.[254] Similarly, suppressing GAP-43 expression in cultured embryonic DRG cells with antisense oligonucleotides inhibited growth cone formation. However, it did not prevent the cells from extending neurites.[255] In transgenic mice, overexpression of GAP-43 leads to the spontaneous formation of new synapses and enhanced sprouting, spontaneously and after injury.[256,257] Because the null mutation of GAP-43 is lethal shortly after birth,[258,259] evidence for the role of GAP-43 in regeneration in vivo is still correlative.[225,260-262] In fact, when GAP-43 was overexpressed in Purkinje's cells in vivo, they showed increased sprouting from axons proximally and from cut axon tips, but no increase in their ability to regenerate either spontaneously or into embryonic neural or Schwann's cell grafts, which are generally growth permissive for other types of axons.[263] Thus, there may be a distinction between the role played by GAP-43 in short-distance axon sprouting and synaptic remodeling and its role, if any, in long-distance regeneration.

Cytoskeletal Proteins

Neurons contain three major cytoskeletal elements:

1. Microtubules, molecularly complex structures that mediate axonal transport of molecules and organelles, whose major structural protein constituents are the tubulins
2. Microfilaments, F-actin strands composed of polymers of G-actin
3. Intermediate filaments, heteropolymers of three neurofilament subunits of different molecular weight, NF-L, NF-M, and NF-H

Transection of axons in peripheral nerve results in decreased synthesis of neurofilament and increased synthesis of actin and tubulin.[264] These changes reverse after the nerve has regenerated to its target,[232,265,266] but do not reverse if regeneration is prevented.[265] In addition, the rates of regeneration of the central and peripheral axons of DRG cells correlated more closely with the transport rates of tubulin than neurofilaments.[267] These and other observations have led to the view that regeneration of peripheral nerve depends on the transport and assembly of actin and microtubules, but not neurofilaments, which participate in the subsequent morphologic maturation and enlargement of the regenerated fibers. Some caution must be taken in interpreting these results. The changes in expression of the various cytoskeletal proteins during regeneration have led to the commonly accepted assumption that regeneration in peripheral nerve involves the same growth cone mechanisms as in development (i.e., elongation of filopodia along an adhesive substrate and pulling of the axon forward by an actin-myosin molecular motor that links the filopodial adhesion sites distally to the microtubule system proximally). This assumption may be reasonable, given the presence of extracellular adhesive molecules in the mature peripheral nerve and the expression of receptors for those adhesion molecules in the regenerating neurons.[268] However, there have been few observations on the structure of regenerating growth cones in peripheral nerve. In fact, immunohistochemical observations have suggested that, after a distal crush lesion, neurofilaments enter the regenerating sprouts several days ahead of microtubules.[269] Moreover, although neurofilament mRNA is down-regulated during regeneration, mRNA levels and immunoreactivity for another intermediate filament, peripherin, are actually increased.[270,271] Because peripherin can both self-assemble and coassemble with NF-L to form intermediate filaments,[272] it is possible that intermediate filaments with an altered subunit composition are important to the mechanism of peripheral nerve regeneration. Caution is even more warranted in assuming that regenerating axons in the CNS use the actin-based filopodial mechanism of elongation, because the CNS lacks extracellular matrix molecules, such as laminin, fibronectin, and collagen that serve as substrates for axon growth in embryonic development, dissociated cell cultures, and peripheral nerve regeneration. Although some cell surface adhesion molecules may be re-expressed after injury to the CNS (e.g., L1), others are not (e.g., neural cell adhesion molecule [NCAM]),[273] and it is not clear that there would be a sufficient basis for adhesive interactions in the regenerating mature spinal cord to support the mechanism of growth cone elongation that is hypothesized for the elongation of axons in the embryo. The most compelling case against the applicability of developmental growth cone mechanisms to regeneration in the CNS derives from work in the lamprey. Observations made in other model systems are consistent with those in lamprey.

Transection of the lamprey spinal cord is followed by functional recovery[153,274] and regeneration of approxi-

mately one-half of the cut axons across the injury site.[155,216] Unlike growth cones of embryonic neurons, the growth cones of lamprey axons regenerating in situ are simple in shape, lacking lamellipodia and filopodia (Figure 27-4). Moreover, although the growth cones of embryonic neurons in tissue culture have abundant F-actin and lack neurofilaments, growth cones of regenerating axons in the lamprey CNS contain abundant neurofilaments, which are packed more densely than in the proximal axon,[275] and have little F-actin.[276] This has suggested the hypothesis that regeneration involves a protrusive force generated by the transport of cytoskeletal elements such as neurofilaments into the growing tip.[218,275] This hypothesis received additional support from observations on the expression of the single lamprey neurofilament subunit NF-180 after spinal cord transection. Lamprey reticulospinal neurons whose axons regenerate well showed only a transient down-regulation of neurofilament mRNA expression, whereas neurons that regenerate poorly showed a permanent down-regulation.[218] This difference was not a consequence of regeneration because blocking regeneration mechanically did not alter the pattern of neurofilament expression. Thus, the ability to re-express neurofilament after a transient down-regulation may be part of an intrinsic program that distinguishes good regenerating from bad regenerating neurons.

Growth cones lacking filopodia and lamellipodia have also been observed in other models of axonal regeneration in the CNS, although the molecular composition of these growth cones has not been studied extensively. Thus far, only two cytoskeletal proteins have been identified as major components—tubulin and neurofilament—and few reports have combined morphologic descriptions of growth cones with identification of their molecular constituents. In goldfish, transection of the optic tract is followed by early development of a bulbous tip.[277] Between 2 hours to 2 days after injury, the bulbous swellings contained bundles of neurofilaments but not microtubules and lacked filopodia and lamellipodia. By 3–4 days, the newly formed sprouts contained both neurofilament bundles and microtubules. Subsequent studies by Schechter and his colleagues suggested that neurofilament protein expression was greatly up-regulated during the course of regeneration, returning to normal by 35 days postcrush.[278] Thus, unlike the situation in peripheral nerve, an early up-regulation of neurofilament mRNA and protein synthesis occurs during regeneration in the goldfish optic nerve. In a more recent study, some growth cones had filopodia, although the precise locations of these are not clear. The majority of examples illustrated had simple profiles, and their cytoskeletal contents were not described.[279] Similarly, in the frog, regenerating optic nerve fibers displayed

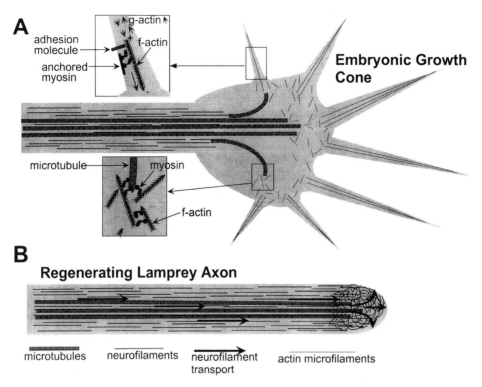

FIGURE 27-4 Role of the neuronal cytoskeleton in axon regeneration. The shape and cytoskeletal contents of growth cones of regenerating axons in the lamprey spinal cord suggest that the mechanism of axon elongation during regeneration is different from that during embryonic development. **A.** Scheme of the embryonic growth cone simplified from the model of Forscher and colleagues.[168] Filopodial elongation is achieved by addition of G-actin subunits to the distal end of F-actin microfilaments. Filopodial position is stabilized by linkage between actin microfilaments and the extracellular matrix via transmembrane adhesion molecules. A myosin molecular motor exerts a retrograde force on the actin microfilaments and links the microfilamentous network to the microtubules in the central region of the lamellipodium. When the actin filaments are stabilized distally, the force generated by actin-myosin interaction applies traction to the microtubular network, pulling the microtubules in the direction of the stabilized filopodia, thereby pulling the axon forward. **B.** Hypothesis for the role of neurofilaments in the mechanism of regeneration of reticulospinal axons in the lamprey. Neurofilaments are transported along microtubules into the growth cone. The pressure generated by this process might result in an increase in the packing density of neurofilaments and a protrusive force that contributes to axon elongation. (Reprinted with permission from A Conti, ME Selzer. The Role of Cytoskeleton in Regeneration of Central Nervous System Axons. In NR Saunders, KM Dziegielewska [eds]. Degeneration and Regeneration in the Nervous System. Amsterdam: Harwood Academic Publishers, 2000;153–169.)

bulbous tips and other simplified tip morphologies without filopodia throughout their course of growth in the optic nerve, chiasm, and tract. Only in the pretectal neuropil and optic tectum were flattened, foliate growth cones similar to those commonly described in vitro observed.[280] The cytoskeletal contents of these growth cones were not described, and it is not clear that any of them had filopodia or actin microfilaments.

In adult rat, as in all mammals, the optic nerve does not ordinarily regenerate, and axotomized retinal ganglion cells undergo different changes in mRNA levels for cytoskeletal proteins than they do in the retinal ganglion cells of fish or in neurons contributing to peripheral

nerves. McKerracher and colleagues found that after optic nerve section, β-tubulin mRNA increased by 140% 1 day after injury,[281] presumably because retinal ganglion cells up-regulated β-tubulin expression. These levels dropped to 70% of control values by 1 week, which probably represents down-regulation of β-tubulin in retinal ganglion cells, since it is unlikely that these cells had died so soon. NF-M mRNA levels decreased to 80% of controls and remained suppressed for at least 6 months. These new levels probably represent the death of most retinal ganglion cells and cannot be interpreted as indicating anything about the physiology of any one neuron type. Twenty to 40% of the retinal ganglion cells are rescued from death when a length of peripheral nerve is grafted to the proximal stump of the severed optic nerve. Of these surviving cells, approximately 20% regenerate an axon into the graft.[146] In this circumstance, the axotomized retinal ganglion cells showed a 50% decrease in NF-M mRNA shortly after injury.[282] In retinal ganglion cells that did not regenerate, β-tubulin mRNA levels decreased to an average of 63% of controls, but in some of the cells whose axons regenerated into the peripheral nerve graft β-tubulin mRNA levels were nearly 300% above control levels. By contrast with mRNA levels, transport rates for both tubulin and neurofilament in the regenerating axons doubled, whereas that for actin decreased to nearly one-third of its normal rate during the period of regeneration.[283] This might suggest that microtubules and neurofilaments are important for the mechanism of regeneration, while actin is not, but clearly this too is overly simplistic.

The interpretation of all these findings is difficult. In the case of structural proteins that turn over slowly, such as neurofilaments, absolute mRNA levels and protein synthesis rates may not be as significant for function as their disposition in the neuron and their rates of transport down the axon. For example, in lamprey reticulospinal neurons axotomized near the brain, 90% of the axoplasm is removed and thus the volume into which neurofilaments must be distributed is only 10% of normal. Under these circumstances, an 80% reduction in neurofilament mRNA and protein synthesis would represent a twofold increase in the volume-specific synthesis of neurofilaments, and this could easily be compatible with the hypothesis of a protrusive force generated by transport of neurofilaments into the axon tip contributing to regeneration. That good regenerating neurons re-express neurofilaments, whereas bad regenerating ones do not, may be more significant than that neurofilament mRNA expression is initially reduced in both. Thus far, it has not been possible to test the effect on regeneration of selectively manipulating the expression or transport of neurofilaments. Thus, as with GAP-43, evidence for the neurofilament hypothesis of regeneration is correlative.

STRATEGIES TO PROMOTE REGENERATION

Reroute Axons (Peripheral Nerve and Artificial Bridges)

Peripheral Nerve Bridges

The discovery of specific molecular mechanisms by which regeneration is inhibited has suggested interventions that may promote regeneration, and some of these are discussed. However, most therapeutic approaches have targeted the inhibitory nature of the mature CNS extracellular environment in a more general way. Aguayo and colleagues have used the ability of CNS axons to regenerate in peripheral nerve grafts to reconnect transected optic nerve to the superior colliculus.[214,284] A few axons reach the tectum and form synapses that mediate electrical responses to illumination of the retina.[285] The nerve grafts appear to supply two important components to the axotomized neurons. First, they provide a substrate permissive for growth, at least in part because Schwann's cells produce extracellular matrix molecules such as laminin. Second, they release trophic factors necessary for the survival of the injured neurons, especially brain-derived neurotrophic factor (BDNF) and neurotrophin 4/5 (NT-4/5).[286–288] Similar nerve grafts were reported to mediate light-dark discrimination in hamsters.[289] Such techniques have potential for enhancing recovery in cases of complete or near complete interruption of long white matter tracts, as in spinal cord injury (Figure 27-5).[144] When grafted into spinal cord, however, peripheral nerve grafts attract axons primarily from neurons situated close to the grafts,[219] and supraspinal neurons necessary for recovery are not among them. Supplementing Schwann's cell grafts with methylprednisolone[290] or with BDNF and NT-3[222] recruits brain stem axons into the grafts, but penetration into host spinal cord, as into the tectum, is limited.

Neutralize Inhibitory Factors

Antibodies to Growth Cone-Inhibiting Molecules

Schnell and Schwab[291] tested the ability of antibodies directed at oligodendrocyte-associated growth cone-collapsing factors to promote regeneration.[291] IN-1–secreting hybridomas were transplanted into the parietal lobes of rats, which were then subjected to spinal cord dorsal hemisection (Figure 27-6). This interrupts both corticospinal tracts, which in rats course in the base of the dorsal columns. Regeneration of corticospinal axons was demonstrated by injecting horseradish peroxidase into the cortex and following its anterograde transport into the growing terminals. In rats with the test hybridomas, corticospinal tract fibers grew up to 15 mm around and beyond the hemisection. Regeneration in control rats did not exceed 1 mm. The antibodies presumably enhanced the growth of axons within white matter, because there is no indication that axons were able to grow through the hemisection scar, and these same antibodies neutralize the growth-inhibiting effect of oligodendrocytes in vitro. It has also been reported that the antibody enhanced regeneration results in behavioral improvement, including the return of contact placing reflexes in the hindlimbs and normalization of stride length.[292] However, only approxi-

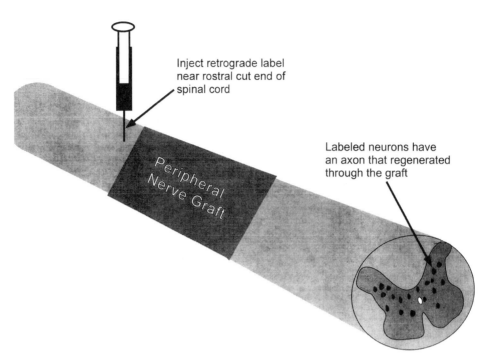

Inject retrograde label
near rostral cut end of
spinal cord

Peripheral
Nerve Graft

Labeled neurons have
an axon that regenerated
through the graft

FIGURE 27-5 Spinal cord axons regenerate into grafts of peripheral nerve. When a piece of peripheral nerve is grafted between two cut ends of the spinal cord, axons of nearby neurons in the caudal stump regenerate into the graft and some grow either very close to the end of the graft or even into the rostral stump. This was demonstrated by injecting the tracer horseradish peroxidase into the rostral stump just rostral to the graft. The horseradish peroxidase is picked up by regenerating axons and transported retrogradely to their neurons of origin, which are identified by a histochemical reaction for horseradish peroxidase. (Diagrammatic representation of work by PM Richardson, UM McGuinness, AJ Aguayo. Axons from CNS neurons regenerate into PNS grafts. Nature 1980;284:264–265.)

mately 10% of corticospinal axons regenerate, probably caused by the limited penetration of the antibody and to the presence of additional inhibitory molecules associated with myelin. Huang and colleagues have immunized mice against several myelin-associated growth inhibitors and demonstrated regeneration of corticospinal axons and recovery of hindlimb motor functions after spinal cord dorsal hemisection.[293] It is possible that similar techniques could be used to overcome additional growth-inhibitory molecules, such as proteoglycans that are associated with reactive astrocytes at the injury site, and other growth-inhibitory molecules that remain to be identified, and that this could enhance growth through a scar.

Enhance Neuronal Survival and Regenerative Capacity

The functional deficits that follow spinal cord injury are largely caused by the death of axotomized neurons and the failure of surviving neurons to regenerate. Although the importance of regeneration for recovery is obvious, increasing the survival of axotomized neu-

rons might also enhance recovery even if the axons of the rescued neurons failed to regenerate. For example, surviving neurons might contribute axons to functionally important circuits that would be interrupted if the neurons died. If the axons of surviving neurons underwent lesion-induced local sprouting (reactive synaptogenesis; see Collateral Sprouting, earlier in this chapter), the contribution of these neurons to residual circuitry and therefore to recovery might even be increased. Neuron survival is also a prerequisite for strategies that are designed to promote regeneration, particularly if these treatments must be delayed after injury. This is likely to be the case if transplants are used to treat patients with spinal cord injury. To avoid worsening the outcome of an evolving injury, the patients who are most likely to receive transplants, at least initially, are those with chronic injuries and stable deficits in whom the natural processes of recovery have reached a plateau.

Earlier in this chapter we discussed treatments that have been used to maintain axotomized neurons after experimental spinal cord injury and emphasized the rescue affected by the exogenous administration of neurotrophic factors. Neurotrophic factors have also been reported to elicit axon outgrowth when delivered to cut intraspinal axons. For example, injection of NT-3 into the site of a dorsal spinal cord hemisection stimulated local sprouting of corticospinal axons, which are located in the dorsal portion of the rodent spinal cord[220]; and nerve growth factor (NGF) infusion into the cut dorsal columns induced dorsal root axons to regenerate 2–3 mm through host white matter.[294] Growth factors have also increased regeneration when applied in combination with different types of intraspinal transplants. For example, both BDNF and NT-3 support the growth of brain stem axons into Schwann's cell grafts placed into the completely transected thoracic spinal cord of adult rats, although supraspinal axons fail to grow into these grafts in the absence of supplemental neurotrophic factors.[222] BDNF, NT-3, and NT-4/5 also increase supraspinal axon growth into fetal spinal cord transplants placed into a unilateral hemisection cavity in adult rats.[143] Important because of its potential clinical applications, exogenously administered growth factors also promote regeneration of brain stem axons into peripheral nerve grafts when they are applied in models of chronic injury.[226] The promotion of process outgrowth by neurotrophic factors is consistent with the classical idea of Cajal[295] that regenerative failure in the CNS is at least partly caused by the low levels of growth-promoting factors normally found there.[295] Exogenous neurotrophic factors, therefore, could make the environment more conducive to growth and exert a chemoattractant effect on regenerating axons.

In most experimental paradigms, the ability of a trophic factor to encourage axons to grow into a certain environment could be caused by a nontropic mechanism. For example, the trophic factor could be transported retrogradely to the nucleus, thereby rescuing the neuron from cell death and activating a more vigorous sprouting effort. Neurons whose axons had not regenerated into the area of trophic support would be less likely to survive or to sprout neurites, and in this way the appearance of directed axon outgrowth could be produced. However, it is clear that neurotrophins also act directly on the growth cone to direct its elongation in a manner similar to that of other guidance molecules.[296] In this action, the binding of a neurotrophin to its specific receptor[297] activates one or more second messenger systems[298,299] that cause axonal elongation in the direction of the source of the neurotrophin. Experimental evidence suggests that neurotrophic factors may also act by a cAMP-dependent mechanism to enhance axonal

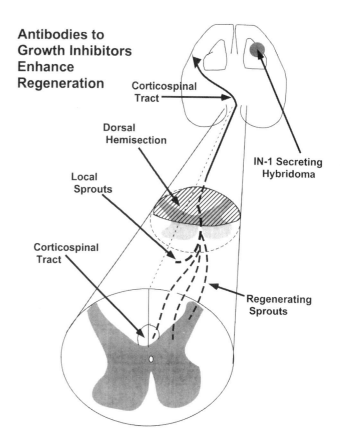

FIGURE 27-6 Enhancement of regeneration by use of antibodies to myelin-associated growth inhibitors. Hybridomas secreting the monoclonal antibody IN-1 were implanted into the brains of rats and their corticospinal tracts were interrupted in the thoracic spinal cord by a dorsal hemisection. The terminals of regenerating corticospinal tracts were located by injection of an anterograde tracer into the cortex. In animals that received a control hybridoma, which did not make IN-1, injured corticospinal axons grew no more than 0.5 mm around the injury scar. However, in animals implanted with the IN-1–secreting hybridoma, some corticospinal axons regenerated more than 10 mm beyond the lesion. (Diagrammatic representation of work by L Schnell, ME Schwab. Axonal regeneration in the rat spinal cord produced by an antibody against myelin-associated neurite growth inhibitors. Nature 1990;343:269–272.)

regeneration of neurons in vitro by blocking the inhibitory effects of myelin-associated glycoprotein and myelin in general.[300] Studies have also shown that DRG neurons exposed to NGF in vitro increase their production of a metalloproteinase that inactivates the growth-inhibiting activity of chondroitin sulfate proteoglycans that are present in the glial scar.[301] Thus, it is possible that part of the mechanism by which NGF promotes axon regeneration is by enabling the neuron to overcome the inhibitory effect of chondroitin sulfate pro-teoglycans in the extracellular environment.

Fetal Transplants

Transplants of fetal spinal cord have been discussed at a symposium designed to plan for their clinical applica-

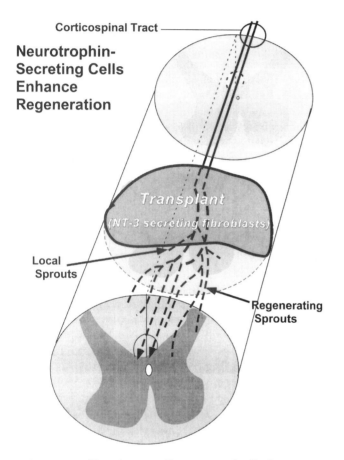

Corticospinal Tract

Neurotrophin-Secreting Cells Enhance Regeneration

Transplant (NT-3 secreting fibroblasts)

Local Sprouts

Regenerating Sprouts

FIGURE 27-7 Use of genetically engineered cells that secrete neurotrophic factors to enhance regeneration of axons in injured spinal cord. The corticospinal tracts were lesioned by a dorsal hemisection and fibroblasts genetically engineered to make the neurotrophin NT-3 were transplanted into the lesion. In animals transplanted with control fibroblasts, corticospinal tract axons did not regenerate around the lesion. However, in animals receiving the genetically engineered NT-3–secreting fibroblasts, corticospinal axons regenerated for several millimeters, and animals showed some evidence of functional recovery. (Diagrammatic representation of work by R Grill, K Murai, A Blesch, et al. Cellular delivery of neurotrophin-3 promotes corticospinal axonal growth and partial functional recovery after spinal cord injury. J Neurosci 1997;17:5560–5572.)

tion,[302] and at least one report of their use to obliterate a posttraumatic cyst has appeared.[303] These transplants may act through several different mechanisms to contribute to functional recovery. For example, they have been reported to reduce both retrograde death of axotomized neurons[41,52,53] and the amount of glial scarring that occurs at the site of a spinal cord injury.[304] In addition, in newborn animals the axons of corticospinal and bulbospinal neurons regenerate through fetal spinal cord transplants and into caudal host spinal cord, where they enhance the development of locomotion and other motor functions.[142,305-308] In adult hosts regeneration of CNS axons derives almost exclusively from neurons close to the transplants, and these axons do not extend into host spinal cord.[309] Exogenous administration of neurotrophic factors, however, increases growth of supraspinal axons into the transplant.[143] In these respects fetal transplants resemble peripheral nerve grafts. Supplementation of fetal spinal cord transplants with neurotrophic factors or with antibodies against myelin inhibitory proteins increases sprouting adjacent to the transplants and long-distance regeneration, which has been associated with recovery of hindlimb locomotor function.[227]

Cell Replacement

Stem Cells and Genetically Engineered Cells

Transplants of fetal spinal cord have elicited only limited regeneration and recovery after experimental spinal cord injury in adult hosts, and their use in humans will inevitably be lumbered with logistical, political, and ethical problems. The available evidence suggests that alternative types of cells, particularly those that are genetically modified to produce growth-promoting molecules, will prove to be both more practical and more efficacious. Cells engineered to express neurotrophic factors have received the most attention (Figure 27-7). For example, fibroblasts that have been engineered to synthesize NT-3 and transplanted into adult rat spinal cord damaged by unilateral hemisection, rescued axotomized Clarke's nucleus neurons as efficiently as transplants of fetal CNS tissues.[310] Schwann's cells engineered to express BDNF promoted supraspinal axon regeneration across a complete spinal cord transection site,[311] and fibroblasts genetically modified to express BDNF or NT-3 increased axon growth and myelination when transplanted into a contusion injury.[228] Several instances have also been reported in which intraspinal transplants of engineered cells supported recovery of locomotor function. Transplants of fibroblasts engineered to express NT-3[312] or leukemia inhibitory factor[313] promoted regeneration of corticospinal axons, and those that expressed NT-3 also supported recovery on a grid-walking task. When transplanted into a cervical lateral fasciculus lesion in adult rats, fibroblasts expressing BDNF appeared both to enhance the regenerative capacity of axotomized red nucleus neurons and to provide a substrate permissive for regeneration of their axons.[230] Rubrospinal axons grew across and around the transplants and continued through caudal host white matter before terminating in regions of gray matter that are the normal targets of rubrospinal axons. The environment provided by the graft contributed to recovery of forelimb and hindlimb motor function as determined by quantitative assays of locomotor performance.

Neural stem cells and progenitor cells have characteristics that make them especially attractive for use as transplants. Stem cells may be defined by their capacity for self-renewal and their ability to generate neurons, astrocytes, and oligodendrocytes. Progenitor cells have a more restricted capacity for differentiation than stem cells.[314] These immature cells have been isolated from the brain and spinal cord of adult as well as developing animals,[315] including humans,[316] and they can be proliferated in an undifferentiated state for long periods of time in culture. In principle, it may, therefore, be possible to obtain adequate numbers of cells for transplantation from an adult patient with a spinal cord injury. Like Schwann's cells and fibroblasts, progenitor cells can be genetically modified to deliver neurotrophic factors and may provide a favorable substrate for regeneration. In addition, stem cells and progenitor cells may be able to generate neurons to replace those lost to trauma and to furnish oligodendrocytes and Schwann's cells that can remyelinate surviving and regenerating axons. Several types of stem cells, including ones isolated from the embryonic human forebrain,[317] have been observed to integrate neatly into the mature, uninjured rat brain and to respond to local cues by adopting the phenotype of neurons present in the area in which they have been grafted.[318–320] Only limited information is available about the effects of transplanting stem cells into injured spinal cord. Progenitor cells isolated from the postnatal rat brain and transplanted into an experimentally demyelinated region of adult rat spinal cord have been reported to differentiate into oligodendrocytes and Schwann's cells that remyelinated denuded axons.[321] Stem-like cells originally isolated from newborn mouse cerebellum and genetically modified to express NT-3 have also been observed to maintain axotomized Clarke's nucleus neurons that otherwise would have been lost after spinal cord hemisection. A great

deal remains to be learned about the normal development of neural cell lineages and about strategies for directing the differentiation of stem cells to optimize their use as transplants, but the response of the normal and injured brain to stem cell grafts encourages hope that these cells will one day make an important contribution to spinal cord repair.[322,323]

Ensheathing Glia

Adult olfactory bulb ensheathing glia have been reported to promote regeneration of brain stem serotonergic axons when added to guidance channels filled with Schwann's cells[324] and of corticospinal axons when placed into a partial cervical spinal cord injury.[324] Rats whose grafts formed continuous bridges across a small electrolytic lesion demonstrated recovery of forelimb reaching.[325] These promising cells are just beginning to be used as intraspinal transplants, and the molecular basis for their support of axon growth has not been described.

Combination Approaches

It is clear from the previously mentioned considerations that multiple regeneration-inhibiting factors are expressed in the mature CNS and that multiple growth-promoting features present in the embryonic intraneuronal and extracellular environment decline with age. It is, therefore, unlikely that any individual treatment will restore function completely. Instead, optimal recovery will require a combination of therapeutic approaches. For example, Schnell and Schwab modified their experiments in animals with dorsal overhemisections and IN-1–secreting hybridomas, inserting fetal spinal cord tissue into the lesion.[326] Although the distances that corticospinal tract axons regenerated were similar to those seen with antibody treatment alone, there was an increase in the number of axon sprouts emanating from the lesioned corticospinal tracts. Of interest, axons grew around the fetal spinal cord transplants and not through them. Thus, the enhancement of neuritic sprouting was attributed to soluble factors released from the transplants. Fetal spinal cord transplants contain several trophic factors, such as BDNF and NT-3. When Schwab's group substituted local injections of NGF, BDNF, or NT-3 for the fetal transplants, they found that NT-3 had the same effect on sprouting of corticospinal tract axons as the embryonic spinal cord transplants, but the other trophic factors did not.[220] A striking example of combination therapy was reported by Olson's group in Sweden.[327] They used multiple peripheral nerve grafts to bridge a gap of 5 mm of spinal cord produced in rats by excision of the T-8 segment. The grafts routed white matter tracts to spinal cord gray matter to avoid contact with myelin-associated growth-inhibiting molecules. The cut ends of the cord were sealed together with fibrin glue mixed with acidic fibroblast growth factor. This factor was selected because it had previously been shown to support the survival of spinal cord neurons in vitro. The apposition of the cut ends of cord was reinforced further by compressive wiring of the dorsal spines in dorsiflexion. Animals were then allowed to recover for 6 months. With this combination of treatments, anterograde tracing demonstrated evidence for anatomic regeneration of ascending and descending pathways. Improvement in open-field walking scores and in more elaborate measures of gait coordination were also seen.[328] Although much work remains to determine the mechanisms underlying the functional improvement and the observations of Olson's group have yet to be replicated, these and other more recent results suggest that combinations of surgical manipulations, trophic factors, and growth inhibitor neutralization measures may provide better results than any single experimental approach.

CONCLUSIONS

Several biological processes participate in the spontaneous partial recovery that often occurs after spinal cord injury. These processes include resolution of edema and related metabolic abnormalities, several forms of synaptic plasticity, denervation supersensitivity, collateral sprouting, and dendritic pruning. We have made significant progress in understanding the molecular mechanisms that underlie these phenomena, and it is likely that ways will be found to manipulate them so as to enhance recovery still more. However, complete recovery will require re-establishing interrupted neural connections. Significant progress has been made in developing methods to replace lost neurons and to overcome the extracellular environmental and intraneuronal factors that currently prevent axons from regenerating in the mature CNS. However, anatomic reconnection is not enough. It will be necessary to devise methods by which to convert regenerated anatomic connections to useful function. This will present rehabilitation professionals with exciting research and therapeutic opportunities.

Acknowledgments
The authors would like to acknowledge the following sources of research grant support: Michael Selzer, Department of Neurology, University of Pennsylvania Medical Center, NIH (NS14837, NS25581), NSF (IBN-9319702), and the University of Pennsylvania Research Foundation; Alan Tessler, Department of Veterans Affairs, NIH (NS24707), Eastern Paralyzed Veterans Association, and International Spinal Research Trust.

REFERENCES

1. Hughes JT. Pathology of the Spinal Cord. Philadelphia: Lippincott, 1966.
2. Kakulas BA, Taylor JR. Pathology of Injuries of the Vertebral Column and Spinal Cord. In H Frankel (ed), Spinal Cord Trauma. Amsterdam: Elsevier, 1992;21–51.
3. Himes BT, Tessler A. Neuroprotection from Cell Death Following Axotomy. In N Ingoglia, M Murray (eds), Nerve Regeneration. New York: Marcel Dekker, 2000;477–503.
4. Ditunno JFJ, Donovan W. International Standards for Neurological and Functional Classification of Spinal Cord Injury. Chicago: American Spinal Injury Association, 1992.
5. Kakulas A. The applied neurobiology of human spinal cord injury: a review. Paraplegia 1988;26:371–379.
6. Bunge RP, Puckett WR, Becerra JL, et al. Observations on the Pathology of Human Spinal Cord Injury. A Review and Classification of 22 New Cases with Details from a Case of Chronic Cord Compression with Extensive Demyelination. In FJ Seil (ed), Advances in Neurology. New York: Raven, 1993;75–89.
7. Ditunno JF Jr, Graziani V, Tessler A. Neurological assessment in spinal cord injury. Adv Neurol 1997;72:325–333.
8. Marino RJ, Ditunno JF Jr, Donovan WH, Maynard F Jr. Neurologic recovery after traumatic spinal cord injury: data from the Model Spinal Cord Injury Systems. Arch Phys Med Rehabil 1999;80:1391–1396.
9. Marino RJ, Crozier KS. Neurologic examination and functional assessment after spinal cord injury. Phys Med Rehabil Clin North Am 1992;3:829–852.
10. Bosch A, Stauffer ES, Nickel VL. Incomplete traumatic quadriplegia: a ten-year review. JAMA 1971;216:473–478.
11. Schneider RC, Cherry G, Pantek H. The syndrome of acute central cervical spinal cord injury. J Neurosurg 1954;11:546–577.
12. Levi AD, Tator CH, Bunge RP. Clinical syndromes associated with disproportionate weakness of the upper versus the lower extremities after cervical spinal cord injury. Neurosurgery 1996;38:179–183; discussion 183–185.
13. Penrod LE, Hegde SK, Ditunno JF Jr. Age effect on prognosis for functional recovery in acute, traumatic central cord syndrome. Arch Phys Med Rehabil 1990;71:963–968.
14. Ingebrigtsen T, Waterloo K, Marup-Jensen S, et al. Quantification of post-concussion symptoms 3 months after minor head injury in 100 consecutive patients. J Neurol 1998;245:609–612.
15. Povlishock JT, Christman CW. The pathobiology of traumatically induced axonal injury in animals and humans: a review of current thoughts. J Neurotrauma 1995;12:555–564.

16. Allen AR. Surgery of experimental lesion of spinal cord equivalent to crush injury of fracture dislocation. JAMA 1911;50:941–952.

17. Blight AR, Decrescito V. Morphometric analysis of experimental spinal cord injury in the cat: the relation of injury intensity to survival of myelinated axons. Neuroscience 1986;19:321–341.

18. Basso DM, Beattie MS, Bresnahan JC. A sensitive and reliable locomotor rating scale for open field testing in rats. J Neurotrauma 1995;12:1–21.

19. Basso DM, Beattie MS, Bresnahan JC. Graded histological and locomotor outcomes after spinal cord contusion using the NYU weight-drop device versus transection. Exp Neurol 1996;139:244–256.

20. Puchala E, Windle WF. The possibility of structural and functional restitution after spinal cord injury. A review. Exp Neurol 1977;55:1–42.

21. Eidelberg E, Straehley D, Erspamer R, Watkins CJ. Relationship between residual hindlimb-assisted locomotion and surviving axons after incomplete spinal cord injuries. Exp Neurol 1977;56:312–322.

22. Eidelberg E, Story JL, Walden JG, Meyer BL. Anatomical correlates of return of locomotor function after partial spinal cord lesions in cats. Exp Brain Res 1981;42:81–88.

23. Guth L, Albuquerque EX, Deshpande SS, et al. Ineffectiveness of enzyme therapy on regeneration in the transected spinal cord of the rat. J Neurosurg 1980;52:73–86.

24. Blight AR. Cellular morphology of chronic spinal cord injury in the cat: analysis of myelinated axons by line-sampling. Neuroscience 1983;10:521–543.

25. Dusart I, Schwab ME. Secondary cell death and the inflammatory reaction after dorsal hemisection of the rat spinal cord. Eur J Neurosci 1994;6:712–724.

26. Tator CH. Update on the pathophysiology and pathology of acute spinal cord injury. Brain Pathol 1995;5:407–413.

27. Lindholm D. Role of neurotrophins in preventing glutamate induced neuronal cell death. J Neurol 1994;242:S16–S18.

28. Schwab ME, Bartholdi D. Degeneration and regeneration of axons in the lesioned spinal cord. Physiol Rev 1996;76:319–370.

29. Sei Y, Fossom L, Goping G, et al. Quinolinic acid protects rat cerebellar granule cells from glutamate-induced apoptosis. Neurosci Lett 1998;241:180–184.

30. Stout AK, Raphael HM, Kanterewicz BI, et al. Glutamate-induced neuron death requires mitochondrial calcium uptake. Nat Neurosci 1998;1:366–373.

31. Wada S, Yone K, Ishidou Y, et al. Apoptosis following spinal cord injury in rats and preventative effect of N-methyl-D-aspartate receptor antagonist. J Neurosurg 1999;91(Suppl 1):98–104.

32. Anderson DK, Braughler JM, Hall ED, et al. Effects of treatment with U-74006F on neurological outcome following experimental spinal cord injury. J Neurosurg 1988;69:562–567.

33. Short DJ, El Masry WS, Jones PW. High-dose methylprednisolone in the management of acute spinal cord injury. A systematic review from a distinct clinical perspective. Spinal Cord 2000;38:223–286.

34. Tator CH, Koyanagi I. Vascular mechanisms in the pathophysiology of human spinal cord injury. J Neurosurg 1997;86:483–492.

35. Imperato-Kalmar EL, McKinney RA, Schnell L, et al. Local changes in vascular architecture following partial spinal cord lesion in the rat. Exp Neurol 1997;145:322–328.

36. Wyllie AH, Kerr JF, Currie AR. Cell death: the significance of apoptosis. Int Rev Cytol 1980;68:251–306.

37. Martin LJ, Al-Abdulla NA, Brambrink AM, et al. Neurodegeneration in excitotoxicity, global cerebral ischemia, and target deprivation: a perspective on the contributions of apoptosis and necrosis. Brain Res Bull 1998;46:281–309.

38. Mori F, Himes BT, Kowada M, et al. Fetal spinal cord transplants rescue some axotomized rubrospinal neurons from retrograde cell death in adult rats. Exp Neurol 1997;143:45–60.

39. Fukuoka T, Miki K, Yoshiya I, Noguchi K. Expression of beta-calcitonin gene-related peptide in axotomized rubrospinal neurons and the effect of brain derived neurotrophic factor. Brain Res 1997;767:250–258.

40. Houle JD, Ye JH. Survival of chronically-injured neurons can be prolonged by treatment with neurotrophic factors. Neuroscience 1999;94:929–936.

41. Himes BT, Goldberger ME, Tessler A. Grafts of fetal central-nervous-system tissue rescue axotomized Clarke nucleus neurons in adult and neonatal operates. J Comp Neurol 1994;339:117–131.

42. Bradbury EJ, King VR, Simmons LJ, et al. NT-3, but not BDNF, prevents atrophy and death of axotomized spinal cord projection neurons. Eur J Neurosci 1998;10:3058–3068.

43. Fischer I, Liu Y. Gene Therapy Strategies in CNS Axon Regeneration. In N Ingoglia, M Murray (eds), Nerve Regeneration. New York: Marcel Dekker, 2000 (in press).

44. Raff MC, Barres BA, Burne JF, et al. Programmed cell death and the control of cell survival: lessons from the nervous system. Science 1993;262:695–700.

45. Adams JM, Cory S. The Bcl-2 protein family: arbiters of cell survival. Science 1998;281:1322–1326.

46. Kinloch RA, Treherne JM, Furness LM, Hajimohamadreza I. The pharmacology of apoptosis. Trends Pharmacol Sci 1999;20:35–42.

47. Green DR. Apoptotic pathways: the roads to ruin. Cell 1998;94:695–698.

48. Thornberry NA, Lazebnik Y. Caspases: enemies within. Science 1998;281:1312–1316.

49. Kermer P, Klocker N, Labes M, Bahr M. Inhibition of CPP32-like proteases rescues axotomized retinal ganglion cells from secondary cell death in vivo. J Neurosci 1998;18:4656–4662.

50. Holtzman DM, Deshmukh M. Caspases: a treatment target for neurodegenerative disease? Nat Med 1997;3:954–955.

51. Takahashi K, Schwarz E, Ljubetic C, et al. DNA plasmid that codes for human Bcl-2 gene preserves axotomized Clarke's nucleus neurons and reduces atrophy after spinal cord hemisection in adult rats. J Comp Neurol 1999;404:159–171.

52. Shibayama M, Hattori S, Himes BT, et al. Neurotrophin-3 prevents death of axotomized Clarke's nucleus neurons in adult rat. J Comp Neurol 1998a;390:102–111.

53. Shibayama M, Matsui N, Himes BT, et al. Critical interval for rescue of axotomized neurons by transplants. Neuroreport 1998b;9:11–14.

54. Chaudhary P, Ahmed F, Quebada P, Sharma SC. Caspase inhibitors block the retinal ganglion cell death following optic nerve transection. Brain Res Mol Brain Res 1999;67:36–45.

55. Crowe MJ, Bresnahan JC, Shuman SL, et al. Apoptosis and delayed degeneration after spinal cord injury in rats and monkeys. Nat Med 1997;3:73–76.

56. Liu XZ, Xu XM, Hu R, et al. Neuronal and glial apoptosis after traumatic spinal cord injury. J Neurosci 1997;17:5395–5406.

57. Beattie MS, Shuman SL, Bresnahan JC. Apoptosis and spinal cord injury. The Neuroscientist 1998;4:163–171.

58. Bondurant FJ, Cotler HB, Kulkarni MV, et al. Acute spinal cord injury. A study using physical examination and magnetic resonance imaging. Spine 1990;15:161–168.

59. Flanders AE, Spettell CM, Tartaglino LM, et al. Forecasting motor recovery after cervical spinal cord injury: value of MR imaging. Radiology 1996;201: 649–655.

60. Carlson SL, Parrish ME, Springer JE, et al. Acute inflammatory response in spinal cord following impact injury. Exp Neurol 1998;151:77–88.

61. Kwo S, Young W, Decrescito V. Spinal cord sodium, potassium, calcium, and water concentration changes in rats after graded contusion injury. J Neurotrauma 1989;6:13–24.

62. Lemke M, Demediuk P, McIntosh TK, et al. Alterations in tissue Mg^{++}, Na^+ and spinal cord edema following impact trauma in rats. Biochem Biophys Res Commun 1987;147:1170–1175.

63. Anderson DK, Demediuk P, Saunders RD, et al. Spinal cord injury and protection. Ann Emerg Med 1985;14:816–821.

64. Demediuk P, Lemke M, Faden AI. Spinal cord edema and changes in tissue content of Na^+, K^+, and $Mg2^+$ after impact trauma in rats. Adv Neurol 1990;52:225–232.

65. Hesse S, Bertelt C, Jahnke MT, et al. Treadmill training with partial body weight support compared with physiotherapy in nonambulatory hemiparetic patients. Stroke 1995;26:976–981.

66. Visintin M, Barbeau H, Korner-Bitensky N, Mayo NE. A new approach to retrain gait in stroke patients through body weight support and treadmill stimulation. Stroke 1998;29:1122–1128.

67. Wernig A, Nanassy A, Muller S. Maintenance of locomotor abilities following Laufband (treadmill) therapy in para- and tetraplegic persons: follow-up studies. Spinal Cord 1998;36:744–749.

68. Edgerton VR, Roy RR, Hodgson JA, et al. Potential of adult mammalian lumbosacral spinal cord to execute and acquire improved locomotion in the absence of supraspinal input. J Neurotrauma 1992;9(Suppl 1):S119–S128.

69. Barbeau H, Chau C, Rossignol S. Noradrenergic agonists and locomotor training affect locomotor recovery after cord transection in adult cats. Brain Res Bull 1993;30:387–393.

70. Dietz V, Colombo G, Jensen L, Baumgartner L. Locomotor capacity of spinal cord in paraplegic patients. Ann Neurol 1995;37:574–582.

71. Harkema SJ, Hurley SL, Patel UK, et al. Human lumbosacral spinal cord interprets loading during stepping. J Neurophysiol 1997;77:797–811.

72. Arshavsky YI, Deliagina TG, Orlovsky GN. Pattern generation. Curr Opin Neurobiol 1997;7:781–789.

73. Grillner S, Ekeberg, El Manira A, et al. Intrinsic function of a neuronal network—a vertebrate central pattern generator. Brain Res Brain Res Rev 1998;26:184–197.

74. De Leon RD, Hodgson JA, Roy RR, Edgerton VR. Retention of hindlimb stepping ability in adult spinal cats after the cessation of step training. J Neurophysiol 1999;81:85–94.

75. Merzenich MM, Kaas JH, Wall JT, et al. Progression of change following median nerve section in the cortical representation of the hand in areas 3b and 1 in adult owl and squirrel monkeys. Neuroscience 1983;10: 639–665.

76. Merzenich MM, Nelson RJ, Stryker MP, et al. Somatosensory cortical map changes following digit amputation in adult monkeys. J Comp Neurol 1984;224:591–605.

77. Calford MB, Tweedale R. Immediate expansion of receptive fields of neurons in area 3b of macaque monkeys after digit denervation. Somat Mot Res 1991;8:249–260.

78. Rausell E, Jones EG. Extent of intracortical arborization of thalamocortical axons as a determinant of representational plasticity in monkey somatic sensory cortex. J Neurosci 1995; 15:4270–4288.

79. Rausell E, Bickford L, Manger PR, et al. Extensive divergence and convergence in the thalamocortical projection to monkey somatosensory cortex. J Neurosci 1998;18:4216–4232.

80. Pons TP, Garraghty PE, Ommaya AK, et al. Massive cortical reorganization after sensory deafferentation in adult macaques. Science 1991;252:1857–1860.

81. Jenkins WM, Merzenich MM, Ochs MT, et al. Functional reorganization of primary somatosensory cortex in adult owl monkeys after behaviorally controlled tactile stimulation. J Neurophysiol 1990;63:82–104.

82. Buonomano DV, Merzenich MM. Cortical plasticity: from synapses to maps. Annu Rev Neurosci 1998;21:149–186.

83. Xerri C, Merzenich MM, Peterson BE, Jenkins W. Plasticity of primary somatosensory cortex paralleling sensorimotor skill recovery from stroke in adult monkeys. J Neurophysiol 1998;79: 2119–2148.

84. Nudo RJ, Milliken GW, Jenkins WM, Merzenich MM. Use-dependent alterations of movement representations in primary motor cortex of adult squirrel monkeys. J Neurosci 1996;16:785–807.

85. Classen J, Liepert J, Wise SP, et al. Rapid plasticity of human cortical movement representation induced by practice. J Neurophysiol 1998;79:1117–1123.

86. Cohen LG, Roth BJ, Wassermann EM, et al. Magnetic stimulation of the human cerebral cortex, an indicator of reorganization in motor pathways in certain pathological conditions. J Clin Neurophysiol 1991;8:56–65.

87. Ziemann U, Hallett M, Cohen LG. Mechanisms of deafferentation-induced plasticity in human motor cortex. J Neurosci 1998;18:7000–7007.

88. Abel T, Kandel E. Positive and negative regulatory mechanisms that mediate long-term memory storage. Brain Res Brain Res Rev 1998;26:360–378.

89. Martin KC, Kandel ER. Cell adhesion molecules, CREB, and the formation of new synaptic connections. Neuron 1996;17:567–570.

90. Lømø T, Rosenthal J. Control of acetylcholine sensitivity by muscle activity in the rat. J Physiol (Lond) 1972;221:493–513.

91. Eken T, Gundersen K. Chronic electrical stimulation resembling normal motor-unit activity: effects on denervated fast and slow rat muscles. J Physiol (Lond) 1988;402:651–669.

92. Rioux L, Gaudin DP, Gagnon C, et al. Decrease of behavioral and biochemical denervation supersensitivity of rat striatum by nigral transplants. Neuroscience 1991;44:75–83.

93. Trugman JM, James CL. Rapid development of dopaminergic supersensitivity in reserpine-treated rats demonstrated with 14C-2-deoxyglucose autoradiography. J Neurosci 1992; 12:2875–2879.

94. Ichise M, Kim YJ, Ballinger JR, et al. SPECT imaging of pre- and postsynaptic dopaminergic alterations in L-dopa-untreated PD. Neurology 1999;52:1206–1214.

95. Benson DM, Blitzer RD, Haroutunian V, Landau EM. Functional muscarinic supersensitivity in denervated rat hip-

pocampus. Brain Res 1989;478:399–402.

96. Perl ER. Causalgia, pathological pain, and adrenergic receptors. Proc Natl Acad Sci U S A 1999;96:7664–7667.

97. Brady LS, Herkenham M, Rothman RB, et al. Region-specific up-regulation of opioid receptor binding in enkephalin knockout mice. Brain Res Mol Brain Res 1999;68:193–197.

98. Bliss TVP, Collingridge GL. A synaptic model of memory: long-term potentiation in the hippocampus. Nature 1993;361:31–39.

99. Gozlan H, Khazipov R, Ben AY. Multiple forms of long-term potentiation and multiple regulatory sites of N-methyl-D-aspartate receptors: role of the redox site. J Neurobiol 1995;26:360–369.

100. Nicoll RA, Malenka RC. Contrasting properties of two forms of long-term potentiation in the hippocampus. Nature 1995;377:115–118.

101. Kimura S, Uchiyama S, Takahashi HE, Shibuki K. cAMP-dependent long-term potentiation of nitric oxide release from cerebellar parallel fibers in rats. J Neurosci 1998;18:8551–8558.

102. Arancio O, Kiebler M, Lee CJ, et al. Nitric oxide acts directly in the presynaptic neuron to produce long-term potentiation in cultured hippocampal neurons. Cell 1996;87:1025–1035.

103. Murphy KP, Bliss TV. Photolytically released nitric oxide produces a delayed but persistent suppression of LTP in area CA1 of the rat hippocampal slice. J Physiol (Lond) 1999;515:453–462.

104. Zhuo M, Laitinen JT, Li XC, Hawkins RD. On the respective roles of nitric oxide and carbon monoxide in long-term potentiation in the hippocampus. Learn Mem 1999;6:63–76.

105. Linden DJ, Connor JA. Long-term synaptic depression. Annu Rev Neurosci 1995;18:319–357.

106. Wang Y, Rowan MJ, Anwyl R. Induction of LTD in the dentate gyrus in vitro is NMDA receptor independent, but dependent on Ca^{2+} influx via low-voltage-activated Ca^{2+} channels and release of Ca^{2+} from intracellular stores. J Neurophysiol 1997;77:812–825.

107. Edds MV Jr. Collateral regeneration of residual motor axons in partially denervated muscles. J Exp Zool 1950;113:517–552.

108. Brown MC, Holland RL, Hopkins WG. Motor nerve sprouting. Annu Rev Neurosci 1981;4:17–42.

109. Son YJ, Thompson WJ. Nerve sprouting in muscle is induced and guided by processes extended by Schwann cells. Neuron 1995;14:133–141.

110. Son YJ, Trachtenberg JT, Thompson WJ. Schwann cells induce and guide sprouting and reinnervation of neuromuscular junctions. Trends Neurosci 1996;19:280–285.

111. Liu CN, Chambers WW. Intraspinal sprouting of dorsal root axons. Arch Neurol Psychiatr 1958;79:46–61.

112. Goldberger ME, Murray M. Restitution of function and collateral sprouting in the cat spinal cord: the deafferented animal. J Comp Neurol 1974;158:37–54.

113. Murray M, Goldberger ME. Restitution of function and collateral sprouting in the cat spinal cord: the partially hemisected animal. J Comp Neurol 1974;158:19–36.

114. Goldberger ME, Murray M, Tessler A. Sprouting and Regeneration in the Spinal Cord: Their Roles in Recovery of Function after Spinal Cord Injury. In A Gorio (ed), Neuroregeneration. New York: Raven, 1993:241–264.

115. Raisman G. Neuronal plasticity in the septal nuclei of the adult rat. Brain Res 1969;14:25–48.

116. Lynch G, Mosko S, Parks T, Cotman CW. Relocation and hyperdevelopment of the dentate gyrus commissural system after entorhinal lesions in immature rats. Brain Res 1973;50:174–178.

117. Lynch G, Stanfield B, Parks T, Cotman CW. Evidence for selective post-lesion axonal growth in the hippocampus. Brain Res 1974;69:1–11.

118. Steward O, Cotman CW, Lynch GS. Growth of a new fiber projection in the brain of adult rats: re-innervation of the dentate gyrus by contralateral entorhinal cortex following ipsilateral entorhinal lesions. Exp Brain Res 1974;20:45–66.

119. McKinney RA, Debanne D, Gahwiler BH, Thompson SM. Lesion-induced axonal sprouting and hyperexcitability in the hippocampus in vitro: implications for the genesis of posttraumatic epilepsy. Nat Med 1997;3:990–996.

120. Fagan AM, Gage FH. Mechanisms of sprouting in the adult central nervous system: cellular responses in areas of terminal degeneration and reinnervation in the rat hippocampus. Neuroscience 1994;58:705–725.

121. Caceres AO, Steward O. Dendritic reorganization in the denervated dentate gyrus of the rat following entorhinal cortical lesions. A Golgi and electron microscopic analysis. J Comp Neurol 1983;214:387–403.

122. Deitch JS, Rubel EW. Afferent influences on the brain stem auditory nuclei of the chicken: the course and specificity of dendritic atrophy following deafferentation. J Comp Neurol 1984;229:66–79.

123. Steward O. Alterations in polyribosomes associated with dendritic spines during the reinnervation of the dentate gyrus of the adult rat. J Neurosci 1983;3:177–188.

124. Steward O, Davis L, Dotti C, et al. Protein synthesis and processing in cytoplasmic microdomains beneath postsynaptic sites on CNS neurons. Mol Neurobiol 1988;2:227–261.

125. Cohen AH, Mackler SA, Selzer ME. Behavioral recovery following spinal transection: functional regeneration in the lamprey CNS. Trends Neurosci 1988;11:227–231.

126. Koppanyi T. Regeneration in the Central Nervous System of Fishes. In WF Windle (ed), Regeneration in the Central Nervous System. Springfield: Thomas, 1955;3–19.

127. Piatt J. Regeneration in the Spinal Cord of Amphibia. In WF Windle (ed), Regeneration in the Central Nervous System. Springfield: Thomas, 1955;20–46.

128. Windle WF. Regeneration in the Central Nervous System. Springfield: Thomas, 1955.

129. Sivron T, Schwab ME, Schwartz M. Presence of growth inhibitors in fish optic nerve myelin: postinjury changes. J Comp Neurol 1994;343:237–246.

130. Lang DM, Rubin BP, Schwab ME, Stuermer CA. CNS myelin and oligodendrocytes of the *Xenopus* spinal cord—but not optic nerve—are nonpermissive for axon growth. J Neurosci 1995;15:99–109.

131. Godsave SF, Anderton BH, Wylie CC. The appearance and distribution of intermediate filament proteins during differentiation of the central nervous system, skin and notochord of *Xenopus laevis*. J Embryol Exp Morph 1986;97:201–223.

132. Fouquet B, Herrmann H, Franz JD, Franke WW. Expression of intermediate filament proteins during development of *Xenopus laevis*. III. Identification of mRNAs encoding cytokeratins typical of complex epithelia. Development 1988;104:533–548.

133. Markl J, Franke WW. Localization of cytokeratins in tissues of the rainbow

trout: fundamental differences in expression pattern between fish and higher vertebrates. Differentiation 1988;39:97–122.

134. Giordano S, Glasgow E, Tesser P, Schechter N. A type II keratin is expressed in glial cells of the goldfish visual pathway. Neuron 1989;2:1507–1516.

135. Rungger-Brandle E, Achtstatter T, Franke WW. An epithelium-type cytoskeleton in a glial cell: astrocytes of amphibian optic nerves contain cytokeratin filaments and are connected by desmosomes. J Cell Biol 1989;109:705–716.

136. Merrick SE, Pleasure SJ, Lurie DI, et al. Glial cells of the lamprey nervous system contain keratin-like proteins. J Comp Neurol 1995;355:199–210.

137. Lurie DI, Pijak DS, Selzer ME. Structure of reticulospinal axon growth cones and their cellular environment during regeneration in the lamprey spinal cord. J Comp Neurol 1994;344:559–580.

138. Forehand CJ, Farel PB. Anatomical and behavioral recovery from the effects of spinal cord transection: dependence on metamorphosis in anuran larvae. J Neurosci 1982;2:654–662.

139. Clarke JD, Tonge DA, Holder NH. Stage-dependent restoration of sensory dorsal columns following spinal cord transection in anuran tadpoles. Proc R Soc Lond B Biol Sci 1986;227:67–82.

140. Beattie MS, Bresnahan JC, Lopate G. Metamorphosis alters the response to spinal cord transection in Xenopus laevis frogs. J Neurobiol 1990;21:1108–1122.

141. Howland DR, Bregman BS, Tessler A, Goldberger ME. Transplants enhance locomotion in neonatal kittens whose spinal cords are transected: a behavioral and anatomical study. Exp Neurol 1995;135:123–145.

142. Miya D, Giszter S, Mori F, et al. Fetal transplants alter the development of function after spinal cord transection in newborn rats. J Neurosci 1997;17:4856–4872.

143. Bregman BS, McAtee M, Dai HN, Kuhn PL. Neurotrophic factors increase axonal growth after spinal cord injury and transplantation in the adult rat. Exp Neurol 1997;148:475–494.

144. Richardson PM, McGuinness UM, Aguayo AJ. Axons from CNS neurons regenerate into PNS grafts. Nature 1980;284:264–265.

145. David S, Aguayo AJ. Axonal elonga-

tion into peripheral nervous system "bridges" after central nervous system injury in adult rats. Science 1981;214:931–933.

146. Villegas-Perez MP, Vidal-Sanz M, Bray GM, Aguayo AJ. Influences of peripheral nerve grafts on the survival and regrowth of axotomized retinal ganglion cells in adult rats. J Neurosci 1988;8:265–280.

147. Chen DF, Jhaveri S, Schneider GE. Intrinsic changes in developing retinal neurons result in regenerative failure of their axons. Proc Natl Acad Sci U S A 1995;92:7287–7291.

148. Li D, Field PM, Raisman G. Failure of axon regeneration in postnatal rat endorhinohippocampal slice coculture is due to maturation of the axon, not that of the pathway or target. Eur J Neurosci 1995;7:1164–1171.

149. Goodman CS. Mechanisms and molecules that control growth cone guidance. Annu Rev Neurosci 1996;19:341–377.

150. Sperry RW. Orderly patterning of synaptic associations in regeneration of intracentral fiber tracts mediating visuomotor coordination. Anat Rec 1948;102:63–75.

151. Gaze RM, Jacobson M. A study of the retino-tectal projection during regeneration of the optic nerve in the frog. Proc R Soc Lond B Biol Sci 1963;157:420–448.

152. Sah DW, Frank E. Regeneration of sensory-motor synapses in the spinal cord of the bullfrog. J Neurosci 1984;4:2784–2791.

153. Selzer ME. Mechanisms of functional recovery and regeneration after spinal cord transection in larval sea lamprey. J Physiol (Lond) 1978;277:395–408.

154. Yin HS, Mackler SA, Selzer ME. Directional specificity in the regeneration of lamprey spinal axons. Science 1984;224:894–896.

155. Lurie DI, Selzer ME. Axonal regeneration in the adult lamprey spinal cord. J Comp Neurol 1991;306:409–416.

156. Mackler SA, Yin HS, Selzer ME. Determinants of directional specificity in the regeneration of lamprey spinal axons. J Neurosci 1986;6:1814–1821.

157. Mackler SA, Selzer ME. Regeneration of functional synapses between individual recognizable neurons in the lamprey spinal cord. Science 1985;229:774–776.

158. Mackler SA, Selzer ME. Specificity of synaptic regeneration in the spinal cord of the larval sea lamprey. J Physiol (Lond) 1987;388:183–198.

159. Vidal-Sanz M, Bray GM, Aguayo AJ. Regenerated synapses persist in the superior colliculus after the regrowth of retinal ganglion cell axons. J Neurocytol 1991;20:940–952.

160. Aubert I, Ridet JL, Gage FH. Regeneration in the adult mammalian CNS: guided by development. Curr Opin Neurobiol 1995;5:625–635.

161. Giger RJ, Pasterkamp RJ, Heijnen S, et al. Anatomical distribution of the chemorepellent semaphorin III/collapsin-1 in the adult rat and human brain: predominant expression in structures of the olfactory-hippocampal pathway and the motor system. J Neurosci Res 1998;52:27–42.

162. Miranda JD, White LA, Marcillo AE, et al. Induction of Eph B3 after spinal cord injury. Exp Neurol 1999;156:218–222.

163. Shifman MI, Selzer ME. Netrin receptor UNC-5 is expressed selectively in poorly regenerating neurons following spinal transection in lamprey. Soc Neurosci Abstr 1999;29:219.

164. Howland DR, Manitt C, Kennedy TE, et al. Netrin and its potential role in the injured spinal cord. Soc Neurosci Abstr 1999;29:495.

165. Shifman MI, Selzer ME. Expression of netrin receptor UNC-5 in lamprey brain: modulation by spinal cord transection. Neurorehabil Neural Repair 2000;14:49–58.

166. Frisen J, Yates PA, McLaughlin T, et al. Ephrin-A5 (AL-1/RAGS) is essential for proper retinal axon guidance and topographic mapping in the mammalian visual system. Neuron 1998;20:235–243.

167. Davenport RW, Thies E, Zhou R, Nelson PG. Cellular localization of ephrin-A2, ephrin-A5, and other functional guidance cues underlies retinotopic development across species. J Neurosci 1998;18:975–986.

168. O'Leary DD, Wilkinson DG. Eph receptors and ephrins in neural development. Curr Opin Neurobiol 1999;9:65–73.

169. Lin CH, Thompson CA, Forscher P. Cytoskeletal reorganization underlying growth cone motility. Curr Opin Neurobiol 1994;4:640–647.

170. Fan J, Mansfield SG, Redmond T, et al. The organization of F-actin and microtubules in growth cones exposed to a brain-derived collapsing factor. J Cell Biol 1993;121:867–878.

171. Conti A, Selzer ME. The Role of Cytoskeleton in Regeneration of Central Nervous System Axons. In NR

Saunders, KM Dziegielewska (eds), Degeneration and Regeneration in the Nervous System. Amsterdam: Harwood, 2000;153–169.

172. Caroni P, Schwab ME. Two membrane protein fractions from rat central myelin with inhibitory properties for neurite growth and fibroblast spreading. J Cell Biol 1988;106:1281–1288.

173. Caroni P, Schwab ME. Antibody against myelin-associated inhibitor of neurite growth neutralizes nonpermissive substrate properties of CNS white matter. Neuron 1988;1:85–96.

174. Spillmann AA, Bandtlow CE, Lottspeich F, et al. Identification and characterization of a bovine neurite growth inhibitor (bNI-220). J Biol Chem 1998;273:19283–19293.

175. Igarashi M, Strittmatter SM, Vartanian T, Fishman MC. Mediation by G proteins of signals that cause collapse of growth cones. Science 1993;259:77–79.

176. Bandtlow CE, Schmidt MF, Hassinger TD, et al. Role of intracellular calcium in NI-35-evoked collapse of neuronal growth cones. Science 1993;259:80–83.

177. McKerracher L, David S, Jackson DL, et al. Identification of myelin-associated glycoprotein as a major myelin-derived inhibitor of neurite growth. Neuron 1994;13:805–811.

178. Mukhopadhyay G, Doherty P, Walsh FS, et al. A novel role for myelin-associated glycoprotein as an inhibitor of axonal regeneration. Neuron 1994;13:757–767.

179. Li M, Shibata A, Li C, et al. Myelin-associated glycoprotein inhibits neurite/axon growth and causes growth cone collapse. J Neurosci Res 1996;46:404–414.

180. Bartsch U, Bandtlow CE, Schnell L, et al. Lack of evidence that myelin-associated glycoprotein is a major inhibitor of axonal regeneration in the CNS. Neuron 1995;15:1375–1381.

181. Niederost BP, Zimmermann DR, Schwab ME, Bandtlow CE. Bovine CNS myelin contains neurite growth-inhibitory activity associated with chondroitin sulfate proteoglycans. J Neurosci 1999;19:8979–8989.

182. Kobayashi H, Watanabe E, Murikami F. Growth cones of dorsal root ganglion but not retina collapse and avoid oligodendrocytes in culture. Dev Biol 1995;168:383–394.

183. Cox EC, Muller B, Bonhoeffer F. Axonal guidance in the chick visual system: posterior tectal membranes induce collapse of growth cones from the temporal retina. Neuron 1990;4:31–37.

184. Ciossek T, Monschau B, Kremoser C, et al. Eph receptor-ligand interactions are necessary for guidance of retinal ganglion cell axons in vitro. Eur J Neurosci 1998;10:1574–1580.

185. Yue Y, Su J, Cerretti DP, et al. Selective inhibition of spinal cord neurite outgrowth and cell survival by the eph family ligand ephrin-A5. J Neurosci 1999;19:10026–10035.

186. Kapfhammer JP, Raper JA. Interactions between growth cones and neurites growing from different neural tissues in culture. J Neurosci 1987;7:1595–1600.

187. Ivins JK, Raper JA, Pittman RN. Intracellular calcium levels do not change during contact-mediated collapse of chick DRG growth cone structure. J Neurosci 1991;11:1597–1608.

188. Raper JA, Kapfhammer JP. The enrichment of a neuronal growth cone collapsing activity from embryonic chick brain. Neuron 1990;4:21–29.

189. Luo YL, Raible D, Raper JA. Collapsin: a protein in brain that induces the collapse and paralysis of neuronal growth cones. Cell 1993;75:217–227.

190. Kolodkin AL, Matthes DJ, Goodman CS. The semaphorin genes encode a family of transmembrane and secreted growth cone guidance molecules. Cell 1993;75:1389–1399.

191. Inagaki S, Furuyama T, Iwahashi Y. Identification of a member of mouse semaphorin family. Febs Lett 1995;370:269–272.

192. Luo Y, Shepherd I, Li J, et al. A family of molecules related to collapsin in the embryonic chick nervous system. Neuron 1995;14:1131–1140.

193. Puschel AW, Adams RH, Betz H. Murine semaphorin D/collapsin is a member of a diverse gene family and creates domains inhibitory for axonal extension. Neuron 1995;14:941–948.

194. Kennedy TE, Serafini T, de la Torre JR, Tessier-Lavigne M. Netrins are diffusible chemotropic factors for commissural axons in the embryonic spinal cord. Cell 1994;78:425–435.

195. Serafini T, Kennedy TE, Galko MJ, et al. The netrins define a family of axon outgrowth-promoting proteins homologous to C. elegans UNC-6. Cell 1994;78:409–424.

196. Wadsworth WG, Bhatt H, Hedgecock EM. Neuroglia and pioneer neurons express UNC-6 to provide global and local netrin cues for guiding migra-tions in C. elegans. Neuron 1996; 16:35–46.

197. Richards LJ, Koester SE, Tuttle R, O'Leary DD. Directed growth of early cortical axons is influenced by a chemoattractant released from an intermediate target. J Neurosci 1997;17:2445–2458.

198. Hedgecock EM, Culotti JG, Hall DH. The unc-5, unc-6, and unc-40 genes guide circumferential migrations of pioneer axons and mesodermal cells on the epidermis in C. elegans. Neuron 1990;4:61–85.

199. Keino-Masu K, Masu M, Hinck L, et al. Deleted in Colorectal Cancer (DCC) encodes a netrin receptor. Cell 1996;87:175–185.

200. Chan SS, Zheng H, Su MW, et al. UNC-40, a C. elegans homolog of DCC (Deleted in Colorectal Cancer), is required in motile cells responding to UNC-6 netrin cues. Cell 1996;87:187–195.

201. Leung-Hagesteijn C, Spence AM, Stern BD, et al. UNC-5, a transmembrane protein with immunoglobulin and thrombospondin type 1 domains, guides cell and pioneer axon migrations in C. elegans. Cell 1992;71:289–299.

202. Hamelin M, Zhou Y, Su MW, et al. Expression of the UNC-5 guidance receptor in the touch neurons of C. elegans steers their axons dorsally. Nature 1993;364:327–330.

203. Culotti JG. Axon guidance mechanisms in Caenorhabditis elegans. Curr Opin Genet Devel 1994;4:587–595.

204. Hong K, Hinck L, Nishiyama M, et al. A ligand-gated association between cytoplasmic domains of UNC5 and DCC family receptors converts netrin-induced growth cone attraction to repulsion. Cell 1999;97:927–941.

205. Meyerhardt JA, Caca K, Eckstrand BC, et al. Netrin-1: interaction with deleted in colorectal cancer (DCC) and alterations in brain tumors and neuroblastomas. Cell Growth Differ 1999;10:35–42.

206. Davies SJ, Field PM, Raisman G. Long fibre growth by axons of embryonic mouse hippocampal neurons microtransplanted into the adult rat fimbria. Eur J Neurosci 1993;5:95–106.

207. Davies SJ, Field PM, Raisman G. Long interfascicular axon growth from embryonic neurons transplanted into adult myelinated tracts. J Neurosci 1994;14:1596–1612.

208. Davies SJ, Fitch MT, Memberg SP, et al. Regeneration of adult axons in

white matter tracts of the central nervous system. Nature 1997;390:680–683.

209. Bovolenta P, Wandosell F, Nieto-Sampedro M. Characterization of a neurite outgrowth inhibitor expressed after CNS injury. Eur J Neurosci 1993;5:454–465.

210. Snow DM, Lemmon V, Carrino DA, et al. Sulfated proteoglycans in astroglial barriers inhibit neurite outgrowth in vitro. Exp Neurol 1990;109:111–130.

211. Silver J. Inhibitory molecules in development and regeneration. J Neurol 1994;242:S22–S24.

212. Bovolenta P, Fernaud-Espinosa I, Mendez-Otero R, Nieto-Sampedro M. Neurite outgrowth inhibitor of gliotic brain tissue. Mode of action and cellular localization, studied with specific monoclonal antibodies. Eur J Neurosci 1997;9:977–989.

213. McKeon RJ, Schreiber RC, Rudge JS, Silver J. Reduction of neurite outgrowth in a model of glial scarring following CNS injury is correlated with the expression of inhibitory molecules on reactive astrocytes. J Neurosci 1991;11:3398–3411.

214. Vidal-Sanz M, Bray GM, Villegas-Perez MP, et al. Axonal regeneration and synapse formation in the superior colliculus by retinal ganglion cells in the adult rat. J Neurosci 1987;7:2894–2909.

215. Schwab ME, Caroni P. Oligodendrocytes and CNS myelin are nonpermissive substrates for neurite growth and fibroblast spreading in vitro. J Neurosci 1988;8:2381–2393.

216. Yin HS, Selzer ME. Axonal regeneration in lamprey spinal cord. J Neurosci 1983;3:1135–1144.

217. Davis GR, McClelland AD. Extent and time course of restoration of descending brainstem projections in spinal cord-transected lamprey. J Comp Neurol 1994;344:65–82.

218. Jacobs AJ, Swain GP, Snedeker JA, et al. Recovery of neurofilament expression selectively in regenerating reticulospinal neurons. J Neurosci 1997;17:5206–5220.

219. Richardson PM, Issa VM, Aguayo AJ. Regeneration of long spinal axons in the rat. J Neurocytol 1984;13:165–182.

220. Schnell L, Schneider R, Kolbeck R, et al. Neurotrophin-3 enhances sprouting of corticospinal tract during development and after adult spinal cord lesion. Nature 1994;367:170–173.

221. Weibel D, Cadelli D, Schwab ME. Regeneration of lesioned rat optic nerve fibers is improved after neutralization of myelin-associated neurite growth inhibitors. Brain Res 1994;642:259–266.

222. Xu XM, Guenard V, Kleitman N, et al. A combination of BDNF and NT-3 promotes supraspinal axonal regeneration into Schwann cell grafts in adult rat thoracic spinal cord. Exp Neurol 1995;134:261–272.

223. Sawai H, Clarke DB, Kittlerova P, et al. Brain-derived neurotrophic factor and neurotrophin-4/5 stimulate growth of axonal branches from regenerating retinal ganglion cells. J Neurosci 1996;16:3887–3894.

224. Blesch A, Tuszynski MH. Robust growth of chronically injured spinal cord axons induced by grafts of genetically modified NGF-secreting cells. Exp Neurol 1997;148:444–542.

225. Kobayashi NR, Fan DP, Giehl KM, et al. BDNF and NT-4/5 prevent atrophy of rat rubrospinal neurons after cervical axotomy, stimulate GAP-43 and Talpha1-tubulin mRNA expression, and promote axonal regeneration. J Neurosci 1997;17:9583–9595.

226. Ye JH, Houle JD. Treatment of the chronically injured spinal cord with neurotrophic factors can promote axonal regeneration from supraspinal neurons. Exp Neurol 1997;143:70–81.

227. Bregman BS, Broude E, McAtee M, Kelley MS. Transplants and neurotrophic factors prevent atrophy of mature CNS neurons after spinal cord injury. Exp Neurol 1998;149:13–27.

228. McTigue DM, Horner PJ, Stokes BT, Gage FH. Neurotrophin-3 and brain-derived neurotrophic factor induce oligodendrocyte proliferation and myelination of regenerating axons in the contused adult rat spinal cord. J Neurosci 1998;18:5354–5365.

229. Iwaya K, Mizoi K, Tessler A, Itoh Y. Neurotrophic agents in fibrin glue mediate adult dorsal root regeneration into spinal cord. Neurosurgery 1999;44:589–595; discussion 595–596.

230. Liu Y, Kim D, Himes BT, et al. Transplants of fibroblasts genetically modified to express BDNF promote regeneration of adult rat rubrospinal axons and recovery of forelimb function. J Neurosci 1999;19:4370–4387.

231. Lankford KL, Waxman SG, Kocsis JD. Mechanisms of enhancement of neurite regeneration in vitro following a conditioning sciatic nerve lesion. J Comp Neurol 1998;391:11–29.

232. Oblinger MM, Lasek RJ Axotomy-induced alterations in the synthesis and transport of neurofilaments and microtubules in dorsal root ganglion cells. J Neurosci 1988;8:1747–1758.

233. Schreyer DJ, Skene JH. Injury-associated induction of GAP-43 expression displays axon branch specificity in rat dorsal root ganglion neurons. J Neurobiol 1993;24:959–970.

234. Chong MS, Reynolds ML, Irwin N, et al. GAP-43 expression in primary sensory neurons following central axotomy. J Neurosci 1994;14:4375–4384.

235. Liuzzi FJ, Lasek RJ. Astrocytes block axonal regeneration in mammals by activating the physiological stop pathway. Science 1987;237:642–645.

236. Carlstedt T. Reinnervation of the mammalian spinal cord after neonatal dorsal root crush. J Neurocytol 1988;17:335–350.

237. Pindzola RR, Doller C, Silver J. Putative inhibitory extracellular matrix molecules at the dorsal root entry zone of the spinal cord during development and after root and sciatic nerve lesions. Dev Biol 1993;156:34–48.

238. Richardson PM, Issa VM. Peripheral injury enhances central regeneration of primary sensory neurones. Nature 1984;309:791–793.

239. Neumann S, Woolf CJ. Regeneration of dorsal column fibers into and beyond the lesion site following adult spinal cord injury. Neuron 1999;23:83–91.

240. Chong MS, Woolf CJ, Haque NS, Anderson PN. Axonal regeneration from injured dorsal roots into the spinal cord of adult rats. J Comp Neurol 1999;410:42–54.

241. Skene JH, Willard M. Characteristics of growth-associated polypeptides in regenerating toad retinal ganglion cell axons. J Neurosci 1981;1:419–426.

242. Goslin K, Schreyer DJ, Skene JH, Banker G. Development of neuronal polarity: GAP-43 distinguishes axonal from dendritic growth cones. Nature 1988;336:672–674.

243. Skene JH, Jacobson RD, Snipes GJ, et al. A protein induced during nerve growth (GAP-43) is a major component of growth-cone membranes. Science 1986;233:783–786.

244. Basi GS, Jacobson RD, Virag I, et al. Primary structure and transcriptional regulation of GAP-43, a protein associated with nerve growth. Cell 1987;49:785–791.

245. Kosik KS, Orecchio LD, Bruns GA, et al. Human GAP-43: its deduced amino acid sequence and chromosomal localization in mouse and human. Neuron 1988;1:127–132.

246. Schaechter JD, Benowitz LI. Activation of protein kinase C by arachidonic acid selectively enhances the phosphorylation of GAP-43 in nerve terminal membranes. J Neurosci 1993;13:4361–4371.

247. LaBate ME, Skene JH. Selective conservation of GAP-43 structure in vertebrate evolution. Neuron 1989;3:299–310.

248. Strittmatter SM, Valenzuela D, Vartanian T, et al. Growth cone transduction: Go and GAP-43. J Cell Sci Suppl 1991;15:27–33.

249. Benowitz LI, Routtenberg A. GAP-43: an intrinsic determinant of neuronal development and plasticity. Trends Neurosci 1997;20:84–91.

250. Namgung U, Matsuyama S, Routtenberg A. Long-term potentiation activates the GAP-43 promoter: selective participation of hippocampal mossy cells. Proc Natl Acad Sci U S A 1997;94:11675–11680.

251. Yankner BA, Benowitz LI, Villa-Komaroff L, Neve RL. Transfection of PC12 cells with the human GAP-43 gene: effects on neurite outgrowth and regeneration. Brain Res Mol Brain Res 1990;7:39–44.

252. Igarashi M, Li WW, Sudo Y, Fishman MC. Ligand-induced growth cone collapse: amplification and blockade by variant GAP-43 peptides. J Neurosci 1995;15:5660–5667.

253. Fournier AE, Beer J, Arregui CO, et al. Brain-derived neurotrophic factor modulates GAP-43 but not T alpha1 expression in injured retinal ganglion cells of adult rats. J Neurosci Res 1997;47:561–572.

254. Shea TB, Perrone-Bizzozero NI, Beermann ML, Benowitz LI. Phospholipid-mediated delivery of anti-GAP-43 antibodies into neuroblastoma cells prevents neurogenesis. J Neurosci 1991;11:1685–1690.

255. Aigner L, Caroni P. Depletion of 43-kD growth-associated protein in primary sensory neurons leads to diminished formation and spreading of growth cones. J Cell Biol 1993;123:417–429.

256. Aigner L, Arber S, Kapfhammer JP, et al. Overexpression of the neural growth-associated protein GAP-43 induces nerve sprouting in the adult nervous system of transgenic mice. Cell 1995;83:269–278.

257. Harding DI, Greensmith L, Mason M, et al. Overexpression of GAP-43 induces prolonged sprouting and causes death of adult motoneurons. Eur J Neurosci 1999;11:2237–2242.

258. Vanselow J, Grabczyk E, Ping J, et al. GAP-43 transgenic mice: dispersed genomic sequences confer a GAP-43–like expression pattern during development and regeneration. J Neurosci 1994;14:499–510.

259. Oestreicher AB, De Graan PN, Gispen WH, et al. B-50, the growth associated protein-43: modulation of cell morphology and communication in the nervous system. Prog Neurobiol 1997;53:627–686.

260. Ng TF, So KF, Chung SK. Influence of peripheral nerve grafts on the expression of GAP-43 in regenerating retinal ganglion cells in adult hamsters. J Neurocytol 1995;24:487–496.

261. Schaden H, Stuermer CA, Bahr M. GAP-43 immunoreactivity and axon regeneration in retinal ganglion cells of the rat. J Neurobiology 1994;25:1570–1578.

262. Chong MS, Woolf CJ, Turmaine M, et al. Intrinsic versus extrinsic factors in determining the regeneration of the central processes of rat dorsal root ganglion neurons: the influence of a peripheral nerve graft. J Comp Neurol 1996;370:97–104.

263. Buffo A, Holtmaat AJ, Savio T, et al. Targeted overexpression of the neurite growth-associated protein B-50/GAP-43 in cerebellar Purkinje cells induces sprouting after axotomy but not axon regeneration into growth-permissive transplants. J Neurosci 1997;17:8778–8791.

264. Bisby MA, Tetzlaff W. Changes in cytoskeletal protein synthesis following axon injury and during axon regeneration. Mol Neurobiol 1992;6:107–123.

265. Tetzlaff W, Bisby MA, Kreutzberg GW. Changes in cytoskeletal proteins in the rat facial nucleus following axotomy. J Neurosci 1988;8:3181–3189.

266. Muma NA, Hoffman PN, Slunt HH, et al. Alterations in levels of mRNAs coding for neurofilament protein subunits during regeneration. Exp Neurol 1990;107:230–235.

267. Wujek JR, Lasek RJ. Correlation of axonal regeneration and slow component B in two branches of a single axon. J Neurosci 1983;3:243–251.

268. Bisby MA. Regeneration in the Peripheral Nervous System. In NR Saunders, KM Dziegielewska (eds), Degeneration and Regeneration in the Nervous System. Amsterdam: Harwood, 2000; 239–262.

269. Alderson K, Yee WC, Pestronk A. Reorganization of intrinsic components in the distal motor axon during outgrowth. J Neurocytol 1989;18:541–552.

270. Oblinger MM, Wong J, Parysek LM. Axotomy-induced changes in the expression of a type III neuronal intermediate filament gene. J Neurosci 1989b;9:3766–3775.

271. Troy CM, Muma NA, Greene LA, et al. Regulation of peripherin and neurofilament expression in regenerating rat motor neurons. Brain Res 1990;529:232–238.

272. Beaulieu JM, Robertson J, Julien JP. Interactions between peripherin and neurofilaments in cultured cells: disruption of peripherin assembly by the NF-M and NF-H subunits. Biochem Cell Biol 1999;77:41–45.

273. Becker T, Bernhardt RR, Reinhard E, et al. Readiness of zebrafish brain neurons to regenerate a spinal axon correlates with differential expression of specific cell recognition molecules. J Neurosci 1998;18:5789–5803.

274. Rovainen CM. Regeneration of Müller and Mauthner axons after spinal transection in larval lampreys. J Comp Neurol 1976;168:545–554.

275. Pijak DS, Hall GF, Tenicki PJ, et al. Neurofilament spacing, phosphorylation, and axon diameter in regenerating and uninjured lamprey axons. J Comp Neurol 1996;368:569–581.

276. Hall GF, Yao J, Selzer ME, Kosik KS. Cytoskeletal changes correlated with the loss of neuronal polarity in axotomized lamprey central neurons. J Neurocytol 1997;26:733–753.

277. Lanners HN, Grafstein B. Early stages of axonal regeneration in the goldfish optic tract: an electron microscopic study. J Neurocytol 1980;9:733–751.

278. Tesser P, Jones PS, Schechter N. Elevated levels of retinal neurofilament mRNA accompany optic nerve regeneration. J Neurochem 1986;47:1235–1243.

279. Strobel G, Stuermer CA. Growth cones of regenerating retinal axons contact a variety of cellular profiles in the transected goldfish optic nerve. J Comp Neurol 1994;346:435–448.

280. Scalia F, Matsumoto DE. The morphology of growth cones of regenerating optic nerve axons. J Comp Neurol 1985;231:323–338.

281. McKerracher L, Essagian C, Aguayo AJ. Temporal changes in beta-tubulin and neurofilament mRNA levels after transection of adult rat retinal ganglion cell axons in the optic nerve. J Neurosci 1993a;13:2617–2626.

282. McKerracher L, Essagian C, Aguayo AJ. Marked increase in beta-tubulin mRNA expression during regeneration of axotomized retinal ganglion cells in adult mammals. J Neurosci 1993b; 13:5294–5300.

283. McKerracher L, Vidal-Sanz M, Aguayo AJ. Slow transport rates of cytoskeletal proteins change during regeneration of axotomized retinal neurons in adult rats. J Neurosci 1990;10:641–648.

284. Carter DA, Bray GM, Aguayo AJ. Regenerated retinal ganglion cell axons can form well-differentiated synapses in the superior colliculus of adult hamsters. J Neurosci 1989;9:4042–4050.

285. Aguayo AJ, Bray GM, Rasminsky M, et al. Synaptic connections made by axons regenerating in the central nervous system of adult mammals. J Exp Biol 1990;153:199–224.

286. Jelsma TN, Friedman HH, Berkelaar M, et al. Different forms of the neurotrophin receptor trkb messenger-RNA predominate in rat retina and optic nerve. J Neurobiol 1993;24:1207–1214.

287. Cohen A, Bray GM, Aguayo AJ. Neurotrophin-4/5 (nt-4/5) increases adult-rat retinal ganglion-cell survival and neurite outgrowth in-vitro. J Neurobiol 1994;25:953–959.

288. Mansour-Robaey S, Clarke DB, Wang YC, et al. Effects of ocular injury and administration of brain-derived neurotrophic factor on survival and regrowth of axotomized retinal ganglion cells. Proc Natl Acad Sci U S A 1994;91:1632–1636.

289. Sasaki H, Inoue T, Iso H, et al. Light-dark discrimination after sciatic nerve transplantation to the sectioned optic nerve in adult hamsters. Vision Res 1993;33:877–880.

290. Chen A, Xu XM, Kleitman N, Bunge MB. Methylprednisolone administration improves axonal regeneration into Schwann cell grafts in transected adult rat thoracic spinal cord. Exp Neurol 1996;138:261–276.

291. Schnell L, Schwab ME. Axonal regeneration in the rat spinal cord produced by an antibody against myelin-associated neurite growth inhibitors. Nature 1990;343:269–272.

292. Bregman BS, Kunkel-Bagden E, Schnell L, et al. Recovery from spinal cord injury mediated by antibodies to neurite growth inhibitors. Nature 1995;378:498–501.

293. Huang DW, McKerracher L, Braun PE, David S. A therapeutic vaccine approach to stimulate axon regeneration in the adult mammalian spinal cord. Neuron 1999;24:639–647.

294. Oudega M, Hagg T. Nerve growth factor promotes regeneration of sensory axons into adult rat spinal cord. Exp Neurol 1996;140:218–229.

295. Ramón y Cajal S. Degeneration and Regeneration of the Nervous System. Translated by RM May. New York: Hafner Press, 1928.

296. Paves H, Saarma M. Neurotrophins as in vitro growth cone guidance molecules for embryonic sensory neurons. Cell Tissue Res 1997;290:285–297.

297. Gallo G, Lefcort FB, Letourneau PC. The trkA receptor mediates growth cone turning toward a localized source of nerve growth factor. J Neurosci 1997;17:5445–5454.

298. Song HJ, Ming GL, Poo MM. cAMP-induced switching in turning direction of nerve growth cones. Nature 1997;388:275–279.

299. Ming G, Song H, Berninger B, et al. Phospholipase C-gamma and phosphoinositide 3-kinase mediate cytoplasmic signaling in nerve growth cone guidance. Neuron 1999;23:139–148.

300. Cai D, Shen Y, De Bellard M, et al. Prior exposure to neurotrophins blocks inhibition of axonal regeneration by MAG and myelin via a cAMP-dependent mechanism. Neuron 1999;22:89–101.

301. Zuo J, Ferguson TA, Hernandez YJ, et al. Neuronal matrix metalloproteinase-2 degrades and inactivates a neurite-inhibiting chondroitin sulfate proteoglycan. J Neurosci 1998;18:5203–5211.

302. Reier PJ, Anderson DK, Young W, et al. Workshop on intraspinal transplantation and clinical application. J Neurotrauma 1994;11:369–377.

303. Falci S, Holtz A, Akesson E, et al. Obliteration of a posttraumatic spinal cord cyst with solid human embryonic spinal cord grafts: first clinical attempt. J Neurotrauma 1997;14:875–884.

304. Houle J. The structural integrity of glial scar tissue associated with a chronic spinal cord lesion can be altered by transplanted fetal spinal cord tissue. J Neurosci Res 1992;31:120–130.

305. Kunkel-Bagden E, Bregman BS. Spinal cord transplants enhance the recovery of locomotor function after spinal cord injury at birth. Exp Brain Res 1990;81:25–34.

306. Bregman BS, Kunkel-Bagden E, Reier PJ, et al. Recovery of function after spinal cord injury: mechanisms underlying transplant-mediated recovery of function differ after spinal cord injury in newborn and adult rats. Exp Neurol 1993;123:3–16.

307. Diener PS, Bregman BS. Fetal spinal cord transplants support the development of target reaching and coordinated postural adjustments after neonatal cervical spinal cord injury. J Neurosci 1998;18:763–778.

308. Kim D, Adipudi V, Shibayama M, et al. Direct agonists for serotonin receptors enhance locomotor function in rats that received neural transplants after neonatal spinal transection. J Neurosci 1999;19:6213–6224.

309. Jakeman LB, Reier PJ. Axonal projections between fetal spinal cord transplants and the adult rat spinal cord: a neuroanatomical tracing study of local interactions. J Comp Neurol 1991;307:311–334.

310. Tessler A, Fischer I, Giszter S, et al. Embryonic spinal cord transplants enhance locomotor performance in spinalized newborn rats. Adv Neurol 1997;72:291–303.

311. Menei P, Montero-Menei C, Whittemore SR, et al. Schwann cells genetically modified to secrete human BDNF promote enhanced axonal regrowth across transected adult rat spinal cord. Eur J Neurosci 1998;10:607–621.

312. Grill R, Murai K, Blesch A, et al. Cellular delivery of neurotrophin-3 promotes corticospinal axonal growth and partial functional recovery after spinal cord injury. J Neurosci 1997;17:5560–5572.

313. Blesch A, Uy HS, Grill RJ, et al. Leukemia inhibitory factor augments neurotrophin expression and corticospinal axon growth after adult CNS injury. J Neurosci 1999;19:3556–3566.

314. McKay R. Stem cells in the central nervous system. Science 1997;276:66–71.

315. Gage FH. Stem cells of the central nervous system. Curr Opin Neurobiol 1998;8:671–676.

316. Eriksson PS, Perfilieva E, Bjork-Eriksson T, et al. Neurogenesis in the adult human hippocampus. Nat Med 1998;4:1313–1317.

317. Fricker RA, Carpenter MK, Winkler C, et al. Site-specific migration and neuronal differentiation of human neural progenitor cells after transplantation in the adult rat brain. J Neurosci 1999;19:5990–6005.

318. Suhonen JO, Peterson DA, Ray J, Gage FH. Differentiation of adult hippocampus-derived progenitors into

olfactory neurons in vivo. Nature 1996;383:624–627.

319. Olsson M, Campbell K, Turnbull DH. Specification of mouse telencephalic and mid-hindbrain progenitors following heterotopic ultrasound-guided embryonic transplantation. Neuron 1997;19:761–772.

320. Takahashi M, Palmer TD, Takahashi J, Gage FH. Widespread integration and survival of adult-derived neural progenitor cells in the developing optic retina. Mol Cell Neurosci 1998;12:340–348.

321. Keirstead HS, Ben-Hur T, Rogister B, et al. Polysialylated neural cell adhesion molecule-positive CNS precursors generate both oligodendrocytes and

Schwann cells to remyelinate the CNS after transplantation. J Neurosci 1999;19:7529–7536.

322. Fisher LJ. Neural precursor cells: applications for the study and repair of the central nervous system. Neurobiol Dis 1997;4:1–22.

323. Pincus DW, Goodman RR, Fraser RA, et al. Neural stem and progenitor cells: a strategy for gene therapy and brain repair. Neurosurgery 1998;42:858–867; discussion 867–868.

324. Ramon-Cueto A, Plant GW, Avila J, Bunge MB. Long-distance axonal regeneration in the transected adult rat spinal cord is promoted by olfactory ensheathing glia transplants. J Neurosci 1998;18:3803–3815.

325. Li Y, Field PM, Raisman G. Repair of adult rat corticospinal tract by transplants of olfactory ensheathing cells. Science 1997;277:2000–2002.

326. Schnell L, Schwab ME. Sprouting and regeneration of lesioned corticospinal tract fibres in the adult rat spinal cord. Eur J Neurosci 1993;5:1156–1171.

327. Cheng H, Cao Y, Olson L. Spinal cord repair in adult paraplegic rats: partial restoration of hind limb function. Science 1996;273:510–513.

328. Cheng H, Almstrom S, Gimenez-Llort L, et al. Gait analysis of adult paraplegic rats after spinal cord repair. Exp Neurol 1997;148:544–557.

28

Peripheral Nerve Regeneration

MAZHER JAWEED

The peripheral nervous system (PNS) was first described by Hippocrates (ca. 460–370 BC), but Galen (ca. 130–200 AD) probably was the first to study the effect of nerve transection on muscle size and power. Between the sixteenth and the nineteenth centuries, massive amounts of information were amassed on nerve excitability and muscle responses. With the invention of the microscope, new knowledge was obtained about the nature of peripheral nerves and myelin. After Galvani (1737–1798) demonstrated that electrical stimulation (ES) evoked responses in nerves and muscles, motor and sensory nerves were identified and associated with the ventral and dorsal roots in the spinal cord, respectively. In 1839, Schwann identified and characterized the nature of Schwann's cell, and Purkinje discovered direct connections between the neuronal cell body and the axon.

In the mid-1800s, Waller reported that injury to the glossopharyngeal and hypoglossal nerves of the frog caused degenerative changes distal to the lesion. He also noted that regeneration was more rapid in younger frogs and was not enhanced by ES. Waller concluded that the neuronal cell body functioned as a trophic center responsible for maintaining the nerve fiber and that an interruption caused by injury resulted in death of the axon.[1]

In 1906, Golgi[2] and Ramon y Cajal[3] separately demonstrated that the nervous system is a network of individual nerve cells and functional connections. In the twentieth century, Sunderland, Sherrington, Seddon, Weiss, and Hoffmann, among others, contributed a great deal to the understanding of nerve-muscle interactions.[4-8] As neurosciences advance, the roles of Schwann's cells; the mechanisms of neural responses to injury, axonal growth, and transport;

and effect of the neural microenvironment continue to be elucidated.[5-8]

ANATOMY AND PHYSIOLOGY OF THE PERIPHERAL NERVOUS SYSTEM

The PNS receives commands from the brain and relays information to target fibers or end organs such as muscle spindle or sympathetic neurons. The PNS comprises a complex composite structure of neuronal cell bodies in the spinal cord, their supportive connective tissue, and cellular elements. The neurons connect to the periphery, with the incoming or afferent nerve endings in the dorsal spinal roots and the outgoing (efferent) nerves originating in the ventral roots (Figure 28-1). Within the spinal cord, the neurons contact one another by their dendrites, but the connection with the periphery is via a single axon that terminates at the neuromuscular junction or sensory receptors. Myelinated efferent fibers innervate both the larger extrafusal fibers (alpha motor neurons) and the smaller intrafusal fibers (gamma motor neurons). Motor innervation to blood vessels and epidermal appendages is through the autonomic nervous system.[1,4,6]

Both afferent and efferent nerve fibers are encased in bundles or fascicles bound by supportive connective tissue, which contributes approximately 25–85% of the bundle volume, depending on the type of nerve.[1] Sherrington[8] compared the composition of afferent and efferent nerves in fascicles of motor and sympathetic nerves and observed that the larger afferent nerves predominated in the nerves innervating muscle. Eccles and Sherrington[9] confirmed this observation and determined that fascicles consist of large and small nerves

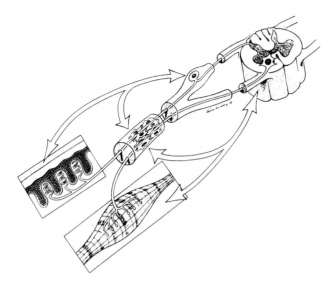

FIGURE 28-1 The peripheral nervous system consists of afferent and efferent nerve endings in the dorsal and ventral roots, respectively. The afferent nerve axons originate from the periphery (e.g., spindle and the Golgi tendon) and terminate at the dorsal root ganglion (*upper arrows*). The efferent nerve axons (*lower arrows*) are the distal extensions of the alpha or gamma motor neurons, which synapse at the periphery (e.g., neuromuscular junction). (Reprinted with permission from G Lundborg, LB Dahlin. Structure and Function of Peripheral Nerve. In RH Gelberman [ed], Operative Nerve Repair and Reconstruction. Philadelphia: Lippincott, 1991.)

of largest diameter are called group I, those of intermediate diameter groups II and III, and those of smaller diameter are identified as unmyelinated group IV fibers. The rates of both degeneration and regeneration of nerve fibers differ significantly in different nerves.

The peripheral nerves are associated with three separate and distinct supportive sheaths, the outer epineurium, the middle perineurium, and the inner endoneurium. These sheaths cover the nerve, nerve fascicle, and nerve axon, respectively (Figure 28-2). The perineurium, a mechanically strong membrane that can sustain intrafascicular pressure of as much as 300–750 mm Hg, acts as a barrier against mechanical trauma and diffusion from extracellular infiltrates. The perineurium blocks diffusion of proteins and ferritin,[11,12] but is permeable to diphosphorus compounds, oxidative enzymes, and adenosine triphosphate.[13] The endoneurium protects the integrity of the axon and other endoneurial contents such as Schwann's cells and axoplasm. Regeneration after injury to the peripheral nerves may depend on the extent of injury to these membranes. For example, if the endoneurial tube is intact after mild compression injury, the axon regenerates smoothly, the synapse is re-established in the area of the degenerated end-plate; by contrast, transection injury, in which a guidance or navigation tube is absent, results in delayed reinnervation of the muscle. Thus, to examine or facilitate nerve regeneration and subsequent reinnervation, it is important to understand the behavior of factors that are linked to degeneration.[14,15]

One of the main factors that contributes to degeneration and regeneration of peripheral nerves is the transport of axoplasm, which carries a wide range of substances, including proteins, membranous vesicles, neurotransmitters, lipids, mitochondria, and RNA. Approximately 70% of these nutrients are lost during transport from the neuronal cell body to the peripheral

and include motor and sensory fibers. Several classifications for the peripheral nerves have been proposed, the most complete of which was advanced by Erlanger and Gasser[10] and later modified by Terzis and associates.[1] According to this classification, myelinated fibers can be grouped into A and B fibers, depending on their fiber diameter, conduction velocity, and function. Nonmyelinated fibers are identified as C fibers (Table 28-1); those

TABLE 28-1
Nerve Fiber Classification

Group	Myelin	Size	Conduction Presence	Fiber and Function
A	Myelinated	Largest	Fastest	Somatic afferents and efferents
Aα	Myelinated	15–20 μm	Fast	Efferent
Aβ	Myelinated	8–15 μm	Fast	Afferent, touch
Aδ	Myelinated	2–5 μm	Fast	Pricking, pain, temperature
B	Myelinated	1–2 μm	Slow	Autonomic afferents and preganglionic
C	Unmyelinated	<1 μm	Slowest	Autonomic efferents and postganglionic; deep, burning pain

Source: Adapted from J Erlanger, H Gasser. Electrical Signs of Nervous Activity. Philadelphia: University of Pennsylvania Press, 1937.

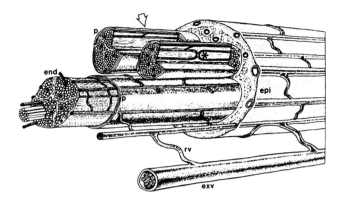

FIGURE 28-2 A peripheral nerve and ensheathing collagenous membranes. The outer epineurium (epi), the middle perineurium (p), and the inner endoneurium (end) encircle the nerve bundle, nerve fascicle, and the nerve axon, respectively. The asterisk represents a node. The nerve is richly vascular with radial vessels (rv) and external vessels (exv). The large arrow on the top shows the perineurium sheath surrounding the fascicle. (Adapted from G Lundborg, LB Dahlin. Structure and Function of Peripheral Nerves. In RH Gelberman [ed], Operative Nerve Repair and Reconstruction, Vol. I. Philadelphia: Lippincott, 1991:3–17.)

TABLE 28-2

Axonal Transport System and Major Components

Transport System	Group	Velocity (mm/day)	Major Components
Anterograde			
Fast	I, II	20–410	Neurotransmitters and related enzymes and amino acids
Fast	III	4–8	Myosin-like actin-binding polypeptides
Slow	IV	2–30	Actin, clathrin
Slow	IV	0.1–15.0	Tubulin, neurofilaments
Retrograde			
Fast	—	≤300	Neurotropic factors, (NGF), lysosomes
Slow	—	3–8	Single protein

NGF = nerve growth factor.
Source: Modified from G Lundborg, LB Dahlin. Structure and Function of Peripheral Nerve. In RH Gelberman (ed), Operative Nerve Repair and Reconstruction. Philadelphia: Lippincott, 1991.

target. The speed of axoplasmic transport contributes to the rate of regeneration of the nerves (Table 28-2). Lundborg and colleagues have identified five groups of anterograde transport.[16,17] The fast axonal transport system (20–410 mm/day, groups I and II) is used to pass membrane-bound materials and depends on the availability of energy; it can be blocked by metabolic and energy system inhibitors.[16,17] Inhibition of fast axonal transport thus interferes with synaptic transmission and, consequently, nerve regeneration of the axon. The slow transport system (0.1–30.0 mm/day), on the other hand, transports substances (mostly proteins) at speeds that vary from nerve to nerve. Retrograde transport from the periphery to the nerve cells in the spinal cord includes both fast (300 mm/day) and slow (4–8 mm/day) components. This system reportedly transports multivesicular and multilamellar organelles such as lysosomes, as well as growth factors and viruses. Retrograde chemotactic factors are also known to play an important role in stimulating or inhibiting peripheral nerve sprouting in partially denervated muscle.[18–20]

PERIPHERAL NERVE DEGENERATION

Peripheral nerve injury can be caused by a variety of lesions, physical injury, or environmental factors. The level of degeneration of the neuron, Schwann's cell,

axon, and target organ can estimate the extent of an injury. Both Seddon[21] and Sunderland[22] developed schemes for classifying peripheral nerve injuries based on the damage to internal structures. The first, mildest degree of injury in this classification is neurapraxia, or nerve conduction block. In this type of injury, axonal continuity is maintained, and nerve conduction proximal and distal to the block is preserved. Recovery is relatively rapid (a few hours to several weeks),[23–25] and neither anterograde nor retrograde transport is interrupted. In this condition, the large fibers (Aα) are affected the most and are narrowed at the nodes of Ranvier. There is reason to believe that pressures as low as 30 mm Hg may impede fast conduction.

Pressures greater than 200 mm Hg may produce a block that can last 2 hours to 3 days, depending on the duration of compression.[1,4,24] Neurapraxic lesions are common in traumatic spinal cord injury (SCI). Prolonged pressure may lead to neural ischemia. Lundborg[24] observed ischemic changes in peripheral nerves with 4–6 hours of compression; compression for such periods resulted in increased intraneural capillary permeability, leading to swelling and intraneural pressure.[25]

Second-degree injury includes all the changes in first-degree lesions plus concomitant degeneration of the axon. Second-degree injuries are produced by crushing as well as by mild traction. The degenerative changes are visible within minutes, both proximally and distally. The pathologic changes depend on the degree and duration of ischemia, fiber size, proximity to cell body, and the age of the patient. In the initial phase of crush injury, organelles and metabolites accumulate in the proximal and distal stumps of the crushed nerve, leading to nerve swelling. The entire length of the distal segment then gradually begins to degenerate. The segment proximal to the lesion undergoes degeneration similar to that after cavitation of the spinal cord. Within 6 hours after injury, the neuronal cell bodies start to change, Nissl bodies disperse, neurofilaments disassemble, and ultimately the nucleus moves from the center of the cell to the periphery. Schwann's cells, perhaps in response to these degenerative changes in the axon and myelin, are released from the nerve axons and begin to multiply, increasing protein synthesis within the basal lamina tube.[26] This process, wallerian degeneration,[27] thus causes the axon to degenerate below the lesion.

Third-degree peripheral nerve injury includes axonotmetic lesion(s), in which the continuity of the basal lamina is significantly disrupted. Hemorrhage, edema, and subsequent ischemia of the nerve axon follow damage to Schwann's cells and their basement membranes. The accumulation of dead cells may complicate and limit the process of regeneration. The regenerated axon, without peripheral guidance, may not be able to form synapses with the appropriate end-organs, particularly in mixed sensory and motor nerves.[1,4,14,15]

Fourth-degree injury involves axonal, endoneurial, and perineurial injury, caused by severe crush or traction damage. The zone of injury is greater, the chance of fascicular organization negligible, and the loss of neurons frequent in this type of injury, leading to failure of regeneration.[1,4]

The fifth and most severe degree of nerve damage is characterized by complete transection of the nerve trunk, and so carries minimal chance of spontaneous recovery. Transection injuries most often result from severe crushing or shearing. In this condition, abortive attempts at regeneration produce a tangled mass of axonal buds and neuromas.[1,4]

In summary, the effect of peripheral nerve injuries is quite variable; different degrees of injury can be associated with a single lesion. The first three degrees of injury can result in subsequent return of function, whereas fourth- and fifth-degree injuries may not. The degree of muscle reinnervation (or synapses with sympathetic neurons) thus depends on the type of injury to the axon.

MECHANISMS OF NERVE DEGENERATION IN DIFFERENT INJURIES

Nerve injuries can result from trauma, compression, stretch, ischemia, electrical shock, radiation, puncture, and laceration. Clinically, diseases such as Charcot-Marie-Tooth disease, diabetes, poliomyelitis, and traumatic spinal cord injuries at the root level, Kugelberg-Welander disease, and several polyneuropathies can cause total and partial denervation. The extent of regeneration depends on the degree of injury. Brief discussions of some common injuries are presented in the following sections and in Table 28-3.

Nerve Compression

Acute nerve compression can be produced by pressures as low as 30 mm Hg. At 60 mm Hg, nerve conduction block may be produced; pressures greater than 90 mm Hg may initiate damage to the internal structures.[28,29] Pressure on the nerve for 30–40 minutes leads to pares-

TABLE 28-3
Peripheral Nerve Injury

Nerve Injury	Symptoms	Tissue and Cellular Changes	Recovery Prognosis
Compressions	Neurapraxia, paresthesia, paralysis	Nerve conduction	Good
Stretch	Tingling, burning sensation, pain	Epineurial and perineurial sheath distention (tear)	Good
Ischemic injury (<6–8 hours)	Pain, paresthesia, hypersensitivity	Vascular damage	Good (>6–8 hours is poor)
Electrical injury	Pain, burning	Nerve tissue coagulation; necrosis of nerve, vessels, skin, muscle	Unpredictable
Radiation injury	Pain	DNA damage, delayed mitosis, fibrosis	Questionable
Injection and laceration	Severe pain	Vascular damage, inflammatory changes	Fair

Source: Adapted from JK Terzis, KL Smith. The Peripheral Nerve. New York: Raven Press, 1990.

thesias, paralysis, and associated pathophysiological changes in the nerve and muscle. More prolonged neurapraxic conditions lead to focal demyelination at the site of injury; the so-called Saturday night palsy results from local demyelination.[30]

Clinically, gunshot wounds and shrapnel cause similar acute nerve compression. Tissue damage is related to the velocity of the projectile (e.g., when the kinetic energy of the shrapnel exceeds the speed of sound [335 m/second] it becomes proportional to the third power of the velocity of the bullet).[1,30] Therefore, the compression produced by a bullet lodged in the muscle or connective tissue adjacent to the nerve may cause partial denervation leading to subsequent peripheral regeneration of the intact axons. This phenomenon is more common in proximal than the distal nerves. It has been proposed that compression-induced anoxia or ischemia could contribute to delayed conduction, loss of oxidative phosphorylation inside the nerve, and inhibition of sodium, potassium, and ATPase.[31-33] Electron microscopic studies of compressed nerves have revealed myofibroblast activation and proliferation in the epineurium and the appearance of small unmyelinated axons, indicating nerve regeneration.[34]

Stretch Damage

Sudden overstretching of joints and muscles may damage superficial nerves. Nerve stretching is common in bone fractures, joint dislocations, obstetric trauma, and inadvertent traction during surgical repair of nerves. Of all stretch injuries, 95% are sustained in upper extremities; 16% in the peroneal nerves, and only 2% in the sciatic nerve.[35] The integrity of the three nerve membrane sheaths is important. One of the common causes of traction injuries is the stretching of the epineurial and perineurial sheaths; however, when only the epineurium is distended, its elasticity protects the nerve. Nerve stretching also may cause proliferation of fibroblasts inside the nerve and hemorrhage in multiple areas, suggesting that stretch injuries may damage the collagen membranes as well as the capillaries and venules inside the nerve. Damaged vessels may form microemboli.[35,36]

Ischemic Injury

Peripheral nerves are supplied with abundant oxygen through an elaborate vascular system to maintain cellular integrity; axoplasmic transport; and the generation, maintenance, and restoration of the membrane potential necessary for nerve conduction. Unlike the CNS,

the PNS is fairly resistant to brief periods of ischemia. However, chronic hypoxia may cause weakness, referred pain, paresthesia, hypersensitivity, and sensory deficits.[1] Ischemia lasting more than 6–8 hours may cause necrosis and abnormal spontaneous potentials.[1,4,37,38] Ischemia can cause first- through fourth-degree nerve injury, as described previously. Asphyxia for 10 minutes or more can result in severe damage in humans, including slowing of the resting potential, decrease in action potential, and ultimately failure of nerve excitability within 30–40 minutes. Reoxygenation can produce complete recovery within 10 minutes, indicating that ischemic changes in the nerve are metabolic rather than anatomic.[39,40]

Electrical Injury

Injuries induced by electricity primarily involve motor nerves and produce immediate neurologic deficits associated with coagulation necrosis, heat production, and burn. This leads to abnormalities of nerve conduction (decrement of approximately 100 mA/mm of nerve diameter) in experimental animals.[41,42] Electrical injuries damage nerves, vessels, skin, or muscle tissue. Consequently, the associated fibrosis and scar formation is considerably greater than that of other injuries, and this impedes regeneration. The degree of recovery after electrical burns is quite unpredictable.

Radiation Injury

The clinical effects of ionizing radiation on nerve and muscle are unknown. Radiation, either directly or indirectly, causes release of free radicals inside cell membranes, which contributes to neurolysis and delayed regeneration.[43] The target site for radiation damage is the DNA, causing genomic alterations followed by imprecise replication. In dividing cells, irradiation causes delayed mitosis, which limits cell division.[44,45] In humans, acute degenerative changes in peripheral nerves are aggravated by repeated or massive doses of radiation. Thus, secondary factors such as fibrosis and vascular impairment might become detrimental to the regeneration and elongation of individual axons.[43-46]

Injection and Laceration Injuries

These types of injuries are associated with severe pain and inflammatory changes in the nerve, the degree of which is related to the degree of injury caused by the substance injected or the tearing produced by the laceration.[47,48]

In summary, a common factor among these different injuries appears to be vascular compromise and associated inflammatory changes. In addition, the collagen and fibroblast proliferation associated with tissue damage may form scar tissue, which significantly delays regeneration.

MOTONEURON DEGENERATION IN SPINAL CORD INJURY AND NEUROPATHIES

The mechanism of degeneration and subsequent regeneration varies significantly in upper and lower motoneurons. SCI may involve both the upper and lower motoneurons depending on the nature and extent of SCI. Motoneuron diseases include the upper and lower motoneuron disorders (amyotrophic lateral sclerosis [ALS]), pure lower motoneuron diseases (spinal muscular atrophies, multifocal motor neuropathies, lumbosacral radiculopathies, postpolio syndrome, hereditary bulbar palsy), and pure upper motoneuron disorders (primary lateral sclerosis, hereditary spastic paraplegia, konzo). Peripheral neuropathies may be manifested in various hormonal deficiencies or disturbances (diabetes and hypothyroidism) and immune suppression diseases (acquired immunodeficiency syndrome [AIDS], cancer).

Spinal Cord Injury

Experimental studies and clinical observations of acute SCI suggest that initial mechanical insult to spinal neurons results in a series of deleterious events that promote progressive damage and ischemia. Although the primary injury is fated by the circumstances of the trauma, the outcome of the secondary injury may be amenable to therapeutic modulations. Unlike lower vertebrates, humans and mammalian experimental animals show only an abortive regeneration of motoneurons after transectional SCI. This is attributed to gap formation after transection, secondary to posttraumatic cell death, and missing guiding channels for sprouting axons.[49] However, studies in experimental animals indicate promising possibilities for regeneration of neurons after SCI and subsequent motor recovery. Various neurotrophic factors, antibodies to inhibitory molecules, electrical and electromagnetic stimulation (EMS), and transplantation of peripheral nerves[50] have been reported to initiate regeneration after SCI. Unlike peripheral nerves, in which there is an immediate onset of regenerative events to promote elongation, the mammalian central motoneurons suffer from a failure of axonal elongation,[51,52] which appears to be regulated by

a proto-oncogene, *Bcl-2*.[53] Schwartz et al.[54] demonstrated that the failure of axonal elongation after SCI is caused by an unfavorable microenvironment as well as the accompanying inflammatory events. Implantation of autologous macrophages from regenerating peripheral nerves and administration of the drug methylprednisolone have been reported to reduce inflammatory changes and enhance motor recovery.[55] Thus, an application of exogenous neurotrophic factors, such as nerve growth factor (NGF), neurotrophin-3, and brain-derived neurotrophic factor, may show well-defined and selective beneficial effects on the survival and phenotypic expression of motoneurons in the spinal cord (see Chapter 27).

Amyotrophic Lateral Sclerosis

ALS is a progressive neurodegenerative disease of unknown origin. The disease is characterized by a loss of motoneurons in the cortex, brain stem, and spinal cord, and symptoms affecting bulbar, limb, and respiratory musculature. Clinically, the disease is diagnosed by symptoms of progressive weakness, muscle atrophy, spasticity, dysarthria, dysphagia, and respiratory compromise. Of all patients with ALS, approximately 5–10% of them have familial ALS disease; whereas most of the others are grouped as having sporadic ALS. Studies suggest that familial ALS may be induced by mutations of a key free radical scavenging enzyme, Cu/Zn superoxide dismutase (Cu/Zn SOD). Kennel et al.[56] showed that the alterations of Cu/Zn SOD lead to a massive loss of functional motor units, which subsequently leads to clinical signs (tremor and shaking) and motoneuron loss. Additionally, serum and CSF of ALS patients have shown an imbalance between excitatory and inhibitory amino acids that contributes to neuronal death. The content of excitatory amino acids such as glutamate and aspartate is increased, whereas the content of inhibitory amino acids such as gamma-aminobutyric acid and glycine is either decreased or not altered.[57] Administration of antioxidant, coenzyme Q10, especially in early stages of the disease, has been known to retard the loss of motoneurons.[58] Pharmacologic treatment of ALS patients with the drug riluzole, glutamate antagonists, and sodium channel blockers appears to slow the degenerative process. To date, attempts to enhance regeneration in ALS have not been fruitful.[59]

Autoimmune Deficiency Syndrome (Acquired Immunodeficiency Syndrome)

The mechanism of extreme weakness and fatigue plus paresis, in patients with AIDS, has not been fully understood. Designed clinical studies indicate that, beside disuse, there is significant neuropathy caused by immune suppression in AIDS patients. Bradley et al.[60] conducted a study with 11 patients with AIDS and 10 control subjects. Compared with the control group, the AIDS patients showed a fivefold accumulation in the so-called nodules of Nageotte in dorsal root ganglia of L-4, L-5, and S-1 and sciatic nerve. In addition, immunohistochemical data indicate considerable axonal degeneration of the sciatic nerves (ninefold), tibial nerves (28-fold), and sural nerves (12-fold). The pathologic process in this neuropathy seems to be associated with an increased density of T cells and macrophage infiltration with cytokine expressions at all levels of PNS, producing segmental multifocal demyelination and degeneration. The reparative process (axonal regeneration and remyelination) occurred only at the most proximal levels. In a study with 18 AIDS patients, Rizzuto et al.[61] noted a distal sensory polyneuropathy accompanied by painful dysesthesias. Motor involvement was not as severe or predominant in occurrence as the sensory component. The human immunodeficiency virus appears to enter the PNS and induce changes in immunocompetent cell populations with activation of macrophages and cytotoxins. Detailed studies are deemed necessary to further elaborate the mechanism of immunosuppressive agents on initiation of neuropathic changes and its relationship to cytokines such as tumor necrosis factors-α and -β and interleukins.

Diabetic Neuropathy

Diabetic neuropathy consists of several clinical syndromes affecting motor, sensory, and autonomic nerves. Of these the most common is distal symmetric sensory polyneuropathy, usually referred to as *diabetic neuropathy*. Two mechanisms are associated with this condition. The first assumes that hypoglycemia induces metabolic changes in structure and function of endoneurial microvessels, causing alterations of the blood-nerve barrier, and induces hypoxia or ischemia or some unknown mechanism(s) responsible for cellular injury. Major pathogenic mechanisms include increased activity of polyol pathway, abnormalities in vasoactive substances, nonenzymatic glycation, increased presence of free radicals, and perturbed neurotrophism.[62] In streptozotocin-treated diabetic rats, a decreased production of nitric oxide, Na/K channel dysfunction, and decreased capacity of sciatic nerve regeneration has been observed. The significance of decreased synthesis of nitric oxide, a potent CNS neurotransmitter, has not been clearly understood. Traditionally, the neuropa-

thies accompanying type I (insulin dependent) and type II (non-insulin dependent) diabetes mellitus have been regarded as identical. However, more recent data suggest distinct differences in functional and structural expressions of the two neuropathies. In proximal diabetic neuropathy, the immunoinflammatory vasculitis induces ischemic nerve fiber degeneration; whereas in truncal radiculopathy, the degeneration may be produced by inflammatory polygangliopathy.[63] In rats, Suh et al.[64] demonstrated that a potent inhibitor of phosphodiesterase enzyme (cilostazol) may significantly slow the progression of neuropathic processes induced by streptozotocin treatment. Treatment of these diabetic rats with high vitamin E doses (70 mg/kg to 12 g/kg of body weight) significantly reduced the sciatic and tibial nerve dysfunction, and attenuated endoneurial lipid peroxidation, as measured by malondialdehyde test.[65] These studies confirm the assertion that diabetic polyneuropathy may be caused by alteration of membranes and reduced cyclic adenosine monophosphate content in motor nerves of the animals.[65-67] Green et al.[68] demonstrated that hyperglycemia and other consequences of insulin deficiency may be ultimately responsible for the pathogenesis in diabetic neuropathy. Thus, emerging data from human and experimental animal studies suggest that glucose-driven oxidative stress may play a central role in activation of aldose reductase and glycation pathways, and consequent degeneration of vascular and neurotrophic support.[69]

PERIPHERAL NERVE REGENERATION

After injury to the peripheral nerve axon, the distal stump starts to undergo wallerian degeneration, whereas the proximal stump begins to regenerate. The changes associated with regeneration begin within 24 hours after the injury (Figure 28-3). It has been reported that the dying axon somehow signals its condition to the neuronal cell body, which responds immediately to re-establish continuity with the periphery. The axonal growth rate and restoration of proper contact with the periphery are regulated by specific biochemical and biophysical factors.[16,17] For example, regeneration is significantly influenced by the integrity of the endoneurial tube. If the endoneurium is not damaged, the regeneration of axon is rather smooth, growing in the intact tube and ultimately finding the end target. In contrast, if the endoneurial wall is severed, the course of regeneration is delayed, possibly because of late neuronal recovery, passage of regenerated axons through the zone of injury or scarred area, elongation, and synapse with the end-

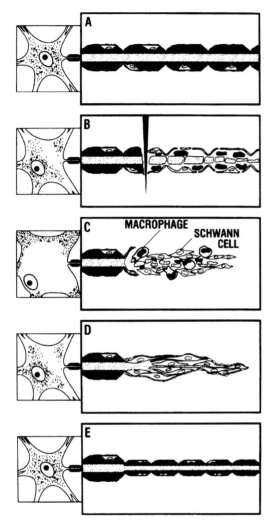

FIGURE 28-3 Diagram describing sequelae of reactions occurring in the distal segment of a peripheral nerve axon after injury to the axon. **A.** Normal myelinated axon shown with intact axoplasm, nodes of Ranvier, and Schwann's cells at the periphery. **B.** Axonal injury, causing wallerian degeneration in the distal segment. Note the beginning of Nissl body rearrangement inside the neuronal cell body. **C.** Total disintegration of the distal segment with microphagic infiltration and multiplication of Schwann's cells. Note maximum rearrangement of Nissl bodies, migration of nucleus, and overall hypertrophy in the cell body. **D.** Growth cone formation and terminal regeneration of the proximal segment. The Schwann's cells start to migrate toward the periphery. **E.** Regenerated and elongated axon exhibits significant thinness. The regenerated axon does not attain the size of the original axon. (Reprinted with permission from G Lundborg, N Danielsen. Injury Degeneration and Regeneration. In RH Gelberman [ed], Operative Nerve Repair and Reconstruction. Philadelphia: Lippincott, 1991.)

organ. Therefore, functional recovery, defined as nerve conduction to the end-organ, is expected to be quicker in axon compression injuries than in traumatic or transection injuries.[1,4,14,15,70,71]

PRIMARY GROWTH VERSUS NERVE REGENERATION

The process of developmental growth and regeneration of nerves appears to be similar. However, there are significant differences. Embryonic nerve cells are *cued* by neurotropic factors, which are used by the axons to initiate growth and attain their targets. The sources of neurotrophic substances, which can stimulate or inhibit synapses with the appropriate targets, include the growth cone of the axon and the matrix of connective tissue or stromal cells, such as glial cells and fibroblasts.[1,4,70–73] The affinity of axons for an inappropriate peripheral target is limited during development, and it is governed by genetic templates to carry out the consequences of growth in a specific order.

Regeneration, on the other hand, is limited in its initiation of growth in an unfavorable environment. Unlike the satellite cells in muscle, fibroblasts in skin, and regenerating hepatocytes in liver, nerves do not contain a reserve of regenerating cells. Degenerating Schwann's cells at the periphery and other chemotactic factors signal a destruction of the axons to the motor neurons via retrograde transport in the spinal cord. Several theories exist about the initiation of regeneration. The most prevalent theory being that the NGF and other chemotactic substances present in the peripheral targets and inside the sheath surrounding the Schwann's cells contribute in some way to the initiation and maintenance of nerve regeneration.[74,75]

Role of Schwann's Cells in Regeneration

The Schwann's and glial cells surrounding the axons of peripheral nerves are heavily laced with collagen fibers, which provide tensile strength to the nerve. Unlike motor neurons in the spinal cord, Schwann's cells can reproduce freely and adapt to environmental demands during degeneration and regeneration of the axon. Schwann's cells and peripheral nerve neurons develop together from neural crest cells. The point at which the two cells separate from each other is unknown, although it is believed to be early, at the time of crest cell migration.[76] The number of Schwann's cells increases with the number of motor and sensory fibers during development; reduction in nerve fibers caused by damage or disease is associated with a decrease in Schwann's cell number.[77] The number of Schwann's cells in the nerve is believed to be regulated by the neuronal cell body. Bunge[78] reviewed tissue culture techniques to isolate Schwann's cells and examine their responses to axonal homogenates, mitogens, and spinal cord explants.[78,79] Biochemical, electron microscopic, and immunocytochemical analyses revealed that the Schwann's cells in contact with axons can generate basal lamina (collagen type IV, laminin, and heparan sulfate proteoglycan). During early neural development and regeneration, each group of unmyelinated axons is harbored within the cytoplasm of a series of ensheathing Schwann's cells; each myelinated fiber is provided with a series of Schwann's cells over its length.[78] The significance of this phenomenon is not fully understood.[79,80]

The roles of Schwann's cells during axonal degeneration, however, have been known for sometime. It appears from tissue culture studies that the proliferation of Schwann's cells after axonal injury results in release of a mitogenic substance that aids the degeneration of myelin.[80] During regeneration, the Schwann's cells also contribute to the ensheathment of sensory axons smaller than 1 μm in diameter and to the myelination of larger fibers. Axonal contacts may regulate the deposition of basal lamina by Schwann's cells, which appear to be capable of forming basal lamina without the aid of fibroblasts. Finally, fibroblasts and Schwann's cells both contribute to fibrous collagen present in the endoneurium. The fibroblasts alone contribute to formation of the perineurium. Regeneration of sensory axons is regulated through the distal segment of a degenerating peripheral nerve.[81]

MECHANISM OF NERVE REGENERATION

Peripheral nerve regeneration involves complex interactions among the nerve cell body, the proximal and distal axon stumps, and neurotrophic, neurite-promoting, and matrix factors. Soon after nerve injury, the neuronal cell body in the spinal cord becomes swollen, the Nissl bodies start to degenerate (chromatolysis), and the nucleus moves to the periphery in preparation for changing the metabolic priority from neurotransmitter synthesis to the production of materials required for axonal growth and elongation.[82] The cell must synthesize new messenger RNA, lipids, and proteins, especially cytoskeletal proteins such as tubulin and actin, neurofilaments, and gap-associated proteins. Gap-associated proteins, which are required to promote regeneration, are transported quickly to the distal end, at a rate of 400 mm per day. Synthesis of these proteins is 20–100 times higher during the early stages of regeneration than during normal growth. Cytoskeletal proteins, on the other hand, are moved much more slowly, at 5–6 mm per day.[83-85] Several investigators have suggested that during early regeneration the neuronal cell body behaves like an embryonic cell, with high growth-promoting activity and accumulation of growth factors.[86,87]

Cajal[88] was the first to demonstrate that viable nerve fibers grow out of the proximal stump of an injured neuron approximately 6 hours after injury, followed approximately 36 hours later by growth at the axon tip. Unlike the normal growth rate of 2–3 mm per day, regenerated axons grow through the scarred area slowly (approximately 0.25 mm/day; see Table 28-4 for rates of regeneration in different nerves).[14] The growth of proximal axon is preceded by formation of a growth cone at the tip of the proximal stump. This is rich in smooth endoplasmic reticulum, microtubules, microfilaments, large mitochondria, lysosomes, and other vacuolar and vesicular structures of unknown function. It was suggested that before the regenerated axons emerge from the proximal stump, the tip of the growth cone

TABLE 28-4
Nerve Regeneration Phases and Events in a Silicone Nerve Chamber

Phases	Days	Events	Promoting Factors
Fluid phase	1	Accumulation of exudates from proximal and distal segments	Neurotropic factors
Matrix phase	2–6	Coalescence to fibrin matrix	Fibrin
Cellular phase	7–14	Migration of cells from distal and proximal segments	Perineurial, endothelial, Schwann's cells
Axonal phase	15–21	Proximal segment growth (1–2 mm/day), myelination, distal segment entry	Capillaries, axons

Source: Data from LR Williams, N Danielsen, H Muller, et al. Influence of the Acellular Fibrin on Nerve Regeneration Success with the Silicone Chamber Model. In T Gordon, R Stein, P Smith (eds), Neurology and Neurobiology: The Current Status of Peripheral Nerve Regeneration. New York: Alan R. Liss, 1988:111–122; and LR Williams, S Varon. Modification of brain fibrin matrix formation in situ enhances nerve regeneration in silicone chambers. J Comp Neurol 1985;231:209–220.

adheres to collagen surrounding the degenerating distal stump. After this the transmembrane events involving internal actin filaments lead to the release of a proteolytic substance that dissolves the matrix, permitting elongation of the axon.[89-91]

Wallerian degeneration of the distal stump causes significant accumulation of collagenous material in and around the degenerating axon. By 28–35 days after injury, when robust regenerative activity is observed in the proximal axon, endoneurial collagen has accumulated in the distal segment, exerting pressure on the regenerated axons, decreasing their diameter and increasing the number of Schwann's cells per unit of length of the regenerated axon. The newly regenerated axons also exhibit short internodal lengths and a vascular supply that is only 60–80% of its original cross-sectional area, even after remyelination.[92,93] This is interpreted to mean that the growth of regenerated axons is significantly influenced by the environment at the distal segment.

In addition to an interaction between the distal and proximal stumps, various neurotrophic factors including NGF and neurite-promoting factors (NPFs) play a significant role in survival, neurite extension, and transmitter production in dorsal root ganglion and sympathetic neurons. The neurotrophic factors are required to regulate cell division, cell death, axonal outgrowth, and synapses during fetal development and to facilitate regeneration after nerve injury.

FACTORS PROMOTING NERVE REGENERATION

Neurotrophic Factors

Axotomy of peripheral nerve results in wallerian degeneration, which creates a microenvironment that allows successful regeneration and regrowth of nerve axons. In addition, neurotrophic factors promote the survival of specific neuronal populations. These include neurotrophins (NGF, NPFs, brain-derived neurotrophic factor, neurotrophin-3, and neurotrophin-4/5), the insulin-like growth factor, ciliary neurotrophic factor (NTF), and glial cell–derived growth factor. Molecular changes in the distal stump include regulation of neurotrophins, neural cell adhesion molecules, cytokines, and other soluble factors and their receptors.

NGF is synthesized in target tissue innervated by sympathetic and sensory neurons and is transported by retrograde transport to the neurons. NGF is a 26-kD polypeptide first isolated by Levi-Montalcini in 1987[94];

it influences neurite navigation, growth cone morphology, regeneration of proximal axons, and axonal elongation. Specific antibodies to NGF have been produced, and its genome has been located.[95-97] Its concentration in the blood is limited, and it is measured primarily in target cells.[68-70] Binding studies with iodine 125 have demonstrated the presence of specific and heterogeneous receptor sites in a variety of cells, including cells of neural crest origin,[96] sympathetic and sensory neuronal cells, and the rat PC-12 cell line.[98,99] The NGF-mediated modulation of PC-12 cell line results in transport of tyrosine hydroxylase and amino acids.[100] The human NGF receptor gene contains approximately 25 kilobases and at least three axons. A better understanding of the biochemistry and physiology of NGF and similar growth factors in peripheral nerves may be necessary before we understand their roles in promoting growth and regeneration of sensory nerves.[100-102]

The role of NGF needs further definition with regard to regeneration in responsive cells. It has been understood that the genome encoding the NGF receptor is the same in the sympathetic and sensory cells[103] and that the signal for gene expression and functional alteration originates from internalization of NGF at the cell surface.[104,105] Therefore, to understand its mechanism of action, it is necessary to determine the effects of NGF on membrane transport, membrane ruffling, and protein phosphorylation in regenerating nerves. Tanuichi,[106] Heumann, and their coworkers[107] reported the largest amounts of NGF and its receptors to be at the terminal ends of the peripheral nerves. Expression of its response appears to be related to the Schwann's cells in the neural sheaths surrounding both NGF-dependent and -independent axons, confirming the belief that the NGF is associated with repair mechanisms.

Similarly, NPFs are substrate-bound glycoproteins that bind to the polycationic substrata in nerve cultures and to the basal lamina of Schwann's cells in vivo. Laminin, for example, a major component of the Schwann's basal lamina, binds to collagen IV type proteoglycan to facilitate target navigation.[108-110] Fibronectin, another NPF, promotes elongation of neurites in tissue culture by enhancing adhesion to the substrata or matrix. Other molecules presumed to enhance neurite growth are cell adhesion molecules. Cell adhesion molecules are also membrane glycoproteins present in the developing nerve cells that promote adhesion.[111,112]

Hormones and Gangliosides

Estrogen, testosterone, insulin, and adrenal and thyroid hormones all reportedly affect nerve regeneration in varied and site-specific ways. For example, estrogen and insulin reportedly facilitate the growth of neurites in explants and tissue culture,[113–115] whereas testosterone and thyroid hormones stimulate regeneration of the sciatic nerve. Protease inhibitors such as glial-derived protease inhibitor[116] and leupeptin[117] inhibit the degeneration of the glial and distal axon, respectively, thus fostering nerve regeneration. Acidic fibroblast growth factor (FGF), a polypeptide present in brain tissue, appears to increase the number of myelinated fibers in the rat and to increase neurite growth in PC-12 cell cultures. Beneficial effects of FGF in vivo are related to Schwann's cell activation and blood supply enhancement. The action of FGF involves membrane-bound adenylcyclase and cyclic adenosine monophosphate and is significantly affected by adding forskolin, which in frog sciatic nerve increases sensory nerve regeneration by 40% or more. Similarly, inhibition of free radicals such as catalase[118,119] appears to enhance nerve regeneration by protecting the neurons from oxidative injury. The organic dye pyronin reportedly accelerates axonal sprouting at the nodes of Ranvier.[120] At present, FGF, forskolin, and leupeptin are being tested for their ability to promote nerve regeneration.

Another group of compounds that has shown significant promise during the last decade is the cerebral gangliosides. These glycolipids are constituents of the neuronal plasma membrane, synthesized in the neural soma and transported to the periphery by fast axonal transport. In vitro preparations of gangliosides, especially GM1 and GM3, have been shown to promote neurite regeneration.[121–123] Gangliosides administered to intact animals enhance the formation of nerve sprouts and neuromuscular junctions and thus improve muscle reinnervation. The clinical utility of these compounds, however, is still controversial.

In summary, peripheral nerve regeneration is a complicated process regulated by interactions between intrinsic factors and the peripheral target. An absence of inputs from the periphery or a disturbance at the spinal cord level would significantly delay or impede the process of regeneration.

Electrical-Electromagnetic Stimulation

The use of physical modalities such as pulsed electromagnetic field and direct current stimulation to promote healing of neural tissue can be traced to the eighteenth century. During the last two decades, interest has been rekindled in the use of ES and EMS to promote nerve regeneration. Despite differences in technique, such as whole body or partial body exposure, types of fields,

and duration of treatment, most studies have demonstrated that pulsed EMS enhances nerve regeneration, particularly axon sprouting.[124–127] Cumulatively, ES and EMS reportedly increase the number of axons below the suture line or guide tube. They promote the rate of axon regeneration, the number of motor axons forming synapses, the recovery of nerve conduction, and functional recovery.

In contrast, Murray and colleagues[128] and Cordiero and coworkers[129] have criticized these reports, noting that in most of them only one of many intrinsic factors was examined. The course of motor or sensory regeneration was not examined in relation to nerve conduction or other functional tests; pain tolerance was not documented; and the confounding role of ES and EMS in promoting collagen synthesis, which may enhance scar formation, was not evaluated.

Direct current ES also has been reported to enhance sciatic nerve regeneration in adult rats. Weak cathode current (10 µamp/cm², field strength 100 mV/cm) or distal placement of cathode increased the reinnervation of hind limb muscles in the rat, as measured by electromyography. Interestingly, weak current was effective only after cut-and-suture techniques[130] and not after crush injuries, which appears to contradict the observation that axon regeneration is smoother when the endoneurium is intact.[131]

Similarly, low-voltage, pulsed ES of partially denervated muscle has been shown to improve the rate of neurotization and thereby improve muscle reinnervation in experimental animals.[131,132] Herbison et al.[133] stimulated partially sectioned sciatic nerves of rats using implanted electrodes and examined the isometric contractile properties of the plantar flexors. ES at 10 Hz for 2–4 hours, five times a week for 6 weeks, produced an increase in muscle mass and tetanic tension; whereas similar stimulation for 8 hours caused a significant decrease in muscle size and tension, suggesting that lengthy ES regimens may actually inhibit axonal sprouting. Similar results were reported by Pestronk and Drachman,[18] who observed inhibition of axon sprouting after continuous ES of muscle. It is also possible that stimulating muscle during axon sprouting may inhibit reinnervation. Jaweed and colleagues[134] observed an inhibited muscle twitch force development in the partially denervated (L-5 sectioned) soleus muscles of adult male rats after whole body EMS at 3 G per day for 4 weeks. Soleus mass was decreased and fatigue was increased, suggesting that ES and EMS procedures must be administered cautiously. It appears that ES enhances nerve regeneration by promoting the matrix bridge formation, Schwann's cell activity, and fibroblast migration and proliferation.[135] The stimulation dosage and stage of nerve regeneration should be monitored carefully, and in treatment of humans, compliance and pain tolerance must be considered.

Surgical Procedures

After a nerve has been severed and the endoneurial tube disrupted, regeneration is poor at best. Several surgical procedures, such as conditioning lesions, sectioning, and resuturing with nerve grafts, have been employed to facilitate nerve regeneration across the gap.[136,137] The rate of nerve regeneration is inversely proportional to the length of the gap produced by a nerve lesion. As shown in Table 28-5, the number of myelinated and nonmyelinated regenerated axons of the rat sciatic nerve declined as the length of the gap between the proximal and distal nerve segments increased from 4 to 8 mm.[138,139] Although axons have been regenerated across a 10-mm gap in the absence of endoneurial tubes,[139-141] Fields and Ellisman[142] found these new axons to be severely impaired. It appears that nerve regeneration and axon elongation are significantly slowed by disturbances in the endoneurial environment, including the presence of endoneurial fibroblasts and associated collagen accumulation plus many minifascicles in place of the original large fascicles. Isolating the regenerating axons from this milieu appears to allow normal elongation to be re-established. Finally, some matrix factors such as fibrin facilitate axonal regeneration by providing a medium for growth and elongation. During nerve repairs, for example, the proximal and distal ends of a cut nerve are passed through a silicone or semipermeable membrane guide laden with fibrin matrix to facilitate nerve regeneration. Fibrin, a product of fibrinogen and fibronectin, interacts with many NPFs in ways that are not clearly understood.[143,144] Experimental and some clinical studies have used silicone tubes coated with laminin-fibronectin, dialyzed plasma, collagen gel, and phosphate buffer solution.[145]

The concept of bridging the gap dates back to 1880, when Gluck[146] used decalcified bone as a neural conduit. New procedures have been developed during the last decade to improve this model, with promising results.[141,142,147] The silicone nerve chambers first proposed by Lundborg and Hansson[17] and subsequently developed by Williams' group[143,144] are considered extremely useful in protecting nerve and fostering nerve regeneration.[15] These chambers offer several advantages. First, the surgical procedures during resuturing and placing the nerve in the nerve chambers probably cause far less trauma to the epineurium than other procedures. Second, the microenvironment is more conducive to regeneration because of the absence of mini-fascicles, scars, and distal nerve stump degeneration. Finally, growth-promoting and adhesion factors can be provided in these chambers. Williams and coworkers[140,144] have demonstrated phase-specific promotion of regeneration in silicone nerve chambers (see Table 28-4).

In summary, a number of new procedures have emerged in recent years that show promise for enhancing nerve regeneration. Although the mechanisms of action of these procedures are not understood completely, a combination of surgical procedures, physical modalities, and biochemical additives may improve nerve repair and regeneration even after traumatic injuries.

TABLE 28-5
Effect of the Length of Gap on Short-Term (8 Weeks) and Long-Term (36 Weeks) Regeneration of Rat Sciatic Nerve Axons

Area of Injury (Gap)	Proximal Segment		Gap		Distal Segment	
	My	Un	My	Un	My	Un
Normal	8,000	15,000	—	—	—	—
4 mm						
8 wk (N = 5)	—	—	9,000	14,000	13,500	10,500
36 wk (N = 6)	—	—	14,000	27,500	13,000	15,000
8 mm						
8 wk (N = 5)	—	—	4,600	10,500	7,000	7,500
36 wk (N = 6)	—	—	8,000	14,500	10,000	13,000

My = myelinated axons; Un = unmyelinated axons.
Source: Modified from C-B Jenq, LL Jenq, HM Bear, et al. Conditioning lesion of peripheral nerve changes regenerated axon numbers. Brain Res 1988;457:63–69.

REINNERVATION OF MUSCLE

The ultimate goal of nerve regeneration is to recreate a synapse with the end-organ. Motor nerve endings normally join the muscle at neuromuscular junctions, where they exert neurotrophic effects. Denervation of muscle causes dramatic changes in morphology, biochemistry, histochemistry, and physiology of the denervated muscle.[148-152] If the motor nerve is crushed, the axons regenerate smoothly and form another synapse, either in the original end-plate area or adjacent to it. Also, the latencies of nerve conduction to the muscle are delayed. Herbison, Jaweed, and others[150-152] demonstrated that crush denervation of rat sciatic nerve produces degenerative changes in the gastrocnemius soleus in accordance with the absence of nerve conduction and appearance of fibrillation potentials. Within 2–3 weeks after denervation, neuromuscular junctions are re-established, after which nerve conduction is normalized and fibrillation disappears (Figure 28-4).

Muscle reinnervation after crush lesions results in 80–90% recovery of the muscle mass, protein content, cross-sectional area, and isometric tension in the slow-twitch and fast-twitch muscle fibers.[150-152] Regeneration of crushed or severed axons may be induced by yet unknown chemotactic factors residing in the muscle. Several investigators have reported that the formation of extrajunctional acetylcholine receptors at the periphery of denervated muscle is one of the stimuli for terminal regeneration of the axon.[18,20] Herbison and colleagues [150,153] demonstrated that overwork induced by synergistic tenotomy of the rat plantaris and gastrocnemius, and daily swimming for 2–4 hours during reinnervation (or synapsis), may delay the recovery of muscle contractile proteins in the soleus. These findings support the hypothesis that physical or electrical activity during neuromuscular synapsis may impair muscle recovery.[133]

After sectioning or trauma, the regeneration of axons is quite slow compared with that after crush denervation. The rate of regeneration, navigation, and subsequent reinnervation is significantly delayed. Polyinnervation of muscle (i.e., multiple nerve endings synapsing with a single end-plate area) persists comparatively longer.

Partial injury to peripheral nerves causes degeneration of some axons while others are left intact. Regeneration of the intact axons causes reinnervation of the adjacent denervated muscle fibers. This process has been called *peripheral reinnervation of the muscle*.[18,20,154] After partial denervation in the rat, the intact axons regenerate within 3–5 days, and neuromuscular synapsis is re-established within 7–14 days. During this period, the neuromuscular junctions are polyinnervated. It normally takes 2–3 months for all synapses to

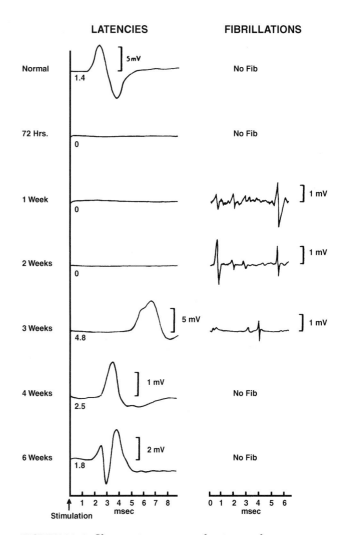

FIGURE 28-4 Changes in nerve conduction to the gastrocnemius muscle and fibrillation potentials after crush denervation of rat sciatic nerve. Note disappearance of nerve conduction for up to 2 weeks and appearance of fibrillation potentials within 72 hours after nerve injury. Nerve conduction to the muscle is re-established with delayed latency between 2 and 3 weeks after nerve crush. This is accompanied by disappearance of fibrillation potentials. By 6 weeks after nerve crush, the action potentials become polyphasic, indicating functional muscle reinnervation. (In this recording, positive wave is upward.) (Reprinted with permission from GJ Herbison, MM Jaweed, JF Ditunno, et al. Effect of over-work during reinnervation of rat muscle. Exp Neurol 1973;41:1–14.)

become completely functional.[153-155] Reinnervation enlarges the innervation field of a motor unit to three to five times its original size.[156,157] Jaweed and colleagues[154] performed bilateral L-5 spinal nerve sectioning and simultaneous unilateral synergistic tenotomy of the rat plantaris and gastrocnemius to induce overwork in the

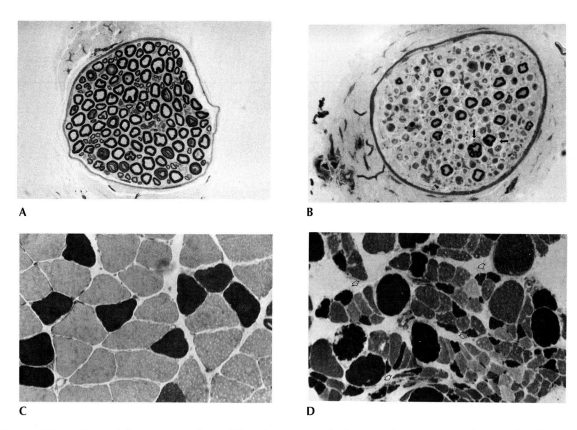

FIGURE 28-5 Effects of partial denervation in the rat. The soleus nerve and soleus muscle were examined 1–3 weeks after sectioning of the L-5 spinal nerve. **A.** Normal rat soleus nerve showing cross-section of the whole nerve and the axons. All of the larger axons are myelinated; whereas the smaller axons consist of both the myelinated and unmyelinated fibers. **B.** L-5 spinal nerve-sectioned rat soleus nerve, 1 week after partial denervation. Note a loss of approximately 90% of innervation caused by spinal nerve sectioning. Some of the intact axons hypertrophy and show myelin abnormalities (*arrows*). **C.** Normal rat soleus muscle showing slow-twitch (*light*) and fast-twitch (*dark*) muscle fibers. The differentiation of muscle fibers was based on the reactivity of myosin adenosine triphosphatase at pH 9.4. There is a normal distribution of the slow-twitch and fast-twitch fibers. **D.** L-5 spinal nerve-sectioned rat soleus muscle 3 weeks after partial denervation. Note significant hypertrophy of the intact slow-twitch and fast-twitch fibers (*rounded fibers*) caused by overwork. The small triangulated fibers are denervated. The medium-sized fibers are presumed to be peripherally reinnervated fibers (*arrowheads*).

soleus. After 7 days, there was no sparing of muscle loss caused by overwork. However, the intact (10–12%) myelinated axons of the soleus nerve showed significant compensatory hypertrophy (22.5% versus control; Figure 28-5). This observation suggests that intact myelinated axons can adapt to overwork-induced stress. It is not clear, however, whether continued stress for prolonged periods might not produce deleterious effects. The significance of this phenomenon can be appreciated in diseases that include partial nerve injuries, such as diabetes, poliomyelitis, and ALS.

Rotshenker[158] outlined three mechanisms for the induction of sprouting and synapse formation during peripheral regeneration of the axon: transneuronal, central, and peripheral. The transneuronal mechanism involves inducing axon sprouting of intact motor neurons within the spinal cord (motor, sensory, or other). The central mechanism, which assumes that the site of regulation of axon growth is the neuronal cell body, proposes that muscle fibers regulate sprouting and synapsis by retrograde axoplasmic transport. The peripheral mechanism implicates neural growth-promoting factors present in the motor neuron extensions, including nerve endings or branches and targets cells. Further investigations are needed to characterize the interaction of these mechanisms in promoting peripheral regeneration.

CONCLUSIONS

Peripheral nerve regeneration is a complex, well-coordinated process involving interactions between the neuron cell body in the spinal cord and its peripheral targets, the muscle or sympathetic neurons. Injury to the nerve induces wallerian degeneration of the axon below the site of the lesion, whereas the proximal stump undergoes immediate remodeling, terminal sprouting, and, ultimately synapsing with the target organ or neuron. The signal for regeneration is believed to be transmitted from either the degenerating axon or the target cell within 24 hours after the lesion. Depending on the degree and type of nerve injury, the nerve regeneration process begins within 36–48 hours after injury. The rate of elongation of the newly regenerated axon depends on the microenvironment surrounding it. Intrinsic factors influencing regeneration reside within and around the neuron: the neuronal cell body, proximal and distal stumps, NGF, NPF, and matrix factors. Optimal interactions among these factors determine the success of regeneration.

Extrinsic factors that can promote nerve regeneration or elongation include biologically active compounds such as hormones, neuroactive peptides, and glycoproteins such as cerebral gangliosides, FGF, forskolin, isoxanine, and pyronin. Inhibitors of wallerian degeneration such as leupeptin may be useful in promoting axon elongation. Pulsed electrical or electromagnetic field stimulation of regenerating nerves or axons has been promising. However, utmost caution must be taken as to when the regenerating nerve and not the muscle should be stimulated to enhance regenera-

tion. ES and EMS procedures may also facilitate regeneration by decreasing fibrosis in the perineurial, epineurial, and endoneurial sheaths. Successful axon regeneration is manifested by synapse with muscle or sympathetic neurons and re-establishment of nerve conduction. Excessive physical or electrical activity imposed on muscle during axonal synapsis (or muscle reinnervation) appears to have a negative influence. Although a suitable replacement for autogenous nerve grafts has not yet been identified, silicone nerve grafts laden with collagen and NGF and NPF are promising tools for protecting and enhancing nerve regeneration during surgery.

Finally, scientific progress during the last decade has brought the field of nerve repair research to the threshold of a new era. It is hoped that, in the future, it would be possible to combine the new surgical manipulations with neurotrophic and other factors or modalities to aid peripheral nerve regeneration. In addition, with the advances in the knowledge of genetic engineering, now it seems possible to design and install complex architectural feats for successful spinal cord repair and regeneration. One of the promising vectors for efficient gene delivery to spinal cord neurons with minimal toxicity is the recombinant herpes simplex virus. Also, a variety of grafted cells (fibroblasts, endothelial cells, Schwann's cells, and neuroprogenitor cells) can be implanted in encapsulated biopolymers to provide focal delivery, a conduit for neurite growth, or both.[159,160]

REFERENCES

1. Terzis JK, Smith KL. The Peripheral Nerve. New York: Raven, 1990.
2. Golgi C. In RK Daniel, JK Terzis (eds), Reconstructive Microsurgery. Boston: Little, Brown, 1977.
3. Cajal RS. Studien uber Nervenregenerationen. Leipzig, 1908. [in Weiss, 1941].
4. Sunderland S. The anatomy and physiology of nerve injury. Muscle Nerve 1990;13:771–784.
5. Seddon HJ, Medawar PB, Smith H. Rate of regeneration of peripheral nerves in man. J Physiol (Lond) 1943;102:191–215.
6. Hoffmann H. Local reinnervation in partially denervated muscle: a histopathological study. Aust J Exp Biol Med Sci 1950;28:383–397.
7. Weiss P. The technology of nerve regeneration: a review. J Neurosurg 1944;1:400–450.
8. Sherrington CS. On the anatomical constitution of nerves of skeletal muscles with remarks on recurrent fibers in

the ventral spinal root. J Physiol (Lond) 1894;17:211.
9. Eccles JC, Sherrington CS. Number and contraction values of individual motor units examined in some muscles of the limb. Proc R Soc Lond B Biol Sci 1930;106:326.
10. Erlanger J, Gasser H. Electrical Signs of Nervous Activity. Philadelphia: University of Pennsylvania Press, 1937.
11. Thomas PK, Jones B. The cellular responses to nerve injury. J Anat 1967;100:45–55.
12. Oldfors A. Permeability of perineurium of small nerve fascicles: an ultrastructural study using ferritin in rats. Neuropathol Appl Neurobiol 1981;7:183–194.
13. Novikoff AB, Quintana N, Villaverde H, et al. Nucleoside phosphatase and choline esterase activities in dorsal root ganglion and peripheral nerve. J Cell Biol 1966;29:525–545.

14. Miller RG. Injury to peripheral motor nerves. Muscle Nerve 1987;10:698–710.
15. Seckel BR. Enhancement of peripheral nerve regeneration. Muscle Nerve 1990;13:785–800.
16. Lundborg G, Dahlin LB. Structure and Function of Peripheral Nerves. In RH Gelberman (ed), Operative Nerve Repair and Reconstruction, Vol I. Philadelphia: JB Lippincott, 1991:3–17.
17. Lundborg G, Hansson H. Regeneration of peripheral nerve through a preformed tissue space. Brain Res 1979;178:573–576.
18. Pestronk A, Drachman DB. Motor nerve sprouting and acetylcholine receptors. Science 1978;199:1223–1225.
19. Kuno M, Miyata Y, Munoz-Martinez EJ. Differential reaction of fast and slow alpha motoneurons to axotomy. J Physiol (Lond) 1974;240:725–739.

20. Brown MC, Holland RC, Hopkins WG. Motor nerve sprouting. Annu Rev Neurosci 1981;4:17–24.

21. Seddon HJ. Three types of nerve injury. Brain 1943;66:237–261.

22. Sunderland S. Nerves and Nerve Injuries. Edinburgh: Churchill Livingstone, 1978;88–132.

23. Simpson JA. Nerve Injuries, General Aspects. In RK Daniel, JK Terzis (eds), Reconstructive Microsurgery. Boston: Little, Brown, 1977;244–264.

24. Lundborg G. Structure and function of the intraneural microvessels as related to trauma, edema formation and nerve function. J Bone Joint Surg 1975; 57:725.

25. Costaldo JE, Ochoa JL. Mechanical injury of peripheral nerves, fine structure and dysfunction. Clin Plast Surg 1984;11:9.

26. Bradley WG. Disorders of Peripheral Nerves. Oxford: Blackwell Scientific, 1974.

27. Waller A. Experiments on the section of glossopharyngeal nerves of frog and observations of the alterations produced thereby in the structure of their primitive fibers. Philos Trans R Soc Lond 1850;140:423.

28. Orgel M, Terzis JK. Epineurial versus perineurial repair: an ultrastructural and electrophysiologic study of nerve regeneration. Plast Reconstr Surg 1977;60:80–91.

29. Lundborg G, Gelberman RH, Minteer-Convery M, et al. Median nerve compression in the carpal tunnel functional response to the experimentally induced controlled pressure. J Hand Surg 1982; 7:252–259.

30. Fowler TJ, Danta G, Gilliatt RW. Recovery of nerve conduction after a pneumatic tourniquet, observations on the hind limb of the baboon. J Neurol Neurosurg Psychiatry 1972;35:638.

31. Swan KG, Swan RC. Gunshot Wound Pathophysiology and Management. Littleton, MA: PSG, 1980.

32. Landon DN, Hall HS. The Myelinated Nerve Fiber. In DN Landon (ed), The Peripheral Nerve. London: Chapman & Hall, 1976.

33. Sunderland S. Nerve lesion in the carpal tunnel syndrome. J Neurol Neurosurg Psychiatry 1976;39:615–626.

34. Mackinnon SE, Dellon AL. Experimental study of chronic nerve compression. Hand Clin 1986;2:639–650.

35. Goodall RJ. Nerve injuries in fresh fractures. Texas State J Med 1956; 52:93.

36. Lundborg G, Rydevik B. Effects of stretching the tibial nerve of the rabbit. J Bone Joint Surg 1973;55B:390–401.

37. Leone J, Ochs S. Anoxic block and recovery of axoplasmic transport and electrical excitability in nerve. J Neurobiol 1978;9:229.

38. Gilliatt RW. Acute Compression Block. In AJ Sumner (ed), The Physiology of Peripheral Nerve. Philadelphia: WB Saunders, 1972;113.

39. Maruhashi J, Wright EB. Effect of oxygen lack in the single isolated mammalian (rat) nerve fiber. J Neurophysiol 1967;30:434.

40. Yates SK, Hurst LM, Brown LF. The pathogenesis of pneumatic tourniquet paralysis in man. J Neurol Neurosurg Psychiatry 1981;44:759–767.

41. Silverside J. The neurological sequelae of electrical injury. J Can Med Assoc 1964;91:195–204.

42. Ponten B, Ericson U, Johansson S. New observations on tissue changes along the pathway of the current in electrical injury. Scand J Plast Reconstr Surg 1970;4:75–82.

43. Cavanaugh JB. Effects of x-irradiation on the proliferation of cells in peripheral nerve during wallerian degeneration in the rat. Br J Radiol 1968;41: 272–281.

44. Little JB. Cellular effects of ionizing radiation. N Engl J Med 1968;278:308–315;369–376.

45. Love S. An experimental study of nerve regeneration after x-irradiation. Brain 1983;106:39–54.

46. Lundborg G, Schildt B. Microvascular permeability in irradiated rabbits. Acta Radiol 1971;10(Suppl):311–320.

47. Gentili F, Hudson AR, Hunter G. Peripheral nerve injection injury: an experimental study. Neurosurgery 1979;4:244–253.

48. Hudson AR. Nerve Injection Injuries. In K Terzis (ed), Microconstruction of Nerve Injuries. Philadelphia: WB Saunders, 1987;173–179.

49. Meuli-Simmen C, Meuli M, Hutchins GM, et al. The fetal spinal cord does not regenerate after in vitro transection in large mammalian model. Neurosurgery 1996;39:555–560.

50. Sims TJ, Durgun MB, Gilmore SA. Transplantation of sciatic nerve segment into normal glia-depleted spinal cords. Exp Brain Res 1999;125:495–501.

51. Borgens RB. Electrically mediated regeneration and guidance of adult spinal axons into polymeric channels. Neuroscience 1999;91:251–264.

52. Longo FM, Yang T, Hamilton S, et al. Electromagnetic field influences NGF activity and levels following sciatic nerve transection. J Neurosci Res 1999; 15:230–237.

53. Chen DF, Tonegawa S. Why do mature CNS of mammals fail to re-establish connections following injury: functions of bcl2. Cell Death Differ 1998; 10:816–822.

54. Schwartz M, Lazarov-Spiegler O, Rapalino O, et al. Potential repair of rat spinal cord injuries using stimulated homologous macrophages. Neurosurgery 1999;44:1041–1045.

55. Amar AP, Levy MI. Pathogenesis and pharmacological strategies for mitigating secondary damage in spinal cord injury. Neurosurgery 1999;44:1027–1039.

56. Kennel PF, Finiels F, Revah F, et al. Neuromuscular functional impairment is not caused by motor neuron loss in FALS mice: an electromyographic study. Neuroreport 1996;7:1427–1431.

57. Niebroj-Dobosz J, Janik P. Amino acids as transmitters in amyotrophic lateral sclerosis. Acta Neurol Scand 1999;100:6–11.

58. Beal MF. Coenzyme Q10 administration and its potential for treatment of neurodegenerative diseases. Biofactors 1999;9:261–266.

59. Francis K, Bach JR, DeLisa JA. Evaluation and rehabilitation of patients with motor neuron disease. Arch Phys Med Rehabil 1999;80:951–963.

60. Bradley WG, Shapshak P, Delgado S, et al. Morphometric analysis of the peripheral neuropathy of AIDS. Muscle Nerve 1998;21:1188–1195.

61. Rizzuto N, Cavallaro T, Monaco S, et al. Role of HIV in the pathogenesis of distal symmetrical peripheral neuropathy. Acta Neuropathol (Berl) 1995;90:244–250.

62. Suzuki T, Mizuno K, Yashima S, et al. Characterization of polyol pathway in Schwann cells isolated from sciatic nerves. J Neurosci Res 1999;57:495–503.

63. Zochodne DW, Nguyen C. Increased peripheral nerve microvessels in early experimental diabetic neuropathy: quantitative studies of nerve and dorsal root ganglia. J Neurol Sci 1999;166:40–46.

64. Suh KS, Oh SJ, Woo JT, et al. Effect of cilostazol on the neuropathies of streptozotocin-induced diabetic rats. Korean J Int Med 1999;14:30–34.

65. Bhardwaj SK, Sandhu SK, Sharma P, et al. Impact of diabetes on CNS: role of signal transduction cascade. Brain Res Bull 1999;49:155–162.

66. van Dam PS, Bravenboer B, van Asbeck BS, et al. High rat food vitamin E content improves nerve function in streptozotocin-diabetic rats. Eur J Pharmacol 1999;376:217–222.

67. Thomas PK. Diabetic neuropathy: mechanism and future treatment options. J Neurosurg Neuropsychiatry 1999;67:277–279.

68. Green DA, Stevenson MJ, Obrosova I, et al. Glucose-induced stress and programmed cell death in diabetic neuropathy. Eur J Pharmacol 1999;375:217–223.

69. Dyck PJ, Giannini C. Pathologic alterations in the diabetic neuropathies of humans: a review. J Neuropathol Exp Neurol 1996;55:1181–1193.

70. Katz B. Nerve Muscle and Synapse. New York: McGraw-Hill, 1966.

71. Peters A, Palay SL, Webster HD. The Fine Structure of the Nervous System: The Neurons and Supporting Cells. Philadelphia: WB Saunders, 1976.

72. Lundborg G, Danielsen N. Injury Degeneration and Regeneration. In RH Gelberman (ed), Operative Nerve Repair and Reconstruction. Philadelphia: JB Lippincott, 1991.

73. Smith J, Baroffio A, Dupin E, et al. Role of Extrinsic Factors in the Development of the Peripheral Nervous System from the Neural Crest. In E Scarpini, MG Fioro, D Pleasure, et al. (eds), Peripheral Nerve Development and Regeneration: Recent Advances and Clinical Applications. Philadelphia: WB Saunders, 1989;3–11.

74. Varon S, Skaper SD, Manthorpe M. Trophic activities for dorsal root and sympathetic ganglionic neurons in media conditioned by Schwann and other peripheral cells. Dev Brain Res 1981;1:73–87.

75. Longo FM, Manthorpe M, Skaper SD, et al. Neurotrophic activities accumulate in vivo within silicone nerve regeneration chambers. Brain Res 1983;261:109–117.

76. LeDourian H. The Neural Crest. London: Oxford University Press, 1982.

77. Aguayo AJ, Epps J, Charron L, et al. Multipotentiality of Schwann cells in cross anatomized and grafted myelinated and unmyelinated nerves. Quantitative microscopy and radioautography. Brain Res 1976;104:1–20.

78. Bunge RP. Tissue culture observations relevant to the study of axon-Schwann cell interactions during peripheral nerve development and repair. J Exp Biol 1987;132:21–34.

79. Slazer JL, Bunge RP, Glaser L. Studies of Schwann cell proliferation. III. Evidence for the surface localization of the neurite mitogen. J Cell Biol 1980;84:767–778.

80. Spencer P. Reappraisal of the model for bulk axoplasmic flow. Nature 1972;240:283–285.

81. Stoll G, Muller HW. Nerve injury, axonal degeneration and neural regeneration. Brain Pathol 1999;9:313–325.

82. Bray D. Isolated Chick Neurons for the Study of Axonal Growth. In G Banker, K Goslin (eds), Culturing Nerve Cells. Cambridge, MA: MIT Press, 1991;137–154.

83. Lasek RJ, Hoffman PN. Neuronal Cytoskeleton, Axonal Transport and Axonal Growth. In R Goldman, T Pollard, J Rosenbaum (eds), Microtubules and Related Proteins: Cell Proteins. Cold Spring Harbor, NY: Cold Spring Harbor Laboratory, 1976;1021–1049.

84. Bisby MA, Redshaw JD, Carlsen RC, et al. Growth-Associated Proteins (GAPS) and Axonal Regeneration. In T Gordon, RB Stein, PA Smith (eds), Neurology and Neurobiology: The Current Status of Peripheral Nerve Regeneration. New York: Liss, 1988;35–52.

85. Stoeckel K, Thoenen H. Retrograde axonal transport of nerve growth factor: specificity and biological importance. Brain Res 1975;85:337–341.

86. Richardson PM, Verge VM. The induction of a regenerative propensity in sensory neurons following peripheral axonal injury. J Neurocytol 1986;15:585–594.

87. Smith PA, Shapiro J, Gurtu S, et al. The response of the ganglionic neurons to axotomy. In T Gordon, RB Stein, PA Smith (eds), Neurology and Neurobiology: The Current Status of Peripheral Nerve Regeneration. New York: Liss, 1988;15–23.

88. Cajal RS. Degeneration and Regeneration of the Nervous System, Vol 1. London: Oxford University Press, 1928.

89. Crockett SA, Kiernan JA. Acceleration of peripheral nerve regeneration in vivo. Attraction of regenerating axons by diffusable factors derived from cells in distal nerve stumps of transected peripheral nerves. Brain Res 1982;253:1–12.

90. Sunderland S. The Future. In S Sunderland (ed), Nerve Injuries and Their Repair: A Critical Appraisal. Edinburgh: Churchill Livingstone, 1991;519–525.

91. Letourneau PC. Cell to substratum adhesion and guidance of axonal elongation. Dev Biol 1975;44:92.

92. Sunderland S, Bradley KC. Denervation atrophy of the distal stump of a severed nerve. J Comp Neurol 1950;93:401–409.

93. Ducker TB, Kempe LG, Hatyes GJ. The metabolic background of peripheral nerve surgery. J Neurosurg 1969;30:270–280.

94. Levi-Montalcini R. The nerve growth factor 35 years later. Science 1987;237:1154–1162.

95. Herrup K, Shooter EM. Properties of the beta nerve growth factor receptor in development. Cell Biol 1975;67:118–125.

96. Johnson EM, Tanuichi M, Clark HB, et al. Demonstration of retrograde transport of nerve growth factor receptor in the peripheral and central nervous system. J Neurosci 1987;7:923–929.

97. Stephani A, Sutter A, Zimmerman A. Nerve growth factor in serum. J Neurosci Res 1987;17:25–35.

98. Vale RD, Shooter EM. Assaying binding of nerve growth factor to cell surface receptors. Meth Enzymol 1985;109:21–39.

99. Schechter AL, Bothwell MA. Nerve growth factor receptors on PC12 cells: evidence for two receptor classes with differing cytoskeletal association. Cell 1981;24:867–874.

100. Rowland EA, Muller TH, Goldstein M, et al. Cell-free detection and characterization of a novel nerve growth factor-activated protein kinase in PC12 cells. J Biol Chem 1987;262:7504–7513.

101. Chandler CE, Parsons LM, Hosang M, et al. A monoclonal antibody modulates the interaction of nerve growth factor with PC12 cells. J Biol Chem 1984;259:6882–6889.

102. Ross AH, Grob P, Bothwell M, et al. Characterization of nerve growth factor receptor in neural crest tumors using monoclonal antibodies. Proc Natl Acad Sci U S A 1984;81:6681–6685.

103. Green SH, Greene LA. A single Mr approximately 103,000 125I-beta-nerve growth factor-affinity-labeled species represents both the low and high affinity nerve growth factor receptor. J Biol Chem 1986;261:15316–15326.

104. Chao MV, Bothwell MA, Ross AH, et al. Gene transfer and molecular cloning of the human NGF receptor. Science 1986;232:518–521.

105. Seeley PJ, Kieth CH, Shelanski ML, et al. Pressure microinjection of nerve growth factor into the nucleus and cytoplasm. J Neurosci 1983;3:1488–1494.

106. Tanuichi M, Clark HB, Johnson EM. Induction of nerve growth factor receptor in Schwann cells after axotomy. Proc Natl Acad Sci U S A 1986;83:4094–4098.

107. Heumann R, Korsching S, Bandtlow C, et al. Changes in nerve growth factor synthesis in non-neuronal cells in response to sciatic nerve transection. J Cell Biol 1987;104:1623–1631.

108. Baron-Van Evercooren A, Kleinman HK, Seppa HE, et al. Fibronectin promotes fast Schwann cell growth and motility. J Cell Biol 1982;93:211–216.

109. Lander AD. Molecules that make axons grow. Mol Neurobiol 1987;1: 213–245.

110. Cornbrooks CJ, Carrey DJ, Timpl R, et al. Immunohistochemical visualization of fibronectin and laminin in adult rat peripheral nerve and peripheral nerve cells in culture. Soc Neurosci Abstr 1982;8:240.

111. Dodd J, Jessell TM. Axon guidance and the pattern of neuronal projections in vertebrates. Science 1987;242:692–699.

112. Dyck PJ, Karnes J, Lais A, et al. Pathological Alterations of Peripheral Alterations of Humans. In PJ Dyck, PK Thomas, EH Lambert, et al. (eds), Peripheral Neuropathy. Philadelphia: WB Saunders, 1984;760–870.

113. Vita G, Dattola R, Girlanda P, et al. Effects of steroid hormones on muscle reinnervation after nerve crush in rabbit. Exp Neurol 1983;80:279–287.

114. Varon S, Bunge RP. Trophic mechanisms in the peripheral nervous system. Annu Rev Neurosci 1978;1:327–361.

115. Bothwell M. Insulin and somatomedin MSA promote nerve growth factor–independent neurite formation by cultured chick dorsal root ganglion sensory neurons. J Neurosci Res 1982;8:225–231.

116. Milesi H. Nerve grafting. Clin Plast Surg 1984;11:105–113.

117. Hurst LC, Badalamente MA, Ellstein J, et al. Inhibition of neural and muscle degeneration after epineural neuropathy. J Hand Surg 1984;9:564–572.

118. Longo FM, Hyman EG, Davis GE, et al. Neurite-promoting factors and extracellular matrix components accumulating in vivo within nerve regeneration chambers. Brain Res 1984; 309:105–117.

119. Muller H, Williams LR, Varon S. Nerve regeneration chamber: evaluation of exogenous applied by multiple injections. Brain Res 1987;413:320–326.

120. Keynes RJ. The effect of pyronin on sprouting and regeneration of mouse motor nerves. Brain Res 1982;253:13–18.

121. Gorio A, Vitadello M. Ganglioside Prevention of Neuronal Functional Decay. In FJ Seil, E Herbert, BM Carlson (eds), Progress in Brain Research, Vol 71. Amsterdam: Elsevier, 1987;289–325.

122. Horowitz SH. Therapeutic strategies in promoting peripheral nerve regeneration. Muscle Nerve 1989;12:314–322.

123. Gorio A, Marini P, Zanoni R. Muscle reinnervation. III. Motoneuron sprouting capacity, enhancement by gangliosides. Neuroscience 1983;8:417–429.

124. Ito H, Bassett CAL. Effect of weak pulsing electromagnetic fields on neural regeneration in rat. Clin Orthop 1983;181:283.

125. Ploitis MJ, Zanakis ME, Albala BJ. Facilitated regeneration in the rat peripheral nerve system using applied electrical fields. J Trauma 1988; 28:1375.

126. Raji ARM, Bowden REM. Effects of high peak electromagnetic fields on degeneration and regeneration of peroneal nerve in rats. J Bone Joint Surg 1983;65:478–492.

127. Wilson DH, Jagadeesh P, Newman PP, et al. The effects of pulsed electromagnetic energy on peripheral nerve regeneration. Ann N Y Acad Sci 1974; 238:575.

128. Murray HM, O'Brien WJ, Orgel MG. Pulsed electromagnetic fields and peripheral nerve regeneration in cat. J Bioelect 1984;3:19.

129. Cordiero PG, Seckel BR, Miller CD, et al. Effects of high intensity magnetic field on sciatic nerve regeneration in the rat. Plast Reconstr Surg 1989;83: 207.

130. McDevitt L, Fortner P, Pomerantz B. Application of weak electrical field to the hind paw enhances sciatic motor nerve regeneration in the adult rat. Brain Res 1987;416:308–314.

131. Borgens RB. Stimulation of neuronal regeneration and development by steady electrical fields. Adv Neurol 1988;47:547–564.

132. Hoffman H. Acceleration and retardation of process of axon sprouting in partially denervated muscles. Aust J Exp Biol Med Sci 1952;30:541–566.

133. Herbison GJ, Jaweed MM, Ditunno JE. Electrical stimulation of sciatic nerve of rats after partial denervation of soleus muscle. Arch Phys Med Rehabil 1986;67:79–83.

134. Jaweed MM, Herbison GJ, Ditunno JF, et al. Effect of electromagnetic stimulation on terminal regeneration-caused peripheral reinnervation of the rat soleus. In Proceedings of the International Symposium on Peripheral Nerve Regeneration. American Association of Electromyography and Electrodiagnosis; August 1989, Washington, DC.

135. Shen N, Zhu J. Experimental study using a direct current electrical field to promote peripheral nerve regeneration. J Reconstr Microsurg 1995; 11:189–193.

136. Carlsen RC. Delayed induction of the cell body response and enhancement of regeneration following a condition/test lesion of frog peripheral nerve at 15 Co. Brain Res 1983;279:9–18.

137. Bisby MA, Keen P. The effect of conditioning lesion on the regeneration rate of peripheral nerve axons containing substance P. Brain Res 1985;336:201–206.

138. Jenq C-B, Jenq LL, Bear HM, et al. Conditioning lesion of peripheral nerve changes regenerated axon numbers. Brain Res 1988;457:63–69.

139. Lundborg G, Dahlin LB, Danielsen N, et al. Nerve regeneration in silicone chambers: influence of gap length and of distal stump components. Exp Neurol 1982;76:361–375.

140. Williams LR, Longo FM, Powell HC, et al. Spatial temporal progress of peripheral nerve regeneration within a silicone chamber: parameters for a bioassay. J Comp Neurol 1983;218: 460–470.

141. LeBeau JM, Ellisman MH, Powell HC. Ultrastructural and morphometric analysis of long term peripheral nerve regeneration through silicone tubes. J Neurocytology 1988;17:161–172.

142. Fields RD, Ellisman MH. Axons regenerated through silicone tube splices. I. Conduction properties. Exp Neurol 1986;92:48–60.

143. Williams LR, Danielsen N, Muller H, et al. Influence of the Acellular Fibrin on Nerve Regeneration Success with the Silicone Chamber Model. In T Gordon, RB Stein, PA Smith (eds), Neurology and Neurobiology: The Current Status of Peripheral Nerve Regeneration. New York: Liss, 1988; 111–122.

144. Williams LR, Varon S. Modification of brain fibrin matrix formation in situ enhances nerve regeneration in silicone chambers. J Comp Neurol 1985;231:209–220.

145. Terris DJ, Cheng ET, Utley DS, et al.

Functional recovery following nerve injury and repair by silicon tubulization: comparison of laminin-fibronectin, dialyzed plasma, collagen gel, and phosphate buffered solution. Auris Nasus Larynx 1999;26:117–122.

146. Gluck T. Uber Neuroplastik auf dem Wege der Transplantation. Arch Klin Chir 1880;25:606–616.

147. Aebischer V, Guenard SR, Winn RF, et al. Blinded semipermeable guidance channel support peripheral nerve regeneration in the absence of a distal nerve stump. Brain Res 1988;454:170–187.

148. Gutmann E, Malichna J, Syrovy I. Contractile properties and ATPase activities in fast and slow muscles of the rat during denervation. Exp Neurol 1972;36:488.

149. Herbison GJ, Jaweed MM, Ditunno JF, et al. Effect of overwork during reinnervation of rat muscle. Exp Neurol 1973;41:1–14.

150. Jaweed MM, Herbison GJ, Ditunno JF. Denervation and reinnervation of fast and slow muscles: a histochemical study in rats. J Histochem Cytochem 1975;23:808–827.

151. Jaweed MM, Herbison GJ, Ditunno JF. Direct electrical stimulation of rat soleus during denervation and reinnervation. Exp Neurol 1982;75:589–599.

152. Lai KS, Jaweed MM, Herbison GJ, et al. Changes in nerve conduction and phosphorus magnetic resonance (^{31}P-NMR) spectra of the gastrocnemius-soleus muscles of rats during denervation and reinnervation. Arch Phys Med Rehabil 1992;73:1155–1159.

153. Herbison GJ, Jaweed MM, Ditunno JF. Effect of swimming on reinnervation of rat skeletal muscle. J Neurol Neurosurg Psychiatry 1974;37:1247–1251.

154. Jaweed MM, Herbison GJ, Ditunno JF. Overwork-induced axonal hypertrophy in the soleus nerve of the rat. Arch Phys Med Rehabil 1989;68:706–709.

155. Coers C, Tellerman-Toppett N, Gerard J-M. Terminal innervation ratio in neuromuscular disease. I. Methods and controls. Arch Neurol 1973;29:210–214.

156. Thompson W, Jansen JKS. Extent of sprouting of remaining motor units in partly denervated immature and adult rat soleus. Neuroscience 1977;5:523–535.

157. Hopkins WG, Brown MC. Distribution of nodal sprouts in paralyzed or partially denervated mouse muscle. Neuroscience 1982;7:37–44.

158. Rotshenker S. Transneural, Peripheral and Central Mechanisms for the Induction of Sprouting. In T Gordon, RB Stein, PA Smith (eds), Neurology and Neurobiology: The Current Status of Peripheral Nerve Regeneration. New York: Liss, 1988;63–75.

159. Breakfield XO. Gene therapy for spinal cord injury. ISRT Res Dig 1994;6:3.

160. Breakfield X, Jacobs A, Wang S. Genetic Engineering for CNS Regeneration. In MH Tuszynski, JH Kordower (eds), CNS Regeneration: Basic Science and Clinical Advances. New York: Academic Press, 1999.

29

Autonomic Function in the Isolated Spinal Cord

Brenda S. Mallory

The most devastating effects of a complete spinal cord injury (SCI) are the complete loss of sensation and voluntary motor activity below the level of the lesion. In contrast, the basic vital functions, such as the circulation, alimentation, defecation, and micturition, appear to be grossly maintained although devoid of supraspinal control. Closer observation confirms that significant dysfunction in these basic homeostatic mechanisms is present in all persons with SCI. In this chapter, the autonomic responses associated with upper motor neuron type lesions of the spinal cord are discussed. In this situation, organization of the neuronal circuitry subserving a given autonomic response is independent of supraspinal control, except of course via the cranial nerves, which by definition are not involved by SCI. The altered autonomic responses may be organized in either the spinal cord or the peripheral autonomic ganglia.

ORGANIZATION OF THE AUTONOMIC NERVOUS SYSTEM

The autonomic nervous system is divided into the parasympathetic and sympathetic nerves. Efferent neuronal cells of the autonomic nervous system, which are located in either the brain stem or the spinal cord, are termed *preganglionic neurons*. These cells project preganglionic fibers, which synapse on postganglionic neurons located in various ganglia and plexuses outside the CNS. The postganglionic neuron, in turn, projects a postganglionic fiber to a specific target organ or effector tissue.

The sympathetic division of the autonomic nervous system has sympathetic preganglionic neurons (SPNs) located in the intermediolateral (IML) cell column of the thoracic and upper lumbar spinal cord, and these project sympathetic preganglionic fibers to postganglionic neurons in either the paravertebral chain or the various prevertebral plexuses. Parasympathetic preganglionic neurons are found in the brain stem and sacral spinal cord. There are four parasympathetic brain stem nuclei: nucleus Edinger-Westphal, superior and inferior salivatory nuclei, and the dorsal vagal complex of the medulla.[1] Sacral parasympathetic preganglionic fibers project to intramural and extramural ganglia of the pelvic viscera.

It is generally assumed that all preganglionic neurons are cholinergic and have nicotinic postsynaptic receptors,[2] but in the cat thoracolumbar intermediate zone there are also neuron cell bodies that are reactive for the peptides enkephalin, neurotensin, somatostatin, and substance P.[3] The presence and release of a variety of substances capable of effecting or modifying neurotransmission have led to the abandonment of the traditional view of "one neurotransmitter for one neuron."[2] Neurotransmitters such as acetylcholine have a duration of action measured in milliseconds, whereas actions of peptides can last minutes.

Most postganglionic sympathetic neurons release norepinephrine (NE) as their primary neurotransmitter.[4] Most of the NE is taken up by the nerve terminal, but some escapes into the plasma, where it can be measured and correlated with activity of sympathetic neurons.[2] Skin sweat glands that subserve thermoregulation are innervated by sympathetic cholinergic postganglionic fibers acting on muscarinic (blocked by atropine) receptors. Postganglionic parasympathetic junctions are also muscarinic cholinergic. Target tissues for postganglionic autonomic fibers include cardiac muscle, sinoatrial and atrioventricular nodes, smooth muscle, secretory glands, and sensory receptors,[1,5,6] fat cells,[7] hepatocytes,[1,8] and lymphoid organs, including thymus, spleen, lymph nodes, and gut-associated lymphoid tissue.[1] There are three different muscarinic receptors (M1, M2, M3).[9] NE receptors are α-receptors and β-receptors. α-Receptors are usually excitatory and β-receptors are inhibitory, with exceptions such as the excitatory effect of the β-receptor to increase myocardial contractility and heart rate. The α_1-receptors are usually postsynaptic excitatory and the α_2-receptors are usually presynaptic inhibitory. Presynaptic sympathetic nerve terminal α_2-receptors inhibit NE release. β-Receptors are divided into β_1- and β_2-receptors. The activation of α_1-, β_1-, and β_2-receptors results in the increased synthesis of cyclic adenosine monophosphate, whereas the activation of α_2-receptors results in a reduction of synthesis of cyclic adenosine monophosphate.[9] It is now recognized that in addition to the previously mentioned classical neurotransmitters, a variety of cotransmitters coexist in single neurons of the autonomic ganglia. In addition, the enteric nervous system contains independent integrative neural circuits controlling complex local activities.

Sympathetic and parasympathetic preganglionic neurons receive afferent fibers from both somatic and visceral sources and projections from the CNS. Some autonomic reflexes are complete at the spinal level, and others have a supraspinal relay (see Chapter 4).

RENOVASCULAR FUNCTION

Afferent renal nerves contain fibers from (1) renal mechanoreceptors that are sensitive to alterations in intrarenal pressure produced by ureteral occlusion, renal vein occlusion, increases in renal arterial perfusion pressure, or application of external mechanical stimuli to the kidney; and (2) renal chemoreceptors: R1 chemoreceptors are activated by renal ischemia and R2 chemoreceptors by renal ischemia and changes in the ion composition of the fluid in the renal interstitium.[10] Afferent renal nerves project to supraspinal structures via the dorsal root ganglion and thoracic spinal cord.[11,12] It is unlikely that afferent renal nerves project via the vagus nerve to the nodose ganglia.[13]

Preganglionic neurons to the human kidney are in spinal cord segments T-5 to L-3.[14] The fibers that make up the renal plexus derive from the celiac plexus, thoracic and lumbar branches of the splanchnic nerves, superior and inferior mesenteric plexus, intermesenteric nerves, and superior hypogastric plexus (also known as the *inferior mesenteric ganglion* [IMG]). Renal nerve

fibers that enter the kidney come from the renal plexus and course along the renal artery and vein to enter the hilus. Postganglionic adrenergic fibers innervate the arteriolar wall and tubular epithelium in both the proximal and distal tubules.[14] Evidence of a vagal efferent parasympathetic innervation of the kidney is lacking.[12]

Retrograde transport of pseudorabies virus injected into the rat kidney has identified infected preganglionic sympathetic neurons in the IML as well as infected neurons in the same segments in the dorsal horn and ventral horn (thought to be labeled via synaptic input from association neurons with shared contact with SPNs).[15] Neurons were also labeled in the rostral ventromedial and ventrolateral medulla, the medullary raphe nuclei, the pontine A5 region, and the paraventricular hypothalamus. Few infected spinal neurons were found outside the levels where SPNs were labeled, suggesting that propriospinal pathways are less important than supraspinal pathways in the regulation of renal function.[15]

Decreases in efferent renal sympathetic nerve activity (ERSNA) result in decreases in renal tubular solute and water resorption, whereas an increase in renal nerve activity results in increases in solute and water resorption.[14] The antidiuretic and antinatriuretic effects of ERSNA are mediated by NE on postjunctional α_1-adrenoceptors on renal tubules.[12]

An increase in efferent renal nerve activity causes renin release via stimulation of postjunctional β_1-adrenoceptors on the renin-containing juxtaglomerular granular cells.[12] Nonneural stimuli also mediate renin release: (1) NaCl sensed at the macula densa, (2) humoral factors with angiotensin II, vasopressin, endothelin, and adenosine inhibiting renin release, and (3) the renal vascular baroreceptor mechanism with increases in renal perfusion pressure decreasing renin secretion and with decreases in renal perfusion pressure resulting in increased prostacyclin synthesis and increased renin secretion.[16]

There are cardiorenal and renorenal reflex mechanisms for the regulation of intravascular volume.[12] Stimulation of renal mechanoreceptors (as occurs with ureteral obstruction) initiates a reflex arc with afferent renal nerve projection to the ipsilateral dorsal root ganglia, a supraspinal CNS relay (including the neurohypophysis for increases in antidiuretic hormone [ADH] and oxytocin), and efferent projection, resulting in inhibition of the contralateral ERSNA.[12] The clinical importance of this renorenal reflex would be the contralateral diuresis and natriuresis in response to ipsilateral urine obstruction resulting in unchanged total urine flow and solute excretion.[12] The afferent limb of the cardiorenal reflex is in the vagus nerve from left atrial Paintal type B receptors, which are activated by left atrial distention.

A central integrative relay involves the brain stem and hypothalamus. The efferent limb consists of a neural pathway, decreasing ERSNA, and a hormonal pathway, decreasing ADH, resulting in diuresis and natriuresis.[12] Supraspinal renorenal and cardiorenal reflexes are lost in SCI; however, there is evidence of arterial baroreceptor reflex regulation of ERSNA at a spinal level in animals.[17] This spinal pathway may eventually compensate for lost supraspinal vagal pathways that occur after spinal cord transection.

SCI has specific effects on urinary excretion of salt and water. Compared with control subjects, quadriplegic subjects have lower urine sodium excretion and lower urine volume[18] but higher urine osmolality. Clinically complete quadriplegic subjects were able to decrease sodium excretion in response to a low-sodium (20 mmol) diet,[19] indicating that central control of the sympathetic nervous system is not required for sodium conservation in response to dietary sodium restriction. There was also a decrease in mean arterial pressure (MAP) and a decrease in plasma water content in response to dietary sodium restriction in quadriplegics. The increase in plasma renin activity in response to salt restriction in quadriplegic subjects was likely caused by the decrease in MAP.

Basal plasma renin activity and plasma aldosterone levels are higher in both paraplegic and quadriplegic persons than in control subjects with intact spinal cords.[18] Paraplegic persons have greater urinary sodium excretion and urinary potassium excretion and urine osmolality than control subjects or quadriplegic persons. The cause of the increased sodium and potassium excretion in paraplegic subjects is unknown. Some 5–10% of persons with SCI have hypo-osmolar hyponatremia, which is generally asymptomatic.[18] The cause of hyponatremia appears multifactorial, including high fluid intake, reset osmostat, and inappropriate ADH.[20,21] It has been suggested that thiazide diuretics be avoided in patients with high SCI as they may have a decreased prostaglandin response, making them more susceptible to thiazide-induced hyponatremia related to renal tubular prostaglandin inhibition.[21]

The effect of renal mechanisms on blood pressure control is discussed in the following section.

CARDIOVASCULAR FUNCTION

Afferent fibers from the heart project via either the sympathetic cardiac nerves or the vagus nerve and are intermingled.[22] Parasympathetic afferent fibers from sensory receptors in the heart have cell bodies in the jugular and nodose ganglia and are conveyed via the cardiac branches of the parasympathetic vagus nerve and project centrally to the nucleus tractus solitarius (NTS). There is also evidence in animals that a portion of vagal afferent neurons in the nodose ganglion project to the upper cervical spinal cord via a supraspinal pathway not involving dorsal root ganglia.[23] The sympathetic afferents course in the inferior cervical and thoracic sympathetic cardiac nerves, then via white rami communicantes to cell bodies in the dorsal root ganglia (T-1 to T-5). The traditional view is that afferent sympathetic cardiac fibers mediate cardiac nociception and afferent vagal cardiac fibers mediate cardiovascular reflexes.[22] However, vagal afferent fibers may have some role in the mediation of cardiac nociception such as pain referred to the head and neck (perhaps via afferent projections to the cervical spinal cord), and afferent sympathetic fibers may also transmit some cardiovascular reflexes.[22]

Baroreceptors are located in the carotid sinuses and in the walls of the aortic arch. A decrease in arterial blood pressure inhibits firing, and an increase in blood pressure increases firing in afferent baroreceptor fibers that are carried in the vagus and glossopharyngeal nerves to the NTS of the medulla.[24] Baroreceptor-mediated sympathoinhibition is predominantly a brain stem reflex mediated via ventral medullary neurons.[25-27] There is also evidence that baroreceptor inhibition of sympathetic activity can be exerted at the spinal cord level, suggesting that some fibers conveying baroceptor afferent information course directly to the spinal cord.[17,28,29]

Peripheral chemoreceptors that sense a decrease in oxygen or an increase in carbon dioxide are located in the carotid bodies and the aorta and have afferent fibers in the glossopharyngeal and vagus nerves.[24] The brain also has chemoreceptors that sense carbon dioxide. In response to systemic hypoxia, perfusion of vital organs needs to be maintained. Hypoxia results in activation of peripheral chemoreceptors, and hypercapnia results principally in activation of central chemoreceptors.[30] Chemoreceptor reflexes result in vasoconstriction, principally in skeletal muscle vascular beds[31] via activation of the sympathetic adrenergic system.

The medulla oblongata is the most important region in the brain that controls blood pressure.[32] Medullary neurons are critical for (1) integration of arterial baroreceptor and chemoreceptor reflexes,[33] (2) arterial pressure elevations associated with excitation of somatic afferent fibers in response to pain[34] or to exercise,[35] and (3) the potent increases in sympathetic discharge and arterial pressure produced by either rendering the brain stem ischemic (the cerebral ischemic reflex)[36] or by mechanical distortion (Cushing's reflex).[32,37]

Cardiac preganglionic sympathetic neurons in humans are found in spinal cord segments T-1 to T-4, whereas the preganglionic neurons for the peripheral vasculature are found mainly in spinal cord segments T-1 to L-2.[38] A small proportion of the neurons in the IML column are interneurons.[39] The cholinergic SPNs innervate the adrenal medulla or noradrenergic neurons in sympathetic ganglia, which in turn innervate blood vessels and the heart. The heart is also innervated by three branches of the vagus nerve (superior cervical cardiac, inferior cervical cardiac, thoracic cardiac). Preganglionic efferent parasympathetic axons in these branches form synapses with neurons in the ganglia of the cardiac plexus.

As the autonomic effects associated with increased carbon dioxide are sympathetic responses, quadriplegic persons would not be expected to show sympathetic responses to increased carbon dioxide because efferent pathways from the brain stem vasomotor center to the SPNs are disrupted. This supposition is supported by the results of a study of mechanically ventilated quadriplegic subjects.[40] No change in heart rate could be detected in the quadriplegic subjects in response to elevation of carbon dioxide[40]; however, in another study, six quadriplegic subjects with complete lesions above the sympathetic outflow responded to breathing carbon dioxide by increased blood pressure, both in the horizontal and the tilted positions, which suggests either a peripheral or spinal cord effect of hypercapnia.[41]

Disorders of cardiovascular regulation are common after SCIs that disrupt supraspinal control of thoracic sympathetic outflow (Table 29-1). Both hypotension and hypertension can occur, depending on the time after injury and associated complications.

Mechanisms of Hypotension

After a high spinal cord transection, systemic arterial pressure decreases,[42] owing to a decrease in cardiac output and in total peripheral resistance. Resistances of the muscle and visceral vascular beds are decreased equally.[43] With no connection between the medullary baroreceptor systems and the spinal cord, sympathetic activity cannot be increased to compensate for postural changes.

In contrast to intact subjects, quadriplegic subjects have a lower resting concentration of catecholamines,[44-46] and there is no significant increase in either NE or epinephrine when quadriplegic subjects change from a lying to a sitting position[44]; this appears to be caused by a reduction in NE release and not to a decrease in NE clearance.[47] Resting skin blood flow is greater in quadriplegic than in control subjects.[44,48] This is in keeping with observations of diminished resting vasoconstrictor tone and much lower plasma NE levels. Submaximal and maximal exercise results in increases in plasma NE in controls and paraplegic subjects but not in quadriplegic subjects.[46]

TABLE 29-1
Cardiovascular Status in Spinal Cord Injury

Item	Control Non–Spinal Cord Injury	Chronic Quadriplegia
Hypercapnic vasoconstriction	Present	Variable
Cardiovascular sympathovagal balance	Normal	Normal
Cardiovascular parasympathetic tone	Normal	Decreased
Cardiovascular sympathetic tone	Normal	Decreased
Resting systolic blood pressure	Normal	Normal or decreased
Resting diastolic blood pressure	Normal	Normal or decreased
Resting heart rate	Normal	Normal
Resting plasma renin	Normal	Increased
Resting plasma aldosterone	Normal	Increased
Resting plasma antidiuretic hormone	Normal	Normal or increased
Nocturnal increase in antidiuretic hormone	Present	Absent
Change in mean arterial pressure with sitting	Increased	Decreased
Change in mean arterial pressure with recumbency	Decreased	Increased
Baseline sympathetic efferent activity	Normal	Decreased
Resting plasma catecholamines	Normal	Decreased
Change in plasma catecholamines with exercise	Increased	None

Immediately after cervical spinal cord transection in animals, discharges of cervical, cardiac, hepatic, gastric, adrenal, renal, and lumbar paravertebral chain sympathetic nerves were reduced,[49-53] whereas discharges of mesenteric and splenic nerves were not.[51,53,54] Subsequent removal of afferent input to the spinal cord did not change the rate of the ongoing neural activity, indicating that the spontaneous activity remaining after SCI was likely generated either within the spinal cord or at ganglionic sites.[55] Pacemaker type potentials that could produce spontaneous activity have not been observed in SPNs; this suggests that the ongoing activity of SPNs seen after spinal cord transection is instead generated by intraspinal systems extrinsic to the SPN.[39]

The activity in mesenteric sympathetic nerves after acute spinal cord transection in anesthetized cats was not as prominent in decerebrate unanesthetized cats. That suggests that the maintained sympathetic activity noted in the study mentioned previously may have been an artifact of anesthesia,[56] but nevertheless, the level of sympathetic activity that remained after acute spinal cord transection in cats was unable to provide significant vasomotor tone.[55] The firing pattern of mesenteric and other sympathetic nerves, however, changed from a rhythmic, synchronized discharge to a less synchronized one when brain stem descending input was disrupted by spinal cord transection.[52,57,58] It may be that the new desynchronized discharge of SPNs could not support vascular tone adequately, regardless of the magnitude of SPN discharge. A less likely explanation is that the maintained mesenteric nerve activity in anesthetized cats after acute spinal cord transection did not subserve vasomotor functions.[43]

Mechanisms of Blood Pressure Normalization

After Spinal Cord Injury

In humans, orthostatic hypotension occurs after SCI,[59] but after a time the ability to maintain blood pressure in a sitting position improves.[24] Improvement may be caused by the development of spinal reflex control of blood pressure or by long-term regulation by renal fluid control. For a review, see Cole.[60]

To investigate the effect of sympathetic activity on blood pressure control, Osborn and coworkers[61] studied spinal cord–transected rats whose (1) sodium and water intake was maintained at pretransection levels, and (2) urine outflow was unobstructed to preserve normal renal function. Arterial pressure was normal by day

9 after the spinal cord transection.[61] Although blood pressure returned to pretransection levels, the heart rate, which had fallen significantly after the spinal lesion, remained low. The normalization of arterial pressure does not appear to be caused by (1) increased vascular sensitivity to a constantly low level of sympathetic activity or (2) a steadily increasing level of sympathetic nerve discharge.[61]

Postsynaptic α_1-adrenoceptor supersensitivity does not appear to contribute to the maintenance of blood pressure or autonomic hyperreflexia after SCI, at least in animals.[61,62] Osborn and coworkers recorded changes in arterial pressure in response to injection of phenylephrine into atropinized rats with either cervical spinal cord transection or ganglionic blockade.[61] The results were similar for both groups, indicating that pressor sensitivity at least to exogenous catecholamines does not increase after chronic spinal cord transection in rats. The development of denervation supersensitivity would have increased pressor sensitivity. This lack of increased pressor sensitivity agrees with investigations of adrenergic receptor density in persons with SCI.[63,64] In contrast, Arnold and coworkers found a left shift of the dose-response curve for local infusions of noradrenaline to reduce dorsal foot vein diameter, suggesting that α-adrenoceptor responsiveness is increased in quadriplegic persons.[65] The enhanced pressor response to NE in humans with cervical SCI reported by Mathias and colleagues[66] may not have been caused by denervation sensitivity, as suggested, but may have resulted from the absence of baroreceptor-mediated sympathoinhibition. Lack of denervation supersensitivity after SCI may be caused by periodic episodes of sympathetic hyperreflexia.[61]

Before, but not after, spinal cord transection in rats, ganglionic blockade resulted in a profound decrease in arterial pressure.[61] This indicates that the normalization of arterial pressure after spinal cord transection in rats cannot be attributed to spinally generated sympathetic activity. This is in agreement with Maiorov et al.,[67] who found low levels of ERSNA in awake rats after spinal transection. Blood pressure and basal ERSNA decreased after cord transection, but by day 6 postspinal transection, the blood pressure had returned to baseline but the ERSNA remained low. This is consistent with evidence in humans of low sympathetic nerve activity in skin and muscle nerves after SCI.[68,69] Normalization of blood pressure may occur because autoregulatory controllers of blood flow completely dominate within 24 hours after spinal cord transection, with the result that any remaining sympathetic vasoconstrictor activity is without effect. Hypotension after spinal cord transection may, therefore, be principally the result of a decrease in sympathetic activity to vascular beds with relatively weak autoregulatory properties, such as skin and skeletal muscle.[61]

The development of spasticity may contribute to the recovery of arterial pressure owing to increased central venous volume resulting from enhanced venous return and to physical compression on the arterial side of the skeletal muscle beds, which would increase vascular resistance.[61]

The vasoconstrictor activity of the renin-angiotensin system and arginine vasopressin (AVP; also known as *ADH*), as well as renal sympathetic nerve activity, may enhance renal retention of sodium and water, which would influence arterial pressure in the long-term. Research findings show that quadriplegic persons have increased plasma renin levels and high normal aldosterone levels,[18,59] probably owing to renin release by the juxtaglomerular cells in response to the decreased renal perfusion that accompanies low arterial pressures.[70] Renin acts on angiotensinogen in the plasma, forming angiotensin, which is converted to angiotensin II, a major vasoconstricting hormone. Increased release of aldosterone is probably a direct effect of the increased serum renin level.[24]

Over a period as short as 12–36 hours after spinal cord transection in dogs, baseline arterial pressure has been shown to be directly related to the level of salt and water intake.[71] After spinal cord transection, rats were in part dependent on angiotensin II vasoconstrictor activity for maintenance of arterial pressure.[61] Long-term quadriplegic individuals exhibit decreased urinary sodium excretion and expansion of the extracellular fluid compartment.[72,73]

The secretion of AVP by the posterior pituitary gland is predominantly controlled by (1) changes in plasma osmolality, which are sensed by osmoreceptors in the hypothalamus, and (2) changes in blood volume and blood pressure relayed from cardiovascular receptors in the carotid sinus and thorax via the glossopharyngeal and vagal cranial nerves to the NTS and thence to the paraventricular and supraoptic nuclei of the hypothalamus.[74] No differences in resting levels of AVP have been identified between control and quadriplegic subjects.[74] Control subjects demonstrate a nocturnal increase in AVP level, which was not seen in quadriplegic or paraplegic individuals.[75] The absence of a nocturnal increase in AVP was associated with an increased urine volume at night relative to controls, although no difference was found between daytime and nighttime urine output in quadriplegic or paraplegic subjects. Kiline et al. hypothesized that daytime

pooling of blood in paralyzed legs with associated reduction of central venous pressure was followed by a redistribution of volume during recumbency, resulting in increased blood pressure, which prevented nocturnal increases in AVP and subsequent nocturnal polyuria. It has been suggested that SCI patients with severe nocturnal polyuria should have AVP levels checked and if necessary be treated with desmopressin acetate (DDVAP) at bedtime.[76]

Infusion of hypertonic saline causes plasma AVP to increase in both control and quadriplegic subjects; however, at any given level of plasma osmolality, plasma AVP tended to be higher in the quadriplegic subjects than in the control subjects.[18] Unlike control subjects, quadriplegic subjects demonstrated an increase in MAP without an increase in heart rate as a result of hypertonic saline infusion. In quadriplegic subjects water loading resulted in normal suppression of urine osmolality, but subnormal free water clearance during maximal water diuresis, despite appropriately suppressed levels of plasma AVP.[18] Plasma AVP increased after head-up tilt in both control and quadriplegic subjects, but the increase was significantly greater in the quadriplegic group.[74] These studies indicate that quadriplegic persons have appropriate cardiovascular and osmotic control of AVP secretion, but increased sensitivity to the pressor effect of AVP. The increase in postural release of AVP may be responsible for the oliguria seen in persons with SCI after prolonged sitting.[74]

Infusion of AVP did not change MAP or heart rate in control subjects, but did result in a marked increase in MAP and bradycardia in quadriplegic subjects. The bradycardic effect of AVP in quadriplegic subjects was probably the result of baroreflex activation of the intact vagal efferents secondary to the increase in MAP. The reason for the pressor response is not clear; it may have been caused by increased sensitivity to peripheral pressor vascular effects of AVP or because baroreflex-mediated inhibition of sympathetic tone was interrupted by the spinal cord lesion.[74]

In control subjects and in persons with SCI below the L-1 level, blood pressure increases with sitting and is lower when they are recumbent. In quadriplegic subjects, blood pressure is lower when sitting than when lying down.[18] This increase in blood pressure during recumbency has been attributed to fluid shifts into the central compartment and subsequent increased venous return and stroke volume. This expansion of central blood volume after recumbency and the accompanying elevation in blood pressure inhibiting the release of AVP may explain the diuresis associated with recumbency in quadriplegic persons.[77]

AUTONOMIC HYPERREFLEXIA

Autonomic hyperreflexia (also known as *autonomic dysreflexia*) is manifested by hypertension, sweating, headache, and bradycardia.[60,78,79] and is most often associated with SCI at or above the T-6 level. This disorder is reported to affect 30–90% of quadriplegic and high paraplegic persons.[80] In individuals with SCI, common sources of afferent stimulation that result in autonomic hyperreflexia include bladder distention, pressure sores, childbirth, and rectal distention.[81] Afferent input enters the spinal cord below the level of the spinal cord lesion and projects to the IML cell column via propriospinal pathways. The spinal sympathetic pathways linking the supraspinal cardiovascular centers with the peripheral sympathetic outflow are interrupted at the level of the injury, but the parasympathetic efferent pathways through the vagus nerve, as well as the afferent arc of the baroreceptor reflex through the glossopharyngeal and vagus nerves, are intact after SCI. Bradycardia results from activation of efferents in the vagus nerve coursing to the sinoatrial node. Descending sympathoinhibitory projections through the spinal cord that would normally result in vasodilatation are disrupted by SCI, and the bradycardia alone is not adequate to reduce blood pressure. Treatment requires that the eliciting cause be eliminated or that pharmacologic treatment be instituted. For reviews see Lee et al.,[82] Naftchi and Richardson,[83] Comarr and Eltorai,[84] Amzallag,[85] and Colachis.[86]

Evidence for Removal of Descending Supraspinal Inhibition in Autonomic Hyperreflexia

Spinal sympathoexcitatory reflexes, which are under such strong supraspinal inhibition that they are not observable in some intact animals, may become evident after spinal cord transection. Studies in rats demonstrated a spinal component of the somatosympathetic reflex in both intact and spinal cord–transected animals. The spinal component of the reflex was sometimes difficult to demonstrate in intact animals, and, in fact, the spinal component of some sympathetic reflexes appeared to be under tonic inhibition by supraspinal systems.[39]

Sympathetic hyperactivity after spinal cord transection might be caused as much by disinhibition of sensory pathways as by direct disinhibition of the sympathetic systems themselves. Supraspinal and propriospinal somatocardiovascular reflexes were dem-onstrated in the rat.[87] In intact rats, noxious mechanical stimulation to any segmental skin area, but particularly from the paws, elicited increases in heart rate, blood pressure, ERSNA, and cardiac sympathetic efferent nerve activity. In animals with acute spinal transections, stimulation of thoracic segments with noxious stimuli elicited even larger increases in heart rate, blood pressure, and sympathetic nerve activity, whereas stimulation applied to other areas such as the paw or perineum resulted in little or no increases. The propriospinal somatocardiovascular excitatory reflex had a strong segmental localization and was under the influence of tonic descending supraspinal inhibition.

Evidence for Altered Reflex Responses in Sympathetic Preganglionic Neurons in Autonomic Hyperreflexia

Spinal cord transection sometimes results in increased sympathetic responses to afferent stimulation or in decreased sympathetic responses to a given afferent stimulation.[39] For example, in intact rats nonnoxious stimulation of the chest wall decreased adrenal nerve activity and adrenal catecholamine secretion, whereas noxious stimulation of the chest elicited increases in adrenal nerve activity and adrenal catecholamine secretion. After spinal cord transection both stimuli increased adrenal nerve activity. Spinal cord transection, therefore, converted a previously sympathoinhibitory response to a nonnoxious stimulus into a sympathoexcitatory one.[39]

Research has shown that activation by capsaicin of chemoreceptors and mechanoreceptors in the small intestine, peripheral vasculature, or urinary bladder of rats produces a depressant response in cardiovascular SPNs.[88] However, bladder distention or intravesical capsaicin, which activates afferent C fibers,[89] in spinal cord–transected rats activated a reflex excitatory response conveyed by pelvic nerve afferents that probably involved activation of SPNs via propriospinal pathways.[88] Altered reflex responses in SPNs may account for the massive autonomic hyperreflexia displayed by quadriplegic persons, particularly responses to stimuli arising from the rectum and urinary bladder.

The afferent pathway that mediates the autonomic hyperreflexia in response to bladder distention in humans is not clear. Complete sacral dorsal rhizotomy reduced but did not eliminate autonomic hyperreflexia in response to intradural sacral ventral root stimulation for bladder emptying.[90] The afferent pathway eliciting autonomic hyperreflexia may have been afferent fibers in the pelvic nerve entering the cord by the ventral roots, as the existence of ventral root afferents has been well established.[91] It is also possible that the afferent pathway was via thoracic and lumbar dorsal roots via afferent fibers in the hypogastric nerve.

Krassioukov and Weaver[92] identified morphologic changes in SPNs after spinal cord transection in rats. SPNs caudal to the spinal transection demonstrated dendritic degeneration and a decrease in soma size within 1 week after transection, which was reversed by 1 month posttransection. Krenz and Weaver[93] found that the time frame of degeneration and recovery of the dendritic arbor of SPNs correlated to the time frame for first reduced and then enhanced vasomotor reflexes in the rat. The SPNs caudal to the SCI appear to be innervated by spinal interneurons after loosing descending synaptic input.

There are problems to consider in studying sympathetic regulation organized in a spinal model.[39] After acute SCI, experimental results may be obscured by spinal shock. In chronic SCI the system the researcher studies may not be the spinal component of normal sympathetic regulation, but a new system formed by regeneration and plasticity.[39]

Spinal Neurotransmitters in Autonomic Hyperreflexia

The excitatory amino acid glutamate may be the neurotransmitter that mediates the viscerosympathetic spinal reflexes involved in generating autonomic hyperreflexia.[94] Maiorov and coworkers demonstrated that the glutamate receptors N-methyl-D-aspartate and alpha-amino-3-hydroxy-5-methyl-4-isoxazolepropionic acid contributed to the increase in MAP secondary to colonic distention in rats after acute and chronic spinal cord transection.[94]

Management of Autonomic Hyperreflexia

Pharmacologic treatment is aimed primarily at producing direct vasodilatation (calcium channel blockers, nitrates, hydralazine, diazoxide), central (spinal) α_2-adrenoceptor agonist activity (clonidine),[95] or ganglionic blockade (mecamylamine).[96] The most frequently used medication is nifedipine.[79] A 10-mg capsule of nifedipine can be bitten and swallowed in a hypertensive emergency and repeated in 30 minutes. Nifedipine can also be given 30 minutes before a pro-

cedure likely to cause autonomic hyperreflexia.[85] In light of reports linking nifedipine to increased mortality in patients with stable angina, caution is recommended when administering nifedipine to elderly patients with SCI and primary hypertension or cardiovascular disease.[95]

α_1-Adrenoceptor blocking agents have been used in the prophylactic management of autonomic dysreflexia. Prazosin, 3 mg twice a day, was effective in reducing the number of severe episodes of autonomic hyperreflexia and in reducing the average increase in systolic and diastolic blood pressure during an episode.[97] Recurrent symptoms of autonomic hyperreflexia such as headache, sweating, and flushing of the face, together with an increase in blood pressure, have been successfully treated with the once-a-day selective α_1-adrenergic blocking drug, terazosin (1–10 mg in adults and 1–2 mg in pediatric patients).[98] Phenoxybenzamine is a longacting α-adrenergic blocker commonly used[97] in a dose of 20–40 mg per day to prevent autonomic hyperreflexia. There are conflicting reports as to the effectiveness of phenoxybenzamine in preventing autonomic hyperreflexia.[97]

OTHER CARDIOVASCULAR DYSFUNCTION

Although the most important sequelae of autonomic cardiovascular dysfunction after SCI are related to disorders of blood pressure control,[60] studies have identified additional alterations in cardiovascular function in persons with high SCI. Those dysfunctions may be attributed to autonomic nervous system dysfunction. For a review of cardiovascular control after SCI see Mathias and Frankel.[99]

In contrast to normal subjects and those with normal variant ST-segment elevation, quadriplegic subjects have been found to have significant multilead ST elevation on electrocardiography[100] that is not altered by exercise. Persons with acute severe injury to the cervical spinal cord have an increased incidence of ventricular and supraventricular arrhythmias and cardiac arrest, but the arrhythmogenic state does not extend into the chronic injury period.[100] The maximal heart rate during arm exercise has been reported to be significantly lower for quadriplegic than for paraplegic subjects.[101] Significantly lower values for stroke volume, cardiac output, and cardiac index were obtained for both paraplegic and quadriplegic groups when compared with the observed values for the control group without SCI. Quadriplegic subjects have even lower values for stroke volume and cardiac output than paraplegic subjects. These differences may have been caused by reduced sympathetic stimulation, but other factors resulting from a lower metabolic rate and smaller active skeletal muscle mass are probably involved.[102]

PULMONARY FUNCTION

Pulmonary problems are common after SCI. They are secondary to impairments in inspiratory and expiratory function, with associated abnormalities in gas exchange that are largely the result of ineffective cough mechanisms. The muscles of respiration are of three groups: (1) the diaphragm, (2) the intercostals and accessory muscles of respiration, and (3) the abdominal muscles.[103] The diaphragm is innervated by the phrenic nerve (C-3 to C-5) and is the principal muscle of respiration. The intercostal muscles are innervated from the corresponding thoracic segments of the spinal cord. Secondary respiratory muscles are the muscles attached to the ribs, such as the sternocleidomastoid and scalene, that do not usually function in respiration but are called on to provide for hyperventilation in healthy subjects or ventilation in subjects with cardiorespiratory dysfunction. Abdominal muscles are predominantly expiratory as far as respiratory function is concerned.

The parasympathetic nervous system via the vagus nerve is the dominant pathway in the control of bronchial smooth muscle tone.[104] Stimulation of cholinergic nerves results in bronchoconstriction, mucus secretion, and bronchial vasodilation.[104] There is also an inhibitory nonadrenergic noncholinergic (i-NANC) pathway that mediates bronchodilitation.[104] The neurotransmitters of the i-NANC pathway are colocalized with acetylcholine in the parasympathetic nerves. The main neurotransmitter of the i-NANC system in human airways appears to be nitric oxide (NO) that may be coreleased with acetylcholine and vasoactive intestinal polypeptide (VIP).[104] Both NO and VIP have potent smooth muscle-relaxing properties. Although β_2-adrenergic receptors are expressed on human bronchial smooth muscle, no innervation from the sympathetic nervous system has been shown.[104] These β_2-adrenoceptors are activated by circulating NE or epinephrine released from the adrenal medulla.[105] The bronchial circulation is controlled by sympathetic vasoconstrictor and parasympathetic vasodilator nerves.[106] It is thought that the bronchial vasculature is under tonic sympathetic influence, resulting in vasoconstriction mediated by α-adrenoceptors.[106] Pulmonary vascular tone is also

regulated by nonadrenergic, noncholinergic neural mechanisms and humoral mechanisms. For a review, see Barnes and Liu.[107]

There are vagal nerve afferents from pulmonary receptors.[108] Slowly adapting receptors and rapidly adapting receptors detect lung volume and changes in lung volume.[109] These afferents terminate in the NTS in the medulla and can reflexly inhibit or excite inspiration.[109] The rapidly adapting receptors in the large bronchi and carina appear to be the most important receptors for the initiation of cough.[110] There is also sensory C-fiber nociceptor innervation of the airways. C-fiber axon stimulation causes bronchial vasodilatation via a peripheral vagal axon reflex mechanism dependent on the release of vasodilator neuropeptides from axon terminals.[111] An axon reflex occurs when the impulse propagated centrally by the stimulation of one branch of the peripheral end of an afferent axon invades a second peripheral branch of the same axon, resulting in the release of neuropeptides from the peripheral end of the second afferent axon branch. Activation of C-fiber afferents in the lungs and airways also causes reflex bronchial vasodilation with afferent and parasympathetic efferent pathways in the vagus nerve.[111] Respiration is also controlled by chemosensors that detect hypoxia and hypercapnia. Peripheral chemoreceptors are located in the carotid and aortic bodies and also project to the NTS.[109] Medullary neurons are also chemosensitive to CO_2.[112]

After SCI, the supraspinal respiratory centers in the brain stem continue to function normally, so that the level of the SCI largely determines impairment in respiratory function. In acute quadriplegia, inspiratory capacity is decreased approximately 40%, and diminished expiratory capacity results in severe impairment of coughing.[113] Long-term quadriplegic patients have been found to have significantly lower values for tidal volume, forced vital capacity, forced expiratory volume in 1 second, and maximum breathing capacity than either paraplegic or control subjects in response to maximal arm exercise.[102] There is some evidence that exercise training can increase forced vital capacity in quadriplegic subjects.[114] Loveridge and coworkers describe changes in breathing patterns during the first year after complete C-5 to C-8 SCI.[115] They identified significantly impaired ventilatory lung function in sitting at 3 months postinjury with improvement between 3 and 6 months. They also found that the sigh reflex is retained in quadriplegic subjects, but they take more big breaths in supine than in sitting.[115]

Several reports describe airway hyperresponsiveness to aerosolized methacholine, histamine, and ultrasonically nebulized distilled water in otherwise healthy subjects with quadriplegia.[116-119] Aerosolized ipratropium bromide blocked airway hyperreactivity associated with aerosolized methacholine and ultrasonically nebulized distilled water, but did not inhibit airway hyperreactivity associated with histamine inhalation.[117] Nebulized β-agonist metaproterenol sulfate blocked both histamine and methacholine-associated airway hyperreactivity.[117] In one report, subjects with high paraplegia (T-1 to T-6) who demonstrated airway hyperresponsiveness to methacholine had significantly lower forced expiratory volume in 1 second than subjects who did not demonstrate hyperreactivity.[119] Singas and coworkers hypothesized that loss of the ability to stretch airways by deep breathing may cause airway hyperresponsiveness in quadriplegic subjects.

The effect of afferent input on parameters of respiration has been investigated in SCI subjects. Normally, ventilatory drive is increased by hypercapnia (primarily via central chemoreceptor stimulation) and hypoxia (primarily via peripheral chemoreceptor stimulation).[30] Conflicting reports exist on the response of quadriplegics to hypercapnia. Several studies have found a blunted ventilatory drive in response to hypercapnia,[120-122] whereas another reports normal ventilatory chemosensory responses to hypercapnia and hypoxia.[123] The later results may have been caused by the inclusion of quadriplegic subjects with incomplete spinal lesions. Manning and coworkers[121] could not attribute the blunted respiratory drive found in quadriplegic subjects to expiratory muscle weakness or altered chest wall mechanics. They hypothesized that the blunted ventilatory drive in response to hypercapnia may be caused by loss of supraspinal control of the sympathetic nervous system as similar blunted responses have been reported previously in individuals with autonomic dysfunction. Unlike Manning and colleagues, Lin and coworkers[122] found that the reduction of minute ventilation (V_E) per increase in PCO_2 was normalized by maximal voluntary ventilation (MVV) (i.e., $\Delta V_E/\Delta PCO_2/\Delta MVV$), suggesting that muscle weakness was the primary factor contributing to the diminished ventilatory response.

The control of a range of ventilatory responses (e.g., tidal volume, respiratory frequency, inspiratory and expiratory durations, and mean inspiratory airflow) does not appear to require afferent pathways from the rib cage and intercostal muscles.[124,125] Quadriplegic subjects were able to modulate the duration, intensity, and timing of the phrenic nerve discharge during the first loaded breath.[124] A group of ventilated quadriplegic

subjects detected changes in tidal volume of as little as 100 ml, just as well as did a group of ventilated control subjects.[126] The sensory information that allowed the quadriplegic group to detect changes in lung volume could arise from visceral lung afferents that project to the CNS in the vagus nerve. Mechanical ventilation is known to inhibit inspiratory muscle activity in humans.[127] In control and C-2 quadriplegic subjects with intact sternocleidomastoid efferents and afferents, inspiratory effort as evidenced by electromyographic activity in the sternocleidomastoid muscle was elicited by increasing end-tidal PCO_2. In both these groups, onset of inspiratory muscle activity occurred at a higher end-tidal PCO_2 when inspiratory activity was elicited by increasing the inspired fraction of CO_2 ($FICO_2$), than when it was elicited by decreasing the tidal volume or frequency during mechanical ventilation. In C-1 quadriplegic subjects with efferent innervation of the sternocleidomastoid muscle via the accessory nerve, but lacking afferent innervation of the sternocleidomastoid, the onset of inspiratory muscle activity occurred at the same level of end-tidal PCO_2, independent of whether end-tidal PCO_2 was increased by increasing $FICO_2$ or by decreasing tidal volume or frequency. Simon and coworkers[127] concluded that afferent feedback from some part of the chest wall was needed to produce a volume- and frequency-dependent inhibition of inspiratory muscle activity during mechanical ventilation.

Sensations of the need to cough and of congestion have been reported to remain after high cervical spinal cord lesions.[126] It has also been shown that ventilated quadriplegic subjects can reliably perceive an increase in PCO_2 in the physiological range as an uncomfortable sense of *air hunger*.[40] Ventilated quadriplegic subjects maintained at a constant but elevated level of end-tidal PCO_2 experienced a similar sensation of air hunger when tidal volume was decreased.[121] The sensation of dyspnea in response to increases in end-tidal PCO_2 is preserved in SCI intact humans, paralyzed with total neuromuscular blockade, suggesting that chemoreceptor activity can lead to discomfort in the absence of any respiratory muscle contraction.[128]

TEMPERATURE REGULATION

The classical cold and warm sensors are located in the hypothalamus and the skin; however, there is evidence of mesencephalic, medullary, spinal, and intra-abdominal temperature sensors.[129] Afferent fibers from peripheral warm and cold receptors with cell bodies in the dorsal root ganglia enter the spinal cord and ascend contralaterally to the medial lemniscus and thalamus and have further projections to the hypothalamus.[130] The preoptic area of the hypothalamus is implicated as the generator of the thermal set point and central integrator of thermoregulatory responses.[130] Efferents from the hypothalamus control thermoregulatory vasomotor and sudomotor tone, as well as nonshivering and shivering thermogenesis via descending noradrenergic and cholinergic fibers. These exit the spinal cord below C-7.[130]

Impairment of temperature regulation is a recognized hazard for persons with SCI.[131] It is most severe for persons with a complete cervical SCI because shivering can only occur above the level of the injury and hypothalamic control of sympathetically mediated vasomotor control and sweating is lost below the level of the lesion. Some degree of thermoregulation via activation of local or spinal vasomotor and sudomotor reflexes has been identified in patients with SCIs. Nonshivering thermogenesis or chemical thermogenesis secondary to increases in cellular metabolism, although important for some animals, has not been clearly demonstrated in humans. Behavioral modification is an important mechanism for thermoregulation, and persons with complete high-level SCIs can avoid environmental temperature extremes[132] (Table 29-2).

Cooling the skin, regardless of whether central body temperature changes, causes increased heat production via shivering.[133] In paraplegic subjects, deep or central temperature receptors sensitive to cold are also able to initiate shivering above the level of the SCI, and these receptors can act independently of the temperature of the skin above the SCI.[133] Researchers have postulated that in healthy humans these central cold receptors may be a backup mechanism that comes into play if there is a loss or diminution of skin cold receptor reflex activity.[133] In humans shivering does not occur below the level of a complete SCI, and, therefore, shivering is thought not to be a spinal reflex.[134] In dogs that had high spinal cord transections, a clearly visible shiver-

like muscle tremor was induced below the level of spinal cord transection by spinal cord cooling, but the tremor was less intense in the spinal cord–transected dog than in the pretransection state.[130] This suggests that spinal cord cold sensors are present in this species and are activated when there is sufficient cooling.

An important mechanism controlling heat transfer from the body core to the surface is the adjustment of cutaneous blood flow.[129] Cooling of peripheral or central areas results in a reduction of skin blood flow and a simultaneous increase in flow to central vascular regions.[129] In control subjects, cooling or warming of one hand elicits a cutaneous vasomotor response of the contralateral hand and both legs.[135] Several investigations[135-137] have failed to observe a similar cutaneous vasomotor response below the level of SCI; others have observed vasomotor responses below the level of SCI in both primates and humans.[138-140] Tsai and coworkers[138] reported that all vasomotor responses to cooling or warming in the paraplegic lower extremities of men were absent after acute SCI (T-5 to T-11). The vasomotor responses in the intact upper extremities were not altered. By 4 months after injury the ipsilateral local vasomotor responses to warming and cooling in the paraplegic lower extremities returned to normal, and by 18 months after injury, the crossed vasomotor reflex to cooling and warming recovered to normal.

The most important mechanisms of heat loss in humans are vasodilatation, sweating, and behavioral aspects, such as choice of posture, amount of clothing, and altering ambient temperature. Conscious control of behavior depends on sensory appreciation of temperature. In one study, paraplegic subjects did feel hot as their oral temperature was raised 1.0–1.5°C by heating insensate skin.[141] However, in the case of one T-8 paraplegic individual, researchers reported that a decrease in central temperature to 36.2°C was not associated with a conscious appreciation of cold.[142] The perception of

TABLE 29-2

Thermoregulatory Mechanisms in Spinal Cord Injury

Mechanisms	Below Level of Spinal Cord Injury	Above Level of Spinal Cord Injury	Effect
Shivering	−	+	Warm
Sweating	±	+	Cool
Vasoconstriction	±	+	Warm
Vasodilatation	±	+	Cool
Behavioral modification	Cold- or heat-seeking behavior	Cold- or heat-seeking behavior	Cool or warm

− = absent, + = present, ± = variable.

warm and cold after SCI appears to depend on the temperature of the sentient skin.

The primary and principal stimulus that elicits the thermoregulatory sweating response is a change in core temperature.[143] Sweat glands receive dual innervation by both cholinergic and adrenergic fibers and are stimulated by cholinergic, α-adrenergic, and β-adrenergic agonists; however, cholinergic stimulation provokes the largest response.[144] Spinal segments T-2 to T-4 supply sweat glands on the head and neck, T-2 to T-8 to glands of the upper limbs, T-6 to T-10 to the trunk, and T-11 to L-2 to the lower extremities.[144] Normell[145] provides an outline of the segmental arrangement of the thermoregulatory vasomotor innervation of the skin of the trunk and lower extremities. Autonomic dermatomes overlap several segments above and below the somatic level. In several reports, spinal lesions are associated with anhidrosis below the level of the lesion.[144,145] Normal evaporative cooling is maintained in persons with spinal injury by increased compensatory sweating from sentient skin.[144,146]

Reflex sweating occurs below the level of lesion in SCI during autonomic hyperreflexia. There is also evidence for thermal reflex sweating below the level of SCI in humans. A 1961 study by Seckendorf and Randall demonstrated low-intensity sweating in five patients with anatomically complete lesions of the spinal cord (T-3 to T-8).[147] In 1991, Silver et al. recorded sweat responses of nine patients with physiologically complete lesions of the spinal cord, including six with cervical lesions.[148] Sweating occurred on the entire cutaneous surface below the level of SCI in every patient in response to environmental heating. However, sweating was not sufficient to prevent an elevation in body temperature in patients with cervical SCI. In one patient with cervical SCI, the amount of sweating was estimated to be approximately 30% of what would be expected in a healthy subject.

Paraplegic men have been shown to have significant differences in skin blood flow response to hyperthermia when compared with intact control subjects.[141] When only insensate skin was heated (to 40°C) in paraplegic subjects, little or no increases in forearm blood flow occurred, even with an elevation of oral temperature of 1.0–1.5°C over 59–71 minutes, although the subjects exhibited mild sweating on the upper body. In contrast, a normal subject exhibited vigorous vasomotor and sudomotor responses to the same pattern of heating that was given to the paraplegic subject. In fact, the thermoregulatory responses of the normal subject were so effective it was impossible to push oral temperature above 37.5°C when lower body skin temperature heating was limited to 40°C. With whole body heating of

paraplegic subjects, all but one exhibited sweating above the level of the spinal cord lesion, and forearm blood flow increased in all subjects. However, the increase in forearm blood flow in the paraplegic subjects was less than that reported for hyperthermic men with intact spinal cords. Freund and coworkers[141] suggested that one reason for the attenuated response of forearm blood flow to whole body heating was diminished thermoregulatory effector outflow resulting from the diminished afferent input that, after SCI, could originate only from above the level of the lesion. Tam and colleagues[149] reached a similar conclusion. They reported that a person with T-6 paraplegia had to achieve a higher core temperature threshold (37.2–37.9°C) to generate sweating and related vasodilatation responses, compared with the core temperature threshold (36.2–37.1°C) of a healthy control subject. It can be concluded that paraplegic men appear to exhibit markedly attenuated skin blood flow in response to hyperthermia and thus are limited in their ability to dissipate excess heat.[141]

Another approach to the study of thermoregulation is to record the activity of vasoconstrictor and sudomotor impulses via microelectrodes in sympathetic skin nerves.[150] In quadriplegic subjects, sympathetic skin nerve recordings from below the level of the lesion made while ambient temperature was varied demonstrated no changes in sympathetic outflow despite cooling that reduced tympanic temperature 2°C.[69] During this study, abdominal pressure over the bladder, as well as mechanical and electrical skin stimulation applied distal to the level of SCI, induced bursts of neural impulses recorded in the sympathetic skin nerve fascicles also below the level of SCI, indicating the presence of spinal vesicosympathetic and somatosympathetic reflexes. It has long been noted that increases in urinary bladder pressure elicit an increase in arterial blood pressure in quadriplegic persons.[151] Of note is that reflex vasoconstriction (below the level of SCI) induced by suprapubic pressure is prolonged during body cooling. The finding of increased vasoconstriction during cooling in persons with SCI may, therefore, not be a thermoregulatory response but simply an artifact induced by facilitation of vesicosympathetic reflexes.[69] This argues against the presence of physiologically significant spinal sympathetic thermoregulatory reflexes (see Chapter 21).

UPPER GASTROINTESTINAL TRACT

The stomach and intestinal wall contain intrinsic neurons that are part of the enteric nervous system, a system that has been referred to as the *third division* of the autonomic nervous system. It is noteworthy that there are as many neurons in the enteric nervous system (10^8) as there are in the spinal cord.[152] The enteric nervous system has two divisions: (1) the submucosal plexus (Meissner's plexus), which innervates the mucosa and regulates secretion, and (2) the myenteric plexus (Auerbach's plexus), which innervates the circular and longitudinal smooth muscle layers and regulates motility. The two plexuses communicate through interconnecting nerves. The enteric nervous system has three types of nerve cells: (1) motor neurons that innervate smooth muscle cells, (2) interneurons that connect different neurons, and (3) intrinsic primary afferent neurons. Although over 20 substances have been identified as putative neurotransmitters in the enteric nervous system, the main neurotransmitters of excitatory motor neurons of the enteric nervous system are acetylcholine and substance P, whereas the main neurotransmitters of inhibitory motor neurons are VIP and NO.[152,153]

In the guinea pig, intrinsic primary afferent neurons (Figure 29-1) have been identified with cell bodies in the wall of the small intestine.[154] The intrinsic primary afferents are thought to be indirectly excited. Luminal chemicals or mechanical stimulation of the mucosa result in the release of serotonin from enteroendocrine cells of the mucosa. Serotonin could be an intermediate substance for intrinsic primary afferent stimulation.[154] Stretching of the intestine also stimulates intrinsic primary afferents. The smooth muscle of the intestine contracts when stretched, and this muscle contraction distorts the intrinsic afferent neuron cell body, thereby activating a mechanosensitive ion channel to generate an action potential.[154] The intrinsic primary afferents synapse with each other as well as with interneurons and motor neurons of the myenteric plexus.[154]

Of the nerve fibers in the abdominal vagus, 80% or more are afferents with cell bodies in the nodose ganglia.[152] Mucosal afferent fibers arise from polymodal as well as selective receptors in the small intestine and stomach that respond to mechanical stimuli such as gentle stroking of the epithelium or chemical stimulation.[155] Thermoreceptors have also been identified in the cat duodenum and stomach.[156] Three types of chemoreceptors found in the small intestine are likely responsible for feedback control of gastric emptying by nutrients; they are osmoreceptors, lipid receptors, and receptors for amino acids.[155] Glucoreceptors and pH receptors are also present in the small intestine. How stimulation of intestinal receptors mediates changes in gastric emptying has not been entirely resolved. In addition to mucosal afferent receptors, there are also vagal afferents with recep-

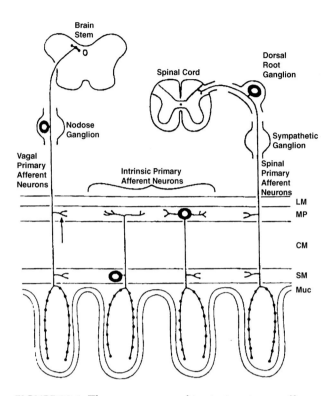

FIGURE 29-1 The arrangement of intrinsic primary afferent neurons, vagal primary afferent neurons, and spinal primary afferent neurons that supply the intestine. Vagal and spinal primary afferent neurons are pseudounipolar and have collaterals that run to enteric ganglia (*arrow*). Vagal primary afferent neurons have cell bodies in the nodose ganglia, and their outputs are via terminals in the nucleus tractus solitarius in the brain stem. The cell bodies of spinal primary afferent neurons are in dorsal root ganglia, their central processes end in the dorsal horns of the spinal cord, and their peripheral axons pass via sympathetic ganglia to the intestine. Intrinsic primary afferent neurons are multipolar, and their terminals are confined within the wall of the intestine. (CM = circular muscle; LM = longitudinal muscle; MP = myenteric plexus; Muc = mucosa; SM = submucosal.) (Reprinted with permission from JB Furness, WAA Kunze, PP Bertrand, N Clerc, JC Bornstein. Intrinsic primary afferent neurons of the intestine. Prog Neurobiol 1998;54:1–18.)

tors in the gastric, duodenal, and jejunal smooth muscle that respond to distention and contraction of the viscus.[156] The splanchnic nerves, which convey afferents from the gut to the spinal cord, are thought to mediate painful sensations, although vagus nerve afferents may also be involved in gut nociception.[156]

The sensation of hunger is reduced in vagotomized patients, but it is not eliminated, perhaps because the hypothalamus monitors the levels of circulating nutrients.[156] A detailed account of abdominal nociception, satiety, and appetite in high SCI patients would provide valuable information on the contribution of spinal afferents to these sensations.

The extrinsic innervation of the stomach and small intestine occurs through the parasympathetic and sympathetic divisions of the autonomic nervous system. In the abdomen, the parasympathetic preganglionic efferent fibers to the stomach are conveyed in the vagus nerve, which in turn gives rise to gastric branches that form synapses with neurons in the myenteric and the submucosal plexuses of the stomach.

Preganglionic sympathetic efferent fibers originate in the mediolateral gray matter of the spinal cord and course through the splanchnic nerves to the celiac and superior mesenteric prevertebral ganglia (plexuses). The stomach receives sympathetic postganglionic fibers principally from the celiac plexus, but also from the left phrenic plexus, bilateral gastric and hepatic plexuses, and the sympathetic trunk. Postganglionic sympathetic efferent nerves emerge from the celiac and superior mesenteric prevertebral ganglia to run along mesenteric blood vessels and innervate the small intestine.

The vagus nerve is important for the motor activity of the stomach. The fundus of the stomach acts as a reservoir to accommodate the meal while the antrum is both a pump and a grinder. Vagal stimulation induces relaxation of the fundus and contraction of the antrum.[155] Mesenteric sympathetic nerve stimulation inhibits contraction in the small intestine.[155]

In the normal interdigestive state of the gastrointestinal tract of humans, a cyclic wave begins in the stomach and duodenum and migrates to the terminal ileum. This activity, characterized by recurring periods of intense regular motor activity, is known as phase III of the interdigestive motor complex (IDMC) and is also referred to as the *migrating myoelectric complex* (MMC).[157,158] The IDMC usually begins in the antrum and migrates to the proximal duodenum in a coordinated manner that is interrupted by feeding. Phase III activity is followed a period of less intense activity (phase IV), then by quiescence (phase I), then by irregular contractions (phase II).[159] The phases of the interdigestive state disappear after a meal and are replaced by the ongoing phasic contractile activity of the fed pattern.[159] The phases of the IDMC and the fed pattern of gastrointestinal contractile activity occur independent of nerves extrinsic to the enteric nervous system.[159] It is thought that in humans the hormone motilin acts on enteric nervous system neurons in the gastric antrum to control gastric emptying and trigger the MMC.[160] Erythromycin has motilin agonist properties and its administration can induce an MMC.[160]

In humans, gastric distention and ileus occur immediately after traumatic spinal cord transection, suggesting abnormal gastrointestinal motility.[161] In long-term quadriplegic persons an intact supraspinal sympathetic pathway is not an absolute requirement for initiation and propagation of antral phase III motor activity,[162] as there are no significant differences in the duration of phases of the IDMC, cycle length of the duodenal IDMC, or the propagation velocity of phase III of the IDMC from the duodenum to the jejunum[162] between subjects with quadriplegia (neurologic level above T-1), low paraplegia (neurologic level below T-10), or an intact spinal cord. In healthy subjects 90% of phase IIIs originated in the antrum and migrated to the duodenum and jejunum, whereas in subjects with high SCI, fewer than 40% of their phase IIIs originated in the antrum. Some 80% of quadriplegic subjects had dissociation between antral and duodenal phase III motility manifested primarily as a pattern of persistent antral activity. In one subject with prominent recurrent autonomic hyperreflexia there was marked antral hypomotility. Antral quiescence was associated with the degree of reflex vascular hypertension resulting from spontaneous and suprapubic pressure-induced autonomic hyperreflexia, whereas duodenal motility was unaffected.[162] This suggests that motility in the antrum is modified by central sympathetic input and that excessive splanchnic sympathetic outflow may delay gastric emptying by inhibiting antral motility.[162] Sympathetic activity may influence gastric motility via a direct neural pathway to the gut wall or via indirect pathways that modulate the release of polypeptide gastrointestinal hormones.[162]

In dogs, after spinal cord transection the only long-term change in the fed and fasted patterns of myoelectric activity in the stomach and small intestine is that the gastric component of the MMC is shorter lived.[163] In the early post–spinal cord transection period there were obvious disruptions of myoelectric activity in both the stomach and duodenum, but not in the jejunum and ileum. In the dog it took an average of 10 (range, 1–36) days after spinal cord transection before normal MMCs returned to the duodenum, and 14 (range, 4–50) days before MMC-like myoelectric activity returned to the stomach. During the first 14 days after spinal cord transection gastric myoelectric activity resembled a fed pattern. There is evidence that the short-term changes seen in dogs persist longer in humans after SCI.[162]

Gastric emptying has been reported as delayed in chronic quadriplegic subjects when data on gastric emptying are collected for at least 2 hours.[162,164] Segal and coworkers[164] identified a biphasic pattern of gastric emptying where the initial (20–30 minutes) gastric emptying, which resembled the patterns seen in control and paraplegic subjects, was followed by a delayed second phase. Lu and coworkers[165] demonstrated a normal cutaneous electrogastrogram result in 12 patients with complete cervical SCI. Abnormalities in the electrogastrogram result have been associated with gastric motor dysfunction, but if there is antral-duodenal motor incoordination after SCI as described by Fealey and coworkers,[162] abnormal gastric myoelectrical activity may correlate poorly with gastric emptying.[165] Paraplegic persons have been reported to have delayed gastric emptying, but this appears to be a nonspecific finding related to prolonged immobilization.[166]

LOWER GASTROINTESTINAL TRACT

Vagal afferents supply the small intestine and the proximal two-thirds of the colon coinciding with the vagal efferent innervation.[156] Vagal afferents respond to distention and contraction of the colon. Other afferent fibers from the colon travel with both sympathetic and parasympathetic axons and have cell bodies in the lumbar and sacral dorsal root ganglia.

The parasympathetic outflow to the colon and anorectum originates from brain stem nuclei and the sacral spinal cord.[167] The ascending and transverse colon receives parasympathetic efferent fibers from the posterior vagus nerve, and the left half of the colon and rectum receives them from the pelvic nerve.[168] Preganglionic parasympathetic neurons project from the sacral segments S-2 to S-5 through the pelvic nerves and pass to the left colon and anorectum via the pelvic plexus.[3]

The sympathetic supply to the right colon arises from T-6 to T-12 and that to the left colon and upper rectum arises from L-1 to L-3.[168] SPNs to the colon and pelvic viscera send fibers through the lumbar splanchnic nerves to the superior and IMG.[3] Postganglionic fibers from the superior mesenteric ganglion innervate the colon from the cecum to the distal transverse colon. Lumbar colonic nerves arise from the IMG and run along the inferior mesenteric artery to innervate the left side of the colon and the hypogastric nerves, which also arise from the IMG, and join the pelvic plexus[3] (known as the *inferior hypogastric plexus*) to innervate the distal colon. Other sympathetic preganglionic axons enter paravertebral chain ganglia and form synapses with postganglionic neurons there.[169]

Preganglionic sympathetic neurons projecting fibers into the lumbar splanchnic nerves are visceral vasoconstrictor neurons and motility-regulating neurons. Elec-

trical stimulation of the sympathetic supply to the colon results in contraction of the internal anal sphincter and relaxation of the colon and rectum.[3] Studies in the rat have shown that the sympathetic inhibition is mediated by postjunctional β-adrenoceptors on colon smooth muscle.[170] In addition, the sympathetic innervation of the rat colon can also cause contractions most prominent in the distal colon (although present in the proximal colon) that are mediated by postjunctional smooth muscle α-adrenoceptors.[170] Transection of the low thoracic spinal cord in cats demonstrates that there is little spinal shock for the motility-regulating neurons, in comparison with the vasoconstrictor system.[3] The patterns of reflex discharge of motility-regulating neurons are determined within the lumbosacral spinal cord.[3]

Some postganglionic neurons directly innervate vascular or visceral smooth muscle. Other postganglionic neurons control the effector organs indirectly by influencing other peripheral neurons such as those in the submucosal ganglia (Meissner's plexus) or myenteric ganglia (Auerbach's plexus) of the enteric nervous system or in the prevertebral ganglia, via presynaptic or postsynaptic mechanisms.[168] The majority of lumbar sympathetic postganglionic neurons is noradrenergic, but many contain a peptide as well.[171] Sympathetic ganglia receive synaptic input from (1) preganglionic neurons with cell bodies in the spinal cord, (2) primary sensory neurons with cell bodies in the dorsal root ganglia, and (3) neurons arising in visceral intramural ganglia (enteric nervous system). The apparent convergence of multiple synaptic inputs onto individual principal ganglionic neurons suggests that the outflow from these neurons is the result of integration of synaptic information from several sources.[172] Therefore, it is reasonable to conclude that the peripheral autonomic nervous system may mediate complex reflex functions of the gastrointestinal system without the involvement of either supraspinal or spinal cord influences.

Research indicates that the lumbar sympathetic outflow exerts a tonic inhibitory influence on the motility of the colon. Studies in rats show that there is differential sympathetic inhibition of the proximal, transverse, and distal colon.[173] The distal colon receives a tonic inhibitory influence with a supraspinal organization, the transverse colon receives a tonic inhibitory influence with a spinal organization, and the proximal colon appears to be influenced by neither spinal nor supraspinal tonic inhibition.

When food is ingested into the stomach there is an increase in colonic motor activity that is called the *gastrocolic reflex*.[174] The afferent limb of this reflex can be blocked by intragastric lidocaine, and the increase in distal colonic spike activity can be blocked by anticholinergics or naloxone, indicating participation of cholinergic and opiate receptors. Colonic cyclical organization in the rat, including enhancement of distal colonic cyclical activity as a secondary response to feeding (gastrocolic reflex), persists after ablation or section of the spinal cord.[173] This demonstrates that, at least for the distal colon, colonic cyclical organization is not initiated by lumbar spinal or supraspinal influences. The local enteric nervous system or the prevertebral ganglionic system, or both, are probably responsible for the cyclical organization of distal colonic motility in rats. However, the gastrocolic reflex in the transverse colon persists in rats after spinal cord transection but not after spinal cord ablation, suggesting that it was organized in the spinal cord.[173]

Analysis of colonic myoelectric spike activity of the rectal mucosa 6–15 cm from the anus revealed that in the fasting state persons with SCI above T-10 who were also more than 3 months postinjury had significantly greater basal colonic myoelectric spike activity than control subjects.[175] Meal stimulation increased basal spike activity (gastrocolic reflex) in the control group compared with the fasting state. In the spinal cord–injured group there was no significant increase in myoelectric spike activity after the meal, compared with the fasting state. Because feeding did not significantly increase the already high basal spike activity of persons with SCI, the gastrocolic reflex could not be demonstrated. The loss of a tonic inhibitory supraspinal influence may cause the increase in basal colonic spike activity after SCI.[175] The absence of a gastrocolic reflex in this study is consistent with studies by Glick and colleagues,[176] who recorded at 12–18 cm from the anus, but the findings differ from those of the study of Connell and associates,[177] who recorded intact gastrocolic reflexes at 15, 20, and 25 cm from the anus.[168]

Fecal material entering the rectum results in relaxation of the internal anal sphincter (rectoanal inhibitory reflex), but contraction of the external anal sphincter to prevent incontinence (holding reflex).[178] Internal anal sphincter relaxation occurs after rectal distention in individuals with SCI above T-12.[179] Complete sacral posterior rhizotomy did not eliminate the internal anal sphincter relaxation induced by rectal distention. However, reflex contraction of the external anal sphincter in response to either rectal distention or increased intra-abdominal pressure was eliminated by sacral posterior rhizotomy, indicating that these contractions are mediated by a spinal reflex.[179] Voluntary relaxation of the external anal sphincter and the puborectalis muscle results in stool elimination.[179]

The most obvious gastrointestinal consequence of SCI is the loss of voluntary control of the initiation of defecation. The most common problems complicating the neurogenic bowel are poorly localized abdominal pain (in 14% of cases studies by Stone's group), difficulty with bowel evacuation (20%), hemorrhoids (74%), abdominal distention (43%), and autonomic hyperreflexia arising from the gastrointestinal tract (43%).[180] As many as 27% of persons with SCI have significant chronic gastrointestinal problems, and those with more complete injuries are more likely to have symptoms (33%) than those with incomplete injuries (6%).[180] In a survey of patients with SCI, 30% regarded colorectal dysfunction as worse than both bladder and sexual dysfunction.[181]

In persons with complete SCI above T-12, transit of contents is slowed throughout the large bowel, regardless of the level of the spinal cord lesion.[182] Studies have identified (1) prolonged rectosigmoid transit times,[182] (2) transit delays more marked in the descending colon, sigmoid, and rectum than in the cecum, ascending colon, and transverse colon,[183,184] or (3) transit delays involving the entire colon.[185] The obvious clinical implication of prolonged transit time throughout the left and right colon is that treatment of colorectal dysfunction in patients with SCI should include not only rectal agents but also prokinetic agents to reduce transit time in the entire colon.[185] Cisapride has been shown to improve chronic constipation and transit times in SCI patients in some studies,[186–188] but not in others.[189]

For reviews of the management of neurogenic bowel dysfunction after SCI see Stiens et al.[190] and Banwell et al.[178]

SEXUAL FUNCTION IN MEN

The penis receives innervation from both somatic and autonomic pathways.[191–194] Somatic afferent innervation to penile skin is carried in a terminal branch of the pudendal nerve called the *dorsal nerve of the penis.*[195] The penile and pelvic nerves also convey part of the sensory innervation to the urethra, rectum, and anus in male rats.[196]

In humans, sympathetic preganglionic fibers from T-11 to L-2 and parasympathetic preganglionic fibers from S-2 to S-4 are involved in erection and ejaculation.[197] Parasympathetic preganglionic fibers from the sacral spinal cord project in the pelvic nerve to the pelvic plexus.[193,195] One pathway for sympathetic preganglionic fibers to the penis is from the thoracolumbar spinal cord through the paravertebral chain ganglia to project via (1) the pelvic nerve and plexus into the penile nerve (also known as the *cavernous nerve*) or (2) the pudendal nerve to the penis.[191–193,195,198] The other pathway for sympathetic preganglionic fibers is through the lumbar splanchnic nerves to the IMG.[193,195] Postganglionic fibers from neurons in the IMG as well as preganglionic fibers project through the hypogastric nerves to the pelvic plexus.[199] Sympathetic and parasympathetic postganglionic efferent fibers project from the pelvic plexus to the penis via the penile nerves.

Physiological activation of afferent pathways in the dorsal nerve of the penis elicits multiple sexual responses, including penile erection, seminal emission, and ejaculation.[200–203] In rats, stimulation of afferent fibers in the dorsal nerve of the penis or pelvic nerve has been shown to elicit reflexes in the penile nerve.[195] These reflexes on the penile nerve were mediated at the spinal cord level, because acute spinal cord transection failed to eliminate the responses.[195] The penile nerve contains a mixture of parasympathetic and sympathetic postganglionic axons that produce vasodilatation of arteries supplying the corpus cavernosum, resulting in penile tumescence.[195,198] This nerve also contains sympathetic vasoconstrictor axons that produce detumescence.[193,194,204] In the male human, the penile nerves travel just lateral to the vascular structures that are located posterolateral to the prostate gland at approximately the 10 o'clock and 2 o'clock positions.[205] Erection involves parasympathetic cholinergic and noncholinergic nonadrenergic mechanisms.[206] Penile flaccidity is maintained by sympathetic efferents and α-adrenoceptors.[207] It is unlikely that acetylcholine causes erection by a direct action on smooth muscle fiber postjunctional muscarinic receptors because isolated human corpus cavernosum smooth muscle cells contract in response to cholinergic stimulation.[207] Acetylcholine may contribute to erection by inhibiting the effects of NE on penile smooth muscle[208] or by modulating NO release by endothelial cells.[207] The NANC neurotransmitter primarily thought to mediate erection is NO, a smooth muscle relaxant and vasodilator.[209] NO relaxation of vascular smooth muscle is mediated through activation of guanylate cyclase to produce cyclic guanosine monophosphate (cGMP).[209] Neurons and endothelial cells in the corpus cavernosum synthesize and release NO.[207] NO is involved in both neural and endothelium-dependent relaxation in human penile arteries[207,210]; however, both neural and endothelium-dependent relaxations seem to involve another factor that is not affected by blocking NO synthase.[210] VIP has also been implicated as a mediator of the noncholinergic nonadrenergic mechanism of erection.[206,211] It is known to relax smooth muscle from the human penis.[199,211] It has been shown that 92% of penile postganglionic neurons are positive

for VIP and 95% of penile postganglionic neurons have high levels of acetylcholinesterase.[199]

Reflex erections are mediated via the sacral parasympathetics with afferent input from the pudendal nerve and efferent output via the pelvic and then penile (cavernous) nerves. Reflex erections are organized in the sacral spinal cord.[197] More than two-thirds of men with complete SCI have some form of reflex penile erection.[212,213] The phenomenon of psychogenic erections in paraplegic men with complete sacral lower motor neuron lesions and abolished reflexogenic erections indicates that a pathway for erection from the sympathetic outflow exists.[197] The sympathetic proerectile outflow may be via the hypogastric to the penile (cavernous) nerves.[207]

Emission of semen and seminal fluid is primarily under sympathetic control. Emission is followed by closure of the bladder neck and contraction of the bulbourethral striated muscles, the latter being mediated by pudendal somatic efferents.[197] Some 5–10% of men with complete SCI experience ejaculation or seminal emission.[197,212,213] For purposes of obtaining semen for artificial insemination, an ejaculation reflex can be obtained by vibratory stimulation of the frenulum and lower surface of the glans penis.[214] The afferent pathway of this ejaculation reflex likely involves the pudendal nerves (dorsal nerve of the penis) and ascending tracts from the sacral spinal cord to the thoracolumbar T-12 to L-1 preganglionic sympathetic nerves.[212,215]

Testosterone levels have been shown to be normal or slightly elevated in men with long-term SCI.[215,216] Levels of follicle-stimulating hormone and luteinizing hormone in young paraplegic subjects did not show evidence of primary testicular failure.[215,217]

Treatment of Erectile and Ejaculatory Dysfunction in Spinal Cord Injury

Sildenafil increases cGMP by inhibition of cGMP-specific phosphodiesterase V, resulting in penile erection.[209] Sildenafil is safe and effective for erectile dysfunction caused by SCI.[218,219] Intracavernosal injection of vasoactive substances such as papaverine, phentolamine, and prostaglandin E_1 are useful for erectile dysfunction after SCI. The medicated urethral system for erection used for administering an intraurethral prostaglandin E_1 suppository can cause hypotension and syncope in SCI patients unless used with a venous constrictive band at the base of the penis before insertion.[209] The vacuum erection device has been effective in up to 93% of SCI patients. The penile prosthesis has been associated with high rates of mechanical failure (43%) and low rates of improved sexual function (41%).[209]

Penile vibratory stimulation and electroejaculation are used to obtain semen in men with SCI.[220-222] Electroejaculation is the electrical stimulation of efferent sympathetic nerves via a rectal probe. Vibratory stimulation to the glans penis triggers an ejaculatory reflex. Penile vibratory stimulation is more successful in lesions above T-10 (81%) than T-10 or below (12%) and is more successful if hip flexion and bulbocavernosus reflexes are present (77%) than absent (14%).[221]

SEXUAL FUNCTION IN WOMEN

Much less is known about sexual function in women with SCI than in men.[223] It is clear that a woman's libido and reproductive capability remain intact after SCI.[224] There is transient anovulation in approximately 50% of women with SCI, but the preinjury menstrual pattern is re-established in 3–6 months.[223-226] Mean menstrual cycle length and the duration of menses have been shown to decrease within the normal range for fertile, able-bodied women, regardless of level or completeness of injury.[225] Menarche is not delayed if the SCI is preadolescent. Anovulation is thought to be a result of the stress of the trauma and is not related to the level of injury or its degree of completeness.

The four components of the sexual response cycle (i.e., excitement, plateau, orgasm, and resolution)[227] are all present, but may vary in degree in women with SCI.[223,224] The normal female sexual excitation phase consists of vaginal lubrication, swelling of the clitoral gland, and congestion of the labia.[223] With complete SCI there is absence of lubrication (reflex or psychogenic) when the injury is situated between T-10 and T-12, indicating that preganglionic neurons at this level of the spinal cord constitute the final efferent pathway for both reflex and centrally mediated lubrication.[223] Reflex lubrication does occur with lesions above T-9, and psychogenic lubrication is present with injuries below T-12.[223] Thirty-six percent of 11 women with complete SCI, 67% of 6 women with incomplete SCI and preserved light touch at T-11 to L-2, and 63% of 8 women with incomplete SCI and preserved pinprick at T-11 to L-2 were able to achieve orgasm in a laboratory-based assessment.[228] Based on animal studies, there are three pathways that convey sensory information from the uterus, cervix, and vagina to the CNS. These pathways are (1) via the hypogastric nerves to the thoracolumbar spinal cord (T-10 to L-1), (2) via the pelvic nerve to the sacral spinal cord (S-2 to S-4), and (3) via the vagal nerve to the nodose ganglia and NTS.[229] Whipple and Komisaruk hypothesize that the orgasms obtained in women with complete SCI in response to genital stimulation are mediated by sensory fibers in the vagus nerve.[230]

The fertility rate and miscarriage rate are the same for women with SCI as for the general population of sexually active women.[224] Pain in the first stage of labor is caused by uterine contraction and cervical dilatation.[224] Since the afferent innervation of the uterus arises from T-10 to L-1, labor is painless for women with an SCI above T-10.[224] In the second stage, labor pain is from the perineum, innervated by the pudendal nerve and spinal cord segments S-2 to S-4. Approximately 25% of pregnant spinal cord–injured women are unable to detect the onset of labor.[224]

Efferent uterine innervation arises from T-10 to T-12.[223] In women with SCI above the T-10 level, uterine contractions are effective and labor progresses normally.[223] The uterus also contracts when its nerve supply is absent by using intermuscular communication.[224] The intensity of uterine contractions is not reduced,[226] and labor is of short duration, often with spasm of the abdominal muscles.[226] Most women with an SCI level above T-6 develop autonomic hyperreflexia with uterine contractions.[224,231] Although an increase in the incidence of premature labor has been suggested,[232] a statistically significant increase in the incidence of premature delivery has not been documented.[224] Women with SCI may be expected to have a reasonably normal pregnancy outcome, provided that specific complications, particularly autonomic hyperreflexia, are anticipated and managed properly.[226,233]

MICTURITION

Bladder mechanoreceptors are activated by bladder distention, mucosal deformation, and a shift in bladder position.[234] Pharmacologic experiments indicate that fluid-induced bladder distention results in the activation of mechanoreceptors, which provide the sensory input needed to facilitate the activation of both supraspinal- and spinal-mediated micturition reflexes.[235-237]

Sensory inputs from the bladder[238] to the human lumbar spinal cord arise from T-11 to L-1, and perhaps as far proximal as T-9; sensory inputs from the bladder to the human sacral spinal cord arise from S-2 to S-4. Afferent fibers in the pelvic nerve projecting to the sacral spinal cord are responsible for the initiation of micturition. Most myelinated Aδ-fiber bladder afferents respond to bladder distention, whereas approximately one-half of unmyelinated C-fiber bladder afferents have no clear mechanoreceptivity but do respond to chemical stimuli.[239]

Preganglionic parasympathetic neurons in the IML of the sacral cord segments S-2 to S-4 project preganglionic fibers in the pelvic nerve to the pelvic plexus.[234] In the human bladder some pelvic plexus neurons are in the bladder wall.[234] Parasympathetic postganglionic nerves excite detrusor smooth muscle via release of acetylcholine or possibly adenosine triphosphate.[240] The parasympathetic input to the urethral smooth muscle is inhibitory and mediated by NO.[239]

SPNs that project to the lower urinary tract are found in spinal cord segments T-10 to L-2 in humans.[234] Most preganglionic sympathetic fibers innervating the pelvic viscera form synapses in the IMG or the pelvic plexus.[3,234] Most preganglionic sympathetic fibers project through the lumbar splanchnic nerves to the IMG, and a smaller number of preganglionic sympathetic fibers project via the sacral paravertebral chain ganglia into the pelvic nerve to the pelvic plexus.[169] The hypogastric nerve (also known as the *presacral nerve*) is composed of both preganglionic and postganglionic sympathetic fibers that pass from the IMG to the pelvic plexus.[3] The sympathetic postganglionic nerves release NE, which (1) inhibits detrusor smooth muscle via β-adrenoceptors, (2) contracts the smooth muscle of the bladder trigone and urethra via α-adrenoceptors, and (3) inhibits (via $α_2$-adrenoceptors) or facilitates (via $α_1$-adrenoceptors) parasympathetic ganglionic transmission.[240,241]

The urethral sphincter mechanism has two parts: the internal and external urethral sphincter (EUS).[242] The internal sphincter is the smooth muscle of the urethra that extends from the bladder outlet through the pelvic floor.[242] The striated muscle of the EUS also has two components: (1) the intrinsic EUS, which lies completely within the urethral wall, and (2) the extrinsic EUS, which is formed by the skeletal muscle fibers of the pelvic floor and urogenital diaphragm.[243] The intrinsic EUS is innervated by somatic pudendal nerve efferents but may have autonomic innervation as well.[242,244] The function of the cholinergic innervation of the EUS is not clear.[245] Adrenergic innervation of the EUS has been suggested, but adrenergic nerves have not been found in the human EUS except when the urinary bladder has been denervated.[245,246] The EUS is the most important active mechanism for maintenance of urinary continence.[242]

Activation of the parasympathetic pathways to the detrusor muscle and inhibition of somatic input to the intrinsic EUS are the essential neuronal events that initiate release of urine. Reflex contractions of the urinary bladder and release of urine that occurs in response to bladder distention are mediated via a parasympathetic reflex pathway consisting of an Aδ-fiber afferent limb and a preganglionic parasympathetic efferent limb in

the pelvic nerve.[247,248] Spinal afferent pathways ascend in the lateral funiculus or the dorsal funiculus of the spinal cord and terminate in the nucleus gracilis and periaqueductal gray. It is thought that neurons in the periaqueductal gray relay information to the pontine micturition center (Figure 29-2) to initiate micturi-

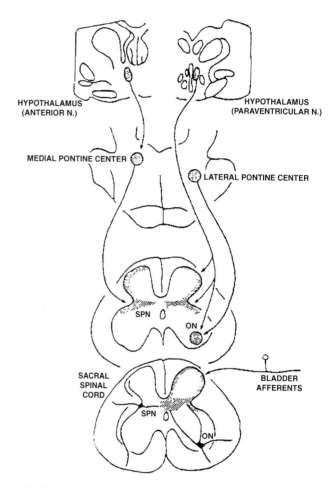

FIGURE 29-2 Neural connections between the brain and the sacral spinal cord that may be involved in the regulation of the lower urinary tract in the cat. Lower section of spinal cord shows the location and morphology of a preganglionic neuron in the sacral parasympathetic nucleus (SPN), a sphincter motoneuron in Onuf's nucleus (ON), and the sites of central termination of afferent projections from the urinary bladder. Upper section of the spinal cord shows the sites of termination of descending pathway arising in the pontine micturition center (medial), the pontine sphincter or urine storage center (lateral), and the paraventricular nuclei of the hypothalamus. Section through the pons shows the projection from the anterior hypothalamic nuclei to the pontine micturition center. (Reprinted with permission from WC de Groat. A neurologic basis for the overactive bladder. Urology 1997;50[Suppl 6A]:36–52.)

tion.[241] Neurons from the nucleus gracilis seem to carry nociceptive information that is relayed to the thalamus and cortex.[241] The descending pathway of the micturition reflex is also in the dorsolateral funiculus, in close proximity to the ascending tracts.[249,250] The spinobulbospinal micturition reflex can be modulated at the spinal level by a variety of afferent inputs from the colon, vagina, penis, or perineum at various sites, including primary afferent terminals, interneurons, or bladder preganglionic neurons.[251]

During continence, the spinal vesicosympathetic reflex pathways allow the urinary bladder to accommodate larger volumes by increasing the tone of the bladder neck,

by depressing impulse transmission from the sacral spinal cord in pelvic vesical ganglia, and by direct inhibition of the detrusor muscle.[252,253] An intersegmental spinal pathway elicits vesicosympathetic reflexes with afferents in the pelvic nerve and efferents in the hypogastric nerve.[240,254] The physiological significance of the sympathetic innervation of the urinary bladder is unclear.

In addition to the spinobulbospinal pathway, which is thought to mediate normal micturition, a spinal micturition reflex pathway (Figure 29-3) has been identified.[255] Research by de Groat and Ryall found that the spinal micturition reflex was present in some intact cats and in all cats with chronic spinal cord transection.[248] It

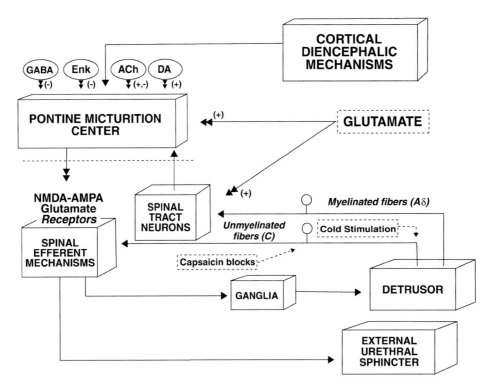

FIGURE 29-3 Central reflex pathways that regulate micturition in the cat. In an animal with an intact neuraxis, micturition is initiated by a supraspinal reflex pathway passing through the pontine micturition center in the brain stem. The pathway is triggered by myelinated afferents connected to tension receptors in the bladder wall. Spinal tract neurons carry information to the brain. During micturition, pathways from the pontine micturition center activate the parasympathetic outflow to the bladder and inhibit the somatic outflow to the urethral sphincter. Corticodiencephalic mechanisms modulate transmission in the pontine micturition center. In spinal cord–transected animals, the micturition reflex is initially blocked. In chronic spinal animals, a spinal micturition reflex emerges that is triggered by unmyelinated bladder afferents. The unmyelinated afferent reflex pathway is usually weak or undetectable in animals with an intact nervous system. Glutamic acid is the principal excitatory transmitter in the ascending and descending limbs of the micturition reflex pathways as well in the reflex pathway controlling sphincter function. Glutamate acts on both N-methyl-D-aspartate (NMDA) and alpha-amino-3-hydroxy-5-methyl-4-isoxazolepropionic acid (AMPA) glutamatergic receptors. Other neurotransmitters that regulate transmission in the micturition reflex pathway include gamma-amino butyric acid (GABA), enkephalins (Enk), acetylcholine (ACh), and dopamine (DA). Acetylcholine has both excitatory and inhibitory effects on the pathway. (+ = Excitatory synapse; – = inhibitory synapse.) (Reprinted with permission from WC de Groat. A neurologic basis for the overactive bladder. Urology 1997;50[Suppl 6A]:36–52.)

is thought that this spinal pathway, which has a C-fiber afferent limb and parasympathetic postganglionic efferent limb in the pelvic nerve, mediates automatic micturition after chronic spinal cord transection.[247] C-fiber afferents, which usually do not respond to bladder distention, may become mechanosensitive after SCI and may elicit the spinal micturition pathway as well as bladder hyperreflexia after SCI. In patients with SCI, intravesical instillation of capsaicin (which is toxic to C fibers) suppresses (1) bladder hyperactivity, (2) autonomic hyperreflexia induced by bladder distention, and (3) cold-induced reflex voiding.[239] In chronic SCI animals, bladder afferent neurons demonstrate morphologic and functional plasticity that may be mediated by the release of neurotrophic factors from hypertrophied bladder muscle. Nerve growth factor, brain-derived neurotrophic factor, and basic fibroblast growth factor are increased in hypertrophied bladder muscle.[239]

Cutaneovesical reflexes have also been described. In rats, cutaneous stimulation resulted in a reflex bladder contraction both before and after spinal cord transection.[256] Neonatal cats exhibit a perineal-bladder reflex mediated in the spinal cord that disappears in adult life,[257,258] and this reflex reappears after spinal cord transection in adult cats.[252,257] Activation of spinal cutaneous somatovesical reflexes may be responsible for voiding elicited by suprapubic tapping or pulling pubic hair in persons with SCI above the sacral outflow.

Complete SCI proximal to the sacral spinal cord results in an upper motor neuron lesion characterized by a hyperreflexic detrusor, whereas injuries involving the sacral cord or cauda equina result in a lower motor neuron lesion characterized by an areflexic detrusor.[259] In a study of 489 persons with spinal cord lesions because of a variety of causes, all those who had suprasacral spinal cord lesions without evidence of additional sacral spinal cord or cauda equina involvement had either detrusor hyperreflexia (defined as involuntary bladder contractions with increased detrusor pressure of at least 6 cm H_2O) or detrusor–EUS dyssynergia.[259] Detrusor–EUS dyssynergia has been defined as the presence of involuntary contractions of the EUS during involuntary detrusor contractions.[260] Detrusor–EUS dyssynergia has been reported to occur during bladder contractions that are evoked either during urodynamic studies or by suprapubic tapping in as many as 86% of persons with SCI.[260,261] In such persons, abrupt discontinuation of suprapubic tapping resulted in brief relaxation of the EUS that was sufficient to result in some urine outflow in 68% of subjects.[261] The loss of reflex inhibition of the EUS during a micturition contraction of the urinary bladder, which occurs after SCI, is a major complicating factor in management of the neurogenic bladder.

The pattern of neurogenic bladder dysfunction after SCI can be identified by urodynamics. For a recent review, see Watanabe et al.[262] (see Chapter 10).

SUMMARY

The function of the autonomic nervous system after injury or damage to the spinal cord cannot be considered only in terms of loss of descending supraspinal control. The neuronal components of the spinal cord, the peripheral autonomic ganglia, and the intrinsic enteric nervous system remain and are capable of complex integrative functions. Furthermore, researchers and clinicians must consider elements of neuronal plasticity and regeneration as contributing to the ultimate pattern of autonomic function after SCI. Plasticity may involve changes in synaptic contacts or physiology, changes in tonic or phasic firing patterns, and changes in neuromodulating peptides.[60]

REFERENCES

1. Felten SY, Carlson SL, Bellinger DL, et al. An Overview of the Efferent Autonomic Nervous System. In RCA Fredrickson, HC Hendrie, JN Hingtgen, et al. (eds), Neuroregulation of Autonomic, Endocrine and Immune Systems. Boston: Martinus Nijhoff, 1986;109–126.

2. Polinsky RJ. Clinical autonomic neuropharmacology. Clin Neuropharmacol 1990;8:77–92.

3. Janig W, McLachlan EM. Organization of lumbar spinal outflow to distal colon and pelvic organs. Physiol Rev 1987;67:1332–1404.

4. Langer SZ, Massingham R, Shepperson NB. α_1 and α_2-Receptor Subtypes: Relevance to Antihypertensive Therapy. In JP Buckley, CM Ferrario (eds), Central Nervous Mechanisms in Hypertension: Perspectives in Cardiovascular Research, Vol 6. New York: Raven, 1981;161–170.

5. Loewenstein W. Modulation of cutaneous mechanoreceptors by sympathetic stimulation. J Physiol 1956;132:40–60.

6. Roberts WJ, Levitt GR. Histochemical evidence for sympathetic innervation of hair receptor afferents in cat skin. J Comp Neurol 1982;210:204–209.

7. Himms-Hagen J. Thermogenesis in brown adipose tissue as an energy buffer. Implications for obesity. N Engl J Med 1984;311:1549–1558.

8. Metz W, Forssmann WG. Innervation of the liver in the guinea pig and rat. Anat Embryol 1980;160:239–252.

9. Shields RW. Functional anatomy of the autonomic nervous system. J Clin Neurophysiol 1993;10(1):2–13.

10. Simon OR, Schramm LP. The spinal and medullary termination of myelinated renal afferents in the rat. Brain Res 1984;290:239–247.

11. Ciriello J, Caverson MM. Central organization of afferent renal nerve pathways. Clin Exper Theory Pract 1987;A9(Suppl 1):33–46.

12. DiBona GF, Kopp UC. Neural control of renal function. Physiol Rev 1997;77(1):75–197.

13. Zheng F, Lawson SN. Immunocytochemical properties of rat renal afferent neurons in dorsal root ganglia: a quantitative study. Neuroscience 1999; 63(1):295–306.

14. DiBona GE. The functions of the renal nerves. Rev Physiol Biochem Pharmacol 1982;94:76–181.

15. Schramm LP, Strack AM, Platt KB, Loewy AD. Peripheral and central pathways regulating the kidney: a study using pseudorabies virus. Brain Res 1993;616(1–2):251–262.

16. Burns KD, Homma T, Harris RC. The intrarenal renin-angiotensin system. Semin Nephrol 1993;13(1):13–30.

17. Coote JH, Lewis DI. The spinal organization of the baroreceptor reflex. Clin Exper Hyperten 1995;17(1–2):295–311.

18. Kooner JS, Frankel HL, Mirando N, et al. Haemodynamic, hormonal and urinary responses to postural change in tetraplegic and paraplegic man. Paraplegia 1988;26:233–237.

19. Sutters M, Wakefield C, O'Neil K, et al. The cardiovascular, endocrine and renal response of tetraplegic and paraplegic subjects to dietary sodium restriction. J Physiol (Lond) 1992;457:515–523.

20. Soni BM, Vaidyanthan MS, Watt JWH, Krishnan KR. A retrospective study of hyponatremia in tetraplegic/paraplegic patients with a review of the literature. Paraplegia 1994;32:597–607.

21. Watson ID, Nathanayan S, Soni B, et al. Profound hyponatremia in quadriplegia. Ann Clin Biochem 1999;36: 673–676.

22. Malliani A, Lombardi F, Pagani M. Sensory innervation of the heart. Prog Brain Res 1986;67:39–48.

23. McNeill DL, Chandler MJ, Fu QG, Foreman RD. Projection of nodose ganglion cells to the upper cervical spinal cord in the rat. Brain Res Bull 1991;27(2):151–155.

24. Groomes TE, Huang C-T. Orthostatic hypotension after spinal cord injury: treatment with fluocortisone and ergotamine. Arch Phys Med Rehabil 1991;72:56–58.

25. Granata AR, Ruggiero AR, Park DA, et al. Brainstem area with C1 epinephrine neurons mediates baroreflex vasodepressor responses. Am J Physiol 1985;248:H547–H567.

26. Yamada KA, McAllen RM, Loewy AD. GABA antagonists applied to the ventral surface of the medulla oblongata block the baroreceptor reflex. Brain Res 1984;297:175–180.

27. McAllen RM. Identification and properties of subretrofacial bulbospinal neurones: a descending cardiovascular pathway in the cat. J Autonom Nerv Syst 1986;17:151–164.

28. Coote JH, Macleod VH, Fleetwood-Walker SM, et al. Baroreceptor inhibition of sympathetic activity at a spinal site. Brain Res 1981;220:81–93.

29. Gebber GL, Taylor DG, Weaver LC. Electrophysiological studies on organization of central vasopressor pathways. Am J Physiol 1973;224:470–481.

30. Somers VK, Mark AL, Zavala DC, et al. Contrasting effects of hypoxia and hypercapnia on ventilation and sympathetic activity in humans. J Appl Physiol 1989;67:2101–2106.

31. Somers VK, Mark AL, Zavala DC, et al. Influence of ventilation and hypocapnia on sympathetic nerve responses to hypoxia in normal humans. J Appl Physiol 1989;67:2095–2100.

32. Reis DJ, Ruggiero DA, Morrison SF. The C1 area of the rostral ventrolateral medulla oblongata. A critical brainstem region for control of resting and reflex integration of arterial pressure. Am J Hypertens 1989;2:363S–374S.

33. Kalia MP. Organization of central control of airways. Annu Rev Physiol 1987;49:595–609.

34. Sato A, Schmidt RF. The modulation of visceral functions by somatic afferent activity. Jpn J Physiol 1987;37:1–17.

35. Mitchell JH, Kaufman MP, Iwamoto GA. The exercise pressor reflex: its cardiovascular effects afferent mechanisms and central pathways. Annu Rev Physiol 1983;45:229–242.

36. Kumada M, Dampney RAL, Reis DJ. Profound hypotension and abolition of the vasomotor component of the cerebral ischemic response produced by restricted lesions of medulla oblongata: Relationship to the so-called tonic vasomotor center. Circ Res 1979;45:63–70.

37. Doba N, Reis DJ. Localization within the lower brainstem of a receptive area mediating the pressor response to increased intracranial pressure (the Cushing response). Brain Res 1972; 47:487–491.

38. Schwaber JS. Neuroanatomical Substrates of Cardiovascular and Emotional-Autonomic Regulation. In A Magro, W Osswald, O Reis, et al. (eds),

Central and Peripheral Mechanisms of Cardiovascular Regulation. New York: Plenum, 1986;353–384.

39. Schramm LP. Spinal Factors in Sympathetic Regulation. In A Magro, W Osswald, O Reis, et al. (eds), Central and Peripheral Mechanisms of Cardiovascular Regulation. New York: Plenum, 1986;303–352.

40. Banzett RB, Lansing RW, Reid MB, et al. "Air hunger" arising from increased PCO_2 in mechanically ventilated quadriplegics. Respir Physiol 1989;76:53–68.

41. Downey JA, Chiodi HP, Miller JM. The effect of inhalation of 5 percent carbon dioxide in air on postural hypotension in quadriplegia. Arch Phys Med Rehabil 1966;47:422–426.

42. Hilton S. The Central Nervous Contribution to Vasomotor Tone. In A Magro, W Osswald, O Reis, et al. (eds), Central and Peripheral Mechanisms of Cardiovascular Regulation. New York: Plenum, 1986;465–486.

43. Yardley CP, Fitzsimons CL, Weaver LC. Cardiac and peripheral vascular contributions to hypotension in spinal cats. Am J Physiol 1989;257:H1347–H1353.

44. Mathias CJ, Christensen NJ, Corbett JL, et al. Plasma catecholamines, plasma renin activity and plasma aldosterone in tetraplegic man, horizontal and tilted. Clin Sci Mol Med 1975;49:291–299.

45. Guttman L, Munro AF, Robinson R, et al. Effect of tilting on the cardiovascular responses and plasma catecholamine levels in spinal man. Paraplegia 1963;1:4–18.

46. Schmid A, Huonker M, Barturen JM, et al. Catecholamines, heart rate, and oxygen uptake during exercise in persons with spinal cord injury. J Appl Physiol 1998;85(2):635–641.

47. Krum H, Brown DJ, Rowe PR, et al. Steady state plasma [3H]-noradrenaline kinetics in quadriplegic chronic spinal cord injury patients. J Autonom Pharmacol 1990;10:221–226.

48. Kooner JS, Birch R, Frankel HL, et al. Hemodynamic and neurohormonal effects of clonidine in patients with preganglionic and postganglionic sympathetic lesions. Circulation 1991;84:75–83.

49. Gootman PM, Cohen MI. Sympathetic rhythms in spinal cats. J Autonom Nerv Syst 1981;3:379–387.

50. Mannard A, Polosa C. Analysis of background firing of single sympathetic preganglionic neurons of cat cer-

vical nerve. J Neurophysiol 1973; 36:398–408.

51. Meckler RL, Weaver LC. Splenic, renal, and cardiac nerves have unequal dependence upon tonic supraspinal inputs. Brain Res 1985;338:123–135.

52. Qu L, Sherebrin R, Weaver LC. Blockade of spinal pathways decreases pre- and postganglionic discharge differentially. Am J Physiol 1988;255:R946–R951.

53. Stein RD, Weaver LC. Multi- and single-fibre mesenteric and renal sympathetic responses to chemical stimulation of intestinal receptors in cats. J Physiol (Lond) 1988;396:155–172.

54. Meckler RL, Weaver LC. Characteristics of on-going and reflex discharge of single splenic and renal sympathetic postganglionic fibers in cats. J Physiol (Lond) 1988;396:139–153.

55. Weaver LC, Meckler RL, Tobey JC, et al. Organization of Differential Sympathetic Responses to Activation of Visceral Receptors and Arterial Baroreceptors. In A Magro, W Osswald, O Reis, et al. (eds), Central and Peripheral Mechanisms of Cardiovascular Regulation. New York: Plenum, 1986; 269–301.

56. Weaver LC, Stein RD. Effects of spinal cord transection on sympathetic discharge in decerebrate unanesthetized cats. Am J Physiol 1989;257:R1506–R1511.

57. McCall RB, Gerber GL. Brain stem and spinal synchronization of sympathetic nervous discharge. Brain Res 1975;89:139–143.

58. Stein RD, Weaver LC, Yardley CP. Ventrolateral medullary neurones: effects on magnitude and rhythm of discharge of mesenteric and renal nerves in cats. J Physiol (Lond) 1989;408:571–586.

59. Johnson RH, Park DM. Effect of change of posture on blood pressure and plasma renin concentration in men with spinal transections. Clin Sci 1973;44:539–546.

60. Cole JD. The Pathophysiology of the Autonomic Nervous System in Spinal Cord Injury. In LS Illis (ed), Spinal Cord Dysfunction Assessment. Oxford: Oxford Medical Publications, 1988;201–235.

61. Osborn JW, Taylor RF, Schramm LP. Determinants of arterial pressure after chronic spinal transection in rats. Am J Physiol 1989;256:R666–R673.

62. Landrum LM, Thompson GM, Blair RW. Does postsynaptic α_1-adrenergic receptor supersensitivity contribute to autonomic dysreflexia. Heart Circ Physiol 1998;274(43):H1090–H1098.

63. Davies IB, Mathias CJ, Sudera D, Sever PS. Agonist regulation of alpha-adrenergic receptor responses in man. J Cardiovasc Pharmacol 1982;4:S139–S144.

64. Rodrigues GP, Clause-Walker J, Kent MC, et al. Adrenergic receptors in insensitive skin of spinal cord injured patients. Arch Phys Med Rehabil 1986;67:177–180.

65. Arnold JM, Feng QP, Delaney GA, Teasell RW. Autonomic dysreflexia in tetraplegic patients: evidence for alpha-adrenoceptor hyper-responsiveness. Clin Auton Res 1995;5(5):267–270.

66. Mathias CJ, Frankel HL, Christensen NJ, et al. Enhanced pressor response to noradrenaline in patients with cervical spinal cord transection. Brain 1976;99:757–770.

67. Maiorov DN, Weaver LC, Krassioukov AV. Relationship between sympathetic activity and arterial pressure in conscious spinal rats. Am J Physiol 1997;272(41):H625–H631.

68. Stjernberg L, Blumberg H, Wallin BG. Sympathetic activity in man after spinal cord injury. Outflow to muscle below the lesion. Brain 1986;109:695–715.

69. Wallin BG, Stjernberg L. Sympathetic activity in man after spinal cord injury. Brain 1984;107:183–198.

70. Mathias CJ, Christensen NJ, Frankel HL, et al. Renin release during head-up tilt occurs independently of sympathetic nervous activity in tetraplegic man. Clin Sci 1980;59:251–256.

71. Mikami H, Bumpus FM, Ferrario CM. Hierarchy of blood pressure control mechanisms after spinal sympathectomy. J Hypertens 1983;1(Suppl 2): 62–65.

72. Cardus D, McTaggart WG. Total body water and its distribution in men with spinal cord injury. Arch Phys Med Rehabil 1984;65:509–512.

73. Osborn JW, Livingstone RH, Schramm LP. Elevated renal nerve activity after spinal transection: effects on renal function. Am J Physiol 1987;253: R619–R625.

74. Poole CJM, Williams TDM, Lightman SL, et al. Neuroendocrine control of vasopressin secretion and its effect on blood pressure in subjects with spinal cord transection. Brain 1987;110:727–735.

75. Kiline S, Akman MN, Levendoglu F, Ozker R. Diurnal variation of antidiuretic hormone and urinary output in spinal cord injury. Spinal Cord 1999; 37:332–335.

76. Szollar SM, North J, Chung J. Antidiuretic hormone levels in spinal cord injury. A preliminary report. Paraplegia 1995;80:271–276.

77. Kooner JS, da Costa DF, Frankel HL, et al. Recumbency induces hypertension, diuresis and natriuresis in autonomic failure, but diuresis alone in tetraplegia. J Hypertens 1987;5(Suppl 5):S327–S329.

78. Kewalramani LS. Autonomic dysreflexia in traumatic myelopathy. Am J Phys Med Rehabil 1980;59:1–21.

79. Braddom RL, Rocco JF. Autonomic dysreflexia. Am J Phys Med Rehabil 1991;70:234–241.

80. Lindan R, Joiner E, Freehafer AA, et al. Incidence and clinical features of autonomic dysreflexia in patients with spinal cord injury. Paraplegia 1980;18: 285–292.

81. Stowe DF, Bernstein JS, Madsen KE, et al. Autonomic hyperreflexia in spinal cord injured patients during extracorporeal shock wave lithotripsy. Anesth Analg 1989;68:788–791.

82. Lee BY, Carmaker MG, Her BL, Strudel RA. Autonomic dysreflexia revisited. J Spinal Cord Med 1995;18:75–87.

83. Naftchi NE, Richardson JS. Autonomic dysreflexia: pharmacological management of hypertensive crises in spinal cord injured patients. J Spinal Cord Med 1997;20(3):355–360.

84. Comarr AE, Eltorai I. Autonomic dysreflexia/hyperreflexia. J Spinal Cord Med 1997;20(3):345–354.

85. Amzallag M. Autonomic hyperreflexia. Int Anesthesiol Clin 1993; 31(1):87–102.

86. Colachis SC. Autonomic hyperreflexia with spinal cord injury. J Am Paraplegia Soc 1992;15(3):171–186.

87. Kimura A, Ohsawa H, Sato A, Sato Y. Somatocardiovascular reflexes in anesthetized rats with the central nervous system intact or acutely spinalized at the cervical level. Neurosci Res 1995;22:297–305.

88. Giuliani S, Maggi CA, Meli A. Capsaicin-sensitive afferents in the rat urinary bladder activate a spinal sympathetic cardiovascular reflex. Naunyn-Schb Arch Pharmacol 1988;338:411–416.

89. Holzer P. Local effector functions of capsaicin sensitive sensory nerve endings: Involvement of tachykinins, calcitonin gene-related peptide and other neuropeptides. Neuroscience 1988;24: 739–768.

90. Schurch B, Knapp PA, Jeanmonod D,

et al. Does sacral posterior rhizotomy suppress autonomic hyper-reflexia in patients with spinal cord injury? Br J Urol 1998;81(1):73–82.

91. Coggeshall RE. Law of separation of function of the spinal roots. Physiol Rev 1980;60:716–755.

92. Krassioukov AV, Weaver LC. Morphological changes in sympathetic preganglionic neurons after spinal cord injury in rats. Neuroscience 1996;70(1):211–225.

93. Krenz NR, Weaver LC. Changes in the morphology of sympathetic preganglionic neurons parallel the development of autonomic dysreflexia after spinal cord injury in rats. Neurosci Lett 1998;243:61–64.

94. Maiorov DN, Krenz NR, Krassioukov AV, Weaver LC. Role of spinal NMDA and AMPA receptors in episodic hypertension in conscious spinal rats. Am J Physiol 1997;273(42):H1266–H1274.

95. Lindan R, Leffler EJ, Kedia KR. A comparison of the efficacy of an alpha$_1$-adrenergic blocker and a slow calcium channel blocker in the control of autonomic dysreflexia. Paraplegia 1985;23:34–38.

96. Apple DF. Autonomic dysreflexia management. ASIA Bull 2000;19(1):3.

97. Krum H, Louis WJ, Brown DJ, Howes LG. A study of the alpha-1 adrenoceptor blocker Prazosin in the prophylactic management of autonomic dysreflexia in high spinal cord injury patients. Clin Auton Res 1992; 2(2):83–88.

98. Vaidyanathan S, Soni BM, Sett P, et al. Pathophysiology of autonomic dysreflexia: long-term treatment with terazosin in adult and pediatric spinal cord injury patients manifesting recurrent dysreflexic episodes. Spinal Cord 1998;36:761–770.

99. Mathias CJ, Frankel HI. Cardiovascular control in spinal man. Annu Rev Physiol 1988;50:577–592.

100. Lehmann KG, Shandling AH, Yusi AU, et al. Altered ventricular repolarization in central sympathetic dysfunction associated with spinal cord injury. Am J Cardiol 1989;63:1498–1504.

101. Coutts KD, Rhodes EC, McKenzie DC. Maximal exercise responses of tetraplegics and paraplegics. J Appl Physiol 1983;55:479–482.

102. VanLoan MD, McCluer S, Loftin JM, et al. Comparison of physiological responses to maximal arm exercise among able-bodied, paraplegics and quadriplegics. Paraplegia 1987;25:397–405.

103. Luce IM, Culver BH. Respiratory muscle function in health and disease. Chest 1982;81:82–90.

104. Van der Velden VHJ, Hulsmann AR. Autonomic innervation of human airways: structure, function, and pathophysiology in asthma. Neuroimmunomodulation 1999;6:145–159.

105. Kamikawa Y. Neurogenic control of airway smooth muscle function. J Pharmacol Toxicol Methods 1994; 31(4):207–213.

106. Coleridge HM, Coleridge JCG. Neural regulation of bronchial blood flow. Respiration Physiology 1994;98:1–13.

107. Barnes PJ, Liu SF. Regulation of pulmonary vascular tone. Pharmacol Rev 1995;47(1):87–131.

108. Widdicombe J. The neural reflexes in the airways. Eur J Respir Dis Suppl 1986;144:1–33.

109. Bianchi AL, Denavit-Saubie M, Champagnat J. Central control of breathing in mammals: neuronal circuitry, membrane properties, and neurotransmitters. Physiol Rev 1995;75(1):1–45.

110. Yu J, Zhang JF, Roberts AM, et al. Pulmonary rapidly adapting receptor stimulation does not increase airway resistance in anesthetized rabbits. Am J Respir Crit Care Med 1999;160:906–912.

111. Coleridge HM, Coleridge JCG. Pulmonary reflexes: neural mechanisms of pulmonary defense. Annu Rev Physiol 1994;56:69–91.

112. Neubauer JA, Gonsalves SF, Chou W, et al. Chemosensitivity of medullary neurons in explant tissue cultures. Neuroscience 1991;45:701–708.

113. McMichan JC, Michel L, Westbrook PR. Pulmonary dysfunction following traumatic quadriplegia. JAMA 1980;243:528–531.

114. Crane L, Klerk K, Ruhl A, et al. The effect of exercise training on pulmonary function in persons with quadriplegia. Paraplegia 1994;32:435–441.

115. Loveridge B, Sanii R, Dubo HI. Breathing pattern adjustments during the first year following cervical spinal cord injury. Paraplegia 1992;30:479–488.

116. Almenoff PL, Alexander LR, Spungen AM, et al. Bronchodilatory effects of ipratropium bromide in patients with tetraplegia. Paraplegia 1995;33:274–277.

117. DeLuca RV, Grimm DR, Lesser M, et al. Effects of a β_2-agonist on airway hyperreactivity in subjects with cervical spinal cord injury. Chest 1999;115:1533–1538.

118. Grimm DR, Arias E, Lesser M, et al. Airway hyperresponsiveness to ultrasonically nebulized distilled water in subjects with tetraplegia. J Appl Physiol 1999;86(4):1165–1169.

119. Singas E, Lesser M, Spungen AM, et al. Airway hyperresponsiveness to methacholine in subjects with spinal cord injury. Chest 1996;110:911–915.

120. Kelling JS, DiMarco AF, Gottfried SB, Altose MD. Respiratory responses to ventilatory loading following low cervical spinal cord injury. J Appl Physiol 1985;59(6):1752–1756.

121. Manning HL, Shea SAK, Schwartzstein RM, et al. Reduced tidal volume increases "air hunger" at fixed PCO_2 in ventilated quadriplegics. Respir Physiol 1992;90(1):19–30.

122. Lin K, Wu H, Chang C, et al. Ventilatory and mouth occlusion pressure responses to hypercapnia in chronic tetraplegia. Arch Phys Med Rehabil 1998;79:795–799.

123. Pokorski M, Morikawa T, Takaishi S, et al. Ventilatory responses to chemosensory stimuli in quadriplegic subjects. Eur Respir J 1990;3(8):891–900.

124. Axen K. Ventilatory responses to mechanical loads in cervical cord-injured humans. J Appl Physiol 1982;52:748–756.

125. O'Donnell DE, Sanii R, Dubo H, et al. Steady-state ventilatory responses to expiratory resistive loading in quadriplegics. Am Rev Respir Dis 1993;147(1):54–59.

126. Banzett RB, Lansing RW, Brown R. High-level quadriplegics perceive lung volume change. J Appl Physiol 1987;62:567–573.

127. Simon PM, Leevers AM, Murty JL, et al. Neuromechanical regulation of respiratory motor output in ventilator-dependent C1-C3 quadriplegics. J Appl Physiol 1995;79(1):312–323.

128. Gandevia SC, Killian K, McKenzie DK, et al. Respiratory sensations, cardiovascular control, kinanesthesia and transcranial stimulation during paralysis in humans. J Physiol 1993;470:85–107.

129. Simon E. Temperature regulation: the spinal cord as a site of extrahypothalamic thermoregulatory functions. Rev Physiol Biochem Pharmacol 1974;71:1–76.

130. Downey RJ, Downey JA, Newhouse E, et al. Hyperthermia in a quadriplegic: evidence for a peripheral action of haloperidol in malignant neuroleptic syndrome. Chest 1992;101:1728–1730.

131. Menard MR, Hahn G. Acute and chronic hypothermia in a man with

spinal cord injury: environmental and pharmacologic causes. Arch Phys Med Rehabil 1991;72:421–424.

132. Schmidt KD, Chan CW. Thermoregulation and fever in normal persons and in those with spinal cord injuries. Mayo Clin Proc 1992;67:469–475.

133. Downey JA, Chiodi HP, Darling RC. Central temperature regulation in the spinal man. J Appl Physiol 1967;22:91–94.

134. Miller JM. Autonomic Function in the Isolated Spinal Cord. In JA Downey, RC Darling (eds), Physiological Basis of Rehabilitation Medicine. Philadelphia: WB Saunders, 1971;265–281.

135. Cooper KE, Ferres HM, Guttman L. Vasomotor responses in the foot to raising body temperature in the paraplegic patient. J Physiol (Lond) 1957;136:547–555.

136. Appenzeller O, Schnieden H. Neurogenic pathways concerned in reflex vasodilatation in the hand with especial reference to stimuli affecting the afferent pathway. Clin Sci 1963;25:413–421.

137. Benzinger TH. Heat regulation: homeostasis of central temperature in man. Physiol Rev 1969;49:671–759.

138. Tsai S-H, Shih C-J, Shyy T-T, et al. Recovery of vasomotor response in human spinal cord transection. J Neurosurg 1980;52:808–811.

139. Corbett JL, Frankel HL, Harris PJ. Cardiovascular reflex responses to cutaneous and visceral stimuli in spinal man. J Physiol (Lond) 1971;215:395–409.

140. Sahs AL, Fulton JR. Somatic and automatic reflexes in spinal monkeys. J Neurophysiol 1940;3:258–268.

141. Freund PR, Brengelmann GL, Rowell LB, et al. Attenuated skin blood flow response to hyperthermia in paraplegic men. J Appl Physiol 1984;56:1104–1109.

142. Johnson RH. Neurological studies in temperature regulation. Ann R Coll Surg Engl 1965;36:339–352.

143. Downey JA, Huckaba CE, Kelley PS, et al. Sweating responses to central and peripheral heating in spinal man. J Appl Physiol 1976;5:701–706.

144. Quinton PM. Sweating and its disorders. Annu Rev Med 1983;34:429–452.

145. Normell LA. Distribution of impaired cutaneous vasomotor and sudomotor function in paraplegic man. Scand J Clin Lab Invest 1974;33(Suppl 138):25–41.

146. Huckaba CE, Frewin DB, Downey JA, et al. Sweating responses of normal, paraplegic and anhidrotic man. Arch Phys Med Rehabil 1976;57:268–274.

147. Seckendorf R, Randall WC. Thermal reflex sweating in normal and paraplegic man. J Appl Physiol 1961;16(5):796–800.

148. Silver JR, Randall WC, Guttmann L. Spinal mediation of thermally induced sweating. J Neurol Neurosurg Psychiatry 1991;54:297–304.

149. Tam HS, Darling RC, Cheh HY, et al. The dead zone of thermoregulation in normal and paraplegic man. Can J Physiol Pharmacol 1978;56:976–983.

150. Stjernberg L, Wallin BG. Sympathetic neural out-flow in spinal man. A preliminary report. J Autonom Nerv Syst 1983;7:313–318.

151. Guttman L, Whitteridge D. Effects of bladder distention on autonomic mechanisms after spinal cord injuries. Brain 1947;70:366–404.

152. Furness JB, Costa M. The Enteric Nervous System. Edinburgh: Churchill Livingstone, 1987.

153. Goyal RK, Hirano I. The enteric nervous system. N Engl J Med 1996;334(17):1106–1115.

154. Furness JB, Kunze WAA, Bertrand PP, et al. Intrinsic primary afferent neurons of the intestine. Prog Neurobiol 1998;54:1–18.

155. Read NW, Houghton LA. Physiology of gastric emptying and pathophysiology of gastroparesis. Gastroenterol Clin North Am 1989;18:359–372.

156. Andrews PLR. Vagal Afferent Innervation of the Gastrointestinal Tract. In F Cervero, JFB Morrison (eds), Progress in Brain Research. Vol 67: Visceral Sensation. Amsterdam: Elsevier, 1986;65–86.

157. Rees WDW, Malagelada JR, Miller LJ, et al. Human interdigestive and postprandial gastrointestinal motor and hormone patterns. Dig Dis Sci 1982;27:321–329.

158. Stoddard CJ, Smallwood RH, Duthie HL. Migrating Myoelectric Complex in Man. In HL Duffy (ed), Proceedings of the Sixth International Motility Symposium. Baltimore: University Park Press, 1978;9–27.

159. Kunze WAA, Furness JB. The enteric nervous system and regulation of intestinal motility. Annu Rev Physiol 1999;61:117–142.

160. Tack J. Georges Brohee Prize 1994. Motilin and the enteric nervous system in the control of interdigestive and postprandial gastric motility. Acta Gastroenterol Belg 1995;58(1):21–30.

161. Guttman L. Spinal Cord Injuries: Comprehensive Management and Research (2nd ed). Oxford: Blackwell Scientific, 1970;237–473.

162. Fealey RD, Szurszewski JH, Merritt JL, et al. Effect of traumatic spinal cord transection on human upper gastrointestinal motility and gastric emptying. Gastroenterology 1984;87:69–75.

163. Telford GL, Go VLW, Szurszewski JH. Effect of central sympathectomy on gastric and small intestinal myoelectric activity and plasma motilin concentrations in the dog. Gastroenterology 1985;89:989–995.

164. Segal JL, Milne N, Brunnemann SR. Gastric emptying is impaired in patients with spinal cord injury. Am J Gastroenterol 1995;90(3):466–470.

165. Lu C, Montgomery P, Zou X, et al. Gastric myoelectrical activity in patients with cervical spinal cord injury. Am J Gastroenterol 1998;93(12):2391–2396.

166. Schuster M. Motor disorders of the stomach. Med Clin North Am 1981;65:1269–1289.

167. Smith T, Sanders KM. Motility of the Large Intestine. In T Yamada, DH Alpers, O Chung, et al. (eds), Textbook of Gastroenterology. Philadelphia: Lippincott, 1995.

168. Longo WE, Ballantyne GH, Modlin IM. The colon, anorectum, and spinal cord patient. A review of the functional alterations of the denervated hindgut. Dis Colon Rectum 1989;32:261–267.

169. Kuo DC, Hisamitsu T, de Groat WC. A sympathetic projection from sacral paravertebral ganglia the pelvic nerve and to postganglionic nerves on the surface of the urinary bladder and large intestine of the cat. J Comp Neurol 1984;226:76–86.

170. Luckensmeyer GB, Keast JR. Activation of α- and β-adrenoceptors by sympathetic nerve stimulation in the large intestine of the rat. J Physiol 1998;510(Pt2):549–561.

171. Lundberg JM, Hokfelt T, Anggard A, et al. Organizational principles in the peripheral sympathetic neurone system. Subdivision by co-existing peptides (somatostatin, avian pancreatic polypeptide, and vasoactive intestinal polypeptide-like immunoreactive materials). Proc Natl Acad Sci U S A 1982;79:1303–1307.

172. Keef KD, Kreulen DL. Comparison of central versus peripheral nerve pathways to the guinea pig inferior mesenteric ganglion determined electro-physiologically after chronic nerve section. J Autonom Nerv Syst 1990; 29:95–112.

173. Du CH, Ferre JR, Ruckebusch Y. Spi-

nal cord influences on the colonic myo-electrical activity of fed and fasted rats. J Physiol 1987;383:395–404.

174. Hertz A, Newton A. The normal movement of the colon in man. J Physiol (Lond) 1913;47:57–65.

175. Aaronson MJ, Freed MM, Burakoff R. Colonic myoelectric activity in persons with spinal cord injury. Dig Dis Sci 1985;30:295–300.

176. Glick ME, Meshkinpour H, Haldeman S, et al. Colonic dysfunction in patients with thoracic spinal cord injury. Gastroenterology 1984;86:287–294.

177. Connell AM, Frankel H, Guttman L. The motility of the pelvic colon following complete lesions of the spinal cord. Paraplegia 1963;1:98–110.

178. Banwell JG, Creasey GH, Aggarwal AM, Mortimer JT. Management of the neurogenic bowel in patients with spinal cord injury. Urol Clin North Am 1993;20(3):517–526.

179. Sun W, MacDonagh R, Forster D, et al. Anorectal function in patients with complete spinal transection before and after sacral posterior rhizotomy. Gastroenterology 1995;108:990–998.

180. Stone JM, Nino-Murcia M, Wolfe VA, et al. Chronic gastrointestinal problems in spinal cord injury patients: a prospective analysis. Am J Gastroenterol 1990;85:1114–1119.

181. Krogh K, Nielsen J, Djurhuus JC, et al. Colorectal function in patients with spinal cord lesions. Dis Colon Rectum 1997;40:1233–1239.

182. Beuret-Blanquart F, Weber J, Gouverneur JP, et al. Colonic transit time and anorectal manometric anomalies in 19 patients with complete transection of the spinal cord. J Auton Nerv Syst 1990;30:199–207.

183. Menardo G, Bausano G, Corrazziari RE. Large bowel transit in paraplegic patients. Dis Colon Rectum 1987;30:924–928.

184. Leduc BE, Giasson M, Favreau-Ethier M, Lepage Y. Colonic transit time after spinal cord injury. J Spinal Cord Med 1997;20:416–421.

185. Keshavarzian A, Barnes WE, Bruninga K, et al. Delayed colonic transit in spinal cord-injured patients measured by indium-111 Amberlite scintigraphy. Am J Gastroenterol 1995;90(8):1295–1300.

186. Binnie NR, Creasey GH, Edmond P, Smith AN. The action of cisapride on the chronic constipation of paraplegia. Paraplegia 1988;26(3):151–158.

187. Longo WE, Woolsey RM, Vernava AM, et al. Cisapride for constipation in spinal cord injured patients: a pre-

liminary report. J Spinal Cord Med 1995;18(4):240–244.

188. Geders JM, Gaing A, Bauman WA, Korsten MA. The effect of cisapride on segmental colonic transit time in patients with spinal cord injury. Am J Gastroenterol 1995;90(2):285–289.

189. Badiali D, Corrazziari E, Habib F, et al. A double-blind controlled trial on the effect of cisapride in the treatment of constipation in paraplegic patients. J Gastro Motil 1991;3:263–267.

190. Stiens SA, Bergman SB, Goetz LL. Neurogenic bowel dysfunction after spinal cord injury: clinical evaluation and rehabilitative management. Arch Phys Med Rehabil 1997;78:S86–S102.

191. de Groat WC, Booth AM. Physiology of male sexual function. Ann Intern Med 1980;92:329–331.

192. de Groat WC, Steers WD. Neuroanatomy and Neurophysiology of Penile Erection. In EA Tanagho, TF Lue, DD McClure (eds), Contemporary Management of Impotence and Infertility. Baltimore: Williams & Wilkins, 1988;3–27.

193. Langley JM, Anderson HR. The innervation of the pelvic and adjoining viscera. Part H: The bladder. J Physiol (Lond) 1896;19:71–84.

194. Semans JH, Langworthy OR. Observation on the neurophysiology of sexual function in the cat. J Urol 1938;40:836–846.

195. Steers WD, Mallory B, de Groat WC. Electrophysiological study of neural activity in penile nerve of the rat. Am J Physiol 1988;254:R989–R1000.

196. Peters LC, Kristal MB, Komisaruk BR. Sensory innervation of the external and internal genitalia of the female rat. Brain Res 1987;408:197–204.

197. Yarkony GM. Enhancement of sexual function and fertility in spinal cord-injured males. Am J Phys Med Rehabil 1990;69:81–87.

198. Lue TF, Zeineh SJ, Schmidt RA, et al. Neuroanatomy of penile erection: its relevance to iatrogenic impotence. J Urol 1984;131:273–280.

199. Dail WG, Minorsky N, Moll MA, et al. The hypogastric nerve pathway to penile erectile tissue: histochemical evidence supporting a vasodilator role. J Autonom Nerv Syst 1986;15:341–349.

200. Bors E, Comarr AE. Neurological disturbance of sexual function with special reference to 529 patients with spinal cord injury. Urol Surg 1960;10:191–222.

201. Hart BL, Melese-D'Hospital PY. Penile mechanisms and the role of the striated

penile muscle in penile reflexes. Physiol Behav 1983;31:807–813.

202. Herbert J. The role of the dorsal nerves of the penis in the sexual behavior of the male rhesus monkey. Physiol Behav 1973;10:292–300.

203. Sachs BD. Role of striated penile muscles in penile reflexes, copulation and induction of pregnancy in the rat. J Reprod Fertil 1982;66:433–443.

204. de Tejada IS, Blanco R, Goldstein L, et al. Cholinergic neurotransmission in human penile corpus cavernosum smooth muscle [Abstract]. Fed Proc 1988;256:454.

205. Lepor H, Gregerman M, Crosby R, et al. Precise localization of the autonomic nerves from the pelvic plexus to the corpora cavernosa: a detailed anatomical study of the adult male pelvis. J Urol 1985;133:207–212.

206. Gu J, Polak M, Probert L, et al. Peptidergic innervation of the human male genital tract. J Urol 1983;130:386–391.

207. Giuiliano FA, Rampin O, Benoit G, Jardin A. Neural control of penile erection. Urol Clin North Am 1995;22(4):747–766.

208. Hedlund H, Andersson K-E, Mattiasson A. Pre- and post-junctional adreno- and muscarinic receptor functions in the isolated human corpus spongiosum urethrae. J Autonom Pharmacol 1984;4:241–249.

209. Monga M, Bernie J, Rajasekaran M. Male infertility and erectile dysfunction in spinal cord injury: a review. Arch Phys Med Rehabil 1999;80:1331–1339.

210. Simonsen U, Prieto D, Hernandez M, et al. Prejunctional alpha 2-adrenoceptors inhibit nitrergic neurotransmission in horse penile resistance arteries. J Urol 1997;157(6):2356–2360.

211. Willis EA, Ottensen B, Wagner G, et al. Vasoactive intestinal polypeptide (VIP) as a putative neurotransmitter in penile erection. Life Sci 1983;33:383–391.

212. Sarkarati M, Rossier AB, Farn BA. Experience in vibratory and electro-ejaculation techniques in spinal cord injury patients: a preliminary report. J Urol 1987;138:59–62.

213. Brindley GS. The fertility of men with spinal injuries. Paraplegia 1984;22:337–348.

214. Brindley GS. Reflex ejaculation under vibratory stimulation in paraplegic men. Paraplegia 1981;19:299–302.

215. Chapelle PA, Roby-Rami A, Yakovleff A, et al. Neurologic correlations of ejaculation and testicular size in men

with a complete spinal cord section. J Neurol Neurosurg Psychiatry 1988;51:197–202.

216. Claus-Walker J, Scurry M, Carter M, et al. Steady-state hormonal secretion in traumatic quadriplegia. J Clin Endocrinol Metab 1977;44:530–535.

217. Young RJ, Strachan RK, Seth J, et al. Is testicular endocrine function abnormal in young men with spinal cord injuries? J Clin Endocrinol Metab 1982;17:303–306.

218. Derry FA, Dinsmore WW, Fraser M, et al. Efficacy and safety of oral sildenafil (Viagra) in men with erectile dysfunction caused by spinal cord injury. Neurology 1998;51(6):1629–1633.

219. Maytom MC, Derry FA, Dinsmore WW, et al. A two-part pilot study of sildenafil (Viagra) in men with erectile dysfunction caused by spinal cord injury. Spinal Cord 1999;37(2):110–116.

220. Seager SWJ, Halstead LS. Fertility options and success after spinal cord injury. Urol Clin North Am 1993;20(3):543–548.

221. Ohl DA, Menge AC, Sonksen J. Penile vibratory stimulation in spinal cord injured men: optimized vibration parameters and prognostic factors. Arch Phys Med Rehabil 1996;77(9):903–905.

222. Brackett NL. Semen retrieval by penile vibratory stimulation in men with spinal cord injury. Hum Reprod Update 1999;5(3):216–222.

223. Berard EJJ. The sexuality of spinal cord injured women: physiology and pathophysiology. A review. Paraplegia 1989;27:99–112.

224. Nygaard I, Bartscht KD, Cole S. Sexuality and reproduction in spinal cord-injured women. Obstet Gynecol Surv 1992;45:727–732.

225. Reame NE. A prospective study of the menstrual cycle and spinal cord injury. Am J Phys Med Rehabil 1992;71:15–21.

226. Young BK, Katz M, Klein SA. Pregnancy after spinal cord injury: altered maternal and fetal response to labor. Obstet Gynecol 1983;62:59–63.

227. Masters WH, Johnson VE. Human Sexual Response. Boston: Little, Brown, 1965;65–130.

228. Sipski ML, Alexander CJ, Rosen RC. Orgasm in women with spinal cord injuries: a laboratory-based assessment. Arch Phys Med Rehabil 1995;76:1097–1102.

229. Collins JJ, Lin CE, Berthoud HR, Papka RE. Vagal afferents from the uterus and cervix provide direct connections to the brainstem. Cell Tissue Res 1999;295:43–54.

230. Whipple B, Komisaruk BR. Sexuality and women with complete spinal cord injury. Spinal Cord 1997;35:136–138.

231. McGregor JA, Meeuwsen J. Autonomic hyperreflexia: a mortal danger for spinal cord-damaged women in labor. Am J Obstet Gynecol 1985;151:330–333.

232. Seftel AD, Oates RD, Krane RJ. Disturbed sexual function in patients with spinal cord disease. Neurol Clin 1991;9:757–778.

233. Baker ER, Cardenas DA. Pregnancy in spinal cord injured women. Arch Phys Med Rehabil 1996;77:501–507.

234. Andersson KE, Sjogren C. Aspects on the physiology and pharmacology of the bladder and urethra. Prog Neurobiol 1982;19:71–89.

235. Maggi CA, Santicioli P, Borsini F, et al. The role of the capsaicin-sensitive innervation of the rat urinary bladder in the activation of micturition reflex. Naunyn-Schb Arch Pharmacol 1986;332:276–283.

236. Santicioli P, Maggi CA, Meli A. Functional evidence for the existence of a capsaicin-sensitive innervation in the rat urinary bladder. J Pharm Pharmacol 1986;38:446–451.

237. Maggi CA, Barbanti G, Santicioli P, et al. Cystometric evidence that capsaicin-sensitive nerves modulate the afferent branch of micturition reflex in humans. J Urol 1989;142:150–154.

238. Janig W, McLachlan EM. Identification of distinct topographical distributions of lumbar sympathetic and sensory neurons projecting to end organs with different functions in the cat. J Comp Neurol 1986;246:104–112.

239. Yoshimura N. Bladder afferent pathway and spinal cord injury: possible mechanisms inducing hyperreflexia of the urinary bladder. Prog Neurobiol 1999;57:583–606.

240. de Groat WC, Booth AM. Physiology of the urinary bladder and urethra. Ann Intern Med 1980;92:312–315.

241. de Groat WC. A neurologic basis for the overactive bladder. Urology 1997;50(Suppl 6A):36–52.

242. McGuire F. The innervation and function of the lower urinary tract. J Neurosurg 1986;65:278–285.

243. Elbadawi A. Neuromorphologic basis of vesicourethral function: histochemistry, ultrastructure, and function of intrinsic nerves of the bladder and urethra. Neurourol Urodyn 1982;1:3–50.

244. Elbadawi A. Ultrastructure of vesicourethral innervation. II. Postganglionic axoaxonal synapses in intrinsic innervation of the vesicourethral lissosphincter: a new structural and functional concept in micturition. J Urol 1984;131:781–790.

245. Crowe R, Burnstock G. A histochemical and immunohistochemical study of the autonomic innervation of the lower urinary tract of the female pig. Is the pig a good model for the human bladder and urethra? J Urol 1989;141:414–422.

246. Lincoln J, Crowe R, Bokor J, et al. Adrenergic and cholinergic innervation of smooth and striated muscle components of the urethra from patients with spinal cord injury. J Urol 1986;135:402–408.

247. Mallory B, Steers WD, de Groat WC. Electrophysiological study of the micturition reflexes in rats. Am J Physiol 1989;257:R410–R421.

248. de Groat WC, Ryall RW. Reflexes to sacral parasympathetic neurones concerned with micturition in the cat. J Physiol (Lond) 1969;200:87–108.

249. Kuru M. Nervous control of micturition. Physiol Rev 1965;45:425–494.

250. Mallory B, Shefchyk SK. Effect of subtotal spinal cord lesions on brainstem evoked and peripheral reflex micturition in cats. Ann R Coll Phys Surg Can 1986.

251. Kruse MN, Mallory BS, Noto H, et al. Modulation of the spinobulbospinal micturition reflex pathway in cats. Am J Physiol 1992;262:R478–R484.

252. de Groat WC. Nervous control of the urinary bladder of the cat. Brain Res 1975;87:201–211.

253. de Groat WC, Booth AM. Autonomic Systems to the Urinary Bladder and Sexual Organs. In PJ Dyck, PK Thomas, EH Lambert, et al. (eds), Peripheral Neuropathy (2nd ed). Philadelphia: WB Saunders, 1984;285–299.

254. Schondorf R, Laskey W, Polosa C. Upper thoracic sympathetic neuron responses to input from urinary bladder afferents. Am J Physiol 1983;245:R311–R320.

255. de Groat WC, Nadelhaft L, Milne RJ, et al. Organization of the sacral parasympathetic reflex pathways to the urinary bladder and large intestine. J Autonom Nerv Syst 1981;3:135–160.

256. Sato A, Sato Y, Shimada F, et al. Changes in vesical function produced by cutaneous stimulation in rats. Brain Res 1975;94:465–474.

257. Thor K, Kawatani M, de Groat WC. Plasticity in the Reflex Pathways to the Lower Urinary Tract of the Cat during Postnatal Development and Following Spinal Cord Injury. In M Goldberger, A Gorio, M Murray (eds), Development and Plasticity of the Mammalian Spinal Cord. Padova: Liviana Press, 1985;105–121.

258. Thor KB, Blais DP, de Groat WC. Behavioral analysis of the postnatal development of micturition in kittens. Dev Brain Res 1989;46:137–144.

259. Kaplan SA, Chancellor MB, Blaivas JG. Bladder and sphincter behavior in patients with spinal cord lesions. J Urol 1991;146:113–117.

260. Blaivas JG, Sinha HP, Zayed AA, Labib KB. Detrusor-external sphincter dyssynergia. J Urol 1981;125:542–544.

261. Wyndaele JJ. Urethral sphincter dyssynergia in spinal cord injury patients. Paraplegia 1987;25:10–15.

262. Watanabe T, Rivas DA, Chancellor MB. Urodynamics of spinal cord injury. Urol Clin North Am 1996;23(3):459–473.

30

Aphasia, Apraxia, and Agnosia

JOHN C. M. BRUST

HANDEDNESS AND CEREBRAL DOMINANCE

Approximately 90% of people are *right-handed*; they have better motor dexterity with their right limbs and prefer to use them in complex motor tasks such as throwing a ball or writing.[1,2] More than 95% of right-handers process language in the left cerebral hemisphere (left cerebral dominance), damage to which causes aphasia. Ten percent of people are left-handed, although among them the degree of left preference varies considerably and some are left-handed as a result of cerebral disease. Approximately one-half of left-handers also have left cerebral dominance for language, and the other half have right dominance. Overall, the hemispheric specialization of left-handers appears to be less pronounced, which may account for the observation that when they develop aphasia it is more likely than in right-handers to be mild or to resolve.

APHASIA: DEFINITION AND HISTORICAL BACKGROUND

Aphasia is a disturbance of language unexplained by articulatory impairment or sensory loss. Abnormal speech (dysarthria) secondary to paresis, spasticity, incoordination, abnormal movements, or dysphonia is not aphasia, and reading difficulty secondary to poor vision is not alexia. Aphasia is a disturbance of higher cortical function resulting from cerebral damage. Although it can occur in isolation, especially after head injury or stroke, aphasia is often a feature of a dementing illness such as Alzheimer's disease, and most severe

aphasics have additional cognitive impairment not related to language.

The modern study of aphasia began in the 1860s with Broca's description of left hemispheric lesions in patients with language disturbance.[3,4] Although details of the neurologic examinations were sparse and the lesions were large (including temporal and frontal lobes and insula), Broca's reports led not only to the recognition that language was usually processed in the left hemisphere but to the notion that the left frontal pars opercularis (Broca's area) was the center for speech, destruction of which caused expressive aphasia (Figure 30-1).

A decade later, Wernicke described infarction of the posterior superior temporal gyrus in patients with impaired speech comprehension.[5] Analogous to Broca's area, this posterior opercular region (Wernicke's area) became regarded as the center for speech comprehension. Wernicke also attributed difficulty in naming and repetition to lesions in the deep white matter tract connecting Wernicke's and Broca's area (the arcuate fasciculus) and called the resulting disorder *conduction aphasia*.

These reports were followed by a spate of clinical and anatomic correlations that attempted to define *centers* not only for particular language skills such as reading and writing but for nonlanguage cognitive activities as well[6] (e.g., as late as the 1920s, Henschen claimed there were centers for musical expression and reception, with a separate center for violin playing[7]). Early skepticism for such compartmentalization was expressed by Hughlings Jackson, who stressed that loss of function after a focal lesion does not necessarily mean that the damaged region is a center for that function.[8] This controversy, between those who sought to understand lan-

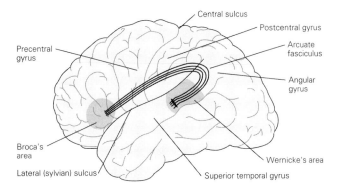

FIGURE 30-1 Lateral surface of the left hemisphere. (Reprinted with permission from ER Kandel, JH Schwartz, TM Jessell. Principles of Neural Science. Originally published by Appleton & Lange. Copyright 1991 by The McGraw-Hill Companies, Inc.)

guage by focusing on anatomic localization and those whose emphasis was psychological or linguistic, persists today, and a consequence has been a bewildering diversity of aphasia classifications.[9–19] In the United States, a classification that has found its way into many current medical and neurologic texts is that of Geschwind.[20,21] Oriented to the concept of centers and disconnections between them, it is as controversial as its historical predecessors. The advantage for clinicians of Geschwind's system, however, is that although it may seem pathophysiologically and linguistically simplistic, it depends on easily assessable symptoms and signs and a relatively unambiguous definition of aphasia subtypes. Geschwind's approach, which lends itself either to brief bedside screening or more formal testing such as the Boston Diagnostic Aphasia Examination,[22] can be said to work practically, even if its ultimate neuropsychological or linguistic validity remains uncertain.

EXAMINATION OF THE PATIENT

Language assessment consists of six parts: verbal expression, auditory comprehension, naming, repetition, writing, and reading. Abnormalities in one sphere obviously influence strategies employed to test others. Equally obvious is that nonlanguage mental abnormalities (e.g., obtundation, delirium, schizophrenia, dementia) can make language assessment difficult or impossible. Conversely, assessment of memory or cognition can be impossible when aphasia is present. The following outline is based on the assumption that the patient is cooperative and that language is impaired out of proportion to any coexisting mental abnormalities.

One assesses verbal expression by posing questions or remarks designed to elicit full-sentence replies. *Fluency* refers to the amount of speech produced over time, normally more than 50 words per minute.[23] Word-finding difficulty can produce nonfluent hesitations, but except with severe anomia the patient is usually able to produce several consecutive words or syllables at a normal rate. By contrast, the speech of so-called Broca's aphasia (defined later) is severely and consistently nonfluent independently of word finding per se and often marked by long delays in initiation and hesitations between words and syllables.

Prosody refers to the musical qualities of speech, including rhythm, accent, and pitch.[24–26] It gives languages and dialects their special oral character. There are different kinds of prosody. That which characterizes the emotional quality of speech (sad, glad, mad) is believed to depend on right hemisphere processing. Prosody also provides propositional information (e.g., the pitch inflections that characterize a sentence as interrogative or imperative, or in languages such as Chinese or Thai, that convey the semantic meaning of words). Propositionally linked prosody is processed in the language hemisphere and can be impaired in some kinds of aphasia.

The term *paraphasia* describes incorrect words unintentionally substituted for correct ones. There are two types of paraphasic errors. In literal or phonemic paraphasia, words produced phonetically resemble the intended word but contain one or more substituted syllables (e.g., *hosicle* for *hospital*). When such alterations have the character of real words, they are called *neologisms*; sometimes ingeniously concocted (e.g., *nork* for a combination of *knife* and *fork*), they are not specific to aphasia, occurring also in psychotic speech. In verbal or semantic paraphasia, real but unintended words are produced (e.g., *hotel* for *hospital*); the substituted word is often semantically close to the intended word. In some patients, paraphasic errors are occasional contaminants of speech. In others, they almost entirely replace it; such speech is called *jargon*.

Even in the absence of paraphasia, the content of aphasic speech may be difficult to grasp. Severely restricted vocabulary may cause logorrheic but empty speech rather than word-finding hesitations. For example, an answer to the question, "Why are you in the hospital?" went, "Well, it was when I did that, that they said I should and so I did here." The term *paragrammatism* refers to the seemingly preserved syntax amidst such profoundly restricted semantic content. By contrast, syntactic or relational words (e.g., prepositions, conjunctions, possessives, verb tenses) are sometimes conspicuously abnormal or absent in aphasic speech, especially with Broca's aphasia; such speech, practically reduced to nouns and verbs, is called *agrammatic* or *telegrammatic*.

Some patients, again especially those with Broca's aphasia, have markedly restricted and nonfluent propositional speech yet produce outbursts of relatively fluent emotional or *inferior* speech. Such dissociation led Jackson to postulate that nonpropositional speech (e.g., amenities or invective cursing) is processed in the nondominant hemisphere. Sometimes aphasic speech is limited largely to a single sentence, cliché, or even syllable, a so-called recurrent utterance.

Having assessed verbal expression, the examiner proceeds to the patient's own auditory comprehension, for if that is impaired, the rest of the examination must be restructured. Strikingly abnormal auditory comprehension may become apparent only on shifting from open-ended conversation to specific testing. Moreover, abnormalities of auditory comprehension (like any neurologic sign) may be mild or severe or may become more severe as the examination progresses.

Assessment of auditory comprehension should be as independent as possible of the patient's own verbal output: A wrong answer to a question could signify a paraphasic error rather than failure to understand the question. Asking the patient to follow spoken commands carries similar potential ambiguities. If a command, simple or complex, is followed, and if the examiner has remembered to avoid nonverbal cues, it can be presumed that it was understood. Failure to follow a command, however, could have different possible explanations (e.g., paralysis, apraxia, pain, or negativism).

A more reliable method of testing speech comprehension is to ask yes or no questions. Even patients whose own speech is so severely restricted that they cannot say the words *yes* or *no* can usually indicate affirmative or negative. The correct answers must of course be known to both the patient and the examiner. Failure to identify a public figure, for example, could signify loss of memory or lack of interest, rather than impaired speech comprehension. Appropriate questions might include, "Is your name Mrs. Jones?" or (if the patient can see), "Am I wearing a hat?" The informational content of questions can be steadily increased (e.g., "Am I wearing a red striped necktie?").

Alternatively, the patient can be asked to point to objects or body parts; motor disability such as apraxia is less likely to interfere with such tasks than with following commands. Again, questions can be made increasingly complex (e.g., from "Where is the ceiling?" to "Where is the source of artificial illumination in this room?" to "Where did we enter this room?") A variant of

the formal Token Test[27] relies on similar identification of increasingly information-laden images; shown an array of drawings the patient might be asked to point first to a circle (not a square), then to a large (not a small) circle, and then to a large red (not a large blue) circle.

These strategies detect disorders of semantic comprehension. As with abnormal speech output, semantic and syntactic or relational comprehension can dissociate.[28] Syntactic or relational comprehension can be assessed (in patients with adequate motor ability) by object manipulation. First identifying, say, a comb, a pen, and a key, the patient is asked to put the key on top of the comb, or the comb between the key and the pen. Alternatively, the patient could be given a statement such as, "Tom's aunt's husband has blue eyes," and then be asked, "Is the person with blue eyes a man or a women?"

Naming ability is tested in patients with adequate vision by showing them objects, body parts, colors, or pictures of actions (*confrontation naming*). Patients with impaired vision can be asked to name body parts being touched or to name from description (e.g., "What do you shave with?" "What is the color of grass?"). Patients with impaired auditory comprehension may not grasp the nature of the task. A variety of abnormal responses indicate anomia. Some patients produce literal or verbal paraphasias, which may or may not then be self-corrected. Some hesitate and effortfully grope for the correct word (tip-of-the-tongue phenomenon); such patients, although unable to come up with the word on their own, may correctly select it from a spoken list or say it correctly after being given its first letter or phoneme or an incomplete sentence that the word would appropriately complete (contextual prompting).[29] Other patients describe rather than name the object (e.g., "It's what you wear around your neck," instead of *necktie*). Infrequently, anomic patients say simply, "I don't know," or "I've forgotten."

In some aphasics confrontation naming may be unexpectedly good compared with the apparent degree of word-finding difficulty in spontaneous verbal expression. Seeing an object may facilitate lexical entry, and so such patients may have much greater difficulty listing names within a category (e.g., articles of clothing, animals, objects of furniture, or words beginning with a particular letter). Not infrequently, only three or four items can be named.

Repetition is tested by having the patient repeat several sentences (e.g., "Today is a sunny day." "In the winter the President lives in Washington."). Syntactically loaded sentences may be especially difficult (e.g., "If he were to come, I would go out."). (The phrase, "No ifs, ands, or buts," has been considered particularly suitable for identifying difficulty with syntax[21]; such an assertion is dubious, because, although the words are all prepositions or conjunctions, they are not being used in a syntactical sense. Moreover, if a sentence is unfamiliar or makes no sense to a patient, difficulty repeating it might have nothing to do with aphasia.) Repetition errors most often consist of paraphasic substitutions.

Testing of writing can begin by having the patient sign his or her name. If that cannot be accomplished, more elaborate tests will almost surely fail. Writing one's name, however, does not necessarily rely on language processing per se; in many people it is an *overlearned motor act* more akin to a golf swing than true graphia. One should therefore proceed to dictated sentences, words, or letters, or to spontaneous writing such as describing what one sees in the room. Right hemiparesis need not deter such testing; most people can write, however awkwardly, with their left hand, and the test here is one of language, not penmanship. Left-handed writing would not explain gross spelling errors or paragraphic substitutions. If writing is abnormal, the patient can be asked to spell aloud, type, or use block or other anagram letters. Abnormalities on such tests signify a disorder affecting more than the mechanism of writing; in other words not only letter production but letter choice.[30] Some patients with severe agraphia on spontaneous or dictated writing are able to copy writing in a slavish fashion.

A number of abnormal writing patterns have been described. For example, in *lexical agraphia* there is impaired spelling of orthographically irregular words with preserved spelling of phonologically regular words or nonwords.[31] In *phonologic agraphia* the reverse occurs.[32] Pure agraphia without other language disturbances can occur with metabolic encephalopathy and with focal lesions affecting the frontal, parietal, or temporal lobes. Agraphia is present in most aphasics, and it may be a prominent residual after recovery of speech.

Reading is tested both orally and for comprehension. Using large print (patients often blame reading difficulty on impaired vision), the patient reads aloud simple sentences, words, or letters. Reading comprehension testing can parallel auditory comprehension testing. Written commands often involve actions that were successfully executed in response to oral commands and yes or no questions or object identification requests can be posed in writing.

Dissociations between oral reading and reading comprehension can be striking.[33] Some patients understand quite well what they read, yet oral reading quickly disintegrates into incomprehensible paralexia. Others can read aloud with astonishing accuracy and yet comprehend little or nothing of what they read. The term *deep dyslexia* refers to loss of the ability to read aloud phonetically with relative preservation of semantic comprehension.[34] Such patients make frequent verbal paralexic substitutions when reading aloud and may appear not to comprehend what they have read, yet they correctly match the seemingly uncomprehended word with an appropriate picture. By contrast, patients with *surface dyslexia* can read phonetically both real words and nonwords, but can no longer attach semantic meaning to what they read.[35]

APHASIC SYNDROMES

Assessing spontaneous speech, speech comprehension, naming, repetition, writing, and reading enables one to determine not only the presence of aphasia but its subtype, the approximate location of the lesion, and the patient's particular functional limitations. Regarding aphasia subtypes, one should keep two concepts in mind. First, the variables that define these subtypes are difficult to quantify beyond such terms as *mild, moderate,* or *severe,* and labels chosen for particular patients really represent points along a continuum. (Some investigators have asserted that as many as 60% of aphasias cannot be subclassified at all into so-called classical syndromes.[36–38]) Second, although the following classification differs from others in terminology and pathophysiological interpretation, the clinical phenomena described are similar for different authors.[39,40]

Broca's aphasia is characterized by such extremely nonfluent and nonprosodic speech that the abnormality is easily recognized, even when the patient speaks only a foreign language. There is often dysarthric slurring as well, and the effortful delivery and incompletely executed words and sentences may be incomprehensible because of combined articulatory distortion and paraphasic substitution. Speech, so far as it is understandable, may be agrammatic, with relatively preserved emotional outbursts or recurrent utterances. The patient appears quite aware of his or her difficulty and is often visibly distressed.

Writing is usually at least as affected as speech, and it may not be executed at all: The patient may grasp the pen but not attempt to use it. Speech comprehension and reading are relatively preserved but not normal; errors can usually be demonstrated with specific testing, and nearly all Broca's aphasic patients have difficulty comprehending syntactically complex sentences. Ability to name or repeat varies. Some patients name unexpectedly well to confrontation. When repetition is relatively intact compared with spontaneous speech, the aphasia is sometimes called *transcortical motor aphasia*; responsible lesions have been observed either superior or anterior to the pars opercularis.[41] Independently of repetition, Broca's aphasics sometimes have remarkably preserved singing ability, with or without words.[42]

Broca's aphasia implies involvement (although not exclusively) of frontal lobe structures. What features of the syndrome are related to the pars opercularis (Broca's area) is still, after more than a century, uncertain.[43] One report correlated nonfluency with computed tomographic lesions affecting the subcallosal fasciculus and periventricular white matter beneath the area of sensorimotor cortex that represents the mouth.[44] In any case, frontal lobe involvement accounts for the observation that the great majority of patients with Broca's aphasia have moderate to severe right hemiparesis. They also frequently have buccolingual apraxia (see the section Apraxia, later in this chapter).

If prerolandic, perirolandic, or subrolandic lesions account for the nonfluency and loss of prosody in Broca's aphasia, then sparing of these regions should predict preserved fluency and prosody. This is the common denominator of several aphasia subtypes caused by lesions restricted to the parietal or temporal lobes. Classification of those subtypes is based on speech comprehension and repetition.

Aphasia characterized by fluent, prosodic speech and moderate or severe impairment of both auditory comprehension and repetition is called *Wernicke's aphasia*. The lesion most often lies in the area originally described by Wernicke, namely the posterior superior temporal gyrus. Speech usually, but not always, is contaminated by paraphasic verbalizations, especially the literal kind; when they are abundant, incomprehensible jargon is produced. The preserved fluency and prosody, however, give the speech a normal sound, so that if the patient speaks only a foreign language, aphasia may be unrecognized. Moreover, patients with severe Wernicke's aphasia often fail to recognize that they have any disability (*anosognosia*) and, preserving paralinguistic aspects of speech (e.g., pausing appropriately for the examiner to speak), participate in a lengthy *conversation*, apparently unaware that they do not understand what is being said to them or that they make no sense to others. When testable, naming, writing, and reading are usually, but not always, severely impaired in Wernicke's aphasia; the types of impairment vary greatly.

When speech is fluent and prosodic, and repetition is much more affected than auditory comprehension, the patient has *conduction aphasia*. Wernicke, and later Geschwind, placed the responsible lesion in the arcuate fasciculus, allegedly disconnecting Wernicke's and Broca's areas. Others have found greater correlation of symptoms with lesions in the inferior parietal lobule (supramarginal and angular gyri). Patients with conduction aphasia usually have impaired naming and writing. Reading ability varies; frequently observed is nearly normal reading comprehension with paralexic oral reading.

Anomic aphasia consists of fluent prosodic speech with normal or nearly normal auditory comprehension and repetition. The major difficulty is word finding, usually apparent on spontaneous speech (sometimes so severe that hesitations compromise fluency), confrontation and list naming, and writing. Restricted vocabulary leads to substitution of phrases for missing words and lengthy, *empty* or *circumlocutory* speech. Manifestations of semantic paraphasia occur; those of literal paraphasia and neologisms are usually infrequent.[39] Reading ability varies. When the anomia is of the tip-of-the-tongue type, the term *amnestic aphasia* has been used. That term is misleading, however, as it implies a true memory dysfunction. In fact, memory is usually normal in patients with this type of aphasia, and conversely, patients with severe amnestic disorders (e.g., Korsakoff's syndrome) have normal naming ability. Anomic aphasia is the least localizable of aphasia subtypes; it is a frequent aftermath of more severe aphasic subtypes (e.g., Wernicke's), and it frequently accompanies diffuse dementing illness (e.g., Alzheimer's disease). When it acutely follows a focal lesion such as stroke or trauma, the inferior parietal lobule is often affected; such patients often have agraphia, alexia, or Gerstmann's syndrome (see discussion later in this section). Anomic aphasia can follow damage to any part of the language areas, or even to the nonlanguage hemisphere.

Persons with *transcortical sensory aphasia* produce fluent prosodic speech; repetition is preserved relative to speech comprehension. Responsible lesions have been parieto-occipital, sparing periopercular parieto-temporal language areas.[45] Transcortical sensory aphasia has also followed lesions of the posterior thalamus.[46] (A frequent, although nonspecific feature of *subcortical* aphasia is a tendency for even a severe language disturbance to improve rapidly. The role of thalamic or basal ganglia damage per se in such aphasias remains controversial.[39])

As might be predicted anatomically, *posterior aphasia syndromes* characterized by fluent prosodic speech are usually accompanied by little or no hemiparesis. Homonymous hemianopia and sensory loss are variable. Ideomotor apraxia, when testable, is not unusual (see discussion later in this section).

The term *expressive aphasia* is usually equated with Broca's aphasia, and receptive aphasia with Wernicke's aphasia. The terms are misleading: Expression is as compromised in severe Wernicke's aphasia as in Broca's aphasia.

Muteness is common in aphasia of sudden onset and has little localizing value (i.e., it does not signify ultimate nonfluency). Whether aphasia is severe or mild, it is unusual for complete muteness to last more than several days.

The aphasia subtypes discussed so far follow damage to particular periopercular areas whereas others are spared; they are frequently the result of middle cerebral artery branch occlusions. When damage extends to the entire perioperculum, the resulting aphasia can have mixed features (e.g., speech of Broca's type plus loss of auditory comprehension). When severe, such mixed aphasias are called *global*. Naming, repetition, writing, and reading are also severely affected. Usually the result of extensive cerebral convexity lesions (e.g., infarction in the entire middle cerebral artery territory, massive head injury, cerebral neoplasm), global aphasia is usually accompanied by hemiplegia, sensory loss, and homonymous hemianopia. (Global aphasia with little or no hemiplegia can follow separate lesions of Broca's and Wernicke's areas, as from embolic strokes.[47]) Global aphasia with preserved repetition is called *mixed transcortical aphasia.* Such patients sometimes repeat what they hear in a compulsive fashion (*echolalia*), and sometimes, even when they have no speech comprehension, they make correct grammatical transpositions (e.g., on hearing the examiner inquire, "How are you today?" the patient might reply, "How am I today?"). Other patients can complete clichés or familiar proverbs or, after getting started with cues, successfully recite serial speech, such as days of the week. Some demonstrate strikingly preserved singing, with or without words.

In an autopsy case of mixed transcortical aphasia, there was infarction of cerebral cortex surrounding the periopercular language areas, which were themselves intact.[48] A proposed formulation for the transcortical aphasias is that they disconnect the periopercular language areas from the rest of the brain, impairing speech output, speech comprehension, or both, yet allowing repetition through the preserved Wernicke's area, arcuate fasciculus, and Broca's area. Accepting such a formulation, Geschwind referred to mixed transcortical aphasia as *isolation aphasia.*[46] Needless to say, not everyone agrees.

As noted, aphasia subtypes represent artificial compartmentalizations. Moreover, it is not unusual during recovery for Wernicke's aphasia to evolve into conduc-

tion and then anomic aphasia, or for global aphasia to evolve into Broca's aphasia.[49,50] Recognizing the oversimplification involved, the clinician can usefully employ aphasia subtypes as guideposts.

A number of other language disturbances do not easily fit into the previously mentioned spectrum. *Aphemia*, or *anarthria*, refers to speech of Broca's type but without the other language abnormalities often seen with Broca's aphasia, including agraphia.[51] It is a disturbance more of speech than of language. The lesion is believed to be frontal, but whether it involves the pars opercularis, the deep white matter, or other structures remains controversial.

Analogously, *pure word deafness* refers to loss of speech comprehension without the other language abnormalities that usually accompany Wernicke's aphasia, including loss of reading comprehension and paraphasic speech. Nonverbal sounds (e.g., a trumpet sounding, a telephone ringing, or a dog barking) are normally identified. The syndrome is rare. Unilateral or bilateral lesions have involved fibers connecting both auditory cortices (Heschl's gyrus) with the language-dominant auditory association cortex (Wernicke's area). What is heard is thus disconnected from periopercular language areas, which themselves are intact and connected to visual pathways.[52]

Pure alexia, or *alexia without agraphia*, describes loss of the ability to read in the absence of any other aphasic features. The patient can write spontaneously or to dictation but is then unable to read what he or she has written.[53,54] Most often the result of left posterior cerebral artery occlusion, the syndrome usually (but not always) includes right homonymous hemianopia; alexia is attributed to posterior corpus callosum damage with disconnection of what is seen (by the right occipital lobe) from the left hemisphere. (When homonymous hemianopia is absent, the lesion is presumed to disconnect both visual cortices from left hemispheric language areas.) Patients with pure alexia can sometimes slowly read individual letters. Color anomia is frequently present.

Unilateral or bilateral damage to the medial frontal lobe (supplementary motor area and cingulate gyrus) can cause difficulty initiating and sustaining speech and writing. Whether such language disturbance should be called *aphasic* is questionable; paraphasias generally do not occur, and the patient is often *abulic* (bradyphrenic, without initiative).[55,56]

Gerstmann's syndrome consists of agraphia, acalculia, left-right confusion, and finger agnosia (failure to recognize, not simply to name). Considerable unresolved speculation has addressed why these features should occasionally be so linked.[57,58] The responsible lesion usually affects the language-dominant inferior parietal lobule.

APRAXIA

The term *apraxia* is problematic, because over the years, it has been used to describe disparate phenomena. In its broadest sense, *apraxia* refers to impaired motor activity not explained by weakness, incoordination, abnormal tone, bradykinesia, movement disorder, dementia, aphasia, or poor cooperation. Failure to perform an act at all is not apractic; it should be performed incorrectly. Parts of the act might be omitted, abnormally sequenced, or incorrectly oriented in space. Any or all components of the act may be performed imprecisely. Heilman and Rothi[59] suggest four types of testing: (1) gesture ("Show me how you would. . . ."), (2) imitation ("Watch how I . . . , then you do it."), (3) use of an actual object ("Here is a. . . . Show me how you would use it."), and (4) imitation of examiner using the object. Tests include limb gestures (e.g., waving goodbye, hitchhiking), limb manipulation (e.g., opening a door with a key, flipping a coin), buccofacial gesture (e.g., sticking out the tongue), buccofacial manipulation (e.g., blowing out a match), and serial acts (e.g., folding a letter, putting it in envelope, sealing the envelope, and placing a stamp on it).

Liepmann classified apraxia as ideational, ideomotor, and limb-kinetic.[60] *Ideomotor apraxia* consisted of the inability to perform learned or complex motor acts although primary executive skills are preserved, as is the *idea* of the act (its engram or physiological memory trace). Affected patients accurately describe what they are supposed to do and correctly perform individual components of the act. Moreover, when the mode of input is switched (e.g., from a spoken command to a visual stimulus), they can sometimes perform the act in its entirety. Liepmann saw ideomotor apraxia as a functional if not an anatomic disconnection between the idea of a motor act and its execution.

Ideomotor apraxia can be demonstrated by asking the patient to pretend to perform a learned act such as striking a match and blowing it out. The act is attempted but done incorrectly. The patient is able to describe the act and to perform the individual motor movements that subserve it. When handed the real objects (match and matchbook) or, less often, after watching the examiner perform the act, the patient correctly executes it.

By contrast, in *ideational apraxia* the patient cannot accurately describe the act, and presentation of the real object produces no improvement; the patient might tear the match in half and chew one end. Here the lesion appears to affect the engram itself. In *limb-kinetic apraxia* the idea is understood, but neither the act itself nor its individual components can be performed, with or without the objects. Presumably, the lesion affects the executive apparatus, not enough to cause frank weakness or ataxia, but enough to prevent accurate motor performance.

It is questionable whether the term *apraxia* is appropriate for the ideational and limb-kinetic types. Ideational apraxia is usually the result of bihemispheric disease and is often associated with obvious dementia. Limb-kinetic apraxia is part of a spectrum of cerebral motor disturbances that include altered tone, power, and coordination. One apractic subtype, so-called gait apraxia, is loosely applied to any impaired gait when strength and coordination of both legs are preserved. The term *constructional apraxia* is even less appropriate.

Ideomotor apraxia is what most neurologists mean when they describe a disturbance as apractic. It most often affects the limbs bilaterally after lesions of the language-dominant parietal or temporal lobe. Such location means that apraxia is often missed, because accompanying aphasia and impaired auditory comprehension make testing difficult. Ideomotor apraxia can also affect the left limbs of patients with left anterior cerebral artery occlusion and right leg weakness (*sympathetic apraxia*); the responsible lesion is presumed to involve the anterior corpus callosum and to disconnect the right motor cortex from left hemispheric language areas or from the motor engram itself.[61] Such patients, for similar reasons, often have left-handed agraphia and tactile anomia. A subtype of ideomotor apraxia, *buccolingual apraxia*, affects lip and tongue movements and is a frequent accompaniment of Broca's aphasia. Probably related, *apraxia of speech* refers to the abnormalities of phonologic selection and sequencing that often accompany aphasia, especially Broca's, although Broca's aphasia and oral apraxia can dissociate.[62,63]

AGNOSIAS AND DISORDERS OF SPATIAL PERCEPTION AND MANIPULATION

Agnosia is a failure of recognition that is not explained by impaired primary sensation (tactile, visual, auditory) or cognitive impairment. It has been described as "perception stripped of its meaning."[64] Agnosia differs from anomia in that the patient cannot name the confronted object or select it from a group or match it to a likeness. In *tactile agnosia* (*astereognosis*), touch threshold is normal, yet the object cannot be tactilely identified. Some patients with tactile agnosia cannot even describe fundamental features of the object such as roundness or smoothness (*apperceptive agnosia*); others can identify the primary features but are unable to synthesize them into full object recognition (*associative agnosia*). Although astereognosis can be the predominant symptom of peripheral lesions (e.g., diabetic sensory neuropathy), when it occurs ipsilaterally, either alone or with other discriminative sensory loss (e.g., proprioception or two-point discrimination), the lesion is likely to affect the contralateral parietal sensory cortex or association areas.

Comparable agnosias exist in the visual and auditory spheres. Responsible lesions are likely to be bilateral, and so *visual agnosia* and *auditory agnosia* are rare. *Simultanagnosia* is the inability to recognize the meaning of a whole scene or object, even though its individual components are correctly perceived and recognized. It is sometimes a feature of so-called Balint's syndrome, defined as an inability to look voluntarily into the peripheral visual field, plus *optic ataxia* (erroneous pointing to objects in space), and decreased visual attention for extrafoveal space. Such patients usually have biparietal lesions.[65,66]

Prosopagnosia is selective inability to recognize familiar faces. The problem seems to be one of fine tuning; affected patients can recognize a face as a face (or a dog as a dog) but are unable to identify which one. To date, all patients examined at autopsy have shown bilateral occipitotemporal lesions; whether unilateral lesions can cause prosopagnosia remains controversial.[67,68]

Posterior cerebral lesions can also cause loss of color vision (*central achromatopsia*), either hemianopic or throughout the visual fields.[69] Unilateral or bilateral lesions usually affect the inferior medial occipital lobe.

Just as the left hemisphere is usually the major processor of language (and related analytic skills), so the right hemisphere processes spatial information. Right hemisphere lesions (especially parietal) cause impairment of spatial perception and manipulation. There may be difficulty reading maps or finding one's way about (*topographagnosia*), copying simple pictures or shapes, or drawing simple objects such as a flower or a clock face (so-called constructional apraxia or apractagnosia). Clothing may be put on backward or upside down (so-called dressing apraxia).

Even more striking is the tendency of a patient with a right hemispheric lesion to ignore the left half of his or her own body or of meaningful or novel objects in left extracorporeal space (*hemineglect*). The patient may fail to recognize severe hemiplegia (*anosognosia*) or even to acknowledge left body parts as his or her own (*asomatognosia*), insisting, for example, that a paralyzed limb belongs to someone else or complaining that his or her own left limbs are missing. Objects or voices in contralateral space are ignored, and grooming or dressing may be restricted to the right half of the body. Asked to bisect a line, the patient indicates a point to the right of midline. Picture copying may omit the left half, and a drawn clock face may have all the numbers neatly arranged on the right side. As with aphasia, when this syndrome is severe there is usually additional cognitive impairment, but not enough to explain the spatial disturbance. Neither is hemineglect the result of homonymous hemianopia.

Constructional apraxia can also follow damage to the language-dominant hemisphere. So can contralateral hemineglect, although the syndrome is usually less obvious in an aphasic patient. Even when aphasia is accounted for, however, hemineglect is more frequently associated with lesions contralateral to the language-dominant hemisphere.[70] As with aphasia, hemineglect also occurs with thalamic and diencephalic lesions.[71]

CALCULATION AND MUSIC

Disorders of calculation (*acalculia*) are of several types, including *alexia* or *agraphia* for numbers, spatial disorganization of numbers, and true anarithmetria.[72] Consequently, acalculia has followed lesions of either hemisphere. The fundamental process of calculation appears to be in the domain of the left hemisphere.[73] Similarly, music involves the processing skills of both hemispheres, and so-called *amusia*, affecting either productive or receptive aspects of music, has been associated with both left- and right-sided brain lesions.[74]

APHASIA TREATMENT

The treatment of aphasia with speech therapy is controversial.[50,75–77] As to whether it helps patients, most agree that it does. Less clear is whether the perceived benefit is the result of the specific strategies employed or of general psychological support, and whether the benefit consists of restored neuropsychological function, of adaptation and compensatory use of preserved function, or simply of improved attention and mood. Treatment techniques include modality specific stimulus-response treatment, language oriented therapy, group therapy, linguistic-specific treatment, functional communication therapy, melodic intonation therapy, visual action therapy, response elaboration therapy, and computerized approaches.[78] Studies include randomized controlled clinical trials, case-control and cohort studies, nonrandomized trials, and case reports.

The fact that aphasia (like other neurologic impairment) can improve, without treatment, for months or even years compounds the problem of assessing speech therapy. Controlled studies have been understandably infrequent. In one study, in which patients were randomly assigned to treatment or no treatment, there was no significant difference in outcome at 24 weeks.[79] In another study, one group of patients began treatment at entry to the study and continued it for 12 weeks; another group began a similar course of treatment 12 weeks after entry. At 12 weeks, the early treated group was significantly more improved than the deferred treatment group, which, however, caught up at 24 weeks.[80] A review of these and other studies concluded ". . . generally, treatment for aphasia is efficacious." Most likely to benefit are younger patients with moderate, not severe, aphasia who receive frequent therapy for several months. Delay in beginning treatment does not preclude benefit.[78]

The efficacy of speech therapy is believed by most workers to reflect training in the use of preserved function. As one investigator put it, "Clinical aphasiologists are not naive enough to believe that they fix damaged brains. Rather, they provide alternative compensatory mechanisms or strategies for approximating adequate (if imperfect) means for meeting daily needs."[81] Studies of the mechanism of recovery after brain damage, how-ever, challenge such a view. Language functions that recover after left hemispheric stroke are sometimes abolished after a new right hemispheric lesion[82] or right intracarotid injection of barbiturate,[83] and after recovery from Wernicke's aphasia, patients performing verbal tasks during positron emission tomographic scanning showed activation of the right superior temporal gyrus.[84] Similar hemispheric shift of activation has been reported using functional magnetic resonance imaging.[85] Negative cortical DC-potential shifts (reflecting postsynaptic depolarization and activation of cortical regions) were studied during a word-generation task in several right-handed patients with different aphasia subtypes.[86] Among Broca's aphasics there was an initial right hemispheric preponderance that over time shifted to the left (where, presumably, it had been prior to their strokes). Among Wernicke's aphasics a shift to the right hemisphere persisted. This study suggests that transcallosal pathways normally inhibit homotopic regions of the nonlanguage hemisphere and that damage to periopercular language areas causes disinhibition of these contralateral regions, analogous to the expansion or shifting of receptive fields that follows damage to sensory or motor areas.[87] Studies have also demonstrated functional shifts within the language hemisphere.[84,88-90]

Technological advances thus demonstrate that recovery from aphasia is far more dynamic than previously suspected, and it is not far-fetched to think that environmental stimuli might influence this plasticity.[91] Speech therapy may turn out to involve more than simply making do with what is still intact.

REFERENCES

1. Subirana A. Handedness and Cerebral Dominance. In PJ Vinken, GW Bruyn (eds), Handbook of Clinical Neurology. Vol 4: Disorders of Speech, Perception, and Symbolic Behavior. Amsterdam: North Holland, 1969;248–272.

2. Springer SP, Deutsch G. Left Brain, Right Brain. San Francisco: WH Freeman, 1981;103–120.

3. Broca P. Perte de la parole. Ramollissement chronique et destruction partielle du lobe antérieur gauche du cerveau. Bull Soc Anthropol Paris 1861;2:235–238.

4. Broca P. Sur la faculté du language articulé. Bull Soc Anthropol Paris 1865;6:337–393.

5. Wernicke C. Der Aphasiche Symptomencomplex. Breslau: Cohn & Weigart, 1874.

6. Lichtheim L. On aphasia. Brain 1885; 7:433–484.

7. Henschen SE. On the function of the right hemisphere of the brain in relation to the left in speech, music, and calculation. Brain 1926;49:110–123.

8. Jackson JH. On the physiology of language. Med Times Gaz 1868;2:275. [Reprinted in Brain 1915;38:59–64.]

9. Marie P. Revision de la question de l'aphasie. Semin Med 1906;26:241–247;493–500;565–571.

10. Pick A. Die Agrammatischen Sprachstörungen. Berlin: Springer, 1913.

11. Head H. Aphasia and Kindred Disorders of Speech. New York: Macmillan, 1926.

12. Weisenberg T, McBride KE. Aphasia. A Clinical and Psychological Study.

New York: The Commonwealth Fund, 1935.

13. Nielsen JM. Agnosia, Apraxia, Aphasia. Their Value in Cerebral Localization. New York: Hoeber, 1946.

14. Goldstein K. Language and Language Disturbances. New York: Grune & Stratton, 1948.

15. Schuell H, Jenkins JJ, Jiminez-Pabon E. Aphasia in Adults. New York: Hoeber, 1964.

16. Bay E. Principles of Classification and Their Influence on Our Concepts of Aphasia. In AVS De Reuk, M O'Connor (eds), Disorders of Language. Boston: Little, Brown, 1964.

17. Brain WR. Speech Disorders. Aphasia, Apraxia and Agnosia. London: Butterworth, 1965.

18. Hecaen H, Albert M. Human Neuropsychology. New York: Wiley, 1978.

19. Luria AR. Higher Cortical Functions in Man (2nd ed). New York: Basic Books, 1980.

20. Geschwind N. Disconnection syndromes in animals and man. Brain 1965;88: 237–294;585–644.

21. Benson DF, Geschwind N. Aphasia and Related Disorders: A Clinical Approach. In M-M Mesulam (ed), Principles of Behavioral Neurology. Philadelphia: FA Davis, 1985;193–238.

22. Goodglass H, Kaplan E. The Assessment of Aphasia and Related Disorders. Philadelphia: Lea & Febiger, 1972.

23. Wagenaar E, Snow C, Prins R. Spontaneous speech of aphasic patients: a psycholinguistic analysis. Brain Lang 1975;3:281–303.

24. Monrad-Krohn GH. Dysprosody or altered melody of language. Brain 1947;70:405–415.

25. Ross ED. The aprosodies: functional-anatomic organization of the affective components of language in the right hemisphere. Arch Neurol 1981;38:561–569.

26. Fromkin VA. The State of Brain/Language Research. In F Plum (ed), Language, Communication, and the Brain. New York: Raven, 1988;1–8.

27. DeRenzi E, Vignolo LA. The token test: a sensitive test to detect receptive disturbances in aphasics. Brain 1962; 85:665–678.

28. Caramazza A, Berndt RS. Semantic and syntactic processes in aphasia: a review of the literature. Psychol Bull 1978;85:898–918.

29. Barton M, Maruszeqski M, Urrea D. Variation of stimulus context and its effect on word-finding ability in aphasics. Cortex 1969;5:351–365.

30. Roeltgen D. Agraphia. In KM Heilman, E Valenstein (eds), Clinical Neuropsychology (2nd ed). New York: Oxford University Press, 1985;75–96.

31. Roeltgen D. Lexical agraphia. Further support for the two-system hypothesis of linguistic agraphia. Brain 1984;107:811–827.

32. Roeltgen D, Sevush S, Heilman KM. Phonological agraphia: writing by the lexical-semantic route. Neurology 1983; 33:755–765.

33. Lytton WW, Brust JCM. Direct dyslexia. Preserved oral reading of real words in Wernicke's aphasia. Brain 1989;112:583–594.

34. Marshall JC, Newcombe F. The Conceptual Status of Deep Dyslexia: An Historical Perspective. In M Coltheart, K Patterson, JC Marshall (eds), Deep Dyslexia (2nd ed). London: Routledge & Kegan Paul, 1987;1–21.

35. Newcombe F, Marshall JC. Reading and Writing by Letter Sounds. In KE Patterson, JC Marshall, M Coltheart (eds), Surface Dyslexia: Neuropsychological and Cognitive Studies of Phonological Reading. London: Lawrence Erlbaum, 1985;35–51.

36. Alexander MP, Fischette MR, Fischer RS. Crossed aphasias can be mirror images or anomalous. Case reports, review and hypothesis. Brain 1989;112(Pt 4):953–974.

37. Albert ML, Goodglass H, Helm-Estabrooks N, et al. Clinical Aspects of Dysphasia. New York: Springer-Verlag, 1981.

38. Basso A, Lecours AR, Moraschim S, et al. Anatomoclinical correlations of the aphasias as defined through computerized tomography: exceptions. Brain Lang 1985;26:201–229.

39. Benson DF. Aphasia. In KM Heilman, E Valenstein (eds), Clinical Neuropsychology (2nd ed). New York: Oxford University Press, 1985;17–47.

40. Brust JCM, Shafer SQ, Richter RW, Bruun B. Aphasia in acute stroke. Stroke 1976;7:167–174.

41. Freedman M, Alexander MP, Naeser MA. Anatomic basis of transcranial motor aphasia. Neurology 1984;34: 409–417.

42. Yamadori A, Osumi Y, Masuhara S, et al. Preservation of singing in Broca's aphasia. J Neurol Neurosurg Psychiatry 1977;40:221–224.

43. Mohr JP, Pessin MS, Finkelstein S, et al. Broca aphasia: pathologic and clinical aspects. Neurology 1978;28:311–324.

44. Naeser MA, Palumbo CL, Helm-Estabrooks N, et al. Severe non-fluency in aphasia. Role of the medial subcallosal fasciculus and other white matter pathways in recovery of spontaneous speech. Brain 1989;112:1–38.

45. Kertesz A, Sheppard A, MacKenzie R. Localization in transcortical sensory aphasia. Arch Neurol 1982;39:475–478.

46. Alexander MP, LoVerme SR. Aphasia after left hemispheric intracerebral hemorrhage. Neurology 1980;30:1193–1202.

47. Legatt AD, Rubin MJ, Kaplan LR, et al. Global aphasia without hemiparesis: multiple etiologies. Neurology 1987;37:201–205.

48. Geschwind N, Quadfasel FA, Segarra J. Isolation of the speech area. Neuropsychologia 1968;6:327–340.

49. Kertesz A, McCabe P. Recovery patterns and prognosis in aphasia. Brain 1977;100:1–18.

50. Vignolo L. Evolution of aphasia and language rehabilitation. A retrospective exploratory study. Cortex 1964;1:344–367.

51. Schiff HB, Alexander MP, Naeser MA, et al. Aphemia. Arch Neurol 1983;40:720–727.

52. Auerbach SH, Alland T, Naeser M, et al. Pure word deafness: analysis of a case with bilateral lesions and a defect at the prephonemic level. Brain 1982;105:271–300.

53. Dejerine J. Contribution a l'étude anatomo-pathologiques et clinique des differentes variétés de cecite verbale. Mem Soc Biol 1892;4:61–90.

54. Damasio AR, Damasio H. The anatomic basis of pure alexia. Neurology 1983;33:1573–1583.

55. Masdeu JC, Schoene WC, Funkenstein H. Aphasia following infarction of the left supplementary motor area. Neurology 1978;28:1220–1223.

56. Brust JCM, Plank C, Burke A, et al. Language disorder in a right-hander after occlusion of the right anterior cerebral artery. Neurology 1982;32: 492–497.

57. Benton AL. Reflection on the Gerstmann syndrome. Brain Lang 1977;4:45–62.

58. Roeltgen DP, Sevush S, Heilman KM. Pure Gerstmann's syndrome from a focal lesion. Arch Neurol 1983;40:46–47.

59. Heilman KM, Rothi LJG. Apraxia. In KM Heilman, E Valenstein (eds), Clinical Neuropsychology (2nd ed). New York: Oxford University Press, 1985; 131–150.

60. Liepmann H. Apraxia. Erbgn Ges Med 1920;1:516–543.

61. Liepmann H, Maas O. Fall von linksseitiger Agraphie und Apraxie bei rechtsseitiger Lähmung. Z L Psychol Neurol 1907;10:214–227.

62. Darley FL, Aronson AE, Brown JR. Motor Speech Disorders. Philadelphia: WB Saunders, 1975;250–269.

63. Heilman KM, Gonyea EF, Geschwind N. Apraxia and agraphia in a right-hander. Brain 1974;96:21–28.

64. Bauer RM, Rubens AB. Agnosia. In KM Heilman, E Valenstein (eds), Clinical Neuropsychology (2nd ed). New York: Oxford University Press, 1985;187–241.

65. Hecaen H, de Arjuriaguerra J. Balint's syndrome (psychic paralysis of visual fixation) and its minor forms. Brain 1954;77:373–400.

66. Levine DN, Calvanio R. A study of the

visual defect in verbal alexia-simultan-agnosia. Brain 1978;101:65–81.

67. Damasio AR, Damasio H, Van Hoesen GW. Prosopagnosia: anatomic basis and behavioral mechanisms. Neurology 1982;32:331–341.

68. Sergent J, Villemure J-G. Prosopagnosia in a right hemispherectomized patient. Brain 1989;112:975–996.

69. Green GL, Lessefl S. Acquired cerebral dyschromatopsia. Arch Ophthalmol 1977;95:121–128.

70. Heilman KM, Van den Abell T. Right hemisphere dominance for attention: the mechanism underlying hemispheric asymmetries of inattention (neglect). Neurology 1980;30:327–330.

71. Healton EB, Navarro C, Bressman S, et al. Subcortical neglect. Neurology 1982;32:776–778.

72. Levin HS, Spiers PA. Acalculia. In KM Heilman, E Valenstein (eds), Clinical Neuropsychology (2nd ed). New York: Oxford University Press, 1985;97–114.

73. Warrington EK. The fractionation of arithmetical skills: single case study. Q J Exp Psychol 1982;34A:31–51.

74. Brust JCM. Music and language. Musical alexia and agraphia. Brain 1980;103:367–392.

75. Darley FL. Aphasia. Philadelphia: WB Saunders, 1982.

76. Sarno MT, Silverman M, Sands E. Speech therapy and language recovery in severe aphasia. J Speech Hear Res 1970;13:607–623.

77. Brust JCM. Neurology. In RM Haller, N Sheldon (eds), Speech Pathology and Audiology in Medical Settings. New York: Stratton Intercontinental Medical Book Corp, 1976;49–57.

78. Holland AL, Fromm DS, DeRuyter F, Stein M. Treatment efficacy: aphasia. J Speech Hear Res 1996;39:S27–S36.

79. Lincoln DB, Mully GP, Jones AL, et al. Effectiveness of speech therapy for aphasic stroke patients. Lancet 1984;1:1197–1200.

80. Wertz RT, Weiss DG, Aten JL, et al. Comparison of clinic, home, and deferred language treatment for aphasia. A Veterans Administration cooperative study. Arch Neurol 1986;43:653–658.

81. Holland AL, Wertz RT. Measuring Aphasia Treatment Effects: Large-Group, Small-Group, and Single-Subject Studies. In F Plum (ed), Language, Communication, and the Brain. New York: Raven, 1988;267–273.

82. Basso A, Gardelli M, Grassi MP, Mariotti M. The role of the right hemisphere in recovery from aphasia. Two case studies. Cortex 1989;25:555–566.

83. Kinsborune M. The minor cerebral hemisphere as a source of aphasic speech. Arch Neurol 1971;25:302–306.

84. Weiller C, Isensee C, Rijntjes M, et al. Recovery from Wernicke's aphasia: a positron emission tomographic study. Ann Neurol 1995;37:723–732.

85. Thulborn KR, Carpenter PA, Just MA. Plasticity of language-related brain function during recovery from stroke. Stroke 1999;30:749–754.

86. Thomas C, Altenmüller E, Marckmann G, et al. Language processing in aphasia: changes in lateralization patterns during recovery reflect cerebral plasticity in adults. Electroencephalogr Clin Neurophysiol 1997;102:86–97.

87. Calford MB, Tweedale R. Interhemispheric transfer of plasticity in the cerebral cortex. Science 1990;248:805–807.

88. Heiss WD, Kessler J, Karbe H, et al. Cerebral glucose metabolism as a predictor of recovery from aphasia in ischemic stroke. Arch Neurol 1993;50:958–964.

89. Lazar RM, Marshall RS, Pile-Spellman J, et al. Anterior translocation of language in patients with left cerebral arteriovenous malformation. Neurology 1997;49:802–808.

90. Frackowiak RJS, Fristo KJ, Frith CD, et al. The Cerebral Basis of Functional Recovery. In RJS Frackowiak (ed), Human Brain Function. San Diego, CA: Academic, 1997;275–299.

91. Musso M, Weiller C, Kiebel S, et al. Training-induced brain plasticity in aphasia. Brain 1999;122:1781–1790.

31

Functional Electrical Stimulation in Persons with Spinal Cord Injury

Kristjan T. Ragnarsson and Lucinda L. Baker

Functional electrical stimulation (FES) may be defined as the application of electrical currents to neural tissue for the purpose of restoring a degree of control over abnormal or absent body functions. Electricity has been applied either experimentally or clinically for many purposes (e.g., to improve hearing and sight, to prevent bladder and bowel incontinence and to control evacuation, to regulate heart rhythm, to reduce spasticity, to allow ventilator-free breathing, to correct scoliosis, and to usefully move paralyzed limbs).

Although FES may be applied successfully for different forms of paralytic conditions caused by upper motor neuron lesions (e.g., stroke, traumatic brain injury, cerebral palsy) in this chapter its application after spinal cord injury (SCI) is principally discussed.

HISTORY

Electricity has been used therapeutically for different human ailments, including treatment of paralysis, for hundreds of years.[1] Gilbert is usually credited with having laid the scientific foundations of electrotherapy with his studies and publications in the sixteenth century on magnetism and electricity,[2] although Krueger, in 1744, may have been the first to use electricity in a scientific fashion for therapeutic purposes. Development of electrostatic generators during the eighteenth century made electricity widely available for experimental and clinical application. During that age, the work of Galvani and Volta[2] led to the clinical use of interrupted direct currents to produce muscle contractions. In the early nineteenth century, Faraday introduced the alternating current generator, which a number of clinicians, most prominently Duchenne, were soon using for therapeutic

purposes. Scientific developments in the fields of electrophysiology and electrical engineering during the second half of the nineteenth century and during the entire twentieth century led to vastly increased knowledge, which, for instance, was useful in promoting the clinical field of electrodiagnosis. The ability to detect and amplify small amounts of electricity in the body was of particular clinical importance, as was the recognition that certain forms of electricity are better suited than others for electrostimulation of neuromuscular structures. A body of work also helped to clarify the limits of the therapeutic and functional use of electricity. For example, it became clear that stimulation of a denervated muscle is difficult, and that electrical stimulation did not significantly change the course of recovery after a peripheral nerve injury. On the other hand, stimulation of an innervated muscle was found to be easy and sometimes even facilitated by the presence of upper motor neuron damage and the resulting hypertonicity.

The first attempts to restore useful movement of limbs by electrostimulation of muscles paralyzed by upper motor neuron lesions are generally credited to Liberson et al.,[3] who reported in 1961 on their work to produce dorsiflexion of the ankle in hemiplegic patients during the swing phase of gait. At the same time, in a little noted report, Kantrowitz described a paraplegic patient who was enabled to stand by electrical stimulation of the quadriceps muscles.[4] Shortly thereafter, Long and Masciarelli reported on their attempts to restore wrist and hand movement for functional grasp and release by using a hybrid system of electrical stimulation and wrist-hand orthosis.[5] These early clinical investigators were hampered in their work by the limitations of the available technology, but during the 1970s improved electronic technology and increased understanding of neuromuscular physiology intensified interest in this field. Kinesiologic electromyography was used to identify clearly all the muscles responsible for completing a given motor task. Researchers claimed that computer-controlled multichannel stimulators using this information would be able to replicate any particular motion accurately by circumducting the lesion in the CNS and thus bypassing the injured upper motor neuron by directly stimulating the peripheral nerve or the motor point of the muscle at the desired preprogrammed times and intensity. Numerous investigators in different countries have since contributed to FES technology and its clinical application; some focused primarily on the lower limbs for ambulation,[6-10] whereas others worked on hand function[11-14] or respiration for ventilator-free breathing.[15-17] Although a number of technical and physiological problems have been overcome, many others remain unsolved.

MOTOR SYSTEM ANATOMY AND PHYSIOLOGY

Although the physiology and anatomy of motion are addressed in Chapters 1, 3, and 17 in this book, it is important to review the basic structure of the motor system to understand all the events related to its electrical excitation. In the simplest terms, the initial motion signal is normally generated by the upper motor neuron in the motor cortex of the brain. This signal travels down the spinal cord, connects with the lower motor neuron at the anterior horn of the cord, and is transmitted through the peripheral nerve to the muscle fibers, which shorten and cause a movement of the body part. Sensory feedback to the spinal cord and brain occurs continuously, in order to control and modify the motions and to accomplish the motor task in a safe and effective manner. The continuous sensory feedback results in constant changes in the number of fibers that is stimulated to contract within each muscle, and in the number of protagonist, antagonist, and synergist muscles that participates in the desired motor task. These constant alterations in fiber contractions occur at a subconscious level, perhaps even at the level of the spinal cord, through a complicated learning process that depends on different parts of the CNS and reciprocal inhibition and facilitation. A voluntary motion is thus considered voluntary only in its purpose, not in the means by which it is accomplished.

Voluntary movements are impaired not only by damage to the efferent neural pathways, which results in paralytic conditions, but whenever there is an interrup-

tion of the afferent channels to the brain from the different sensory organs. The countless normal physiological events that continuously occur with even the simplest motor task are clearly far more complex than what can currently be accomplished by artificially stimulating the neuromuscular system, even with the most sophisticated technology, computer-controlled multichannel stimulators, and closed-loop sensory feedback.

Completion of a motor task, whether by voluntary effort, reflex action, or FES, is accomplished by activation of the intact motor unit, which consists of the alpha motor neuron, located in the anterior horn of the spinal cord, its axonal nerve fiber, the myoneural junction, and the group of muscle fibers that it innervates. The number of muscle fibers innervated by a single but branching axonal nerve fiber varies inversely with the precision of the movement performed by the muscle (e.g., a motor unit may contain hundreds of muscle fibers in the limb muscles, but in the eye muscles it may contain less than five). A single muscle thus consists of many motor units, the exact number of which depends on the size of the muscle and its specific function. Within the muscle the fibers from different motor units lie intermingled with each other. All the efferent nerve fibers to a striated skeletal muscle are excitatory (i.e., they always produce contraction of the muscle, but never relaxation by inhibition), in contrast to efferent nerve supply to smooth and cardiac muscle, which may also cause relaxation on stimulation. On excitation, all the muscle fibers of a single motor unit are activated to contract.

An electrical stimulus of threshold strength theoretically may activate only one motor nerve fiber and all the muscle fibers it innervates, whereas a maximal stimulus strength may activate all the nerve fibers with consequent contraction of all the muscle fibers. The activation of an increasing number of motor units within a muscle on contraction is referred to as *recruitment*. A succession of maximal stimuli produces different results depending on the firing rate (i.e., rate of activation). A second maximal stimulus given during the latent period (the first milliseconds of the first stimulus) produces no additional contraction, as the muscle is in its refractory state, whereas if the stimulus is given slightly later, the muscle tension generated is greater than that generated by the first stimulus. A series of maximal stimuli applied at progressively shorter intervals, at low rates (10–20 stimuli per second), produce a tremulous response, whereas at higher rates (60 per second) full tetanus results, with greater tension of the muscle fibers and a steadier pull. The increased firing rate of active motor units is referred to as *temporal sum-*

mation. During voluntary activation, recruitment and temporal summation are the two mechanisms that regulate the strength of muscle contraction, and usually these mechanisms act simultaneously. Asynchronous activation of a large number of different motor units results in a smooth, voluntary contraction of a muscle. Although modern FES systems strive toward achieving precise control that results in smooth muscle contraction, this has not been entirely successful because neuromuscular stimulation relies exclusively on increasing recruitment of motor units, rather than also altering the temporal excitation of asynchronously driven motor units.

Not all alpha motor neurons are identical, and neither are the muscle fibers. The alpha motor neurons differ in both size and function. Small alpha motor neurons usually innervate slow muscle fibers, and the large neurons innervate fast fibers. The small motor neurons physiologically have the lowest activation threshold. All the muscle fibers within a single motor unit are usually thought to be histologically identical, whereas within a whole muscle they are not.

Muscle fibers are usually considered to be of two different types, referred to as *type I* (red, slow, aerobic) and *type II* (white, fast, anaerobic) (see Chapter 5). Histologically, the type I muscle fibers are of relatively small diameter, as they have relatively small amounts of contractile proteins. Their smaller diameter facilitates oxygen diffusion from the surrounding capillaries into the fiber. These fibers are rich in glycolytic and oxidative enzymes, substances that give them their dark or red appearance, and metabolically provide them with aerobic capacity for different endurance tasks (e.g., maintenance of posture, walking, distance running, bicycling). Physiologically, type I fibers have a slow twitch speed on activation and are naturally driven at low electrical frequencies for tonic contraction. They are recruited first on physiological excitation and can continue to contract for prolonged periods. Type II muscle fibers, in contrast, are larger, have less glycolytic and oxidative enzymes, appear pale or white, have low aerobic capacity and fast speed of twitch, and are activated at higher electrical frequency levels for phasic but relatively strong contractions of short duration.

Clearly, type I and type II muscle fibers are metabolically suited to perform different tasks. Normally, type I and type II muscle fibers are recruited in sequence by the CNS in order to perform different tasks, but with recruitment by electrical stimulation such differentiation is not possible. On sustained or repeated contractions, muscle fatigue occurs, apparently because of changes in the muscle fiber induced by anoxia and accumulation of metabolites, regardless of the type of fiber. Fatigue may be offset or delayed by exclusive activation of type I fibers and maintenance of adequate blood supply. The blood flow and oxygenation of the muscle fiber, however, are reduced during a sustained contraction of the muscle, and in the presence of impaired physiological response of the cardiovascular and respiratory systems.

Ample evidence exists for the transformation of type I muscle fibers into type II fibers with inactivity and paralysis and for the reversibility of this process with appropriate external stimulus (e.g., endurance exercise or regular prolonged electrical stimulation of the paralyzed muscle[18-22]). Similarly, endurance training may improve the physiological responses and work capacity of the healthy but deconditioned cardiovascular system, a process that is necessary to sustain the desired work of the muscles.

The function of a skeletal muscle is to generate force with or without visible movement. The muscle's ability to generate force and movement depends on two different relationships: the length-tension relationship and the force-velocity relationship.[23] The *length-tension relationship* means that isometric (static) muscle force varies as a function of muscle length. The length-tension force may be assessed by measuring the force generated by maximal stimulation at different muscle lengths. The *force-velocity relationship* means that isotonic (dynamic) velocity (contraction velocity against a constant force) varies as a function of muscle force. The force-velocity relationship may be assessed by subjecting the muscle to a constant force, stimulating maximally, and measuring the initial contraction velocity at each force level. The length-tension, as well as the force-velocity relationship, is related to the histochemical properties of the muscle fibers (i.e., type I or type II), which, in turn, are affected by and may be altered by appropriate external stimuli.[19,20,24] Although electrical stimulation of the isolated muscle under experimental circumstances can produce different and predictable length-tension and force-velocity relationships, this is much more difficult during clinical application of FES in the human body.

COMPONENTS OF FUNCTIONAL ELECTRICAL STIMULATION SYSTEMS

The FES systems that are currently used are fundamentally quite similar. They are designed to deliver pulses of electrical currents at predetermined frequencies and amplitudes to nerves or the myoneural junctions. The main components of such systems include a portable power source for the electrical stimulation device, control mechanism, lead wires, electrodes, and, in the more sophisticated systems, peripherally placed sensors and microprocessor (computer) for preprogrammed or automatic control (Figure 31-1). Most FES systems remain external to the body at the present time, with electrodes applied to the skin and the stimulator and power source carried by the user. Implanted stimulation, in which the electrodes and stimulator are implanted while the power source is maintained externally, has been in restricted use for more than 20 years. Partially implanted systems are becoming more common as stimulation technology improves.

Electrical Stimulation Device

Muscle contraction by electrical stimulation is usually achieved by activation of a peripheral motor nerve, either well before or near the point at which the nerve connects with the muscle (at the motor point). Electrical activation of the muscle itself is not practical because the muscle's membrane properties are different from those of nerves and would require an approximately 100 times greater level of current and charge injection.[25] Preservation of the entire lower motor neuron is therefore essential for all forms of FES. A muscle that is paralyzed by damage to the lower motor neuron has no motor point. The motor point of a muscle is a relatively

small area where the motor nerve ending connects with the muscle and where sensitivity to stimulation is high. A denervated muscle (one without a motor point) responds only to long pulse durations (i.e., duration of at least 1–10 msec), compared with less than 1 msec for an innervated muscle. The current must pass through each denervated muscle fiber in order to generate an effective contraction. Such high current levels may be both dangerous and painful for a subject with preserved sensation. For these reasons, a muscle denervated by a lower motor neuron lesion cannot be subjected to FES, given the current state of technology and knowledge.

The magnitude of the electrical stimulus delivered in terms of its pulse amplitude and pulse duration determines the number of nerve fibers activated and consequently the force of the muscle contraction. Additionally, it should be noted that large nerve fibers are easier to activate through electrical stimulation than small fibers. The electrical stimulus used most frequently for FES to generate depolarization and action potentials is a pulsed monophasic waveform. A predictable relationship exists between the stimulus pulse amplitude and the pulse duration that is necessary to reach the threshold required for nerve excitation and muscle contraction (Figure 31-2). When the pulse is long, the excitation thresholds for muscle and nerve are nearly equal, but for short pulses, which are usually used for FES, the nerve has a much lower threshold than the muscle. Therefore, on stimulation of the nerve or of the motor point, when using short electrical pulse durations, there is little direct activation of the muscle fibers, and contraction occurs mostly by nerve excitation.

For implanted electrodes, a series of short-duration (i.e., 10–100 μsec) charge-balanced biphasic stimuli are

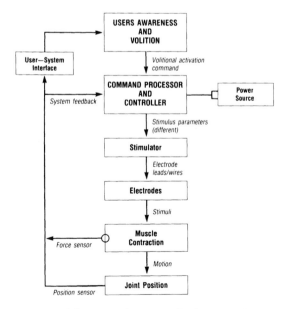

FIGURE 31-1 Schematic drawing of a functional electrical stimulation system's main components and sequence of action.

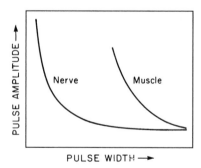

FIGURE 31-2 The relationship between the electrical stimulus pulse amplitude and the pulse width necessary to reach the threshold required for nerve excitation and muscle contraction. When the pulse width is long, the thresholds are almost equal, but for the more commonly used short pulse widths, the nerve has a much lower threshold than the muscle.

used,[26,27] with pulse amplitudes no greater than 50 mA.[28] These are the most common parameters used at this time with implanted electrodes (i.e., 300 μsec and up to 100 mA, respectively),[29] although stimuli of longer duration and amplitude have been used experimentally.

A biphasic waveform is preferable to monophasic wave (Figure 31-3), as it may provide better control of recruitment and thus muscle contraction force.[30] Control may be further improved by decreasing pulse duration.[30,31] Biphasic waveforms also provide a greater measure of safety to the underlying tissues, because some level of balance of positive and negative charges exists under each stimulating electrode. Implanted nerve cuff electrodes require the least electrical current and charge to elicit contraction. It is clear, however, that some tissue damage may result from long-term electrical stimulation of implanted electrodes, especially nerve cuff electrodes. Such damage is related to the total charge of the stimulus, as well as to the current intensity used to drive the desired response. By maintaining equal charge in both the negative and positive phases of a waveform, which can be achieved with biphasic waveforms, a greater peak charge may be used without causing tissue damage.[32,33]

Researchers have observed that a muscle fatigues more rapidly when stimulated by artificial means than when activated voluntarily, the cause apparently being the different order in which motor units are recruited.[34,35] By voluntary contraction, the slow and aerobic type I muscle fibers are recruited first and the rapidly fatiguing type II fibers last. This order of recruitment is largely reversed during FES because the threshold of excitation varies inversely with the diameter of the nerve fiber when electrical currents are applied externally. The small diameter nerve fibers within a bundle of nerve fibers have the highest threshold to electrical stimulation, which tends to activate the largest nerves first, recruiting the fast, type II muscle fibers preferentially. Special stimulation techniques have been tested in animals to recruit first the slow, type I muscle fibers by using high currents and additional electrodes, but they have not yet been tried in humans.[36]

Muscle endurance can be increased to a certain extent by restricting the electrical stimulation frequency, which is usually in the range of 15–50 Hz.[29,37,38] In general, low-frequency stimulation is clearly preferred in order to minimize stimulated fatigue. Muscle endurance can also be increased experimentally by sequentially stimulating different groups of motor units within each muscle by means of multipolar nerve electrode designs.[39] Finally, endurance may be increased by altering the contractile properties of the muscle by regular electrical stimulation training, which results in an alteration of muscle fibers from type II to type I.[38]

Electrodes

The selection of electrode design for FES systems depends on the specific purpose of the application and on availability of equipment, clinical experience, and other variables. Four main electrode designs are currently available: skin surface, epimysial (muscle surface), intramuscular with percutaneous leads, and surgically implanted nerve cuff electrodes (Figure 31-4). No single electrode type meets all the ideal criteria for safety, reliability, efficiency, specificity, durability, low cost, ease of application, and minimal maintenance. Although surface electrodes clearly are the safest, least invasive, easiest, and simplest to apply, they do not always provide adequate selectivity of excitation, particularly not for excitation of deep muscles, which the electrical stimulus may not reach, nor can they provide accurate repeatability in muscle responses. Minor displacement of such electrodes on the skin surface may result in a major alteration in the muscle response. Electrical stimulation by surface electrodes may be painful because afferent cutaneous nerves may be stimulated before sufficient numbers of efferent motor nerve fibers. Nonetheless, surface electrodes may be adequate for therapeutic purposes or for a short-term trial of FES, which employs a system with relatively few stimulation channels, usually eight or fewer. For long-term application of FES systems with a greater number of channels, researchers generally prefer implanted electrodes.[11]

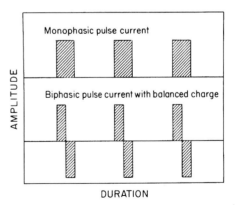

FIGURE 31-3 Pulsed direct current waveforms with either monophasic (*above*) or biphasic (*below*) action potentials are used for neuromuscular electrical stimulation. To minimize tissue damage, a biphasic pulsed current with equal positive and negative charge is preferred.

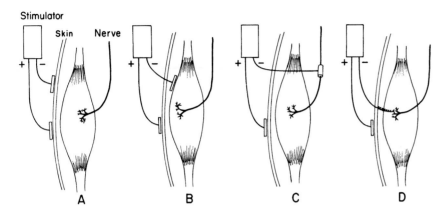

FIGURE 31-4 Electrode designs for functional electrical stimulation systems: **(A)** skin surface electrode, **(B)** implanted epimysial (muscle surface) electrode, **(C)** implanted nerve cuff electrode, and **(D)** intramuscular electrode with percutaneous lead.

Despite their inherent shortcomings, skin surface electrodes have improved in quality and now may provide excellent skin contact and can be left in place for days without causing irritation. In the clinical setting, individual electrodes are usually used, but for long-term FES participation the electrodes may be sewn into skin-tight garments for the subject to wear when stimulation is desired.[40]

Intramuscular electrodes with percutaneous leads have only been used experimentally and are not part of any approved FES system. They are usually fabricated from a fine multifilament stainless steel wire with Teflon insulation in a coiled configuration with an exposed tip. These electrodes may be inserted through the skin with a large-gauge hypodermic needle (i.e., gauge 19–26) and placed subcutaneously, epimysially on the surface of the muscle, or into the muscle itself.[11,41,42]

Implanted Electrodes

Implanted electrodes are inserted surgically and then placed either epimysially[13,43] or directly over or around the nerve by a cuff. Although nerve cuff electrodes were used for activation of limb muscles in the past,[13,44] their clinical use currently appears to be more restricted to diaphragmatic pacing by stimulation of the phrenic nerve[15] or to bladder evacuation by stimulation of the sacral anterior nerve roots.[44] Although implanted cuff electrodes provide good muscle specificity and allow stimulation with relatively low current, the implantation is invasive, and surgical insertion is difficult without damaging the nerve. Although the experience of some clinicians has shown that properly implanted electrodes using correct stimulation parameters do not appear to damage the nerve functionally,[6] other clinicians have expressed concern that the nerve may be damaged either by the electrical stimulation itself or mechanically by the electrodes'

attachment to the stimulated tissues.[42,45] Continuous stimulation at frequencies of 50 Hz or greater for constant periods of 8–16 hours daily may damage the nerve irreversibly.[45]

More recent implanted electrodes designed to activate skeletal muscle to provide limb movement have been epimysial, being sewn directly onto the muscle over the motor point. The epimysial electrodes provide the advantage of minimal damage to the underlying tissue, a problem with some of the nerve cuff electrodes. The disadvantage to the epimysial electrodes is the even greater surgical exposure of each muscle requiring a stimulating electrode, as well as the time necessary to identify the best placement for the electrode. Only a restricted number of electrodes have been attempted, partially because of the laborious surgical procedure. A new form of implanted electrode, which will be injectable but requires no external wires to drive it, is beginning clinical trials.[46,47]

Materials for implanted electrodes and the leads must be carefully selected. There must be minimal biological reaction to the material, which should be strong, flexible, resistant to fatigue and corrosion, and of low impedance. Metals such as stainless steel or platinum or alloys of platinum and iridium or of nickel, cobalt, chromium, and molybdenum have been used in the fabrication of such electrodes and leads.[32]

Sensors

Sensors are essential parts of all sophisticated FES systems and are necessary for proper interaction between the stimulator, the user, and the environment. Normally, the five senses provide the brain and the spinal cord with information about the external and internal environment of the body through innumerable sensory nerve end-organs, in order to make motor activity accurate and effective. Without such sensory feedback, motor activity becomes grossly uncoordinated and essentially useless. Coordinated motor activity requires accurate sensory information on the positions and motions of individual joints, as well as of whole limbs, in addition to sensory feedback on impact force, pressure, and tendon tension. The tiny signals from the sensory nerve end-organs can be detected by percutaneous intraneural electrodes, but use of this information for FES systems would require a large number of implantable microelectrodes and a highly intelligent microprocessor.[48] Neither is currently available.[49] The types of sensors required for FES systems are similar to the transducers used in industry for measurement and control of manufactured devices. These sensors, however, must meet the additional criteria of reliability, ease of use, small size, low mass, easy mounting, flexibility, and cosmesis, and they should not interfere with normal joint function.[49] Currently, sensory feedback signals from the limbs are obtained primarily from externally mounted goniometers or potentiometers on ankles and knees. They allow measurement of joint position and, from the absolute sense of position, velocity and acceleration of movement to be calculated by the systems microprocessor, which in turn controls the stimulator.[48] At present, no sensors can monitor from their placement on the body surface the tension developed by a contracting skeletal muscle, although such capability would be ideal for sensory feedback.

Control of Functional Neuromuscular Stimulation Systems

FES systems are frequently described as *user-interactive devices*, with which the user is able to control the electrical stimulation to the muscles by different means, including a joystick, push-button switches, voice recognition, breath force, myoelectric signals, or motion sensors. A display, either by visible liquid crystal or by an audible sound, may inform the user of the system's status. A computer may provide additional automatic control either by an open-loop or closed-loop mechanism. In an *open-loop control system*, preprogrammed patterns of electrical stimulation are generated for a specific function and for a specific individual, but without automatic correction for changes in the external environment, in the mechanical function of the system, or in muscle contraction. In a *closed-loop control system*,[50] the computer receives feedback information from sensors about a particular motion and institutes a remedial action or gives a warning if motion is not possible or should be altered.

FUNCTIONAL ELECTRICAL STIMULATION AFTER SPINAL CORD INJURY

SCI results in numerous degenerative physiological changes that to some extent affect most, if not all, organ systems of the body. Many of these physiological changes result in diminished work capacity and physical fitness, which may not only impair the person's ability to use FES systems, but may also negatively affect general health and well-being. Although some of these changes are unalterable and directly related to the loss of supraspinal control over voluntary and autonomic motor functions, the enforced sedentary lifestyle and lack of exercise programs for the pursuit of physical fitness further compound the problem. Major degenerative physiological changes that can diminish work performance after SCI occur in many organ systems.

Skeletal Muscles

During the initial areflexic state of SCI, rapid and progressive atrophy of the paralyzed muscles occurs, which appears to continue for several months. When reflex activity and tone return to muscles that are paralyzed by an upper motor neuron lesion, further atrophy may not develop, but even in the presence of significant spasticity, muscle bulk usually is not restored to normal. On external excitation of the muscle, maximum contraction strength and endurance are diminished. Morphologic studies have shown that after SCI, as with other causes of paralysis and immobilization, many muscle fibers change from type I (slow, aerobic) to type II (fast, anaerobic).[22,51,52] This change is accompanied by reduction in mitochondria concentration, glycolytic and oxidative enzyme level, and the number of capillaries in the muscle. As type II fibers become preponderant, the contractile properties of the muscle change dramatically. There is increased speed of muscle contraction and relaxation, and the muscle becomes unable to generate prolonged contractions (i.e., the type of contractions that are normally required of most antigravity muscles in the lower limbs during standing and locomotion). Strength of individual muscle fibers, as measured by maximum tetanic tension, may not decrease,[52] although it appears clinically that on electrical stimulation of an entire muscle the strength is significantly diminished compared with that of a muscle contracting voluntarily. Muscle endurance (the ability of the muscle to contract repeatedly against little or no resistance) is clinically reduced, as fatigue is usually observed after relatively few contractions that are elicited by electrical stimulation. Skeletal muscle has remarkable adaptability, and many of the changes associated with disuse are reversible, although perhaps not completely.

Cardiovascular System

Cardiovascular fitness, expressed as physical work capacity and maximum oxygen consumption (VO_2max), is diminished in most individuals with SCI, particularly those with high cord lesions.[53-62] Two major factors may be responsible for this reduction: The muscle mass available for voluntary exercise is diminished, and responses of the autonomic nervous system are altered. Both are the result of lost supraspinal control. Secondarily, there is loss of cardiovascular fitness as a result of the sedentary lifestyle.

VO_2max is customarily used as a measure of cardiovascular fitness (i.e., endurance or aerobic capacity). In able-bodied persons obtainable VO_2max is influenced by many factors, including gender, age, genetics, endurance training, type of exercise, organ health, and environment. SCI typically results in extensive muscle paralysis, and consequently the muscle mass that remains under voluntary control is significantly decreased. It is thus clear that a person with high-level tetraplegia is not capable of substantially increasing VO_2max through exercise of the few residual functional muscles, whereas a paraplegic person may be able to increase VO_2max considerably through upper extremity endurance exercise.[63,64] Physical work and aerobic exercise capacity after SCI are reduced proportionally with the muscle mass available for voluntary exercise.[65-69] It is not clear if involuntary FES exercise can significantly increase VO_2max, but it appears that such a potential increase may depend to a certain degree on the level of the lesion and autonomic control of the cardiovascular system.

The extent of autonomic dysfunction after SCI depends on the level of the cord lesion. Persons with tetraplegia lose all supraspinal control of the sympathetic nervous system and of the sacral parasympathetic efferent flow, while retaining essentially normal and uninhibited vagal parasympathetic function. Individuals with high-level paraplegia (i.e., T-5 or above) similarly experience severe loss of supraspinal sympathetic control, primarily control over the splanchnic nerve supply rather than that for cardiopulmonary functions. Paraplegia with a cord lesion lower than T-5 seems to affect autonomic dysfunction less. It has been reasonably argued that loss of supraspinal sympathetic control limits maximum heart rate, contractility of the heart muscle, stroke volume, and cardiac output during strenuous physical exercise.[70] Further, loss of supraspinal sympathetic control predictably may impair effective dilatation of arterioles supplying working muscles and compensatory vasoconstriction to resting organs such as intestines, kidneys, and skin. As a consequence, maximum work capacity may be limited for both voluntary upper limb exercise and electrically stimulated lower limb endurance activities. Several studies have shown that the cardiac output of persons with SCI, both at rest and during maximum arm exercise, is lower than that of able-bodied persons, that the arteriovenous oxygen gradient is high, and that serum lactate levels are elevated.[53,54,56] Oxygen pulse (milliliters of oxygen consumed per heart beat), a parameter frequently used as a noninvasive measure of stroke volume, has been shown to be decreased to a greater extent in persons with high cord lesions than in those with lower levels of paraplegia.[68,71-74] It is obvious that if neurologic recovery does not occur, the individual with high-level cord injury will not regain supraspinal sympathetic control and exercise performance will be limited. There is evidence, however, that in response to a different form of physical stress (i.e., head-up tilt), a limited reflex sympathetic activity occurs, as seen by an increase in serum dopamine-beta-hydroxylase and plasma renin.[75] Additionally, there may be increased vascular reactivity to normal levels of norepinephrine and other vasoconstricting agents.[76] Both the reflex sympathetic activity and increased sensitivity to the neurotransmitters may have some beneficial effect on circulatory response during physical exercise in persons with tetraplegia.

Thermoregulation during rest and exercise is, to a large extent, a sympathetically mediated process that consists of vasoconstriction or vasodilatation, as well as sweating and shivering. Concern may be expressed that persons with high spinal cord lesions subjected to strenuous exercise may experience an excessive increase of body temperature, but no such increase has been reported.

SCI may impair both venous and arterial circulation in the peripheral areas of the paralyzed parts. Paralysis of muscles in the lower limbs and abdominal wall, along with decreased venomotor tone, may contribute to peripheral pooling of venous blood and consequently cause reduced venous return to the heart. The reduced return of venous blood to the heart may further contribute to reduction in stroke volume and cardiac output during physical exercise, especially during exercise performed in an upright position, as during ambulation by means of FES or with orthoses, arm cranking, and FES cycle ergometry.

Arteries in the chronically paralyzed lower limbs become small and atrophic, perhaps owing to lack of muscle activity and chronically reduced blood flow. Although this condition does not lead to frank ischemia except in the presence of other risk factors, such as cigarette smoking and diabetes, it is possible that atrophic arteries may limit oxygen supply to muscles subjected to endurance exercise by FES after years of inactivity. This would contribute to early development of muscle fatigue. Narrowed lower limb arteries, however, may prevent excessive shunting of blood to these body parts, a condition that may be helpful during upper limb voluntary exercise.

Respiratory Function

Paralysis of the intercostal and abdominal muscles impairs the respiratory capacity of persons with SCI. Several studies have shown that with each ascending level of the spinal cord lesion there is a progressive reduction of vital capacity.[65,77-79] This impairment, however, does not appear to affect exercise capacity significantly, which is primarily limited by the available muscle mass and cardiac reserve. Thus, respiration and oxygenation of blood seem to be sufficient for most endurance exercises[65] that persons with SCI are capable of performing with the residual voluntary muscles. Reduced respiratory capacity may only limit exercise capacity in some highly trained paraplegic athletes during high-level endurance activities.

Endocrine Function

Normally, several hormones are secreted in response to strenuous exercise. These are primarily hormones that increase the rate of lipolysis, glycolysis, and gluconeogenesis (i.e., epinephrine, norepinephrine, growth hormone, adrenocorticotropin, cortisol, glucagon, thyroid-stimulating hormone, thyroid hormone), and hormones that are important for regulation of body fluids and electrolytes (aldosterone, antidiuretic hormone). In contrast, there is decreased secretion of hormones that increase synthesis of fat and glycogen. Insulin is the most important of these. The first and most significant hormonal response to sudden exercise is sympathetically mediated secretion of catecholamines (epinephrine and norepinephrine), both from nerve endings and the adrenal medulla, in amounts that are proportional to the increase in workload and the duration of the exercise.[80] It is probable that secretion of catecholamines during such exercise may be impaired with high cord lesions and a dysfunctional sympathetic nervous system. In general, however, secretion of different hormones in response to sudden vigorous exercise or

prolonged exercise training program after SCI has not yet been adequately studied. Currently, it does not appear that endocrine imbalance significantly affects exercise response in this condition.

CLINICAL APPLICATIONS

Clinicians have long practiced the application of controlled currents of electricity to nerves or to motor points of muscles in order to generate a contraction for therapeutic purposes. Earlier in this chapter, brief reference was made to the use of relatively simple systems of FES to generate ankle dorsiflexion during the swing phase of gait in subjects with stroke, usually with a single stimulation channel. The discussion here addresses the clinical application of computer-controlled multi-channel FES systems in persons with SCI for the purposes of restoring prehension to the hand; allowing ventilator-free breathing; regaining the ability to stand, walk, and leg pedal; or regaining certain control over bladder, bowel, and sexual functions.

Upper Limb Control

Injury to the cervical spinal cord usually causes paralysis of the upper and lower limbs. The paralysis of the upper limbs most consistently involves the hands and thus reduces the person's self-care skills and vocational potential. Depending on the extent and distribution of the cord damage, the paralysis is caused in varying proportions by both upper and lower motor neuron destruction. Rehabilitation interventions to improve upper limb function after such paralysis have traditionally consisted of maintaining joint range of motion, strengthening residual muscles, teaching new skills, providing orthoses and adaptive equipment, and surgically reconstructing the hand. FES systems have been successfully developed for persons with tetraplegia and cord lesions at C-5 and C-6, but whose lower motor neurons are preserved for the C-7 and C-8 segments.[11,13,81-86]

Restoration of upper limb function by FES aims at re-establishing the ability of the person to position the arm in space and to grasp or to release objects from the hand. Either one or both of these key components of upper limb function may be impaired or lost after cervical SCI, and traditional rehabilitation methods may not provide adequate functional restoration. Because persons with C-5 and C-6 tetraplegia have voluntary control of shoulder muscles and elbow flexors, they are generally capable of positioning their arms and hands over a working surface in front of them; however, they do not have functional prehension of the hands, owing to paralysis of the more distal muscles. Consequently, functional restoration by means of FES for these persons has focused on achieving opening and closing of the hand by means of stimulating flexors and extensors of the fingers and thumb. Systems have been developed for simultaneous FES control of both the hand muscles and the more proximal upper limb muscles paralyzed by cord lesions at C-4 or above.[14] The task is complicated, and extensive research and development are needed before clinical application can be attempted.

Long first described a hybrid upper limb FES system,[5] in which an orthosis provided stability of the wrist, thumb, and the interphalangeal joints of the fingers, an electrical stimulation device generated finger extension, and a spring across the metacarpophalangeal joints generated flexion torque. Most users rejected this crude device because of its unsightly appearance and the rapid muscle fatigue they experienced when using it. Subsequent work by Peckham and associates has led to the development of a portable FES hand neuroprosthesis for persons with C-5 and C-6 tetraplegia.[11,13,83] In a retro-

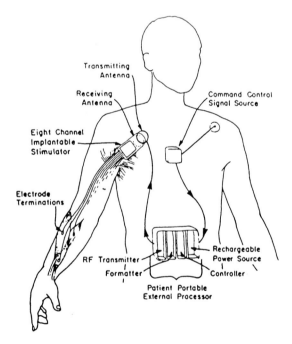

FIGURE 31-5 A multichannel hand functional electrical stimulation system (neuroprosthesis) with implanted motor and sensory electrodes, lead wires, and receiver stimulator, but with external power source and controlled by radiofrequency (RF) and an external control unit. (Reprinted with permission from MW Keith, PH Peckham, GB Thrope, et al. Functional neuromuscular stimulation, neuroprosthesis for the tetraplegic hand. Clin Orthop 1988;233:25–33.)

spective study, this device was shown to have measurably increased the function of the users, although the relative improvement was greater for persons with C-5 than with C-6 tetraplegia.[81,84]

This neuroprosthesis consists of both implanted and external components as described by Kilgore et al.[81] (Figure 31-5). The *implanted* components are an eight-channel receiver stimulator, eight epimysial electrodes, leads, and connectors. Seven electrodes are placed on the muscles used to control thumb and finger movements, but one electrode is placed in the supraclavicular region to provide sensory feedback. A radiofrequency inductive link provides the communication and power to the implanted stimulator receiver. The *external* components consist of a shoulder position sensor control unit placed on the contralateral shoulder, a battery-powered and portable external control unit, usually mounted on the wheelchair, and a transmitting coil taped on the ipsilateral chest directly over the implanted stimulator receiver. The external control unit receives control signals from the shoulder position sensor, processes these, and is programmed to generate appropriate stimulus outputs for each muscle through the transmitting coil to the stimulator receiver. The shoulder control unit consists of a position sensor and joystick mounted on the contralateral shoulder and chest and a logic switch, but occasionally a similar mechanism can be attached to the ipsilateral wrist to control opening and closing of the hand.[87] The implanted stimulator receiver, the size of a pacemaker, has eight fine lead wires, seven of which are tunneled subcutaneously to the humeral connector site where a spring connector is used to connect these to the distal lead wires that are attached to the epimysial electrodes sutured on the desired muscles.

In some persons with tetraplegia, upper limb surgical reconstruction with tendon transfers and anastomoses and fusions of certain finger joints has long been shown clinically to increase hand function.[88,89] Such reconstruction has also been used in combination with FES, particularly when FES of the usual muscles cannot elicit suitable finger motion and no adjacent voluntary muscles can be used for transfer.[82] Under these circumstances, spastic hand muscles, which are paralyzed by upper motor neuron lesions and lie close to flaccid paralyzed muscles or their tendons, may be used for transfers in a fashion identical to the traditional transfers of tendons from voluntarily contracting muscles.[13] Thumb and finger joints to be fused, as well as the tendons to be transferred, are selected individually based on availability of excitable muscles and the biomechanics of the hand. The transferred spastic muscles are subsequently stimulated for functional purposes in a manner similar to that of the other muscles.

Functional evaluation done retrospectively on 22 patients with tetraplegia who used a hand neuroprosthesis has shown that performance of 10 different functional hand tasks was 89% successful with the use of the FES neuroprosthesis, but only 49% successful without it. The improvement in performance with the neuroprosthesis was significantly greater in those with C-5 tetraplegia than with C-6 tetraplegia.[84] Another study on five users of such a neuroprosthesis showed improved pinch force, grasp-release, functional independence, and use of the device at home.[81]

Stimulation of the Diaphragm

Persons with tetraplegia caused by cord lesions at C-3 or higher lose the phrenic nerve control of the diaphragm, become unable to breathe on their own, and for survival usually require mechanical ventilation by negative or positive pressure. When the lesion in the spinal cord is at C-1 or C-2 and spares the lower motor neurons for the phrenic nerve at the third, fourth, and fifth cervical segments, it is possible to stimulate the nerve anywhere between the neck and its motor points in the diaphragm, and thus reduce or eliminate the need for mechanical ventilation.[15,16] Electrophrenic respiration (EPR), or *diaphragmatic/phrenic nerve pacing*, as this technique is often called, was initially used at night for persons with sleep apnea who were otherwise healthy. It has since proven to be a reliable mode of ventilation for some persons with tetraplegia. It is an attractive alternative to mechanical ventilation, because the tracheostomy can be plugged, the ventilator tubing can be eliminated, and the transmitter box can be inconspicuously attached to the wheelchair.[90] Solving clinical problems associated with mechanical ventilation may subsequently improve anxiety, including physical discomfort, speech impediment, mobility restriction, and transfer difficulties.[91]

Candidates for electrostimulation of the diaphragm must be chosen carefully. The cervical cord injury must have happened at least 6 months earlier to allow spontaneous improvement to have occurred, and all respiratory complications must have been effectively treated. There should be no evidence of atelectasis, pneumonitis, bronchiectasis, chronic obstructive pulmonary disease, or significant stenosis of the trachea. The patient must have adequate sitting tolerance and be able to tolerate room air without supplemental oxygen. Children younger than 6 years of age generally are not considered good candidates. Family members must not only be

emotionally supportive but able to learn how to use and maintain the equipment. Careful evaluation of the viability of the phrenic nerve is most important.[92] This usually involves fluoroscopic assessment of diaphragm motions, both during voluntary effort and during electrical stimulation of the phrenic nerve in the neck with a recording electrode attached to the chest wall just below the insertion of the diaphragm (Figure 31-6). The diaphragmatic excursions on fluoroscopy should normally measure 4–6 cm, and the latency of the phrenic nerve on stimulation should average 6–9 μsec,[90] although less optimal values have occasionally been associated with good results with EPR.[91]

Three commercial EPR systems are available.[91] Ordinarily, stimulating electrodes are surgically implanted bilaterally at or around the phrenic nerve, either at the base of the neck or more preferably along the route of the phrenic nerve in the chest. The radiofrequency receiver and electrical stimulator are surgically implanted in a subcutaneous pocket on the anterior chest or abdominal wall just below the costal border (Figure 31-7). Subcutaneous lead wires connect the device with the stimulating electrodes. An external transmitter with a circular antenna controls the stimulation parameters. Synchronous activation of the phrenic nerves causes the diaphragm to contract bilaterally, intrathoracic pressure to decrease, and inspiration to occur. When stimulation ceases, the reverse occurs. Stimulation is usually provided 8–14 times per minute to generate adequate ventilation, but total volume and respiratory rate may be altered by adjusting the amplitude and rate of the stimulus. Postoperatively, a carefully incremented program of electrical stimulation is initiated to recondition the diaphragm while minimizing

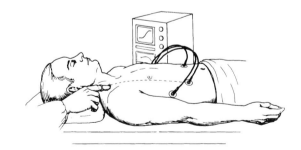

FIGURE 31-6 Stimulation of the phrenic nerve in the neck by an external electrode with recording electrodes attached to the chest wall at approximately the eighth intercostal space, close to where the diaphragm inserts on the chest wall. (Reprinted with permission from RK Shaw, WWL Glenn, JF Hogan, et al. Electrophysiological evaluation of phrenic nerve function in candidates for diaphragm pacing. J Neurosurg 1980;53:345–354.)

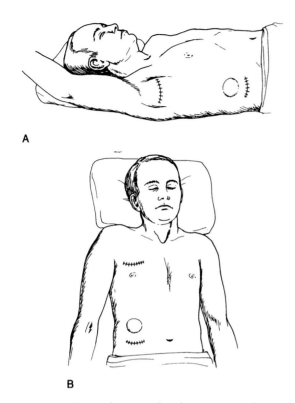

FIGURE 31-7 Surgical approaches for insertion of intrathoracic phrenic nerve stimulation electrodes **(A)** through the axilla at the third intercostal space or **(B)** through the anterior chest wall at the second intercostal space. The receiver is placed subcutaneously, either **(A)** anteriorly on the lower chest wall or **(B)** in the abdominal wall below the costal border.

muscle fatigue. Because stimulation of one-half of the diaphragm is usually adequate for ventilation while resting in the supine position, alternate stimulation of each half of the diaphragm may be desirable to avoid muscle fatigue. Unfortunately, such stimulation is not adequate while the patient is sitting. Blood gases are carefully monitored during the reconditioning phase, which may last 2–4 months or until the user is able to breathe without any other ventilatory support except as a safety backup.

More than 20 years of clinical experience has demonstrated the efficacy and safety of EPR for appropriate candidates.[15,90,93] It is clear that continuous stimulation of the phrenic nerve bilaterally can be safely applied if the stimulation frequencies are low (8–12 Hz).[15] Excessive stimulation may damage the nerve, as can physical contact between the nerve and the electrode, localized infection, or fibrosis. It has, therefore, been suggested that electrodes that are implanted intramuscularly into

the diaphragm may prove safer and require a less invasive implantation procedure,[94] but apparently, clinical implementation of this system has not reached realization. Many persons with tetraplegia who are ventilator dependent are not candidates for EPR because of damage to either the phrenic motor neurons in the cervical spinal cord or the phrenic nerves. It has been suggested that electrical stimulation of the inspiratory intercostal muscles or intercostal to phrenic nerve grafting may provide an alternative to EPR in some cases.[95,96]

Lower Limb Control

Restoration of lower limb function by FES has received much attention in recent years. Research projects have demonstrated that with FES paraplegic persons can stand and walk short distances; negotiate stairs, curbs, and inclines; and pedal exercise cycles for physical fitness training. Despite promising results in the laboratory and improved technology, clinical application of FES for ambulation has been slow. Only one commercially available system has been introduced in the United States, and no paraplegic persons have reported using this technology as their primary means for mobility. In contrast to the limited clinical application of FES ambulation systems, a FES ergometer has been available commercially for more than a decade, and many persons with tetraplegia or paraplegia have used it regularly to exercise paralyzed limbs for physical fitness and potential health benefits.

Standing and Ambulation

The early clinical attempts to use FES involved electrical stimulation of the ankle dorsiflexors in a hemiplegic limb in order to obtain foot clearance during the swing phase of gait[3,97] and stimulation of the quadriceps muscles in paraplegic limbs to maintain a standing position.[4] For the last 25 years extensive research and development efforts in different countries have been directed toward enabling paraplegic individuals to functionally stand and ambulate by means of FES. Additionally, it has been suggested that FES systems can be used to restore gait after stroke or traumatic brain injury.[9] Despite the extensive work, currently no FES system for ambulation adequately meets all the requirements; this partly accounts for their limited clinical application and commercial availability.

In concept, FES systems for ambulation and standing may differ in several ways with respect to their purposes and to the components used. The simplest systems have a single channel for muscle stimulation.

One such system, which stimulates the peroneal nerve to correct the foot drop of hemiplegia caused by stroke, has been rejected clinically because similar correction may be obtained by wearing a regular ankle-foot orthosis.[7,97] A simple two-channel device for bilateral stimulation of the quadriceps muscles with the hips positioned in hyperextension has been shown to be adequate for standing, and it might be useful for more SCI patients than the more complex systems used for ambulation.[98,99] The first FES ambulation system for paraplegic persons to be commercially available in the United States[100] uses a four-channel stimulator for surface stimulation of the quadriceps muscles bilaterally, and a second pair of electrodes located distally over the dermatomes of the peroneal, sural, or saphenous sensory nerves (Figure 31-8).[101] Standing is maintained by simultaneous activation of both quadriceps muscles while a stride is produced by maintaining activation of the quadriceps muscle on the stance side while creating a flexion reflex on the opposite limb. A partially implantable lower limb neuroprosthesis has been developed using essentially the same basic components as described previously for the upper extremity (i.e., consisting of implanted eight-channel receiver stimulator, epimysial electrodes, lead wires and connectors, as well as external control unit and transmitting coil).[101] This FES system is not yet commercially available, but may reportedly be useful for various mobility tasks (i.e., transfers; standing; stepping forward, sideways, and backwards), as well as for ascending and descending stairs.[101]

Electrodes For practical clinical reasons, FES systems using skin surface electrodes should have no more than four stimulation channels. Surgically implanted electrodes are generally preferred for multiple channel systems, owing to their greater accuracy in stimulating deep or small muscles, greater effectiveness in producing repeated muscle responses, and less irritation to the skin. Intramuscular electrodes with percutaneous leads have a considerable failure rate[9] and occasionally even cause a burn or an infection and are generally not used for clinical purposes.

Control FES systems that are designed for accomplishing a relatively simple task, such as stimulation of one or two groups of muscles for ankle dorsiflexion or knee extension, are best preprogrammed with an open-loop control, whereas the more complicated multi-channel systems are designed with peripherally placed sensors and a closed-loop control. The stimulation patterns for different lower limb tasks are evaluated individually for each subject and are properly adjusted

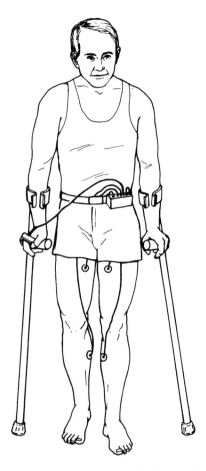

FIGURE 31-8 Four-channel functional electrical stimulation system for ambulation, which is open loop and user controlled.

before the patterns are programmed and transferred into the portable computer stimulator's memory. The number of such preprogrammed activities may vary greatly, depending on the system and number of muscles that can be individually activated.[101] The user operates a manual switch to select the desired programmed activity (e.g., standing up from sitting, sitting down, prolonged standing, walking on a level surface, negotiating stairs, performing different exercises). A visual display on the computer stimulator may provide the user information on the activated function. In an open-loop control system, sensory feedback is obtained simply by using residual sensory functions (visual, auditory, vestibular), but in elaborate experimental systems with closed-loop controls, artificial sensors have been placed in the paralyzed limbs to provide the computer-stimulator with information on joint position and pressure on the limb, which in turn may institute a remedial action or give a warning signal.

Ideally, an FES system for ambulation should allow the paralyzed person to walk without any other assistive devices, but currently this is not possible, because standing and ambulation balance cannot be provided even with experimental FES systems, which were equipped with multiple sensors and closed-loop control. All users of FES ambulation systems require arm support from canes, crutches, or a walker. Additionally, lower limb orthoses of different designs are used with many, if not most, FES systems to provide joint stability, prevent joint injuries, reduce oxygen consumption, provide mounting for sensors, increase limb control, reduce the number of electrodes and stimulation channels required, and minimize the degree of joint freedom requiring control by electrical stimulation. These orthoses may vary in design from a simple ankle-foot orthosis to a knee-ankle-foot orthosis with trunk extensions (i.e., a reciprocating gait orthosis) (see Chapter 18).[102]

Despite advances in biomechanical technology and better understanding of the pathophysiology of SCI, numerous obstacles must be overcome before FES systems for ambulation become widely used. Electrodes must be made that are reliable for long-term stimulation, safe, and easily implantable. Currently used surface electrodes may occasionally produce skin burns, and implanted nerve cuff electrodes may cause nerve damage. To date, epimysial electrodes have been relatively free of complications, and the new injectable electrode is unknown as far as both safety in humans and efficacy in large muscles requiring activation. A totally implantable eight-channel receiver stimulator with electrodes is now available,[101] but must be further tested. Current FES systems demand a high level of attentiveness on the part of the user, whereas, optimally, the sensory feedback should result in automatic correction of limb movement to control posture and gait. Preliminary work on FES control has relied on computer simulation models, which consist of nonlinear muscle-tendon dynamics, nonlinear body segment dynamics, and linear output-feedback control law.[103] The physiology of muscle contraction and aerobic metabolism during chronic electrical stimulation needs to be better understood, and methods must be developed to effectively restore adequate strength and endurance to muscles atrophied by disuse. Undesirable spinal reflexes and spasticity elicited or aggravated by the electrical stimulation and consequent sensory neuron discharge must be suppressed or better used for functional purposes. Interventions must be identified to

restore optimal cardiovascular function during prolonged ambulation, especially for persons with high-level SCI who have limited supraspinal control, if any, over the sympathetic nervous system. In order to ambulate functionally, the user has to be able to obtain an acceptable speed of gait and be able to travel significant distances and negotiate different surfaces (e.g., stairs and inclines). FES ambulation speed has been reported to be slow (between 12 and 18 m/minute[8]; maximum in the best subjects is 50–60 m/minute). The usual distance traveled on level surfaces is 100–200 m; the maximum distance approximately 400 m.[9] Most FES systems are preprogrammed for ambulation on level surfaces only, although the more sophisticated systems allow the patient to ascend and descend stairs and inclines. Energy cost of FES ambulation has been found to be similar to that measured for persons with paraplegia using bilateral knee-ankle-foot orthoses and crutches for ambulation, which is two or three times higher than oxygen consumption per minute during walking for persons without disabilities.[104] There are indications, however, that as the speed of FES ambulation increases with training and improved skills, there is no further increase in oxygen consumption,[104] leading to an increased efficiency over time. Another study showed a smaller energy cost during ambulation with a hybrid reciprocating gait orthosis and FES system than with the orthosis alone,[102] but this may not be clinically significant.

From the patient's perspective, an FES system must be easy to manage. Intensive training for at least 4–6 weeks is required before the system can be used safely. Application of the system takes an average of 15 minutes. The external stimulator, leads, and electrodes are quite conspicuous and are generally found to be cosmetically unacceptable.

The safety of FES systems for ambulation has not yet been adequately documented. Skin burns and infections associated with use of electrodes are relatively rare,[9] but it may easily be anticipated that extensive clinical use may cause injuries to anesthetic joints, resulting in the development of neuropathic joint disease (Charcot's joints), and that with minor trauma or as a result of falls, osteoporotic bones in the paralyzed limbs may fracture.

Clearly, not all SCI patients are candidates for even the most ideal yet-to-be-designed FES ambulation. Those with thoracic cord lesions are the ideal users, but they represent only approximately 25% of all SCI patients. In addition, different health problems may reduce this number significantly. Those with lower motor neuron paralysis in general would not qualify.

One study refers to 500 persons with SCI, who over a 9-year period were admitted and evaluated for FES system use. The system was prescribed and implemented when the application criteria were met,[8] but only 76 persons, 15% of the entire group, met the criteria. Fifty had neurologically complete cord lesions, and all were followed and evaluated regularly. Only 25% of the 50 subjects with complete cord lesions were able to ambulate effectively with the FES system, and for various reasons nine subjects soon stopped using the system. Thus, only 16 subjects remained ambulatory by this means, a small percentage of the 500 patients originally evaluated. Given the current state of technology and training, it appears that for the near future only the exceptional person with SCI will be able to use FES systems for ambulation.

Lower Limb Exercise

FES systems have been designed and commercially marketed to provide strengthening and endurance exercise for lower limb muscles that have been paralyzed by upper motor neuron lesions in the spinal cord (Figure 31-9). Hundreds of such devices have been sold, and it is probable that thousands of persons with SCI have used this clinical intervention. The systems were first developed as a by-product of research and development on FES systems for ambulation. During the early clinical experiments with FES systems for ambulation, it was recognized that considerable training of the paralyzed muscles was necessary if functional ambulation was to be obtained with synchronized electrical stimulation by subjects who were significantly deconditioned owing to disuse and immobilization. Preparation for ambulation thus required strengthening exercises by regular stimulation of the key lower limb muscles (quadriceps and gluteus maximus), or preferably by isotonic or dynamic muscle contraction in which the knee was raised against gravity and some degree of resistance. To further improve the oxidative capacity of the muscles, the subjects trained by pedaling an exercise cycle against different degrees of resistance. Although only a few of the subjects involved in such training programs eventually progressed to experimental FES ambulation, most indicated that subjectively their physical and mental condition had improved during this preparatory therapy. Although such subjective observations do not have a ready scientific explanation, speculative and hypothetical explanations abound. It has long been recognized that immobilization for any reason, including the sedentary lifestyle forced by SCI, results in many adverse physiological changes[105] and that many of these changes may be reversed by regular and sustained physical exer-

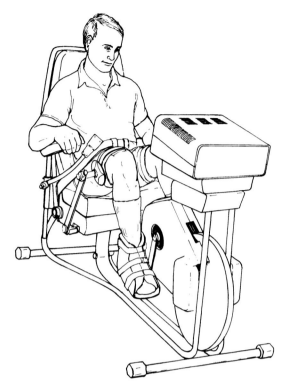

FIGURE 31-9 Multichannel functional electrical stimulation system for lower limb cycle ergometry.

cise. Additionally, numerous scientific studies[57,106,107] have demonstrated various beneficial effects of regular physical exercise on health and longevity in able-bodied persons.

Earlier in this chapter, some of the degenerative physiological changes secondary to SCI, including those caused primarily by disuse and a sedentary lifestyle were described. Clinicians have speculated that many of the symptoms and signs noted during long-term follow-up evaluation of SCI patients may be related to, or aggravated by, the lack of physical exercise, both for nonparalyzed upper limb muscles and in particular for the large muscle mass of the paralyzed lower limbs.[108] Clinicians speculate further that these symptoms and signs, often refractory to customary interventions, may be reduced through fitness training of upper and lower limb muscles.[109] Sedentary lifestyle and the consequent reduced cardiovascular fitness after SCI[67,110] have been linked hypothetically[109] to the high reported mortality from cardiovascular conditions after SCI,[111] a rate that may be exceeded only by that of pulmonary complications. Although numerous forms of wheelchair sports and upper limb exercise programs exist for upper body fitness training, FES provides the only means of actively exercising the large mass of paralyzed muscles in the lower limbs. In more recent years a large number of persons with SCI have participated in FES ergometry training programs. As a result, a considerable body of clinical and research data has been gathered on its effects. Description of the FES ergometer and some of the reported results from this application are summarized in this section.

The most commonly used FES exercise ergometers (see Figure 31-9) consist of a remote-control keyboard for the computer, a stimulus control unit, six channels for sequential muscle stimulation through skin surface electrodes, position and resistance sensors, and the patient's chair. By proper programming and by closed-loop control through feedback from the sensors, the exact stimulus amplitude is provided to generate a constant pedaling speed of 35–50 revolutions per minute against a precise prescribed resistance. The amount of resistance provided by this ergometer is much lower than that of a conventional exercise cycle: 0–7/8 kilopond (kp) (1 kp = 9.80665 Newton units of force) compared with 0–10 kp for conventional exercise cycles.[112] Judging from the relative dearth of reports on adverse effects, this treatment appears to be relatively safe; nonetheless all users must meet defined clinical criteria (Table 31-1) to further ensure safety, comfort, and suitability for this form of exercise. The therapeutic effects of FES ergometry, hypothetically, are many, although only relatively few have been confirmed scientifically. Some of these are discussed in the following paragraphs.

Muscles   FES has repeatedly been shown to reverse to a certain extent the reduced bulk, strength, and endurance of muscles paralyzed by SCI.[18,112-114] As noted previously, chronic low-frequency electrical stimulation and other forms of increased muscle use have been shown to reverse the biochemical, morphologic, and functional changes that occur during muscle disuse (i.e., to change a muscle from a predominantly type II [fast, anaerobic] to type I [slow, aerobic] fiber type).[18,19,24] To examine whether such alteration in muscle fibers does occur during FES ergometry, comparison of muscle biopsy specimens taken before and after training would be needed. No such studies on SCI subjects have been completed and reported. An alternative method of measuring the relative contributions of type I and type II fibers during muscle contraction may be done by comparing quadriceps twitch time before and after FES strengthening and endurance training. Such evaluation has shown a significant decrease in the initial slope of quadriceps twitch time with training, which suggests increased contributions from type I fibers to muscle contraction.[115]

Cardiovascular System   Although no amount of FES-induced exercise can alter the SCI patient's reduced exercise capacity, which largely results from lost supraspinal control over the sympathetic nervous system, both voluntary exercise of the nonparalyzed muscles and FES exercise of paralyzed muscles may significantly increase VO_2max. Many studies have shown that with upper limb exercise alone even patients who have a high-level spinal lesion can increase VO_2max and other corresponding measured parameters by as much as 50%.[68,74] Similarly, people with cervical and high thoracic cord lesions who participated in FES ergometry programs have become able to pedal the ergometer for increasingly longer periods and against progressively greater resistance[115] while demonstrating improved peak work performance and aerobic capacity (i.e., increased VO_2, VCO_2, minute ventilation, and so forth). The aerobic capacity appeared to increase rapidly during the early phase of training, but after a point a number of relevant exercise stress test parameters remained relatively constant, although pedaling time continued to improve. This suggests that the maximum effect on the cardiovascular system may have been obtained early and that peripheral muscle strength and oxidative capacity continued to increase. It is probable that the exercise quickly becomes anaerobic and that the serum lactate levels increase owing to poor return of venous blood to the heart, which in turn is caused by inadequate vasoconstriction to nonworking muscles and organs, weak venomotor tone, ineffective muscle pump, and lower intra-abdominal pressure. This in turn results in insufficient stroke volume, cardiac output, and delivery of

TABLE 31-1
Selection Criteria for Functional Electrical Stimulation Ergometry

Upper motor neuron lesion
Impaired sensation to tolerate stimulus
Minimal to moderate spasticity
Joint range of motion in lower extremities is within functional limits
Roentgenographic examination of lower extremities is unremarkable
Health generally good
Emotionally stable, reliable, and realistic

oxygen to the exercising muscles.[116] This exercise response in persons with high cord lesions is not restricted to FES exercise; similar results are noted during performance of maximum upper limb exercises.[65] Although this modest exercise response, which is significantly below normal values, may prevent persons with high cord lesions from performing work that requires sustained high output, it is possible that such exercise may be adequate to secure certain cardiovascular health benefits.[116]

No reports exist on quantitative assessment of peripheral arterial and venous circulation during FES training. Single-channel electrical stimulation of the gastrocnemius muscle during the early phases of SCI, especially when combined with administration of subcutaneous low-dose heparin, has been reported to reduce the incidence of deep venous thrombosis and pulmonary embolism,[117] and it may be speculated that FES exercise in the chronic phase of SCI may help to increase both venous and arterial circulation of the exercising lower limbs with similar preventive effect. Anecdotal reports describe clinically reduced acrocyanosis of the lower limbs with FES exercise and reduction of pedal edema.[118]

Clinicians speculate that FES exercise may have another indirect beneficial effect on the cardiovascular system, especially the coronary arteries, by raising the serum levels of high-density lipoproteins (HDL).[116,119] It is well-documented that serum HDL levels are significantly lower in SCI patients than in the nondisabled population, which may in part be because of their sedentary lifestyle. It has also been shown that although wheelchair athletes have relatively low serum HDL levels, their levels are higher than those of inactive SCI patients.[60] No studies, however, exist that show any change in serum HDL with FES exercise.

Although the incidence of obesity during the chronic phase of SCI is not well documented, body composition studies have shown that even in the absence of clinical obesity lean body mass decreases and total body fat increases, especially with higher cord lesions.[120] This change in body composition is attributed to physical inactivity and oversupply of energy relative to energy expenditure. Although obesity is known to be a major risk factor for coronary heart disease and development of adult onset diabetes mellitus, it is not known whether the reduced lean body mass after SCI is clinically harmful or, if so, whether regular FES or voluntary muscle exercise and modifications of diet would have a beneficial effect on this condition.

Respiratory System   As noted previously in this chapter, respiratory capacity, although diminished by SCI, has been found to be sufficient for whatever voluntary exercise a person with an SCI is capable of performing. Similarly, no reports demonstrate that respiratory capacity may be inadequate for FES exercise, even during simultaneous voluntary upper limb exercise by arm cranking.

Endocrine Function   The sedentary lifestyle after SCI may affect secretion of insulin as well as the sensitivity to the hormone itself of insulin receptor sites in the muscles. It has been well documented in able-bodied people that insulin sensitivity at its receptor sites increases as physical fitness improves,[121] with consequent reduction in insulin secretion, and that the reverse process may occur with inactivity and physical deconditioning. Research also confirms that persons with chronic SCI have an increased prevalence of abnormal carbohydrate metabolism (i.e., abnormal glucose tolerance test, hyperinsulinemia, insulin resistance).[122-124] Although it may be hypothesized that increased physical fitness through both upper limb voluntary exercise and lower limb FES ergometry may improve carbohydrate metabolism after SCI and insulin sensitivity, no studies exist to support this hypothesis.

Although patients' altered self-image and depression in both the acute and chronic phases of SCI are primarily an emotional reaction to the disability, the depression may be aggravated by neuroendocrine dysfunction (i.e., excessive secretion of cortisol and inadequate secretion of β-endorphin [BEP]). BEP is a peptide with opium-like properties that is normally secreted in the brain and other body tissues and appears to influence a number of physiological and psychological functions.[125-127] Plasma levels of BEP and its precursor β-lipotropin have been shown to be increased by physical exercise, and fitness training reportedly augments the effects of these natural chemicals.[126,128] The majority of SCI patients who participated in a clinical FES ergometry program reported improved self-image and perceived that their appearance was better after participation in this program.[129] It has since been shown that SCI is associated with a decreased level of BEP and flattened circadian rhythm, as well as dysregulated cortisol serum level.[130] The same study showed that regular FES exercise caused a significant and sustained increase in BEP, along with regulation of the cortisol level and improved depression scores.[130] The efficacy of upper limb endurance exercise in stimulating BEP secretion after SCI has not been reported.

Skeletal System   SCI is followed by immediate and significant loss of bone minerals and bone mass in the paralyzed body parts. This bone loss continues for many months and may not come to a halt until 2–3 years after the injury.[131,132] The evidence for this prolonged bone catabolism is found in the increased excretion of calcium and hydroxyproline in the urine.[133] The mechanisms for this pathogenic bone loss are generally believed to be immobilization and inadequate bone stress, which is normally generated by active muscle contraction and longitudinal weight bearing. Endocrine dysfunction does not seem to play a major role in the bone loss, as the nonparalyzed limbs are not affected, but dysfunction of the sympathetic nervous system resulting in inadequate trophic support and blood flow regulation has been thought to have some effect.[134,135] Although bone loss eventually halts, no known interventions increase the rate of bone formation. In contrast, able-bodied persons can reverse immobilization osteoporosis if they resume physical activity after a period of disuse.[136-138] The persistent osteoporosis increases the risk of long bone fractures, which can occur with minor injury.[139] Concern has been expressed that FES of the paralyzed and osteoporotic lower limbs, either during ambulation or ergometry exercise, may cause fractures of the bones, and, indeed, anecdotal reports of such injuries exist. In general, however, the degree of osteoporosis found in most persons with SCI does not appear to present a significant clinical risk during FES.

The osteoporosis observed in paralyzed body parts is thought to be unalterable by any known clinical means (chemical treatment, daily standing with orthoses) or the development of spasticity.[131] Lower limb FES for ambulation or ergometry exercise has frequently been mentioned hypothetically as an effective therapy for osteoporosis after SCI,[140] but investigators who have evaluated the effect of this technology on bone mineral density have failed to show any increase in bone density.[109,141]

Control of Bladder

The neuroanatomy and physiology of bladder and sexual functions and how these are affected by SCI are described in detail elsewhere in this book (see Chapters 10 and 29). In brief, the urinary bladder, rectum, internal sphincters, and erectile tissue obtain parasympathetic innervation from the sacral segments of the spinal cord through the pelvic nerves, but the external sphincters and the striated pelvic floor muscles receive somatic innervation from the same segments through the pudendal nerves. Additionally, sympathetic innervations of these organs are received from T-10 to L-2 segments of the spinal cord through the lumbar sympathetic chain, presacral plexus, and hypogastric nerves.

Damage to the spinal cord above the sacral segments (i.e., to the upper motor neuron) usually results in loss of voluntary control over bladder and bowel evacuation and

sexual dysfunction. If the lower motor neurons in the sacral segments of the cord are intact, hyperreflexia of the bladder's detrusor muscle and of the external urethral sphincter usually occurs, variably resulting in urinary reflex incontinence or detrusor-sphincter dyssynergia. In such dyssynergia, failure of the external sphincter to relax on detrusor contraction usually results in abnormally high intravesical pressures and elevated residual postvoiding urinary volumes, predisposing the person to reflux of urine to the ureter, development of hydroureter, hydronephrosis, and urinary tract infections.[142] Evacuation of stools may be slowed by the hyperreflexic anal sphincter, and involuntary evacuation may occur with a hyperreactive rectum. In men, reflex penile erections are usually possible although frequently poorly sustained, but ejaculation is most difficult to obtain. The preservation of intact lower motor neurons in the sacral segments of the cords permits the use of electrical stimulation to restore a degree of function to the bladder, bowel, and sexual organs.

Damage of the parasympathetic and somatic lower motor neurons in the sacral segments of the spinal cord results in areflexia of the bladder detrusor muscle, urethral external sphincter, rectum, anal sphincter, erectile tissue, and muscles for ejaculation, clinically apparent, respectively, as urinary overflow incontinence, constipation, fecal incontinence, erectile dysfunction, and inability to ejaculate. In such instances, electrical stimulation for restoration of function cannot be done.

Electrical stimulation of the parasympathetic nerve fibers in the anterior roots of S-2, S-3, and S-4 can reliably cause contraction of the detrusor muscle of the bladder.[44,142-147] However, because the somatic efferent nerves to the external sphincter are present in the same nerve roots, contraction of the external sphincter may occur simultaneously with inadequate micturition. Early efforts to produce micturition by electrical stimulation of the sacral anterior roots, therefore, met with limited success,[148] and incontinence was frequent because of spontaneous or reflex parasympathetic stimulation. During the 1980s, it was reported[149] that continence could be much improved by performing S-2 to S-4 posterior sacral rhizotomies at the time of the implantation of electrodes to the sacral anterior roots. This approach has since become common. The major advantages and disadvantages of performing sacral posterior rhizotomies have been described by Creasey.[142] It is considered advantageous that uninhibited bladder contractions are abolished with increased bladder capacity and reduced bladder incontinence, that bladder compliance is restored, which protects upper urinary tracts from hydroureter and hydronephrosis, and that detrusor sphincter dyssynergia and autonomic dysreflexia triggered by bladder or rectal problems are eliminated. On the other hand, the disadvantages of sacral posterior rhizotomies include loss of reflex erection and ejaculation, reflex micturition, and reflex defecation as well as loss of perineal sensation if present. However, erection can still be produced by injection of papaverine or prostaglandin into the corpora cavernosa or by the use of external devices or by penile implant, and electrical stimulation of the sacral anterior roots can still cause erection, ejaculation, micturition, and defecation.

Worldwide, more than 1,500 people with SCI have received implantable sacral anterior root electrical stimulating systems during the last two decades.[142] One such system has been approved in the United States by the Food and Drug Administration for humanitarian use in properly selected individuals with SCI who also will undergo sacral posterior rhizotomy at the time of implantation. Users must have neurologically complete SCI (American Spinal Injury Association [ASIA] classification A) with intact parasympathetic innervation of the bladder; be free of septic infections, pressure sores, and implanted cardiac pacemakers; and be reliable and emotionally stable. The primary indication for such an implantable system is to provide micturition on demand and to reduce postvoiding residual urine volumes, with a secondary indication to aid in bowel evacuation.

The system consists of a receiver stimulator, surgically implanted under the skin of the abdomen, and electrodes that are implanted either intradurally on the sacral anterior roots in the cauda equina or extradurally on the mixed sacral nerves within the sacral spinal canal. Lead wires tunneled subcutaneously connect the electrodes and the receiver stimulator. An external controller that is operated by the user provides command signals and power to an external radio transmitter that sends signals through the skin to the receiver stimulator.

Follow-up studies[44,142-147] have shown that most individuals use the system regularly for bladder evacuation and 73–86% report complete continence,[142,146] reduced postvoiding residual urine volumes, decreased incidence of symptomatic urinary tract infection and of episodes of autonomic dysreflexia,[142,144,146,147] less constipation, and better fecal continence.[142] The electrical stimulation patterns used for micturition usually do not cause defecation, but a different pattern can be used for bowel evacuation program.[142] Penile erection reportedly occurs in approximately 70% of individuals with intradural electrical stimulation of the sacral anterior roots, but results with extradural stimulation reportedly are less successful.[142] Reported adverse events have been few but include implant infections, CSF leak, and implant failures.[144,145,147]

CONCLUSION

The clinical use of electricity allows physiatrists and other rehabilitation specialists to diagnose neuromuscular disorders, prevent and manage disease, and enhance function. In more recent years, a better understanding of the physiology of the neuromuscular system and of physical exercise, along with rapid progress in electronic technology, has enhanced the use of electricity for functional restoration in persons with disease or disability. At times it is difficult to distinguish between the use of electricity for therapeutic purposes and its application for functional restoration. Indications and contraindications for prescribing different forms of FES have been described in the literature and in this chapter. Promising results of this intervention have raised hopes that in the near future FES technology may dramatically change the lives of many persons with physical disability, but caution is advised. Compared with performance of the intact human body, that produced by the current FES technology is crude and cannot be described as well-coordinated movement. The maximum success of FES as a clinical intervention depends on the solution of innumerable technological problems, better understanding of neuromuscular physiology, and improved training methods. Such developments may then afford more accurate control over paralyzed but otherwise essentially intact body parts by methods that effectively bypass the damaged motor and sensory pathways in the CNS.

The application of FES systems for the purposes of improving upper limb function, allowing respirator-free ventilation, inducing lower limb exercise, and increasing control over bladder and bowel evacuation has been well established clinically. FES systems for ambulation have received much public attention, but if everyday ambulation in the community by FES is to become a practical reality, the stimulation of individual muscles must be highly selective, contraction must be uniform throughout the muscle, incremental activation of muscle must be reproducible, complete reconditioning of the muscle must occur with training, metabolic requirements must be fully met, muscle fatigue on repeated artificial stimulation must be reduced, spasticity must be controllable, balance with canes and crutches must be good, and full miniaturization of more accurate devices for total body implantation must be developed. Eventually, FES systems for different purposes may produce valuable clinical alternatives to wheelchairs, orthoses, and other forms of assistive devices now prescribed to improve the health, mobility, and self-care skills of many paralyzed persons.

REFERENCES

1. Licht S. Therapeutic Electricity and Ultraviolet Radiation (2nd ed). New Haven, CT: Elizabeth Licht, 1967;1–70.

2. Krusen FH. Physical Medicine: The Employment of Physical Agents for Diagnosis and Therapy. Philadelphia: WB Saunders, 1941.

3. Liberson WT, Holmquest HJ, Scot D, et al. Functional electrotherapy: stimulation of the peroneal nerve synchronized with the swing phase of gait of hemiplegic patients. Arch Phys Med Rehabil 1961;42:101–105.

4. Kantrowitz A. Electronic Physiologic Aids. Brooklyn, NY: Maimonides Hospital, 1960;4–5.

5. Long C, Masciarelli VD. An electrophysiologic splint for the hand. Arch Phys Med Rehabil 1963;44:499–503.

6. Waters RL, McNeal D, Tasto J. Peroneal nerve conduction velocity after chronic electrical stimulation. Arch Phys Med Rehabil 1975;56:240–243.

7. Waters RL, McNeal DR, Perry J. Experimental correction of footdrop by electrical stimulation of peroneal nerve. J Bone Joint Surg 1975;57A:1047–1054.

8. Kralj A, Bajd R, Turk R. Enhancement of gait restoration in spinal-injured patients by functional electrical stimulation. Clin Orthop 1988;233:34–43.

9. Marsolais EB, Kobetic R. Development of a practical electrical stimulation system for restoring gait in a paralyzed patient. Clin Orthop 1988;233:64–74.

10. Petrofsky JS, Phillips CA. Computer controlled walking in the paralyzed individual. Neurol Orthop Surg 1983; 4:153–164.

11. Peckham PH. Functional electrical stimulation: current status and future prospects of applications to the neuromuscular system in spinal cord injury. Paraplegia 1987;25:279–288.

12. Keith MW, Peckham PH, Thrope GB, et al. Functional neuromuscular stimulation, neuroprosthesis for the tetraplegic hand. Clin Orthop 1988;233:25–33.

13. Keith MW, Peckham PH, Thrope GB, et al. Implantable functional neuromuscular stimulation in the tetraplegic hand. J Hand Surg 1989;3:524–530.

14. Nathan RH. Generation of Functional Arm Movements in C4 Quadriplegics by Neuromuscular Stimulation. In FC Rose, R Jones, G Vrbova (eds), Comprehensive Neurologic Rehabilitation. Vol 3: Neuromuscular Stimulation: Basics, Concepts and Clinical Implications. New York: Demos, 1989;273–284.

15. Glenn WWL, Hogan JF, Loke JS, et al. Ventilatory support by pacing of the conditioned diaphragm in quadriplegics. N Engl J Med 1984;310:1150–1155.

16. Glenn WWL. The treatment of respiratory paralysis by diaphragmatic pacing. Ann Thorac Surg 1980;30:106–109.

17. Nochomowitz ML, Hopkins M, Brodkey J, et al. Conditioning of the diaphragm with phrenic nerve stimulation following prolonged disuse. Am Rev Respir Dis 1984;130:686–688.

18. Lieber RL. Comparison between animal and human studies of skeletal muscle adaptation to chronic stimulation. Clin Orthop 1988;233:19–24.

19. Salmons S, Henriksson J. The adaptive response of skeletal muscle to increased used. Muscle Nerve 1981;4:94–105.

20. Munsat TL, McNeal D, Waters R. Effects of nerve stimulation on human muscle. Arch Neurol 1975;33:176–182.

21. Grimby G, Nordwall A, Hulten B, et al. Changes in histochemical profile of muscle after long-term electrical stimulation in patients with idiopathic scoliosis. Scand J Rehabil Med 1985; 17:191–196.

22. Peckham PH, Mortimer JT, Marsolais EB. Alterations in the force and fatigability of skeletal muscle in quadriplegic humans following exercise induced by chronic electrical stimulation. Clin Orthop 1976;114:326–334.

23. Lieber RL. Skeletal muscle adaptability I. Review of basic properties. Dev Med Child Neurol 1986;28:390–397.

24. Jolesz F, Sreter FA. Development, innervation and activity pattern-induced changes in skeletal muscle. Annu Rev Physiol 1981;43:531–552.

25. Peckham PH. Principles of electrical stimulation. Top Spinal Cord Inj Rehabil 1999;5:105.

26. Van den Honert C, Mortimer JT. The response of the myelinated nerve fiber to short duration biphasic stimulating currents. Ann Biomed Eng 1979;7:117–125.

27. Van den Honert C, Mortimer JT. A technique for collision block of peripheral nerve: single stimulus analysis. IEEE Trans Biomed Eng 1981;28:373–378.

28. Thrope GB, Peckham PH, Crago BE. A computer controlled multichannel stimulation system for laboratory use in functional neuromuscular stimulation. IEEE Trans Biomed Eng 1985;32:363–370.

29. McNeil DR, Baker LL. Stimulating the quadriceps and hamstrings with surface electrodes. Proc 8th Annu Conf RESNA 1985;651–653.

30. Gorman PH, Mortimer JT. The effect of stimulus parameters on the recruitment characteristics of direct nerve stimulation. IEEE Trans Biomed Eng 1983;30:407–414.

31. McNeil DR, Baker LL, Symons J. Recruitment data for nerve cuff and epimysial electrodes. Proc 10th Annu Conf RESNA 1987;651–653.

32. Peckham PH. Functional neuromuscular stimulation. Phys Technol 1981; 12:114–121.

33. Mortimer JT. Motor Prosthesis. In JM Brookhart, VB Mountcastle (eds), Handbook of Physiology. Sec I: The Nervous System. Bethesda, MD: American Physiological Society, 1981; 155–187.

34. Peckham PH. Electrical Excitation of Skeletal Muscle: Alterations in Force, Fatigue and Metabolic Properties [Dissertation]. Cleveland, OH: Case Western Reserve University, 1972.

35. Campbell J. Efficacy of volitional versus electrically evoked knee extension exercise. Proc 10th Annu Conf RESNA 1987;648–650.

36. Fang ZP. Presented at the Engineering Foundation Conference on Neuroprosthesis: Motor System. July 17–22, 1988, Potosi, MO.

37. Petrofsky JS, Phillips CA. Microprocessor-controlled simulation in paralyzed muscle. IEEE NAECON Rec 1979;79:198–210.

38. Kralj AR, Bajd T. Functional Electrical Stimulation: Standing and Walking after Spinal Cord Injury. Boca Raton, FL: CRC, 1989.

39. Petrofsky JS. Sequential motor unit stimulation through peripheral motor nerves in a cat. Med Biol Eng Comput 1979;17:87–93.

40. Patterson RP, Lockwood JS, Dykstra DD. A functional electric stimulation using an electrode garment. Arch Phys Med Rehabil 1990;71:340–342.

41. Marsolais EB, Kobetic R. Functional electrical stimulation for walking in paraplegia. J Bone Joint Surg 1987; 69A:728–733.

42. Mortimer JT, Kaufman D, Roessmann U. Intramuscular electrical stimulation: tissue damage. Ann Biomed Eng 1980;8:235–244.

43. Waters RL, Campbell JM, Nakai R. Therapeutic electrical stimulation of the lower limb by epimysial electrodes. Clin Orthop 1988;233:44–52.

44. Brindley GS, Rushton DN. Long-term follow-up of patients with sacral ante-

rior root stimulators. Paraplegia 1990;28:469–475.

45. Agnew WF, McCreery DB, Yuen TG, et al. Histologic and physiologic evaluation of electrically stimulated peripheral nerve: considerations for the selection of parameters. Ann Biomed Eng 1989;17:39–60.

46. Cameron T, Loeb GE, Peck RA, et al. Micromodular implants to provide electrical stimulation of paralyzed muscles and limbs. IEEE Trans Biomed Eng 1997;44:781–790.

47. Cameron T, Richmond FJ, Loeb GE. Effects of regional stimulation using a miniature stimulator implanted in feline posterior biceps femoris. IEEE Trans Biomed Eng 1998;45:1036–1043.

48. Loeb GE, Walmsley B, Duysens J. Obtaining Proprioceptive Information from Natural Limbs: Implantable Transducers versus Somatosensory Neuron Recordings. In MR Neuman, et al. (eds), Solid State Physical Sensors for Biomedical Applications. Boca Raton, FL: CRC, 1980.

49. Crago PE, Chizeck HJ, Neuman MR, et al. Sensors for use with functional neuromuscular stimulation. IEEE Trans Biomed Eng 1986;33:256–268.

50. Petrofsky JS, Phillips CA, Stafford DE. Closed-loop control for restoration of movement in paralyzed muscle. Orthopaedics 1984;7:1289–1302.

51. Grimby G, Broberg C, Krotkiewska I, et al. Muscle fiber composition in patients with traumatic cord lesions. Scand J Rehabil Med 1976;8:37–42.

52. Lieber RL. Skeletal muscle adaptability II: muscle properties following SCI. Dev Med Child Neurol 1986;28:533–542.

53. Heigenhauscher GF, Ruff GL, Miller B, et al. Cardiovascular response of paraplegics during graded arm ergometry. Med Sci Sports Exerc 1976;8:68.

54. Hjeltnes N. Oxygen uptake and cardiac output in graded arm exercise in paraplegics with low-level spinal lesions. Scand J Rehabil Med 1977;9:107–113.

55. Hjeltnes N. Cardiorespiratory capacity in tetra- and paraplegia shortly after injury. Scand J Rehabil Med 1986;18:65–70.

56. VanLoan M, McCluer S, Loftin JM, et al. Comparison of maximal physiological responses to arm exercise among able-bodied paraplegics and quadriplegics. Med Sci Sports Exerc 1985;17:250.

57. Glaser RM, Sawka MN, Brune MF, et al. Physical responses to maximal effort wheelchair and arm crank ergometry. J Appl Physiol 1980;48:1060–1064.

58. Knutsson E, Lewenhaupt-Olsson E, Thorsen M. Physical work capacity and physical conditioning in paraplegic patients. Paraplegia 1973;11:205–216.

59. Blair SN, Kohl HW, Pattenbarger RS, et al. Physical fitness and all-cause mortality. A prospective study of healthy men and women. JAMA 1989;262:2395–2401.

60. Brenes G, Dearwater S, Shapera R, et al. High density lipoprotein cholesterol concentrations in physically active and sedentary spinal cord injured patients. Arch Phys Med Rehabil 1986;67:445–450.

61. Ferrara MS, Davis RW. Injuries to the elite wheelchair athletes. Paraplegia 1990;28:335–341.

62. DeBoer LB, Kallal JE, Longo MR. Upper extremity prone position exercise as aerobic capacity indicator. Arch Phys Med Rehabil 1982;63:467–471.

63. Wicks JR, Oldridge NB, Cameron BJ, et al. Arm cranking and wheelchair ergometry in elite spinal cord injured athletes. Med Sci Sports Exerc 1983;15:224–231.

64. Drory Y, Ohry A, Brooks ME, et al. Arm crank ergometry in chronic spinal cord injured patients. Arch Phys Med Rehabil 1990;71:389–392.

65. Coutts DK, Rhodes EC, McKenzie DC. Maximal exercise responses of tetraplegics and paraplegics. J Appl Physiol 1983;55:479–482.

66. Davis GM, Kofsky PR, Kelsey JC, et al. Cardiorespiratory fitness and muscular strength of wheelchair uses. Can Med Assoc J 1981;125:1317–1323.

67. Figoni SF. Spinal cord injury and maximal aerobic power. Am Correct Ther J 1984;38:44–50.

68. Gass GC, Watson J, Camp EM, et al. Effects of physical training on high-level spinal lesion patients. Scand J Rehabil Med 1980;12:61–65.

69. Hass F, Axen K, Pineda H. Aerobic capacity in spinal cord injured people. Cent Nerv Syst Trauma 1986;3:77–91.

70. Freyschuss U, Knuttson E. Cardiovascular control in man with transverse cervical cord lesions. Life Sci 1969;8:421–424.

71. Coutts KD. Prediction of oxygen uptake from power output in tetraplegics and paraplegics during wheelchair ergometry. Med Sci Sports Exerc 1983;15:181.

72. Gass GC, Camp EM. The maximum physiological responses during incremental wheelchair and arm cranking

exercise in male paraplegics. Med Sci Sports Exerc 1984;16:355–359.

73. Sawka MM, Glaser RM, Laubach LL, et al. Wheelchair exercise performance of the young, middle-aged and elderly. J Appl Physiol 1981;50:824–828.

74. Whiting RB, Dreisinger TE, Dalton RB, et al. Improved physical fitness and work capacity in quadriplegics by wheelchair exercise. J Cardiac Rehabil 1983;3:251–255.

75. Kamelhar DL, Steele JM, Schact RG, et al. Plasma renin and serum dopamine-beta-hydroxylase during orthostatic hypotension in quadriplegic man. Arch Phys Med Rehabil 1978;59:212–216.

76. Naftchi NE, Ragnarsson KT, Sell GH, et al. Increased digital vascular reactivity to L-norepinephrine in quadriplegics. Arch Phys Med Rehabil 1975;56:554.

77. Fugl-Meyer AR. Effects of respiratory muscle paralysis in tetraplegia and paraplegia patients. Scand J Rehabil Med 1971;3:141–150.

78. Kokkola K, Moller K, Lehtonen T. Pulmonary function in tetraplegia and paraplegia patients. Ann Clin Res 1975;7:76–80.

79. Rhodes EC, McKenzie DC, Coutts KD, et al. A field test for the prediction of aerobic capacity in male paraplegics and quadriplegics. Can J Appl Sports Sci 1981;6:182–186.

80. Bunt JC. Hormonal alterations due to exercise. Sports Med 1986;3:331–345.

81. Kilgore KL, Peckham PH, Keith MW, et al. An implanted upper-extremity neuroprosthesis. Follow-up of five patients. J Bone Joint Surg 1997;79A:533–541.

82. Keith MW, Kilgore KL, Pechkahm PH. Tendon transfers and functional electrical stimulation for restoration of hand function in spinal cord injury. J Hand Surg 1996;21A:89–99.

83. Peckham PH, Keith MW, Freehafer AA. Restoration of functional control by electrical stimulation in the upper extremity of the quadriplegic patient. J Bone Joint Surg 1988;70A:144–148.

84. Wijman CAC, Stroh KC, Van Doren CL, et al. Functional evaluation of quadriplegic patients using a hand neuroprosthesis. Arch Phys Med Rehabil 1990;71:1053–1057.

85. Smith B, Peckham PH, Roscoe DD, et al. An externally powered multichannel implantable stimulator for versatile control of paralyzed muscles. IEEE Trans Biomed Eng 1987;34:499–508.

86. Brindley GS, Donaldson N, Perkins TA, et al. Two-stage key grip by joy

stick from an eleven-channel upper limb FES implant in C6 tetraplegia. Proc Biol Eng Soc 1989;41.

87. Hart RL, Kilgore KL, Peckham PH. A comparison between control methods for implanted FES hand grasp system. IEEE Trans Rehabil Eng 1998;6:1–11.

88. Moberg E. The Upper Limb and Tetraplegia: A New Approach to Surgical Rehabilitation. Stuttgart: George Thieme, 1978.

89. House JH, Shannon MA. Restoration of strong grasp and lateral pinch in tetraplegia: a comparison of two methods of thumb control in each patient. J Hand Surg 1985;10:22–29.

90. Carter RE. Available Respiratory Options. In G Whiteneck, et al. (eds), The Management of High Quadriplegia. New York: Demos, 1989.

91. DiMarco AF. Diaphragmatic pacing in patients with spinal cord injury. Top Spinal Cord Inj Rehabil 1999;5:6–20.

92. Shaw RK, Glenn WWL, Hogan JF, et al. Electrophysiological evaluation of phrenic nerve function in candidates for diaphragm pacing. J Neurosurg 1980;53:345–354.

93. Dobelle WH, D'Angelo MS, Goetz BF, et al. 200 cases with a new breathing pacemaker dispel myths about diaphragm pacing. ASAIO J 1994;40:M244–M252.

94. Nochomovitz ML, DiMarco AF, Mortimer JT, et al. Diaphragm activation with intramuscular stimulation. Am Rev Respir Dis 1983;127:325–329.

95. DiMarco AF, Supinski GS, Petro JA, Takaoka Y. Evaluation of intercostal pacing to provide artificial ventilation in quadriplegics. Am J Respir Crit Care Med 1994;150:934–940.

96. Krieger AF, Gropper MR, Adler RJ. Electrophrenic respiration after intercostal to phrenic nerve grafting in a patient with anterior spinal artery syndrome: technical case report. Neurosurgery 1994;35:760–763.

97. Merletti R, Andina A, Galante N, et al. Clinical experience of electrical peroneal stimulators in fifty hemiparetic patients. Scand J Rehabil Med 1979;11:111–121.

98. Jaeger RJ, Yarkony GM, Roth EJ, et al. Estimating the user population of a simple electrical system for standing. Paraplegia 1990;28:505–511.

99. Yarkony GM, Jaeger RJ, Roth EJ, et al. Functional neuromuscular stimulation for standing after spinal cord injury. Arch Phys Med Rehabil 1990;71:201–206.

100. Technological Advancements in Rehabilitation: Independent Standing and Short Distance Walking for the Spinal Cord Injured. An Overview of the Parastep. Northfield, IL: System Sigmedics, Inc, 1991.

101. Triolo RJ, Bogie K. Lower extremity applications of functional neuromuscular stimulation after spinal cord injury. Top Spinal Cord Rehabil 1999;5:49–65.

102. Nene AB, Patrick JH. Energy cost of paraplegic locomotion using the parawalker/electrical stimulation hybrid orthosis. Arch Phys Med Rehabil 1990;71:116–120.

103. Khang G, Zajac FE. Paraplegic standing controlled by functional neuromuscular stimulation. Part I and Part II: Computer model and control system design; computer stimulation studies. IEEE Trans Biomech Eng 1989;36:873–894.

104. Marsolais EB, Edwards BG. Energy cost of walking and standing with functional neuromuscular stimulation and long leg braces. Arch Phys Med Rehabil 1988;69:243–249.

105. Dietrich JE, Whedon GD, Shorr E. Effects of immobilization upon various metabolic and physiological functions of normal man. Am J Med 1948;4:3–36.

106. Rippe JM, Ward A, Porcari JP, et al. Walking for health and fitness. JAMA 1988;259:2720–2724.

107. Harris SS, Caspersen CJ, DeFriese GH, et al. Physical activity counseling for healthy adults as primary preventive intervention in a clinical setting: report for the US Preventive Service Task Force. JAMA 1989;261:3590–3598.

108. Ragnarsson KT. Spinal cord injury: old problems, new approaches. Bull N Y Acad Med 1986;62:174–181.

109. Ragnarsson KT. Physiologic effects of functional electrical stimulation-induced exercises in spinal cord injured individuals. Clin Orthop 1988;233:53–63.

110. Figoni SE. Perspectives on cardiovascular fitness and SCI. J Am Parapleg Soc 1990;13:63–71.

111. Stover SL, Fine PR. Spinal Cord Injury: Facts and Figures. Birmingham, AL: University of Alabama, 1986.

112. Ragnarsson KT, Pollack S, O'Daniel W, et al. Clinical evaluation of computerized functional electrical stimulation after spinal cord injury: a multicenter pilot study. Arch Phys Med Rehabil 1988;69:672–677.

113. Gruner JA, Glaser RM, Feinberg SD, et al. A system for evaluation and exercise conditioning of paralyzed muscles. J Rehabil Res Dev 1983;20:21–30.

114. Faghri PD, Glaser RM, Figoni SF, et al. Feasibility of using two FNS exercise modes for spinal cord injured patients. Clin Kinesiol 1989;43:62–68.

115. Pollack SF, Axen K, Spielholtz N, et al. Aerobic training effects of electrically induced lower extremity exercises in spinal cord injured people. Arch Phys Med Rehabil 1989;70:214–219.

116. Ragnarsson KT, Pollack SF, Twist D. Lower limb endurance exercise after spinal cord injury: implications for health and functional ambulation. J Neurol Rehabil 1991;5:37–48.

117. Merli GJ, Herbison GJ, Ditunno JF, et al. Deep vein thrombosis: prophylaxis in acute spinal cord injured patients. Arch Phys Med Rehabil 1988;69:661–664.

118. Twist DF. Acrocyanosis in spinal cord injured patients: effects of computer-controlled neuromuscular electrical stimulation. A case report. Phys Ther 1990;70:45–49.

119. Brenes G, McDermott AL, Sikora JM. The effect of computerized functional electrical stimulation on lipoprotein cholesterol in the spinal cord injured. Proc 15th Annu Sci Meet Am Spinal Inj Assoc 1989;78.

120. Nuhlicek DNR, Spurr GB, Barboriak JJ, et al. Body composition of patients with spinal cord injury. Eur J Clin Nutr 1988;42:765–773.

121. Mondon CE, Dolkas CB, Reaven GM. Site of enhanced insulin sensitivity in exercise-trained rats at rest. Am J Physiol 1980;239:E169–E177.

122. Duckworth WC, Solomon SS, Jallpalli P, et al. Glucose intolerance due to insulin resistance in patients with spinal cord injuries. Diabetes 1980;29:906–910.

123. Duckworth WC, Jappalli P, Solomon SS. Glucose intolerance in spinal cord injury. Arch Phys Med Rehabil 1983;64:107–110.

124. Bauman WA, Yalow RS, Zhang RL, et al. Glucose intolerance in diabetes mellitus in paraplegic veterans. J Am Parapleg Soc 1991;14:195.

125. Byck R. Peptide transmitters: a unifying hypothesis for euphoria, respiration, sleep and the action of lithium. Lancet 1976;2:72–73.

126. Carr DB, Bullen BA, Skrinar GS, et al. Physical conditioning facilitates the exercise induced secretion of beta-endorphin and beta-alipotropin in women. N Engl J Med 1981;305:560–563.

127. Pasternak GW. Multiple morphine and encephalon receptors and the relief of pain. JAMA 1988;259:1362–1367.

128. Harber VJ, Sutton JR. Endorphins and exercise. Sports Med 1984;1:154–171.

129. Sipski ML, DeLisa JA, Schweer S. Functional electrical stimulation by cycle ergometry: patient perceptions. Am J Phys Med Rehabil 1989;68:147–149.

130. Twist DJ, Culpepper-Morgan JA, Ragnarsson KT, et al. Neuroendocrine parameters in spinal cord injured involved in a computerized functional electrical stimulation exercise program. Am J Phys Med Rehabil 1992;71:156–163.

131. Biering-Sorensen F, Bohr H, Schaadt O. Bone mineral content of the lumbar spine and lower extremities years after spinal cord lesion. Paraplegia 1988;26:293–301.

132. Naftchi NE, Viau AT, Sell GH, et al. Mineral metabolism in spinal cord injury. Arch Phys Med Rehabil 1980;61:139–142.

133. Claus-Walker J, Comporse RJ, Carter RE, et al. Calcium excretion in quadriplegia. Arch Phys Med Rehabil 1972;53:14–20.

134. Dietz FR. Effect of peripheral nerve on limb development. J Orthop Res 1986;5:576–585.

135. Gillis BJA. The nature of the bone changes associated with nerve injuries and disuse. J Bone Joint Surg 1954;36B:464–473.

136. Donaldson CL, Hulley SB, Vogel JM, et al. Effect of prolonged bedrest on bone mineral. Metabolism 1970;19:1071–1084.

137. Uhtoff HK, Jaworski ZFG. Bone loss and response to long term immobilization. J Bone Joint Surg 1978;60B:420–429.

138. Ruben CT, Lanyon LE. Regulation of bone formation by applied dynamic loads. J Bone Joint Surg 1984;66A:397–402.

139. Ragnarsson KT, Sell GH. Lower extremity fractures after SCI: a retrospective study. Arch Phys Med Rehabil 1981;62:418–422.

140. Phillips CA, Petrofsky JS, Hendershot DM, et al. Functional electrical exercise: a comprehensive approach for physical conditioning of the spinal cord injured patient. Orthopaedics 1984;7:1112–1123.

141. Leeds EM, Klose KJ, Ganz W, et al. Bone mineral density after bicycle ergometry training. Arch Phys Med Rehabil 1990;71:207–219.

142. Creasey GH. Restoration of bladder, bowel and sexual functions. Top Spinal Cord Inj Rehabil 1999;5:21–32.

143. Brindley GS. Emptying the bladder by stimulating sacral ventral roots. J Physiol 1993;237:15–156.

144. Brindley GS. The first 500 patients with sacral anterior root stimulator implants: general description. Paraplegia 1994;32:795–805.

145. Brindley GS. The first 500 sacral anterior roots stimulators: implant failures and their repair. Paraplegia 1995;33:5–9.

146. Van Kerrebroeck EV, van der Aa HE, Bosch JL, et al. Sacral rhizotomies and electrical bladder stimulation in spinal cord injury. Part 1: Clinical and urodynamic analysis. Dutch Study Group on sacral anterior root stimulation. Eur Urol 1997;31:263–271.

147. Egon G, Barat M, Colombel P, et al. Implantation of anterior sacral root stimulators combined with posterior sacral rhizotomies in spinal cord injury patients. J Urol 1998;16:342–349.

148. Brindley GS, Polkey CE, Rushton DN. Sacral anterior root stimulator for bladder control in paraplegia. Paraplegia 1992;l20:365–381.

149. Brindley GS, Polkey CE, Rushton DN, Cardozo L. Sacral anterior root stimulators for bladder control in paraplegia: the first 50 cases. J Neurol Neurosurg Psychiatry 1986;49:1104–1114.

32

Biofeedback

STEVEN L. WOLF

Since its first conceptualization in 1969, biofeedback has been viewed as both a clinical revelation and a misplaced enigma. This disparity is best attributed to the variability in biofeedback's reputed effectiveness when applied to different clinical problems. In the field of rehabilitation, however, the literature is replete with studies demonstrating biofeedback's clinical efficacy for a host of neuromuscular and musculoskeletal disorders. In fact, the accumulated evidence of the benefits of feedback in reducing spasms and hyperactive muscle responses has been convincing, even to most third-party payers of medical costs. This chapter reviews historic and contemporary perspectives on biofeedback, discusses clinical findings, explores the notion of kinesiologic electromyography (EMG), and discusses mechanisms to account for changes in movement control subsequent to EMG biofeedback interventions.

EXAMINING THE CONCEPT OF FEEDBACK

Biofeedback describes the use of instrumentation to make a covert physiological process obvious to the user by providing timely and specific visual, auditory, or both representations of that process.[1] For rehabilitation, EMG, position, or force feedback is most commonly provided. The visual and auditory cues are supplied virtually instantaneously, and the information is specified by the proximity of the signal transducers (e.g., surface electrodes, potentiometers, strain gauges, force plates) to the signal source.

The behavior of the user (patient) appears stereotypic. At first, most patients are intently attuned to both visual and auditory feedback cues. With time and practice, patients direct their visual attention toward the limb segment while still being mindful of auditory signals. Eventually, patients may abandon both auditory and visual cues, but still demand that they be available as a reference.[2] An integral aspect of this typical scenario is the need for the clinician to withdraw all feedback cues from the patient periodically. Then, the patient is asked to produce an output that approaches a known threshold or target level. Once this attempt has been made, the patient may then view the stored response to determine how accurately the target level was reproduced. Inevitably, success at these tasks must be linked to a relearned appreciation of internal cues, perhaps even representative of a recalibrated proprioceptive system.[3]

The foregoing perspective contrasts with the interest in motor control theory appropriately manifested by clinicians specializing in the rehabilitation of patients with neurologic lesions. Winstein[4] has provided an excellent account of feedback in the context of knowledge of results (KR). Most clinical applications of feedback are extrinsic, and, in most settings, the feedback would be verbal and not instrumented. In fact, most feedback is more attuned to performance than to discrete selection of individual muscles or muscle groups.[5] Motor learning theorists have divided the learning of a movement into acquisition and transfer phases.[6] Data have shown that for normal persons, providing periodic KR rather than continuous KR enhances learning and retention.[7,8] Explanations for these results include (1) a guidance hypothesis, which suggests that too much reliance on guidance properties might retard response-produced feedback, thereby preventing improvement in error detection capability, and (2) a consistency hypothesis predicated on the belief that too much feedback leads to maladaptive cor-

TABLE 32-1
Comparing the Notion of Feedback

Component	Motor Learning Therapy	Clinical Biofeedback
Type	Extrinsic	Extrinsic
Source	Usually verbal	Instrumental
Timing	Delayed when verbal	Instantaneous
Specificity	Nonspecific	Specific, defined by transducer and its placement
Best frequency of feedback	Occasional (50%)	100%
Application	Nonpatient	Patient
Task	Movement pattern	Joint or muscle specific

rections and heightened response variability.[9] The validity of these explanations to account for performance changes in patients has been questioned.[4,10]

Table 32-1 contrasts the notion of feedback in motor learning and biofeedback contexts. Contrary to the perception of many clinicians and motor theorists, although verbal feedback is continuous (and helpful), it is delayed. In the context of motor relearning, any delay impedes the relearning process. Additionally, verbal feedback inevitably lacks informational specificity. For example, how much *harder* is contextually conveyed in the command, "That's good; now try harder"? As noted earlier, clinical experience dictates that patients with disrupted control of the peripheral nervous system voraciously *consume* specificity of feedback in the early relearning phase. Removal of feedback must be continuously graded, in terms of the unique sensory or motor deficits of each patient. Undoubtedly, controlled research paradigms, such as those expressed by Mulder,[11] will have to be tested to validate this point. In the interim, clinicians must remember an inherent distinction when interpreting data from most motor control studies and from clinical muscle biofeedback investigations. For many motor control studies, subjects possess an intact sensorium and reasonably controlled movement patterns. Among studies on patients, sensory, motor, or both systems may be disrupted, and specific muscle activity, rather than patterns of movement, may be measured. Within the past few years, however, biofeedback practitioners have been encouraged to quantify more functional and limb-specific activities rather than emphasizing individual muscle responses.[12]

RETHINKING THE CONCEPTUAL FRAMEWORK FOR BIOFEEDBACK

Since the 1970s, biofeedback has been viewed as a procedure or as a modality, depending on the orientation of the clinician. This oversimplification has been challenged in a series of position statements.[13] Perhaps the conceptualization of biofeedback has become outdated. After all, the feedback derived from a machine-based signal provides valuable information for the clinician as well as the patient. By observing the timing and magnitude of patient muscle responses to instruction, the clinician can change his or her subsequent instruction, manual positioning, patient positioning, or any host of options in order to affect a more meaningful response. Thus, if a goal of muscle biofeedback is to change procedural memory or processes, just whose procedures are changed: those of the patient, the clinician, or both? One could argue that this family of questions is worthy of exploration and that the effect of what has been called *physiological biofeedback* may be far more profound than previously realized; we may be changing behaviors and actions of clinicians as well as behaviors and motoric responses of patients. Little or no study has been undertaken about the extent to which the process of self-exploration of physiological control through feedback has motivated or altered the subsequent behaviors and attitudes of all who become engaged with this modality.

OTHER FEEDBACK OPTIONS

KR need not be limited to information derived from muscle. Figure 32-1 shows an electrogoniometer applied to an interphalangeal joint. The leads are attached to a potentiometer through which a small current is passed. The parallelogram arrangement moves as the finger is extended, causing the potentiometer to rotate about its axis. As this rotation occurs, a small amount of current is passed through a strip of linearly placed resistors, each having progressively greater resistance. In keeping with Ohm's law,

$$I = V/R$$

the current (I) remains constant but the resistance value (R) changes, and the voltage (V) varies linearly with the resistance. This voltage change is reflected on the lead-emitting diode display in Figure 32-1, which has been arranged to correspond to joint angles. By incorporating a level detector or threshold, the clinician can add

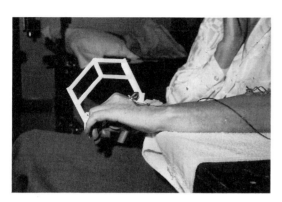

FIGURE 32-1 Electrogoniometric positional feedback device placed about metacarpal-phalangeal joint of left index finger. Note potentiometer at base of modified goniometer.

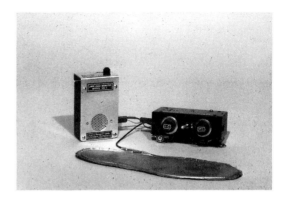

FIGURE 32-2 Shoe insert housing force plate to convey voltage signal proportional to force exerted through plate placed in a properly fitted shoe.

an audio tone that changes in quality when the threshold or desired joint angle is achieved.

Another form of feedback, force or pressure feedback, is represented in Figure 32-2. Force transducers, housed within the shoe inserts, produce a linear voltage change proportional to the force exerted through the foot. Once again, a tone may be emitted through an audio amplifier (see Figure 32-2, background). This application is relevant to training an amputee to transfer weight onto the prosthesis,[14] training older patients for postural stability,[15] or assessing gait characteristics.[16] The construction and application of these devices is presented in detail elsewhere.[17,18]

TOWARD NEW APPLICATIONS OF FORCE FEEDBACK

Considerable interest has been directed toward center of pressure feedback over the past 10 years. New computerized machine systems allow for transducers embedded in the floor of moveable platforms to resolve vertical forces directed against the feet into a cursor whose location appears on a monitor positioned at the patient's eye level. The output is sensitive to even the most subtle shifts in center of pressure under conditions of quiet standing or linear or angular perturbations in the platform. Often, the platform can be programmed to move at different velocities or displacements. Several companies manufacture variations on this concept, but essentially all devices are intended to train patients with varying diagnoses to control postural sway. A comprehensive, updated review of literature is on the web site created by NeuroCom, International, Inc. (www.onbalance.com).

Clinicians should, however, be cautious about claims made regarding the outcome resulting from treatment on computerized balance machines. Fundamentally, the most important question that must be posed is whether patients have improved control over balance during functional tasks as a result of center of pressure feedback training. Such tasks can be quantified by walking speed, specificity in the direction of the path, duration of single limb support during walking, and number of stumbles or stops per distance unit, and so forth. For example, our group has used center of pressure feedback training as an intervention to delay the onset of falls among older adults.[19] Numbers of falls or onset of fall events was not reduced substantially, perhaps because the application of this feedback form was limited to bipedal stance. Because many falls occur during single limb support, such as trips and slips,[20] it makes sense that some training with center of pressure feedback might be undertaken during single limb support. This approach can be applied during quiet standing or *paced* ambulation when patients are asked to walk more slowly and spend more time on a single limb.

Another interesting variation of center of pressure feedback has been introduced.[21] In this case patients were given feedback about their loading responses to dynamic toes-up (angular) perturbations in the form of a bar graph, the height of which was proportional to the loading force from the previous perturbation. Responses could be *shaped* upward or downward by giving an auditory cue, or reward, each time the magnitude of change exceeded (up-training) or went below (down-training) specified levels from baseline. The question to be answered is the extent to which such deliberate training to induce load changes during angular perturbations influences clinical outcome events, such as falls. Remarkably, older adults constrain their loading responses to rapid angular perturbations on a computerized balance machine no matter whether the goal is to up-train or to down-train the response.

APPLICATIONS OF MUSCLE BIOFEEDBACK

More than 300 clinical studies addressing feedback applications in physical rehabilitation have been published, excluding publications that address feedback or behavior modification approaches to patients whose primary symptom is pain. The number of articles on that one problem exceeds the total number of biofeedback articles for all other problems involving limitation of movement. Here the focus is on information about common musculoskeletal and neuromuscular disorders. For more historic perspectives, the reader is referred to several classic texts.[22-27] The interested reader may also want to consult a text on the use of surface EMG to treat clinical problems for which pain is a major symptom.[28]

Musculoskeletal Disorders

Most patients with musculoskeletal disorders need to restore strength and mobility without being excessively concerned about proprioceptive and cutaneous loss or cognitive dysfunction precipitated by CNS trauma or demyelinating disease.[29] Sensorimotor impairment may not necessarily deter biofeedback interventions for patients with peripheral nerve injury provided there is percutaneous evidence of volitional motor unit return. During the time volitional control is returning, however, impaired kinesthesia cannot be discarded as a contributor to reduced motor drive, even with the provision of muscle feedback. In retrospect, the paucity of clinical research using feedback interfaces for musculoskeletal injury could probably be attributed to a collective belief in the obvious benefits of immediate quantification of muscle signals during strengthening programs.

Several hundred papers describe the interface between EMG biofeedback and functional recovery among patients with low back pain. The reality is, however, that the data are rather equivocal, and one is not sure the degree to which improved function is precipitated by targeted feedback training, biobehavioral interventions, the healing process, environmental alternations, or a combination of these factors. We have concluded that simply balancing paraspinal back muscle responses is not a fundamental determinant for recovery from back pain, particularly in light of the multiple etiologies of this problem.[28] More important, the Agency for Health Care Policy and Research has concluded that treatment approaches and assessment of effectiveness may be age dependent, and that no one conservative treatment is superior to another.[30] It seems reasonable to believe that combined physical and behavioral interventions that may include EMG biofeedback cannot be harmful, but the degree to which improvement can be attributed to a behavioral approach is unclear.[31]

In the treatment of extremity-based impairments, EMG feedback may serve some fundamentally important roles. One of the first documented studies to support this contention was reported by Lucca and Recchiuti,[32] who showed that women performing isometric contractions with visual EMG feedback gained more peak torque than an exercise group or a nontreatment group. In a similar study, Croce[33] demonstrated that integrated EMG levels from the quadriceps muscle showed significantly greater increases over a 5-week training period under conditions of isokinetic exercise (at a speed of 30 degrees/second) for subjects who received feedback compared with groups that received no feedback.

Another variation on a similar theme addressed whether normal subjects could differentially activate vastus medialis and lateralis, both muscles of the quadriceps mass innervated by the femoral nerve.[34] Under precise and specified training controls, subjects were able to down-train the vastus lateralis and up-train the vastus medialis. Because it has now been proven that patients with patellofemoral pain have abnormal vastus medialis to vastus lateralis EMG ratios during specific functional tasks[35] it is time to ascertain (1) whether targeted biofeedback training to these two muscles can properly alter this ratio and (2) whether the change affects patellofemoral pain and knee function.

Following the suggestion by Fernie and coworkers[36] that above-knee amputees might gain better prosthetic knee control if given force feedback, controlled clinical trials have been completed by other investigators. The results have demonstrated that feedback can augment control in both upper[37] and lower[38] extremity amputees. In the former study, subjects who used a prosthetic limb performed most accurately when audio-augmented feedback was concurrent with the elbow joint movement response as compared with no feedback or postural feedback. Lower extremity amputees showed equal improvement in sway reduction whether with mirror feedback or feedback through pressure exerted on a force plate in the prosthetic foot; however, force feedback provided better quantification and control of weight bearing.

The prospects for using force feedback are limited only by the imagination of the user. As an example of exceptional inventiveness, Clarkson and coworkers[39] demonstrated that force feedback from a transducer placed on the instep reduced excessive foot pronation more than control or sham conditions. Force feedback can also be derived from assistive devices such as a feedback cane. Strain gauges can be placed along the shaft of the cane, producing a tone when the torque generated through the shaft exceeds a preset threshold.[40] In essence, the patient is obliged to bear more weight through the limbs and less through the cane as the audio threshold is lowered and the patient is instructed to prevent the sound from occurring.

Draper[41] applied muscle feedback to the quadriceps of 11 patients with anterior cruciate ligament (ACL) repair within 1 week of reconstructive surgery. Compared with a matched group of 11 ACL patients who served as feedback controls, the group that received feedback showed a significant improvement in peak torque at 45-, 60-, and 90-degree joint angles over the 12-week rehabilitation period. The degree to which surface EMG feedback should be used to instruct ACL patients to engage in coactivation of muscles about the knee joint after ACL repair has been discussed by several investigators.[42,43] Sinkjaer and Arendt-Nielsen[44] demonstrated that training for recruitment of the medial gastrocnemius muscle during heel strike among ACL patients with poor clinical outcomes produced improved walking capability by fostering knee joint stiffening. This form of feedback training, although potentially beneficial, could even be augmented further through the inclusion of muscle feedback soon after arthroscopic surgery.[45]

Feedback may be beneficial from other perspectives as well. Lee and colleagues[46] showed that feedback of force through the hands of students learning spinal mobilization techniques yielded more *ideal* forces at training and at 1-week follow-up than those seen in a control group of students given no feedback on the manual forces used in their applications. These data support the use of feedback as a teaching tool and as a technique to train musculoskeletal injury patients. Awkward hand positioning during manual labor can be assessed through feedback in an effort to improve motions and reduce carpal tunnel syndrome,[47] and to reduce exaggerated thumb usage during piano performance.[48] EMG feedback also has a distinct history in efforts to enhance athletic performance[49] or reduce ataxia.[50] Each of these examples shares in common the

observation that repetitive use can lead to exaggerated muscle responses that can be retrained with muscle biofeedback.

On the other hand, more compelling evidence indicates that a key component to pain relief among patients with cumulative trauma disorders may be in relaxation training rather than the contribution from EMG biofeedback.[51] Undoubtedly, the growing use of computer keyboards has led to a greater amount of repetitive activation of muscle groups with resulting tissue compression, cumulative trauma, and postural aberrations. This reality brings into focus the importance of exploring the benefits from on-line muscle monitoring in the workplace to reduce the frequency of these injuries. The growth of sedentary jobs, including keyboard-based activities with high-technology but intense concentration, inevitably leads to prolonged static posturing, which, in the absence of ergonomically sound engineering, may produce musculoskeletal difficulties, such as the increasing incidence of reflex sympathetic dystrophy. This diagnosis may be precipitated by prolonged neck flexion and working with arms overhead or with scapulae elevated. This combination could cause an overuse of the anterior scalene muscles and compression of the underlying subclavian artery, leading to vascular muscle spasm and upper extremity pain. If so, then EMG feedback training to reduce activity in the scalene muscles could be beneficial.[52] This approach awaits systematic evaluation.

In 1978, Keefe and Surwit[53] issued an admonition that was judiciously recalled 10 years later by John Basmajian.[54] In essence, a note of optimism was sounded over the myriad applications of biofeedback for the rehabilitation community. The major proviso was that the outcome studies being undertaken were rigorously designed and used appropriate control groups. In the area of many musculoskeletal disorders, this concern has been addressed since Basmajian's 1988 comment. The underlying optimism is well founded when the interface between biofeedback and diseases of neuromuscular origin is considered.

Neuromuscular Disorders

Perhaps no single biofeedback application in rehabilitation has been researched as much as the relationship between EMG feedback and motor improvement among stroke patients.[55] Numerous examples of treatment strategies and controlled clinical trials of biofeedback treatments for other neuromuscular disorders such as spinal cord injury, multiple sclerosis, and cerebral palsy are available; this chapter concentrates on the feedback-stroke patient interface.

The pioneering work of Basmajian et al.[56] and Brudny et al.[57] drew particular attention to the prospects for chronic stroke patients learning to walk with few or no assistive devices. Presumably, by training such patients to recruit anterior leg compartment muscles while inhibiting the triceps surae with the use of muscle biofeedback, control of ankle movement during the swing phase of gait would be improved more than it would be by a conventional exercise program. Although encouraging, the early work did not account for ankle inversion and eversion control, nor were other factors that contribute to successful ambulation, including cutaneous or proprioceptive integrity or degree of cognitive impairment, evaluated. Through systematic study of lower extremity performance among chronic stroke patients receiving muscle feedback training, we learned that proprioception and cognitive integrity were essential to maximizing ambulatory independence.[58,59] Subsequent controlled clinical trials[60-62] revealed that muscle feedback training was superior to no treatment or relaxation training alternatives. More recent data corroborate the value of feedback to enhance ambulatory control in healthy subjects[63] and in stroke patients given positional feedback.[64]

The value of muscle feedback to improve upper extremity movement control has also been studied vigorously. Initial results, however, were more equivocal.[55,65,66] This fact was probably attributable to variations in method and discrepancies in what constituted upper extremity improvement, especially in light of limitations in manual skills. Ultimately, in the absence of reacquisition of manual dexterity, the ability to use the upper extremity in an assistive capacity (e.g., carrying an object under the arm) is of limited functional value and such behaviors rarely persist in the presence of learned nonuse. Ince and coworkers[67] have thoughtfully reviewed these problems, but as noted by Basmajian[68] in his more recent review, the provision of controlled studies has changed this perspective dramatically.

One paper by Basmajian's group[69] demonstrated that biofeedback applications to stroke patients classified as "early mild" resulted in major upper extremity improvement, whereas those to patients labeled as "late severe" did not. Among many measures of function, patients who received EMG biofeedback with physical therapy showed greater quantitative improvement than those who received only a standard exercise program. Wolf and Binder-Macleod[61] examined quantified EMG values, range of motion, and quantified timed functional tasks among groups of chronic stroke patients who received either exclusive EMG feedback training or no treatment at all. Blind evaluations revealed that most patients' capacity to assist the contralateral limb

improved. Among the subgroup that regained independent use of the hemiparetic hand, all subjects had the pretreatment ability to initiate some voluntary extensor activity in the wrist or fingers. This factor was the single best predictor of total upper limb return with biofeedback training. Control patients showed no improvement; but once placed into a treatment group, the two subjects who had isolated finger or wrist extension activity subsequently gained independent manual use.

We took these criteria to suggest that chronic stroke or head-injured patients could improve their upper extremity and hand use. In a subsequent study,[70] we demonstrated that these new patients were able to improve to the same extent as the former group, whether they received conventional targeted feedback training or a new technique called *motor copy*. In the latter treatment, homologous muscles of the upper extremities were used to produce matched outputs from the less impaired and involved limb, using only differences in amplifier gain to shape responses. Since that time, similar approaches[71] have been applied. Other investigators have undertaken specific training of shoulder muscles among patients with hemiplegia. Mathieu and coworkers[72,73] have shown that EMG biofeedback applied to patients with subacute stroke can increase torque and EMG outputs about the shoulder, and training of the deltoid muscle produces strategies that may engage even more shoulder muscles.

But just how is the role of EMG biofeedback for the treatment of patients with stroke perceived today and have feedback applications to stroke patients expanded in the past decade? At least two meta-analyses have been undertaken to assess the value of biofeedback therapy in poststroke rehabilitation. In one review, Glanz and colleagues[74] concluded, after examining eight studies, that the main effect size for lower extremity treatment was 1.50 (95% confidence interval: –0.59, 3.59) and 2.30 (95% confidence interval: –1.06, 5.66) for upper extremity treatment. Although it was believed that the available evidence did not support the utility of EMG biofeedback to restore joint motion in patients with hemiplegia, the main effect sizes were large and had wide confidence intervals, posing the possibility of a type II error masking the value of the clinical benefits. On the other hand, using slightly different evaluation criteria, the meta-analysis on lower extremity feedback studies among patients with stroke, performed by Moreland et al.,[75] yielded far more substantial effect sizes, especially for muscle strength and gait quality. Perhaps the most comprehensive analysis came from a task force configured by the Agency for Health Care Policy and Research, which in 1995 concluded that the results of biofeedback applications to improve function in chronic stroke patients are inconclusive.[76] For lower extremity EMG biofeedback training among patients with acute stroke, this notion was substantiated by Bradley and coworkers[77] who found no difference in functional outcomes between the feedback group and those patients receiving conventional rehabilitation. Further controlled studies are needed to resolve this issue.

Regarding the emerging use of pressure feedback, in the 1990s this form of KR was studied extensively. Preliminary data speak to the prospects for achieving at least transient benefits in loading of the predominantly impaired limb with center of pressure feedback. The feedback source can be visual cueing of pressure as a cursor on a screen,[78-81] a bathroom scale,[82] vibratory sensation caused by lower extremity forces,[83] auditory feedback related to the magnitude of lower extremity force production,[84] or even use of angular feedback to improve sitting balance.[85] The degree to which this form of training can yield substantial improvement in balance among patients with stroke has been questioned recently.[86]

TREATMENT STRATEGY

The task of treating musculoskeletal injuries or reinnervating peripheral nerve injuries is relatively straightforward: to increase EMG output and shape responses by reducing the amplifier gain and elevating the threshold at any one sensitivity setting. Success has been reported with facial nerve palsy patients.[87] In treating patients with CNS involvement, the training strategy is much more complex. Table 32-2 summarizes the general approach, sometimes referred to as *conventional* or *targeted* biofeedback training.

The progression stems from assumptions derived from the teachings of Bobath,[88] specifically, that muscles should be treated in a proximal-to-distal manner and that hyperactive muscles should be relaxed (inhibited) before weak antagonists are recruited. As a result, the typical muscles or muscle groups shown in Table 32-2 are trained by presuming that the upper extremity possesses predominantly flexor synergy and the lower extremity extensor synergy.

The notion that hyperactive muscles should be inhibited and weak muscles recruited has met with some opposition. Many clinicians[89-91] now suggest that treatment orientation should be geared toward function. This thought suggests some unique possibilities that can be systematically explored through clinical research efforts. For example, might better results with EMG feedback be obtained through direct training of the

weaker muscle group without first down-training spastic muscles? Is there a need to select muscles by synergy groupings or joint specifications as opposed to simple choice of muscle monitoring based on requirements to accomplish a specific task?

CONCEPT OF KINESIOLOGIC ELECTROMYOGRAPHY

Several years ago we suggested that, in addition to training patients with EMG biofeedback, the informa-

TABLE 32-2

Typical Conventional Electromyographic Training Strategies in the Treatment of Stroke Patients

Location	Movement	Inhibit	Recruit
Upper extremity			
Scapula	Adduction	—	Serratus anterior
Shoulder	Elevation	Upper trapezius	—
	Internal rotation	Pectoralis major	—
	External rotation	—	Infraspinatus
	Flexion	—	Anterior deltoid
	Abduction	—	Middle deltoid
Elbow	Flexion	Biceps	—
	Extension	—	Triceps
Wrist	Flexion	Flexor mass	—
	Extension	—	Extensor mass
Fingers	Flexion	Finger flexors	—
	Extension	—	Finger extensors
Thumb	Abduction	Thenar eminence	—
	Extension	—	Wrist dorsum
Lower extremity			
Hip	Abductor	—	Gluteus medius
	Extension	—	Gluteus maximus
	Flexion	—	Sartorius
	Adduction	Adductor mass	—
Knee	Extension	Quadriceps	—
	Flexion	—	Biceps femoris
Ankle	Plantar flexion	Triceps surae	—
	Dorsiflexion	—	Anterior leg compartment
	Eversion	—	Extensor digitorum brevis

tion could be processed and quantified on line, so that direct evidence of treatment effectiveness could be obtained or an immediate change could be made in treatment plan or patient handling. The issue no longer was one of proving or disproving the usefulness of a treatment approach, but rather of altering a given aspect of that intervention via feedback to the clinician and the patient simultaneously. No longer would the clinician be dependent only on vision and palpation. We coined the acronym CAMA, for concurrent assessment of muscle activity.[92]

An example of concurrent assessment of muscle activity can be seen in Figures 32-3 and 32-4. A stroke patient is being asked to recruit the weaker left hamstring muscles during a sit-to-stand task. Not only does the patient observe the response, but the clinician, by keying on the feedback signal, can offer guidance or suggestions to the patient to help activate this muscle group. A foot switch

engaged by the clinician defines the interval of the training and the response. On activating the switch a second time, the duration of the task and the quantification of the response are recorded for the patient's record (see Figure 32-4). Since then, other investigators have used this approach or variations thereof.[93]

Integrating quantified EMG values into the treatment assessment or recording procedure is beneficial, as these data offer one more piece of evidence to support the value of a clinical intervention. This validation factor is becoming progressively more important as third-party payers seek proof of rehabilitation treatment benefits before a reimbursement is rendered. In addition, although EMG values themselves may not be conclusive in confirming the efficacy of treatment, combined with other measures (e.g., range of motion, torque, time to complete tasks), they help to complete the picture. In this regard, EMG biofeedback instrumentation is of particular interest because such equipment combines treatment capability with evaluation through quantification.

HOW MIGHT MUSCLE FEEDBACK WORK?

One major benefit of EMG feedback, particularly if it is adopted after more traditional therapy has been offered, is that it promotes expanded discussions about the possibilities for patients to improve, especially those with long-standing limitations. We pondered this question previously.[1,55] Based on the stereotypic nature of patient responses, clearly the speed with which information is provided to the patient and the specificity of that information, defined by the locus of electrode placements, constitute the unique attributes of the modality.

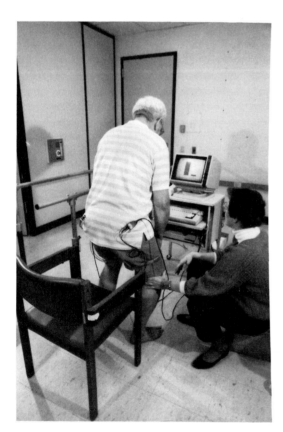

FIGURE 32-3 Monitoring bilateral hamstring activity as stroke patient practices sit-to-stand activity with effort designed to provide electromyographic feedback in weaker muscle group while quantifying muscle activity for the duration of the task.

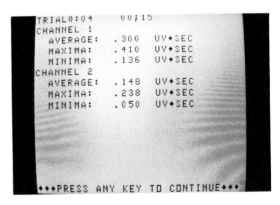

FIGURE 32-4 Representative output of electromyographic effort from each hamstring muscle group in tasks shown in Figure 32-3.

The neurophysiological factors that allow processing of a visual or auditory representation of a biofeedback signal are complex and poorly understood.[94] Undoubtedly, for patients whose CNS is intact, the timing of feedback serves to create a *feedforward* mechanism designed to augment motor drive. This situation is most prevalent in training for strength or mobility after disturbances that cause muscle weakness and limit joint range of motion.

With diseases that have affected the CNS so that the continuity of sensory inflow and motor output has been disrupted, our understanding of the relationship of instrumented feedback signals to enhanced movement performance is exceptionally vague. If one observes patient interaction with feedback devices, however, there appears to be an effort at recalibrating sensorimotor timing. At first, patients tend to focus compulsively on both forms of feedback; only later do they observe the limb segment under training while attending to auditory cues. Over time, it appears that patients no longer attend to either cue but insist they be available. This consistently reproducible behavior suggests that with practice and training patients grow to rely more on proprioceptive and interoceptive cues and less on the original exteroceptive cues, which, in reality, were only representations of self-generated muscle activity. In short, the patient may have regained an appreciation or sensitivity to length changes caused by eccentric or concentric muscle efforts.

Many patients with neurologic diseases are aware of the tasks they should accomplish but fail to execute them. This implies that the specific sensory engram is intact and the disorder must lie in the motor system or between the sensory cortex and the motor command system (i.e., in the sensory association cortex). Ostensibly then, the feedback loops in the brain would be incapable of successfully modifying the temporal-spatial requirements for appropriate motor behavior. Desired use of the feedback signals probably rests on the capacity for using these inputs to activate subsidiary functional sets of motor cells through either direct or reflex loops. Such mechanisms should not be construed to demonstrate true neuroplasticity; rather, central synapses previously unused in the execution of specific motor commands are now accessed in a way that conventional rehabilitation could not achieve. This phenomenon has been referred to as *unmasking* by Bach-y-Rita and colleagues.[95]

As biofeedback retraining progresses, available and responsive motor cells are called into play. With continued training, patients are able to improve performance. It is interesting to speculate that the sensory engram has established an increasingly reliable linkage with functional transmitting cells, thus making the patient more reliant on proprioceptive feedback and less dependent on an artificial form of information, biofeedback.

Our understanding of how the feedback signal is processed into meaningful movement is still fragmentary. We do not yet fully comprehend the circumstances that permit this instrumented effort at relearning to be completed successfully by some patients and not by others, even when all ostensibly have the same diagnosis and lesion site. Furthermore, we have yet to determine whether feedback training that is totally goal oriented yields better function than single movement-directed training or individual muscle training, especially among patients with neurologic deficits. Should clinicians favor one approach over another? Is there merit in viewing muscles as having subcompartments, each of which possesses unique retraining requirements? Answers to these and other questions await investigation, which, unquestionably, will be easier to conduct with future generations of more sophisticated instruments.

NOVEL APPROACHES: EXPANDING DISCIPLINES

The use of biofeedback has not been restricted to rehabilitationists, even within the context of rehabilitation applications. Inevitably other professionals, most often psychologists, perceive biofeedback not only as a modality but as a behavioral procedure. Consequently, efforts to use physiological monitoring for relaxation and stress reduction have become a segment of the treatment strategy used by many behaviorists. At times these approaches progress to neuromuscular retraining, particularly for patients with pain. These efforts can be perceived as infringements on the treatment domains of physical or occupational therapists or as attempts to expand the scope of practice among such individuals. In either event, the interface between psychologists and therapists using biofeedback exists and will continue to do so.

Despite this apparent expansion in the use of biofeedback, some exceptionally creative approaches can spawn new ideas and applications among rehabilitation professionals seeking new ways to explore treatment options. For example, Walker and colleagues have created a novel way of assisting diabetic patients with peripheral neuropathy to improve gait by substituting auditory cues to shape limb loading, particularly at faster velocity walking speeds.[96] Hirvonen and colleagues[97] are among a multitude of investigators seeking to expand the limits of center of pressure feedback to enhance postural control. They demonstrated that patients with vestibular disease can be trained to improve the displacement and accuracy of their center of pressure efforts. The question still open to evaluation among this type of studies remains the extent to which such training produces functional improvements, most importantly reductions in falls and in fear of falling.

An exciting area worthy of exploration is the use of biofeedback after muscle transfer. One such procedure involves retraining the gracilis muscle after transposition of a portion of it as a new external anal sphincter. Woolner[98] reported success in retraining the remaining portion of the intact muscle so that the patient thinks about adduction of the thigh when contracting the remaining half of the muscle as a sphincter. These approaches hold great promise for all muscle transfers, particularly in the absence of CNS pathology. Other successful applications for EMG biofeedback have been reported for certain dystonias, such as writer's cramp[99] and to control voice pitch[100] in the presence of aprosody.

One of the more disappointing applications for EMG biofeedback has been in the area of spinal cord injury.

Although biofeedback can be helpful with patients who have some form of cord compression thus rendering them quadriparetic or paraparetic, virtually no evidence suggests that this approach is successful with more impaired spinal cord–injured patients. Although less impaired patients may be able to augment muscle output with EMG feedback alone[101] or in the presence of functional electrical stimulation,[102] few data indicate that the application of the modality among profoundly impaired spinal-injured patients has functional ramifications.

On the other hand, one of the more exciting avenues under exploration is the use of EEG feedback to help patients with extreme movement limitations to control their environment.[103-105] The issue here is not to train rehabilitation specialists to become electroencephalographers or to understand brain activity beyond their basic training, but to explore the possibility of seeking trace muscle activity or joint movement and providing feedback of those physiological events to drive enhanced cognitive ability or as a substitute physiological system to control the environment. The technology to explore these possibilities exists and will surely be exploited early in the twenty-first century.

REFERENCES

1. Wolf SL. Electromyographic Biofeedback: An Overview. In RM Nelson, DP Currier (eds), Clinical Electromyography (2nd ed). Norwalk, CT: Appleton & Lange, 1991;361–384.
2. Wolf SL, Binder-Macleod SA. Electromyographic Biofeedback in the Physical Therapy Clinic. In JV Basmajian (ed), Biofeedback: Principles and Practice for Clinicians (3rd ed). Baltimore: Williams & Wilkins, 1989;91–103.
3. Wolf SL. EMG biofeedback applications in rehabilitation. Physiother Can 1979;31:65–72.
4. Winstein CJ. Motor Learning Consideration in Stroke Rehabilitation. In PW Duncan, MB Badke (eds), Stroke Rehabilitation: The Recovery of Motor Function. Chicago: Year Book Medical Publishers, 1987;109–134.
5. Gentile AM. A working model of skill acquisition with application to teaching. Quest 1972;17:3–23.
6. Adams JA, Reynolds B. Effect of shift on distribution of practice conditions following an interpolated rest. J Exp Psychol 1954;47:32–36.
7. Schmidt RA, Young DE, Swinnen S. Summary knowledge of results for skill

acquisition: support for the guidance hypothesis. J Exp Psychol Learn Mem Cogn 1989;15:352–359.
8. Winstein CJ, Schmidt RA. Reduced frequency of knowledge of results enhances motor skill learning. J Exp Psychol Learn Mem Cogn 1990; 10:677–691.
9. Lee TD, White MA, Carnahan H. On the role of knowledge of results in motor learning: exploring the guidance hypothesis. J Motor Behav 1990; 22:191–208.
10. Winstein CJ. Knowledge of results and motor learning—implications for physical therapy. Phys Ther 1991;71:140–149.
11. Mulder T. The Learning of Motor Control Following Brain Damage: Experimental and Clinical Studies. Berwyn, PA: Swets North America, 1985.
12. LeCraw DE, Wolf SL. Contemporary Perspectives on Electromyographic Feedback for Rehabilitation Clinicians. In MR Gersh (ed), Electrotherapy. Philadelphia: FA Davis, 1991.
13. Wolf SL. Commentary on biofeedback. Appl Psychophysiol Biofeedback 1999;24:39–40,43–54.
14. Wannstedt GT, Herman RM. Use of augmented sensory feedback to

achieve symmetrical standing. Phys Ther 1978;58:553–559.
15. Woollacott MH. Gait and Postural Control in the Aging Adult. In W Bles, T Brandt (eds), Disorders of Posture and Gait. New York: Elsevier, 1986;325–336.
16. Wolf SL, Binder-Macleod SA. Use of the Krusen limb load monitor to quantify temporal and loading measurements of gait. Phys Ther 1982;62:976–984.
17. Wolf SL. Biofeedback Applications in Rehabilitation Medicine: Implications for Performance in Sports. In JH Sandweiss, SL Wolf (eds), Biofeedback and Sports Science. New York: Plenum, 1985;159–180.
18. Brown DM, Nahai E. Biofeedback Strategies of the Occupational Therapist in Total Hand Rehabilitation. In JV Basmajian (ed), Biofeedback: Principles and Practice for Clinicians (3rd ed). Baltimore: Williams & Wilkins, 1989;123–135.
19. Wolf SL, Barnhart HX, Kutner NG, et al. Exercise training and subsequent falls among older persons: comparison of Tai Chi and computerized balance training. J Amer Geriatr Soc 1996; 44:489–449.

20. Pavol MJ, Owings TM, Foley KT, Grabiner MD. The sex and age of older adults influence the outcome of induced trips. J Gerontol 1999;54A: M103–M108.

21. Wolf SL, Catlin PA, Bonner B, et al. Up-training loading responses in older adults. Appl Psychophysiol Biofeedback 1999;24:179–195.

22. Brown BB. Stress and the Art of Biofeedback. New York: Harper & Row, 1977.

23. Yates AL. Biofeedback and the Modification of Behavior. New York: Plenum, 1980.

24. Olton DS, Noonberg AR. Biofeedback: Clinical Applications in Behavioral Medicine. Englewood Cliffs, NJ: Prentice Hall, 1980.

25. Ince LP. Behavioral Psychology in Rehabilitation Medicine: Clinical Applications. Baltimore: Williams & Wilkins, 1980.

26. Sandweiss JH, Wolf SL. Biofeedback and Sports Science. New York: Plenum, 1985.

27. Marcer D. Biofeedback and Related Therapies in Clinical Practice. Gaithersburg, MD: Aspen, 1986.

28. Kasman GS, Cram JR, Wolf SL. Clinical Applications in Surface Electromyography: Chronic Musculoskeletal Pain. Gaithersburg, MD: Aspen, 1998.

29. Wolf SL, Fischer-Williams M. The Use of Biofeedback in Disorders of Motor Function. In JP Hatch, JG Fisher, JD Rugh (eds), Biofeedback: Studies in Clinical Efficacy. New York: Plenum, 1987;153–177.

30. Bigos SJ (chair). Clinical Practice Guideline Number 14: Acute Low Back Problems in Adults. Rockville, MD: US Department of Health and Human Services, Public Health Service, Agency for Health Care Policy and Research, 1994.

31. Vlaeyen JW, Haazen IW, Schuerman JA, et al. Behavioural rehabilitation of chronic low back pain: comparison of an operant treatment, an operant-cognitive treatment and an operant-respondent treatment. Br J Clin Psychol 1995;34(Pt 1):95–118.

32. Lucca JA, Recchiuti SJ. Effect of electromyographic biofeedback on an isometric strengthening program. Phys Ther 1983;63:200–203.

33. Croce RV. The effects of EMG biofeedback on strength acquisition. Biofeedback Self Regul 1986;11:299–310.

34. LeVeau BF, Rogers C. Selective training of the vastus medialis muscle using EMG biofeedback. Phys Ther 1980;60:1410–1415.

35. Souza DR, Gross MT. Comparison of vastus medialis obliques: vastus lateralis muscle integrated electromyographic ratios between healthy subjects and patients with patellofemoral pain. Phys Ther 1991;71: 310–319.

36. Fernie G, Holden J, Soto M. Biofeedback training of knee control in the above-knee amputee. Am J Phys Med 1978;57:161–166.

37. Patterson P, Shea CH. Augmented auditory information in the control of upper-limb prostheses. Arch Phys Med Rehabil 1985;66:243–245.

38. Gauthier-Gagnon C, St Pierre D, Drouin G, et al. Augmented sensory feedback in the early training of standing balance of below-knee amputees. Physiother Can 1986;38:137–142.

39. Clarkson PM, James R, Watkins A, et al. The effect of augmented feedback on foot pronation during barre exercise in dance. Res Q 1986;57:33–40.

40. Baker M, Hudson J, Wolf SL. A "feedback" cane to improve the hemiplegic patient's gait. Phys Ther 1979;59:170–171.

41. Draper V. Electromyographic biofeedback and recovery of quadriceps femoris, muscle function following anterior cruciate ligament reconstruction. Phys Ther 1990;70:11–17.

42. Draganich LF, Jaeger RJ, Krajl AR. Coactivation of the hamstrings and quadriceps during extension of the knee. J Bone Joint Surg Am 1989; 71:1071–1081.

43. Gryzlo SM, Patek RM, Pink M, Parry J. Electromyographic analysis of knee joint exercises. J Orthop Sports Phys Ther 1994;20:36–43.

44. Sinkjaer T, Arndt-Nielsen L. Knee stability and muscle coordination in patients with anterior cruciate ligament injuries: an electromyographic approach. J Electromyogr Kinesiol 1991;1:209–217.

45. Levitt R, Deisinger JA, Redondet WJ, et al. EMG-assisted postoperative rehabilitation of minor arthroscopic knee surgeries. J Sports Med Phys Fitness 1995;35:218–223.

46. Lee M, Moseley A, Refshauge K. Effect of feedback on learning a vertebral joint mobilization skill. Phys Ther 1990;70:97–104.

47. Thomas RE, Vaidya SC, Herrick RT, Congleton JJ. The effects of biofeedback on carpal tunnel syndrome. Ergonomics 1993;36:353–361.

48. Montes R, Bedmar M. EMG biofeedback of the abductor pollicis brevis muscle in piano performance. Biofeedback Self Regul 1993;18:67–77.

49. Blumenstein B, Bar-Eli M, Tenenbaum G. The augmenting role of biofeedback: effects of autogenic, imagery and music training on physiological indices and athletic performance. J Sports Sci 1995;13:343–354.

50. Guercio J, Chittum R, McMorrow M. Self-management in the treatment of ataxia: a case study in reducing ataxic tremor through relaxation and biofeedback. Brain Inj 1997;11:353–362.

51. Spence SH, Sharp L, Newton-John T, Champion D. Effect of EMG biofeedback compared to relaxation training with chronic, upper extremity cumulative trauma disorders. Pain 1995; 63:199–206.

52. Cram JR (ed). Clinical EMG for Surface Recordings, Vol 2. Nevada City, CA: Clinical Resources, 1990.

53. Keefe FJ, Surwit RS. Electromyographic biofeedback: behavioral treatment of neuromuscular disorders. J Behav Med 1978;1:13–24.

54. Basmajian JV. Research foundations of EMG biofeedback in rehabilitation. Biofeedback Self Regul 1988;13:275–298.

55. Wolf SL. Electromyographic biofeedback applications to stroke patients: a critical review. Phys Ther 1983;63:1448–1455.

56. Basmajian JV, Kukulka CG, Narayan MG. Biofeedback treatment of footdrop after stroke compared with standard rehabilitation technique: effects on voluntary control and strength. Arch Phys Med Rehabil 1975;56:231–236.

57. Brudny J, Korein J, Grynbaum B, et al. Sensory feedback therapy as a modality of treatment in central nervous system disorders of voluntary movement. Neurology 1974;24:925–932.

58. Wolf SL, Baker MP, Kelly JL. EMG biofeedback in stroke: effect of patient characteristics. Arch Phys Med Rehabil 1979;60:96–102.

59. Wolf SL, Baker MP, Kelly JL. EMG biofeedback in stroke: a 1-year follow-up on the effect of patient characteristics. Arch Phys Med Rehabil 1980; 61:351–355.

60. Middaugh SJ, Miller MC. Electromyographic feedback: effects on voluntary contractions in paretic patients. Arch Phys Med Rehabil 1980;61:24–29.

61. Wolf SL, Binder-Macleod SA. Electromyographic biofeedback applications to the hemiplegic patient: changes in lower extremity neuromuscular and

functional status. Phys Ther 1983;63:1404–1413.

62. Binder SA, Moll CB, Wolf SL. Evaluation of electromyographic biofeedback as an adjunct to therapeutic exercise in treating the lower extremities of hemiplegic patients. Phys Ther 1981;61: 886–893.

63. Colborne CR, Olney SJ. Feedback of joint angle and EMG in gait of able-bodied subjects. Arch Phys Med Rehabil 1990;71:478–483.

64. Mandel AR, Nymark JR, Balmer SJ, et al. Electromyographic versus rhythmic positional biofeedback in computerized gait training with stroke patients. Arch Phys Med Rehabil 1990;71:649–654.

65. Brudny J, Korein J, Grynbaum BB, et al. Helping hemiparetics to help themselves. Sensory feedback therapy. JAMA 1979;241:814–818.

66. Prevo AJH, Visser SL, Vogelaar TW. Effect of EMG feedback on paretic muscles and abnormal co-contraction in the hemiplegic arm, compared with conventional physical therapy. Scand J Rehabil Med 1982;14:121–131.

67. Ince LP, Leon MS, Christidis D. EMG biofeedback for improvement of upper extremity function: a critical review of the literature. Physiother Can 1985;37:12–17.

68. Basmajian JV. Biofeedback for neuromuscular rehabilitation. Crit Rev Phys Med Rehabil 1989;1:37–58.

69. Basmajian JV, Gowland C, Brandstater ME, et al. EMG feedback treatment of upper limb in hemiplegic stroke patients: pilot study. Arch Phys Med Rehabil 1982;63:613–616.

70. Wolf SL, LeCraw DE, Barton LA, et al. A comparison of motor copy and targeted feedback training techniques for restitution of upper extremity function among neurologic patients. Phys Ther 1989;69:719–735.

71. Wissel J, Ebersbach G, Gutjahr L, et al. Treating chronic hemiparesis with modified biofeedback. Arch Phys Med Rehabil 1989;70:612–617.

72. Mathieu PA, Sullivan SJ. Changes in the hemiparetic limb with training. I. Torque output. Electromyogr Clin Electrophysiol 1995;35:492–502.

73. Mathieu PA. Changes in the hemiparetic limb with training. II. EMG signal. Electromyogr Clin Electrophysiol 1995;35:503–513.

74. Glanz M, Klawansky S, Stason W, et al. Biofeedback therapy in poststroke rehabilitation: a meta-analysis of the randomized controlled trials. Arch Phys Med Rehabil 1995;76:508–515.

75. Moreland JD, Thomson MA, Fuoco AR. Electromyographic biofeedback to improve lower extremity function after stroke: a meta-analysis. Arch Phys Med Rehabil 1998;79:134–140.

76. Clinical Practice Guideline Number 16: Post-Stroke Rehabilitation. Rockville, MD: US Department of Health and Human Services, Public Health Service, Agency for Health Care Policy and Research, 1995.

77. Bradley L, Hart BB, Mandana S, et al. Electromyographic biofeedback for gait training after stroke. Clin Rehabil 1998;12:11–22.

78. Lee MY, Wong MK, Tang FT. Clinical evaluation of a new biofeedback standing balance training device. J Med Eng Technol 1996;20:60–66.

79. Simmons RW, Smith K, Erez E, et al. Balance retraining in a hemiparetic patient using center of gravity biofeedback: a single-case study. Percept Mot Skills 1998;87:603–609.

80. Sackley CM, Lincoln NB. Single blind randomized clinical trail of visual feedback after stroke: effects on stance symmetry and function. J Disabil Rehabil 1997;19:536–546.

81. Nichols DS. Balance retraining after stroke using force platform biofeedback. Phys Ther 1997;77:553–558.

82. Gray FB, Gray C, McClanaham JW. Assessing the accuracy of partial weight-bearing instrument. Am J Orthop 1998;27:558–560.

83. Kitamura J, Nakagawa H. Visual influence on contact pressure of hemiplegic patients through photoelastic sole image. Arch Phys Med Rehabil 1996;77:14–18.

84. Petersen H, Magnusson M, Johansson R, Fransson PA. Auditory feedback regulation of perturbed stance in stroke patients. Scand J Rehabil Med 1996;28:217–223.

85. Dursun E, Hamamci N, Donmez S, et al. Angular biofeedback device for sitting balance of stroke patients. Stroke 1996;27:1354–1357.

86. Walker C, Brouwer BJ, Culham EG. Use of visual feedback in retraining balance following acute stroke. Phys Ther 2000;80(9):886–895.

87. Brach JS, Van Swearingen JM, Lenert J, et al. Facial neuromuscular retraining for oral synkinesis. Plast Reconstr Surg 1997;99:1922–1931.

88. Bobath B. Adult Hemiplegia: Evaluation and Treatment (2nd ed). London: Heinemann, 1978.

89. Lord JP, Hall K. Neuromuscular reeducation versus traditional programs for stroke rehabilitation. Arch Phys Med Rehabil 1986;67:88–91.

90. Sivenius J, Pyorala K, Heininen OP, et al. The significance of intensity of rehabilitation of stroke-controlled trial. Stroke 1985;16:928–931.

91. Ballantyne B. Factors contributing to voluntary movement deficit and spasticity following cerebral vascular accidents. Neurol Rep 1991;15: 15–18.

92. Wolf SL, Edwards DI, Shutter LA. Concurrent assessment of muscle activity (CAMA): a procedural approach to assess treatment goals. Phys Ther 1986;66:218–224.

93. Anderson PA, Hobart DJ, Danoff JV (eds). Electro-Myographical Kinesiology. New York: Excerpta Medica, 1991.

94. Wolf SL, Binder-Macleod SA. Neurophysiological Factors in Electromyographic Feedback for Neuromotor Disturbances. In JV Basmajian (ed), Biofeedback: Principles and Practice for Clinicians (3rd ed). Baltimore: Williams & Wilkins, 1989;17–36.

95. Bach-y-Rita P, Balliet R. Recovery from Stroke. In PW Duncan, M Badke (eds), Stroke Rehabilitation. New York: Year Book, 1987;79–108.

96. Walker SC, Helm PA, Lavery LA. Gait pattern alteration by functional sensory substitution in healthy subjects and in diabetic subjects with peripheral neuropathy. Arch Phys Med Rehabil 1997;78:853–856.

97. Hirvonen TP, Aalto H, Pyykko I. Stability limits for visual feedback posturography in vestibular rehabilitation. Acta Otolaryngol 1997;529(Suppl): 104–107.

98. Woolner B. Biofeedback reeducation in gracilis muscle transposition after rectal trauma: a case presentation. J Wound Ostomy Continence Nurs 1997;24:38–50.

99. O'Neill MA, Gwinn KA, Adler CH. Biofeedback for writer's cramp. Am J Occup Ther 1997;51:605–607.

100. Stringer AY. Treatment of motor aprosopia with pitch biofeedback and expression modelling. Brain Inj 1996;10:583–590.

101. Brucker BS, Bulawva NV. Biofeedback effect on electromyographic responses in patients with spinal cord injury. Arch Phys Med Rehabil 1996;77:133–137.

102. Kohmeyer KM, Hill JP, Yarkony GM,

Jaeger RJ. Electrical stimulation and biofeedback effect on recovery of tenodesis grasp: a controlled study. Arch Phys Med Rehabil 1996;77:702–706.

103. Wolpaw JR, Flotzinger D, Pfurtscheller G, McFarland DJ. Timing of EEG-based cursor control. J Clin Neuophysiol 1997;14:529–538.

104. Mohr B, Pulvermuller F, Schleichert H. Learned changes in brain states alter cognitive processing in humans. Neursci Lett 1998;253:159–162.

105. Kubler A, Kotchoubey B, Hinterberger T, et al. The thought translation device: a neurophysiological approach to communication in total motor paralysis. Exp Brain Res 1999; 124:223–232.

33

Manual Modalities

ROBERT S. GAILEY, JR., AND MICHELE A. RAYA

Manual modalities are the oldest, most widely used form of treatment throughout history. For the purpose of this chapter, *manual modalities* are defined as treatments performed with the hands for the purposes of affecting the skeletal, neuromuscular, and circulatory systems. The three most common forms of such treatment are massage, stretching, and joint mobilization.

Rehabilitation medicine recognizes that increased stress causes greater cellular activity and that any alteration in the degree or type of physical loading changes cellular metabolism, matrix morphology, and functional capacity.[1,2] Manual forces influence the tissues to which they are applied. Therapy is designed to permit clinicians to provide the stress necessary to affect the bone and soft tissue structures involved in musculoskeletal dysfunction that have resulted in pain, loss of motion, adaptive connective tissue shortening, and inflammation.

The long history of manual modalities is replete with treatment methods based solely on the clinical experience of the advocate of the particular protocol. The need for evidence-based practice compels subjecting traditional beliefs to impartial, clinically based trials. This chapter explores scientific research on contemporary manual modalities.

MASSAGE

Massage is one of the oldest and most widely accepted forms of treatment. Today more than 75 types of massage are practiced. Some forms date back as early as 3000 BC according to documentation from China.[3] Since the 1980s a considerable increase in popularity of massage techniques has been seen, some falling under the generic heading of *alternative therapies*. Surprisingly, although massage has such a venerable history and is used in a vast array of clinical settings, relatively few scientific reports have been published.

The physiological and therapeutic effects of massage have been credited with promoting healing, restoring function, and enhancing physical performance. Specifically, *massage* has been described as assisting with circulation and lymphatic drainage, enhancing the elastic and inelastic properties of connective tissue and muscle, fostering relaxation, counteracting edema, and alleviating muscle pain.[4-8] Contraindications to massage are few but include malignancy, infection, and unusually fragile skin.[9]

The five most widely accepted massage strokes are effleurage (stroking), pétrissage (kneading), longitudinal and transverse friction, tapotement (percussion, hacking), and vibration (shaking).[3,4,7,10,11] Table 33-1 describes the treatment rationale and clinical applications for each stroke.

Physiological Effects

Blood Flow

From the earliest writings to modern texts, the single most positive effect attributed to massage is the assumption that manual forces applied to the body enhance blood flow.[4-8,10] Many positive physiological effects associated with massage have been attributed to the altered movement of fluids through the body.

Historically, alteration in blood flow presumed to be caused by massage was studied with venous occlusion plethysmography, in which changes in blood flow are inferred from changes in limb circumference. Plethysmography, however, does not distinguish blood flow

TABLE 33-1
Massage Techniques and Indications

Techniques	Treatment Rationale	Description of Application
Effleurage (stroking)	Often used in preparation for additional soft tissue treatments and to apply lubricant if necessary. Gradual compression reduces muscle tone, induces relaxation, relieves muscle spasm, accelerates blood and lymph flow, thus reducing swelling.	Slow rhythmic superficial stroking hand movements over the skin, frequently applied at the beginning and end of treatment. Light gliding movements over the skin without attempting to move or manipulate the deeper tissues.
Pétrissage (kneading)	Promotes flow of blood and fluids causing reflexive vasodilatation, hyperemia, and a reduction in swelling caused by injury and abnormal inactivity. This action may also help to free adhesions.	Kneading manipulations, which use compression, rolling, grasping, and lifting, creating a *milking* action of the muscles and soft tissues.
Friction	Adhesions and scar tissue are disrupted, while the parallel organization of new collagen fibers is mechanically assisted, promoting optimal movement and elongation of healing soft tissues.	Deep perpendicular movements are performed across soft tissue fibers.
Tapotement (percussion)	Contrary to most massage that is relaxing, this technique is used to stimulate or prepare an athlete for competition.	A series of brisk blows applied in rapid succession with specific hand techniques such as hacking, cupping, slapping, beating, and tapping.
Vibration (shaking)	Rarely used manually, but often performed using electronic vibrators, this technique has the ability to facilitate or inhibit and therefore is used both for simulation and relaxation.	The hands, fingers, or an electromechanical device are used to create small rhythmic, tremulous movements.

Source: Adapted from E Cafarelli, F Flint. The role of massage in preparation for and recovery from exercise. An overview. Sports Med 1992;14:1–9; and FM Tappan. Healing Massage Techniques: A Study of Eastern and Western Methods. Reston, VA: Reston Publishing, 1980.

through muscle from cutaneous circulation. The latter provides no nutritive benefit to the muscle inasmuch as blood bypasses the muscle capillary beds via the superficial arteriovenous shunt.[12] Additionally, the results of blood flow studies using venous occlusion plethysmography varied tremendously. Wakim et al.[13] reported a 50% increase in blood flow after vigorous massage, whereas Ebel and Wisham[14] did not find that massage had any effect on blood flow in the resting limb. Hansen and Kristiansen,[15] Wakim,[16] and Hovind and Neisen[17] reported 5%, 20%, and 35% increases in venous occlusion plethysmography results, respectively. Cafarelli and Flint[12] estimated the average changes in resting blood flow to be approximately 25%; however, this change amounts to only a few milliliters per minute per 100 ml. If these changes do occur within the muscle, some benefit could be realized before or after exercise. If, however, changes are restricted to the skin flow, then the effect on muscle is of little consequence.

Arkko et al.[18] examined blood chemistry after a 1-hour whole body massage. Blood drawn before treatment, immediately after, and after 2, 24, and 48 hours revealed an increase in creatine kinase, lactate dehydrogenase, and its isoenzymes LDH_4 and LDH_5 and in the

concentration of serum potassium, which are indicative of increased permeability of muscle cells. The investigators suggested that the most probable reason for the increase in serum enzyme activities was that mechanical trauma initiated an inflammatory response leading to the natural increase of the cell membrane permeability. The permeability typically associated with muscle hypoxia caused by work was not at issue because muscles were relaxed and passive during testing. Massage produced no changes in blood hematocrit readings and only minimal increases in serum total protein concentration. Other hematologic parameters remained essentially unchanged.

Hovind and Nielsen[17] found that pétrissage produced insignificant increases in blood flow that quickly leveled off, whereas tapotement caused an immediate increase in blood flow comparable with that of active muscular contractions. The interpretation was that hacking massage applied over skeletal muscle causes minute repetitive muscular contractions in the treated area; consequently changes in blood flow are similar to voluntary muscular contractions.

Shoemaker et al.[19] reviewed the literature regarding the effect of massage on increasing blood flow. Studies involving smaller muscle groups such as in the forearm and calf supported the benefit of massage.[15,17] In contrast, studies of massage on larger muscle groups failed to reveal any appreciable changes in blood flow.[20-22] Three common forms of massage, effleurage, pétrissage, and tapotement, were applied to the forearm and anterior thigh. Beat-by-beat measures of arterial mean blood velocities were obtained from the brachial and femoral arteries. Arterial diameters were obtained by echo Doppler at the beginning and end of each treatment. Mean blood velocity and arterial diameter in both areas remained essentially unchanged. The research refuted the hypothesis that massage increases blood flow to small and large muscles. After testing, subjects were asked to perform light exercise in the form of a voluntary handgrip and gentle quadriceps contractions. Mean blood velocity changed significantly in both the forearm and quadriceps, suggesting that voluntary contractions of skeletal muscle may be more beneficial than massage to promote increased blood flow. Although some evidence suggests that massage increases blood flow, which, in turn, aids muscle healing, nevertheless, light exercise appears more beneficial than massage.[15,17,19,21,23]

Autonomic Nervous System

The general feeling of well-being and relaxation typically associated with massage has been attributed to autonomic nervous system activity, in particular, to an increase in parasympathetic stimulation that produces deep relaxation.[4] Barr and Taslitz[24] administered three 20-minute massages and three control sessions on 10 women. The investigators found just the opposite of what was expected. Sympathetic activity increased during the massage followed by a delayed increase in systolic blood pressure, heart rate, sweat gland activity, peripheral skin temperature, body temperature, and pupil diameter and a decrease in respiration rate. Isolated instances of parasympathetic activity during the massage periods were observed with an initial decrease in systolic and diastolic blood pressure.

Likewise, Reed and Held[25] described autonomic nervous system responses to serial connective tissue massage in 14 healthy middle-aged subjects. Nine separate treatments over 3 weeks were administered with no change observed in skin temperature, galvanic skin response, mean arterial pressure, and heart rate. The results suggested that connective tissue massage has no consistent immediate or long-term effects on the autonomic nervous system.

These studies do not support the supposition that relaxing effects or the therapeutic effects attributed to massage are related to the autonomic nervous system.

The question remains regarding how massage produces the soothing properties so often achieved.

Range of Motion

Increased extensibility of soft tissue, including muscle, tendon, fascia, joint capsule, and ligaments, has been described as an effect of massage.[26] Crosman et al.[27] examined the effects on range of motion (ROM) of a single massage treatment to the hamstring group. The authors administered a 9- to 12-minute combination of effleurage, pétrissage, and friction massage and measured ROM pretreatment, immediately posttreatment, and 7 days afterward. A significant increase in ROM occurred after treatment; however, subjects returned to pretreatment ROM at the 7-day posttreatment measurement. The authors concluded that some immediate improvement of ROM occurred directly after treatment, but there appears to be little long-term effect from a single massage treatment.

When warm-up exercise, massage, and stretching were compared with respect to their effects on ROM and strength of the hamstrings and quadriceps, Wiktorsson-Moller et al.[28] reported that stretching increased ROM, whereas massage and warmup employed either separately or in combination had no effect.

Performance

Massage to prepare athletes for training and competition is a long-standing tradition. Ask et al.[29] reported an 11% increase in maximal muscle power output during leg extension when massage was applied before exercise. Viitasalo et al.[30] reported slightly better performance using 20–30 minutes of warm underwater jet massage in increased serum enzyme activities after treatment. However, the positive effects could be related to the warm water (38°C) heating the muscle.

In contrast, Boone et al.[31] examined the effects on subjects who had a 30-minute massage before running at 80% intensity on a treadmill. No differences were found in cardiac output and oxygen uptake. Massage was determined not to have an effect on energy exchange during exercise or to improve performance. Moreover, Wiktorsson-Moller et al.[28] found a negative effect of massage before activity in which the maximum voluntary contraction force was reduced by 9%.

Athletes often report feeling relaxed and refreshed after massage with the sense of being able to perform better. Harmer[32] found no statistically significant change in maximal stride frequency during simulated sprinting exercise. Three of the four sprinters did experience a 2.4–3.1% higher mean stride frequency under postmassage conditions. Theoretically, this would improve the sprinter's 100-yard time by 0.5 seconds. Although not statistically significant, in a sport where 0.01 seconds can determine winners, these results could be considered positive.[32]

Massage to accelerate recovery from athletic competition or between events has been offered as possible mechanism to decrease fatigue and improve recovery time.[3] The effects of massage on muscle recovery have yet to be established. As discussed earlier, increasing blood flow, thereby returning more oxygen to injured muscle tissue to speed healing, has been offered as a possible benefit of massage.[6,33] Because muscle strength is at the core of improved performance, a brief review of the effects of exercise on muscle and the physiological mechanisms occurring before the ready state for exercise is warranted (see Chapter 16).

Strength in untrained muscle reduces after intense eccentric exercise, with effects lasting 5–10 days.[34-36] High-intensity exercise, particularly that involving eccentric contractions, produces a loss of muscle force generation immediately after activity. The change is believed to be related to a nonuniform overstretching of sarcomeres.[34,37] Muscle injury involves several components of the sarcomere, interrupting muscle cell calcium homeostasis. An increase in the intracellular calcium concentration increases protein levels and reduces phosphocreatine levels within the muscle and thereby causes membrane degeneration.[34,38] The intercellular changes may persist for several days to a week, producing evidence of muscle damage and membrane disruption with the presence of creatine kinase in the blood. Damage to sarcomeres and subsequent contractile structures and the altered chemical state of proteins and calcium may be the cause of reduced muscle strength caused by overexertion.[39,40] If massage were to enhance removal of hydrogen ions from muscle cells or to improve recovery of lost muscle potassium, high-energy phosphates, or glycogen, it could conceivably improve the rate of recovery of muscle function immediately postexercise.[40] The literature, however, provides little support for this contention.[12,23]

Caferelli et al.[41] found that electromechanical percussive vibratory massage produced no short-term recovery from repeated maximal contractions. Drews et al.[33] administered 30 minutes of massage daily to elite cyclists during a four-stage race. They reported no difference between the placebo, prerace, postrace, and posttreatment, or 3 days after postrace groups of cyclists. Likewise, Tiidus and Shoemaker[21] provided daily deep and superficial massage for 4 days after

intense eccentric exercise to the quadriceps and used pulsed Doppler velocimetry to study femoral arterial and venous blood flow. They concluded that massage was not an effective modality for enhancing long-term restoration of postexercise muscle strength, nor was there any appreciable increase in blood flow. Light exercise in the form of gentle quadriceps contractions did elevate arterial and venous blood flow, but did not demonstrate a difference in exercise peak torque values.

Weber et al.[42] also found no benefit for massage, microcurrent electrical neural stimulation, or upper body ergometry after exercise. They reported similar results with respect to isometric force production at 24 and 48 hours after initial exercise bouts. The maximal voluntary isometric contraction deficits reported in this study were similar to other studies in which massage was not introduced.[39,43]

Overall objective evidence to support the use of massage for the enhancement of performance before, during, or after intense training or athletic competition is exceedingly sparse.

Psychological Effects

Beard and Wood[10] extolled the psychological effects of massage: "Most persons are familiar with the soothing effect of gentle massage, even when there is no pathology or physical disability present." The psychological effects of massage have been described as possibly being more beneficial than its physiological effects.[31] Few would disagree that the sense of well-being, the value of therapeutic touch, or the simple hands-on stimulation experienced through tactile contact has some psychoemotional component. Touch is probably the oldest form of comfort. Since the beginning of time the ill have been comforted by even the simplest therapeutic gesture of bedside hand holding. Although the psychological benefits derived from massage have yet to be investigated in terms of measurable outcomes on specific diagnoses, the intangible value should not be summarily dismissed.

Classically, massage therapy has been credited with reducing stress and anxiety through relaxation of the body and mind.[3] Relaxation leads to a sense of well-being, positive mood change, greater energy, increased participation, and faster recovery from other diagnoses.[44] Other benefits relate to calming attention deficit hyperactive disorder, improving body image, satisfying needs for intimacy, enhancing self-esteem, increasing mental alertness, and assisting with recovery from clinical depression.[3] Most clinicians would agree that the hands-on effect helps patients feel as if someone is helping them.[6]

In spite of abundant anecdotal testimony and clinical declarations, the effects of massage on psychological parameters are supported by relatively few empirical data. Most studies are weakened by poor design, small sample size, and methodologic and statistical limitations.[12] Of special importance is the work of Weinberg et al.,[45] who explored the relation between positive mood effects with exercise and massage. They randomly assigned 183 physical education students to swimming, jogging, racquetball, or tennis classes, a rest control, and a massage condition. Instruments included the Profile of Mood States,[46] the State of Anxiety Inventory,[47] and the general and high activation subscales from the Adjective Checklist[48] condition. The results indicated that massage repeatedly demonstrated positive effects with respect to mood states and psychological well-being. More specifically mood state subscale score changes that were observed included decreased tension, anger, fatigue, depression, anxiety, and confusion. Alteration in mood states might have a positive effect on athletic performance; however, the investigators did not test athletes in a competitive environment.

Conversely, when Drews et al.[33] administered the Profile of Mood States and Perceived Exertion Feeling Scale to six elite cyclists, they found no significant differences between massage and placebo trials, suggesting that massage fostered no psychological enhancement with respect to performance capacity.

Hemming et al.[49] had eight amateur boxers complete two performances on a boxing ergometer on two occasions after receiving either a massage or passive rest. Each boxer gave a perceived recovery rating at the conclusion of each trial. Heart rates, blood lactates, and glucose levels were assessed. The massage intervention significantly increased perception of recovery when compared with passive rest, although no difference in blood lactate or glucose occurred after either intervention. The investigators concluded that some psychological advantage of massage might be present in the absence of physiological benefits.

Effects on Impairments

Pain

Massage has been described as an effective treatment for disrupting the pain cycle by improving circulation and inducing mechanical and reflex effects.[4,26,50] Day et al.[51] studied 21 healthy subjects divided into two groups: One rested while the others received a 30-minute back massage. The study investigated the analgesic effects afforded by massage. The hypothesis was that pain relief would result with the release of the endogenous

opiates β-endorphin and β-lipotropin, which have been demonstrated to increase after exercise.[52,53] This effect is based on a premise similar to the use of transcutaneous electrical stimulation as an analgesic; studies have suggested that endogenous opiates released with the use of transcutaneous electrical stimulation reduce pain.[54,55] The results achieved by Day and associates[51] were not consistent with this theory because the massage did not significantly change the measured serum levels of β-endorphin and β-lipotropin, thus bringing into question the analgesic effect of massage. Kaada and Torsteinbo[56] in a later study did find a moderate increase of 16% in β-endorphin levels lasting approximately 1 hour after a 30-minute session of connective tissue massage, thus suggesting that pain relief may be linked to massage.

Muscle Soreness

Massage has been applied after exercise not only as a means of increasing blood flow, but also to reduce the effects of muscle soreness and as a result, potentially speed recovery and improve future performance. Delayed muscle soreness is associated with intense exercise, particularly eccentric strengthening, and generally becomes evident 8–24 hours after the cessation of exercise, peaks 48–72 hours postexercise, and disappears 3–7 days later.[57] This sequence supports Armstrong's theoretical model of exercised-induced muscle fiber injury in which increased muscle tension related to eccentric contractions interrupts the calcium homeostasis, as the normal permeability barrier provided by the cell membrane and basal lamina is disrupted. The eccentric exercise–induced injury to muscle fibers is frequently accompanied by loss of contractile force.[34,58] The sensation of soreness is similar to the effects related to acute inflammation and the associated edema produced by increased lysosomal activity and macrophage invasion.[40]

Other common assumptions regarding delayed soreness suggest damage to muscle connective tissue.[59] Wheat[60] contested this theory. The once popular thinking that lactate and hydrogen ion accumulation produces soreness has been refuted.[12,40] Regardless, it does not appear that massage administered before exercise with the purpose of increasing blood flow has any effect on the magnitude of lactic acid accumulation after steady-state exercise.[31]

Gupta et al.[61] compared passive recovery (sitting for 40 minutes), active recovery (light 30% maximum ergometry for 40 minutes), and massage recovery (effleurage and pétrissage for 10 minutes). They found no significant difference in lactate values between passive and massage recovery; however, active exercise did produce a much better recovery process with significantly faster lactate elimination.

Rodenburg et al.[62] applied warmup, stretching, and massage to determine if the negative effects of eccentric exercise, specifically muscle soreness, could be diminished. Subjects received a 15-minute warmup, passive stretching before and after exercise, and 15 minutes of superficial effleurage and deep pétrissage to the arms. Functional and biomechanical measurements were obtained. Maximal isotonic force of the biceps brachii and brachialis muscles, elbow flexion angle, and creatine kinase were found to have significant main effects, whereas soreness on pressure, extension angle, and myoglobin concentration in the blood did not change between groups. The inconsistent results raise questions about the efficacy of warmup and stretching. It was postulated that massage probably does not have as significant a contribution to postexercise effect as did stretching and warmup because massage only affects blood flow. During eccentric exercise, the metabolic load on the muscle fibers is relatively low, and lactate production does not influence the onset of soreness.

Smith et al.[44] found that, by administering massage within 2 hours after isokinetic eccentric exercise, soreness was reduced, creatine kinase was reduced, neutrophils displayed a prolonged elevation, and cortisol showed a diminished diurnal reduction. The investigators concluded that to be effective in reducing the physiological response of muscle damage, massage would have to be administered within 2 hours after exercise.[44] Tiidus[40] pointed out that, contrary to the Smith's conclusion, muscle damage may have been reduced by massage because of the reduction in serum creatine kinase, suggesting that changes in blood creatine kinase activities can be highly variable and not necessarily reflective of, or proportional to, muscle damage alone.[63,64]

Other forms of treatment have been used in combination with massage in an attempt to reduce soreness. Weber et al.[42] produced soreness with high-intensity eccentric exercise in four groups of untrained women, including a control group and three treatment groups who received either massage, microcurrent electrical neural stimulation, or upper body ergometry. Treatments were administered immediately after exercise, and pain scale measurements were performed immediately, 24, and 48 hours after exercise. Contrary to Smith's findings, no significant differences were observed among the groups, and all treatments were determined to be ineffective in reducing soreness.

The value of massage as a means of reducing muscle soreness has come under scrutiny, for practitioners must consider the merit of such a time-consuming and expensive practice that has demonstrated no relief of soreness whether administered before or after exercise.[42,65,66] Warmup, stretching, and light exercise are easily performed independently and may be more practical in situations in which the individual or athletic team does not have access to massage.

Connective Tissue Injury

Inflammation, the body's primary response to injury, is an imperative first step toward the restoration of normal cellular functioning.[67] The process allows the body to rid itself of invading bacteria and the resultant cellular debris and to begin the reparative process.[1,67] Therapeutic interventions should not be aimed at stopping the inflammatory process but rather be directed at maximizing the conditions for tissue regeneration. Early, controlled motion of the injured tissue is recognized as an important step in the formation of strong, compacted scar tissue.[1,2,67] Scar tissue is initially laid down haphazardly but as stresses are applied to the tissue, the fibers become parallel and more resistant to the forces applied to them.[1,2,67] It is the scar tissue response in this remodeling phase that is dependent on mechanical stimuli.[1,2,67]

Cyriax's[68] earliest description of friction massage offered two forms of treatment. The first is the longitudinal in which the application of force runs parallel to the fibers of the soft tissue structures. The second is transverse friction massage or deep friction massage (DFM) in which the forces are applied perpendicular to the fibers in an attempt to separate each fiber, mechanically assisting in the alignment of newly formed collagen during healing. DFM has been used to promote local hyperemia, analgesia, and reduction of adherent scar tissue to ligament, tendon, and muscle structures.[11] Pathologic conditions successfully treated by DFM include tendinitis, adhesions, fibromyositis, sprains, and tears.[11,69]

Walker[70] was the first to examine the effect of DFM on the healing of a minor sprain of the medial collateral ligament of the knee in rabbits. He administered 10 treatment sessions on alternate days, beginning with a 3-minute duration and progressing to 10 minutes during the last five treatments. Histologic observations were made after sacrificing selected animals at intervals of 22–34 days after spraining. Thickening and organization of new collagen fibers in skin were evident; however, inconsistent new collagen fibers were observed with the treated and untreated fibers, making it difficult to distinguish healed from uninjured tissue. The investigators concluded that DFM did not promote repair of sprained ligaments, as the longitudinal arrangement of collagen as well as the random orientation of collagen fibers were similar between the treated and untreated ligaments.

Davidson et al.[71] described a technique similar to DFM, called *augmented soft tissue mobilization* (ASTM), in which specifically designed solid instruments, rather than the fingers of the therapist, are used to provide the mobilizing force to the soft tissue structure. The theory assumes that the instrument would permit greater control of the amount of microtrauma that could augment the healing process. Davidson's study on rats demonstrated increased fibroblast recruitment suggesting ASTM does promote healing, even though there was an absence of inflammatory cells, such as mononuclear blood cells and lymphocytes, at the injury site.

Gehlsen[72] demonstrated that ASTM not only stimulates fibroblast proliferation but that this proliferative response apparently depends on the magnitude of applied pressure. Fibroblast proliferation and activation have a major contribution in tendon healing, stimulating production of cellular mediators of healing and proteinaceous synthesis of collagen fibers.[72-74] These results support Cyriax and Russell's[11] contention that movement, whether mechanical (DFM or ASTM) or intrinsic (stretching or muscular contractions) would facilitate realignment and healing of soft tissue fibers. Mechanical force appears to be a critical component of transverse friction treatments. Light and moderate pressures are not as productive in promoting fibroblast proliferation as is heavy pressure.

Hypertonicity

The reduction of hypertonicity has long been a goal of therapeutic rehabilitation, specifically with neurologically impaired persons such as those with traumatic brain injury, stroke, spinal cord injury, and multiple sclerosis. A series of studies by Sullivan and colleagues have demonstrated that pétrissage decreases peak-to-peak Hoffman reflex (H-reflex) amplitude as reflected by a significant decrease in mean inhibitory response in the triceps surae muscle motor neuron excitability.[75-79] When massage was used in subjects with spinal cord injury a reduction in H-reflex amplitude during treatment was observed in eight of ten subjects. The reduced level of motor neuron excitability remained in some individuals for periods that could prove clinically beneficial. However, no sustainable decrease in H-reflex amplitude was observed.[77]

Unfortunately, the inhibitory responses produced by massage are limited only to the muscle being treated[75] and for the duration of the massage with no lasting effects.[77,79] Moreover, the inhibitory effects are specific to the muscle being examined and not caused by the effects of reciprocal inhibition, temperature change, changes in nerve conduction velocity, or gender differences.[75,78,80]

Deep massage produces a 49% reduction in H-reflex amplitude as compared with light massage, which produces a 39% reduction.[78] Earlier studies have demonstrated as much as a 71% reduction in H-reflex reduction.[79] Morelli et al. applied two treatment conditions, the first was 3 minutes of pétrissage, and the second included the application of ethyl chloride topically before 3 minutes of pétrissage. On H-reflex testing, both groups exhibited a reduction in H-reflex amplitude during massage; however, no differences were observed between the two groups. The authors concluded that cutaneous receptors do not play any significant role in the inhibitory responses achieved during deep muscle massage. The inhibitory effects of massage do not appear to originate from mechanical stimuli of cutaneous mechanoreceptors. Rather, inhibition appears to be produced by the deep mechanoreceptors.[81] Evidence that increased muscle tone, such as spasms and cramps, would benefit from massage has yet to be published. Furthermore, Travell's belief that the skin overlying tense muscle should be primed before relaxation techniques for optimal effect is still lacking scientific scrutiny.[82]

STRETCHING

The ability of connective tissue and muscle to absorb force is related to its resting length; thus, the greater the flexibility, the greater the ability to absorb forces and avoid strain.[67] Preventing muscle injury and maintaining optimal functional efficiency are important rehabilitative goals that should govern treatment plans, thus making a good flexibility program pertinent to the well-being of our patients.

Stretching techniques are widely used (Table 33-2).[76,83-85] *Flexibility*, a component of mobility, has been described as "The maximal passive angle mobility compared with corresponding anatomical zero positions."[86] Zachazewski, expounding on the definition of flexibility, divided it into the motion available at a joint secondary

TABLE 33-2
Benefits of Stretching and Flexibility

Improved flexibility
Allows tissues to accommodate more easily to stress
Allows for greater dissipation of shock during impact
Improved efficiency and effectiveness of movement
Protects against and minimizes injury

to the inherent arthrokinematics and the surrounding tissue's ability to lengthen about that joint.[87]

Many elements (muscle, tendon, ligaments, and connective tissue) contribute to articular flexibility. Cyriax[88] divided these elements into active (contractile) and passive components. The contractile elements include the muscle sarcomeres with the myofilament cross-bridges and the myotatic stretch reflex derived from spinal reflex activity within the muscle.[89] Thus, the contractile components would provide resistance to stretch either by reflexogenic or volitional contraction of the muscle.[90] The passive elements are the inert connective tissue, joint capsule, ligament, and fascia; they provide mechanical resistance to muscle stretch.[89] Research attempting to determine which structure plays the greatest role in limiting flexibility is inconclusive.[76,89,90]

Zachazewski[87] stated that the primary limiting factor to movement at end range is the muscle and its fascial sheath, the capsule, and the tendon in that order. When the muscle is taken into consideration as a limiting factor in ROM, the contribution of the peripheral receptors must be considered. The muscle spindle and Golgi tendon organ have an important role in a muscle's ability to lengthen adequately in response to imposed tension.[91] When a muscle is stretched, the muscle spindle also stretches, exciting the Ia afferent fibers. This results in alpha–gamma coactivation, which is also present during a voluntary contraction. The Golgi tendon organ is sensitive to the tension changes within the muscle as it stretches or contracts. The resulting reflex is inhibitory and acts to inhibit its own muscle and excite the antagonist muscle.[92]

These principles form the rationale for proprioceptive neuromuscular facilitation (PNF) stretching. These techniques use volitional contractions to increase ROM by minimizing the resistance to stretch by the active components attributed to spinal reflex pathways.[93] PNF stretching techniques include hold-relax, contract-relax, contract-relax agonist contract, and hold-relax agonist contract. The hold-relax agonist contract technique is performed by contracting the muscle to be stretched (antagonist), allowing the muscle to relax briefly and then performing a concentric contraction of the agonist muscle. It is believed this results in reciprocal inhibition of the antagonist through the principle of successive inductions.[94] The basic premise of PNF stretching is founded on the muscle's ability to relax further through inhibitory influences, allowing greater ROM to be achieved. Increase in muscle compliance, denoted by a decrease in electromyographic (EMG) activity, allows for the elongation of the active contractile components.

The H-reflex is a monosynaptic reflex from the Ia afferents to the alpha motor neuron and is considered a measure of motor pool excitability.[91,95] Measuring this reflex allows us to determine the level of inhibitory or excitatory effects that the spindles and Golgi tendon organ might be having on a muscle as it is elongated. Thus, the lower the level of excitation of the motor pool, the greater the ability of the muscle to relax as it is being elongated.[95]

Condon and Hutton,[94] looking at both EMG levels and H-reflex amplitudes in the soleus muscle, compared static stretching with three forms of PNF stretching. They found no significant difference in the amount of ankle dorsiflexion gained during each procedure; however, they did note higher H-reflex amplitudes and lower EMG activity during the static stretching and hold-relax procedures. They determined that muscle relaxation was unrelated to the amount of dorsiflexion gained and that static stretching may be the method of choice because of its uncomplicated nature.

In contrast, Etnyre and Abraham,[91] also looking at H-reflex changes during static and PNF stretching, determined that there were several inhibitory neural influences producing a reduction in motor pool excitability seen during the PNF technique, specifically contract-relax agonist contract (CRAC), and thus concluded that PNF techniques provide the greatest potential for muscle elongation. They concluded that the reduction in EMG activity was a result of cross-talk between the surface electrodes.

Osternig et al.[96] examined EMG levels during different PNF stretching techniques and reported findings similar to those of Condon and Hutton. Maximum ROM gains were made with the PNF methods; however, subjects exhibited significant elevations in muscle EMG levels. Consequently, static stretching might be a safer method with less chance of producing residual muscle soreness or muscle strain caused by the greater relaxation of the muscle fibers.

Static stretching differs from PNF techniques in that a primary goal is to address the viscoelastic components, specifically the connective tissue that may be responsible for limiting range about a joint (Table 33-3).[90,94] The

TABLE 33-3

Factors Affecting Deformation of Connective Tissue

Magnitude of stretch
Duration of stretch
Velocity of force applied
Tissue temperature
Immediate past history of tissue

passive components of flexibility must be dealt with differently than the active components, which exhibit time- and rate-dependent changes. Zachazewski referred to the *creep response* as the ability of the viscoelastic tissue to undergo plastic deformation over time while a constant force is being applied to it.[97] Many investigators have asserted that, to achieve a permanent lengthening of the musculotendinous structures, passive components must be targeted.[94,98–100] Webright et al., citing Gajdosik, stated that the deep fascia and soft tissues of the pelvis and leg combine to limit ROM obtained during the performance of a straight leg raise. If passive components were the main factor limiting ROM, then the best method to address them would be static stretching techniques (Table 33-4).[99,101] Comparison between passive hamstring stretching and nonballistic repetitive active knee extension in a neutral slump position (sitting with legs extended while the trunk and head achieve maximum flexion) resulted in no significant difference in ROM gained between the methods.[99] Unfortunately, their use of the slump position made it impossible to determine whether the hamstring muscle was ever elongated past resting length, thus stretching the active elements about the joints. One may speculate that passive elements are responsible for flexibility gains in both methods, thus supporting the belief that a major limiting factor in flexibility is the connective tissue.

Some of the principal underlying mechanisms for static stretching are the same as for PNF stretching, but with greater emphasis on connective tissue contributions to stiffness.[99] Whereas PNF stretching has been shown to be an effective method for achieving improved flexibility, static stretching has been reported to be equal to or slightly better than PNF techniques (Table 33-5).[94,98–100]

The rationale behind static stretching is based on minimizing excitatory responses of spindle afferents to stretch, allowing the muscle fibers to achieve greater length while maintaining passive components in an elongated position.[91] Muir et al.[90] attempted to identify the variables responsible for passive resistance about a joint in an effort to quantify the ability of the connective tissue to deform throughout the ROM of the ankle. They hypothesized that static stretching of the calf muscles would produce a significant reduction in the passive resistance to stretch of the connective tissue. Because their results did not support the hypothesis, they concluded that neuromuscular changes might have been responsible for improvements in ROM. Subjects in their study did not have any limitations in ROM before stretching; thus the connective tissue may not have been at a compromised length.

To achieve maximum effectiveness, the duration and frequency of static stretching must also be considered. Bandy and Irion,[98] in an attempt to determine the optimal length of time to maintain a static stretch, compared durations of 15, 30, and 60 seconds. They found that maintaining a stretch for 15 seconds did not produce significant changes in flexibility, unlike stretches maintained for 30 and 60 seconds. No significant difference was noted between the 30- and 60-second durations. He concluded that 30 seconds was the optimal time to maintain a static stretch.

Wallin et al.,[86] comparing PNF with ballistic stretching, noted that one session a week of flexibility exercises was enough to maintain flexibility once gained, and three to five sessions were needed to increase flexibility.

Improvements in flexibility are attributed to a decrease in the muscle's resistance to stretch secondary to motor neuron inhibition.[95,99,102] Muscle inhibition allows the joint to be taken through a greater ROM, thus applying an even greater stretch to the viscoelastic components. Although this appears to be a valid assumption, it must be remembered that the ability to produce lasting change in the viscoelastic components is time dependent.[87]

TABLE 33-4
Stretching Techniques and Effects

Technique	Advantages	Disadvantages
Static stretching	Low energy cost; low risk of injury; minimal muscle soreness	Does not address dynamic flexibility
Proprioceptive neuromuscular facilitation techniques	Minimizes resistance to stretch attributed to spinal reflex pathways	Requires a highly trained stretching partner
Active isolated stretching	Appears to achieve large gains in range in short period	Complicated technique; high energy cost to perform technique
Ballistic	Effective for patients requiring high levels of dynamic flexibility	High risk of injury; muscle soreness

TABLE 33-5
Types of Stretching

Type	Technique	Physiological Effect
Static stretching	Agonist maintained in lengthened position and held for period of time	Stretch of the viscoelastic structures; alpha-gamma coactivation; reflex inhibition
Proprioceptive neuromuscular facilitation techniques		
HR	Limb brought to end range, patient holds position against practitioner's resistance	Autonomic inhibition: Golgi tendon organ inhibits agonist, allowing for greater lengthening
CR	Same as HR but practitioner holds against patient's resistance	Reciprocal inhibition: relaxation of agonist as antagonist contracts (reflex loop mediated by muscle spindle)
HRAC	Same as HR with active contraction of agonist muscle to achieve greater ROM	Same as HR
CRAC	Contraction of antagonist, followed by contraction of agonist to achieve greater ROM	Same as CR
Ballistic stretching	Dynamic rapid bouncing motion initiated by antagonist muscle to the muscle being stretched	Elicits stretch reflex; associated with high rates of muscle soreness and injury
Active isolated stretching	Repetitive contractions of the antagonist using extremity positions to isolate different aspects of the agonist	Acts to inhibit elicitation of stretch reflex

CR = contract-relax; CRAC = contract-relax agonist contract; HR = hold-relax; HRAC = hold-relax agonist contract; ROM = range of motion.

Active isolated stretching (AIS), a relatively new stretching technique, relies on many of the same principles as PNF.[103] As the hamstring muscle is stretched, secondary to the contracting quadriceps, the muscle spindle Ia afferents are excited, which results in excitation of the alpha motor neurons, which in turn results in hamstring contraction. If adequate flexibility is not available for a movement, then the stretch reflex exerts force against that movement. This results in additional energy being required to overcome the stretch reflex, thus increasing the likelihood of injury. AIS routines are "based on a continued program of flexibility that avoids the activation of this defense mechanism."[103] Additionally, stretching exercises increase the ability of the tissues to lengthen, enabling joints to move through a greater range before meeting resistance from tension and muscle contraction activated by the stretch reflex. Research confirming the ability to neutralize the stretch reflex and thus achieve greater range through the use of AIS is not yet forthcoming.

Newham and Lederman[104] examined mediation of the stretch reflex using manual therapy techniques. Changes in the excitability of the stretch reflex have been reported after a voluntary contraction of the muscle, but there is no consensus as to what mediates this change. Four possible explanations for the mechanism are mechanical viscoelastic changes to the receptors of surrounding connective tissue, history of previous muscle activity resulting in weakly engaged intrafusal cross-bridges, increase in temporal and spatial summation from proprioceptors, and central influences depressing motor neuron excitability. Whether any of these mechanisms is responsible for the success of AIS cannot be determined as there is little more than anecdotal evidence to support the theory.

Avela et al.[95] tested the effect of prolonged and repeated passive stretching on the triceps surae muscle on reflex sensitivity. They theorized that repetitive passive stretching would result in a direct fatigue effect on the muscle spindle. Their results suggest that repeated passive stretching of a muscle renders it more compliant, resulting in an impaired external force response of the muscle to stretch that leads to reduced stretch response of the muscle spindle.

Another explanation for ROM improvements seen after stretching is found in the phenomenon termed *thixotropy*. Thixotropy refers to the stiffness of a material based on its immediate past use.[89,104] Possibly, connective tissue is in a gel state caused by cross-bridge stiffness, and movement transforms it into a much more mobile solvent state.[89] Thixotropic theory states that when the movement is discontinued, the tissue returns to its original state.[89] Perhaps the more mobile solvent state lasts long enough to allow the muscle to achieve greater length and thus increase its permanent resting length. AIS may evoke a thixotropic response as it would affect the immediate past use of the tissue because of the repeated antagonistic contractions.

When sufficient flexibility is not present, movement economy suffers as a result of compensatory mechanisms from the surrounding structures acting to achieve normal movement patterns. With limitation of ROM about a joint, one experiences a diminished efficiency when performing functional activities.[105] Surrounding joints compensate for the decreased range, thus disrupting the normal movement pattern. Godges et al.[106] showed that improving hamstring flexibility in individuals demonstrated to have inflexibility resulted in a decrease of inefficient compensations occurring in the joints above and below the pelvis. Subjects had decreased submaximal oxygen consumption while walking at three different work loads after achieving ROM gains through the use of static stretching. It would then follow that improving flexibility about a joint enables restoration of balance to that joint, which, in turn, would allow it to function efficiently and thus restore movement economy to that extremity.[105]

Worrell et al.[85] compared static and PNF stretching of the hamstring muscle to determine if either had any effect on muscle performance. Flexibility gains were made with no difference noted in type of stretch used. Performance increased during isokinetic testing after flexibility had been improved. Unfortunately, the study suffered from low statistical power and large intersubject variations in responses.

JOINT MOBILIZATION AND MANIPULATION

Manual mobilization and manipulative techniques are used extensively in the treatment of vertebral and extra-

vertebral joint dysfunction. Mennell[107] first described the etiology of joint dysfunction as being a loss in the mechanical play within a synovial joint, producing pain and dysfunction through structural compensation. Mechanical joint play is the short, rectilinear, passive movement between bones that cannot be produced independently by volitional movement.[108] The loss of arthrokinematic motion or joint play results in compensatory movement dysfunction that eventually may lead to degradation of the articular joint surfaces, pain, and decreased mobility. The clinician assesses arthrokinematic motion to determine where restrictions may be present and then attempts to correct the restriction by using techniques directed at regaining motion in the direction of the restriction.

Manual therapy is the term used to describe different forms of mobilization techniques that address soft and articular tissue lesions.[109] Joint mobilizations, including traction (separation of joint surfaces) and glides (movement across joint surfaces), occur as a passive movement of varying amplitude performed within or beyond the pathologic limit of motion, but within the anatomic limit and can be prevented by the patient.[108,109] In contrast, a manipulation is small-amplitude, high-velocity thrust performed beyond the limit of available range that cannot be controlled by the patient.[109] These techniques are thought to decrease pain, provide reflex inhibition to muscle, increase circulation, increase nutrition to articular cartilage, and increase mobility.[108,110]

One mechanism by which these techniques are thought to work is by stimulation of articular mechanoreceptors (Table 33-6). Three varieties of mechanoreceptors found within synovial joints (types I, II, and III) function to produce reflexogenic effects, perceptual effects, and pain suppression.[111] The fourth mechanoreceptor (IV) is responsible for nociceptive input and responds to abnormally high stresses and chemical irritants within the tissue.[111]

TABLE 33-6
Articular Mechanoreceptors

Type	Location/Behavior	Response	Function
I	Superficial layers of joint capsule; tonic reflexogenic effects	Postural and kinesthetic sensation; low threshold, slow adapting	Static and dynamic, inhibition of pain
II	Deep layers of joint capsule; phasic reflexogenic effects	Dynamic sensation; low threshold, fast adapting	Dynamic, inhibition of pain
III	Deep and superficial layers of ligaments	Dynamic sensation, slow adapting; responds to stretch at end range	Dynamic, reflex inhibition of muscle tone
IV	Free unmyelinated nerve endings in joint capsule, blood vessels, articular fat pads	High threshold, nonadapting; responds to deforming stretch, abnormal tissue metabolites	Nociceptive mechanoreceptors; pain provoking

Manual therapy in general has not been studied scientifically.[112] The exception to this is in the use of mobilizations and manipulations in the treatment of low back pain. A review of the literature in this area reveals mixed results. Terret et al.[113] attempted to demonstrate pain inhibition using manipulation in healthy subjects. They received 60 Hz of interrupted direct current to determine individual pain thresholds. One-half of the subjects were then treated with manipulation, while the other half were not. Those having manipulation demonstrated significantly higher pain thresholds on subsequent delivery of the 60-Hz direct current than those who did not. Sherkelle et al.[114] reviewed the efficacy of spinal manipulation in treating low back pain. They determined that it was an appropriate short-term treatment in acute low back pain but was inconclusive for chronic pain. Pope et al.,[97] in a prospective randomized trial, compared the treatment of low back pain using spinal manipulation, transcutaneous muscle stimulation, massage, and corsets. After the 3-week trial, the manipulation group showed the greatest improvements in flexion range and pain reduction, the massage group had the best extension effort and least fatigue, whereas the muscle stimulation group had the best extension range. There were no significant differences between groups with regard to physical outcome measures (range, strength, fatigue, and pain). Interestingly, the authors considered the massage group to act as a placebo, even though this group did demonstrate improvement. The authors also expected the group treated with corsets to show significant decreases in ROM, but this did not occur either. Farrell et al.[112] reviewed several studies, concluding that manipulation, mobilization, or both produce significant reduction in acute back pain and accelerate the recovery process; the effect of these techniques on chronic symptoms was not determined.

The same investigators considered treatment of low back pain without neurologic signs by comparing two groups (n = 48) that received conservative treatments of passive mobilization, manipulation, diathermy, ergonomic assessment, and isometric abdominal exercises. The group receiving the manipulation and mobilization techniques demonstrated shorter recovery times in fewer sessions than groups receiving the other treatments. Treatment in general was noted to be the single most important factor in predicting recovery time in both patient groups.

Nwuga[115] studied the effects of spinal mobilizations in a group of subjects suffering from back pain for 2 weeks or less. All subjects had evidence of unilateral disk protrusion and nerve root compression. Subjects treated with two lumbar mobilization techniques showed better outcomes than a control group that received short-wave diathermy and flexion exercises.

In summary, it appears that manipulation and mobilization of the low back are of some value and have their greatest beneficial effect when applied in the acute and subacute stages of the disorder. Much more research is needed in this area as the type of manual therapy and outcome measurements used were not consistent across studies.

Another purported benefit of joint mobilization techniques is the application of Wolff's law, which states that the internal architecture of bone changes in response to stresses applied to it. Mobilization stresses load-bearing joints across the bone as well as the articular cartilage, joint capsule, and accompanying ligaments.[116,117] These stresses are known to be important for the maintenance of the structural integrity of the joint involved.[117] Immobilization of these structures has profound effects, causing deterioration of cartilage through deprivation of nutrients, weakening tendon and ligament attachment sites, inducing muscular atrophy and inhibition, fostering contracture of the joint capsule, and enabling osteoporotic changes in the involved bone.[116,117] Joint mobilizations may provide the necessary stimulus to counteract the negative sequelae.[2,108]

Wilson et al.[118] examined the ability of manual therapy techniques to stimulate bone metabolism and induce changes in the internal architecture of bone as well as maintenance of bone mass. The animal-based study revealed that manual levered bending techniques were associated with creation of levels of compressive strain that might be sufficient to induce osteogenesis in 3-year-old sheep.

The importance of movement and weight-bearing to the health of articular cartilage has been well documented.[119] The avascular extracellular matrix of cartilage receives its nutrition by being bathed in synovial fluid. Synovial fluid cannot pass through the chondrosynovial membrane when a joint is passive. Movement causes a decrease in the viscosity of the synovial fluid, thereby increasing the flow of nutrients from the synovial fluid into the extracellular matrix.[120] Mobilization, or more specifically, compression and distraction of the joint surfaces, may provide the necessary loading and movement needed to maintain the health of the articular cartilage in an otherwise immobilized joint.

Articular cartilage is not the only structure to be adversely affected by joint immobilization. The changes that result from insufficient stresses placed on the connective tissue of the joint capsule are similar to those seen in acute injury.[2] Common connective tissue changes include lower water content and increased cross-linkage between fibers resulting in significantly more joint stiffness and lessened ability of tissues to adapt to stresses.[2,117] The ensuing sequelae result in shortening in the joint capsule and decreased ROM. Joint mobilizations are commonly employed to address joint stiffness by breaking fiber cross-linkage and inducing plastic deformation of the connective tissue with the goal of changing the length of the connective tissue.[2,108] The forces needed to produce these changes need to be safe, effective, reproducible, and of sufficient magnitude.[2] To date, little research has documented the actual forces needed or produced during manual therapy techniques, whether cross-fiber friction, massage, stretching, or joint manipulation/mobilization.

CONCLUSION

It may be true that as the fervent debate regarding the effects of massage, stretching, and joint mobilization continues, the suggestion that the outcome of a treatment is frequently influenced by nonmeasurable factors such as the mind-body connection, subtle healing energies, and interaction between the patient and the therapist should be noted.[4] However, the paucity of objective evidence-based research regarding manual modalities raises questions about the efficacy and physiological basis of employing such treatments. This is not to say that such treatments should be eliminated; yet, in today's cost-conscious health care environment the time invested in treating patients with these modalities as compared with the functional outcome of the treatment must be considered.

REFERENCES

1. Injeyan HS, Fraser IH, Peek WD. Basics of Soft Tissue Examination. In WI Hammer (ed), Functional Soft Tissue Examination and Treatment by Manual Methods: New Perspectives (2nd ed). Gaithersburg, MD: Aspen, 1999;13–31.

2. Threlkeld JA. The effects of manual therapy on connective tissue. Phys Ther 1992;72:61–70.

3. Salva SG. Massage Therapy: Principles and Practice. Philadelphia: WB Saunders, 1999.

4. Cassar MP. Handbook of Massage Therapy. Oxford: Butterworth–Heinemann, 1999.

5. Goats GC. Massage—the scientific basis of an ancient art: part 2. Physiological and therapeutic effects. Br J Sports Med 1994;28:153–156.

6. Prentice WE. Therapeutic Modalities for Allied Health Professionals. New York: McGraw-Hill, 1998.

7. Tappan FM. Healing Massage Techniques: A Study of Eastern and Western Methods. Reston, VA: Reston Publishing, 1980.

8. Werner R. A Massage Therapist's Guide to Pathology. Philadelphia: Lippincott Williams & Wilkins, 1998.

9. Goats GC. Massage—the scientific basis of an ancient art: part 1. The techniques. Br J Sports Med 1994;28:149–152.

10. Beard G, Wood EC. Massage: Principles and Techniques. Philadelphia: WB Saunders, 1964.

11. Cyriax J, Russell G. Textbook of Orthopedic Medicine, Vol 2 (10th ed). Baltimore: Williams & Wilkins, 1980;15–21.

12. Cafarelli E, Flint F. The role of massage in preparation for and recovery from exercise. An overview. Sports Med 1992;14:1–9.

13. Wakim KG, Martin GM, Terrier JC, et al. The effects of massage on the circulation in normal and paralyzed extremities. Arch Phys Med Rehabil 1949;30:135–144.

14. Ebel A, Wisham LH. Effect of massage on muscle temperature and radiosodium clearance. Arch Phys Med Rehabil 1952;33:399–405.

15. Hansen TI, Kristiansen JH. Effect of massage, short-wave diathermy and ultrasound upon ^{133}Xe disappearance rate from muscle and subcutaneous tissue in the human calf. Scand J Rehabil Med 1973;5:179–182.

16. Wakim KG, Martin GM, Krusen FH. Influence of centripetal rhythmic compression on localized edema of an extremity. Arch Phys Med Rehabil 1955;36:98–103.

17. Hovind H, Nielsen SL. Effect of massage on blood flow in skeletal muscle. Scand J Rehabil Med 1974;6:74–77.

18. Arkko PJ, Pakarinen AJ, Kari-Koskinen O. Effects of whole body massage on serum protein, electrolyte and hormone concentrations, enzyme activities, and hematological parameters. Int J Sports Med 1983;4:265–267.

19. Shoemaker JK, Tiidus PM, Mader R. Failure of manual massage to alter limb blood flow: measures by Doppler ultrasound. Med Sci Sports Exerc 1997;29:610–614.

20. Linde B. Disassociation of insulin absorption and blood flow during massage of a subcutaneous injection site. Diabetes Care 1986;9:570–574.

21. Tiidus PM, Shoemaker JK. Effleurage massage, muscle blood flow and long-term post-exercise strength recovery. Int J Sports Med 1995;16:475–483.

22. Wyper DJ, McNiven DR. Effects of some physiotherapeutic agents on skeletal muscle blood flow. Physiotherapy 1976;62:83–85.

23. Callahan MJ. The role of massage in the management of the athlete: a review. Br J Sports Med 1993;27(1):28–33.

24. Barr JS, Taslitz N. The influence of back massage on autonomic functions. Phys Ther 1970;50:1679–1691.

25. Reed BV, Held JM. Effects of sequential connective tissue massage on autonomic nervous system of middle-aged and elderly adults. Phys Ther 1988;68:1231–1234.

26. Jacobs M. Massage for the relief of pain anatomical and physiological considerations. Phys Ther Rev 1960;40:93–98.

27. Crosman LJ, Chateauvert SR, Weisberg J. The effects of massage to the hamstring muscle group on range of motion. J Orthop Sports Phys Ther 1984;6:168–172.

28. Wiktorsson-Moller M, Oberg B, Ekstrand J, et al. Effects of warming up, massage, and stretching on range of

motion and muscle strength in the lower extremity. Am J Sports Med 1983;11:249–252.

29. Ask N, Oxelbeck U, Lundeberg T, et al. The influence of massage on quadriceps function after exhaustive exercise [Abstract]. Med Sci Sports Exerc 1987;19:53.

30. Viitasalo J, Miemela K, Kaapola R, et al. Warm underwater water-jet massage improves recovery from intense physical exercise. Eur J Appl Physiol 1995;71:431–438.

31. Boone T, Cooper R, Thompson WR. A physiologic evaluation of the sports massage. Athletic Train J Natl Athletic Train Assoc 1991;26:51–54.

32. Harmer PA. The effect of pre-performance massage on stride frequency in sprinters. Athletic Train J Natl Athletic Train Assoc 1991;26:55–59.

33. Drews T, Kreider RB, Drinkard B, et al. Effects of post-event massage therapy on repeated ultra-endurance cycling [Abstract]. Int J Sports Med 1990; 11:407.

34. Fitts RH. Cellular mechanisms of muscle fatigue. Physiol Rev 1994;74:49–94.

35. Howell JN, Chleboun G, Conatser R. Muscle stiffness, strength loss, swelling and soreness following exercise-induced injury in humans. J Physiol 1993;464:183–196.

36. Kuipers H. Exercise-induced muscle damage. Int J Sports Med 1994;15:132–135.

37. Friden J, Leiber RL. Structural and mechanical basis of exercise-induced muscle injury. Med Sci Sports Exerc 1992;24:521–530.

38. Armstrong RB, Warren GL, Warren JA. Mechanisms of exercise-induced muscle fiber injury. Sports Med 1991;12:184–207.

39. Newham DJ, Jones DA, Clarkson PM. Repeated high-force eccentric exercise: effects on muscle pain and damage. J Appl Physiol 1987;63:1381–1386.

40. Tiidus PM. Manual massage and recovery of muscle function following exercise: a literature review. J Orthop Sports Phys Ther 1997;25:107–112.

41. Cafarelli E, Sim J, Carolan B, et al. Vibratory massage and short term recovery from muscular fatigue. Int J Sports Med 1990;11:474–478.

42. Weber MD, Servedio FJ, Woodall WR. The effects of three modalities on delayed onset muscle soreness. J Orthop Sports Phys Ther 1994;20:236–242.

43. Francis KT, Hoobler T. Effects of aspirin on delayed muscle soreness. J Sports Med 1987;27:333–337.

44. Smith LL, Keating MN, Holbert D, et al. The effects of athletic massage on delayed onset muscle soreness, creatine kinase, and neutrophil count: a preliminary report. J Orthop Sports Phys Ther 1994;19:93–99.

45. Weinberg R, Jackson A, Kolodny K. The relationship of massage and exercise to mood enhancement. Sport Psychologist 1988;2:202–211.

46. McNair DM, Lorr M, Droppleman LF. Profile of Mood States Manual. Educational and Industrial Testing Service, San Diego, 1971.

47. Speilberger C, Gorsuch R, Lushene R. State-trait Anxiety Inventory Manual. Consulting Psychologist Press. Palo Alto, CA, 1970.

48. Thayer RE, Measurement through self-report. Psychological Reports 1967;20:663–678.

49. Hemmings B, Smith M, Graydon J, Dyson R. Effects of massage on physiological restoration, perceived recovery and repeated sports performance. Br J Sports Med 2000;34(2):109–114.

50. Licht S (ed). Massage Manipulation and Traction (4th ed). Huntington, NY: Krieger, 1976.

51. Day JA, Mason RR, Chesrown SE. Effect of massage on serum level of beta-endorphin and beta-lipotropin in healthy adults. Phys Ther 1987;67: 926–930.

52. Carr DB, Bullen BA, Skrinar GS, et al. Physical conditioning facilitates the exercise-induced secretion of beta-endorphin and beta-lipotropin in women. N Engl J Med 1981;305:560–563.

53. Gambert SR, Hagen TC, Garthwaite TL, et al. Exercise and the endogenous opioids. N Engl J Med 1981;305:1590–1591.

54. Chapman CR, Benedetti C. Analgesia following transcutaneous electrical stimulation and its partial reversal by a narcotic antagonist. Life Sci 1977;21:1645–1648.

55. Hughes GS Jr, Lichstein PR, Whitlock D, et al. Response of plasma beta-endorphins to transcutaneous electrical nerve stimulation in healthy subjects. Phys Ther 1984;64:1062–1066.

56. Kaada B, Torsteinbo O. Increase of plasma beta-endorphins in connective tissue massage. Gen Pharmacol 1987;20:487–489.

57. Armstrong RB. Mechanisms of exercise-induced delayed onset muscular soreness: a brief review. Med Sci Sports Exerc 1984;16:529–538.

58. Friden J, Sjostrom M, Ekblom B. Myofibrillar damage following intense eccentric exercise in man. Int J Sports Med 1983;4:170–176.

59. Stauber WT. Eccentric action of muscles: physiology, injury and adaptation. In KB Pandolf (ed), Exercise and Sport Sciences Review, Vol 17. Baltimore: Williams & Wilkins, 1989;157–186.

60. Wheat M, McCoy S, Barton E, et al. Hydroxylysine excretion does not indicate collagen damage with downhill running in young men. Int J Sports Med 1989;10:155–160.

61. Gupta S, Goswami A, Sadhukhan AK, et al. Comparative study of lactate removal in short term massage of extremities, active recovery and a passive recovery period after supramaximal exercise sessions. Int J Sports Med 1996;17:106–110.

62. Rodenburg JB, Steenbeck D, Schiereck P, et al. Warm-up, stretching and massage diminish harmful effects of eccentric exercise. Int J Sports Med 1994;15:414–419.

63. Hortobagyi T, Deneham T. Variability in creatine kinase: methodological, exercise and clinically related factors. Int J Sports Med 1989;10:69–80.

64. Rodenburg JB, Bar PR, De Boer RW. Relations between muscle soreness and biochemical and functional outcomes of eccentric exercise. J Appl Physiol 1993;74:2976–2983.

65. Rodenburg JB, De Boer RW, Jeneson JA, et al. 31P-MRS and simultaneous quantification of dynamic human quadriceps exercise in a whole body MR scanner. J Appl Physiol 1994;77:1021–1029.

66. Wenos JZ, Brilla LR, Morrison MJ. Effect of massage on delayed onset muscle soreness. Med Sci Sports Exerc 1990;22:S34.

67. Quillen WS, Magee DJ, Zachazewski JE. The Process of Athletic Injury and Rehabilitation. In JE Zachazewski, DJ Magee, WS Quillen (eds), Athletic Injuries and Rehabilitation. Philadelphia: WB Saunders, 1996;3–7.

68. Cyriax J. Deep Massage and Manipulation Illustrated. London: Hoeber, 1944.

69. Chamberlain GJ. Cyriax's friction massage: a review. J Orthop Sports Phys Ther 1982;4:16–22.

70. Walker JM. Deep transverse frictions in ligament healing. J Orthop Sports Phys Ther 1984;6:89–94.

71. Davidson CJ, Ganion LR, Gehlsen GM, et al. Rat tendon morphologic and functional changes resulting from soft tissue mobilization. Med Sci Sports Exerc 1997;29(3):313–319.

72. Gehlsen GM, Ganion LR, Helfst R. Fibroblast responses to variation in soft tissue mobilization pressure. Med Sci Sports Exerc 1999;31:531–535.

73. Gross M. Chronic tendinitis: pathomechanics of injury, factors affecting the healing response, and treatment. J Orthop Sports Phys Ther 1992;16:248–261.

74. Leadbetter W. Cell-matrix response in tendon injury. Clin Sports Med 1992;11:533–577.

75. Sullivan SJ, Williams LRT, Seaborne DE, et al. Effects of massage on alpha motor neuron excitability. Phys Ther 1991;71:555–560.

76. Sullivan MK, Dejulia JJ, Worrell TW. Effects of pelvic position and stretching method on hamstring muscle flexibility. Med Sci Sports Exerc 1992;24:1383–1389.

77. Goldberg J, Seaborne DE, Sullivan SJ, et al. The effect of therapeutic massage on H-reflex amplitude in persons with a spinal cord injury. Phys Ther 1994;74:728–737.

78. Goldberg J, Sullivan SJ, Seaborne DE. The effect of two intensities of massage on H-reflex amplitude. Phys Ther 1992;72:449–457.

79. Morelli M, Seaborne DE, Sullivan SJ. Changes in H-reflex amplitude during massage of the triceps surae in healthy subjects. J Orthop Sports Phys Ther 1990;12:55–59.

80. Morelli M, Seaborne DE, Sullivan SJ. H-reflex modulation during manual muscle massage of human triceps surae. Arch Phys Med Rehabil 1991;72:915–919.

81. Morelli M, Chapman CE, Sullivan SJ. Do cutaneous receptors contribute to the changes in the amplitude of the H-reflex during massage? Electromyogr Clin Neurophysiol 1999;39:441–447.

82. Travell J. Ethyl chloride spray for painful muscle spasm. Arch Phys Med Rehabil 1952;33:291–298.

83. Kroll PG, Raya MA. Hamstring muscles: an overview of anatomy, biomechanics and function, injury etiology, treatment, and prevention. Crit Rev Phys Rehabil Med 1997;9:191–203.

84. Malone TR, Garrett WE, Zachazewski JE. Muscle: Deformation, Injury, Repair. In JE Zachazewski, DJ Magee, WS Quillen (eds), Athletic Injuries and Rehabilitation. Philadelphia: WB Saunders, 1996;71–91.

85. Worrell TW, Perrin DH. Hamstring muscle injury: the influence of strength, flexibility, warm-up, and fatigue. J Orthop Sports Phys Ther 1992;16.

86. Wallin D, Ekblom B, Grahn R, et al. Improvement of muscle flexibility: a comparison between two techniques. Am J Sports Med 1985;13:263–268.

87. Zachazewski JE. Improving Flexibility. In RM Scully, MR Barnes (eds), Physical Therapy. Philadelphia: JB Lippincott, 1989;698–738.

88. Cyriax JH, Cyriax PJ. Illustrated Manual of Orthopaedic Medicine. London: Butterworth, 1984;1–26.

89. Carey JR, Burghardt TP. Movement dysfunction following central nervous system lesions: a problem of neurologic or muscular impairment? Phys Ther 1993;73:538–547.

90. Muir IW, Chesworth BM, Vandervoort AA. Effect of a static calf-stretching exercise on the resistive torque during passive ankle dorsiflexion in healthy subjects. J Orthop Sports Phys Ther 1999;29:106–115.

91. Etnyre BR, Abraham LD. H-reflex changes during static stretching and two variations of proprioceptive neuromuscular facilitation techniques. Electromyogr Neurophysiol 1986;86:174–179.

92. Brooks VB. Motor control: how posture and movements are governed. Phys Ther 1983;63:664–673.

93. Voss DE, Ionta MK, Myers BJ. Proprioceptive Neuromuscular Facilitation (3rd ed). Philadelphia: Harper & Row, 1985;1–8.

94. Condon SM, Hutton RS. Soleus muscle electromyographic activity and ankle dorsiflexion range of motion during four stretching procedures. Phys Ther 1987;67:24–30.

95. Avela J, Heikki K, Komi PV. Altered reflex sensitivity after repeated and prolonged passive muscle stretching. J Appl Physiol 1999;86:1283–1291.

96. Osternig LR, Robertson RN, Troxel RK, et al. Differential responses to proprioceptive neuromuscular facilitation (PNF) stretch techniques. Med Sci Sports Exerc 1990;22:298–307.

97. Pope MH, Phillips RB, Haugh LD, et al. A prospective randomized three-week trial of spinal manipulation, transcutaneous muscle stimulation, massage and corset in the treatment of subacute low back pain. Spine 1994;19:2571–2577.

98. Bandy WD, Irion JM. The effect of time on static stretch on the flexibility of the hamstring muscles. Phys Ther 1994;74:845–850, discussion 850–852.

99. Webright WG, Randolph BJ, Perrin DH. Comparison of nonballistic active knee extension in neural slump position and static stretch techniques on hamstring flexibility. J Orthop Sports Phys Ther 1997;26:7–12.

100. Zito M, Driver D, Parker C, Bohannon R. Lasting effects of one bout of two 15-second passive stretches on ankle dorsiflexion range of motion. J Orthop Sports Phys Ther 1997;26:214–221.

101. Gajdosik RL. Effects of static stretching on the maximal length and resistance to passive stretch of short hamstring muscles. J Orthop Sports Phys Ther 1991;14:250–255.

102. Lamotagne A, Malouin F, Richards CL. Viscoelastic behavior of plantar flexor muscle-tendon unit at rest. J Orthop Sports Phys Ther 1997;26:244–252.

103. Mattes AL. Active Isolated Stretching. Sarasota, FL: Mattes, 1995.

104. Newham DJ, Lederman E. Effect of manual therapy techniques on the stretch reflex in normal human quadriceps. Disabil Rehabil 1997;19:326–331.

105. Lakie M, Robson LG. Thixotropy: the effect of stimulation in frog muscle. Q J Exp Physiol 1988;73:627–630.

106. Godges JJ, MacRae H, Longdon C, et al. The effects of two stretching procedures on hip range of motion and gait economy. J Orthop Sports Phys Ther 1989;10:350–357.

107. Mennell JM. Joint Pain Diagnosis and Treatment Using Manipulative Techniques. Boston: Little, Brown, 1964;1–30.

108. Kaltenborn FM. Manual Mobilization of the Extremity Joints: Basic Examination and Treatment Techniques (4th ed). Oslo, Norway: Olaf Norlis Bokhandel, 1989;1–48.

109. Di Fabio RP. Efficacy of manual therapy. Phys Ther 1992;72:21–32.

110. Ombregt L, Bisschop P, ter Veer HJ, et al. A System of Orthopaedic Medicine. London: WB Saunders, 1995;3–71.

111. Wyke BD. Articular Neurology and Manipulative Therapy. In EF Glasgow, LT Twomey, ER Scull, et al. (eds), Aspects of Manipulative Therapy (2nd ed). Edinburgh: Churchill Livingstone, 1985;72–77.

112. Farrell J, Twomey L. Acute low back pain comparison of two conservative treatment approaches. Med J Australia 1982;20:160–164.

113. Terret ACJ, Vernon H. A controlled study of the effect of spinal manipulation on paraspinal cutaneous pain tolerance levels. Am J Phys Med 1984;63:217–225.

114. Sherkelle P, Adams A, Chassin M, et al. Spinal manipulation in low back pain. Ann Intern Med 1992;117:590–598.

115. Nwuga VCB. Relative therapeutic efficacy of vertebral manipulation and conventional treatment in back pain management. Am J Phys Med 1982;61:273–278.

116. Loitz-Ramage BJ, Zernicke RF. Bone Biology and Mechanics. In JE Zachazewski, DJ Magee, WS Quillen (eds), Athletic Injuries and Rehabilitation. Philadelphia: WB Saunders, 1996;99–117.

117. Woo SL-Y, Maynard J, Butler D, et al. Ligament, Tendon, and Joint Capsule Insertions to Bone. In SL-Y Woo, JA Buckwalter (eds), Injury and Repair of the Musculoskeletal Soft Tissues (2nd ed). Park Ridge, IL: American Academy of Orthopedic Surgeons, 1991;133–166.

118. Wilson AW, Davies HMS, Edwards GA, et al. Can some physical therapy and manual techniques generate potentially osteogenic levels of strain within mammalian bone? Phys Ther 1999;79:931–938.

119. Buckwalter J, Rosenberg L, Coutts R, et al. Articular Cartilage: Injury and Repair. In SL-Y Woo, JA Buckwalter (eds), Injury and Repair of the Musculoskeletal Soft Tissues (2nd ed). Park Ridge, IL: American Academy of Orthopedic Surgeons, 1991;465–482.

120. Mow V, Rosenwasser M. Articular Cartilage: Biomechanics. In SL-Y Woo, JA Buckwalter (eds), Injury and Repair of the Musculoskeletal Soft Tissues (2nd ed). Park Ridge, IL: American Academy of Orthopedic Surgeons, 1991;427–463.

34

Complementary Therapies in Rehabilitation

CAROL M. DAVIS

"Rehabilitation medicine is the area of specialty concerned with the management of patients with impairments of function due to disease or trauma." So begins the preface of the previous edition of this text. With the advent of the new millennium, the practice of medicine and health care, especially rehabilitation of chronic illness, has changed. Inclusion of this chapter reflects one of the most dramatic changes—the increasing prevalence of patients seeking complementary therapies for acute and chronic illness, and the increasing numbers of rehabilitation professionals practicing holistic therapies. This chapter describes the nature of this movement in health care, explores more fully what is meant by *mind/ body* health care, explains (as comprehensively as the author dares) the science that suggests the theories that seem to account for what we observe, and provides reports of the best evidence for efficacy.

Complementary and holistic therapies do not lend themselves to study by the randomized controlled trial. When we stray from the reductionist model, we open ourselves to harsh criticism and accusations of practicing quackery or witchcraft. And it is true that the theory on which holistic approaches are based cannot be proven with traditional science. But science never stands still, and some of the most frequent and compelling events in health care today (e.g., spontaneous regression of space-invading tumors, near death experiences, and medical intuition) fall outside the explanations offered by traditional Newtonian Cartesian thought. Theory is only adequate when it admits few exceptions. All theories have exceptions that cannot be explained, but when the exceptions become more prevalent and relevant, theory must be revisited, expanded, and altered. From the dialectic that is framed, a higher level of synthesis should emerge and a new, more encompassing theory created. We are living through such a time today, and for many in rehabilitation, it is very exciting.

The scientific paradigm for evaluating traditional systems of health has been called into question and a search has begun, including an important endeavor by the United States National Institutes of Health, to identify and develop methodologies that, according to the mission statement of the NIH's Office of Alternative Medicine (now the Center for Complementary and Alternative Medicine) "respect the paradigms" of traditional (holistic) medicine.[1]

HOLISTIC HEALTH

The World Health Organization defined *holistic approaches to care* as provision of care wherein people "are viewed in totality within a wide ecological spectrum, and emphasizes the view that ill health or disease is brought about by an imbalance, or disequilibrium, of a person in his or her total ecological system and not only by the causative agent and pathogenic evolution."[2] The totality of the person is often referred to in holistic health care as incorporating four quadrants of need and function: (1) the *physical* (traditionally the body and movement), (2) the *intellectual* (the brain and the mind), (3) the *emotional* (referring to feelings), and (4) the *spiritual* (referring to the eternal questions such as, "Who am I?" and "Why have I lived?" and "What am I to do?"). How one then applies these functions while interrelating in the world refers to the *social* aspect of need and function. In rehabilitation, we focus on helping heal disorders of function that are primarily physical, but are strongly influenced by the intellectual, emotional, and spiritual quadrants. One who practices holistically questions the patient in such a way, most pointedly while taking the history, that brings to the surface problems and unmet needs in all four areas, and then advocates to see that all those needs are addressed.

In the main, complementary and alternative therapies can be termed *holistic* and focus on using to advantage the inextricable link between mind and body. These therapies are administered in an effort to help the person get well and stay healthy by facilitating the flow of a person's human energy or *ch'i*. Holistic theory posits that when human energy is balanced and flowing freely, it contributes to homeostasis, but when blocked, it interferes with health and renders the body and mind together vulnerable to pathogens or biochemical imbalance. Blocks to ch'i can occur from disruptions in each of the four quadrants of function. Ideally, once a block in homeostasis occurs, we would be able to detect it and reverse it without the need for medications or major interventions. And this does, indeed, happen. Evidence that people often heal themselves is the basis for the traditional double-blind, placebo-based clinical trial.

In 1993, Eisenberg[3] published a study of 1,539 adults. One-third reported that they had used at least one alternative therapy in the previous year. Middle-aged (25–49) respondents were most apt to use unconventional medicine. The most frequent complaints for which alternative therapies were used are of special interest to rehabilitation—headaches, back problems, anxiety, and depression. Therapies most often used included chiropractic, relaxation, imagery, and self-help groups. Seventy-two percent of the respondents did not inform their physicians that they were using these therapies. Of the $14 billion spent for alternative therapies, an estimated $10 billion was paid out of pocket. Although this study reported data collected in 1989, it is likely that an increasing proportion of patients will seek alternative and complementary therapies. The use of complementary therapies is widespread in the United States, but even more prevalent in Europe and Asia. In 1994, Fisher and Ward[4] reported between 20% and 50% of Europeans use complementary therapies; in the Netherlands and Belgium, use was as high as 60%, and in Great Britain, 74% of subjects questioned were willing to pay extra for insurance that covered complementary therapies.[5] Astin proposed that a majority of people seeking alternative therapies did so largely because these therapies are more aligned with "their

own values, beliefs, and philosophical orientations toward health and life."[6] Krauss et al. reported the use of alternative health care by individuals with physical disabilities[7]:

> More of this sample of individuals with physical disabilities than a randomized, national sample of the general population used alternative therapies (51.1% vs. 34%) and saw providers of those therapies (22% vs. 10%). Alternative therapies were chosen more often than conventional therapies by those with physical disabilities for pain (51.8% vs. 33.9%), depression (33.9% vs. 25%), anxiety (42.1% vs. 13.1%), insomnia (32.2% vs. 16.1%), and headaches (51.4% vs. 18.9%).

Thus, an increasingly larger number of people are turning to holistic approaches. Micozzi stated:

> I have likened the recent "discovery" of alternative medicine to Columbus' discovery of the Americas. Although his voyage was a great feat that expanded the intellectual frontiers of Europe, Columbus could not really discover a world already known to millions of indigenous people who enjoyed complex systems of social organization and subsistence activities. Likewise, the definitional statement that alternatives are "not within the existing US health care system" is a curious observation for the millions of Americans who routinely use them today.[8]

In 1992 the National Institutes of Health (NIH) created the Office of Alternative Medicine. Although roadblocks and criticisms from the prevailing science bias against alternative and complementary approaches made the initial 2 years of maintaining this office quite difficult,[9] in 1999 the office was upgraded to a full-fledged center, renamed the *Center for Complementary and Alternative Medicine*, and is now funding research at several medical centers. In 1997, a panel convened by the NIH held a consensus conference on the use of acupuncture and, among its results, was the directive for third-party payers to reimburse for use of acupuncture that achieved the level of scrutiny reported in the articles that were reviewed, and called for further research investigating what is termed as the *flow of body energy*, or *qi* or *ch'i*.[10]

The eastern concept of ch'i is reminiscent of the *vitalist* principle, an idea that has come and gone in western science, that people have a flow of energy.[11] The theory is rejected by most traditional scientists who espouse the seventeenth century mechanistic, linear philosophies of Decartes and Newton, termed the *new science*. The notion of a continuity between psyche and soma reflected in vitalism was deemed too interrelated with theology to be acceptable. Indeed, it did not serve the common good to use the rationale, for example, that God was purposely punishing those who died of bubonic plague and sparing those who did not.[11] Today's prevailing paradigm of science remains locked into the 200-year-old reductionistic model. Nonetheless, a shift is occurring toward the unmistakable unity of the mind and body. Health care would be wise to take this into account to be maximally responsible to those it serves. Facilitating the flow of human energy is the hallmark of most complementary and alternative therapies. Investigating the concept of bioenergies, biomicroelectropotentials, and energy *fields* of consciousness is predicated on the idea that consciousness might be causal. Researchers in the area of distance healing studies maintain that one (or many) can bring about change (e.g., healing) by the effort of directing attention or directing conscious thought to that change.[12-17] The rather substantial body of evidence on the effects of prayer on healing speaks to this issue.[12]

WHAT ARE COMPLEMENTARY AND ALTERNATIVE THERAPIES?

Complementary and alternative therapies are nontraditional interventions that can be administered either as a substitute to (alternative to) traditional allopathic therapies or in conjunction with (complementary with) traditional therapies. They can be classified as *systems*, *approaches*, or *techniques* within approaches.[18] Examples of health care *systems* include chiropractic, Ayurveda, traditional Chinese medicine, homeopathy, and naturopathy. Within systems are found *approaches* such as acupuncture and acupressure, qi gong, yoga, herbal remedies, myofascial release, craniosacral therapy, Rolfing, Pilates, Rosen method, Hellerwork, soma, Alexander technique, Feldenkrais Awareness through Movement and Functional Integration, neuromuscular therapy, and reflexology. Even more basic is a *technique within an approach*, such as auricular acupuncture, found within the system of traditional Chinese medicine, and the approach of acupuncture; transcendental meditation and sesame seed oil massage, both found within the system of Ayurveda, can also be classified in this category. Although today it is out of date, one of the first categorizations of holistic approaches was found in *The Chantilly Report of the NIH*,[19] which listed the following categories of alternative therapies in 1992. (The interested reader is directed

to the extended list of references in this document for specifics on the research completed on each of these therapies at the time of that publication. For more recent research on many of these therapies, refer to Spencer and Jacobs' text, *Complementary/Alternative Medicine—An Evidenced Based Approach*.)[20]

- Alternative systems of medical practice (70–90% of all health care worldwide): Popular health care, community-based care, professionalized health care, traditional oriental medicine (including acupuncture and Ayurveda), homeopathy, anthroposophically extended medicine (elements of homeopathy and naturopathy), naturopathic medicine[19,20]
- Mind-body interventions: psychotherapy, support groups, meditation, imagery, hypnosis, biofeedback, dance and music therapies, art therapy, prayer, mental healing[19,20]
- Bioelectromagnetics application to medicine: thermal applications of nonionizing radiation; radiofrequency hyperthermia, laser and radiofrequency surgery, and radiofrequency diathermy; nonthermal applications of nonionizing radiation for bone repair; nerve stimulation; wound healing[19,20]
- Manual healing methods: touch; manipulation; osteopathy; chiropractics; massage therapy; biofield therapeutics including healing touch, noncontact therapeutic touch, and specific human energy nexus therapy—a biofield method of treating psychosomatic disorders by releasing repressed and suppressed debilitating emotions[19]
- Pharmacologic and biological treatments (medications and vaccines not accepted in 1992 by mainstream medicine): antineo-plastons (peptide fractions originally derived from normal human blood and urine and thought to be a natural form of anticancer protection), cartilage products, chelation therapy (using ethylenediaminetetraacetic acid), the highly controversial immunoaugmentative therapy (experimental form of cancer immunotherapy consisting of daily injections of processed blood products designed to rid the body of proteins that prevent the patient's immune system from detecting the cancer), 714-X (a mixture of camphor and nitrogen designed to turn cancer cells deficient in nitrogen into normal cells), Coley's toxins (a mixture of killed cultures of bacteria designed to improve the immune systems of patients with cancer, no longer in use in the United States but used in China and Germany), MTH-68 (a modified attenuated strain of the Newcastle's disease virus of chickens, harmless to humans but shown in randomized controlled trials with placebo to exhibit promise

for cancer patients), neural therapy (injection of local anesthetics into autonomic ganglia, peripheral nerves, scars, glands, acupuncture points, and trigger points for pain control), apiotherapy (medicinal use of various products of the common honeybee for alleviating chronic pain, inflammation, and symptoms of neurologic disease), iscador (liquid extract from the mistletoe plant used to treat tumors), biologically guided chemotherapy[19]

- Herbal medicines: folk remedies that rely on botanical knowledge of the effects of herbs on the body/mind[19,20]

- Diet and nutrition for the prevention of chronic disease, including Dean Ornish's program and the Pritikin plan[19,20]

An overview of the most prevalent contemporary interventions used in rehabilitation follows.

ALTERNATIVE SYSTEMS OF MEDICAL PRACTICE

Traditional Chinese Medicine

Acupuncture, Acupressure, and Laser Acupuncture

Acupuncture is perhaps the oldest holistic approach. Archeological findings suggest the possibility that the early roots of acupuncture date from the primitive Stone Age clan society in ancient China, where people used sharpened stones for medical purposes 5,000 years ago. "Acupuncture is the insertion of slender, sterile needles into specific anatomic locations at specific angles and depths to influence the flow of ch'i, or a vital force in the body, thereby assisting the body to self-regulate or adjust, promoting circulation and healing and reducing pain."[21] These specific anatomic locations, or acupuncture points, lie along pathways, or *meridians*, and respond not only to needles, but also to pressure and to neuroprobe stimulus and laser. Twenty pathways are charted: 12 regular meridians or channels that correlate to and connect with an organ, and eight extra meridians. Meridian channels are energetic pathways that flow through fascia and connective tissue, although no Western anatomic verification of these pathways exists. Just as an air travel route from New York to Paris exists on charts, one cannot find any representation in nature that verifies its existence. Acupuncture is one small part of the practice of traditional Chinese medicine, based on a theory of the causes of disease, nutrition and lifestyle, diagnosis of symptoms,

and the therapeutic effect of herbs.[21] Acupuncture is one of the most researched and documented holistic therapies used for a variety of illnesses, especially useful in the presence of pain. An estimated 137 randomized clinical trials on 10 painful conditions have been reported, providing evidence, although not statistically conclusive, of the efficacy of acupuncture in patients with osteoarthritis, fibromyalgia, back pain, tennis elbow, painful menstruation, and migraine headaches.[22]

Polarity

Developed by Randolph Stone, naturopath, chiropractor, and osteopath, in the mid-1900s, polarity is also based on the concept of a flow of energy along pathways or meridians that can be influenced by a transfer of energy from the practitioner.[23] Polarity makes special mention that the practitioner must come to the treatment centered and balanced in his or her own energy. Polarity therapy views energy as flowing from positive to negative. The purpose of polarity manipulation is to locate blocked energy and release it. The techniques of polarity therapy involve bipolar contacts: A positive contact (right-hand finger) pushes energy and is stimulating, whereas a negative contact (left-hand finger) is relaxing and receiving energy.[23]

Jin Shin Do

A form of acupressure, jin shin do was developed in the 1970s by psychotherapist Iona Marsaa Teeguarden.[24] It is a combination of an ancient Japanese self-help technique, traditional Chinese medicine, and body-oriented psychology as practiced by Wilhelm Reich and Alexander Lowen. Reich was one of the first psychotherapists to touch his patients for assessment, and he described a form of muscle holding that accompanies an unbearable excess of emotion that he termed *armorings*. For example, for some patients, holding the breath and pulling up the shoulders become an automatic defensive response. To release tension from the armorings, the jin shin do practitioner tries to establish a safe place where the recipient can dare to feel and, with gentle, specific touch, become aware again and relive the original feeling in slow motion to the intensity that he or she desires. Then the patient has an obvious choice, whether to modify or continue with the reaction, whichever feels appropriate.[25] Soft touch or pressure with the fingertips is applied to acupressure points along the meridians, focusing on parts of the body with an excess of energy with the goal of releasing undesired blocked energy, restoring balance to body, mind, and spirit. As with other holistic energy techniques, practitioners are required to take good care of themselves, balance and center their energy, and use compassion, honesty, empathy, and a willingness to be honestly present with all qualities and deficits.[25] Therapists learn to avoid the common tendency to want to *fix* patients and replace that feeling with the role of amplifying catalyst, simply supporting redistribution of blocked energy, releasing muscular tension, and helping to free the flow of qi. This, in turn, opens emotions and supports natural healing.[25] Publications on the efficacy of this treatment in rehabilitation are not found.

Herbal Treatment

Homeopathy Based on the principle of like treats like and first reported in ancient Greek medicine, homeopathy was developed into a practice by physician Samuel Hahnemann (1755–1843). Natural remedies were developed from plant, animal, and mineral tinctures that induced similar symptoms as that of the disease manifested. Water-based solutions are prepared by soaking the plant or other substance in pure alcohol, and then placing a drop of the solution into either a 1 to 10 or 1 to 100 ratio of distilled water. Successive dilutions of one drop of each proceeding solution is placed into a fresh container. The water molecule appears to hold a memory of the substance, even when dilutions have diminished the chance that any of the active substance remains.[26,27] Homeopathic practitioners believe that they are preserving and magnifying the energetic signature or frequency of the substance in the dilution process. They maintain that they are matching the *vibrational properties* of the remedy to the vibrational properties of the symptom complex. Research evaluating the efficacy of homeopathy, widely reported in the literature, has been evaluated as *weak* by traditional scientific standards.[20,28]

Naturopathy Naturopathy is more than a system of health care; it is a way of life.[29] It traces its roots back thousands of years to the Hippocratic school of medicine, circa 400 BC. Benedict Lust is credited with bringing naturopathy to the United States from Germany in 1896 and founding the first school of naturopathy in New York City. The 4-year training includes education in hydrotherapy, botanical medicine, nutritional therapy, psychology, homeopathy, manual manipulative techniques, and some principles of physical therapy. Naturopathic physicians are trained and licensed as primary care providers with preparation in prevention and natural therapeutics, as well as diagnosing, managing, and treating chronic degenerative disease. The key principle is a system for curing disease based on a "return to nature in regulating the diet, breathing, exercising, bathing and the use of various forces to eliminate the poisonous products in the system, and so to raise the vitality of the patient to a proper standard of health."[30] Naturopaths work well with allopathic physicians and see themselves as complementary to them. The therapeutic approach of helping patients heal themselves, and then using the opportunity to guide and educate patients to develop more healthy lifestyles, has begun to be researched for efficacy.[29,30] A comprehensive compilation of the scientific documentation of this research can be found in Pizzorno and Murray's *Textbook of Natural Medicine.*[31]

Mind/Body Interventions

Biofeedback

One of the oldest methods used in rehabilitation, biofeedback (see Chapter 32) is a "process of electronically utilizing information from the body/mind to teach an individual to recognize what is going on inside of his or her own brain, nervous system, and muscles."[32] Its efficacy in rehabilitation of neuromuscular problems providing muscle re-education and relaxation is unquestioned and well documented in the literature.[32,33] The fact that it is a tool that assists the mind to have an energetic and relaxation effect on the body places it among holistic approaches. The documented effects of biofeedback-assisted relaxation on cell-mediated immunity, cortisol, and white blood cell count locate this approach clearly in a holistic category.[34]

Hypnosis, Hypnotherapy, and Relaxation

In 1843, James Braid, an English physician, proposed to shed light on the negative view of the concept of *mesmerism* or mesmeric vital energy by postulating that its effects stemmed from a mental force rather than a mysterious fluid. He changed its name to *hypnosis*, after the Greek god for sleep. Soon after, hypnosis became a major concern in psychology, until Freud's writings reduced it to merely a way of seeing into the unconscious.[19] Hypnosis, hypnotherapy, and relaxation currently are widely used by psychiatrists and psychologists to treat behavior that is harmful or nonproductive, such as smoking, alcohol abuse, eating disorders, and obsessive compulsive disorders, as well as such problems as nausea and vomiting with pregnancy, allergies and asthma, and headaches from spinal cord injury.[20] Hypnotic techniques "induce states of selective attentional focusing or diffusion, combined with enhanced imagery; and are often used to induce relaxation."[35] They seem to work by fostering relaxation and allowing a measure of control over the body by way of the breath, images, and attentional focusing, altering negative thoughts and behaviors. They are a widely used alternative in pain management, and their efficacy is well documented.[20]

Yoga

Seated in the Hindu tradition, the teachings of yoga are reported to be more than 5,000 years old.[36] The teachings of yoga are thought to have been spread from Egypt to India, based on analysis of Egyptian carvings showing figures sitting in the traditional cross-legged lotus pose associated with yoga. The commonly known postures of hatha-yoga, or *asanas*, are believed to assist the natural flow of ch'i or prana throughout the body. Critical to the success of the postures is proper breathing and the meditative assumption of the pose. Deep relaxation and a special awareness are used to help clients and patients improve the quality of their lives. Yoga has been documented to assist in health care with patients with alcohol abuse, anxiety, cancer, diabetes, hot flashes with menopause, neurologic disorders, narcotic addiction, osteoarthritis, and stress.[26]

T'ai Chi

T'ai chi is an ancient physical art form, first developed as a martial art, in which the defendant actually uses his or her attacker's own energy against the assailant by drawing the attack, sidestepping the attacker, and throwing the opponent off balance.[37] The benefits of t'ai chi in improving balance, posture, coordination, integration of movements, endurance, strength, flexibility, and relaxation are well documented in the literature.[20,37-40] Behind the t'ai chi movements is the philosophy of yin and yang from Taoist philosophy. The purpose is to use the ultimate energy of t'ai chi to create a balance between the positive and negative energies of nature. T'ai chi has been called a *movement meditation technique* and is used to enable one to reach the ultimate level of health and physical and mental well-being.

Qi Gong: Subtle Energy Manipulation

Qi gong is an ancient Chinese practice dating back more than 5,000 years, involving the regulation of the body's energy through control of the mind and breath, posture, and movement and self-massage.[41] Ch'i (qi) is seen as the link between the mind and the body, and qi gong attempts to open the ch'i channels permanently so that self-healing can take place continually. Each day a person goes through a sequence of movements in learning the feeling of ch'i that includes action, visualization, and affirmations, with or with-

out a qi gong master. Eventually, the mind and the body connect and illnesses disappear. In the presence of a qi gong grandmaster, every word and gesture become healing ch'i as the student consciously delivers them into where it is needed in the body. The student's belief turns into healing. Healings also take place when a group of people come together with love and compassion. The qi gong master, through resonance and induction, reinforces the overall resonant field of the patient by identifying diseased resonant patterns of specific organs and *harmonizing* the energy by sending healthy ch'i.[41] Improving the quantity and quality of energy flow tends to decrease tension in connective tissue, thus enhancing rehabilitation. Most of the research on qi gong has been carried out in China over the past 20 years, since 1980. Reports of miraculous cures of cancerous tumors and of patients with spinal cord injury paraplegia being able to walk have made qi gong a common practice and household word in China.[42] English translations of most of the clinical and experimental research are available in abstracts (with detailed research protocols) from the Qi Gong Institute.[43]

Meditation

Several forms of meditation exist, but perhaps the form most documented in the literature for its positive effects on stress is transcendental meditation,[44] which is seated in the Ayurvedic system. The object is to control the *runaway* nature of a person's thought process by calming the mind through focusing on the breath. Breathing and tracking the breath as it flows in and out in the present moment transfer attention from the future of fears of what might happen and anxiety from the past about what has already happened. In addition, one might be instructed to focus on a word (a mantra, or a syllable such as *ooomm*) or a picture of spiritual significance in one's mind's eye. Concentrating in this way has proven benefits to blood pressure, cortisol levels, and other common measures of stress.[44]

Prayer and Mental Healing

Prayer and mental healing have been shown to be positive forces for healing in double-blind studies.[12,14,15] Even so, contemporary conventional science views the mind and consciousness as entirely local phenomena (i.e., localized to the brain and body and confined to the present moment). The mind cannot stray outside the here and now to cause a remote event. The underlying mechanism may lie in the theory of nonlocality in quantum physics. Studies in mental healing that takes place over long distances challenge conventional assumptions.[14,15] Current research on consciousness as *causal* is taking place at Duke, Stanford, Princeton, and other major research universities. The mind can bring about changes in faraway physical bodies, "even when the distant person or organism is shielded from all known sensory and electromagnetic influences."[14,17] These studies imply that the mind and consciousness may not always be localized or confined to our brains and bodies, or confined in time such as the present moment.

Psychotherapy

Psychotherapy first began with Freud in the late 1800s and early 1900s.[11] Psychological interventions, as practiced by psychiatrists, psychologists, mental health and rehabilitation counselors, social workers, and occupational therapists, include the practice of altering the mind/body's harmful beliefs through the use of counseling and interpersonal interactive techniques designed to facilitate insight on the part of the client or patient. Sometimes in conjunction with medication, relaxation, and dream analysis, negative and harmful beliefs and actions are brought to conscious awareness and challenged. Positron emission tomographic scan technology has documented change in synaptic flow as the harmful ideas and beliefs are transformed into more life-affirming and positive beliefs and behaviors. This form of therapy is firmly seated in the category of treatments that illustrate the mind/body connection.

Music Therapies, Art Therapies, and Dance Therapies

Music, art, and dance therapies are designed to affect energy flow holistically. Each therapy brings about a positive effect by promoting physical, emotional, intellectual, spiritual, or several such responses for analgesia, relaxation, communication, and the evoking of memories facilitating the client's ability to talk about whatever might be blocking healing. Self-awareness is fostered, and frequently unconscious concerns are brought to the surface and dealt with for a positive healing effect.[45]

Support Groups

One of the first documented studies that revealed the clinical significance of the positive effects of the mind on the body was the research conducted by David Spiegel, reported in 1992, that suggested that breast cancer patients randomly assigned to weekly support groups lived markedly longer than control patients assigned only to regular care.[46] The opportunity for people with illnesses to verbalize their feelings and give support to one another as they struggle to search for meaning and hope seems to have a positive effect on the ability to heal from life-threatening illness in ways that are not fully understood.

Bioelectromagnetics

Transcutaneous Nerve Stimulation

Well known to rehabilitation professionals, transcutaneous electrical nerve stimulation (TENS) units are electroanalgesic devices that control pain by activating large-diameter afferent fibers by transmitting microvoltage. Units are usually pocket sized and battery powered and contain an electronic pulse generator that transmits pulses to electrodes placed on the skin. TENS is most useful with acute pain in the early stages of reflex sympathetic dystrophy and postoperative incisional pain, diminishing the need for narcotics.[47,48] TENS has shown inconsistent significant benefit for chronic pain and low back pain. Deyo[47] pointed out that such unproved use had a detrimental effect when results were generalized so that third-party payers and the public assumed that TENS was ineffective for relieving any pain. TENS has been used to great benefit along with acupuncture and exercise in reducing chronic low back pain,[20] however, and has also been used to stimulate the secretion of serotonin in treatment for depression.

Magnets

Magnets appear to increase blood flow to an area of pain or inflammation, bringing more oxygen to the area and removing toxic substances.[49] Magnets seem to affect the positive and negative charges of sodium and potassium ions within the membranes that line blood vessels and nerves and to relax small smooth muscle valves in the capillaries, which promote blood flow. Several brands of magnets are currently available on the market. Neodymium magnets (*neos*) from rare earth metals have been shaped into dime and 50-cent piece sizes and emit a stronger field called *gauss strength*. Magnets seem most effective when placed over acupuncture points. They envelop the target zone with a magnetic field in the range of 500–3,500 G. The Earth's magnetic field is only approximately 0.5 G. The south or negative pole should be placed against the skin to produce analgesia, vasodilation, and relaxation. The north or positive pole produces stimulation. Magnets reduced knee pain of 50 patients with postpolio syndrome, with active magnets significantly outperforming placebo magnets.[49] Flexible magnets are ineffective in decreasing pain perception in muscle microinjury.[50] Magnets are not considered *medical* and thus are not regulated by the U.S. Food and Drug Administration, and no prescriptions are required.

Manual Therapies

Myofascial Release

Myofascial release has been most well developed by physical therapist John F. Barnes since the 1980s. It is based on the myofascial theories of Janet Travell and calls for influencing the length of the fascia by manual techniques that facilitate *flow* of the collagen layer. Unlike other soft tissue mobilization techniques that are mechanistic, this approach facilitates a unique form of *release*, that results from a combination of the pressure of body weight through the hands in gravity and human energy. The therapist takes the slack out of the tissue under the hands, waiting for 90–120 seconds for a feeling of flow, in which the collagenous barrier is engaged energetically, and then following the flow for an extended period as it flows and stops, flows and stops, thereby releasing the collagenous barriers at the level of the ground substance of the fascia. Using cross-hands release, plus partial and whole body *unwinding* to influence what is thought to be trapped energy in tissues, the therapist energetically engages the collagenous barrier, allowing the muscle and fascia unit to return to its original shape and length to operate most efficiently. Although published reports are lacking, Barnes and colleagues have accumulated many case reports indicating that this approach has been shown to correct postural deviations, and, hypothetically, facilitate the flow of ch'i.[51] Myofascial release also uses craniosacral and soft tissue mobilization techniques to influence the fascia of the body including the cerebral spinal column and the dura (see Chapter 33).[51,52]

Rosen Method

The Rosen method is a hands-on, nonintrusive body work developed by physical therapist Marion Rosen, a German therapist who studied physical therapy in Sweden during World War II.[53] After the war she emigrated to the United States and studied physical therapy further at the Mayo Clinic. The goal is to help the client relax and increase emotional awareness, facilitating the body/mind's ability to heal itself. The client learns how to relax muscle-holding patterns, thereby releasing tension, enabling freer movement with fewer symptoms, "allowing the full range of possibilities for movement and expression in life to come forth."[53] The quality of touch is sensitive, specific, and noninvasive and meets the client's tension with equal pressure. The muscle thus has the opportunity to stop holding as it is ready. The diaphragm is also worked with to help the body relax with the breath. Rosen body work training can be completed in 2 years of part-time classes followed by a 1- to 2-year internship. Prerequisite to this work, one must complete an introductory weekend workshop.

Rolfing, Hellerwork, and Soma

Rolfing, or structural integration, was developed in the 1950s by Ida P. Rolf.[54] The concept is based on the theory that the optimal structure of the body, which facilitates optimal function, is one in which the body has a vertical relationship with gravity. When the body is not in balance with gravity, tissue constantly wears and function diminishes. When the body is properly aligned, the force of gravity flows through with minimal work required by the muscles to keep the body upright. In this position, the body can facilitate a smooth energy flow, and thus homeostasis or healing is enhanced. Rolfing, or deep connective tissue or fascial massage, helps maintain a balanced structure without physical or conscious effort. The basic Rolfing series involves ten 1-hour sessions of myofascial mobilization and movement re-education aimed at establishing the vertical line of the body. Hellerwork, created by Joseph Heller, a trained Rolfer, in the 1970s, is identical to Rolfing except it incorporates movement lessons into the sessions rather than addressing them separately.[55] Soma body work, developed in 1978 by Bill M. Williams, who studied under Dr. Rolf, also involves 10 sessions, and addresses psychological facilitation, right/left hemisphere integration, and mind/body integration.[55]

Noncontact Therapeutic Touch

Delores Krieger and Dora Kunz, clairvoyant and healer, respectively, are credited with being the first to introduce noncontact therapeutic touch to health professionals in the 1970s, and it is the only holistic therapy that has been taught for years in university nursing curricula.[56] Touch is widely accepted as being therapeutic. The therapist attempts to relax the patient by manipulating the energy field around the patient, never placing hands directly on the body. A critical factor in understanding this approach is the belief that the body/mind is surrounded by an energy field that is a continuation of the electromagnetic energy within the tissues of the person. The energy field of the practitioner interacts with that of the patient or client, with the therapist holding a conscious intent to help or heal in a spirit of unconditional love. A large body of literature on the efficacy of this approach exists,[57] but the validity of noncontact therapeutic touch has been questioned for decades. The recent article in the *Journal of the American Medical Association* (volume 279)[58] that seemed to discredit this approach has brought this technique to the forefront of discussion.

Reflexology

Reflexology, thought to first be used around 2300 BCE in Egypt, is best known today for physical therapist Eunice Ingham's Foot Reflexology Method developed in the early 1930s.[23] She related zones of the hands and feet to the organs and other body parts. Five zones on each side of the body, and one for each finger and toe, run from the top of the head to the tips of the toes. An organ, gland, or other body part in a specific zone has its reflex in the corresponding zone of the foot via nerve endings. Sensitivity of an area on the foot signals that there could be something abnormal taking place in the corresponding body part.[23]

> Therapy consists of using the thumbs, fingertips, or knuckles to apply a firm, constant, deep massaging pressure to the sensitive area on the foot for 1–2 minutes, so that working the whole foot affects the entire side of the body of that foot. In this way the practitioner is stimulating the circulation, unblocking nerve impulses and raising the vitality of the body, ridding toxins from the system and assisting the body's own healing mechanisms.[23]

Craniosacral Therapy

Developed by John Upledger in the late 1970s, craniosacral therapy attempts to unblock the flow of ch'i so that the body can heal itself spontaneously through the light touch of the therapist's hands on the head as well as other parts of the body.[52] Craniosacral therapy is a combination of manual therapies, myofascial release and mobilization, osteopathic-type manipulation, and light touch. Some work is done off the body in the human energy field. Energy is thought to be trapped in tissue or energy cysts, and, after a whole body diagnosis, the skilled therapist can locate these places and release the trapped energy with the techniques listed. Manipulation of the craniosacral rhythm, and facilitation of the body/mind's unleashing of trapped energy by way of somatoemotional release, or unwinding, allows the energy to flow freely again.[52]

Chiropractic

Started by Daniel David Palmer in Davenport, IA, in 1895, chiropractic is founded on the principles that vertebral subluxation is the cause of virtually all disease, and the body's ability to heal itself spontaneously requires the proper alignment of the vertebral bodies and other joints through which the nervous system passes, so that the

flow of ch'i is unimpeded.[59] Few, if any, modern day chiropractors would espouse the "one cause–one cure" philosophy, yet their reason for existing is to detect and correct *spinal subluxations*,[60] defined as spinal misalignments causing abnormal nerve transmission. Manipulation of the vertebrae and pelvis for proper alignment is carried out by practitioners who study for 4 years for the Doctor of Chiropractic degree. Some use procedures other than manipulation of vertebrae to assist in meeting goals; these may include physical agents, massage, exercise, and nutritional counseling.[60]

Manual Lymphatic Drainage

Emil Vodder perfected manual lymphatic drainage in the 1930s as a holistic approach to reducing edema. Precise and complex pumping, circular and spiral, flat and pushing hand movements follow pathways of the lymph vessel system to create an increase of pressure followed by a release of pressure.[61] This technique is designed to move fluid from the loose connective tissues into the prelymph vessels, along the vessel pathways culminating at the clavicular fossa. The entire process of edema treatment includes manual lymphatic drainage, bandaging, movement and breathing exercises, and skin care and is called *complex physical therapy* or *combined decongestive therapy*. Intensive therapy takes place over 4 or 5 weeks. Practitioners must be certified in the Vodder technique after many weeks of training. Outcomes research demonstrates the superiority of this approach over mechanical compression.[61,62]

Massage Implemented from a Holistic Perspective

When a therapist applies massage strokes to the body with the intention of mechanically moving fluid from one area of the body, such as the arm or leg, to another, the trunk, the therapeutic approach is termed *traditional* or *allopathic*. However, when the therapist applies manual stroking or touch in such a way as to influence the flow of body energy, or ch'i, then massage becomes a holistic approach that is designed to facilitate the body's ability to heal itself. Tiffany Field used holistic massage or stroking with neonatal infants, which resulted in their discharge home 6 days sooner than control subjects who were not stroked.[63] In addition, they gained 47% more weight, became more responsive, and 8 months later were still showing an advantage on weight, mental, and motor development.

Movement Awareness

Alexander Technique   When a recurrent hoarseness and loss of voice threatened the career of renowned Shakespearean elocutionist, Frederick Matthias Alexander

(1869–1955), he observed his behavior to develop a process of using his body in a way that changed his habit of pulling his head down and back when he performed. In a single case research design method, he published his discoveries about his faulty use of his body, which negatively affected his function, and went on to develop an entire technique of describing the organization of the head to the neck and to the back for maximal function.[64] The Alexander technique is used in many arts to instruct musicians and vocalists in the proper integration of awareness and intention in using the body to perform by bringing the mind and body into harmony. The technique is also used in rehabilitation, mostly through nonverbal kinesthetic cues, to give patients new ways to manage their own bodies and their movements and thus facilitate more efficient and pain-free function. An Alexander technique teacher has at least 1,600 hours of teacher training over a period of 3–4 years.[64]

Feldenkrais Approach The Feldenkrais approach grew out of the observations and writings of physicist Moshe Feldenkrais in the early 1970s, who, when faced with a severe knee injury, realized by observing his own adaptation to the knee problems that human beings have a choice about how to move.[65,66] Feldenkrais practitioners help clients to choose to be involved in awareness of how their movements are counterproductive to efficient function, and verbally help them to choose to let go of habitual ways of moving that interfere with pain-free, efficient function. In this process of mental and physical attention, the client begins more clearly to observe restrictive habitual thoughts and feelings, which then allows for new ways of thinking, feeling, and moving that assist in the flow of the body's own natural energy. This facilitates a return to more efficient movement and function. The Feldenkrais practitioner is a teacher, facilitator, and guide who helps the individual learn through discovery, using verbal, visual, and kinesthetic information. Touch is not a central part of the Feldenkrais approach.[66] Feldenkrais practitioners are certified after 4 years of training.

Trager Approach Developed by Hawaiian physician, Milton Trager, the Trager approach

uses a series of gentle, non-invasive, passive movements of joints, muscles, and the entire body, through fully available (pain free) range of motion. This work conveys positive, pleasurable feelings which enter the central nervous system and begin to trigger tissue changes by means of many sensory-motor-feedback loops between the mind and the muscles. The therapist does not try to fix or change the tissues with his/her hands, but merely feeds the mind with an attitude of how these tissues should feel.[67]

The Trager approach provides a safe environment for allowing a release of blocks or holding patterns that have resulted from physical or emotional trauma, disease, or illness that have inhibited free movement and disrupted normal function. Trager is an approach, not a technique; there is no set formula. It targets the unconscious mind rather than local tissue and gives the body freedom to experience in a totally different way. The therapist maintains relaxed hands, and, in so doing, the patient's mind is *reminded* of how it feels to be free, moving, and soft. Gentle rhythmic rocking, elongation, traction, and jiggling of the tissue may be included. Trager is about "not trying." "The goals include decreased muscular tension, improved body alignment, renewed and greater ease of movement, the experience of total relaxation and peace, and a sense of a functionally integrated body/mind."[67]

Pilates Most frequently associated with dance rehabilitation, Pilates was developed by Joseph Pilates in the 1920s. Exercises feature hundreds of movements that focus on strengthening and flexibility with a primary emphasis on dynamic trunk and abdominal stabilization. Various apparatus are used in *studios* and clinics to support parts of the body while other parts are assisted in moving. All exercises center around an awareness of the breath. Control precision, natural flow, and rhythm support a unique movement pattern for each exercise. The result is the development of greater efficiency of movement with an emphasis on trunk control and strength. Posture is enhanced as is the flow of body energy and increased body awareness.[68]

Exercise Implemented from a Holistic Perspective
Exercise prescribed for holistic purposes (e.g., to bring about a shift in emotions for people with depression, or to enhance immune system T-cell function) is being used as a complementary therapy. The traditional outcomes of exercise of increased strength, flexibility, and endurance have been supplemented with the growing awareness of the effect of exercise on the immune system and the endocrine system.[69] Much of traditional physical therapy, including exercise, manual therapy, and the use of physical agents, can be administered with the intention of facilitating the flow of body energy, thus encouraging self-regulation and homeostasis.

CONNECTION BETWEEN MIND AND BODY IS PRIMARILY PHYSIOLOGICAL

The world of traditional medicine is a biological science entity in which parts define the whole, and research strives to discern cause and effect. Control is paramount. People are viewed as machines and when they become sick, the effort all too often focuses on relieving their symptoms. Now it is more commonly appreciated that reality is not made of what we can experience with our five senses plus unconscious perceptions. According to quantum physics, the material aspect of what we can experience is only a fraction of reality.[70] People are not machines; that which we cannot see or measure (e.g., the mind and consciousness) plays critical roles in health and healing.

Each time one awakens in fear to a strange noise in the middle of the night and lies awake trying to figure out what could be causing it, as heart rates elevate, pupils dilate, and hair stands on end, one recognizes that the mind affects the body as a matter of everyday experience. Although the physiology of the sympathetic nervous system response is well known, not enough attention has been paid to the foundational question, "How does our fearful thought, or our emotion, get translated into our biochemistry?" This is the influence of the mind, thought, and emotions on the body. What is thought? What is mind? What is emotion? What is consciousness? How are they interrelated physically, physiologically?

In 1971, Benson and colleagues published results of research that seemed to point toward a mind/body link and coined the phrase, *relaxation response.*[71] At the same time, Ader and Cohen at the University of Rochester were investigating the phenomenon of anticipatory nausea in women receiving chemotherapy for breast cancer. They hypothesized that their clients were experiencing nausea in advance of the active medication as a result of a Pavlovian conditioned response. They fed rats saccharine water mixed with cyclophosphamide. The rats experienced nausea, and their blood indicated an immune system depression, which was the expected medication effect. When the chemotherapeutic agent was withdrawn, the rats experienced nausea again, and their immune systems continued to be depressed. Somehow, the rats learned by conditioning to suppress their immune systems. The biochemical result offered strong evidence of the effect of the mind on the body. Ader coined the word *psychoneuroimmunology,* the effect of the mind on the immune system, as mediated by the autonomic nervous system and the nonadrenergic, noncholinergic neurotransmitters and neuropeptides.[72] Felten and colleagues[73] maintained that these pathways innervate bone marrow, thymus, spleen, and mucosal surfaces where immune cells develop, mature, and encounter foreign substances. "Each [of the two nerve systems] communicates with the immune cells directly

through the release of chemical messages which range from adrenaline, noradrenaline, and acetylcholine to small proteins called neuropeptides . . . and cause an inflammatory or anti-inflammatory effect on the immune system."[74]

Pert,[74,75] at Johns Hopkins University, discovered the opiate receptor and revealed with bench research results how "molecules of emotion run every system in our body." She coined the term *psychoimmunoendocrinology.*[75] The fact that mind and emotions directly affect disease and illness is no longer speculative.

Some scientists are replacing the biomedical model with a new model, the *infomedical model.*[76]

> In this model, the organism is redescribed in multi-modal, informational terms, as a self-organizing system that maintains dynamic equilibrium by a circular flow of information among all its levels and between itself and the environment. . . . Information is carried in the form of symbols conveying messages that are decoded at the appropriate level of the organism. At lower levels information is carried by hormones and neurotransmitters. At the level of the whole organism, it is carried by stimuli reaching the special senses, among which are the word and other symbols by which meaning is expressed in human relationships.[76]

The key concept is meaning. What an illness means to a person or, in large part, what meaning a person attributes to any experience determines the cascade of neurochemicals that share information with cells throughout the entire body/mind.[77]

Pert described the interaction of the receptor on the surface of the cell, which she compares to a water lily floating on the surface of the pond, with roots reaching deep into the interior of the cell, and the ligand, the natural or human-made substance that binds selectively to its own receptor. Receptors are composed of a single molecule, and ligands are usually much smaller molecules than the receptors to which they bond. Three natural chemicals bind with receptors in the fluid nervous system: neurotransmitters (dopamine, acetylcholine, norepinephrine, histamine, glycine [gamma-aminobutyric acid], and serotonin), corticosteroids (cortisol, testosterone, progesterone, and estrogen), and peptides, the largest category of ligands, regulating not only the emotions, but all life processes.[75]

The discovery of the fluid nervous system has expanded the idea that the nervous system was essentially an electrical network of axon, dendrite, and neurotransmitter connections. Even more difficult for western science to accept was the realization that the fluid nervous system was even more ancient to the organism. Peptides, such as endorphins, were being made inside cells long before there were dendrites, axons, or even neurons; long before the brain itself evolved.[75]

The *key fitting in the lock* is the standard metaphor used to describe the ligand and receptor binding process. Pert described the action of binding as more dynamic: ". . . two voices—ligand and receptor—striking the same note and producing a vibration that rings a doorbell to open the doorway to the cell."[75]

> What happens next is quite amazing. The receptor, having received a message, transmits it from the surface of the cell deep into the cell's interior, where the message can change the state of the cell dramatically. A chain reaction of biochemical events is initiated as tiny machines roar into action and, directed by the message of the ligand, begin any number of activities—manufacturing new proteins, making decisions about cell division, opening or closing ion channels, adding or subtracting energetic chemical groups like the phosphates—to name just a few. . . . On a more global scale, these minute physiological phenomena at the cellular level can translate to large changes in behavior, physical activity, even mood.[75]

Thus, receptors and their ligands have come to be known as *information molecules*,

> the basic units of a language used by cells throughout the organism to communicate across systems such as the endocrine, neurological, gastrointestinal, and even the immune system. Overall, the musical hum of the receptors as they bind to their many ligands, often in far-flung parts of the organism creates an integration of structure and function that allows the organism to run smoothly, intelligently.[75]

Pert and colleagues discovered that immune cells make, store, and secrete neuropeptides. In sum, the brain and the immune system are responsible for activity that, in part, controls mood. Neuropeptides, 95% of all ligands, "unify the classically separated areas of neuroscience, endocrinology, and immunology, with various respective organs—the brain; the glands; and the spleen, bone marrow and lymph nodes."[75] The continual discovery of peptide receptors throughout the entire body has led Pert to propose: "I can no longer make a strong distinction between the brain and the body—white blood cells are bits of our brain floating around in our body."[78]

Thus, the work of Ader, Cohen, Benson, and Pert and associates have clarified how thought and emotions become translated into physical events, and how the mind and body are inextricably linked. When we feel fear, anger, or rage, phenomenologically we know that we feel it in our whole body, not just in our minds. We hyperventilate, we shiver, we blush, we experience *goosebumps* and butterflies in our stomachs, because the meaning we have attributed to an event results in an instantaneous communication with the cells throughout our body/mind. Peptides have the unifying function of coordinating physiology, behavior, and emotion toward what seems to be a coherent, meaningful end.[75]

Wisneski and colleagues[79] are clarifying the role of the endocrine system in interpreting meaning from interaction with other human energy fields. Endocrine glands, particularly the pineal gland, may act as energy transducers that convert external energy impinging on the human energy field by way of light, sound, and electromagnetism into electrical and then chemical energy in the form of hormones and peptides. Wisneski et al. commented that our bodies are both reflective and generative energy fields,[79-81] and that we absorb and are affected by energy fields that surround us, such as light and heat from the sun, the warmth of air, water, the push of the wind, and the sting of the rain. We also produce our own internal electrical energy fields.[81]

THEORETIC BASIS FOR HOLISTIC COMPLEMENTARY THERAPIES: SYSTEMS THEORY AND QUANTUM PHYSICS

Atoms are sometimes referred to as the *building blocks* of all that we know as real. The periodic chart of the elements categorizes atoms according to their number of electrons, or atomic weight. Newtonian physics, the foundation of biomedical science, states that what is real is solid, material, and made of atoms joining to form molecules. These form solid, discrete bits of matter with clearly differentiated boundaries. What is *real* is thus what we can measure and observe with our senses.

Newtonian physics also posits several seemingly inviolate laws that govern what we believe is reality. For example, two objects cannot occupy the same space at the same time, or energy dissipates as it travels away from its source. These and other theorems, proven on paper sometimes even before experimentally verified, were developed and refined in the late 1600s, and remain for most as the inviolate description of the true nature of reality. Newtonian physics remains the foundation for medical science and research today, which strives for evidence of cause and effect ideally by way of the reductionistic double-blind, placebo-based, randomized controlled trial. From the time of Newton until the early part of the twentieth century, the whole of the study of physics was based on this materialistic view. However, discoveries at the turn of the century have challenged this world view.[82] By focusing attention on the characteristics of electrons and subatomic particles, quantum physics has described an expanded view of reality. At the center of this view is the function of electron interaction, energy flow, and the role of nonmaterial consciousness in the physical world. Hari Sharma, a researcher in Ayurveda, describes the consciousness model of medicine this way.[83]

The four basic principles that support the common sense view of reality, or materialistic view, are as follows:

- Solid matter—the world is composed fundamentally of solid matter.
- Strict causality—change in motion of one object can only be caused by direct interaction with another object.
- Locality—interactions between particles can occur only through collisions or through influences radiated through the electromagnetic or gravitational fields at the speed of light, or less. No nonlocal interaction can occur.
- Reductionism—large systems, including people and the universe, can only be understood by examining the parts that make up the system. Understanding of the whole is gained by carefully examining the properties and local, causal interactions of their smallest discrete components.[83]

In materialist theory, the consciousness of the examiner is considered separate from any part of what is being examined. The knower (consciousness) and the known (object) are thought to exist in completely separate domains. This separation is the very foundation of objective science.

Subatomic particles, that make up atoms, molecules, and the solid bits of matter, do not appear to be composed of solid matter, however. In some experiments, electrons behaved like particles, but in others, they behaved like waves, which were invisible. In some experiments, electrons took instantaneous, discontinuous quantum jumps from one atomic orbit to another with no intervening time and no journey through space, an impossible act for a particle. The uncertainty principle stated that electrons cannot have both a precise position and a precise momentum simultaneously, which would also not apply to a solid particle. Finally, electrons were

observed to, with predictable regularity, pierce through a solid barrier that would be classically impenetrable.[84,85]

This research, first made public in the famous Copenhagen conference interpretation by physicist Niels Bohr, rejects the model of Newtonian physics[86] and challenges the traditional materialistic world view with the following findings:

- No such thing as *solid* matter exists—This interpretation accepted the research findings described previously (wave/particle, quantum jumps, uncertainty, and piercing through solids) that contradicted the notion that atoms, and thus all matter, are solid.
- No strict causality—precise predictions for individual subatomic particles are actually impossible. Quantum mechanics thus loses the ability to trace causal relations among individual particles.
- No locality—quantum mechanical equations indicate that two particles, once they have interacted, are instantaneously connected, even across astronomical distances. This defies the strictly local connections allowed in classical materialism.
- No reductionism—if apparently separate particles actually are connected nonlocally, a reductionistic view based on isolated particles is untenable.[83]

Sharma went on to say that the Copenhagen interpretation was not put to experimental tests for decades, leaving some physicists unconvinced that solidity, causality, locality, and reductionism had to be abandoned. In the 1980s, however, a number of different experiments produced results that consistently contradicted the theories of materialism (often called *local realism*) and consistently confirmed the predictions of quantum mechanics.[84–86] These studies found that once two particles have interacted, they are instantaneously correlated nonlocally, over arbitrarily vast distances, an impossibility in materialism. These results do not invalidate materialism altogether. In the everyday world of *large* objects, the mechanistic causation of Newtonian physics is approximately correct, which is why much of medicine has been able to rely on it without apparently ill consequences. But at the fundamental, subatomic level, materialism conflicts both with theory and with frequently replicated experimental evidence. This gives rise to a fundamentally different world view. Many physicists now argue that nature is composed of probability waves that are a function of intelligence alone, not of discrete physical particles. The equations of quantum mechanics thus describe a world made of abstract patterns of intelligence.[83]

Quantum is defined as a subatomic *discrete* indivisible packet of energy transfer with a wave-like frequency.[87]

The theory of nonlocality indicates that, once two electrons or photons (light particles) have interrelated with each other, once they are joined and then separated, they exhibit instantaneous *knowing* of the other. Nonlocal means "information or influence transfer without local signals," without the usual physical means of transferring information.[13] But to describe the instantaneous knowing as a "transfer of information" is erroneous, for there is no distance between the two quanta. Physicist John Haaland stated, "At a distance . . . means that the information or influence transfer without local signals" effect is *not* a function of distance. Strictly speaking, describing a nonlocal effect as information transfer is not accurate, since instantaneous information transfer at a distance would violate the speed of light. Quantum coherent states imply a state of oneness where instant knowing occurs, giving rise to the property of nonlocality.[13]

Researchers at Princeton, Stanford, and the University of Nevada have discovered an instantaneous knowing or nonlocal effect among human interaction and living systems using random processes.[13,14] In other words, distant healing, or distant mental influence on biological systems, is an attempt to find a way to objectively describe the outcome of what others call psychic healing or prayer.[16]

> Apparently some kind of nonlocal "wave" or "field" is generated by some aspect of some living systems which is not constrained to the properties of electromagnetic waves, and under certain conditions, this "wave" can alter the physical reality with which it becomes *coherent*, or . . . oscillations at different places beat time with each other.[16]

This becomes relevant as we try to understand how the mind-body communicates or exchanges information with parts of itself and as we try to understand phenomena like extrasensory perception and consciousness transfer of knowing.

Distance Healing Studies

Current research in consciousness has focused on verifying the possibility that one person's thoughts (or prayers) can influence the experience of another person, even at a distance. Harvard University and the Institute of Noetic Sciences in Sausalito, CA, cosponsored a 3-day conference in December, 1998, to examine and evaluate data on nonlocal or distant effects of consciousness. According to Targ, "preliminary data presented at this conference suggested that we are on the verge of an explosion of evidence to support the efficacy of distant healing."[14]

The term now used by the National Institutes for Health for this category of phenomena is "distant mental influence on biological systems" and refers to what is commonly known as *psychic healing, energy healing*, or *prayer*. Since 1960, more than 150 formal, controlled studies of distance healing have been published, more than two-thirds of them showing significant effects at the $P < .05$ level.[15] That there is an effect at a distance is clearly indicated by the data. Certainly, consciousness seems to be showing *field-like* effects, but no coherent theory exists currently to account for this. De Quincy suggests, "All we have are anomalous data . . . unless, following A. N. Whitehead, we take the radical step of shifting from 'space-talk' to 'time-talk,' that is, recognizing that both the ontological nature and relationship between consciousness and matter grow out of *process* rather than substance."[16]

Research Evidence

The common comment about complementary and alternative therapies is that they are not proven by way of research, specifically, the randomized controlled trial with placebo. However, a review of the literature suggests that a great deal of research has taken place to establish the effectiveness of most of the therapies listed, and in some cases rather substantial bodies of evidence exist. The task remains to read critically the existing research for evidence of efficacy and to continue to contribute good science in peer-reviewed journals for the benefit of clinicians and patients.

CONCLUSION

Complementary and alternative therapies are holistic approaches in health care. A growing body of research-based evidence suggests that many of these therapies have a great deal to offer in rehabilitation. Psychoneuroimmunology and psychoendocrineimmunology are new basic sciences that help explain how the body and mind are all one system that cannot be separated and be fully understood or described. This body of inquiry of holistic therapies represents the growing edge of the science of health care and promises to yield rich rewards for patients and professionals alike as we enter the next century of health care. Perhaps it will be through the research and application of holistic therapies that further light will be shed on the mysteries of quantum physics, and we will more fully come to understand the mystery of the work of subatomic particles in the macroscopic world.

REFERENCES

1. Bodeker GC. Global Health Traditions. In MS Micozzi (ed), Fundamentals of Complementary and Alternative Medicine. New York: Churchill Livingstone, 1996;279–290.

2. World Health Organization. Traditional Medicine. Geneva: WHO Publications, 1978.

3. Eisenberg DM. Unconventional medicine in the United States: prevalence, costs and patterns of use. N Engl J Med 1993;328:4.

4. Fisher P, Ward A. Complementary medicine in Europe. BMJ 1994;309(6947):107.

5. Spencer JW. Essential Issues in Complementary/Alternative Medicine. In JW Spencer, JJ Jacobs (eds), Complementary/Alternative Medicine—An Evidence-Based Approach. St. Louis: Mosby, 1999;3–36.

6. Astin JA. Why patients use alternative medicine: results of a national study. JAMA 1998;279:1548–1553.

7. Krauss HH, Godfrey C, Kirk J, Eisenberg DM. Alternative health care: its use by individuals with physical disabilities. Arch Phys Med Rehabil 1998;79:1440–1447.

8. Micozzi MS. Characteristics of Complementary and Alternative Medicine. In MS Micozzi (ed), Fundamentals of Complementary and Alternative Medicine. New York: Churchill Livingstone, 1996;5.

9. Kolata G. In quests outside the mainstream, medical projects rewrite the rules. New York Times National 1996;CXLV(50,462):A1,A14.

10. National Institutes of Health. Acupuncture Consensus Statement and Literature Review. Integrative Med Consult 1999;1(3):23–29.

11. Kaptchuk T. Historical Context of the Concept of Vitalism in Complementary and Alternative Medicine. In MS Micozzi (ed), Fundamentals of Complementary and Alternative Medicine. New York: Churchill Livingstone, 1996;35–48.

12. Jahn RG. Information, consciousness and health. Altern Ther Health Med 1996;2:3.

13. Nelson RD, Bradish GJ, Dobybs BJ, et al. Field REG anomalies in group situations. J Scientific Explor 1996;10(1):111.

14. Targ E. Distance healing. IONS Noetic Sci Rev 1999;Aug–Nov:24–31.

15. Benor DJ. Healing Research, Vol 1. Deddington, England: Helix Editions, 1992.

16. de Quincy C. Past matter, present mind. J Consciousness Stud 1999;6:28–30.

17. Jahn RG, Dunne BJ. Precognitive Remote Perception. In RG Jahn (ed), Margins of Reality: The Role of Consciousness in the Physical World. New York: Harcourt Brace, 1987;149–191.

18. Davis CM. Introduction. In CM Davis (ed), Complementary Therapies in Rehabilitation—Holistic Approaches for Prevention and Wellness. Thorofare, NJ: SLACK, 1997;xxxvi.

19. Alternative medicine: expanding medical horizons. A report to the National Institutes of health on alternative medical systems and practices in the United States. September 14-16, 1992. Chantilly, VA.

20. Spencer JW, Jacobs JJ. Complementary/Alternative Medicine—An Evidence-Based Approach. St. Louis: Mosby, 1999.

21. Gordon K. Acupuncture in the Physical Therapy Clinic. In CM Davis (ed), Complementary Therapies in Rehabilitation—Holistic Approaches for Prevention and Wellness. Thorofare, NJ: SLACK, 1997;217–232.

22. Taylor AG. Complementary Alternative Therapies in the Treatment of Pain. In JW Spencer, JJ Jacobs (eds), Complementary/Alternative Medicine—An Evidence-Based Approach. St. Louis: Mosby, 1999;282–330.

23. Sharp MMB. Polarity, Reflexology and Touch for Health. In CM Davis (ed), Complementary Therapies in Rehabilitation—Holistic Approaches for Prevention and Wellness. Thorofare, NJ: SLACK, 1997;235–256.

24. Teeguarden M. Acupressure Way of Health, Jin Shin Do. Tokyo: Japan Publications, 1982.

25. Mik GH, Treppmann U. Jin Shin Do. In CM Davis (ed), Complementary Therapies in Rehabilitation—Holistic Approaches for Prevention and Wellness. Thorofare, NJ: SLACK, 1997; 267–278.

26. Jacobs J, Morkowitz R. Homeopathy. In MS Micozzi (ed), Fundamentals of Complementary and Alternative Medicine. New York: Churchill Livingstone, 1996;67–78.

27. Collinge W. Homeopathy: The Grand Provocateur. In W Collinge (ed), The American Holistic Health Association Complete Guide to Alternative Medicine. New York: Warner Books, 1996;134–166.

28. Kleijnen J, Knipschild P, Rietter G. Clinical trials of homeopathy. BMJ 1991;302(316):23.

29. Pizzorno JE. Naturopathic Medicine. In MS Micozzi (ed), Fundamentals of Complementary and Alternative Medicine. New York: Churchill Livingstone, 1996;163–181.

30. Collinge W. Naturopathic Medicine: The Great Cornucopia. In W Collinge (ed), The American Holistic Health Association Complete Guide to Alternative Medicine. New York: Warner Books, 1996;96–113.

31. Pizzorno JE, Murray MT. A Textbook of Natural Medicine. Seattle: John Bastyr College Publications, 1985–1995.

32. Bottomley JM. Biofeedback—Connecting the Body and Mind. In CM Davis (ed), Complementary Therapies in Rehabilitation—Holistic Approaches for Prevention and Wellness. Thorofare, NJ: SLACK, 1997;101–120.

33. Collinge W. Mind/Body Medicine: The Dance of Soma and Psyche. In W Collinge (ed), The American Holistic Health Association Complete Guide to Alternative Medicine. New York: Warner Books, 1996;182.

34. Steggles S, Fehr R, Aucoin P, Stam HJ. Relaxation, biofeedback training and cancer: an annotated bibliography. 1960-1985. Hospice J 1987;3:1–10.

35. Diamond BJ, Shiflett SC, Schoenberger NE, et al. Complementary/Alternative Therapies in the Treatment of Neurological Disorders. In JW Spencer, JJ Jacobs (eds), Complementary/Alternative Medicine—An Evidence-Based Approach. St. Louis: Mosby, 1999;170–199.

36. Laseter J. Untying the Knot—Yoga as Physical Therapy. In CM Davis (ed), Complementary Therapies in Rehabilitation—Holistic Approaches for Prevention and Wellness. Thorofare, NJ: SLACK, 1997;125–131.

37. Bottomley JM. T'ai Chi—Choreography of Body and Mind. In CM Davis (ed), Complementary Therapies in Rehabilitation—Holistic Approaches for Prevention and Wellness. Thorofare, NJ: SLACK, 1997;133–156.

38. Collinge W. The American Holistic Health Association Complete Guide to Alternative Medicine. New York: Warner Books, 1996.

39. Wolf SL, Barnhart H, Ellison GL, Coogler CE. The effect of Tai Chi Quan

and computerized balance training on postural stability in older subjects. Phys Ther 1997;77(4):371–381.

40. Wolf SL, Coogler CE, Tingsen X. Exploring the basis for Tai chi Chuan as a therapeutic exercise approach. Arch Phys Med Rehabil 1997;78:886–892.

41. Selby P. Subtle Energy Manipulation and Physical Therapy. In CM Davis (ed), Complementary Therapies in Rehabilitation—Holistic Approaches for Prevention and Wellness. Thorofare, NJ: SLACK, 1997;267–278.

42. McGee CT, Sancier K, Chow EPY. Qigong in Traditional Chinese Medicine. In MS Micozzi (ed), Fundamentals of Complementary and Alternative Medicine. New York: Churchill Livingstone, 1996;225–230.

43. Qi Gong Data Base. Qi Gong Institute, 561 Berkeley Avenue, Menlo Park, CA 94025, 1999.

44. Bloomfield HH, Cain MO, Jaffe DT. Transcendental Meditation—Discovering Inner Energy and Overcoming Stress. New York: Delacorte, 1975.

45. Lest'e A, Rust J. Effects of dance on anxiety. Percept Mot Skills 1984;58(3):767.

46. Spiegel D. Use of support groups in treatment of women with breast cancer receiving chemotherapy. Sci News 1992;317(19):141.

47. Deyo RA. A controlled trial of transcutaneous electrical nerve stimulation (TENS) and exercise for chronic low back pain. N Engl J Med 1990;322:23.

48. Lehmann TR. Efficacy of electroacupuncture and TENS in rehabilitation of chronic low back pain patients. Pain 1986;26:277.

49. Vallbona C, Hazelwook CF, Jurida G. Response of pain to static magnetic fields in postpolio patients: a double-blind pilot study. Arch Phys Med Rehabil 1997;78:1200–1203.

50. Borsa P, Liggett C. Flexible magnets are not effective in decreasing pain perception and recovery time after muscle microinjury. J Athl Train 1998;33(2):150–154.

51. Barnes JF. Myofascial Release—The Missing Link in Traditional Treatment. In CM Davis (ed), Complementary Therapies in Rehabilitation—Holistic Approaches for Prevention and Wellness. Thorofare, NJ: SLACK, 1997;21–47.

52. Upledger JE, Vredevoogd JD. Craniosacral Therapy. Seattle, WA: Eastland, 1983.

53. Berger D. Rosen Method Bodywork. In CM Davis (ed), Complementary Therapies in Rehabilitation—Holistic Approaches for Prevention and Wellness. Thorofare, NJ: SLACK, 1997; 49–66.

54. Rolf I. Rolfing and Physical Reality. Rochester, VT: Healing Arts Press, 1978.

55. Tavrazich HJ. Rolfing, Hellerwork and Soma. In CM Davis (ed), Complementary Therapies in Rehabilitation—Holistic Approaches for Prevention and Wellness. Thorofare, NJ: SLACK, 1997;70–80.

56. Krieger D. The Therapeutic Touch: How to Use Your Hands to Help or to Heal. Englewood Cliffs, NJ: Prentice Hall, 1979.

57. Quinn JF. Building a body of knowledge: research on therapeutic touch, 1974–1986. J Holistic Nurs 1988; 6(1):37.

58. Rosa L, Rosa E, Sarner L, Barrett S. A close look at therapeutic touch. JAMA 1998;279:1005–1010.

59. Palmer DD. Textbook of the Science, Art and Philosophy of Chiropractic. Portland, OR: Portland Printing House, 1910.

60. Redwood D. Chiropractic. In MS Micozzi (ed), Fundamentals of Complementary and Alternative Medicine. New York: Churchill Livingstone, 1996;91.

61. Casley-Smith JR, Casley-Smith JR. Modern treatment of lymphoedema. I. Complex physical therapy: the first 200 Australian limbs. Aust J Dermatol 1992;33:61–68.

62. Foldi E, Foldi M, Clodius L. The lymphedema chaos: a lancet. Ann Plastic Surg 1989;222:505–515.

63. Field T. Massage therapy for infants and children. J Devel Behav Pediatr 1995;16(20):105.

64. Zuck D. The Alexander Technique. In CM Davis (ed), Complementary Therapies in Rehabilitation—Holistic Approaches for Prevention and Wellness. Thorofare, NJ: SLACK, 1997;161–187.

65. Feldenkrais M. Awareness Through Movement: Health Exercises for Personal Growth. New York: Harper & Row, 1972.

66. Jackson-Wyatt O. Feldenkrais Method and Rehabilitation. In CM Davis (ed), Complementary Therapies in Rehabilitation—Holistic Approaches for Prevention and Wellness. Thorofare, NJ: SLACK, 1997;189–197.

67. Stone A. The Trager Approach. In CM Davis (ed), Complementary Therapies

in Rehabilitation—Holistic Approaches for Prevention and Wellness. Thorofare, NJ: SLACK, 1997;199–212.

68. Morrill Ramsey S. Pilates: a well kept secret. Adv Phys Therapist PT Assist 1998;1:5,30.

69. Simon H. The immunology of exercise: a brief review. JAMA 1984;252:381.

70. Bohm D. Wholeness and the Implicate Order. New York: Routledge & Kegan Paul, 1980.

71. Wallace RK, Benson H, Wilson AF. A wakeful hypometabolic physiologic state. Am J Physiol 1971;221(3):795–799.

72. Ader R, Cohen N. The Influence of Conditioning on Immune Responses. In R Ader, DL Felten, N Cohen (eds), Psychoneuroimmunology (2nd ed). San Diego, CA: Academic, 1991;611–646.

73. Felten SY, Felten DL, Olschowka JA. Nonadrenergic and peptide innervation of lymphoid organs. Chem Immunol 1992;52:25–48.

74. Pert CB, Ruff, M, et al. Neuropeptides and their receptors: a psychosomatic network. J Immunol 1985;135:2.

75. Pert CB. Molecules of Emotion. New York: Scribner, 1997.

76. Foss L. The necessary subjectivity of body-mind medicine : Candace Pert's Molecules of Emotion. Adv Mind Body Med 1999;15:122–134.

77. Mc Whinney JR. The importance of being different. Br J Gen Prac 1996;46L:433–436.

78. Pert CB. Healing ourselves and our society. Presentation to the Elmwood Symposium. Boston, 1989.

79. Wisneski LA. A unified energy field theory of physiology and healing. Stress Med 1997;13:259–265.

80. Becker RO, Selden G. The Body Electric—Electromagnetism and the Foundation of Life. New York: William Morrow, 1985.

81. Hunt V. Infinite Mind—The Science of the Human Vibrations of Consciousness. Malibu, CA: Malibu Publishing Co, 1989.

82. Stapp HP. Mind, Matter and Quantum Mechanics. New York: Springer-Verlag, 1994.

83. Sharma HM. Maharishi Ayurveda. In MS Micozzi (ed), Fundamentals of Complementary Medicine. New York: Churchill Livingstone, 1996;244–245.

84. Aspect A, Grangier P, Roger G. Experimental tests of realistic local theories via Bell's theorem. Phys Rev Lett 1981;47:460.

85. Rarity JG, Tapster PR. Experimental

violation of Bell's inequality based on phase and momentum. Phys Rev Lett 1990;64:2495.

86. Bohm D. A Physics Perspective. In N Freidman (ed), Bridging Science and Spirit. St. Louis: Living Lake Books, 1994.

87. Aspect A. Bell's inequality test: more ideal than ever. Nature 1999;398:188–190.

35

Diagnostic and Therapeutic Injections

CURTIS W. SLIPMAN, CHRISTOPHER W. HUSTON, AND
CARL SHIN

To understand the physiological basis of diagnostic and therapeutic injections, it is necessary to re-examine the premise behind these procedures. It is likewise important to review basic peripheral neuroanatomy, neurophysiology, and the physiological effects of local anesthetic agents and glucocorticoids.

PREMISE OF DIAGNOSTIC INJECTIONS

Diagnostic injections are performed to confirm or rule out a clinical suspicion. They may be performed as a prelude to surgery or for definitive interventional clinical management.[1-5] Examples of these instances include a patient with upper extremity pain and multilevel cervical foraminal stenosis with seemingly atypical dermatomal symptoms, or a competitive athlete with an acute lumbar focal protrusion and correlative radicular pain.

Three clinical requirements must be met before recommending a diagnostic block. First, the diagnosis must be unclear after performing less invasive diagnostic tools, including physical examination, imaging, or neurophysiological testing.[6] Second, the result of a block will alter the treatment plan, and third, the diagnostic intervention should have a high sensitivity, specificity, and accuracy. North et al. suggest that spinal diagnostic blocks do not meet these criteria.[7] Unfortunately, North et. al. used a large volume (3.0 ml) of local anesthetic for each block, causing spreading of the injectant to adjacent nerve roots, thus diminishing the strength of the study design. In contrast, van Akkerveeken reported the sensitivity, specificity, and positive predictive value of selective nerve root block to be 100%, 90%, and 95%, respectively.[8,9]

PREMISE OF THERAPEUTIC INJECTIONS

The primary concept underlying the use of therapeutic injections is the abatement of the inflammatory process. The most potent anti-inflammatory agents available are glucocorticoids. It is reasonable to assume that using corticosteroids requires the presence of inflammation. However, corticosteroids may be used and can be effective in conditions with questionable or even without a demonstrable inflammatory mechanism. This issue is discussed in greater detail in the sections Zygapophyseal Joint Syndrome and Spinal Stenosis.

Local anesthetic agents are frequently injected concurrently with glucocorticoids as an adjunctive medication in order to provide immediate pain relief. Interestingly, there seems to be an added benefit because local anesthetics possess anti-inflammatory properties as well.

The beneficial effect of a therapeutic injection does not depend solely on its ability to halt the inflammatory process. A *therapeutic cure* is achieved when the desired outcome results from the block. When only a partial reduction of pain results, the result is classified as a *therapeutic window*. This window allows for the performance of noninvasive rehabilitation techniques. An example is the patient with hip or knee pain secondary to mild osteoarthritis, who is unable to progress in physical therapy despite oral nonsteroidal anti-inflammatory drugs. A corticosteroid injection may offer partial relief, but the complete relief from pain may depend on the performance of specific joint-stabilizing exercises.

PERIPHERAL NEUROANATOMY

The cell bodies of sensory and motor neurons are located within the dorsal and ventral ganglia, respectively. Projecting from these ganglia are the axons, which are essentially axoplasms enclosed by axoplasmic membrane. Each axon has a unique relationship with the surrounding Schwann's cells. The Schwann's cells may form myelin sheaths, which wrap around an axon or an axon may be simply enveloped by a Schwann's cell. Myelin sheaths arise from the Schwann's cell plasma membrane. Myelin is present in 0.25- to 3-mm segments with varying numbers of folds or lamina. The interface between adjacent myelin segments is called the *node of Ranvier*. Although a gap exists between adjacent sections of myelin, there is no direct contact between the axon and the surrounding endoneurium. The basal cell membrane of the Schwann's cell, the neurolemma, serves as a relative barrier. Unmyelinated nerves rest within the Schwann's cell cytoplasm. In myelinated nerves, one Schwann's cell is responsible for a segment of myelin. In contrast, multiple unmyelinated nerves can be found coursing through a single Schwann's cell.

Surrounding each of the motor and sensory nerve axons and their Schwann's cells is the endoneurium (Figures 35-1 and 35-2). Also located within the endoneurium are capillaries, fibrocytes, and collagen fibrils. The perineurium is a squamous cellular sheath of closely approximated cells,[10] which encase bundles of axons. The perineurium serves as a physical barrier to local anesthetic penetration.[11] The epineurium may cover one or more bundles of perineurium. Nutrient arteries coalesce in the epineurium to form a vascular lattice of arterioles and capillaries that penetrates to the perineurium.

The axoplasmic membrane is a layer of double rows of lipid molecules consisting primarily of phospholipids. Glycolipids and cholesterol are present in lesser amounts. The two outer layers contain the hydrophobic portion of the lipid molecule, whereas the inner layers consist of the hydrophilic component. Interspersed among the glycolipids are numerous proteins, many of which are glycosylated. These fixed proteins form pores, which traverse the entire axoplasmic membrane. It is through these pores or channels that sodium (Na^+) and potassium (K^+) flow. These selective channels allow the preferential egress of either Na^+ or K^+. While the Na^+ channels are concentrated at the nodes of Ranvier, the K^+ channels are interspersed between nodes.[12] For unmyelinated axons, the Na^+ and K^+ channels are not selectively distributed.[13] Inflow or outflow of ions is dependent on numerous variables including the concentration gradient, the voltage gradient, and most importantly, the configuration of its respective channel. Each transmembrane channel can assume an open, closed resting, or closed inactivated state. Using the Na^+ channel as an example will demonstrate the difference between these three channel states. In the open configuration, Na^+ freely travels through the channel. This occurs during depolarization. In the closed resting state, Na^+ is unable to traverse the channel, but the Na^+ channel can be opened by a wave of depolarization. In the closed inactivated state, Na^+ cannot traverse the channel and the channel cannot be opened by a wave of depolarization. The channel assumes this configuration in the presence of local anesthetic agents.

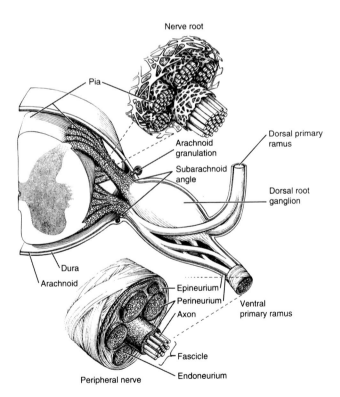

FIGURE 35-1 Structure of nerve roots and peripheral nerve and the continuity of various layers. (Reprinted with permission from T Hogan. Regional Anesthesia & Analgesia: Re-Examination of Anatomy in Regional Anesthesia. Rochester, MN: Mayo Foundation 1996;690.)

NEUROPHYSIOLOGY

An axon in the resting state is electrically charged. This is generated by the distribution of Na^+ and K^+ within and just surrounding the axoplasmic membrane. Within the axon, the concentration of K^+ is 10 times greater than outside. In comparison, Na^+ is 10 times more concentrated outside the axon. These concentration gradients are created by an energy-dependent transport mechanism. An adenosine triphosphate–driven pump allows K^+ to distribute within the cell and relocates Na^+ outside in a ratio of approximately 2 to 3, respectively. In addition to this active mechanism, the distribution of Na^+ and K^+ depends on the relative permeability of the axoplasmic membrane to these ions. In general, the axoplasmic membrane is 50–100 times more permeable to K^+ than Na^+. The Na^+/K^+ pump creates a concentration gradient, allowing K^+ to flow from the intracellular to the extracellular compartment, causing some leakage of K^+ outside of the axon. This seepage creates an axonal negative resting voltage potential. Essentially, the inner axon has a negative charge of approximately –70 mV, compared with the immediate surrounding area. Chloride (Cl⁻) responds to this electrical current by moving from within the axon to the extracellular compartment. Cl⁻ can easily complete this relocation, as the axon membrane is as permeable to Cl⁻ as it is to K^+. Consequently, Cl⁻ tends to concentrate extracellularly during the resting state.

The ability to maintain an electrical charge is as important as creating one. Such a state is achievable because of the double-layer phospholipid construction of the axon membrane, thus allowing it to function as a capacitor. The outer hydrophobic bilayer phospholipid membrane acts as an electrical insulator. In between the two lipid bilayers is an aqueous ionic solution. It is through this lipid barrier that an uncharged local anesthetic must pass and within the ionic solution that the cation moiety exerts its conduction block.

It is the resting electrical potential previously described that allows for the propagation of electrical current along the length of an axon. After a nerve is depolarized, the action potential is transmitted segmentally along the nerve. Na^+ influx through opened Na^+ channels diminishes the resting negative electrical current within the axon. Once the firing threshold of approximately –55 mV is reached, a full depolarization transpires and the rate of Na^+ entry increases. This flow of Na^+ down its concentration gradient transpires as the axoplasmic membrane suddenly allows an influx of Na^+. This sudden spike in Na^+ influx is mediated through the now open Na^+ channels. This process is self-limited by virtue of the inevitable decrement in the Na^+ concentration gradient, change in intracellular charge from negative to neutral and then positive, closure of the Na^+ channels, opening of the K^+ channels, and resumption of Na^+/K^+ pump activity. These fac-

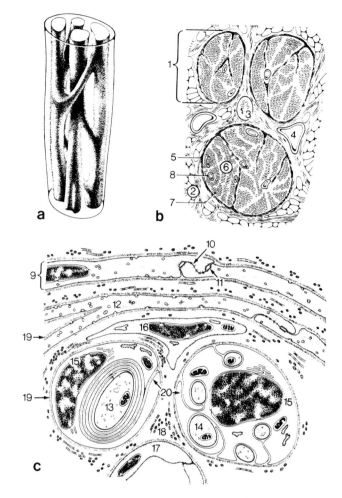

FIGURE 35-2 Peripheral nerve (schematic representation). **A.** Under the magnifying glass, note the arrangement of the nerve fascicles in the form of a plexus. **B.** Light microscopic magnification. Near the nerve fascicles (1), which are contained in a common epineurium (2) rich in fat tissue and connective tissue, the vasa nervorum (3 = arteries; 4 = veins) can be seen. Septa projecting from the perineurium (5) separates the fascicles. In the endoneurium (6), one can recognize myelinated fibers (7) and capillaries (8). **C.** Electron microscopic magnification. The picture shows a section of a fascicle close to the perineurium. The flattened perineural cells (9) are densely interconnected through tight junctions (10 = zonula occludens) and desmosomes (11). The cytoplasm of the perineural cells contains numerous pinocytotic vesicles (12). In the endoneurium, one can recognize myelinated (13) and unmyelinated axons (14). Schwann's cells (15), a fibrocyte (16), and a capillary (17 = endothelial cell). The endoneural interstitial tissue contains numerous collagen fibrils (18). Perineural, endothelial, and Schwann's cells are covered with a basal membrane (19). (20 = mesaxon.) (Reprinted with permission from M Mumenthaler, H Schliach. Peripheral Nerve Lesions: Anatomy of the Peripheral Nerve—Diagnosis and Therapy. New York: Thieme, 1991;8.)

TABLE 35-1
Fiber Type, Myelination, Conduction Velocity, and Function

Fiber Type	Myelin	Diameter Range (mm)	Conduction Velocity Range (mean) (m/second)	Function
A α	Yes	12–20	70–120 (100)	Proprioception, large motor, skeletal muscle
A β	Yes	5–15	30–70 (50)	Touch, pressure, small motor
A γ	Yes	3–8	15–30 (20)	Motor tone (muscle spindle)
A δ	Yes	1–5	12–30 (15)	Sharp pain, temperature
B	Yes	1–4	3–15 (7)	Preganglionic autonomic
C	No	0.3–1.5	0.5–2 (1)	Touch, temperature, dull pain, postganglionic autonomic

tors lead to a restoration of the baseline negative axoplasmic charge, also termed *repolarization*. This sequence of events unfolds within successive segments of axon, creating a wave of depolarization.

Depolarization occurs at segments of the axon covered by sheaths of myelin. In myelinated nerves, the wave of depolarization is triggered at sequential nodes of Ranvier. This process is termed *saltatory conduction*. For unmyelinated nerves, depolarization occurs in successive segments of axon. An electrical impulse travels faster by saltatory conduction than by depolarization of the entire axon. Therefore, myelinated nerves conduct impulses faster than unmyelinated ones. Faster conduction velocity is also associated with larger diameter nerves. This results from the increased number of myelin lamella, and the longer internodal distances associated with larger circumference nerves (Table 35-1) (see Chapter 13).

PHYSIOLOGICAL EFFECTS OF LOCAL ANESTHETIC DRUGS

Local anesthetics are primarily used for diagnostic purposes because of their direct nerve-blocking properties, but therapeutic benefits from these agents have been reported as well. In 1930, Evans postulated that infusing a large volume of fluid could disrupt perineural adhesions,[14] which seems unlikely given Burn's radiologic finding that contrast flows down the path of least resistance.[15]

Winnie,[16] el Mahdi,[17] and coinvestigators suggested that the therapeutic effect may be achieved by impeding sympathetic output. Cullen and Haschke,[18] Hoidal et al.,[19] and Goldstein and colleagues[20] reported on the anti-inflammatory effect of local anesthetics by inhibiting phagocytosis, decreasing phagocytic oxygen consumption, reducing polymorphonuclear leukocyte lysosomal enzyme release, and diminishing superoxide anion production. MacGregor, in 1980, demonstrated a reversible

inhibition of granulocyte adherence, thereby minimizing the delivery of polymorphonuclear cells to an inflammatory foci.[21] Other researchers have later corroborated the anti-inflammatory effects caused by anesthetic agents.[22–27]

Another potential explanation for the therapeutic effect of local anesthetic agents involves the restoration of blood flow. In 1995, Yabuki and Kikuchi, using an animal model, observed that nerve root block leads to improved intraradicular blood flow.[28] If the basis of pain is caused by diminished blood flow, as has been hypothesized for spinal stenosis[29,30] or a herniated disk,[31] then this effect could be therapeutic. This hypothesis is applicable to disorders mediated by the presence of chemical inflammogens. The increased blood flow may serve to *wash them away*. Although increased intraradicular blood flow has been demonstrated in an animal model, two concerns must be addressed before accepting these experimental observations as explanations for the therapeutic effect of local anesthetics. First is whether the increased intraradicular flow is sustained after the local anesthetic effect has subsided. The second issue is to question whether this increased intraradicular blood flow translates into a measurable clinical effect. Hayashi et al., using an animal model that caused a chemical radiculitis, was unable to establish a sustained clinical effect after local anesthetic infiltration.[32] However, using a different model to simulate an inflammatory radiculopathy, Yabuki found a seemingly protective effect of local anesthetics, postulating that this observation resulted from enhanced intraradicular blood flow and direct local anesthetic anti-inflammatory effects.[33]

There are potential *central processing* theories to explain the therapeutic benefits of local anesthetic agents. One theory postulates a placebo response, which has been reported in one-third of all interventions.[34,35] Another concept involves the "temporary block of a pain cycle."[36] This theory suggests that a neural engram of a painful sensation has been established in the brain, or repetitively firing nerves of the wide dynamic type have been created in the spinal column. Each of these areas is incited by afferent information, thereby triggering activity. Through peripheral blockade, these central processing zones are shut off, thereby achieving a therapeutic benefit.

NEUROPHYSIOLOGICAL EFFECTS OF LOCAL ANESTHETIC DRUGS

Local anesthetics block the transmission of electrical impulses by exerting their effect on the Na^+ channels that are concentrated at the node of Ranvier. The charged cation moiety of the local anesthetic binds to the Na^+ channel, altering its configuration to assume the open state. Local anesthetics have been observed to attach to the axoplasmic rather than the extracellular side of the axon membrane[37-40] and that they bind to a specific protein receptor site.[41,42] By preventing access of extracellular Na^+ to the Na^+ channel, the cascade of events leading to depolarization and subsequent action potential propagation is hindered. Local anesthetics, therefore, prevent depolarization, while maintaining the resting state of the nerve, thereby stabilizing the nerve membrane.[43] This effect is not an all or none phenomenon, but rather, a dose-dependent response. As the concentration of local anesthetic increases, a commensurate alteration in the ability of the nerve to depolarize occurs. According to Raymond and Strichartz, as the action potential height is lowered, the rates of rise of the action potential and impulse conduction are slowed, while the firing threshold is increased.[44] The electrical current is eventually diminished to such an extent that the firing threshold is not reached, and the action potential is blocked from propagation.

A blockade at the node of Ranvier is not sufficient to bring the action potential to a halt. Because depolarization at one node of Ranvier can cause depolarization of one or two successive nodes,[45] local anesthetic blockade must include two and preferably three nodes of Ranvier. This is termed the *critical blocking length*. Because the internodal distance is directly proportional to the diameter of the nerve, the critical blocking length is also directly proportionate to nerve thickness.

Numerous factors affect the rapidity, density, and duration of action of local anesthetic neural blockade. As previously noted, conduction block occurs at the protein receptor site of the Na^+ channel. Local anesthetic preferentially binds to that site when it is in the open state. Because a firing axon has a greater percentage of open state channels than an axon at rest, it is the firing axon that demonstrates a shorter temporal onset.

Thus, any local anesthetic affecting a nerve fiber has a different onset latency that is dependent on whether the axon is at rest or not. Because the outer axon membrane is composed of lipids, there is a direct relationship between onset of action and lipid solubility of the local anesthetic.[46] It is the neutral form of a local anesthetic that can diffuse through the lipid bilayer rather than its cation.[47] Each local anesthetic has a fixed dissociation constant or pKa (Table 35-2), which is a measure of when it is in equal ionic and nonionic forms. The pH of the environment in which the local anesthetic is injected influences the concentration of the cation and base state according to the following formula:

$$Log\left(\frac{[cation]}{[base]}\right) = pKa - pH$$

Because the neural environment has a pH of approximately 7.4, a local anesthetic with pKa close to that value will have a greater concentration of the nonionic state as compared with one with a higher pKa. As expected, the onset of anesthesia is faster for those with a lower pKa.[42,48] Once the nonionic form of local anesthetic crosses the phospholipid barrier, it disassociates into its base moiety. The positively charged ion binds to the Na^+ channel receptor site and thereby alters its configuration to an inactive state. The duration of binding to the protein receptor site depends on the protein-binding ability of a particular local anesthetic. As the affinity for protein binding increases, the duration of blockade commensurately lengthens (see Table 35-2). The amount of local anesthetic available affects the manifestation of blockade. In highly vascularized regions, local anesthetic clears more effectively, thereby decreasing the density and duration of its effects. Adding a vasoconstrictor such as epinephrine has the opposite effect. In the epidural space, an unexpected rapid

TABLE 35-2
Local Anesthetic pKa, Duration of Effect, and Affinity for Protein Binding

Agent	pKa	Duration (hours)	Protein Binding (%)
Amide			
Lidocaine	7.8	1–3	65
Bupivacaine	8.1	4–12	95
Etidocaine	7.9	3–12	95
Ester			
Procaine	8.9	0.5–1.0	6
Tetracaine	8.4	2–4	85

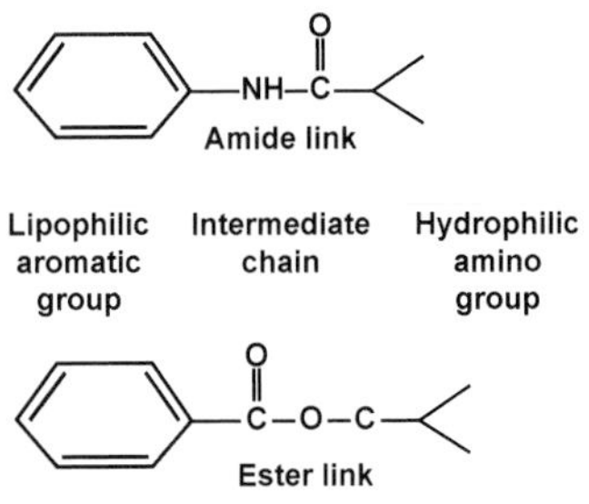

FIGURE 35-3 Chemical structural template of organic amide local anesthetic drugs.

onset may occur because of an undefined rapid transport pathway connecting the epidural space to the endoneurial space.[49]

There are two broad categories of local anesthetics defined by the link between their lipophilic aromatic head and middle chain (Figure 35-3). Esters (Figure 35-4) are hydrolyzed by circulating pseudocholinesterase. One of the metabolic by-products of ester anesthetic agents is para-amino benzoic acid, which is responsible for its common association with allergic reactions. Amides (Figure 35-5) do not form para-amino benzoic acid and are metabolized in the liver.

Both groups of local anesthetics have varying properties that are related to their biochemical structure. For example, substituting a butyl group for methane on the amine end enhances the protein-binding capacity of mepivacaine. When this substitution occurs, bupivacaine is created. As expected, bupivacaine has a longer duration of action than mepivacaine because of its increased ability to bind to the specific protein receptor

site at the base of the Na^+ channel. Changes on the aromatic head affect lipid solubility. As the primary determinant of onset latency is lipid solubility, any alteration in this property affects how quickly that local anesthetic can block a wave of depolarization.

The desired effect in treating painful musculoskeletal disorders is the depolarization block. Knowledge of the physiology of this blockade is essential before performing an injection procedure. Equally critical is an appreciation of the technique of the injection. Although not a focus in this chapter, a few thoughts must be conveyed. A limited and specific region is affected in diagnostic blocks. For example, when a single spinal nerve root is infiltrated, it is the peripheral impulses carried by Aδ, C fibers, or both that must be blocked.[50] These are the nerve fibers of interest because they transmit the signals of acute sharp pain and the delayed onset dull aching or burning pain, respectively.[51] Diagnostic blockade of a knee joint or the sacroiliac joint would involve blocking of the Aδ and C fibers as well as the Aα and Aγ fibers.[52] If pain relief is achieved after either of these diagnostic injections, then a positive block is recorded, meaning that the nociceptive source has essentially been identified. This assumes (1) the amount of local anesthetic used was small enough to avoid blockade of nearby structures, (2) the amount was sufficient to create a conduction block, (3) the needle was situated in a manner that limited the diffusion of local anesthetic to the targeted site, and (4) the vascular system was not inadvertently injected. In the axial skeleton or for deep joints, such as the hip, using fluoroscopic guidance and injecting contrast minimize the probability of these factors influencing the reliability of a diagnostic injection.[6,53-55]

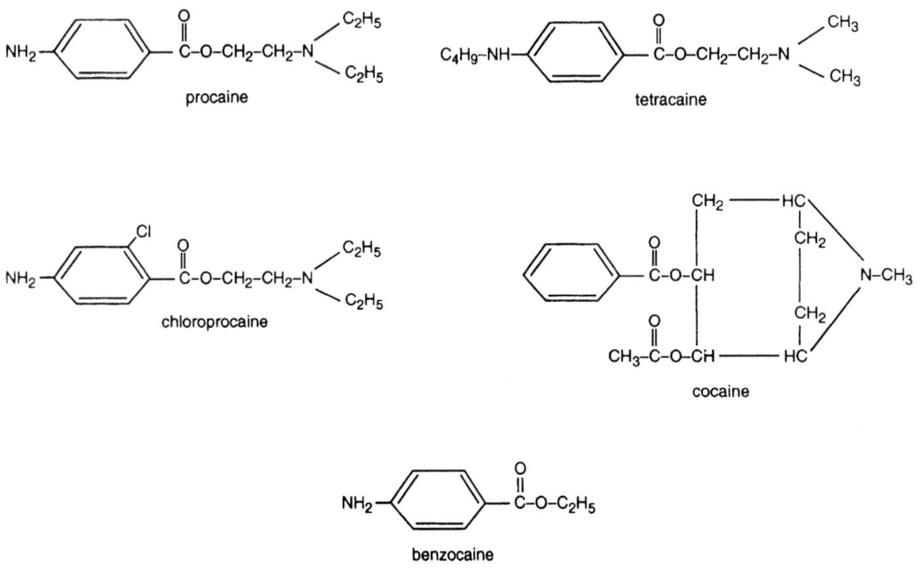

FIGURE 35-4 Representative ester-linked local anesthetics. (Reprinted with permission from deJong. Local Anesthetics: Biotransformation. St. Louis: Mosby, 1994;178.)

MECHANISM OF ACTION OF GLUCOCORTICOIDS

Glucocorticoids are used in a variety of musculoskeletal and neurologic disorders for anti-inflammatory and immunosuppressive reactions. Glucocorticoids are 21 carbon steroid molecules with activity dependent on a hydroxyl group at carbon 11 (Figure 35-6).[56] Cortisol is the normal human circulating glucocorticoid. Cortisol is secreted by the adrenal gland and under the regulation of adrenocorticotropic hormone (ACTH). ACTH is secreted from the anterior pituitary gland, with diurnal variation (i.e., higher in the morning). ACTH results in increased release of cortisol, which has negative feedback on ACTH release. With stress, the hypothalamus increases release of corticotropin-releasing hormone. Corticotropin-releasing hormone travels in the hypophyseal-portal system to the anterior pituitary gland with increased release of ACTH.

Cortisol exhibits glucocorticoid and mineralocorticoid activities. Synthetic derivatives vary in their individual expression of glucocorticoids and mineralocorticoid activity (Table 35-3).[56] In the treatment of inflammatory and immunologic disorders, it is glucocorticoid activity that is desirable. Glucocorticoids affect glucose transport, inflammation, and immune reactions. Mineralocorticoid activity results in Na^+ retention, extracellular fluid volume expansion, hypokalemia, and metabolic alkalosis.[57] Cortisol and cortisone have significant mineralocorticoid activity and are, therefore, less desirable therapeutic agents.

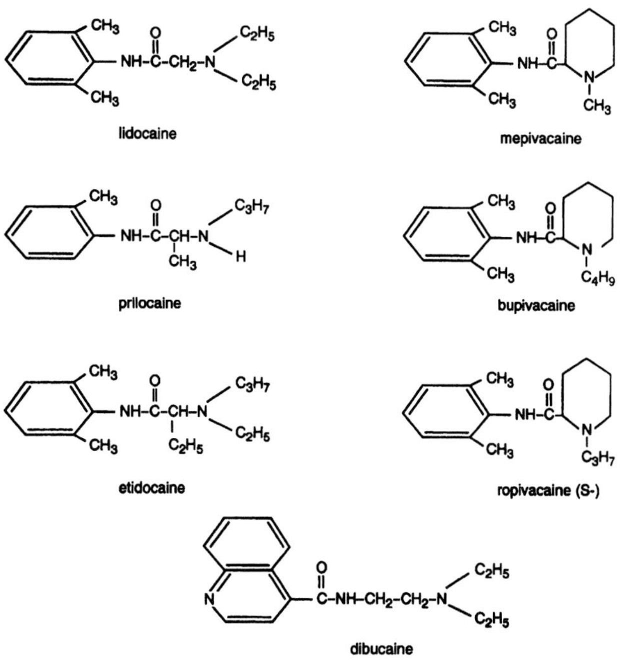

FIGURE 35-5 Representative amide-linked local anesthetics. (Reprinted with permission from deJong. Local Anesthetics: Biotransformation. St. Louis: Mosby, 1994;186.)

FIGURE 35-6 Commonly used glucocorticoids, which are 21 carbon molecules with activity dependent on hydroxyl group at carbon 11. Bold arrows represent differences from cortisol. (Reprinted with permission from L Axelrod. Glucocorticoid therapy. Medicine 1976;55:39–65.)

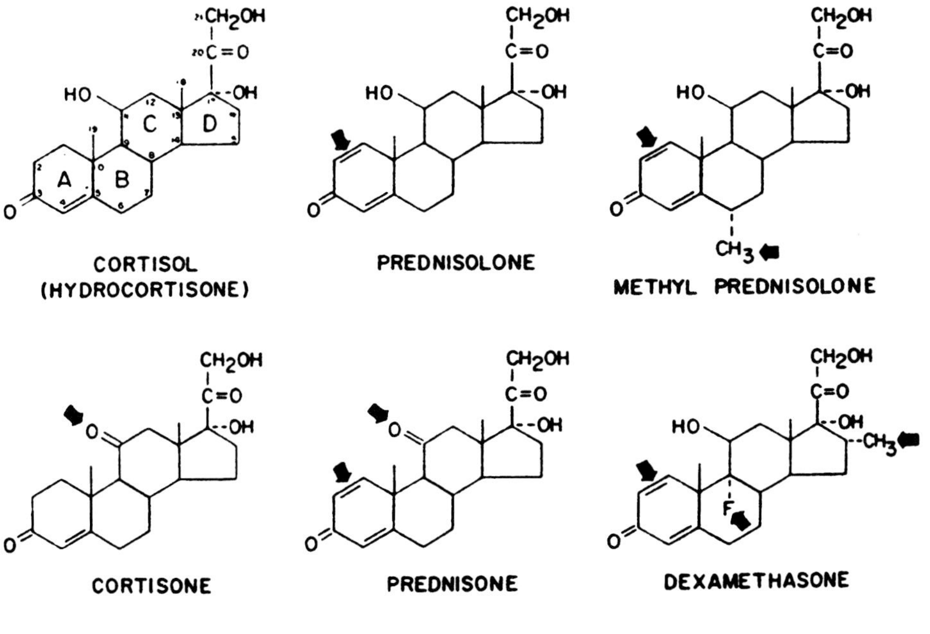

TABLE 35-3
Commonly Used Glucocorticoids

Duration of Action	Glucocorticoid Potency	Equivalent Glucocorticoid Dose (mg)	Mineralocorticoid Activity
Short-acting			
Cortisol (hydrocortisone)	1	20	Yes
Cortisone	0.8	25	—
Prednisone	4	5	Yes
Prednisolone	4	5	No
Methylprednisolone	5	4	No
Intermediate-acting			
Triamcinolone	5	4	No
Long-acting			
Betamethasone	25	0.60	No
Dexamethasone	30	0.75	No

Source: Adapted with permission from L Axelrod. Glucocorticoid therapy. Mineralocorticoid effects are dose related. Medicine 1976;55:39–65.

Synthetic glucocorticoids vary in potency and duration of action. The glucocorticoids are categorized into short- (24–36 hours), intermediate- (24–48 hours), and long- (>48 hours) acting agents based on ACTH suppression.[58] Short-acting agents include cortisone, hydrocortisone, prednisone, prednisolone, and methylprednisolone. Triamcinolone is an intermediate agent. Dexamethasone and betamethasone are long-acting agents. Cortisone and prednisone are 11-keto compounds and require hepatic biotransformation into 11-β-hydroxyl form to be active (see Figure 35-6). Ninety percent of glucocorticoids are bound in the circulation to corticosteroid-binding globulin or albumin.[57] Glucocorticoids are metabolized in the liver and excreted in the urine.[57]

Our understanding of glucocorticoid effects in humans is based on numerous animal and human studies. Caution must be exercised when extrapolating results of animal studies to potential effects on humans, as conflicting conclusions may occur. These conflicts typically arise when comparing studies between different species or if suprapharmacologic glucocorticoid dosages are used. Species have been divided into corticosteroid sensitive and corticosteroid resistant. Corticosteroid-sensitive species (rat, mice, and rabbit) exhibit lympholysis with corticosteroids not typically seen in corticosteroid-resistant species (human, monkey, and guinea pig).[59] Also, in vitro studies using suprapharmacologic dosages need to be interpreted with caution. With these limitations in mind, the effects of glucocorticoids on leukocyte distribution, leukocyte function, protein synthesis, and neural tissues are reviewed in greater detail.

Administration of prednisone in normal adults results in granulocytosis in 4–6 hours.[60] Neutrophilia occurs from release from bone marrow and inhibition of egress from circulation. This results in higher intravascular counts, with less available at the site of inflammation. The differences between prednisone and dexamethasone in granulocyte mobilization have been reported.[61] Compared with prednisone, dexamethasone resulted in increased extravascular granulocytosis. Peters et al. concluded there may be more than just potency and duration of activity differences between glucocorticoids.[61]

Pharmacologic dosages of prednisone in human adults result in lymphopenia, peaking at 4–6 hours and returning to normal by 24[60,62] to 48 hours.[62] Although T and B lymphocytes are affected, a greater decline in T lymphocytes occurs.[60,62] Lympholysis is seen in corticosteroid-sensitive species, but is not the main mechanism for lymphopenia observed in humans.[62] Lympholysis has been described in one study of a small subset of activated T lymphocytes, but the majority is resistant to lympholysis.[63] Lymphopenia probably results from sequestration of recirculating lymphocytes to other body compartments.[62,64] Lymphocytes are divided into nonrecirculating and recirculating lymphocytes. Nonrecirculating lymphocytes spend their entire life in the intravascular space.[65] Recirculating lymphocytes travel between intravascular and extravascular spaces. The extravascular spaces include thymus, bone marrow, thoracic duct, spleen, lymphatics, and lymph nodes.[59] Glucocorticoids cause lymphopenia by redistributing recirculating lymphocytes into the extravascular spaces. Nonrecirculating lymphocytes are not affected and probably not involved in distant target inflammatory or immune responses.[65]

The overall effect of glucocorticoids on leukocytes is to decrease availability of these cells at inflammatory sites. Prednisone administered to humans resulted in monocytopenia within 2 hours, with return to normal counts by 12 hours.[66] It has been postulated that mono-cytopenia occurs as a result of delayed release of bone marrow precursors and the disappearance of mature monocytes from circulation.[65] Glucocorticoids also cause transient eosinopenia.[65]

Cell Function

Glucocorticoids inhibit chemotaxis and vascular endo-thelium adherence of neurophils.[59,65] Lysosomal stabili-zation has been observed with in vitro animal studies, but does not seem to occur in vivo in humans because suprapharmacologic dosages are required.[65]

Glucocorticoids suppress cell-mediated activity in corticosteroid-resistant species when administered in prolonged and large dosages.[59] Exposure of mitogens to lymphocytes results in elevation of various proteins to include lymphocyte glucocorticoid receptors.[67] Leukocytes stimulated by mitogens or antigens pro-duce T-cell growth factor. Glucocorticoids suppress T-cell growth factor.[67] Depressed levels of T-cell growth factor suppress proliferation of specific mito-gen or antigen-responsive lymphocytes.[67] Glucocorti-coids result in depression of mitogen T lymphocytes blastogenesis[59] and mixed leukocyte reactions.[64] The immune response is subsequently delayed or reduced. Already established immune responses in which clones of antigen-responsive lymphocytes exist would not be affected by glucocorticoids.[67]

Transient inhibition of bactericidal and fungicidal activity of monocytes occurs for 48 hours[66] after gluco-corticoid administration. Glucocorticoids affect chemo-taxis of macrophages in vitro by antagonistic effects on macrophage migration inhibitory factor and macro-phage-aggregating factor.[65]

Glucocorticoids reduce the number of Fc receptors on phagocytic cells.[67] This effect occurs within 24 hours of glucocorticoid exposure and returns to normal 48 hours after removal. The affinity of IgG for Fc receptors is not affected.[67] Lack of IgG binding to Fc receptors on phagocytic cells inhibits phagocytosis. Also, macro-phage-antigen complexes are required for T lymphocyte recognition.[65,68]

After 3 or 5 days of methylprednisolone adminis-tration in humans, IgG levels are depressed, with nadirs observed at 2 weeks and 3–4 weeks. Rate of recovery is inversely related to rate of decline.[69] In general, glucocorticoids modulate early immuno-genic reactions as opposed to established reac-tions.[64] Immune complexes passage across basement membranes and reticuloendothelial clearance are inhibited.[65,70]

Glucocorticoids affect a variety of cell functions pri-marily involved in inflammation and cell-mediated immunity. Humoral immunity is affected but to a lesser extent. Many of these effects are postulated to occur through alteration of cell protein synthesis and secretion of active substances.

Protein Synthesis

Cytokines, previously termed *lymphokines*, are polypeptide products of cells involved in regulation of various cellular responses, which include the inflammatogenic and immunologic. The name was changed to *cytokines* when the proteins were found to be secreted by other cells and were not exclusive to lymphocytes.[68]

Glucocorticoids can be perceived as having primary and secondary targets. Primary targets have glucocorti-coid receptors and are directly affected by glucocorti-coids. Secondary targets are influenced by cytokines produced by primary target cells under the regulation of glucocorticoids.[71]

Glucocorticoids bind to cytoplasmic receptors. The activated complex translocates into the nucleus to a tar-get genome. In the nucleus, production of RNA and tran-scription of mRNA occurs. Protein synthesis ensues, with subsequent secretion of polypeptides with specific effects on target tissues.[64,65,70,71] Which genes and proteins glu-cocorticoids regulate depends on the cell type.

Glucocorticoids inhibit monocyte release of inter-leukin-1 and plasminogen activator, macrophage tumor necrosis factor, and granulocyte colony-stimulating factor.[64,70-72] These polypeptides are involved in a wide variety of inflammatory and cell-mediated immune reactions. These effects are depen-dent on the presence of glucocorticoid receptors on leukocytes. Glucocorticoids receptor are regulated to control inflammatory and immune responses. Gluco-corticoid receptors may be down-regulated by syn-thetic glucocorticoids and hypothalamic dopamine.[71] Increased receptors have been observed in the pres-ence of mitogens.

The wide variety of glucocorticoids effects cannot be explained solely by receptor density or affinity.[64] Increased levels of cAMP with increased sensitivity to catecholamines occur within minutes of glucocorticoid administration.[73] This effect occurs quicker than one would expect for synthesis of new proteins. As gluco-corticoids affect protein synthesis, time is required for this process to occur. In glucocorticoid inhibition of glucose transport, nuclear complexes appear within a minute and inhibition within 30 minutes.[71]

Direct Effects

Rat neuromas injected with glucocorticoids reduce the incidence of spontaneous discharges in A fibers.[74] Because the interval during which the study was conducted occurred before development of C-fiber discharges, any comment about glucocorticoid effects on C fibers was obviated. Glucocorticoids prevented the development of ectopic hyperexcitability when applied at the time of nerve sectioning. Glucocorticoids did suppress already active neuromas postoperatively.[74] Nerve conduction of A and C fibers was normal in glucocorticoid-treated nerves. Also, no histologic difference in the glucocorticoid-treated neuromas to untreated was found. Devor et al. concluded the mechanism of action is a direct drug effect of glucocorticoids on the neuroma impulse generator. Glucocorticoids were postulated to affect membrane ion conductance inhibiting impulse generation.[74] Intravenous methylprednisolone administered to cats caused hyperpolarization of the lumbar spinal neuron.[75] Glucocorticoids may affect Na/K ATPase pump, thereby influencing membrane ion conductance and depolarization.[76]

The effect of glucocorticoids on C fibers has been investigated. Methylprednisolone application to rat C fiber suppressed transmission. The effect was reversed when glucocorticoids were removed. Suppression of transmission was hypothesized to be caused by direct action on nerve membranes.[77] Johansson et al. further concluded this may explain why glucocorticoids work in chronic pain when inflammation is not present.[77]

PATHOPHYSIOLOGY OF COMMON SPINAL DISORDERS AND BASIS FOR INJECTION PROCEDURES

Discogenic Conditions

The intervertebral disk may produce extremity pain by nerve root or dorsal root ganglion (DRG) involvement. The effect of mechanical compression on the nerve root and DRG has been studied in rabbits and cats.[78] Compression of the DRG results in repetitive electrical discharge, which potentially explains radicular pain in the presence of a foraminal disk protrusion or stenosis. However, many disk herniations occur posterolaterally, thereby compressing the nerve root rather than the DRG. Nerve root compression causes only a single burst of electrical discharge with no repetitive firing.

Disk herniation with nerve root compression alone does not completely explain continuous radicular pain. Howe et al.[78] placed chromic suture around the nerve root, resulting in inflammation and compression, and in turn, causing repetitive firing. Kawakami and co-investigators[79] found severe thermal hyperalgesia in rats treated with chromic suture as opposed to silk ligature or clip placed around the nerve root. The chromic suture resulted in inflammation whereas the silk ligature and clip did not. Thermal hyperalgesia was found to correspond with radicular pain. They postulated that inflammation, not compression, was important in the development of radicular pain.

A variety of studies have been performed to understand the role of inflammation in radicular pain. Leukocytes, macrophages, and lymphocytes have been found at the site of surgically created porcine disk protrusions in vivo.[80] McCarron and coinvestigators[81] injected nucleus pulposus or saline into the epidural space of dogs. Histologic analysis demonstrated edema, fibrin deposition, marked neutrophil infiltrate, and minimal histiocytic-lymphocytic infiltration in the 5- and 7-day specimens. The 14- and 21-day specimens demonstrated regional fibrosis and vascularity with marked histiocytic-lymphocytic infiltration. Marked granulation tissue was present. These findings were seen in the nucleus pulposus group, but not in the saline group.

Disk materials obtained during surgery for disk herniation in humans have shown inflammatory cells with predominance of macrophages.[82] Nucleus pulposus has been found to induce leukotaxis in pigs implanted with a titanium chamber containing nucleus pulposus, but not with fat.[83] The study concluded that either the nucleus pulposus or a substance liberated by tissue reaction to nucleus pulposus resulted in the leukotaxis.

Olmarker and investigators[84] evaluated the effect of methylprednisolone on porcine cauda equina exposed to nucleus pulposus. The corticosteroid-treated animals got a dose of intravenous methylprednisolone at 5 minutes, 24 hours, or 48 hours after exposure. Animals were studied 7 days after exposure. They found the untreated cauda equina to be red and swollen. The corticosteroid-treated subjects' cauda equina were not swollen and were pale in appearance. Histologic analysis demonstrated the presence of inflammatory cells in all groups, but in less than 50% of nerve fibers. Nerve conduction velocity was slowed in the untreated group. Olmarker et al.[84] determined that subcellular processes account for the difference in nerve conduction velocity because there was no significant difference on histology.

Kayama et al.[85] placed autologous porcine nucleus pulposus cells on to pig cauda equina and reported slowing of nerve conduction on electrophysiological testing. The authors postulated that membrane structures in the nucleus pulposus cells were responsible for the effect.

Saal and coinvestigators[86] found elevated levels of phospholipase A_2 in disk material obtained from patients surgically treated for radiculopathy caused by herniation. Phospholipase A_2 is the rate-limiting step in the liberation of arachidonic acid and the generation of prostaglandins and leukotrienes involved in inflammation.[87] Phospholipase A_2 has been shown to be neurotoxic.[88]

Wilburger and Wittenberg[89] found elevated levels of prostaglandin E_2 and prostaglandin E_1 in disk material obtained at surgery. Prostaglandin E_2 is involved in sensitizing nociceptors to bradykinins.

The role of various cytokines in inflammation and development of radicular and low back pain has gained attention. Takahashi and investigators[90] assayed and cultured disk material obtained at surgery in human subjects. The assays were divided in three groups: disk protrusion, extrusion, or sequestration. Although the cytokines between groups did not differ, the cell types producing the cytokines were different. Disk protrusion had elevated counts of chondrocytes, whereas disk extrusion and sequestration groups contained histiocytes, fibroblasts, and endothelial cells with few chondrocytes. Betamethasone added to cell cultures of disk material inhibited cytokine production and prostaglandin E_2 levels. In another study,[91] disk samples were obtained from surgical patients with disk extrusions or sequestrations. In two-thirds of the samples, granulation tissue and monocellular infiltrates were found. The mononuclear cells expressed interleukin-1, which is involved in stimulating inflammatory mediators and proteolytic enzymes such as collagenase, stromelysis, and plasminogen activators. These studies demonstrate cytokines are present at the site of disk herniation and probably play an important role in radicular and low back pain.

Studies have also shown interrelations with cytokines and components of disk degeneration. Kang and coinvestigators[92] assayed disk material obtained at surgery in patients being treated for herniated disk or scoliosis. Compared with the scoliosis disks, herniated disk material had statistically elevated levels of matrix metalloproteinase activity, nitric oxide, prostaglandin E_2, and interleukin-6. Interleukin-1, tumor-necrosing factor, interleukin-1 receptor antagonist protein (IRAP), and substance P were not found at appreciable levels in either group. Matrix metalloproteinase is involved in disk degeneration. Nitric oxide is involved in immune regulation and inflammation.

Kanemoto[93] evaluated surgical disk specimens for matrix metalloproteinase-3 and tissue inhibitor of metalloproteinase-1, both of which are involved in disk degeneration. Higher levels of tissue inhibitor of metalloproteinase-1 and matrix metalloproteinase-3 were found in disk extrusions and sequestrations compared with protrusions. The precise role of matrix metalloproteinase-3 in discogenic low back pain, other than its degenerative effects, is unclear.

Various neuropeptides have been found in disk specimens. Ashton and investigators[94] found elevated levels of calcitonin gene-related peptide (CGRP) and substance P in the outer annulus fibrosis. Nerve fibers immunoreactive to vasoactive intestinal peptide (VIP) and C-flanking peptide of neuropeptide were also found in the majority of annulus fibrosis specimens. VIP is involved in vasodilation and possibly in sensory transmission. CGRP is involved in nociception, whereas C-flanking peptide of neuropeptide is a vasoconstrictor. Besides involvement in nociception, substance P also increases prostaglandins, interleukin-1, collagenase, and tumor-necrosing factor. Substance P and CGRP were also found in annulus and posterior longitudinal ligament in human specimens obtained at the time of surgery.[95] Elevated levels of substance P, but not VIP, were found in DRG in porcine compressed nerve root.[96] An elevated level of both substance P and VIP was found in DRG of dogs who underwent diskography.[97] The authors postulated compressive forces applied to disk can pump fluids into vertebral body, annulus, or posterior longitudinal ligaments with stimulation of nociceptive fibers. Mechanical stimulation of DRG in rats resulted in higher concentrations of substance P in DRG, Lissauer's tract, and substantia gelatinosa laminae I–III.[98] Substance P is a neurotransmitter for nociception. Increased substance P in classic pain pathways is one mechanism for possible nerve root pain.

Immune responses to nucleus pulposus have been hypothesized as causes of chronic inflammation.[99] Nucleus pulposus exposed to the vascular space results in an immune response with subsequent antibody formation. To explain this theory, Gertzbein[99] evaluated 10 patients with sequestered disks or disk protrusion contained by annulus or posterior longitudinal ligament. He hypothesized that an immune response occurs when a sequestered disk is exposed to the vascular system. His study showed significant elevation of lymphocyte transformation test results, a measure of cellular immune response. Marshall et al.[100] also found elevated titers of IgM in six of nine subjects suffering from discogenic back pain or sciatica.

Jayson[101] obtained cadaver intervertebral foramen specimens in nonoperated chronic back pain sufferers.

Frequently found were perineural fibrosis with compression of epidural veins and dilation of noncompressed veins. Direct compression of nerve root by disk or osteophyte was rarely found. The author hypothesized mechanical damage led to venous obstruction and dilation with anoxia, fibrosis, and neuronal atrophy. The tissue injury leads to fibrin deposition. Tissue plasminogen activator activates plasminogen in the fibrinolytic system to cleave fibrin for clearance. Tissue plasminogen activator inhibitor balances this response. The author reported increased levels of tissue plasminogen activator antigen and inhibitor in some severe low back pain sufferers, but concluded that further research needed to be done.

Zygapophyseal Joint Syndrome

The zygapophyseal joint (z joint) contains nociceptive fibers rendering the joint a potential cause of low back pain.[102-104] Immunohistochemical staining of z joint from human surgical samples demonstrated substance P–positive nerve fibers.[103,105] Experiments have been performed demonstrating pain referral patterns from the z joint.[106-108] Z joint injection of local anesthetics under fluoroscopic guidance has provided relief of low back pain.[109] How the z joint causes pain in various clinical situations is not understood. The z joint is a synovial joint. As a synovial joint, it is subject to rheumatologic disorders such as gout and rheumatoid arthritis. The joint may also be subject to inflammation from trauma and degenerative osteoarthritis. However, this has not been adequately evaluated. Ozaktay and investigators[88] isolated nerve fibers from rabbit z-joint capsules. The nerve fibers were then exposed to phospholipase A_2. Phospholipase A_2 induced an inflammatory reaction histologically with subsequent neurotoxicity as measured electrophysiologically. Lumbar facet joint material obtained at the time of surgical fusion in humans demonstrated increased levels of prostaglandin E_2 and prostaglandin $F_1\alpha$.[94] Assay for neuropeptides on human z joint obtained at surgery has been performed in 14 subjects.[110] Elevated levels of substance P, VIP, CGRP, and C-flanking peptide of neuropeptide were found. C-flanking peptide of neuropeptide is a potent vasoconstrictor, but its role is unclear at this time. The presence of substance P, VIP, and CGRP suggest potential mechanisms of pain production through chemical or mechanical irritation of the z-joint capsule.[110]

Spinal Stenosis

The pathophysiology of neurogenic claudication is currently not known. Various studies have been performed evaluating blood flow. Porter[111] proposes that neurogenic claudication arises from venous pooling with resultant decreased blood flow, resulting in metabolite buildup and decreased nutrients, causing nerve dysfunction. Walking increases spinal canal pressures from arteriole dilation, and the upright position in stenosis patients increases epidural pressure. Both situations negatively affect venous flow. Walking also results in increased venous return from the lower extremities into the pelvic veins with engorgement of Batson's plexus, which further impairs venous flow from the spine. The impaired flow eventually results in nerve dysfunction and symptoms. Postmortem study of spinal stenosis patients with neurogenic claudication has shown nerve root compression from central stenosis, various vascular pathologies, demyelination, and loss of neurons.[112] Watanabe and associates[112] hypothesized that neurogenic claudication arises from avascular atrophy of nerve fibers with constriction of the pia arachnoiditis at the nerve root. The nerve root becomes fixed and more susceptible to mechanical excursions of the spine. Additionally, the thickened pia arachnoid tissue decreases permeability of nerve root to CSF nutrients. Exercise induces increased metabolic demands and neural activity, resulting in nerve root dysfunction.

The delivery of nutrients to the nerve roots in the cauda equina depends on the vascular system as well as CSF. To evaluate the CSF delivery system, methylglucose was injected and its uptake was measured in the cauda equina.[113] In this study, porcine cauda equina was subjected to various compression protocols and no compression (control). Surprisingly, even low compression from sham compression had a statistically significant decrement in methylglucose transport as compared with the control group, although not as severe as with balloon compression.[113] For venous flow to be impaired, at least two adjacent levels need to be involved.[114]

Takahashi and co-investigators[90] evaluated epidural pressures in humans with lumbar spinal stenosis and normal control subjects. In the upright position the lumbar spinal stenosis subjects had significantly increased pressures (82 mm Hg) versus lumbar spinal stenosis flexed posture (37 mm Hg) and normal control upright (34 mm Hg). There was no statistical significance in normal upright and lumbar spinal stenosis flexed posture pressures. The authors concluded that increased epidural pressures in lumbar spinal stenosis in the upright position may lead to nutritional compromise with nerve dysfunction.

The previously mentioned studies suggest a role of impaired venous flow and elevated CSF pressures in the pathophysiology of neurogenic claudication from spinal stenosis. However, these morphologic models do not account for asymptomatic individuals with radiologic evidence of spinal stenosis.[115] Furthermore, the previously mentioned mechanism does not explain the successful treatment of neurogenic claudication from spinal stenosis with the use of selective nerve root block or epidural glucocorticoids.[116,117] Biochemical studies are required to gain further insight into the role of cytokines, neuropeptides, and inflammatory mediators in symptomatic spinal stenosis.

PATHOPHYSIOLOGY OF MYOFASCIAL DYSFUNCTION AND BASIS FOR TRIGGER POINT INJECTIONS

A trigger point is a discrete and hyperirritable focus in skeletal muscle fibers, which manifests as a palpable, tender, and taut band.[118,119] Two important features of trigger points are referred pain elicited on percutaneous compression and a local twitch response or a brisk contraction of a group of muscle fibers on mechanical stimulation.[120-127] Other characteristics include a restricted range of stretch for that muscle; painful weakness without discernible atrophy; and associated autonomic phenomena including vasoconstriction, sweating, pilomotor response, ptosis, and hypersecretion.[124,127,128] Trigger points are termed *active* when spontaneously painful and *latent* when painful with palpation only.[120]

Identification of a trigger point is based on clinical palpation of tender foci. There is no satisfactory laboratory or imaging test currently available for making the diagnosis of myofascial pain syndrome.[129] Four studies have investigated the interrater reliability of clinical examination in identifying a trigger point.[130-134] Wolfe et al., Nice et al., and Njoo and Van der Does found poor reliabilities for identifying palpable band and twitch response, and moderate reliabilities were found for identifying spot tenderness of trigger points.[132,133,135] Gerwin and coworkers reported excellent interrater reliability for identifying local tenderness and taut band, moderate reliability for identifying referred pain, and poor reliability for identifying local twitch response.[130] This study was interesting in that physicians experienced in diagnosing and treating patients with trigger points underwent a supplementary 3-hour training session immediately before the study. The investigators concluded that a hands-on training was essential to achieve a reliable trigger point examination.

To date, there are no biopsy studies assessing the histology of the trigger points taken from patients with myofascial pain syndrome. However, histopathologic studies have been performed of tender spots in fibromyalgic patients that demonstrated type II fiber atrophy and moth-eaten appearances, and electron microscopy revealed segmental muscle fiber necrosis and glycogen and lipid deposition suggestive of ischemic changes.[136,137] These findings are nonspecific and showed no significant differences from control samples.[137] Various biochemical abnormalities have been reported including reduced high-energy muscle substrates and low subcutaneous oxygen tension, implying altered cellular metabolism and local, temporary hypoxia.[138,139] De Blecourt et al. failed to demonstrate any changes in muscle metabolism of fibromyalgic patients,[140] and Simms et al. showed similar levels of maximum oxygen consumption when compared with sedentary control subjects.[141] There is no broad base of evidence to suggest that the biochemical abnormalities, if present, can account for muscular pain.[120] Similarly, histologic studies have not demonstrated inflammation or evidence that prostaglandins may play a role in the development of trigger points.[142,143] Although there is a paucity of studies evaluating the histology or biochemical composition of trigger points, there are numerous conflicting studies assessing the electrophysiological properties of trigger points. Although some studies demonstrate no electrical activity within a trigger point,[144-148] others have identified both spikes and continuous low-amplitude action potentials,[149] in both active and latent trigger points,[150-152] and frequent or increased discharge of motor activity when twitch response was elicited.[153-157] Bohr's review of Hubbard and Berkoff's recordings made him believe that these were end-plate noise.[158] Gerwin also concluded that the low-amplitude activity observed by Hubbard and Berkoff was end-plate noise as defined by Jones and Wiederholt.[120] In a personal communication with Gerwin, Hubbard and Berkoff revealed an interesting finding that was not reported in the original study.[120] They found that the spontaneous activity was abolished when a sympathetic blocking agent (phentolamine) was injected but not abolished with an alpha-motor neuron blocking agent, (curare), which normally suppresses end-plate activity. This nonpublished observation is substantiated by Chen et al.,[159] who reported similar findings. Bengtsson et al. reported a significant reduction in the number of palpated trigger points after stellate ganglion injection.[138] These studies implicate involvement of the sympathetic system in the maintenance of a trigger point. In animal studies, the low-amplitude, continuous discharges in trigger points have been identified as abnormal end-plate potentials by neurophysiologists.[160,161] Ito et al. demonstrated excessive release of acetylcholine packets in the end-plates to account for this abnormality. The results of these aforementioned studies have led Simons to theorize that the locus of the trigger point is a dysfunctional end-plate.[129]

The pathophysiology of the spinal cord pathways[120,123,162] of referred pain from muscle has been better elucidated since its first description by Kellgren in 1957. The theory of convergence of afferent pathways[163] in which branching of unmyelinated peripheral sensory nerves provide input from two separate sites into one dorsal horn neuron is generally accepted.[164] Neurons receiving input from skeletal muscles always receive input from skin or other deep tissues and none from skeletal muscle exclusively.[120] Hoheisel et al. showed that a painful stimulus in muscle could induce widespread changes in receptive fields without requiring a noxious stimulus of the specific dorsal horn neuron whose field is altered.[165] There appear to be latent connections between dorsal horn and peripheral receptors that can be activated with an appropriate stimulus, which may explain the referred pain zone described in myofascial trigger points.[120]

The underlying precept supporting the use of injections in discogenic, facetogenic, and neurogenic spinal disorders is the ability to abate an inflammatory process, suppression of neuronal firing, or both. Inactivation of trigger points by injections on the other hand relies on mechanical disruption of muscle fibers and nerve endings. The trigger point is believed to be most responsive when needled at the locus maximal pain[119,166-168] and when a local twitch response is elicited on needle insertion.[124,125,169-171] The nature of the injected substance is not a critical factor. Efficacy has been demonstrated with sterile water,[172] saline,[173] lidocaine,[174-176] procaine,[173,177] etidocaine,[173] bupivacaine,[178] diclofenac,[142,179] prednisolone,[142,176] botulinum A toxin,[171-182] and dry needling without any injectate.[167,170,183] One study demonstrated superior results with local anesthetic.[173] Currently, the use of local anesthetic is preferred, as it seems to decrease postinjection local soreness.[125]

The mechanism of injection to inactivate a trigger point is unknown.[125] Travell and Simons have suggested several mechanisms: mechanical disruption of the self-sustaining trigger point mechanism, depolarization block of the nerve fibers by the released intracellular potassium, removal of the nerve-sensitizing substances by the injected fluid or local hemorrhage, interruption of the central feedback mechanism, and focal necrosis of the area of the trigger point by the injected drug.[120] However, these hypotheses have not been supported through scientific inquiry.[125]

A study by Fine et al. found that, compared with placebo, naloxone reverses the analgesic effect of the injection.[184] Thus, an endogenous opioid system may be involved in the mechanism of pain relief. Because pain relief can occur within seconds after dry needling, Hong theorizes either mechanical disruption locally or central interruption reflexively that break the vicious cycle of the trigger point phenomena.[173] Interruption of the peripheral nociceptive input to the central control mechanism has been proposed to break the vicious cycle of pain.[185] He favored the central mechanism because animal studies demonstrated decreased or abolished electrical activity in local twitch response when the muscle fiber was denervated.[125] A needle stimulation to a trigger point, via local twitch response, may deliver a strong counterirritation stimuli to the CNS to induce a strong reflex and subsequently relieve the CNS control of the trigger point.[125]

CONCLUSION

The ability of local anesthetics and glucocorticoids to affect the inflammatory pathway and inhibit nerve impulse transmission provides a rationale for their use in the treatment of various spinal conditions. Additionally, glucocorticoids also modulate cytokines and neuropeptides. Although trigger point injections are routinely used in musculoskeletal practice, there remains a large gap in our ability to explain how they work. Numerous studies have investigated tender points, but whether their results can be extrapolated to trigger points is unproven. Much remains to be investigated, and as more information is acquired, our ability to properly select patients will be enhanced.

REFERENCES

1. Kikuchi S, Hasue M. Combined contrast studies in lumbar spine disease: myelography (peridurography) and nerve root infiltration. Spine 1988;13:1327–1331.
2. Macnab I. Negative disc exploration: an analysis of the causes of nerve root involvement in sixty-eight patients. J Bone Joint Surg Am 1971;53A:5891–5903.
3. Dooley JF, McBroom RJ, Taguchi T, Macnab I. Nerve root infiltration in the diagnosis of radicular pain. Spine 1988;13:79–83.
4. Stanley D, McLaren MI, Euinton HA, Getty CJM. A prospective study of nerve root infiltration in the diagnosis of sciatica: a comparison with radiculography, computed tomography, and operative findings. Spine 1990;6:540–543.
5. Slipman CW. Diagnostic Nerve Root Blocks. In E Gonzalez, R Matterson

(eds), Non Surgical Management of Acute Low Back Pain. New York: Demos, 1998;115–122.

6. Slipman CW, Palmitier RA. Diagnostic Selective Nerve Root Blocks. In EJ Henley, M Grabois (eds), Critical Reviews in Physical and Rehabilitation Medicine. New York: Begell House, 1998;123–146.

7. North RB, Kidd DH, Zahurak M, Piantadosi S. Specificity of diagnostic nerve blocks: a prospective, randomized study of sciatica due to lumbosacral spine disease. Pain 1996;65:77–85.

8. van Akkerveeken PF. Lateral Stenosis of the Lumbar Spine [Thesis]. Netherlands: University of Utrecht, 1989.

9. van Akkerveeken PF. The diagnostic value of nerve root sheath infiltration. Acta Orthop Scand 1993;64:61–63.

10. Akert K, Sandri C, Weibel R, et al. The fine structures of the perineural endothelium. Cell Tissue Res 1976;165:281–295.

11. Ritchie JM, Ritchie B, Greengard P. The effect of the nerve sheath on the action of local anesthetics. J Pharmacol Exp Ther 1965;150:160.

12. Chiu SY, Ritchie JM. Potassium channels in nodal and internodal axonal membrane of mammalian myelinated fibres. Nature 1980;284:170.

13. Bostock H, Sears TA. The internodal axon membrane: electrical excitability and continuous conduction in segmental demyelination. J Physiol (Lond) 1978;280:273.

14. Evans W. Intrasacral epidural injection in the treatment of sciatica. Lancet 1930;2:1225–1229.

15. Burn JM, Guyer PB, Langdon L. The spread of solutions injected into the epidural space. Br J Anaesth 1973;45:338.

16. Winne AP, Hartman JT, Meyers HL Jr, et al. Pain Clinic II: Intradural and extradural corticosteroids for sciatica. Anesth Analg Curr Res 1972;51:990–1003.

17. El Mahdi MA, Abdel Latif FY, Janko M. The spinal nerve root "innervation" and a new concept of the clinico-pathological interrelations in back pain and sciatica. Neurochirurgia 1981;24:137–141.

18. Cullen BF, Haschke RH. Local anesthetic inhibition of phagocytosis and metabolism of human leukocytes. Anesthesiology 1974;40:142.

19. Hoidal JR, White JG, Repine JE. Influence of cationic local anesthetics on the metabolism and ultrastructure of human alveolar macrophages. J Lab Clin Med 1979;93:857.

20. Goldstein IM, Lind S, Hoffstein S, Weissmann G. Influence of local anesthetics upon human polymorphonuclear leukocyte function in vitro. J Exp Med 1977;146:483–494.

21. MacGregor RR, Thorner RE, Wright DM. Lidocaine inhibits granulocyte adherence and prevents granulocyte delivery to inflammatory sites. Blood 1980;56(2):203–209.

22. Cassuto J, Nellgard P, Stage L, Jonsson A. Amide local anesthetics reduce albumin extravasation in burn injuries. Anesthesiology 1990;72:302–307.

23. Peck SL, Johnston RB, Horwitz LD. Reduced neutrophil superoxide anion release after prolonged infusions of lidocaine. J Pharmacol Exp Ther 1985;235:418–422.

24. Rimback G, Cassuto J, Wallin G, Weslander G. Inhibition of peritonitis by amide local anesthetics. Anesthesiology 1988;69:881–886.

25. Martinsson T, Haegerstrand A, Dalsgaard C. Ropivacaine and lidocaine inhibit proliferation of non-transformed cultured adult human fibroblasts, endothelial cells and keratinocytes. Agents Actions 1993;40:78–85.

26. Ohsaka A, Saionji D, Sato N, et al. Local anesthetic lidocaine inhibits the effect of granulocyte colony-stimulating factor on human neutrophil functions. Exp Hematol 1994;22:460–466.

27. Ramus GV, Cesano L, Barbalonga A. Different concentrations of local anesthetics have different modes of action on human lymphocytes. Agents Actions 1983;13:333–341.

28. Yabuki S, Kikuchi S. Nerve root infiltration and sympathetic block. Spine 1995;20(8):901–906.

29. Olmarker K, Rydevik B, Holm S, Bagge U. Effects of experimental graded compression on blood flow in spinal nerve roots. A vital microscopic study on the porcine cauda equina. J Orthop Res 1989;7(6):817–823.

30. Takahashi K, Olmarker K, Holm S, et al. Double-level cauda equina compression: an experimental study with continuous monitoring of intraneural blood flow in the porcine cauda equina. J Orthop Res 1993;11(1):104–109.

31. Yabuki S, Kikuchi S, Omarker K, Myers RR. Acute effects of nucleus pulposus on blood flow and endoneurial fluid pressure in rat dorsal root ganglia. Spine 1998;23(23):2517–2523.

32. Hayashi N, Weinstein JN, Meller ST, et al. The effect of epidural injection of betamethasone or bupivacaine in a rat model of lumbar radiculopathy. Spine 1998;23(8):877–885.

33. Yabuki SH, Kawaguchi Y, Nordborg C, et al. Effects of lidocaine on nucleus pulposus-induced nerve root injury. Spine 1998;23(22):2383–2389.

34. Beecher HK. The powerful placebo. JAMA 1955;159:1602.

35. Benson H, Epstein MD. The placebo effect. A neglected asset in the care of patients. JAMA 1975;232:1225.

36. Raj PP. Prognostic and Therapeutic Local Anesthetic Blockade. In MJ Cousins, PO Bridenbaugh (eds), Neural Blockade. Philadelphia: Lippincott, 1988;899.

37. Wang HW, Jay ZY, Narahashi T. Interaction of spin-labeled local anesthetics with the sodium channel of squid axon membranes. J Mem Biol 1982;66:227–233.

38. Narahashi T, Frazier DT, Yamada M. The site of action and active form of local anesthetics. I. Theory and pH experiments with tertiary compounds. J Pharmacol Exp Ther 1970;171:32–44.

39. Frazier DT, Narahashi T, Yamada M. The site of action and active form of local anesthetics. II. Experiments with quaternary ammonium compounds. J Pharmacol Exp Ther 1970;171:45–51.

40. Strichartz GR. The inhibition of sodium currents in myelinated nerve by quaternary derivatives of lidocaine. J Gen Physiol 1973;62:37.

41. Radsdale DS, McPhee JC, Schever T, Cattaerall WA. Molecular determinants of state-dependent block of Na^+ channels by local anesthetic. Science 1995;265:1724.

42. Covino BG. Pharmacology of local anaesthetic agents. Br J Anaesth 1986;58:701.

43. Shanes AM. Electrochemical aspects of physiological and pharmacological action in excitable cells. Part I. The resting cell and its alteration by extrinsic factors. Pharmacol Rev 1958;10:59–164.

44. Raymond SA, Strichartz GR. Further comments on the failure of impulse propagation in nerves marginally blocked by local anesthetics. Anesth Analg 1990;70:121.

45. Tasaki I. Conduction of the Nerve Impulse. In J Field (ed), Handbook of Physiology, Vol 1. Sec 1: The Nervous System. Washington, DC: American Physiological Society, 1959.

46. Courtney KR, Kendig JJ, Cohen EN. Frequency-dependent conduction block. Anesthesiology 1978;48:111.

47. Ritchie JM, Ritchie B, Greengard P.

The active structure of local anesthetics. J Pharmacol Exp Ther 1965;150: 152.

48. Ohki S. Permeability of axon membranes to local anesthetics. Biochim Biophys Acta 1981;643:495.

49. Byrod G, Olmarker K, Konno S, et al. A rapid transport route between the epidural space and the intraneural capillaries of the nerve roots. Spine 1995;20(2):138–143.

50. Slipman CW, Palmitier RA, DeDianous DK. Physical Medicine and Rehabilitation: The Complete Approach. In M Grabois, SJ Garrison, KA Hart, et al. (eds), Injection Techniques. Malden, MA: Blackwell Science, 2000;458–486.

51. Nygaard OP, Mellgren SI. The function of sensory nerve fibers in lumbar radiculopathy. Spine 1998;23(3):348–352.

52. LaMotte RH, Campbell JN. Comparison of responses of warm and nociceptive C-fiber afferents in monkey with human judgments of thermal pain. J Neurophysiol 1978;41:509–528.

53. Kaplan M, Dreyfuss P, Halbrook B, Bogduk N. The ability of lumbar medial branch blocks to anesthetize the zygapophysial joint. Spine 1998; 23(17):1847–1852.

54. Slosar PJ, White AH, Wetzel FT. The use of selective nerve root blocks: diagnostic, therapeutic, or placebo? Spine 1998;23(20):2253–2256.

55. Renfrew DL, Moore TE, Kathol MH, et al. Correct placement of epidural steroid injections: fluoroscopic guidance and contrast administration. AJNR Am J Neuroradiol 1991;12:1003–1007.

56. Axelrod L. Glucocorticoid therapy. Medicine 1976;55:39–65.

57. Haynes RC Jr, Murad R. Adrenocorticotropic Hormone: Adrenocortical Steroids and Their Synthetic Analogs. Inhibitors of Adrenocortical Steroid Biosynthesis. In LS Goodman, A Gilman (eds), The Pharmacological Basis of Therapeutics (6th ed). New York: Macmillan, 1980;1466–1496.

58. Harter JG. Corticosteroids: their physiologic use in allergic diseases. N Y State J Med 1966;66:827.

59. Claman HN. Corticosteroids and lymphoid cells. N Engl J Med 1972;287(8): 388–397.

60. Yu DTY, Clements PJ, Paulus HE, et al. Human lymphocyte subpopulations. Effect of corticosteroids. J Clin Invest 1974;53:565–571.

61. Peters WP, Holland JF, Senn H, et al. Corticosteroid administration and

localized leukocyte mobilization in man. N Engl J Med 1972;282:342–345.

62. Fan PT, Yu DTY, Clements PJ, et al. Effect of corticosteroids on the human immune response: comparison of one and three daily 1 gm intravenous pulses of methylprednisolone. J Lab Clin Med 1978;91:625–634.

63. Galili N, Galili U, Klein E, et al. Human T lymphocytes become glucocorticoid-sensitive upon immune activation. Cell Immunol 1980;50:440.

64. Cupps TR, Fauci AS. Corticosteroid-mediated immunoregulation in man. Immunol Rev 1982;65:133–155.

65. Fauci AS, Dale DC, Balow JE. Glucocorticoids therapy: mechanisms of action and clinical considerations. Ann Intern Med 1976;84:304–315.

66. Rinehart JJ, Sagone AL, Balcerzak SP, et al. Effects of corticosteroid therapy on human monocyte function. N Engl J Med 1975;292:236–241.

67. Crabtree GR, Gillis S, Smith KA, Munck A. Glucocorticoids and immune responses. Arthritis Rheum 1979;22:1246–1256.

68. Dinarello CA, Mier JW. Lymphokines. N Engl J Med 1987;317:940–945.

69. Butler WT, Rossen RD. Effects of corticosteroids on immunity in man. I. Decreased serum IgG concentration caused by 3 or 5 days of high doses of methylprednisolone. J Clin Invest 1973;52:2629–2640.

70. Kehrl JH, Fauci AS. The clinical use of glucocorticoids. Ann Allergy 1983;50:2–8.

71. Munck A, Mendel DB, Smith LI, Orti E. Glucocorticoid receptors and actions. Am Rev Respir Dis 1990; 141:S2–S10.

72. Kern JA, Lamb RJ, Reed JC, et al. Dexamethasone inhibition of interleukin 1 beta production by human monocytes. J Clin Invest 1988;81:237–244.

73. Parker CW, Huber MG, Baumann ML. Alterations of the cyclic AMP metabolism in human bronchial asthma. III. Leukocyte and lymphocyte responses to steroids. J Clin Invest 1973;52:1342.

74. Devor M, Govrin-Lippmann R, Raber P. Corticosteroids suppress ectopic neural discharge originating in experimental neuromas. Pain 1985;22:127–137.

75. Hall ED. Acute effects of intravenous glucocorticoid on cat spinal motor neuron electrical properties. Brain Res 1982;240:186–190.

76. Hall ED. Glucocorticoid effect on central nervous excitability and synaptic transmission. Int Rev Neurobiol 1982;23:165–195.

77. Johansson A, Hao J, Sjolund B. Local corticosteroid application blocks transmission in normal nociceptive C-fibres. Acta Anaesthesiol Scand 1990;34:335–338.

78. Howe JF, Loeser JD, Calvin WH. Mechanosensitivity of dorsal root ganglia and chronically injured axons: a physiological basis for the radicular pain of nerve root compression. Pain 1977;3:25–41.

79. Kawakami M, Weinstein JN, Spratt KF, et al. Experimental lumbar radiculopathy. Immunohistochemical and quantitative demonstrations of pain induced by lumbar nerve root irritation of the rat. Spine 1994;19:1780–1794.

80. Habtemariam A, Virri J, Gronblad M, et al. Inflammatory cells in full-thickness anulus injury in pigs. An experimental disc herniation animal model. Spine 1998;23:524–529.

81. McCarron RF, Wimpee MW, Hudkins PG, Laros GS. The inflammatory effect of nucleus pulposus. A possible element in the pathogenesis of low back pain. Spine 1987;12:760–764.

82. Gronblad M, Virri J, Tolonen J, et al. A controlled immunohistochemical study of inflammatory cells in disc herniation tissue. Spine 1994;19:2744–2751.

83. Olmarker K, Blomquist J, Stromberg J, et al. Inflammatogenic properties of nucleus pulposus. Spine 1995;20:665–669.

84. Olmarker K, Byrod G, Cornefjord M, et al. Effects of methylprednisolone on nucleus pulposus-induced nerve root injury. Spine 1994;19:1803–1808.

85. Kayama S, Olmarker K, Larsson K, et al. Cultured autologous nucleus pulposus cells induce functional changes in spinal nerve roots. Spine 1998;23: 2155–2158.

86. Saal JS, Franson RC, Dobrow R, et al. High levels of inflammatory phospholipase A2 activity in lumbar disc herniations. Spine 1990;15:674–678.

87. Franson RC, Saal JS, Saal JA. Human disc phospholipase A2 is inflammatory. Spine 1992;17:S129–S132.

88. Ozaktay AC, Cavanaugh JM, Blagoev DC, King AI. Phospholipase A2 induced electrophysiologic and histologic changes in rabbit dorsal lumbar spine tissues. Spine 1995;20:2659–2668.

89. Wilburger RE, Wittenberg RH. Prostaglandin release from lumbar disc and facet joint tissue. Spine 1994;19:2068–2070.

90. Takahashi H, Suguro T, Okazima Y, et

al. Inflammatory cytokines in the herniated disc of lumbar spine. Spine 1996;21:218–224.

91. Doita M, Kanatani T, Harada T, Mizuno K. Immunohistologic study of the ruptured intervertebral disc of the lumbar spine. Spine 1996;21:235–241.

92. Kang JD, Gergescu HI, McIntyre-Larkin L, et al. Herniated lumbar intervertebral discs spontaneously produce matrix metalloproteinases, nitric oxide, interleukin-6, and prostaglandin E$_2$. Spine 1996;21:271–277.

93. Kanemoto M, Hukada S, Komiya Y, et al. Immunohistochemical study of matrix metalloproteinase-3 and tissue inhibitor of metalloproteinase-1 in human intervertebral discs. Spine 1996;21:1–8.

94. Ashton IK, Roberts S, Jaffray DC, et al. Neuropeptides in the human intervertebral disc. J Orthop Res 1994;12:186–192.

95. Konttinen YT, Gronblad M, Antti-Poika I, et al. Neuroimmunohistochemical analysis of periodical nociceptive neural elements. Spine 1990;15:383–386.

96. Cornefjord M, Olmarker K, Farley DB, et al. Neuropeptide changes in compressed spinal nerve roots. Spine 1995;20:670–673.

97. Weinstein J, Claverie W, Gibson S. The pain of discography. Spine 1988;13:1344–1348.

98. Badalamente MA, Dee R, Ghillani R, et al. Mechanical stimulation of dorsal root ganglia induces increased production of substance P: a mechanism for pain following nerve root compromise? Spine 1987;12:552–555.

99. Gertzbein SD. Degenerative disk disease of the lumbar spine. Clin Orthop Rel Res 1977;129:68–71.

100. Marshall LL, Trethewie ER, Curtain CC. Chemical radiculitis. Clin Orthop Rel Res 1977;129:61–67.

101. Jayson MIV. The role of vascular damage and fibrosis in the pathogenesis of nerve root damage. Clin Orthop Rel Res 1992;279:40–48.

102. Hirsch C, Ingelmark BE, Miller M. The anatomical basis of low back pain. Studies on the presence of sensory nerve endings in ligamentous, capsular, and intervertebral disc structures in the human lumbar spine. Acta Scand Orthop 1963;33:1–17.

103. Giles LGF, Harvey R. Immunohistochemical demonstration of nociceptors in the capsule and synovial folds of human zygapophyseal joints. Br J Rheum 1987;26:362–364.

104. Yamashita T, Cavanaugh JM, El-Bohy AA, et al. Mechanosensitive afferent units in the lumbar facet joint. J Bone Joint Surg 1990;72A:865–870.

105. Beaman DN, Graziano GP, Glover RA, et al. Substance P innervation of lumbar spine facet joints. Spine 1993;18:1044–1049.

106. Mooney V, Robertson J. The facet syndrome. Clin Orthop Rel Res 1976;115:149–156.

107. McCall IW, Park WM, O'Brien JP. Induced pain referral from posterior lumbar elements in normal subjects. Spine 1979;4:441–446.

108. Bogduk N. Lumbar dorsal ramus syndrome. Med J Aust 1980;2:537–541.

109. Schwarzer AC, Aprill CN, Derby R, et al. Clinical features of patients with pain stemming from the lumbar zygapophysial joints. Is the lumbar facet syndrome a clinical entity? Spine 1994;19:1132–1137.

110. Ashton IK, Ashton BA, Gibson SJ, et al. Morphological basis for back pain: the demonstration of nerve fibers and neuropeptides in the lumbar facet joint capsule but not in ligamentum flavum. J Orthop Res 1992;10:72–78.

111. Porter RW. Spinal stenosis and neurogenic claudication. Spine 1996;21:2046–2052.

112. Watanabe R, Parke WW. Vascular and neural pathology of lumbosacral spinal stenosis. J Neurosurg 1986;64:64–70.

113. Olmarker K, Rydevik B, Hansson T, Holm S. Compression-induced changes of the nutritional supply to the porcine cauda equina. J Spinal Disord 1990;3:25–29.

114. Olmarker K, Holm S, Rydevik B. Single versus double level nerve root compression: an experimental study on the porcine cauda equina with analyses of nerve impulse conduction properties. Clin Orthop 1992;6:35–39.

115. Boden SD, Davis DO, Dina TS, et al. Abnormal magnetic-resonance scans of the lumbar spine in asymptomatic subjects. J Bone Joint Surg 1990;72A:403–408.

116. Saal JS, Saal JA, Parthasarathy R. The natural history of lumbar spinal stenosis: the results of nonoperative treatment. Proc Tenth Annu Conf North Am Spine Soc, 1995.

117. Ciocon JO, Galindo-Ciocon D, Amaranath L, Galindo D. Caudal epidural blocks for elderly patients with lumbar canal stenosis. JAGS 1994;42:593–596.

118. Yunus MB. Fibromyalgia Syndrome and Myofascial Pain Syndrome: Clinical Features, Laboratory Tests, Diagnosis and Pathophysiologic Mechanisms. In ES Rachlin (ed), Myofascial Pain and Fibromyalgia: Trigger Point Management. St. Louis: Mosby, 1994;3–29.

119. Travell JG, Simons DG. Myofascial Pain and Dysfunction: The Trigger Point Manual, Vol 1–2. Baltimore: Williams & Wilkins, 1983.

120. Gerwin RD. Neurobiology of the myofascial trigger point. Bailliere Clin Rheum 1994;8(4):747–762.

121. Han SC, Harrison P. Myofascial pain syndrome and trigger-point management. Reg Anesthes 1997;22(1):89–101.

122. Hong CZ, Simons DG. Pathophysiologic and electrophysiologic mechanisms of myofascial trigger points. Arch Phys Med Rehabil 1998;79:863–872.

123. Hong CZ. Pathophysiology of myofascial trigger points. J Formos Med Assoc 1996;95(2):93–104.

124. Hong CZ. Myofascial trigger point injection. Crit Rev Phys Rehab Med 1993;5:203–217.

125. Hong CZ. Considerations and recommendations regarding myofascial trigger point injection. J Musculoskel Pain 1994;2(1):29–59.

126. Fricton JR. Myofascial pain: clinical characteristics and diagnostic criteria. J Musculoskel Pain 1993;1:37–47.

127. Fricton JR. Myofascial pain syndrome. Neurol Clin 1989;7(2):413–427.

128. Campbell SM. Regional myofascial pain syndrome. Rheum Dis Clin North Am 1989;15(1):31–44.

129. Simons DG. Clinical and etiological update of myofascial pain from trigger points. J Musculoskel Pain 1996;4:93–121.

130. Gerwin RD, Shannon S, Hong CZ, et al. Identification of myofascial trigger points: interrater agreement and effect of training. Pain 1997;69:65–73.

131. Lew PC, Lewis JL, Story I. Inter-therapist reliability in locating latent myofascial trigger points using palpation. Man Ther 1997;2(2):87–90.

132. Nice DA, Riddle DL, Lamb RL, et al. Intertester reliability of judgments of the presence of trigger points in patients with low back pain. Arch Phys Med Rehabil 1992;73:893–898.

133. Njoo KH, Van der Does E. The occurrence and inter-rater reliability of myofascial trigger points in the quadratus lumborum and gluteus medius: a prospective study in non-specific low back pain patients and controls in general practice. Pain 1994;58:317–323.

134. Tunks E, McGain GA, Hart LE, et al. The reliability of examination for ten-

derness in patients with myofascial pain, chronic fibromyalgia and controls. J Rheumatol 1995;22:944–952.

135. Wolfe F, Simons DG, Fricton J, et al. The fibromyalgia and myofascial pain syndromes: a preliminary study of tender points and trigger points in persons with fibromyalgia, myofascial pain syndrome and no disease. J Rheumatol 1992;19(6):944–951.

136. Yunus MB, Kalyan-Raman UP, Kalyan-Raman K. Primary fibromyalgia syndrome and myofascial pain syndrome: clinical features and muscle pathology. Arch Phys Med Rehabil 1988;69:451–454.

137. Yunus MB, Kalyan-Raman UP, Masi AT, Aldag JC. Electron microscopic studies of muscle biopsy in primary fibromyalgia syndrome: a controlled and blinded study. J Rheumatol 1989;16:97–101.

138. Bengtsson A, Bengtsson M. Regional sympathetic blockade in primary fibromyalgia. Pain 1988;33(Suppl):161–167.

139. Lund N, Bengtsson A, Thorborg P. Muscle tissue oxygen pressure in primary fibromyalgia. Scand J Rheumatol 1986;15:165–173.

140. De Blecourt AC, Wolf RF, van Rijswizk MH, et al. In vivo 31P magnetic resonance spectroscopy (MRS) of tender points in patients with primary fibromyalgia syndrome. Rheumatol Int 1991;11:51–54.

141. Simms RW, Roy SH, Hrovat M, et al. Lack of association between fibromyalgia syndrome and abnormalities in muscle energy metabolism. Arthritis Rheum 1994;37:794–800.

142. Drewes AM, Andereasen A, Poulsen LH. Injection therapy for treatment of chronic myofascial pain: a double-blind study comparing corticosteroid versus diclofenac injections. J Musculoskel Pain 1993;1:289–294.

143. Kalyan-Raman UP, Kalyan-Raman K, Yunus MB, Masi AT. Muscle pathology in primary fibromyalgia syndrome: a light microscopic, histochemical and ultrastructural study. J Rheumatol 1984;11:808–813.

144. Durette MR, Rodriguez AA, Agre JC, Silverman JL. Needle electromyographic evaluation of patients with myofascial or fibromyalgic pain. Am J Phys Med Rehabil 1991;70:154–156.

145. Kraft GH, Johnson EW, Laban MM. The fibrositis syndrome. Arch Phys Med Rehabil 1968;9:155–162.

146. Svebak S, Angia R, Karstad S. Task-induced electromyographic activation

in fibromyalgia subjects and controls. Scand J Rheumatol 1993;22:124–130.

147. Zidar J, Backman E, Bengtsson A, et al. Quantitative EMG and muscle tension in painful muscles in fibromyalgia. Pain 1990;40:249–254.

148. Brucini M, Duranti R, Galletti R, et al. Pain thresholds and electromyographic features of periarticular muscles in patients with osteoarthritis of the knee. Pain 1981;10:57–66.

149. Hubbard DR, Berkoff GM. Myofascial trigger points show spontaneous needle EMG activity. Spine 1993;18:1803–1807.

150. Simons DG, Hong C-Z, Simons LS. Nature of myofascial trigger points: active loci [Abstract]. J Musculoskel Pain 1995;3(Suppl 1):62.

151. Simons DG, Hong C-Z, Simons LS. Spontaneous electrical activity of trigger points [Abstract]. J Musculoskel Pain 1995;3(Suppl 1):124.

152. Simons DG, Hong C-Z, Simons LS. Spike activity in trigger points [Abstract]. J Musculoskel Pain 1995;3(Suppl 1):125.

153. Fricton JR, Auvinen MD, Dykstra D, Schiffman E. Myofascial pain syndrome: electromyographic changes associated with local twitch response. Arch Phys Med Rehabil 1985;66:314–317.

154. Dexter JR, Simons DG. Local twitch response in human muscle evoked by palpation and needle penetration on a trigger point. Arch Phys Med Rehabil 1981;62:521–522.

155. Hong CZ, Simons DG, Stathana L. Electromyographic analysis of local twitch responses of human extensor digitorum communis muscle during ischemia compression over the arm. Arch Phys Med Rehabil 1986;67:680.

156. Elliott FA. Tender muscles in sciatica. Lancet 1944;1:47–49.

157. Simons DG, Dexter JR. Comparison of local twitch responses elicited by palpation and needling of myofascial trigger points. J Musculoskel Pain 1995;3:49–61.

158. Bohr T. Fibromyalgia syndrome and myofascial pain syndrome: Do they exist? Neurol Clin 1995;1(2):365–384.

159. Chen JT, Chen SM, Kuan TS, et al. Phentolamine effect on the spontaneous electrical activity of active loci in a myofascial trigger spot of rabbit skeletal muscle. Arch Phys Med Rehabil 1998;79:790–794.

160. Liley AW. An investigation of spontaneous activity at the neuromuscular junction of the rat. J Physiol 1956;132:650–666.

161. Ito Y, Miledi R, Vincent A. Transmitter release induced by a "factor" in rabbit serum. Proc R Soc Lond B Biol Sci 1974;187:235–241.

162. Mense S. Considerations concerning the neurological basis of muscle pain. Can J Physiol Pharmacol 1991;69(5):610–616.

163. Ruch TC. Pathophysiology of Pain. In TC Ruch, HD Patton (eds), Physiology and Biophysics: The Brain and Neural Function. Philadelphia: WB Saunders, 1979;272–324.

164. McMahon SB, Wall PD. Physiological evidence for branching of peripheral unmyelinated sensory afferent fibers in the rat. J Comp Neurol 1987;261:130–136.

165. Hoheisel U, Mense S, Simons DG, Yu X-M. Appearance of new receptive fields in rat dorsal horn neurons following noxious stimulation of skeletal muscle: a model for referral of muscle pain? Neurosci Lett 1993;133:9–12.

166. Fricton JR. Myofascial Pain Syndrome: Characteristics and Epidemiology. In JR Fricton, EA Awad (eds), Myofascial Pain and Fibromyalgia. Advances in Pain Research and Therapy, Vol 17. New York: Raven, 1990;107–127.

167. Lewit K. The needle effect in relief of myofascial pain. Pain 1979;6:83–90.

168. Wolens D. The myofascial pain syndrome: a critical appraisal. State of the Art Rev: Phys Med Rehabil 1998;12(2):299–316.

169. Hong CZ, Simons DG. Response to standard treatment for pectoralis minor myofascial pain syndrome after whiplash. J Musculoskel Pain 1993;1:89–131.

170. Hong CZ. Trigger point injection: dry needling vs. lidocaine injection. Am J Phys Med Rehabil 1994;73:256–263.

171. Chu J. Dry needling (intramuscular stimulation) in myofascial pain related to lumbar radiculopathy. Eur J Phys Med Rehabil 1995;5:106–121.

172. Byrn C, Olsson I, Falkheden L, et al. Subcutaneous sterile water injections for chronic neck and shoulder pain following whiplash injuries. Lancet 1993;341:449–452.

173. Jaeger B, Skootsky SA. Double blind, controlled study of different myofascial trigger point injection techniques. Pain 1987;4(Suppl):560.

174. Garvey TA, Marks MR, Wiesel SW. A prospective, randomized, double-blind evaluation of trigger point injection therapy for low-back pain. Spine 1989;14:962–964.

175. Carlson CR, Okeson JP, Falace DA, et al. Reduction of pain and EMG activity in the masseter region by trapezius trigger point injection. Pain 1993;55:397–400.

176. Bourne IHJ. Treatment of chronic back pain comparing corticosteroid-lignocaine injections with lignocaine alone. Practitioner 1984;228:333–338.

177. Delin C. Treatment of sciatica with injection of novocain into tender points along the sciatic nerve, 132 cases. J Trad Chin Med 1994;14:32–34.

178. Hameroff SR, Crago R, Blitt CD, et al. Comparison of bupivacaine, etidocaine, and saline for trigger-point therapy. Anesth Analg 1981;60:752–755.

179. Frost A. Diclofenac versus lidocaine as injection therapy in myofascial pain. Scand J Rheumatol 1986;15:153–156.

180. Acquadro MA, Borodic GE. Treatment of myofascial pain with botulinum A toxin. Anesthesiology 1994;80:705–706.

181. Yue SK. Initial experience in the use of botulinum toxin A for the treatment of myofascial related muscle dysfunctions [Abstract]. J Musculoskel Pain 1995;3(Suppl 1):22.

182. Cheshire W, Abashian SW, Mann DJ. Botulinum toxin in the treatment of myofascial pain syndrome. Pain 1995;59:65–69.

183. Gunn CC, Milbrandt WE, Little AS, Mason KE. Dry needling of muscle motor points for chronic low-back pain: a clinical trial with long-term follow-up. Spine 1980;5:279–292.

184. Fine PG, Milano R, Hare B. The effects of myofascial trigger point injections are naloxone reversible. Pain 1988;32:15–20.

185. Bonica JJ. The Management of Pain. Beckenham, KY: Lea & Febiger, 1990.

36

Pain and Emotion

W. Crawford Clark

The purpose of this chapter is to review all aspects of our current knowledge of the mechanisms and treatment of acute and chronic pain. The title emphasizes the view taken throughout this chapter that the emotional and psychosocial aspects of pain are often as important as the sensory component. The chapter begins with an introduction to the evaluation of the sensory and emotional aspects of clinical pain. This is followed by a section on experimentally induced pain. Next, the neuroanatomic, neurophysiological, and neurohumoral mechanisms of pain and its modulation are described. A section on what is coming to be known about the genetics of pain follows. This is followed by a brief description of pharmacologic, surgical, and behavioral treatments. The influence of ethnic and cultural differences and personality on the patient's report of pain (i.e., the psychosocial aspects) is outlined. The chapter concludes with a discussion of the relation between the patient's beliefs and the effectiveness of more controversial treatment approaches, including acupuncture and hypnosis. Relevant examples from the clinic appear throughout the chapter.

INTRODUCTION TO CLINICAL PAIN

Pain is an unpleasant subjective experience familiar to all of us. Most of the time it signals that something is wrong: Some tissue has been injured or has become inflamed, or our bodies are being assaulted by extremes of heat, cold, pressure, or other noxious stimuli. We can infer its presence in others by their vocalizations and behavior. When an injured or inflamed part is touched, the patient winces or writhes and withdraws from the stimulus. In addition, autonomic symptoms such as pal-

lor, flushing, or perspiration may be apparent, and the general pattern of activity may be altered; the patient becomes restless or, alternatively, relatively immobile and passive. The emotional (anxiety, depression) and psychosocial (job loss, marital difficulties, social isolation) effects of pain not only are as important as the pain sensations themselves, but may be more devastating. Most important, the patient's behavior appears to center on pain, as if the experience has pre-empted consciousness and altered motivation.

The practitioner bases the initial assessment of pain on observable behavior and a physical examination of the patient. The patient's subjective report is useful, because different pain qualities are associated with specific disorders. For example, a report of chronic burning pain could support a diagnosis of causalgia, whereas paroxysmal facial pain touched off by pressure could support a diagnosis of trigeminal neuralgia. Variations in intensity, locus, and persistence are also important. Pain may be dull or sharp, diffuse or localized, deep or superficial, continuous or intermittent. Migraine headaches throb; tension headaches typically do not. Cutaneous pain tends to be sharp and well localized, whereas internal pain originating in muscles and viscera tends to be diffuse, aching, and poorly localized. The patient's report can also aid diagnosis by indicating what circumstances initiate, ease, or exacerbate the pain or change its quality. As with other symptoms, observation and inquiry are essential aspects of the diagnostic work-up. Important as the patient's pain report is, the practitioner must constantly keep in mind that what we know is only what the patient says; what the patient is experiencing remains forever unknown to the outside observer. The report of pain is not the sensation of pain.

The patient always must be viewed as a whole person. Although a specific treatment relieves the pain itself, a physician's failure to comprehend the emotional focus of the patient's suffering can increase the total suffering. Cassel[1] emphasizes the following three points:

1. Suffering is experienced by persons, not minds or bodies; it is the person that must be treated.
2. Suffering occurs when the impending disintegration of the person is perceived. Suffering may occur in the presence of pain and other physical symptoms, but not necessarily; the meaning of the symptom to the patient is all important.
3. Suffering can occur with respect to altered social and career roles, loss of loved ones, loss of a perceived future, or changed spiritual values. Recovering from suffering is enhanced by help from family, friends, and health care professionals.

To accomplish this, it is often more important that the patient be seen as a total person than that the immediate physical distress be treated.

ATTEMPTS TO DEFINE PAIN

A complete classification of chronic pain syndromes has been prepared by Merskey and Bogduk.[2] It describes the following five major axes for coding pain:

1. Regions
2. Organ systems
3. Temporal characteristics
4. Patient's statement of intensity
5. Etiology

Pain has been defined by the International Association for the Study of Pain Subcommittee on Taxonomy[2] as "an unpleasant sensory and emotional experience associated with actual or potential tissue damage, or described in terms of such damage." Thus, emotion is fundamental to the pain experience and not a reaction after the sensation of pain. Nevertheless, this definition is oversimplified and presents immediate difficulties. Not only can damage occur without pain, as it does in some malignancies, mild sunburn, or tooth decay, but pain also can continue long after the initial injury has healed, as in phantom limb pain or sympathetically maintained pain. Psychological intervention may ameliorate pain, although the tissue damage remains the

same. Further, the same amount of tissue damage, insofar as this can be determined, may produce quite different intensities of pain in different persons or in one person at different times. Objective and detectable tissue damage, although it usually produces pain, represents only a part of the total complex of conditions that produce the experience of pain. In many instances of chronic pain, the pain and suffering persist long after healing of the initial site is complete.

Pain describes a broad spectrum of unpleasant sensory and emotional experiences and pain behaviors. At one end are the brief, localized, protective sensations such as those produced by noxious heat, cold, pinch, pin prick, and chemical stimuli. Without these warning sensations, survival would be difficult. At the other end of the spectrum are the nonprotective, pathologic, persistent pains associated with chronic disease states. Here, pain is not a symptom but part of the disease itself. Such pain and suffering experiences provoke emotional disturbances including anxiety, fear, and depression, which activate the autonomic nervous system and the hypothalamic-pituitary-adrenal (HPA) axis.

EVALUATING THE COMPLAINT OF PAIN

Evaluating a patient's pain is difficult. The practitioner cannot share the patient's urgent experience of pain; it must be inferred. The initial assessment of pain is most frequently based on the medical history, in combination with objective findings and an evaluation of the patient's psychological status.[3] Interpretation of the patient's description is particularly difficult in cases in which the physical findings provided by radiography, computerized imaging techniques, and other objective medical tests do not explain the patient's complaints. We ask ourselves, "How valid is the report of pain? Is the patient expressing mental anguish rather than physical pain? Is he or she by nature stoic or not?" The primary problem here is not the patient's veracity, but the manifold meanings that people attach to the word *pain*. Patients have enough difficulty interpreting and conveying their experiences, but clinicians are faced with an even more arduous task: They must attempt to unravel the sensory, psychological, and other components of the patient's message. The interpretation is not always accurate. Briones and coworkers[4] compared the ratings of patients undergoing sigmoidoscopy with ratings by health professionals. Health providers were found to underestimate the patients' ratings of pain, anxiety, and depression.

Tailoring treatment to individual patients requires accurate diagnosis and assessment of their physical and mental status. Pain frequently compromises movement and task performance and contributes to the patient's disability and emotional distress. This complex interrelationship is now recognized as a multidimensional biopsychosocial problem to which the relative contributions of pain and the seriousness of the disability vary.

Physical impairment is assessed by instrumented and noninstrumented performance tests and by the patient's report of physical activities. Pain is generally assessed by observation and the patient's responses to statistically validated pain, emotion, and quality-of-life questionnaires. The information obtained has two functions: to guide treatment and to establish a baseline level of pain and physical function to which treatment outcome may be compared.

ASSESSMENT OF PHYSICAL FUNCTION

Magee[5] has described commonly used tests of physical impairment, such as range of motion and muscle strength, but the reliability and validity of many of these measures have been questioned.[6,7] However, Keefe and Block[8] have developed objective protocols for assessing pain behaviors. In these videotaped sessions, the patient engages in a standardized set of activities (standing, sitting, walking, and reclining) that are likely to elicit pain behaviors. The pain-related behaviors include guarding, stiff movement, bracing, pain-avoiding posturing (rubbing, holding), grimacing, and so forth. These studies demonstrated high reliability, significant correlations with patients' ratings of their own pain, and excellent discrimination between patients and healthy controls and reflected the decrease in pain behaviors after successful treatment.

Objective tests should be supplemented by the patient's self-report. However, self-report measures are often subject to bias. There may be a discrepancy between actual function and the patient's perception, or in compensation cases the patient's report of function. Accordingly, the clinician's observations and objective tests of function are important. An example of a superior questionnaire is the Roland and Morris Disability Questionnaire for lower back pain.[9] The patient checks items describing various everyday activities such as lifting, walking, and dressing that are difficult because of pain and disability.

It is also important to assess the patient's therapeutic goals, which may be quite different from those of the practitioner. Is the patient's criterion for successful treatment playing soccer or being able to walk a block? One must determine the level of recovery that would be satisfactory to the patient. On the Patient Specific Questionnaire[10] the patient rates his or her present status and specifies his or her recovery goals with respect to five activities that are important to the patient, but difficult to perform. Throughout the course of treatment, the patient rates his or her ability to perform each activity. The gap between present performance and goals can thus be monitored continuously.

In an attempt to increase the objectivity of disability assessment, various instruments have been used to measure muscle strength and movement precision. For instance, electromyograms recorded during various movement tasks have been studied. Although the relationships between test scores on these instruments and the ability to function in real-world tasks has been questioned, further research may demonstrate their usefulness.[11]

PATIENT MOTIVATION

Treatment success is dependent on personal and psychosocial variables. The patient's therapeutic goals and the determination to reach them depend on the patient's belief that he or she has the personal ability to work through pain and to reduce disability through specific behaviors. Those include the will to maintain physical activity despite persistent pain or to control pain itself. These qualities exemplify what has been termed *self-efficacy*.[12] A self-efficacy scale for patients with rheumatic diseases has been developed.[13] Patients who report an increase in self-efficacy over the course of treatment have better long-term outcomes.[14] On the other hand, patients who lack self-efficacy avoid exercise because of the mistaken belief that it will increase chronic pain and cause reinjury. A questionnaire to assess the strength of fear and avoidance beliefs has been developed by Waddell et al.[15]

The patient's beliefs about pain itself are important and should be assessed. Williams and Thorn[16] developed the Pain Beliefs and Perceptions Inventory, which identifies three kinds of beliefs: temporal characteristics of pain, nature of pain (mysteriousness), and whether the patient blames him- or herself. Another patient belief that can affect treatment outcome concerns *controllability*, which may be measured by one of the *locus of control* questionnaires.[17] Patients' beliefs regarding pain and treatment outcome are typified as one of three loci of control: *internal* (cure is in the hands of the patient), *powerful other* (cure will come from the caregiver), and external (nothing can be done; cure is in the hands of fate). The latter two loci of control foster the belief that the patient does not have an active role in treatment. The caregiver must address this problem and instill in the patient the belief that therapeutic outcome is the responsibility of the patient (see Chapter 37).

NEW THERAPEUTIC APPROACHES

Early postinjury movement therapy for pain reduction and healing has replaced the traditional medical approach of enforced rest and immobilization. Next day ambulation has greatly decreased mortality and morbidity for hip fractures. Soft tissue injuries such as sprained ankles are immediately treated with ice, compression to prevent edema, and gentle movement instead of rest, crutches, and perhaps a plaster cast. The Melzack-Wall gate theory[18] provides theoretical support for the advantages of movement therapy. The model suggests that increased Aβ fiber input arising from mechanoreceptor stimulation occasioned by rubbing, shaking, vibration, massage, and passive movement could close the *gate* (i.e., inhibit painful afferent Aδ and C-fiber input).

To increase the patient's motivation as well as to provide information, the patient should be asked to keep a diary that indicates on a daily, or even hourly, basis how much time was spent in various activities (walking, sleeping, socializing). Also, a record of how much medication was taken, as well as ratings of pain, mood, and so forth, could be kept. Keefe and Caldwell[19] note that a daily pain-coping inventory that assesses pain-reduction efforts and various relaxation strategies is beneficial. A diary is helpful because it motivates the patient to pursue the treatment regimen for those long periods of time when she or he is not at the clinic. A diary also avoids the problem of relying on the patient's memory of how the patient has felt since the last visit.

MEMORY FOR PAIN

Accurate reports of past pains, emotions, and related behaviors are important for diagnosis and treatment. The medical history taken at the initial visit is largely dependent on memory. When did the pain start? How intense was it? What was its diurnal pattern? A study by Salovey and coworkers[20] compared real-time diary entries with subsequent recall; they found few significant differences between the two sources of information. In contrast, Eich and coworkers (cited in Salovey and coworkers[20]) found that when the present pain level

was high, the recalled pain levels were higher than when the present pain level was low. Although Salovey et al. found that the best predictor of recalled pain was mean pain level during the diary period, they also found that subjects who were in greater pain at the time of recall were apt to inflate the intensities of the previous pains. Kent[21] demonstrated the influence of psychological variables on memory for dental pain. He found that the memory at recall (1 or 2 weeks after surgery) was more closely related to the pain that the patient expected to experience (as rated before surgery) than to the patient's rating of the actual pain. Such findings suggest that memory for past pains may be poor, and that further research is needed.

Clark and Bennett-Clark,[22] in a review of pain memory studies, criticized researchers in the field of pain for failing to use modern approaches to the study of painful memories. These methods involve the simultaneous assessment of two, not one, indices of memory: recall and recognition. Statistical decision theory is now commonly used to measure response bias (*B*) effects, and to obtain a pure measure of recognition memory [*P(A)*], the ability to discriminate previously used pain descriptors from new ones. Application of the statistical decision theory model would permit the comparison of stored memory [measured by *P(A)*] with the patient's ability to access that stored memory (measured by recall). Nor is attention paid to exactly what is recalled. Is it, as some maintain,[20] the actual physical sensory and emotional experience itself, or, as seems more likely, is it only the verbal label that had been used to describe that event?

It is often reported that "correlations between recalled pain and *actual* pain were obtained." Surely, the correlation is between the recalled pain report and the earlier pain report. The initial self-assessment is mistakenly reified as the pain itself, and only the recall report is considered an abstraction influenced by psychological variables. As a result, the literature devotes considerable attention to the influence of psychological state and pain intensity on the pain report made during recall, but ignores the influence of these variables when the initial pain report was made. On both occasions we know only that the patient reported a particular level of pain; what the patient experienced remains forever unknown to the outside observer.

DIMENSIONS OF PAIN AND SUFFERING

If we are to understand and relieve pain and associated emotions we must be able to measure it, but, quantitation is difficult because pain is a multidimensional experience that varies over a wide range of intensities and possesses an almost infinite number of qualities. Although thousands of words have been used to describe pain and emotion, our ability to understand and treat pain would be much enhanced if these words could be reduced to a smaller number of dimensions or clusters. Because the number and the characteristics of the dimensions are currently in dispute, the first step toward the quantitation of pain and emotion is a better understanding of its dimensions.[23]

The history of speculation concerning the dimensions of pain and emotion has been reviewed by Melzack.[24] He noted that while Aristotle thought of pain as an emotion, not a sensation, nineteenth century physiologists thought of pain as a sensory modality devoid of emotion. Sherrington combined these views and held that pain had two dimensions: sensory and affective. Melzack and Casey[25] argue for three dimensions. The sensory-discriminative dimension is the sensory aspect of pain, including intensity, temporal, and spatial properties and somatosensory qualities. The affective-motivational dimension reflects the emotional and aversive aspects of pain and suffering. The cognitive-evaluative dimension reflects the patient's evaluation of the meaning and possible consequences of the pain, including the quality of life and even death itself. This three-dimensional model is widely accepted, because it succeeds in integrating much of what is known about the physiology and psychology of pain and suffering.

A view that expands on Melzack and Casey's by placing even greater emphasis on the emotional and behavioral dimensions is presented by Loeser[26] and Fordyce.[27] They describe four aspects of pain and suffering: nociception, the activation of Aδ and C fibers by tissue-damaging stimuli; pain, the sensation that usually, but not always, follows nociceptive stimulation; suffering, which includes the affective or emotional response of the CNS and includes anxiety, depression, and fear; and pain behaviors, the observable muscular and autonomic activities of patients experiencing pain or suffering. The Melzack-Casey and Loeser-Fordyce views, which are complementary, are now widely accepted, but more recent multidimensional scaling research suggests there may be additional dimensions.

MULTIDIMENSIONAL SCALING

Multidimensional scaling represents an objective approach to discovering the number and kinds of dimensions of pain and suffering.[23] The view that pain

and emotion may be represented by specific dimensions and that individual patients are located at different points along these dimensions represents an important advance toward the understanding of pain and emotion. Fernandez and Turk[28] question the separability of what are held to be independent sensory pain and emotional dimensions. (Dimensions may be envisioned as axes in space, such as compass directions.) Clark and coworkers[29] used Individual Differences Scaling (INDSCAL), a multidimensional scaling technique, to analyze similarity judgments of descriptors of painful experiences. They found four dimensions, but failed to isolate separate, independent painful sensory and emotion dimensions at right angles to each other (orthogonal). The dimensions found were intense pain and emotion, moderate pain and emotion, pain and arousal-apathy (or motivational state), and pain and somatosensory qualities. Thus, painful sensations appeared as an attribute on each dimension and painful emotions were entangled within a single dimension. In particular, painful sensations and painful emotions were merged within a single dimension. In addition to confirming Fernandez and Turk's conjecture, this study amplifies the definition of pain given earlier, by adding arousal-apathy (i.e., motivation) to the unpleasant sensory and emotional experience. The brain-imaging data described later also lend support to the inseparability of pain, emotion, and motivational state.

Another INDSCAL study[30] asked the question, what kind of space, or map, is obtained from pairwise similarity judgments made between physical stimuli (in this instance electrical) and verbal descriptors of pain and emotion, both of which range in intensity from innocuous to noxious? One might expect two orthogonal dimensions (e.g., north-south and east-west), one for the physical stimuli and one for the verbal descriptors. On the other hand, a single dimension might emerge with the physical stimuli and the descriptors systematically interdigitated with respect to intensity along a single dimension (e.g., northeast-southwest). The single dimension solution was obtained. Thus, words describing pain are indeed closely related to the physical experience of pain. This finding provides a rationale for the administration of questionnaires to patients suffering clinical pain.

PAIN QUESTIONNAIRES

Theories about the dimensions of pain have influenced the construction of pain scales and questionnaires. These standardized tests are used in research as well as clinically because unlike a relatively unstructured doctor–patient interview, answers to the questionnaire items yield a circumscribed data set that allows analyses by a wide variety of statistical procedures.[31,32] The most elementary approach to pain assessment is to have the patient rate his or her pain on a single scale anchored at one end by "no pain" and at the other by "as much pain as I can bear." On the visual analog scale the anchors appear at the ends of a horizontal line. The numeric rating scale is defined by numbers, usually 0–10, and the category rating scale includes a series of pain descriptors ordered with respect to intensity. These single-item *pain* scales are commonly used, especially with hospitalized patients on analgesics; unfortunately, there is no way to determine how much of the pain intensity rated on the scale is sensory in nature and how much of it is based on emotion. If the sensory and emotional components of the pain rating were each known, medication could be tailored more accurately to the patient's needs. Perhaps an anxiolytic medication could partially substitute for a prescribed narcotic.

More sophisticated questionnaires have been developed to replace or augment the single-item scale.[33-36] The McGill Pain Questionnaire (MPQ) with 88 descriptors is far superior to the simple pain scale; it has been used extensively and is well validated.[35] However, two major drawbacks to the MPQ are its lack of emotional words such as *anxious*, *depressed*, and *angry*, and the subjective rather than mathematically determined assignment of descriptors into 21 subgroups and 4 major groups (sensory, affective, evaluative, and miscellaneous). When evaluating patients, the paucity of emotional words in the MPQ is often remedied by adding a psychometric test such as the Derogatis Brief Symptom Inventory[37]; unfortunately, since the tests were designed to evaluate psychiatric patients, they contain questions that are often irrelevant and even offensive to pain patients.

The development of mathematical modeling techniques, such as multidimensional scaling and cluster analysis, which were not available when the MPQ was designed, now permit descriptors to be located in their objectively determined dimensions and clusters. Hierarchical cluster analysis of 270 descriptors of pain and emotion evidenced a discrepancy between the clusters and the MPQ groups.[38] In particular, the MPQ Evaluative Group was not a homogeneous group as had been thought; cluster analysis demonstrated that each MPQ evaluative descriptor belonged to a different cluster.

Cluster analysis was used to design a new, mathematically objective questionnaire that places greater emphasis on pain-associated emotions. The procedure is described

here because it represents a new objective way to construct questionnaires of any kind. To construct the Multidimensional Affect and Pain Survey (MAPS), 104 healthy female and male college students of Puerto Rican, Euro-American, and African-American background sorted and resorted 189 descriptors (selected from the original 270) into 20 to 40 piles that in their individual opinions contained closely related words. The similarity data were analyzed by the average-linkage-between-groups algorithm, an agglomerative, hierarchical clustering technique. Eighty-eight descriptors were eliminated because men and women of the various ethnocultural groups did not agree on their meanings. The 101 descriptors of the MAPS questionnaire are grouped into three superclusters and 30 clusters. Supercluster I, Sensory Qualities, contains descriptors of painful sensory qualities. Supercluster II, Negative Emotions, contains descriptors of negative emotional responses. Supercluster III, Well-Being, contains descriptors of positive affect and health. A translation of the MAPS has been used to study the influence of presurgical expectation of pain and suffering on postsurgical morphine demand in Chinese patients underlying colorectal surgery for cancer.[39] High scores on the 101 MAPS descriptors rated before surgery correlated with higher morphine consumption during recovery: This demonstrates that psychological variables (expectation and emotional state) as well as pain influence morphine demand.

EXPERIMENTALLY INDUCED PAIN IN HUMANS

Clinical pain and suffering are almost hopelessly complex subjects. Accordingly, a number of investigators take the view that the understanding of pain in humans can best be made by first investigating simpler types of pain, such as that induced in the laboratory by precisely calibrated noxious stimuli of different sensory modalities and of varying intensities. Experimental or laboratory pain procedures have been used to study the effects of culture, personality, age, sex, drugs, hypnosis, acupuncture, and clinical pain itself on the pain threshold. Much has been learned from the responses of volunteers and patients to precisely calibrated noxious stimulation that could not be learned from the study of clinical pain, in which the intensity of the noxious stimulus cannot be determined with any degree of precision, and biopsychosocial factors greatly influence the pain response.

Most experimental approaches to sensation, including vision, audition, and pain, emphasize the application of graded intensities of the physical stimulus and require the subject (the observer) to make some judgment about the presence, absence, or intensity of the stimulus. For pain, the major methodologic approaches include pain detection and pain tolerance thresholds obtained by a variety of psychophysical procedures: the method of serial exploration or *limits*, magnitude estimation, sensory decision theory (SDT), and multidimensional scaling. Procedural and statistical controls, designed to minimize error in these reports, are usually elaborate and include careful control of stimulus and test conditions, placebo controls, and the use of single- or double-blind controls. (In the latter, neither subject nor the assessor of treatment outcome knows which treatment has been given.)

For ethical reasons, experimental pain stimuli must produce short-term and reversible effects. Electrical stimulation of tooth pulp or skin, immersion of a limb in ice water, stimulation of the skin with cold, heat, pressure over superficial bony structures, pinch, and the tourniquet procedure that produces ischemic pain by obstructing circulation are options. Internal stimuli include esophageal, lower bowel, and rectal distension by a pressurized balloon and infusion of dilute acids into the lower esophagus.

Many different response modes to noxious stimulation have been investigated. Some investigators have sought pain indicators that would be more objective than verbal report, which is easily influenced by attitudes, expectations, and social norms. Tests that use a variety of physiological responses not ordinarily considered to be under voluntary control have been thought to be more objective. These include pulse rate, blood pressure, shift of blood flow from viscera to striated muscles, inhibition of salivary and gastric secretions, pupil dilation, blood glucose, corticosteroid and epinephrine levels, and palmar skin potential. Although these physiological measures provide information, they are not more valid than verbal report, as none is truly specific to pain, as opposed to stress or arousal. For example, the palmar skin potential may show a greater increase in response to an unexpected soft sound than to an expected noxious electrical pulse. Like verbal report, these so-called objective indicators are influenced by psychological variables, including fear, stress, and social demand characteristics. Orne[40] originated the term *social demand characteristics* to refer to the compelling influence on subjects of what is expected of them by the investigator or of the social imperatives implicit in the situation.

Method of Serial Exploration

In the method of limits or serial exploration, the observer responds to each of a series of brief, physically calibrated thermal, pressure, pinch, or electrical stimuli that are gradually increased in intensity. The pain sensitivity or detection threshold is the intensity at which the subject first reports pain; the pain tolerance threshold is the intensity at which the subject elects to terminate stimulation.

Although the threshold was once thought to be a pure measure of sensory function, it is now clear that it is heavily influenced by nonsensory factors, especially the subject's expectations and attitudes. When the subject is in doubt about the sensation, he or she may repeat the previous response, an *error of habituation*, or because he or she knows that the series is increasing in intensity, the subject may commit the *error of anticipation*. Also, other nonsensory factors such as the subject's idiosyncratic definition of pain and propensity to stoicism or squeamishness distort the pain threshold and mask the true neurosensory sensitivity. The serial forced-choice version of the method of limits described later circumvents these problems.

Method of Constant Stimuli

In this procedure the stimuli are presented randomly with respect to intensity, thus avoiding errors caused by the subject's expectations. However, the threshold is just as affected by nonsensory variables as that of the method of limits.

Sensory Decision Theory Measures

A major problem in measuring the pain threshold is the seemingly inseparable mixture of sensory and psychological variables. Fortunately, a resolution to this problem is offered by developments in measurement, based on the statistical decision theory model, known in its various guises as the *medical decision-making model*, *signal detection theory*, or *SDT*. These procedures separate the sensory component of the traditional method of limits threshold from its otherwise hidden psychological or attitudinal component. Clark[41-43] has reviewed the application of SDT to the measurement of responses to noxious stimulation and its advantages over other psychophysical procedures. SDT can be used with untrained subjects and has been applied not only to verbal report but also to physiological and motor indicators of pain.

The advantage of SDT is that it yields two measures of perceptual performance. $P(A)$ is a pure measure of discrimination, the ability to distinguish between stimuli of higher and lower intensities. Nonsensory variables such as expectation do not influence this measure. The other index, pain report criterion, *B*, is independent of *P(A)*; it indexes the propensity or bias of the observer to report pain. In the one-interval rating procedure, the subject rates each stimulus on an intensity scale to yield the discrimination index, *P(A)*. Earlier studies used a related measure, *d'*, but *P(A)*, a nonparametric measure, is considered superior. High values suggest that neurosensory functioning is normal; low values that afferent neurosensory activity has been attenuated, as it might be by an analgesic. Discrimination has been shown to be decreased by analgesics such as morphine and by nerve blocks, which attenuate neural activity and, hence, the amount of information that reaches higher centers.[44]

That the SDT discrimination measure reflects the amount of neurosensory information transmitted to higher centers has been demonstrated by Gybels and coworkers.[45] They found a close relation between values of *d'*, based on subjective intensity rating reports, and the discharge rate of human peripheral nociceptive nerve fibers responding to noxious thermal stimulation; higher intensities yielded higher values of *d'*. Unlike the pain threshold, *P(A)* has been shown to be essentially independent of changes in the subject's expectation, mood, and motivation.[43]

The other SDT measure of perceptual performance is the report criterion, L_x or *B*; it indexes response bias, which is the willingness or reluctance of a subject to use a particular response. The criterion is influenced by nonsensory, psychosocial factors such as anxiety, personality, and culture. A high criterion reflects stoicism, whereas a low criterion indicates that the subject readily reports pain even to relatively innocuous stimulus intensities. Many studies[42,43] have used SDT to demonstrate the effect of attitudinal and emotional variables on the pain report criterion. For example, a placebo described and accepted by the subject as a powerful analgesic raised the pain threshold (i.e., it apparently decreased pain sensitivity according to the traditional method of limits). Analysis by SDT, however, demonstrated that only the pain report criterion had been raised (fewer pain reports); discrimination, *d'*, did not change. Thus, the placebo-induced reduction in pain report was caused not by an analgesic effect of the placebo on neurosensory function, but by a criterion shift made in response to the social demand characteristics of the situation.

The two-interval forced-choice variant of SDT also yields a pure measure of discrimination. In this procedure the subject must choose which of two stimuli, of slightly different intensities, was the more intense. The discrimination or sensitivity measure is the percentage of correct responses. It completely eliminates the response bias and linguistic problems associated with pain report. The subject's ability to discriminate intensity differences, not pain, yields the sensitivity measure *percent correct* (after correction for chance success; even when guessing the subject would be right half the time). Forced choice is the only psychophysical procedure that can score each response as right or wrong, hence its power.

Serial-Forced Choice

The ascending method of limits described earlier has the advantage that the investigator can stop a series at any time. This is important in testing patients who may have abnormally low pain thresholds. However, it has been noted that to avoid the effect of expectation on the threshold, stimuli must be presented randomly. As a compromise, the nonrandomness inherent in the method of limits can be avoided by increasing the stimulus intensities in a semirandom way, so that although overall the stimuli increase in intensity, at any step the next stimulus may be just above or just below the previous one (determined randomly). The patient rates the subjective intensity of each of two stimuli presented in succession (single interval procedure); next the patient decides whether the first or the second (most recent) stimulus was more intense (forced-choice procedure). The semirandom, gradually increasing series can be stopped at any time, thus avoiding any possibility of upsetting or injuring the patient. The data obtained can be analyzed by both SDT and traditional methods.

Magnitude Estimation

With the magnitude estimation, or ratio scaling, procedure, the subject is assigned a simple number, such as 10, to describe a calibrated stimulus (the modulus) of an intensity in the mildly painful range. The subject then assigns proportional numbers to subsequently presented variable stimulus intensities that range above and below the modulus value. These numbers reflect the ratios between the sensations produced by the modulus and the variable stimulus intensities. Gracely and coworkers[46] reported an interesting study that demonstrated that subjects could separately rate electrocutaneous stimuli with respect to sensory (pain) and affect (unpleasantness) dimensions. An anxiety-reducing drug (diazepam) reduced intensity ratings on the affect, but not on the sensory dimension. In another study,[47] they found that a narcotic reduced sensory pain intensity ratings but did not, surprisingly, influence the affect intensity ratings. The results of these studies are generally in accord with the known tranquilizing and analgesic effects of these drugs and support the concept of separate sensory and emotional components of pain and suffering. In spite of the results of these well-designed experiments, other studies have raised questions about the validity of results obtained with the magnitude estimation procedure[28] and of the subjective assignment of words to the various dimensions of pain.[37] Further, unlike the SDT procedures, it has not been demonstrated that poorly educated people or members of other cultures can master the complex rating scale procedure.

Multidimensional Scaling

The pain and suffering dimensions associated with laboratory and clinical pain have been investigated by a new technique, multidimensional scaling.[23] An important advantage of this method is that, unlike the laboratory procedures just described, it is equally applicable to verbal descriptors of pain and suffering as it is to physical stimuli. In the mathematical model, both are *stimulus objects*.

INDSCAL is a multidimensional scaling procedure that yields the *group stimulus space*, a geometric configuration of points in the pain, emotion, and motivation space, as on a map, in which each point corresponds to one of the stimulus objects. This map allows inferences to be made about the structure or dimensions of the pain and suffering universe. Unlike the dimensions described in the literature, which are based on ad hoc opinions, these dimensions are obtained in an objective manner, because the subject, not the experimenter, determines the type and number of dimensions. INDSCAL also generates a *subject weight space*; the coordinates (location) of each patient in this space represent the relative importance or salience of each dimension to that particular individual.

Clark and colleagues[48] used multidimensional scaling to study a group of patients suffering cancer-related pain and a matched group of healthy pain-free volunteers. The subjects made pair-wise similarity judgments between all possible pairings of the following cancer-related pain words: burning, cramping, shooting, annoying, miserable, sickening, mild pain, intense pain, and unbearable pain. Three dimensions emerged in the group stimulus space, namely, pain intensity, emotional quality, and somatosensory quality. The subject weight space revealed that, although there were individual differences, on average the pain intensity dimension was most important for the patients, whereas the emotional quality dimension was most important for the healthy

volunteers. If the multidimensional scaling approaches fulfill their promise, we should soon be nearing a better understanding of the variables that affect clinical pain and suffering.

NOCICEPTORS AND NERVE FIBERS

Abundant experimental and clinical evidence indicates that, up to a point, the pain system is organized and responds in much the same way as other sensory systems. At mild to moderate levels of calibrated noxious stimulation, for which the emotional component is minimal, reports of pain intensity can be obtained that systematically relate subjects' judgments of pain to the intensities of the physical stimuli (i.e., a close relation exists between noxious stimulus intensity and reported magnitude of sensation). To this limited degree, a *specificity theory* of pain can be entertained, namely, a relatively direct pathway conducts stimulus-related neural activity from the periphery to pain centers in the brain. However, when the pain is intense, various mechanisms are recruited to modulate the pain, and the simple sensory model no longer applies.

Primary afferent neurons extend from the axon tip in the periphery (skin, viscera, and so forth) where they transduce the stimulus into neural activity, to the dorsal horn in the spinal column. Second-order neurons extend from the dorsal horn to the thalamus, and third-order neurons from thalamus to cortex and subcortical structures. It will soon become clear that this is a gross oversimplification, although it is true in some instances. The receptors for pain are usually fine, unmyelinated nerve endings, the axon tips of the first-order neurons. These endings are present in a variety of tissues that are sensitive to pain: skin, viscera, joints, muscles, teeth, bones, and blood vessels. Pain sensibility on the body's surface is not uniformly acute. Each sensory area, which may be smaller than 1 cm in diameter, transmits a unique pattern of excitation to higher centers, permitting localization and two-point discrimination. Individual receptive fields are innervated by several nerve fibers, which ensure multiple projections to the neuraxis. The various fibers that serve temperature, touch, and pain sensibility in a given region come together as a peripheral nerve on their way to the spinal cord. The sensory territory of any peripheral nerve widely overlaps that of adjoining nerves. Thus, several peripheral nerve trunks or dorsal roots usually must be cut to eliminate pain in a particular area. The amount of overlap varies from region to region in the body, but every locus on the skin appears to be supplied by at least two dorsal roots.

Skin receptors are sensitive to a variety of stimuli. Skin cooling (30–16°C) is mediated by Aδ fibers, painful cold (<10°C) by polymodal C fibers. Warm stimuli (34–42°C) are mediated by C fibers, painful heat (>44°C) by Aδ fibers. Sharp, pinch pain is mediated by mechanical nociceptors and Aδ fibers, burning pain by heat mechanical nociceptors and Aδ fibers, freezing pain by cold mechanical nociceptors and C fibers, and burning pain and toothache by polymodal heat-pinch-cold (HPC) nociceptors and C fibers. Thinly myelinated Aδ fibers conduct signals at 3–30 m per second. Small diameter, unmyelinated C fibers conduct signals at 0.1–2.5 m per second. Nonpainful stroking, pressure, and vibratory sensations are mediated by mechanoreceptors with specialized end organs: Meissner's corpuscle and Merkel's disk in glabrous skin and the hair receptor in hairy skin. Free nerve endings and other receptor structures underlie both glabrous and hairy skin. Large myelinated Aα and Aβ fibers transmit mechanical information at 36–120 m per second. Except for specialized receptors for touch and pressure, most receptors are bare (*free*) nerve endings.

In diabetic neuropathy, degeneration of the large fibers causes a loss in the vibration sense, whereas the Aδ fibers retain their function, so that the warmth threshold remains normal. Sensory testing can aid diagnosis at an early stage.

Tissue injury or inflammation releases a variety of substances that produce pain: bradykinin, histamine, prostaglandins, acetylcholine, serotonin, and substance P. Many of these act to *sensitize* (i.e., to lower the nociceptive threshold). Others, such as histamine and bradykinin, directly activate nociceptors.

ASCENDING SPINAL TRACTS

The primary afferent nerves from skin, muscle, joints, viscera, and so forth project to the spinal cord gray matter, which is organized into anatomically distinct layers (Rexed laminae) of the dorsal horn. They project contralaterally and synapse with secondary neurons and ascend in the anterolateral quadrant in five major pathways: spinothalamic, spinoreticulothalamic, spinomesencephalic, cervicothalamic, and spinohypothalamic (Figure 36-1). These tracts carry information about noxious and innocuous thermal stimulation from dorsal roots to the brain. The tactile and proprioceptive fibers ascend through the ipsilateral dorsal column–medial lemniscal system to the brain stem where they terminate in the cuneate

nucleus. Transmission after this nucleus is contralateral. Basbaum and Jessell[49] have published an excellent review. Willis[50] also provides descriptions in much greater detail of the ascending pain system in a number of mammalian species.

Spinothalamic Tract

The two main bundles of the spinothalamic tract (STT), lateral and anterior STT, project contralaterally and ascend somatotopically to the thalamus in the anterolateral column (see Figure 36-1). More than 85% of these fibers project contralaterally. This tract is often referred to as the *neospinothalamic tract*, because it appeared later in evolution. The lateral STT mediates mostly pain and temperature sensations. It is composed of the axons of cells in lamina I and receives Aδ and C fiber terminals from primary neurons innervating skin, joint, muscle, and viscera. Lamina I contains three classes of STT cells: nociceptive-specific cells that respond to mechanical, thermal, or both stimuli; polymodal nociceptive (HPC) cells that respond to noxious heat, pinch, or cold; and specific cool cells that are excited by innocuous cooling. The specific cool cells, which are the only ones known to respond to a single sensory modality, are inhibited by warm stimuli.

The main lamina I projection site in the thalamus is the ventral medial nucleus; lesions there alter pain and temperature sensation and can cause central pain. The ventral medial nucleus projects via third-order neurons to the insular cortex and to area 3a in the postcentral sulcus, which may be responsible for discriminative and motor aspects of pain. The second lamina I projection site is the ventral posterior lateral nucleus, which in turn projects to the somatosensory cortex and associated insular and opercular cortex. These structures may be related to the various somatosensory qualities that accompany pain. The input to the thalamus is arranged somatotopically and also projects somatotopically to the somatosensory cortex. Lesions of the ventral posterior lateral and medial thalamic nuclei, made electively in humans to control intractable pain, have reduced acute pain, whereas electrical stimulation of these sites has provoked burning sensations. Thus, these nuclei, as well as those that receive projections originating in the contralateral laminae I and IV through VII, are clearly related to the Melzack-Casey sensory-discriminative dimension. The third projection site of lamina I is the medial dorsal nucleus of the thalamus, which in turn projects to the anterior cingulate cortex and plays an important role in the emotional aspect of pain.

FIGURE 36-1 Three of the five major ascending nociceptive pathways from the laminae of the dorsal root to the brain. (Reprinted with permission from E Kandel. Principles of Neuroscience [4th ed]. New York: McGraw-Hill, 2000;482.)

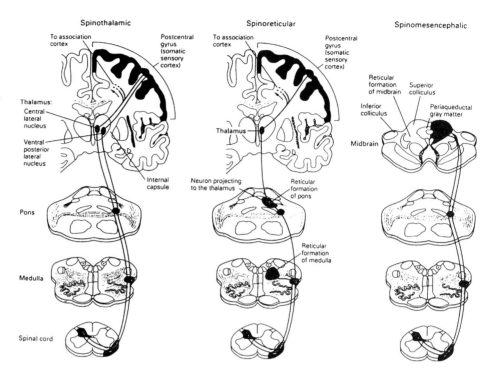

The anterior STT also carries axons from laminae IV, V, VII, and VIII. Laminae IV and V cells receive Aβ and Aδ fibers and contain low-threshold cells that respond to non-noxious mechanical cutaneous stimulation (touch) and wide dynamic range nociceptive cells that respond to both low- and high-intensity pinch and heat stimulation. Lamina V cells receive input from visceral, muscle, and joint tissues. Lamina VII and VIII wide dynamic range cells respond to a wide range of stimulus modalities and intensities over large regions; they have large inhibitory fields and are polymodal, including both proprioceptive and visceral inputs. Many of the laminae V and VII cells project to ventral lateral and intralaminar nuclei related to motor activity and to the same cortical sites that receive lamina I projections. It should be borne in mind that these cortical structures interact with subcortical sites that are also involved in the experience of pain, and in addition may be crucial for forebrain processing of pain behavior and pain memory.

Spinoreticulothalamic Tract

The second major afferent sensory route is the spinoreticulothalamic tract. It consists of the axons of neurons in laminae VII and VIII of the dorsal horn (see Figure 36-1). It is mainly ipsilateral and terminates in both the reticular formation of the pons and medulla

and in the medial thalamus. This path appeared early in evolution and is known as the *paleospinoreticulothalamic tract* because it includes a polysynaptic path via the brain stem reticular formation.

Spinomesencephalic Tract

The third route is the spinomesencephalic tract. Its fibers from laminae I and V project to the mesencephalic reticular formation and the periaqueductal gray matter, a key endogenous opioid center. This tract also projects to the parabrachial nuclei, which, in turn, project to the hypothalamus, amygdala, and insular and cingulate cortices. Thus, the lateral cortical target of these lamina I projections may be considered a system involved in the control of autonomic function, because some lamina V–VII cells project to the reticular formation of the brain stem, and these brain stem regions are involved with autonomic integration and homeostasis.

Cervicothalamic Tract

The fourth pathway, the cervicothalamic tract, arises from the lateral cervical nucleus, which receives input from nociceptive neurons in laminae III and IV. The axons ascend contralaterally to nuclei in the midbrain and to ventroposterior lateral and posteromedial nuclei of the thalamus. Some of these axons travel together in the dorsal columns (with axons of the large Aα and Aβ fibers) to the medulla.

Spinohypothalamic Tract

The fifth pathway, the spinohypothalamic tract, consists of fibers from laminae I, V, and VIII; it projects directly to supraspinal autonomic control centers including the hypothalamus, where it activates the autonomic nervous system and the neuroendocrine system.

CENTRAL PAIN

Central pain is chronic pain caused by a lesion or dysfunction in the CNS. A variety of lesions in the brain or spinal cord can cause central pain; these include stroke, trauma, tumors, and inflammatory processes. Central pain thus differs from neuropathic pain, which involves primary afferent neurons. The location of the lesion is more important than its size or type. Lesions at any level of the neuraxis (dorsal and cranial nerve roots, ascending spinal pathways, thalamus, and some subcortical and cortical regions) can cause central pain. The prevalence of major central pain disorders is as follows: spinal cord injury (30%), multiple sclerosis (28%), and stroke (8%). Location of the perceived pain varies with the type of lesion. In stroke, the pain is typically unilateral; in spinal cord injury, usually bilateral in the body below the lesion; in syringomyelia, unilateral in arm, thorax, or both; and in multiple sclerosis, often in the lower half of body, leg, arm, or all three. The onset of central pain is typically delayed, commonly for 1–3 months, but 2–3 years is possible. The most common pain quality is a severe burning sensation, but aching, pricking, pressing, lacerating, other sensations, or mixtures may be reported. The quality and intensity of sensation vary greatly from patient to patient, even among those with the same diagnosis and seemingly identical lesions. Central pain is usually constant, but some patients have paroxysmal attacks; central pain may be exacerbated by sensory or emotional stimulation.

Somatosensory abnormalities in response to calibrated innocuous and noxious sensory stimuli are always present, both within and outside the painful region. These abnormalities include decreased detection sensitivity, hyperalgesic response to moderate innocuous stimuli (allodynia), hypoalgesia, hyperalgesia, delayed response, radiation to unstimulated sites, and persistence of the sensation. Central pain is accompanied by abnormal heat, cold, and pin-prick pain thresh-olds. The tactile system is often thought to be spared, but according to Boivie,[51] vibration and touch thresholds are abnormal in almost 50% of the cases.

A lateral medullary infarction produces the central pain of Wallenberg's syndrome in approximately 25% of patients. McGowan and coworkers,[52] in a study of patients with Wallenberg's syndrome, determined that almost all patients with central pain had normal sensory thresholds to innocuous and noxious heat and pressure stimuli in the cheek contralateral to the infarct, whereas all patients without central pain had abnormal thresholds in the contralateral cheek. They concluded that abnormalities in the face contralateral to the infarct are referable to the crossed trigeminal tract in the medullary reticular formation medial to the infarcted lateral medulla. They concluded further that central pain in these patients is caused by lesions of the STT that spare the spinoreticulothalamic system and result in a form of denervation sensitivity of the paleospinoreticulothalamic tract caused by a selective neospinothalamic lesion.

A lesion in the ventroposterolateral thalamus can produce the central pain of the Dejerine-Roussy syndrome. The anatomic substrates for pain sensation suggest an explanation for the burning pain reported by patients with thalamic lesions and by those with spinal cord injuries. Craig[53] hypothesizes that central pain (often described as burning or freezing pain) is related to the decrease in thermal sensitivity found in virtually all central pain patients. He suggested that a lesion that interferes with the output of the thermosensory area in the insula disinhibits a limbic network involving the anterior cingulate that generates the pain and affect associated with disturbed homeostatic thermoregulatory function. A cold-evoked burning sensation is produced by stimuli of less than 10–15°C. However, when A fibers are blocked by pressure on a peripheral nerve so that both touch and noxious cold sensitivity is eliminated, then a non-noxious cool stimulus (approximately 24°C) provokes the intense burning sensation of a stimulus less than 15°C. This sensation is caused by the activation of polymodal C nociceptors and HPC neurons (even though noxious intensities are absent). The pain that can be produced by this neural activity is normally blocked centrally by activity in Aδ receptors responsible for non-noxious cool sensations. In the thermal grill illusion,[54] alternating warm (40°C) and cool (24°C) bars reduce the activity of the cool cells by spatial inhibition. However, the cold-evoked activity of the HPC neurons remains unchanged. The result is an intense burning pain produced by innocuous stimuli. Brain imaging studies have demonstrated that the thermal grill activates the same cortical areas, including the anterior cingulate, that are activated by noxious cold and heat intensities. Thus, an infarct that causes the loss of the cool cell (specific cool) pathway could produce the burning pain of thalamic origin.

Treatment of central pain is difficult; opioids are usually ineffective. Tricyclic antidepressants such as amitriptyline have had a 60% success rate in clinical trials. Their action is more than simply psychotherapeutic, because they diminish pain in patients who are not depressed. Selective serotonin reuptake inhibitors tested to date have proven less effective than the tricyclics. An antiepileptic drug, such as carbamazepine, should be considered if the central pain is paroxysmal (sometimes referred to as *lancinating pain*) in nature. Antiepileptic drugs are rarely effective for most forms of central pain, but some spinal cord injury and multiple sclerosis patients have benefited. The pattern of response to medication in central pain parallels that of neuropathic pain. The pharmacologic basis of this similarity remains a mystery. Spinal cord and brain stimulation have been tried as treatments for central pain, but the results have been disappointing according to Tasker.[55]

The fact that pain and touch fibers travel in separate tracts, the anterolateral and dorsal columns, respectively, has led to a controversial treatment for lower body pain. The procedure involves long-term implantation of electrodes over the dorsal columns. Mild electrical stimulation of the dorsal column elicits neural impulses that travel to the dorsal column nuclei as well as antidromically to the dorsal horn. According to the Melzack-Wall gate hypothesis, this should have an inhibitory effect on the pain transmission neurons. A large proportion of patients do report pain relief initially, but the long-term results are generally disappointing.[56] However, transcutaneous electrical nerve stimulation (TENS) has proven more successful with a small proportion of patients who have close to normal touch and vibration thresholds and presumably functioning dorsal column pathways.

Our present knowledge of what TENS in combination with cognitive restructuring can do is best reflected by a study by Lehman and coworkers.[57] All inpatients received 3 weeks of education and exercise training; in addition, in three separate groups they received electroacupuncture, TENS, or TENS with a dead battery (placebo). There were no significant differences among the three groups: All improved with respect to their overall rehabilitation. Most important, all three treatment groups ranked the contribution of education as

greater than that of the electrical stimulation. Clearly, psychological variables and their interaction with a physical treatment (even the placebo treatment) proved effective, and electrical stimulation itself failed to enhance improvement.

DESCENDING SPINAL ANALGESIC TRACTS

Morphine-induced analgesia results from excitation of descending pathways that inhibit nociceptive neurons in the spinal cord (Figure 36-2). These paths are activated by endogenous opioids that act on the same receptors as morphine. The descending pathway includes the periaqueductal gray matter and its connections to the rostroventral medulla, in particular the serotonergic neurons in the raphe magnus, which make inhibitory connections with neurons in laminae I, II, and V of the dorsal horn. Other descending inhibitory systems originate in the noradrenergic locus ceruleus and other nuclei of the medulla and pons.

The brain contains three major specific receptors for endogenous opiates: μ, δ, and κ. The three classes of endogenous opioid peptides are enkephalins (active at both μ and δ receptors), dynorphins (active at the κ receptor), and β-endorphin. β-Endorphin is released into the circulation in response to stress and produces stress-induced analgesia. The stress does not have to reach painful levels for β-endorphin to be released; heavy exercise is sufficient.

Opioid receptors are located at sites associated with the modulation of pain and are found in the periaqueductal gray matter, rostral ventral medulla, and in laminae I and II of the dorsal horn, but opioid receptors are also widely distributed throughout the body including skin, joints, and muscle, and opioids do much more than produce analgesia. The endogenous opioid system is involved in food consumption, temperature regulation, pituitary hormone release, respiration, and cardiovascular regulation. Opioid receptors in the gut, for example, are responsible for the constipation produced by morphine. Their presence in the spinal cord permits the treatment of cancer pain by intrathecal injection, which, because receptors in the brain are avoided, prevents many of the side effects (e.g., drowsiness) produced by systemic administration.

The action of both endogenous opioids and morphine is blocked by naloxone, a synthetic drug that preferentially occupies the μ receptor site without stimulating it. Thus, upon administration of naloxone, a drug user taking narcotics rapidly experiences symptoms of withdrawal because the narcotic has effectively disappeared.

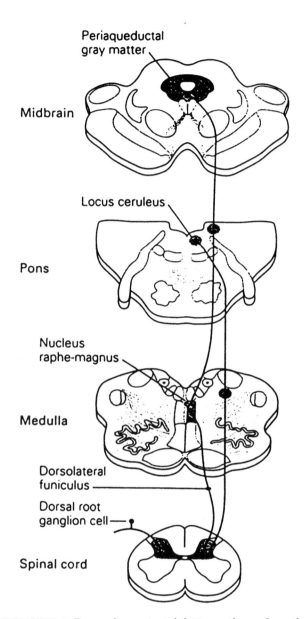

FIGURE 36-2 Descending pain–inhibiting pathway from the periaqueductal gray to the laminae of the dorsal root. (Reprinted with permission from E Kandel. Principles of Neuroscience [4th ed]. New York: McGraw-Hill, 2000;486.)

Drug tolerance after repeated administration of narcotics for chronic pain causes a decrease in the number of receptor sites, a reduction in their binding affinity, or both. Accordingly, tolerant subjects require increasingly larger doses of opiates. Considering the action of naloxone at the opioid receptor, one would expect that the administration of naloxone to someone in pain would greatly increase his or her

pain. Convincing evidence for a dramatic hyperalgesic effect under these circumstances has not been obtained. The reason for this is unknown. Perhaps nonopioids play a greater role in pain modulation than is presently suspected.

MODULATION OF PAIN

Attenuation of pain by arousal, stress, counter-irritant stimulation, and various psychological factors is well known. It is common knowledge that injuries sustained during strenuous physical activity may go unnoticed at the time or be perceived as not especially painful. Goals, purposes, and general activity levels appear to modulate the pain experience. In some circumstances reactions to ordinarily painful tissue damage may be surprisingly slight, as in painless childbirth or in primitive puberty rites (e.g., penile incision among Polynesians). A football player who cracks an ankle bone in an active scrimmage may not feel a great deal of pain until later, when the excitement has subsided and he is physically inactive. Here, sensory inputs that might ordinarily be perceived as painful signify the achievement of valued goals. Activity and excitement are at a high pitch. The physiological and cognitive responses to this acute stress combine to limit sharply the perception of pain.

The effect of stress on pain and pain-suppressing mechanisms has been the object of intensive investigation.[58] Stress mobilizes a defense system that involves the CNS, endogenous analgesics, and the HPA axis. Other endocrine secretions also can modulate pain sensitivity; Goolkasian,[59] using SDT methods, demonstrated reduced discrimination of calibrated noxious thermal stimulation during the ovulatory phase of the menstrual cycle.

Janal and coworkers[60] studied a group of marathon runners before and after a 10-km run and observed analgesic effects after the run, namely, decreased discrimination, $P(A)$, of noxious thermal stimulation and decreased sensitivity to tourniquet ischemic pain. In addition, the runners were in a euphoric mood. Elevated plasma levels of β-endorphin, adrenocorticotropic hormone, prolactin, and growth hormone were found, thus demonstrating the effect of exercise stress on HPA axis activity. The analgesia and the euphoria suggest increased central endogenous opioid activity. The hypothesis that the action was central was confirmed when the analgesia and euphoria were absent on another occasion when the runners were administered naloxone, which blocks the central effects of opioids.

Animal studies have shown that nonopioid mechanisms also contribute to the analgesic effect. Thus, naloxone, which blocks opioid receptors, does not reverse all stress-induced analgesic effects. Endogenous nonopioid mechanisms may be involved in the analgesia claimed to be induced by acupuncture and other types of counter-irritant stimulation such as TENS.

Activation of endogenous pain-inhibitory circuits is adaptive, because an injured but analgesic animal is better able to cope with an emergency situation. Once the emergency has passed, however, the animal must become aware of, and immediately attend to, its injuries if it is to survive. Wiertelak and associates[61] demonstrated an endogenous analgesia inhibitory system in rats that is activated by environmental safety signals. They found that a safety signal reversed morphine analgesia by initiating processes that act at the spinal cord. Moreover, the administration of a cholecystokinin antagonist prevented the safety signal from abolishing the morphine analgesia (i.e., the antianalgesia system was inhibited). Their work suggests that in nature a safety signal at the level of the cerebral cortex releases cholecystokinin in the spinal cord via descending fibers that synapse on enkephalinergic islet cells. The authors concluded that pain depends on the complex interplay of pain-inhibitory and anti–pain-inhibitory processes.

Endogenous opioid changes induced by chronic stress in humans may explain the results obtained by Yang and associates.[62] They used the SDT procedure to study the responses of chronic back pain patients to brief, calibrated thermal stimuli. Compared with healthy volunteers, patients were less able to discriminate among the stimuli (lower d') and set a higher criterion (L_x) (i.e., reported less pain to the thermal stimuli). These findings, a lower d' and a higher L_x, were the same as those produced by analgesics and suggest that an endogenous analgesic system had been activated. Apparently, the endogenous analgesic response triggered by the pain was sufficient to blunt the response to the relatively low-intensity noxious thermal stimuli, but was insufficient to ameliorate the more intense back pain. The stoical criterion suggests that, in comparison with their clinical pain, the pain induced by the brief thermal stimuli appeared relatively innocuous.

Arousal by pleasurable stimulation can also inhibit pain responses. Whipple and Komisaruk[63] demonstrated in a group of college students that vaginal self-stimulation increased the threshold of noxious finger compression. No change was found in the ability to detect innocuous touch stimuli, demonstrating that the decreased sensitivity to pain was not caused by distraction.

FUNCTIONAL BRAIN IMAGING

New findings from functional imaging studies have caused a sea change in our understanding of the supraspinal processing of acute pain, in identifying neural systems mediating pain, and in some of the poorly understood aspects of clinical pain. This new knowledge, along with the discovery of the descending opioid pain inhibitory system, has led to a modification of the 1965 Melzack-Wall gate model. The interactions governing neural transmission in the dorsal horn, midbrain, thalamus, and brain are far more complex than was originally envisioned.

Melzack's latest model,[18] although explaining a number of diverse phenomena, does not offer a detailed neurophysiological account for the preservation of pain after lesions at various spinal and supraspinal levels. For example, lesions of the primary somatosensory cortex produce a permanent loss of the ability to discriminate innocuous tactile and thermal stimulation, but not a permanent loss of the ability to discriminate the intensity of noxious stimulation. Sensory-discriminative aspects of pain are generally thought to be processed contralaterally; however, brain-imaging studies of *split brain* patients with complete transection of the corpus callosum demonstrate that pain intensity information from a unilateral noxious stimulus is processed in both hemispheres. Furthermore, affective responses to pain are preserved after lesions to some brain regions that mediate emotion. It has been generally believed that patients who underwent prefrontal lobotomy for chronic pain experienced pain, but did not find it distressing. However, later when "lobotomized" patients were studied in greater detail, they were able to discriminate the intensity of the stimuli.

Functional imaging has demonstrated that the anterior cingulate cortex and prefrontal cortex are activated by noxious stimulation. Along with clinical findings after cingulotomies and lobotomies, imaging studies suggest that these structures are involved in emotional responses to pain. In contrast to prefrontal lobotomy, which often produced drastic personality changes, contemporary brain surgical techniques entail lesioning small selected areas of brain tissue. Corkin and colleagues[64] demonstrated that bilateral anterior cingulotomy relieves persistent, often life-long, non-neoplastic pain, as well as the accompanying depression. In meticulous, well-designed studies of cognitive function, these investigators found no evidence of lasting neurologic or behavioral deficit; in fact, there were significant gains on tests of general intelligence.

The medial thalamic nuclei, once thought to be involved in processing only affect because of their projection to the reticular and limbic systems, have been found to encode sensory intensity information with a precision sufficient for behavioral discrimination. Functional imaging studies with calibrated noxious stimuli in humans demonstrate that the vast majority of pain-processing areas receives intensity information. These include the cerebellum, putamen, thalamus, primary and secondary somatosensory cortex, insula, and anterior cingulate cortex. Thus, affective, motoric, attentional, and autonomic aspects of pain respond to gradations in the intensity of noxious stimuli. Both innocuous and noxious stimuli produce somatically consistent localization in the primary and secondary somatosensory cortex and in adjacent insular regions. Therefore, these regions must contribute to stimulus localization. Conscious awareness probably involves the participation of other brain regions such as the prefrontal cortex and posterior parietal cortex, which imaging studies have shown to be activated by painful stimulation. These regions are, of course, not solely pain-processing areas.

The complexity of the cognitive, affective, and motoric interactions is illustrated on those occasions when withdrawal from a painful stimulus must be inhibited. One does not drop an expensive, but painfully hot, teacup. Functional imaging studies[64] have shown that tasks involving the suppression of highly learned motor responses evoke increased activation of the anterior cingulate cortex. Thus, brain-imaging techniques have made it clear that the scheme of two parallel, essentially serial, sensory and affect pathways must be replaced by a distributed system that embraces multiple brain regions and paths.

PHANTOM PAIN

Most recent amputees experience a complex of sensations patterned in a way that makes them feel as if they still had limbs of normal size, shape, and mobility. Usually, this phantom limb gradually shrinks and eventually disappears, but in a small proportion of cases, particularly when the limb was painful before the amputation, severe pain continues to be felt in the phantom limb. Some causes are understandable. Neuromas may develop at the severed nerve endings at the amputation site, and these can be stimulated accidentally.

Neurosurgery or local anesthetic injected at the site eliminates this peripheral source of pain, although often only temporarily. Patients whose pain is not improved by surgery pose a problem. What is the source of the spontaneously recurring pain? Even dorsal root resections that remove all pain sensibility from the stump itself may not eliminate phantom limb pain.

The brain activity revealed in imaging studies makes the case of phantom pain introduced by Melzack[18] somewhat less mysterious. Although it is now recognized that pain may arise from activity at any level in the nervous system, this was not always understood. Nineteenth century specificity theory held that the intensity of the pain experience was directly related to the intensity of the noxious stimulus and the resulting afferent input from primary neurons. The early gate theory maintained that the afferent input could be modulated by secondary neurons at the spinal level, but not above. Melzack has described a case of phantom pain that persisted even without spinal input. This striking case of central pain without any spinal input poses a problem for theories of peripheral pain modulation. After an accident that rendered him paraplegic, the patient underwent cordectomy (complete removal of a section of the spinal cord) for the intractable pain that radiated from his legs and body below the lesion. The operation gave complete relief for 11 years, until he again reported daily shooting pains in both legs and the back. To explain this case of phantom pain, Melzack postulated a widespread network of positive and negative feedback, in third-order neurons and above, with loops between thalamus, cortex, and limbic systems. He postulated further that this neural network is normally activated and modulated by non-noxious inputs from the periphery. The brain can drive itself.

Melzack's model is compatible with much of the more recent brain-imaging data. Centrally mediated pain may play a role in other types of chronic pain (e.g., approximately three-fourths of patients with low back pain continue to suffer in spite of a variety of therapies, including disk surgery, trigger-point injection of analgesics or corticosteroids, physical therapy, and behavior therapy). These treatments may fail because the pain is maintained at least in part by independent, self-contained brain mechanisms.

Another puzzle is that some patients suffer intense pain and others experience little pain from the same injury or condition. This may be explained by the findings of brain imaging investigators who report wide individual differences in the amount of activity induced in various brain structures by calibrated noxious stimuli. This suggests that anatomic or functional distribution differences might account in part for individual differences in pain sensitivity.

The potential of brain imaging to resolve controversy and to illuminate mechanisms that modulate pain is illustrated by a study of the effects of hypnosis. Rainville and coworkers[65] used hypnotic suggestion to exaggerate or to minimize the affect associated with noxious heat stimulation during positron emission tomographic scans. They demonstrated that the activity of the anterior cingulate was significantly related to the subject's hypnotic state, which was reflected in the subject's responses to an affective pain-rating scale. They also found that the somatosensory cortex was not influenced by the hypnotic manipulation of affect, thus demonstrating the different functional properties of these structures.

One might expect that functional imaging studies of patients suffering central pain or chronic pain could have yielded the locus of the clinical pain-related activity. However, unlike the findings with calibrated noxious stimuli in healthy volunteers, brain imaging studies of clinical pain have produced inconsistent results.[66]

Another pain puzzle is the restriction of analgesia to specific regions of the body. Stress-related activation of the endogenous opioid system or the HPA axis would be expected to produce an analgesic response throughout the body. Thus, central pain-inhibitory mechanisms must be invoked to account for the specificity of some responses to injury. For example, Beecher[67] described how wounded soldiers complained little of pain from their wounds but bitterly about inept venipuncture. Thus, the general excitement of the situation and the relief of leaving battle with a *good* wound did not make them generally hypoalgesic. Rather, the perception of pain was highly selective. The site specificity of these analgesic effects demonstrates that the higher centers in the brain discovered by brain imaging are involved in pain suppression.

VISCERAL PAIN

Visceral pain is one of the most frequent reasons for patients to seek medical attention. Until relatively recently our knowledge of basic mechanisms of pain has come from studies of somatic, especially cutaneous stimulation. Although there are some similarities, visceral and somatic pain differ in a number of ways.

The viscera do have pain sensibility, particularly when the whole organ is involved and a sufficient number of the sparsely distributed stretch receptors are stimulated. Adequate stimuli include rapid distension or

contraction of hollow organs, distension of the capsule of solid organs such as the liver, damage to blood vessels, and ischemia. Intense pain from deep somatic structures and viscera often produces such autonomic symptoms as nausea, decreased blood pressure, and syncope. Pain fibers from deep tissues, such as viscera, muscles, and periosteum are more sparsely distributed than somatic pain fibers. These visceral afferents are anatomically associated with sympathetic efferent fibers to smooth muscles and glands, but they do not differ from other somatic afferents and are not part of the sympathetic system. Meticulous neurophysiological studies in animals and psychophysical measurement of responses by humans to calibrated stimuli, such as balloon distention pressures in the gut by Cervero,[68] Gebhart and Randich,[69] and Cervero and Morrison,[70] have done much to increase our knowledge of visceral pain.

There are a number of differences between somatic and visceral pain: Visceral pain is poorly localized, some organs lack sensory receptors, pain or distress can occur without tissue injury, and pain often is referred to somatic structures. There are two biochemical types of unmyelinated visceral afferents. One, which terminates in laminae I, II, and V, contains neuropeptides (e.g., substance P). The other contains nonpeptide groups and terminates in inner lamina II. The view that pain signals from the viscera are transmitted solely in the anterolateral columns has been questioned. There is evidence that the dorsal columns, the spino-parabrachial-amygdaloid system, and the spinohypothalamic path transmit nociceptive information from the viscera. Brain imaging studies have shown that noxious rectal stimulation evokes brain activity in a region of the anterior cingulate that is not activated by somatic stimuli.

Berkley[71] discusses in detail the viscerosomatic convergence of cutaneous, muscle, and visceral afferent inputs in the laminae of the dorsal horn. This convergence suggests the basis of referred pain. Diagnosing the cause of visceral pain on the basis of symptom report is extremely difficult. For example, pain resulting from myocardial ischemia or from gastric acid reflux in the esophagus can cause referred pain to the chest, arm, shoulder, face, or teeth. Moreover, the warning signs do not always work.

Silent myocardial ischemia is a coronary artery disease syndrome in which cardiac ischemia fails to provoke angina (i.e., the warning signs of oxygen insufficiency are absent). Vagal afferents have long been known to play a role in cardiopulmonary and gastrointestinal function. Gebhart and Randich[69] discuss work in which vagal afferent and spinopetal (descending) systems modulate pain. Whether the absence of pain report in silent myocardial ischemia is caused by a sensory deficit (demonstrated by a decrease in *P[A]*) or to a stoic pain report criterion (*B*) was studied by Glusman and colleagues.[72] They used the SDT model described earlier. Electrocardiograms were recorded while the patient exercised, and, on cue, rated the presence or absence of any weak sensations in the chest, arm, or face. An ST-segment depression greater than 0.05 mV was defined as a *signal*, and less than 0.05 mV as a *blank*. Analysis of the resulting hit and false affirmative rates yielded the SDT parameters, *P(A)* and (*B*). The symptomatic patients were able to discriminate between the two levels of ST-segment depression; the silent patients could not. It was concluded that the cardiac sensory system failed to transmit painful sensory information that should have been initiated by the ischemia. The alternative view that the patients were in denial and not reporting the pain they felt was not supported. Nor did naloxone infusion demonstrate that the absence of pain was caused by endogenous opioidergic mechanisms.

SYNAPTIC TRANSMISSION

Knowledge of the mechanisms mediating synaptic transmission is essential to understanding the pharmacologic action of analgesics and other drugs. Transmission at the first synapse (in the dorsal horn) is mediated by the amino acid glutamate, released by Aδ, Aβ, and C fibers, which activates glutamate receptors. In addition, C fibers release the neuropeptide substance P, which persists longer and diffuses more widely than glutamate. Synaptic transmission between central neurons is complex, but it is clearly explained by Kandel et al.[73] These cells receive connections from hundreds of bundles of excitatory and inhibitory neurons. Neurotransmitters, released in packets from the presynaptic neuron into the synaptic cleft, bind to postsynaptic receptors that alter the membrane potential, after which a reuptake mechanism returns the transmitters to the presynaptic neuron. One type of receptor, the *ionotropic* receptor, gates ion channels directly through the action of a single molecule; their synaptic action is fast and brief. The main excitatory transmitter in the CNS is glutamate. Glutamate binds to non–*N*-methyl-aspartate receptors, which form channels permeable to both Na$^+$ and K$^+$ ions, as well as to the *N*-methyl-aspartate receptor, which forms a channel permeable to Ca^{++} as well as Na$^+$ and K$^+$ ions. The main inhibitory transmitters are gamma-aminobutyric acid and glycine; they increase permeability to permit the influx of Cl$^-$ ions that hyperpolarize

the membrane and inhibit excitatory currents. Alcohol, barbiturates, and benzodiazepines, which affect emotion, memory, and to some extent pain, bind to certain gamma-aminobutyric acid receptors, enhance Cl$^-$ inflow, and hence neural inhibition.

The second type of glutamate receptor acts indirectly on channels through second messengers. The first type of *metabotropic* receptor requires the activity of an additional molecule, of which there are two classes. The guanine nucleotide-binding (or G) protein-coupled receptors activate ion channels indirectly through a protein that initiates a second messenger cascade. This G group contains α- and β-adrenergic, acetylcholine, neuropeptide, and serotonin receptors. A second type of metabotropic receptor modulates the activity of membrane channels indirectly through a series of protein phosphorylation reactions. This type of receptor is activated by hormones, growth factors, and neuropeptides. The second messenger actions may last up to minutes and underlie states of negative and positive affect and arousal. Metabotropic receptors also activate second messenger pathways in synaptic transmission. Nongaseous second messengers include cyclic adenosine monophosphate and intracellular Ca^{++}, whereas the best known gaseous messengers are nitric oxide and carbon monoxide. They act by stimulating the synthesis of cyclic guanosine monophosphate, a cytoplasmic second messenger that activates a specific protein kinase. These gases have unique properties as messengers. They diffuse readily into cells without acting through a receptor and can diffuse in a retrograde manner to the presynaptic terminal. The slower metabotropic receptors, because they recruit diffusible gaseous intracellular second messengers, can act throughout the cell: dendrites, axons, and presynaptic terminals. Thus, metabotropic receptors are well suited to modulate the threshold and temporal characteristics of transmission.

In addition to the ionotropic and metabotropic receptors, a third type acts through second messengers on transcriptional regulatory proteins that activate gene expression to induce the synthesis of new proteins. This mechanism is responsible for a centrally mediated hyperalgesia that sometimes follows persistent noxious stimulation. The repetitive firing of C fibers increases the response of dorsal horn neurons, known as *wind-up*. Wind-up is readily reproduced in the laboratory. Price[74] has demonstrated that when a brief, innocuous, warm stimulus is presented as a train of 10 stimuli at 0.3 Hz, a painful sensation is provoked. Wind-up pain depends on the release of the excitatory transmitter glutamate followed by the opening of polysynaptic ion channels gated by *N*-methyl-aspartate receptors.

NEURAL PLASTICITY

Persistent pain and other sensory abnormalities are often reported after peripheral nerve injury.[75] These abnormalities include paresthesias, dysesthesias, allodynia, and hyperalgesia. In some cases a partial explanation of symptoms that follow nerve injury lies in the fact that the nociceptive afferents have a greater capacity to regrow into the denervated region than do the larger axons that mediate touch (thus, the dysesthesia). This imbalance would cause loss of large-fiber inhibition of the nociceptive neurons (i.e., it would open the Melzack-Wall gate). This problem may disappear after some months, when the larger, Aβ nerves have regrown and can once again transmit impulses that close the gate.

But often cases of pain persist for months or years after complete regrowth of the large fibers. Dubner[76] reviewed the latest findings on the causes of long-term allodynia and hyperalgesia after tissue damage, inflammation, edema, and erythema. Neuropathic hyperalgesia (frequently with burning, causalgic pain) may appear after nerve injury by trauma (sympathetic dystrophy), infection (postherpetic neuralgia), or metabolic disease (diabetic neuropathy). After injury to the skin, previously innocuous stimuli can provoke activity in myelinated and unmyelinated mechanical, thermal, and polymodal nociceptive afferent fibers. Surprisingly, both inflammatory and neuropathic allodynia appear to be mediated by input from large myelinated afferents, which, when the tissue is healthy, signal tactile sensations, not pain. Both inflammatory and neuropathic hyperalgesias are associated with prolonged hyperexcitability of the spinal dorsal horn wide dynamic range and nociceptive-specific neurons and are maintained by both peripheral input and local circuit activity. The hyperexcitability probably involves both increased activity in excitatory fibers and reduced activity of inhibitory neurons, including descending inputs from supraspinal sites.

Long-term changes in neural function responsible for persistent pain involve changes in gene expression. The *c-fos* proto-oncogene (oncogene indicates that it is involved in cell growth, as in cancer) is rapidly induced by various normal and pathologic stimuli. The *c-fos* protein (FOS) binds to DNA, where it acts as a transcription regulator; it is thought to mediate long-term changes in neural responsivity. Noxious stimulation has been shown to increase, and morphine to reduce, neuronal levels of FOS in laminae I, II, and V. The action of FOS is to increase the intracellular calcium ion flow induced by substance P and glutamate. The up-regulation of neurotransmitters and receptors can lead to pain that continues long after healing at the original site of injury is complete. Such mechanisms probably underlie the puzzling persistence of sympathetic dystrophy and phantom limb pain.

The devastating effect of hyperactivity within neural systems that mediate pain forces a shift in the way we think about pain. Pain is not only a manifestation of an underlying disease; pain can be a disease itself, one that can profoundly alter the functioning of the nervous system and delay healing and recovery, and, at its worst, can kill. With this realization, there is now considerable discussion of premedication with local anesthetics at the surgical site to prevent intense nociceptive stimulation and the FOS synthesis that may follow.

EMOTIONS AND FEELINGS

A noxious stimulus evokes emotional as well as sensory experiences. *Emotion* may be considered to refer to the bodily response to biopsychosocial stimuli, whereas *feeling* refers to conscious awareness.[73] Emotional bodily states involve endocrine, cardiac, vasomotor, respiratory, and skeletal motor responses. These involve mainly subcortical structures: the HPA system and brain stem. Feelings include fear, anxiety, hostility, euphoria, and arousal. They are mediated mainly by cerebral cortex, including cingulate cortex and frontal lobes. Autonomic and behavioral responses are closely integrated in all behaviors. For example, stimulation of a specific site in the hypothalamus of the rat leads to coordinated autonomic (heart rate, blood pressure) and behavioral responses (aggression, placidity) characteristic of a variety of emotional states. Because of this close integration, it is not surprising that a painful stimulus administered to one animal in a group will provoke it to attack another.

Electrical stimulation, brain imaging, and surgical studies have established the role of the *limbic circuit* involving the amygdala, frontal, cingulate, and parahippocampal cortices in emotion and feeling. Lesions of the anterior cingulate in humans often reduce chronic pain (e.g., in the painful form of Briquet's syndrome, a psychiatric somatization disorder).[64] The amygdala, a subcortical structure, appears to be involved in both the emotional and feeling systems. The somatic responses to emotional state involve connections from the amygdala to the hypothalamus and autonomic nervous system, whereas the conscious feeling responses involve projections from the amygdala to the cortical structures.

AUTONOMIC NERVOUS SYSTEM

Pain and other types of stress mobilize the autonomic nervous and endocrine systems. The autonomic system responds to external and internal sensory input. A penetrating wound activates local circuits that produce local vasoconstriction, as well as more general circuits in the STT to the medulla that increase heart rate, stroke volume, and general vasoconstriction.

The two major divisions of the autonomic nervous system are the sympathetic and parasympathetic. Generally, the sympathetic nervous system governs the emergency responses to blood loss, drastic temperature changes, and emotional stress. The parasympathetic system maintains basal heart rate, metabolism, and regulation under normal conditions. The two systems are actually much more synchronized than once thought; both are tonically active and operate in conjunction with the somatic nervous system to regulate both resting and emergency behavior. Sympathetic activation of mainly adrenergic neurons increases blood pressure by increasing heart rate and stroke volume and by constricting arterioles. Reduced sympathetic and increased parasympathetic activity leads to vasodilatation. Norepinephrine released in response to pain-induced stress increases stroke volume and heart rate via β-adrenergic receptors on cardiac muscle and by decreasing the threshold of cardiac pacemaker cells in the sinoatrial node of the heart muscle. Stress-induced epinephrine released from the adrenal medulla greatly augments the effects of norepinephrine. In relaxed circumstances the parasympathetic system releases acetylcholine, which slows the heart rate by acting on receptors in the sinoatrial and atrioventricular nodes. Parasympathetic inputs increase activity of salivary, lacrimal, and gastrointestinal glands by increasing local blood flow. Sympathetic input has the opposite effect in glands, with the exception that sympathetic stimulation increases sweating.

Autonomic input from the CNS and the periphery is primarily transmitted by acetylcholine and norepinephrine, although neuropeptides such as calcitonin gene-related peptide, substance P, enkephalins, neurotensin, and somatostatin are also involved.

HYPOTHALAMUS

The hypothalamus plays a major role in the stress response; it integrates autonomic and endocrine functions with behavior. It regulates blood pressure and osmolarity, body temperature, metabolism (including glucose levels), and reproduction. Further, it regulates the hormonal and immunologic responses to stress. Projections from the hypothalamus to the posterior pituitary stimulate the release of vasopressin and oxytocin into the general circulation. In addition, hypothalamic neurons secrete a wide range of releasing hormones that are carried to the anterior pituitary by hypophysial portal veins. Hormones released by the anterior pituitary into the general circulation include the stress-related hormones adrenocorticotropin, β-lipotropin, β-endorphin, as well as others such as thyrotropin, growth hormone, luteinizing, and follicle-stimulating hormones.

IMMUNE SYSTEM

The immune system and the brain communicate with each other. Stress hormones in response to pain and psychosocial stimuli can alter the immune response. If these hormonal levels are too high, the immune system is suppressed and one becomes more susceptible to infection. However, if stress hormonal levels are too low, the immune system is not suppressed enough by glucosteroids that should act to turn it down, and one becomes more susceptible to inflammation and arthritic disease.

The etiology of immune disease is multifactorial, resulting from a combination of genetically predetermined host characteristics and environmental exposures. Sternberg[77] notes that an important role in susceptibility to inflammatory disease is played by interaction between the central components of the stress response and the immune system. Immune system products (e.g., cytokines) activate the HPA axis, which in turn regulate immune response through the immunosuppressive effects of glucocorticoids.

Pain, acting via the immune system, can kill. One group of patients suffering pain from inoperable pancreatic cancer received standard treatment, which did not completely block the pain. Another group received an alcohol block that was much more successful at eliminating pain. Unexpectedly, the second group's survival time was much longer. Apparently, the greater pain-induced stress in the first group caused an immune response that suppressed natural killer cell activity and thereby permitted more rapid tumor growth.

Fibromyalgia, characterized by complaints of chronic diffuse musculoskeletal aching and stiffness and by tender points at specific anatomic sites (myalgia), fatigue, and unrefreshing sleep, has baffled physicians for a long time. Other terms for related disorders with this complex of symptoms include *fibrositis, neurasthenia, masked depression, chronic fatigue syndrome,* and *somatoform pain disorder.* Theories of causation include a pathologic immune system response. In the absence of any specific cause, doubts have been raised about the diagnostic legitimacy of this syndrome. However, Moldofsky[78] argues that the illness is characterized by an alpha-delta frequency electroencephalographic non–rapid eye movement sleep anomaly that is absent in healthy controls and in insomniacs. Although the electroencephalographic sleep anomaly is frequently correlated with the fibromyalgia syndrome, it has relatively low specificity, being found in some 15% of asymptomatic patients. Moldofsky postulates a close relation between the immune system, immunologically active peptides, and the brain, particularly the serotoninergic pain-inhibitory system. This conclusion is supported by the study by Crofford and associates,[79] who found fibromyalgia patients to have adrenal hyporesponsiveness compared with controls. Obviously, the relationship between pain-induced stress and the immune system is an important one.

GENETICS

Before considering the exciting findings related to the genetics of pain, a few commonly used terms are discussed. The pain threshold, which can vary with nongenetic psychosocial variables, is not inherited. What is inherited is DNA, which encodes proteins and is arranged in a precise configuration on chromosomes. Genes direct the manufacture of specific proteins. The reason cells differ in various organs is that a different set of genes is expressed in each type of cell. Each gene is located at a characteristic locus on a specific chromosome. During mitosis the chromosomes are portioned equally. The two copies of the gene at corresponding loci on a pair of homologous chromosomes usually differ slightly. These alternate versions are referred to as *alleles.* If the two alleles differ in their nucleotide sequence, the organism is termed *heterozygous* at that site, and *homozygous* if the two alleles are identical. If a mutant phenotypic trait is expressed only when both alleles of a gene are mutated, then the phenotype is recessive; if the mutant phenotype is the result of a combination of a mutant allele with a normal allele, then the phenotypic trait is dominant.

Individual differences in the response to analgesics are common, but disappointing to the clinician. A patient who fails to respond to, or has excessive side effects to ibuprofen, for example, may have a good result with acetaminophen, or the reverse may occur. It is now recognized that genetic variability may be a source of idiosyncratic responses. Some of the ethnic differences in response to drugs undoubtedly have a genetic basis. These differences can occur because of differences in the rate of drug disposition (e.g., metabolism) or in drug sensitivity (e.g., receptors). Zhou and coworkers[80] found that morphine depressed the respiratory response, leading to doubling the carbon dioxide retention, and reduced blood pressure to a greater extent in white Americans than in Chinese patients. This faster disposition of morphine in the Chinese was caused by an increase in the partial metabolic clearance of morphine by glucuronidation. These results suggest that Chinese patients may be undermedicated, and Western patients overmedicated with morphine. Interestingly, Chinese patients complained much more about nausea. This suggests that Chinese may have more μ receptors in the gut, which also could represent a genetic difference. Ethnic differences have also been found in response to adrenergic and cholinergic antagonists as well as other substances. Because it is well-established that specific genes control enzymes and receptors, it is possible that individual differences in gene expression within a group could explain some of the differences in response to drugs. Approximately 8% of Westerners are unable to metabolize codeine into morphine, the metabolite responsible for the analgesic effect of codeine. The inherited allele is easily typed, and this error in treatment could thereby be avoided.

Even when the physical source of clinical pain appears the same, there is wide individual variation in the pain response. With the same injury, some people develop dystrophy, back pain, neuropathic and central pain, and others do not. Some of this variability may be related to genotype. A number of inherited painful syndromes such as familial hemiplegic migraine, painful congenital myotonia, as well as congenital insensitivity to pain, have been shown to have a genetic basis. Psychosocial factors play a role in the experience of pain, but some of the variability can be explained by multiple pain-relevant genes interacting with each other and the environment.

Animal studies offer the clearest evidence for the role of genes in pain sensitivity. In the mouse, Mogil and coworkers[81,82] found large strain differences in the response to 12 different thermal, chemical, and mechanical nociceptive assays. They found that genotype significantly affected threshold performance in all of these pain measures. Analysis of the number of genetic loci led them to conclude that relatively few, rather than many genes, were mediating these pain responses.

Two chromosomal regions associated with variability in morphine analgesia in the mouse have been found. One gene encodes the μ opioid receptor and the other a serotonin receptor subtype. The genes encoding the μ, δ, and κ opioid receptors have been found to be members of the G protein–coupled class of receptors. Morphine is a potent agonist at the μ receptor; deletion of the gene for that receptor produces mice that are insensitive to the analgesic effects of morphine. It is clear that future investigation into the interaction between the psychosocial, pharmacologic, and genetic aspects of pain will greatly facilitate our understanding and treatment of pain.

MEDICATION

A variety of drugs used to treat pain are discussed here with respect to what is known about their mechanisms of action, rather than rules for their therapeutic use. Drugs that are used to ameliorate pain and suffering include the opioids and the nonsteroidal anti-inflammatory drugs (NSAIDs), sedatives, antidepressants, anticonvulsants, and antihistamines, as well as adjuvants such as caffeine. Injection of local anesthetics produces temporary local nerve blocks; alcohol and phenol injections have more permanent effects. Local injection of corticosteroids reduces inflammation, and so, pain.

Opioids

Drugs of the opioid family are the most effective substances available for the management of severe pain such as postsurgical and cancer pain. Their use for severe chronic nonmalignant pain is now being advocated.[82] Their mechanisms of action have been discussed.

Nonsteroidal Anti-Inflammatory Drugs

Salicylates, such as aspirin and other NSAIDs, are useful for the treatment of moderate pain from a number of causes, including surgery, inflammation (e.g., arthritis), and cancer at an early stage. They are less effective for intense, sharp pains, which respond only to narcotics. NSAIDs now are known to act centrally as well as peripherally. In the periphery, pain is caused by prostaglandins, which induce inflammation and directly facilitate C fiber activity. Prostaglandins are produced by the action of the enzyme cyclo-oxygenase on arachidonic acid. NSAIDs reduce prostaglandin levels by inhibiting the action of cyclo-oxygenase. Malmberg and

Yaksh[83] demonstrated that NSAIDs also act centrally at the spinal level. Activation of C fiber afferents by noxious stimulation causes spinal release of the excitatory amino acids glutamate and aspartate, as well as substance P. These substances activate pharmacologically distinct receptor sites to produce hyperalgesia and, in some way still unknown, to increase spinal levels of arachidonic acid, which augments the hyperalgesia.

Antidepressants

Tricyclic antidepressants (e.g., amitriptyline and imipramine) and selective serotonin reuptake inhibitors, although not classified as analgesics, are used to treat neuropathic pain such as diabetic neuropathy, postherpetic neuralgia, tension and migraine headaches, rheumatoid arthritis, low back pain, malignant nerve infiltration, and central pain after stroke and spinal injury. In many instances, part of the effect may be related to the amelioration of depression, but, at least in the instances of neuropathy and central pain, there appears to be a specific analgesic effect, since pain relief can occur regardless of whether patients are depressed or not. Moreover, the analgesic effect is much faster than the 2 or more weeks it takes for the antidepressant action. On the other hand, many patients fail to show any pain relief after antidepressant medication. One possible mechanism of action implicates the increase in the concentrations of the biogenic amine transmitters serotonin and norepinephrine that occur when reuptake of these substances at the synapse is blocked by the antidepressant medication. As outlined earlier, both serotonergic and noradrenergic neurons originating in the brain stem project to nociceptive transmission cells in the spinal cord.

An evaluation of the effectiveness of antidepressant medication for pain was conducted by Onghena and Van Houdenhoue.[84] They performed a meta-analysis of 39 placebo-controlled studies and concluded that the average chronic pain patient who received an antidepressant was "better off" than 74% of those who received a placebo. The effect appeared to be, in most cases, a specifically analgesic action and not a secondary response to successful treatment of the depression.

Anticonvulsants

Anticonvulsants (e.g., carbamazepine) may relieve lancinating pain, which is typically described as a paroxysmal, shooting, stabbing pain associated with peripheral nerve syndromes such as trigeminal neuralgia and spinal cord injury. Their mode of action appears to be related to their ability to suppress massive, synchronous neural discharges in compressed or otherwise damaged nerves.

SURGERY

Ablation of nociceptive pathways, including dorsal root ganglia, ascending columns, and thalamic nuclei, is seldom practiced for a number of reasons: improved analgesic medication, better understanding of the contribution of emotion to pain and suffering, and, most important, the growing awareness that in addition to serious and irreversible side effects, surgery provides only transient relief or may fail entirely. The usual indication for ablative procedures is for patients with uncontrollable pain and limited life expectancy. However, as neural structures mediating pain become better known, surgery may play a greater role. Note the cingulotomies described earlier.

PSYCHOSOCIAL ASPECTS OF PAIN AND EMOTION

The previous section has provided a cursory overview of what is currently understood about the neurophysiological basis of pain and suffering. We turn now to a large body of scientific information that describes the psychological and psychosocial aspects of pain and suffering. Besides providing guidance for treatment, this body of knowledge integrates the psychological mechanisms underlying pain and suffering behavior. A thorough introduction to this literature, plus a discussion of the roles of the physician, anesthetist, physical therapist, nurse, psychologist, social worker, and others in the management of chronic pain has been published.[85]

Personality Differences

Many studies have found that anxiety tends to increase sensitivity to calibrated experimental pain stimuli. Clark[86] studied a group of anxiety-prone psychiatric patients who suffered from a variety of atypical pains of unknown origin such as muscle pain, headaches, facial pain, and abdominal pain. The pains were often diffuse, migratory, and episodic rather than localized and continuous. The patients appeared to be far more concerned with the possible medical significance of the pain than with the pain itself. All had been referred for psychiatric evaluation after two or three subspecialty medical workups proved inconclusive, and various treatment attempts

had produced mixed results. The patients commonly had a history of disturbed interpersonal relationships. On psychological tests such as the Brief Symptom Inventory,[37] they scored high on the anxiety scale. They were independently diagnosed as suffering from a well-defined, chronic, generalized anxiety disorder. These atypical pain patients were remarkably over-responsive to noxious stimuli, including thermal pain, cold pressor pain, and ischemic tourniquet pain. SDT analysis of their responses to thermal stimulation revealed that they set an extremely low pain report criterion, often reporting as painful a stimulus that was merely warm. In this respect they differed from a group of chronic back pain patients (described later), who were experiencing physical pain and who set a high, that is, stoical pain report criterion. The low pain report criterion of anxious patients probably reflects the fact they that are overly fearful of injury and report as painful low-intensity stimuli, in an attempt to discourage the investigator from increasing the intensity of the stimulus. It seems likely that patients who describe these relatively innocuous physical stimuli as painful may also be *amplifying* their reports of clinical pain. Such patients are not necessarily deliberately misleading the physician; indeed, they are probably unaware of their motivation. That anxiety and not pain is the main problem of these patients is also supported by their response to treatment. Many of them, including some who had not responded to analgesics or to antidepressants, responded well to anxiolytic medication.

Sex Differences

Possible differences in the amount of pain experienced by women and men remain controversial.[87] This long-standing question applies not only to complex instances of clinical pain, but even to the much more precisely controlled studies of laboratory pain, in which the strength and sensory modality of the noxious stimulus is known exactly. The considerable disagreement among investigators is probably caused by the use of traditional psychophysical procedures, such as the method of limits and constant stimuli. A number of studies using traditional procedures have found women to be more sensitive to noxious stimulation. On the other hand, Clark and Yang[43] used SDT to compare responses by men and women to calibrated noxious heat stimuli. They found that the sexes did not differ in their ability to discriminate, $P(A)$, between intensities. Thus, as reflected in the neurosensory information transmitted, the sensory input was the same for men and women, and, accordingly, the sexes presumably experienced the same pain. Women did, however, set a lower criterion,

B, more pain responses, which traditional psychophysics would mistakenly treat as greater sensitivity. Because anxiety is known to lower both the criterion, *B,* and pain threshold, it is likely that some test situations (e.g., an unsympathetic male investigator) cause women to respond with more pain reports.

Sex differences in the language of pain (i.e., in the different meanings that men and women attach to some descriptors of pain and emotion) probably account for differences in pain report even when the sensory experiences are the same. Studies of language are essential to the understanding of a patient's description of pain and for the construction of gender-free (and culture-free) pain questionnaires. According to the clinical literature,[88] women report more severe, frequent, and longer duration pain over a larger number of sites than do men. Women also differ in other ways; Bendelow[89] showed that women were more likely to give "holistic, integrated" reports of pain (pain and emotional descriptions tend to be grouped together), whereas men tend to group pain and somatosensory descriptors together. Men also were more reluctant to classify pain associated with emotional suffering as *real* pain.

Clark and coworkers,[38] using hierarchical cluster analysis of similarity data obtained for 189 descriptors of pain and emotion, found 30 clusters of descriptors. A notable finding was that men of various ethnocultural groups interpreted the mental distress cluster (containing descriptors such as *uncomfortable, bothersome,* and *troublesome*) as belonging to the sensory qualities supercluster, whereas the women interpreted the same descriptors as belonging to the negative emotions supercluster. Thus, men interpreted the descriptors as being related to pain sensations, whereas the women treated the same descriptors as having an emotional meaning in the various ethnocultural groups. Also, the sexes differed on individual descriptors: the descriptor *agitated* was included in the anger cluster by men, but in the anxiety cluster by women; *insensible* was in the cold/numb cluster for men, but in the depression cluster for women; *tender sensation* (in spite of the inclusion of *sensation* in the descriptor) was in the positive affect cluster for women, but in the muscle pain cluster for men. Thus, women tended to stress the emotional meaning and men the sensory meaning of these descriptors. Ethnocultural differences were also found in the meaning of words. The reason for the belief that women suffer greater clinical pain may be because when they respond to a scale that asks for a single pain rating women are rating emotional pain, and men are rating sensory pain.

Yang and coworkers[39] studied sex differences in pain ratings by Chinese patients recovering from surgery for colorectal cancer. Patients rated their pain and emotions on the 101-item MAPS questionnaire. No sex differences were found in the patient ratings on the 30 sensory and emotional clusters. As explained earlier, the MAPS contains only those descriptors that had been demonstrated to have the same meaning for men and women. These results suggest the possibility that when sex differences in pain report are found, it is because words that differ in meaning for men and women have been included in the questionnaires used.

It is known that women require less morphine for postoperative pain. The reason for this may be the greater number, sensitivity, or both, of κ receptors in women. This has been demonstrated in female rats.[90] The experimental κ-opioid drug kappa opioid has been shown to produce a strong analgesic effect in women, but not in men. There are clear gender differences in responses to drugs; whether there also is a difference in pain itself remains to be seen.

It may be concluded that many of the gender and ethnocultural differences found in clinical and laboratory pain studies are linguistic instead of (or, as well as) sensory in nature. However, the physiological response of the sexes to analgesics, and probably other medications, is not the same.

Ethnocultural Differences

Numerous studies have documented ethnic and cultural differences in pain expression, but whether these differences are caused by differences in pain sensation, or simply to differences in pain report, is difficult to establish. Zatzick and Dimsdale[91] concluded in a review that there is little evidence for ethnocultural differences in the discrimination of noxious stimuli, but that there are cultural differences in reporting pain. This view is supported by Lipton and Marbach,[92] who found interethnic differences in 35% of the items on a pain questionnaire; however, these differences were concerned only with stoicism versus expressiveness and interference with daily functioning. The pain experiences reported by African American, Italian, and Jewish patients were mostly similar; but, Irish and Puerto Ricans differed from each other and from the other three groups. The specific variables that were most influential were for African Americans, degree of medical acculturation; for Irish, degree of social assimilation; for Italians, duration of pain; and for Jewish and Puerto Rican patients, level of psychological distress. Thus, the groups were generally similar in their sensitivity to pain, but emotional and ethnocultural variables influenced their pain response.

Wolff and Langley[93] cite a number of studies that demonstrate that attitudinal factors influence the response to pain among ethnocultural groups. For example, in laboratory studies with calibrated noxious stimulation, members of minority groups who were told that they could not stand as much pain as the majority group significantly increased their tolerance of noxious stimulation. Also, if the experimenter came from a different ethnic group than the subjects, the subjects reported pain at higher intensities than if the experimenter and subject were from the same ethnic group.

Moore[94] used multidimensional scaling to demonstrate cultural differences in the use of words that describe either the pain itself (e.g., burning) or the cause of pain (e.g., heart pain, backache). He also found that Euro-Americans preferred pills or injections to stop their pain, whereas Chinese patients preferred external agents such as salves, compresses, or massage. Payer[95] has found striking differences in the particular body organ that a culture focuses on as a source of pain. Germans are much more apt to complain of heart pain (and German cardiologists are more likely to read an electrocardiogram as abnormal), the French focus on the liver (and refer to a migraine headache as a "liver crisis"), whereas the English are most concerned about the gastrointestinal tract.

People from nonwestern cultures have been thought to be more tolerant of pain because of possible physiological differences. However, using SDT methods, Clark and Bennett Clark[96] found that the ability of Nepalese Sherpas to discriminate among noxious electrical stimuli was the same as that of westerners, suggesting that their nociceptive sensory systems were the same. However, the Sherpas had a much more stoical pain report criterion, probably owing to cultural and climatic factors.

In summary, probably most of the differences in pain thresholds reported among various ethnocultural and religious groups are caused by cultural differences in the criterion for reporting pain and not to differences in the sensory experience of pain itself. It is possible, of course, that there may be some slight genetic differences, but this remains to be established. In spite of the evidence that there are few, if any ethnocultural differences, it is well-established that members of minority groups are undertreated with analgesics.

BEHAVIORAL TREATMENT OF PAIN AND SUFFERING

Analgesic medication is the primary treatment approach for most physicians, because it is effective, available, and convenient for the patient. Nevertheless, both patients and physicians are dissatisfied with long-term use of analgesics for nonmalignant pain. The pain, although attenuated, remains in the background, and unpleasant side effects such as drowsiness, impaired memory, and gastric upset usually occur. The patient must weigh the positive and negative effects of the medication. Problems like these have led to nonpharmacologic approaches to pain control, such as behavioral-cognitive restructuring, psychotherapy, carefully supervised exercise regimens, acupuncture, and TENS.

Two approaches to the behavioral treatment of pain and suffering have evolved within the past 20 years. Behavior modification focuses on changing the behavior itself, whereas cognitive restructuring focuses on altering the psychosocial attitudes, or cognitions, of patients. The two approaches are being used increasingly to treat chronic pain, especially when surgery is contraindicated, when patients are depressed because they have lost their normal social life, or when patients have become overdependent on, or addicted to, medication.

Behavioral Modification

Fordyce's[97,98] method is designed to modify maladaptive pain behaviors such as overmedication, poor sleep habits, and social isolation by making social and environmental rewards and punishments contingent on the patient's behavior. In this model, pain behavior is determined by the psychosocial context in which it occurs. Thus, it is important that the people who constitute the psychosocial environment, especially the spouse, become actively involved in the treatment program.

The behavioral approach seeks to mobilize central control mechanisms through specific reward contingencies; it seeks to control behavior by manipulating its consequences. The patient is rewarded or reinforced for beginning and maintaining initially painful physical therapy and for reducing drug intake and illness behavior. Operant conditioning techniques have proven helpful in these circumstances. Specific tasks and goals are set forth in a mutually agreed upon, signed contract. The patient is rewarded with concrete information concerning progress and by social reinforcers such as praise, appreciation, and attention. Maladaptive behaviors, such as crying and generally acting in a sick role, are ignored. This mild negative reinforcement technique is difficult for many therapists and requires considerable training.

To produce the greatest and most durable behavior changes, the pattern of reinforcements is carefully scheduled. The amount of work required for each reward varies randomly around some suitable average value. These intermittent schedules resemble the random payoff schedules used to keep gamblers in the casino, and they produce stable, high rates of the desired behavior that are resistant to extinction through nonreward. Visual and auditory displays also should be available (on an exercise apparatus, for example) to provide the necessary information to allow the patient to control his or her behavior and to reward progress. Unfortunately, in busy rehabilitation centers, patient motivation is poor and behavior-sustaining immediate reinforcing feedback is often left to chance.

Clearly, beneficial behaviors such as reduction of medication, dieting, exercise, and desisting from complaining about pain and life in general can be induced by behavioral methods. It is even possible that some patients feel as much pain as before, but if they complain less and become more active, they can live more normal, socially rewarding, less depressed lives. Thus, pain therapy can prove effective in improving the quality of life, even if, as is sometimes the case, the sensory component of pain itself has not changed. What has improved is the emotional component of pain and suffering.

Cognitive Restructuring

The second approach[99] focuses on the cognitive and emotional components of the pain experience, in addition to reinforcing medically desirable behaviors. This approach places more emphasis on cognitive strategies for coping with pain and suffering. Here the therapist must gain a thorough understanding of the patient's beliefs about the pain and illness (its causes, probable duration, and controllability).

Various cognitive strategies help ameliorate pain. *Coping strategies* refer to the diverse set of techniques that a person may use to modulate pain and suffering (attention focusing, self-instruction, behavioral relaxation). Various coping strategies used by patients who suffer chronic pain have been extensively studied with the Coping Strategies Questionnaire. Keefe and colleagues[100] studied patients with low back pain and found, for example, that higher ratings on the helplessness factor of the Coping Strategies Questionnaire were related to increased psychological distress and depression, whereas higher ratings on the diverting-attention and praying factors were related to the amount of pain reported. They suggested ways in which such knowledge may be used to teach patients more adaptive coping strategies. The extent to which patients actively attempt to cope with chronic pain and suffering depends

on their sense of control over their destiny. Crisson and Keefe[17] observed that chronic pain patients who had high *external locus of control* scores (i.e., who relied on fate) exhibited more maladaptive pain coping strategies and greater psychological distress.

Marbach and coworkers[101] found that patients with temporomandibular joint pain and dysfunction were more oriented toward external locus of control, were far more distressed, and had fewer sources of emotional support than healthy controls. Jensen and associates,[102] after an extensive review of the literature, concluded that patients who believe that they are able to control their pain, who do not catastrophize about their condition, and who believe that their disability is not severe, appear to function better. One of the goals of therapy is to lead patients to the belief that they can improve their health by taking control of health-related behaviors and by increasing social activities.

Teaching coping skills to patients can be aided by knowledge gained from studies of volunteers who experience experimental pain. Wack and Turk[103] speculate that individual differences in pain tolerance reflect different coping strategies. They used multidimensional scaling procedures to uncover latent coping strategies used by subjects experiencing cold pressor pain. Analysis revealed three dimensions. Dimension 1, *sensation focusing*, encompassed sensation avoidance at one pole ("I sang 'Yellow Submarine'") and sensation acknowledgment at the other ("I viewed the cold sensations as being separate from the pain"). Dimension 2, *coping relevance*, ranged from directed coping ("I did breathing exercises") to undirected activity "(I examined the equipment in the room"). Dimension 3, *behavioral/cognitive*, distinguished between behavioral ("I bit my fingers") and fantasy strategies ("I imagined sitting on the beach in Hawaii").

Turk and coworkers[104] attempted to discover dimensions that might underlie various pain behaviors. Subjects sorted 20 descriptors of pain behavior into as many different groups of similar items as they wished. Multidimensional scaling yielded two dimensions. The first dimension, with the behaviors clenching teeth and facial grimacing at one pole and taking analgesic medication and lying down frequently at the other, could be interpreted as an *Active–Passive* or *Do something—Wait it out* dimension. The second dimension, with limping and moving in a guarded fashion at one pole and irritability and "Why me?" at the other, was interpreted as a *behavioral/affective* dimension. Knowledge of which dimension is most salient for a particular patient, which can be determined by multidimensional scaling procedures, should prove useful therapeutically. These studies demonstrate that patients' attempts to control pain differ considerably. Clearly, the therapist must understand where a patient stands on each of these various dimensions and tailor the treatment plan accordingly.

One can argue that behavioral and cognitive treatment approaches are not as antithetical as their proponents so often maintain. The behavioral approach holds that if the clinician changes the patient's behavior, the patient's thoughts and attitudes are restructured. The cognitive approach holds that if the clinician changes the patient's way of thinking about the illness, the patient's behavior will change. In practice, both cognitively and behaviorally induced changes can occur in concert, each influencing the other.

PATIENTS' BELIEFS AND PAIN TREATMENT

Placebo Effect

Suggestion, direct or indirect, can exert powerful effects. It is not always clear how much of the effect is caused by a change in pain report to please the caregiver and how much to a change in the pain sensation itself. Clark and Yang[43] found that a placebo described and accepted as a powerful analgesic markedly raised the pain threshold (i.e., it apparently decreased the sensitivity to noxious thermal stimulation). Application of SDT to the same data demonstrated that this decrease in the report of pain was caused by a raised pain report criterion, B, and not by a decrease in thermal discrimination, $P(A)$. It was concluded that the analgesia typically believed to be produced by a placebo in a laboratory pain situation was entirely a psychological response to the social demand characteristics of the experimental situation and was not caused by decreased neurosensory activity, which would be expected to reduce discrimination. The large number of adverse side effects induced by the placebo in healthy volunteers was remarkable. The following symptoms were reported (prevalence of each symptom in parentheses): numbness (50%), slight nausea (14%), headache (41%), light-headedness or euphoria (32%), nervousness (32%), tingling sensations (36%), and inability to concentrate (18%).

In another study using SDT,[43] a subtle hint (no pill was given) that previous thermal stimulation had *anesthetized* the skin caused subjects to set a high, stoical pain report criterion. During a second session, a hint that the previous stimulation had *sensitized* the skin caused subjects to set a liberal (low) pain report criterion (more pain reports). Schweiger and Parducci[105]

demonstrated that even without any aversive stimulation, two-thirds of a group of college students reported mild headaches when told that a (nonexistent) electric current was passing through their heads. Clearly, a placebo can produce dramatic psychological and physiological effects.

The placebo effect may include physiological as well as subjective changes. Inert substances, properly packaged, often have startling effects. Beecher[106] reviewed studies of patients who suffered severe pain and found that approximately two-thirds obtained relief with 10 mg of oral morphine. However, one-third of this group received satisfactory relief from placebos. The placebo effect does not require the administration of an inert pill; it is a component of any therapeutic intervention and derives from the beliefs and expectations of physician and patient. Faith in the success of the intervention plays a significant role and explains why novel treatments (often later demonstrated to have no specific physiological effect) are successful initially but fail later. In contrast, the placebo effect has been hailed as "the one constant in the long history of medical practice." Certainly, many of the substances administered over the centuries have now been proven to have no specific therapeutic effect.

Although placebo responses involve a wide variety of psychological factors, such as the personalities of the physician and the patient, their motivations, expectations, and anxieties, no clear fixed personality type appears to characterize the placebo respondent. The mechanism of the placebo response is unclear, but reduced anxiety and improved willingness to cope with difficult personal situations may be important. Also, placebo responses are more prevalent in clinical than in experimental pain situations, suggesting the importance of motivational and affective factors in the patient–therapist interaction. For this interaction to occur, a common set of beliefs about the optimal therapeutic approach must be shared.

A reaction as powerful as a placebo response deserves more careful study than it has received. It is a mistake to dismiss the placebo effect as something in the patient's imagination. If the patient is made to feel more optimistic, and as a result is more active, undertakes exercise, improves diet, and makes other positive changes, there is nothing mysterious about an improvement in health. Much effort has been devoted to removing this *artifact*, which interferes with *real effects* of a treatment regimen. Perhaps the trend should be reversed and a greater effort made to learn more about its mode of action. The endorphins[76] and the response of the immune system to stress have also been implicated in the placebo response.

There are rational physical explanations for the mystery of the placebo effect.

COMPLEMENTARY THERAPIES

The strength of the placebo effect, which can produce general physiological changes as a result of psychological changes, makes it difficult to evaluate the effectiveness of treatments such as TENS and acupuncture. In some instances these procedures are clearly beneficial, at least for a while, but the question remains: Are these improvements caused by a specific analgesic effect or by a general improvement in psychological well-being (see Chapter 34)?

Acupuncture

Acupuncture is a controversial treatment that exemplifies the problems of evaluating the effectiveness of certain therapies. Acupuncture treatment for pain has always been a subject of much controversy. Reports of its success in the clinic (where careful scientific controls are difficult to implement) have not always been matched in the laboratory. Clark and Yang[107] found that acupuncture delivered to traditional sites did, indeed, decrease the report of pain in response to thermal stimulation, but only in the acupunctured arm. No reduction of pain was reported in the contralateral arm. This result contradicted traditional Chinese medical theory, which holds that stimulation of the Ho-Ku point for 20 minutes should have rendered the entire body analgesic. Thus, the subjects' expectation that only the acupunctured arm would become analgesic appears to have played a large role in what they reported. (The subjects did not know traditional Chinese medical theory about the Ho-Ku point.) Furthermore, SDT analysis of the data revealed only an increase in the pain report criterion, B; this shift followed the expectations of the subject. The failure to find any change in discrimination, $P(A)$, such as would have been produced by an analgesic or by a peripheral nerve block, was a decisive finding. Contrary to reports from the People's Republic of China, the subjects in this study said they certainly would not undergo surgery with acupuncture as the sole analgesic. This failure to find acupunctural analgesia has been confirmed by Li and colleagues,[108] who found that hypnosis but not acupuncture produced analgesia to noxious electrical stimulation. They also found no difference between results of accepted-site and placebo (off-site) acupuncture.

What is to be made of reports of surgery performed with acupuncture that once filled western newspapers?

First, Chinese patients are screened for positive responses to acupuncture; this leaves only a small portion of the population (fewer than 15%) who are acceptable candidates for surgery under acupuncture analgesia. Second, the acupuncture procedure is often supplemented with analgesic substances such as intravenous procaine. Third, even in the People's Republic of China, acupuncture now is seldom used for surgery; it is, however, used with apparent success for chronic pain. These observations are based on two trips made by the author in the People's Republic of China.

Although the effectiveness of acupuncture in surgery may be questioned, it has proven successful in the treatment of chronic pain. The explanation for this success confirms once again the far-reaching importance of the psychological component of pain. A study of the effect of acupuncture on patients suffering back and neck pain has proven more rewarding than the search for acupuncture anesthesia.[109] This study emphasizes the importance of carefully controlled experiments and detailed statistical analyses. Western patients suffering cervical or low back pain were randomly assigned to one of three study groups: *on-site* acupuncture (needles placed at recognized acupuncture points); *off-site* or placebo acupuncture (needles inserted superficially 1 cm from the correct site, which according to traditional Chinese medicine should not produce analgesia); and conventional western physiotherapy. After 2 weeks' treatment by one of these three methods, the patients received a blind evaluation from a rheumatologist. Both acupuncture groups were significantly improved compared with the group that received western physiotherapy, but there was no difference between the on-site and off-site groups. Patients in the failed physiotherapy group also improved when they subsequently received acupuncture treatment. The results suggest that acupuncture works, but not in the traditional way that postulates an anatomic basis for a specific analgesic effect. Instead, the improvement in both acupuncture groups probably was caused by psychological factors. These patients were positively disposed toward acupuncture and were dissatisfied with western medicine, which had previously failed them.

This study demonstrated that patients who receive the treatment they want and believe in profit from it. This is probably true whether the treatment be drugs, acupuncture, or psychotherapy. In addition, acupuncture is mildly painful, and the well-known mild analgesic effects produced by counterirritant stimulation and stress-induced analgesia (described earlier) may account for some of the effect. Another interesting finding was that the best predictor of outcome was not the type of treatment but the patient's mental status; patients who before treatment were rated as depressed by a psychiatrist did not improve, regardless of which treatment they received.

ASSESSING THE RELATIVE PHYSIOLOGICAL AND PSYCHOLOGICAL CONTRIBUTIONS TO TREATMENT SUCCESS

The placebo effect is real and so are the effects of medication. Psychotherapy works and can alter physiological function; why should not a placebo, which may be regarded as a type of psychotherapy?

The next step is to examine the relative contributions of each to the therapeutic outcome. Clark[110] has suggested a way by which this could be accomplished by asking patients which treatment they believed they had received. The table entries (proportion of successfully treated patients) in this contingency table (Table 36-1) allow the relative strength of the physiological and psychological contributions to successful outcome to be evaluated. The accepted treatment could be accepted-site acupuncture, drugs, and so forth. The comparison or placebo treatment could be off-site acupuncture, placebo, and so forth. After the study is completed, the patient is asked to rate on a scale how confident he or she was that the accepted treatment or the placebo treatment had been administered. The cells A, B, C, and D represent the proportion of patients reaching a defined level of improvement. Comparison among the cells in this contingency table would permit the evaluation of the relative strengths of the medical and psychological contributions to successful outcome.

Congruence of Treatment and Patients' Beliefs

The acupuncture study[109] illustrates the importance of understanding and sharing the patient's pain beliefs. Patients did best when they received the treatment they wanted. Williams and Thorn[16] point out that when the patient's beliefs about the source and proper treatment of the pain are discordant with those of the health caregiver, the results are poor because the patient is not emotionally engaged and may not comply with the treatment plan, or may unconsciously sabotage it.

Many studies demonstrate that the patient's emotional state and how it is treated psychologically are important determinants of outcome, even for what are regarded as purely physical diseases. For example,

TABLE 36-1

Successful Outcome Contingent on Type of Treatment and Patient's Belief

	Patient's Belief in Type of Treatment Received	
	Real Treatment	Comparison Treatment
Accepted treatment	A	B
Comparison or placebo treatment	C	D

The number or proportion of patients reaching a predetermined criterion of successful outcome is entered into each of the cells, A, B, C, D of the Contingency Table (see text).
Source: Adapted with permission from WC Clark. Pin and pang: research methodology for acupuncture and other "alternative medicine" therapies. A commentary on: two decades after ping-pong diplomacy. Is there a role for acupuncture in American pain medicine by M Belgrade. Am Pain Soc J 1994;3:84–88.

elderly patients who received psychiatric consultation during recovery from hip fractures were discharged 2 days sooner than a control group.[111] In another study of patients undergoing bone marrow transplants for leukemia, a larger proportion of depressed patients died within 1 year of the transplant. These findings are dramatic and may even seem mysterious, but, as in the case of the placebo effect, there are rational explanations. Compliance with the treatment regimen may be poorer in depressed patients, or stress and depression may interfere with the function of the immune system.[112] Dworkin[113] presents an excellent review of the possible psychological origins of chronic pain and it should be consulted on many of the points raised here.

Hypnosis

Hypnosis, and even simple suggestion, clearly alter pain-related behavior in a significant proportion of patients: Reports of pain decrease, sympathetic activity is reduced, and requests for analgesics decline. Such phenomena pose serious problems for the concept that pain is a simple function of the amount and kind of sensory input. Indeed, they pose problems for those who view pain thoughtfully in any way at all. The modern approach to the problem investigates what hypnotic and other procedures are necessary, sufficient, and important for producing effective analgesia. An excellent review of the scientific approaches to hypnosis in the relief of pain may be found in Hilgard and Hilgard[114] and Hart and Alden.[115]

Investigators' ideas of the essential nature of hypnosis differ greatly.[116] Barber[117] takes the view that the hypnotic trance may be extraneous and that the important factor is the suggestion of pain relief in a close, interpersonal setting, which produces a stoical response set (i.e., a marked increase in the pain report criterion, as defined by SDT). In this view, hypnotic phenomena can be observed in the performance of unhypnotized subjects who are given similar, but forceful, task-motivating instructions.

Orne[118] takes a more moderate view. He readily admits the importance of *social demand characteristics* (he originated the term), but he argues that something else is operating as well. He has identified objective differences in the behavior of hypnotized subjects and those who are simulating the hypnotic state. Only hypnotized subjects tolerate perceptual inconsistencies (e.g., the subject is not concerned when a person who has been hypnotically imaged to be in one part of the room simultaneously appears in the flesh elsewhere). Hypnotized subjects report both the image and the real person, but the simulator reports only one. Hypnotized subjects differ from unhypnotized subjects in other ways. They appear to lack internal, spontaneous motivation; they are relatively immobile; and they have a narrow focus of attention. For an explicit discussion of simulation controls, see O'Connell and colleagues.[119]

Much of the controversy surrounding hypnotic analgesia, including the failure of investigators to replicate each others' work, arises from the fact that subjects differ in their susceptibility to hypnosis, and hypnotists vary in their ability to induce trance. Although standardized scales for measuring susceptibility and depth of trance exist, they are not always used. Finally, laboratories and workers may differ in subtle but important ways with respect to expectations, implicit definitions of appropriate performance, and careful engineering of the social context of the experiment to produce maximum effects.

Many well-documented studies demonstrate that hypnotic analgesia relieves clinical pain, as indicated by changes in verbal report, motor activity, and physiological indicators.[118] Definitive studies of hypnotically induced relief of experimental pain are much rarer. A study by McGlashan and colleagues[120] is worth examining in detail, because it demonstrates remarkable attention to experimental control and scientific objectivity. The response to ischemic tourniquet pain was studied in two groups of subjects: Those who were rated highly susceptible to hypnosis by clinical tests and objective ratings, and those who were extremely resistant. The

two groups of subjects were studied under analgesic hypnosis and placebo conditions. Hypnosis-resistant subjects' pain reports decreased equally under analgesic hypnosis and placebo hypnosis conditions, whereas hypnosis-susceptible subjects' pain reports decreased more under analgesic hypnosis than under the placebo condition. The authors concluded that hypnotic analgesia had two components. One, found in insusceptible subjects, was essentially a placebo response to the demand characteristics of the situation, which caused a shift in the pain report criterion. The other component of the decrease in pain report, which was evidenced in subjects who were susceptible to hypnosis and entered a deep trance, may be regarded as a true analgesic effect. Described from the viewpoint of SDT, the susceptible hypnotic subjects behaved as though they had received morphine: decreased discrimination, $P(A)$, and increased pain response criterion, B. The resistant subjects showed only a criterion increase, as reported in the placebo study by Clark.[42] Hilgard and Hilgard[114] note that, whereas indicators of pain that are under voluntary control (verbal report, grimacing, withdrawal, catching breath) are consistently reduced by hypnosis, involuntary responses (heart rate, blood pressure) usually remain unaffected. Some have argued that the persistence of the involuntary responses means that hypnotic analgesia has not been induced, but this position is invalid, because it implies that physiological responses define pain and verbal reports do not. There is no evidence to support this opinion. The decrease in voluntary pain indicators is sufficient to demonstrate a state of hypnotically induced analgesia in susceptible patients.

Although brain imaging has shown that hypnosis modifies activity in the anterior cingulate region, the mechanisms that produce this effect are unknown. Perhaps relabeling of sensation (a normal coping skill that may be amplified by hypnosis) contributes. Changes in states of consciousness are frequently reported in the absence of formal hypnosis, particularly during strong emotional stress. Effective autosuggestion and informal, partial autohypnosis may be much more frequent than we realize. Occasionally, sophisticated observers report dramatic instances of deliberately induced analgesia without hypnosis in any formal sense. For example, Reis[121] reported undergoing major surgery with neither formally induced hypnosis nor chemical anesthesia. Reasoning that she could manage the problem of operative pain by autosuggestion, she did so, requiring no physical restraints on the operating table and reporting only slight cutaneous sensations, but no pain or discomfort.

As a closing comment, we present an interesting case study by Kaplan[122] that dramatizes the interpretive dilemma of hypnotic analgesia. A highly trained subject was placed in a deep trance and given two suggestions: (1) that his left arm was analgesic and insensitive and (2) that his right hand would perform automatic writing continuously throughout the experiment. The analgesic left arm was pricked four times with a hypodermic needle. During the reception of this stimulus, the subject's right hand wrote, "Ouch, damn it, you're hurting me." A few minutes later, the subject turned to the experimenter and asked when he was going to begin the experiment, apparently unaware that he had already received the painful stimuli. Kaplan interpreted these findings to indicate that hypnotic suggestions of analgesia produce artificial repression and denial of pain but that pain is experienced "at some level." The brain imaging study by Rainville and associates,[65] who found that hypnosis inhibited the response at the anterior cingulate but not at the primary sensory cortex, suggests that something indeed happened at some level.

FUTURE DIRECTIONS

In spite of the truly amazing progress of the past 10 years in our understanding of pain and suffering, much remains to be done. The wide individual differences revealed by brain imaging studies in many of the excitatory and inhibitory structures in the brain that mediate pain and emotion remain to be explained. Much more remains to be learned about neurotransmitters and plasticity in the nervous system, including factors that influence the expression of neurotransmitter receptors. More detailed knowledge of difficult-to-find, minor neural pathways mediating pain may lead to new neurosurgical approaches for pain control. The many mechanisms through which pain affects the psychoneuroimmune system need to be elucidated. There is a need for analgesics without harmful side effects such as drowsiness, decreased motivation, and memory impairment. There is a need for improved evaluation of the sensory, emotional, and other aspects of the patient's pain; a number of approaches, such as verbal report, autonomic and musculoskeletal responses, sensory-evoked potentials, brain imaging, and genetic profiling, need further study. Finally, the management of chronic pain and suffering could be improved by developing procedures that are more successful at integrating behavioral and pharmacologic treatment approaches.

Acknowledgments
I wish to thank Mieko Hobara, Germaine Griswold, John Kuhl, and Dr. Susanne Bennett Clark for their enthusiastic assistance with the preparation of this manuscript. This chapter was supported in part by grants from the National Institute of Dental and Craniofacial Research (DE-12725) and The Nathanial Wharton Fund for Research and Education in Brain, Body, and Behavior.

REFERENCES

1. Cassel E. The Nature of Suffering and the Goals of Medicine. New York: Oxford University Press, 1991.
2. Merskey H, Bogduk N (eds). Classification of Chronic Pain (2nd ed). Seattle, WA: IASP Press, 1994.
3. Kanner R (ed). Pain Management Secrets. Philadelphia: Hanley & Belfus, 1997.
4. Briones A, Chokhavatia S, Bennett-Clark S, Clark WC. Is flexible sigmoidoscopy painful? Am J Gastroenterol 1999;94:2749.
5. Magee DM. Orthopaedic Physical Assessment (2nd ed). Philadelphia: WB Saunders, 1992.
6. Simmonds MJ, Kumar S. Health care ergonomics. Part I: The fundamental skill of palpation: a review and critique. Int J Ind Ergonomics 1993;11:135–143.
7. Simmonds MJ, Kumar S. Health care ergonomics. Part II: Location of body structures by palpation: a reliability study. Int J Ind Ergonomics 1993; 11:145–151.
8. Keefe FJ, Block AR. Development of an observation method for assessing pain behavior in chronic low back pain patients. Behav Ther 1982;13:363–375.
9. Roland M, Morris R. A study of the natural history of back pain. Part I: Development of a reliable and sensitive measure of disability in low-back pain. Spine 1983;8:141–144.
10. Stratford PW, Gill C, Westaway M, et al. Assessing disability and change on individual patients: a report of a patient specific measure. Physiother Can 1995;47:258–263.
11. Pope MH. A Critical Evaluation of Functional Muscle Testing. In JN Weinstein (ed), Clinical Efficacy and Outcome in the Diagnosis and Treatment of Low Back Pain. New York: Raven, 1992;101–113.
12. Bandura A. Self-efficacy: towards a unifying theory of behavioral change. Psychol Rev 1977;84:191–215.
13. Lorig K, Chastain RL, Ung E, et al. Development and evaluation of a scale to measure perceived self-efficacy in people with arthritis. Arthritis Rheum 1989;32:37–44.
14. Keefe FJ, Caldwell DS, Baucom D, et al. Spouse-assisted coping skills training in the measurement of osteoarthritis knee pain. Arthritis Care Res 1996;9:279–291.
15. Waddell G, Newton M, Henderson I, et al. A fear-avoidance belief questionnaire (FABQ) and the role of fear avoidance in chronic low back pain and disability. Pain 1993;52:157–168.
16. Williams DA, Thorn BE. An empirical assessment of pain beliefs. Pain 1989; 36:351–358.
17. Crisson JE, Keefe FJ. The relationship

of locus of control to pain coping strategies and psychological distress in chronic pain patients. Pain 1988; 35:147–154.

18. Melzack R. The Gate Control Theory 25 Years Later: New Perspectives in Phantom Limb Pain. In MR Bond, JE Charlton, CJ Woolf (eds), Proceedings of the Sixth World Congress on Pain. Amsterdam: Elsevier, 1991;9–21.

19. Keefe FJ, Caldwell DS. Cognitive behavioral control of arthritis pain. Med Clin North Am 1997;81:277–290.

20. Salovey P, Smith AF, Turk DC, et al. The accuracy of memory for pain: not so bad most of the time. Am Pain Soc J 1993;2:184–191.

21. Kent G. Memory of dental pain. Pain 1985;21:187–194.

22. Clark WC, Bennett-Clark S. Remembrance of pain past? A commentary on "The accuracy of memory for pain: not so bad most of the time" by Salovey P, et al. Am Pain Soc J 1993;2:195–200.

23. Clark WC, Janal MN, Carroll JD. Multidimensional Pain Requires Multidimensional Scaling. In JD Loeser, CR Chapman (eds), Issues in Pain Measurement. New York: Raven, 1989; 285–325.

24. Melzack R. The Puzzle of Pain. New York: Basic Books, 1973.

25. Melzack R, Casey KL. Sensory, Motivational and Central Control Determinants of Pain: A New Conceptual Model. In D Kenshalo (ed), The Skin Senses. Springfield, IL: Thomas, 1968; 423–435.

26. Loeser JD. Perspectives on Pain. In Proceedings of the First World Conference on Clinical Pharmacology and Therapeutics. London: Macmillan, 1980;313–316.

27. Fordyce WE. Pain and suffering: a reappraisal. Am Psychol 1988;43:276–283.

28. Fernandez E, Turk DC. Sensory and affective components of pain: separation and synthesis. Psychol Bull 1992; 112:205–217.

29. Clark WC, Janal MH, Hoben E, Carroll JD. How distinct are the sensory, emotional and motivational dimensions of pain? Somatosens Motor Res 2001.

30. Janal MN. Concerning the homology of painful experiences and pain descriptors: a multidimensional scaling analysis. Pain 1995;64:373–378.

31. Williams RC. Toward a set of reliable and valid measures for chronic pain assessment and outcome research. Pain 1988;35:239–251.

32. Turk DC, Melzak R (eds). Handbook of Pain Assessment. New York: Guilford, 1992.

33. Chapman CR, Loeser JD (eds). Advances in Pain Research and Therapy, Vol 12: Issues in Pain Measurement. New York: Raven, 1989.

34. Melzack R (ed). Pain Measurement and Assessment. New York: Raven, 1983.

35. Bromm B (ed). Pain Measurement in Man: Neurophysiological Correlates of Pain. Amsterdam: Elsevier, 1984.

36. Bromm B, Desmedt JE (eds). Pain and the Brain: From Nociception to Sensation. New York: Raven, 1995.

37. Derogatis LR, Melisaratos N. The brief symptom inventory: an introductory report. Psychol Med 1983;13: 595–605.

38. Clark WC, Fletcher JD, Janal MN, Caroll JD. Hierarchical Clustering of 270 Pain/Emotion Descriptors: Toward a Revision of the McGill Pain Questionnaire. In B Bromm, J Desmedt (eds), Pain and the Brain: From Nociception to Sensation. New York: Raven, 1995;319–330.

39. Yang JC, Clark WC, Tsui SL, et al. Pre-operative multidimensional affect and pain survey (MAPS), scores predict post-colectomy analgesia requirement. Clin J Pain 2000;10.

40. Orne MT. On the social psychology of the psychological experiment. Am Psychol 1962;17:776–783.

41. Clark WC. Pain, Emotion, and Drug Induced Subjective States: Analysis by Multidimensional Scaling. In G Adelman, B Smith (eds), Encyclopedia of Neuroscience (2nd ed). Amsterdam: Elsevier, 1999.

42. Clark WC. The Psyche in the Psychophysics in Pain: An Introduction to Sensory Decision Theory. In J Boivie, P Hansson, U Linblom (eds), Touch, Temperature, and Pain in Health and Disease: Mechanisms and Assessment. Vol 3: Progress in Pain Research and Management. Seattle, WA: International Association for the Study of Pain Press, 1994.

43. Clark WC, Yang JC. Applications of Sensory Decision Theory to Problems in Laboratory and Clinical Pain. In R Melzack (ed), Pain Measurement and Assessment. New York: Raven, 1983; 15–25.

44. Yang JC, Clark WC, Ng SH, et al. Analgesic action and pharmacokinetics of morphine and diazepam in man: an evaluation by sensory decision theory. Anesthesiology 1979;51:495–502.

45. Gybels J, Handwerker HO, Van Hees J. A comparison between the discharges of

human nociceptive nerve fibers and the subject's ratings of his sensations. J Physiol 1979;292:193–206.

46. Gracely RH, McGrath PA, Dubner RE. Validity and sensitivity of ratio scales of sensory and affective verbal pain descriptors: manipulation of affect by diazepam. Pain 1978;5:19–29.

47. Gracely RH, McGrath PA, Dubner R. Narcotic analgesia: fentanyl reduces the intensity but not the unpleasantness of painful tooth pulp sensations. Science 1979;203:1261–1263.

48. Clark WC, Ferrer-Brechner T, Janal MN, et al. The dimensions of pain: a multidimensional scaling comparison of cancer patients and healthy volunteers. Pain 1989;37:23–32.

49. Basbaum AI, Jessell TM. The Perception of Pain. In ER Kandel, HS James, MJ Thomas (eds), Principles of Neural Science (4th ed). New York: McGraw-Hill, 2000;472–491.

50. Willis WD Jr. The Pain System: The Neural Basis of Nociceptive Transmission in the Mammalian Nervous System. Basel: Kager, 1985.

51. Boivie J, Johansson I. Central post-stroke pain: a study of the mechanism through analyses of the sensory abnormalities. Pain 1989;37:173–185.

52. McGowan DJL, Janal MN, Clark WC, et al. Central post-stroke pain and Wallenberg's lateral medullary infarction: the frequency, character and determinants in 63 patients. Neurology 1997;122:120–125.

53. Craig AD. A new version of thalamic disinhibition hypothesis of central pain. Pain Forum 1998;7:1–14.

54. Craig AD, Bushnell MC. The thermal grill illusion: unmasking the burn of cold pain. Science 1994;265:252–255.

55. Tasker R. Pain Resulting from Central Nervous System Pathology (Central Pain). In JJ Bonica (eds), The Management of Pain (2nd ed). Philadelphia: Lea & Febiger, 1990;264–280.

56. Nashold BS. Dorsal column stimulation for the control of pain: a three-year follow-up. Surg Neurol 1975;4:146–147.

57. Lehman TR, Russell DW, Spratt KF, et al. Efficacy of electroacupuncture and TENS in the rehabilitation of chronic low back pain patients. Pain 1986;26:277–290.

58. Kelly DD (ed). Stress-Induced Analgesia. New York: New York Academy of Science, 1986;467.

59. Goolkasian P. Cyclic changes in pain perception: an ROC analysis. Percept Psychophys 1980;27:299–504.

60. Janal MN, Glusman M, Kuhl JP, Clark WC. Are runners stoical? An examination of pain sensitivity in habitual runners and normally active controls. Pain 1994;58:109–116.

61. Wiertelak EP, Maier SE Watkins LR. Cholecystokinin antianalgesia: safety cues abolish morphine analgesia. Science 1992;256:830–833.

62. Yang JC, Richlin D, Brand L, et al. Thermal sensory decision theory indices and pain threshold in chronic pain patients and healthy volunteers. Psychosom Med 1985;47:461–468.

63. Whipple B, Komisaruk BR. Elevation of pain threshold by vaginal stimulation in women. Pain 1985;21:357–367.

64. Corkin S, Twitchell TE, Sullivan EV. Safety and Efficacy of Cingulotomy for Pain and Psychiatric Disorder. In E Hitchcock (ed), Alteration in Brain Function. Amsterdam: Elsevier, 1979.

65. Rainville P, Duncan GH, Price DD, et al. Pain affect encoded in human anterior cingulate but not somatosensory cortex. Science 1997;277:968–971.

66. Schott GD. From thalamic syndrome to central post-stroke pain. J Neurol Neurosurg Psychiatry 1995;61:560–564.

67. Beecher HK. Measurement of Subjective Responses. New York: Oxford University Press, 1952.

68. Cervero F. Physiology and Physiopathology of Visceral Pain. In M Mitchell (ed), Pain 1999: An Updated Review. Seattle, WA: International Association for the Study of Pain Press, 1999; 39–47.

69. Gebhart GF, Randich A. Vagal modulation of nociception. Am Pain Soc J 1992;1:26–32.

70. Cervero F, Morrison JFB. Visceral sensation. Prog Brain Res 1986;67:1–324.

71. Berkley KJ. On the significance of viscerosomatic convergence. Am Pain Soc J 1993;2:239–247.

72. Glusman M, Clark WC, Coromilas J, et al. Pain sensitivity in silent myocardial ischemia. Pain 1996;64:477–483.

73. Kandel ER, Schwartz JH, Jessell TM (eds). Principles of Neural Science (4th ed). San Francisco: McGraw-Hill, 2000.

74. Price DD. Psychological and Neural Mechanisms of Pain. New York: Raven, 1988.

75. Kinnman E, Aldskogius H, Wiesenfeld-Hallin Z, et al. Expansion of Sensory Enervation after Peripheral Nerve Injury. In MR Bond, JE Charlton, CJ Woolf (eds), Proceedings of the Sixth World Congress on Pain. Amsterdam: Elsevier, 1991;277–282.

76. Dubner R. Neuronal Plasticity and Pain Following Peripheral Tissue Inflammation or Nerve Injury. In MR Bond, JE Charlton, CJ Woolf (eds), Proceedings of the Sixth World Congress on Pain. Amsterdam: Elsevier, 1991;263–276.

77. Sternberg EM. Neuroendocrine factors in susceptibility to inflammatory disease: focus on the hypothalamic-pituitary-adrenal axis. Horm Res 1995; 43:159–161.

78. Moldofsky H. Nonrestorative sleep and symptoms after febrile illness in patients with fibrositis and chronic fatigue syndromes. J Rheumatol 1989; 16(Suppl 19):150–153.

79. Crofford LJ, Pillemer SR, Kalogeras KT, et al. Hypothalamic-pituitary-adrenal axis perturbations in patients with fibromyalgia. Arthritis Rheum 1994;37(11):1583–1592.

80. Zhou HH, Sheller JR, Nu H, et al. Pharmacodynamics and drug action: ethnic differences in response to morphine. Clin Pharmacol Ther 1993;54(5):507–513.

81. Mogil JS, Willson SG, Bon K, et al. Heritability of nociception. II. "Types" of nociception revealed by genetic correlation analysis. Pain 1999;80:82–83.

82. Portenoy RK. Chronic opioid therapy for nonmalignant pain: from models to practice. Am Pain Soc J 1992;1:285–288.

83. Malmberg AB, Yaksh TL. Hyperalgesia mediated by spinal glutamate or substance P receptor blocked by spinal cyclooxygenase inhibition. Science 1992;257:1276–1279.

84. Onghena P, Van Houdenhove B. Antidepressant-induced analgesia in chronic non-malignant pain: a meta-analysis of 39 placebo-controlled studies. Pain 1992;49(2):205–219.

85. Burrows GD, Elton D, Stanley GV (eds). Handbook of Chronic Pain Management. Amsterdam: Elsevier, 1987.

86. Clark WC. Quantitative Models for the Assessment of Clinical Pain: Individual Differences Scaling and Sensory Decision Theory. In GD Burrows, D Elton, GV Stanley (eds), Handbook of Chronic Pain Management. Amsterdam: Elsevier, 1987;57–67.

87. Berkley KJ. Sex differences in pain. Behav Brain Sci 1997;20:371–380.

88. Unruh AM. Gender variation in clinical pain experience. Pain 1996;65:123–164.

89. Bendelow G. Pain perceptions, emotions, and gender. Soc Health Illness 1993;15:273–294.

90. Tershner SA, Mitchell JM, Fields HL. Brainstem pain modulating circuitry is sexually dimorphic with respect to mu and kappa opioid receptor function. Pain 2000;85:153–160.

91. Zatzick DF, Dimsdale JE. Cultural variations in the response to painful stimuli. Psychosom Med 1990;52:544–557.

92. Lipton JA, Marbach JJ. Ethnicity and the pain experience. Soc Sci Med 1984;19:1279–1298.

93. Wolff BB, Langley S. Cultural factors and the response to pain: a review. Am Anthropol 1968;70:494–501.

94. Moore R. Ethnographic assessment of pain coping perceptions. Psychosom Med 1990;52:171–181.

95. Payer L. Medicine and Culture. New York: Holt, 1988.

96. Clark WC, Bennett SC. Pain responses in Nepalese porters. Science 1980;209:440–442.

97. Fordyce WE. Behavioral Methods for Chronic Pain and Illness. St Louis: Mosby, 1976.

98. Fordyce WE. The behavioral management of chronic pain: a response to critics. Pain 1985;22:113–125.

99. Turk DC, Meichenbaum D, Genest M. Pain and Behavioral Medicine: A Cognitive-Behavioral Perspective. New York: Guilford, 1983.

100. Keefe FJ, Crisson J, Urban BJ, et al. Analyzing chronic low back pain: the relative contribution of pain coping strategies. Pain 1990;40:293–301.

101. Marbach JJ, Lennon MC, Dohrenwend BP. Candidate risk factors for temporomandibular pain and dysfunction syndrome: psychosocial, health behavior, physical illness and injury. Pain 1988;34:139–151.

102. Jensen MP, Turner JA, Romano JM, et al. Coping with chronic pain: a critical review of the literature. Pain 1991;47:249–283.

103. Wack JT, Turk DC. Latent structure of strategies used to cope with nociceptive stimulation. Health Psychol 1984;3:27–43.

104. Turk DC, Wack JT, Kerns RD. An empirical examination of the "pain-behavior" construct. J Behav Med 1985;8:119–130.

105. Schweiger A, Parducci A. Nocebo: the psychologic induction of pain. Pavlov J Bio Sci 1981;16:140–143.

106. Beecher HK. The powerful placebo. JAMA 1955;159:1602–1606.

107. Clark WC, Yang JC. Acupunctural analgesia? Evaluation by signal detection theory. Science 1974;184:1096–1098.

108. Li CL, Ahlberg D, Lansdell H, et al. Acupuncture and hypnosis: effects on

induced pain. Exp Neurol 1975;49:272–280.

109. Lewin H, Yue SJ, Clark WC. Basic concepts in signal detection theory and its clinical application for the evaluation of the pain threshold. Acupunct Electrother Res 1978;3:319–322.

110. Clark WC. Pin and Pang: research methodology for acupuncture and other "alternative medicine" therapies. A commentary on: "Two decades after ping-pong diplomacy. Is there a role for acupuncture in American pain medicine?" by Belgrade M. Am Pain Soc J 1994;3:84–88.

111. Strain JJ, Lyons JS, Hammer JS, et al. Cost offset from a psychiatric consultation-liaison intervention with elderly hip fracture patients. Am J Psychiatry 1991;148:1044–1049.

112. Adler R, Felten DL, Cohen N (eds). Psychoneuroimmunology (2nd ed). New York: Academic, 1991.

113. Dworkin RH. What do we really know about the psychological origins of chronic pain? Am Pain Soc Bull 1991;1:7–11.

114. Hilgard ER, Hilgard JR. Hypnosis in the Relief of Pain. Los Altos, CA: W Kauffman, 1975.

115. Hart BB, Alden PA. Hypnotic Techniques in the Control of Pain. In HB Gibson (ed), Psychology, Pain and Anesthesia. London: Chapman and Hall, 1993;121–145.

116. Barber TX. The effects of hypnosis on pain: a critical review of experimental and clinical findings. Psychosom Med 1963;25:303–333.

117. Barber J. Hypnosis and Suggestion in the Treatment of Pain. New York: WW Norton, 1996.

118. Orne MT. The nature of hypnosis: artifact and essence. J Abnorm Psychol 1959;58:277–299.

119. O'Connell DN, Shor RE, Orne MT. Hypnotic age regression: an empirical and methodological analysis. J Abnorm Psychol 1970;(Pt 2):1–32.

120. McGlashan TH, Evans FJ, Orne MT. The nature of hypnotic analgesia and placebo responses to experimental pain. Psychosom Med 1969;31:227–246.

121. Reis M. Subjective reactions of a patient having surgery without chemical anesthesia. Am J Clin Hypn 1966;9:122–124.

122. Kaplan EA. Hypnosis and pain. Arch Gen Psychiatry 1960;2:567–568.

37

Adaptation, Learning, and Motivation

EDWARD M. PHILLIPS AND JULIE M. BRODY

One of the distinguishing characteristics of rehabilitation is the degree to which individuals are expected to participate actively in their own care. Patients should be involved in setting appropriate goals. They acquire new skills and repeat specific movements through a process of motor learning. Simultaneously, these individuals adapt to their impairment or disability and to the rehabilitation process itself. An essential ingredient for navigating this difficult terrain is motivation.

Whether the patient is an 89-year-old woman with a stroke or a 29-year-old professional athlete with a rotator cuff strain, these individuals do not self-select into the rehabilitation process. They may have poor adaptation and coping skills, little experience in motor learning, and decreased motivation to participate actively in the rehabilitation process. Therefore, the purpose of this chapter is to present (1) an understanding of the psychological adaptation process, (2) elements of motor learning to treat and educate patients, and (3) an overview of motivation. Finally, specific attention is paid to common impediments to adaptation, learning, and motivation to allow rehabilitation professionals to better recognize and mitigate these hindrances. These insights actualize the science described elsewhere in this volume and maximize the success of the rehabilitation process.

ADAPTATION

Adaptation or *adjustment* is the psychological process by which individuals accommodate to their new circumstances. Psychological coping and adaptation often begin acutely postinjury or illness, before formal rehabilitation is even contemplated. The process of adapting to the acute and long-term effects of the presenting illness and to the

rehabilitation program and impairment or disability differs from person to person. Adjustment can depend on a multitude of variables, including intrinsic strengths, preexisting coping skills, overall personality, and intelligence. Moreover, the nature of the illness, level of mobility limitation, availability of support systems, developmental stage, and cognitive abilities have a significant effect on the adaptation process. Rehabilitation professionals should be able to identify nonproductive coping mechanisms or inappropriate adaptation in order to maximize rehabilitation. Poor adaptation may manifest as a clinically significant psychological problem such as depression or anxiety, which in turn can impair motivation and learning in the rehabilitation program.

Stage Theories

Various theories regarding stages of adjustment to injury or disability have been postulated. For example, Livnik and Antonak's theory[1] described stages of shock, denial, anger and depression, and ultimately acceptance and integration. According to Rohe,[2] most stage theories have three underlying assumptions: (1) people respond to the onset of disability in specific and predictable ways, (2) a series of stages occur over time, and (3) there is an eventual acceptance or resolution to the emotional crisis. Such theories have been based on anecdotal information, however, and with no empirical evidence to support the notion that specific sequential stages occur in patients who have similar impairments or disabilities. There is also no indication that every individual ultimately gains acceptance of his or her situation in a predictable manner. The common beliefs presented in stage theories may be secondary to rehabilitation professionals' need to be able to negotiate "unpredictable and emotionally charged situations,"[3] which may prompt the labeling of patients in certain stages and the propensity toward overdiagnosis of pathology. Furthermore, the popularity of stage theories may represent staff's wishes that, over time, everyone resolves the problems they encounter as a result of disabilities.[2] In reality, it appears that patients cope with injury and disability in personal ways that may involve vacillating between different emotional reactions. Several mitigating factors (i.e., premorbid coping skills, cognitive abilities, perceived availability of social support, and so forth) may determine outcome.

Variables Associated with Successful Coping and Adjustment

Several studies have focused on personal variables associated with adaptive coping and successful outcomes. Green et al.[4] found that after a spinal cord injury (SCI), positive self-concept, which includes "body image, self-esteem, perceptions, cognitions, and feelings about the self," was correlated with living at home and not at a residential treatment facility, being more educated, believing oneself to be as physically independent as possible, and being able to drive a motor vehicle.[5] Interestingly, this study also revealed that receiving assistance with activities of daily living was positively related to good self-concept, probably secondary to supportive social interactions with caretakers.[6]

The process of adjustment or adaptation is largely contingent on perceptions of the meaning and effects of the injury or disability. Emotional responses depend on an appraisal process, which involves personal meaningfulness, level of possible control, expectations for future change, and potential to influence adjustment through coping.[3,7] It is important to note that the appraisal of the event, and not the event itself, has been identified as the most crucial factor. An individual's prior experiences, personality, sociocultural background, and cognitive functioning inform this appraisal. Consistent with the personal appraisal theory, Taylor[7] found that some patients derived a sense of positive personal change in response to life-threatening illness. This manifested as reordered priorities, increased time spent on important relationships, seeing a need for enhanced enjoyment in life, becoming more focused on living in the present, and viewing life as precious and fragile.[8,9]

Locus of Control

Locus of control[10] is a construct that is frequently cited in the cognitive and health psychology literature regard-

ing perceptions of internal or external attributions to events or actions. Individuals with an internal locus of control tend to believe that their "well-being can be controlled by their own actions, (whereas), those with an external locus of control believe that their well-being is controlled by fate or powerful others."[5,10] Research has shown that an internal locus of control promotes optimal adjustment, both emotionally and functionally.[11,12] Locus of control is also closely tied to the concept of hardiness, or strong, solid coping during stressful times. "Hardy individuals a) believe they can control events; b) are committed to the activities of their lives; and c) perceive change as a challenge to further their development." Hardiness has been correlated with better psychological adjustment but not physiological adaptation in individuals with chronic illness.[5,13]

Successful coping includes seeking information and education regarding the diagnosis, related procedures, and prognosis. Furthermore, the establishment of concrete and attainable goals that can be easily self-reinforced promotes feelings of self-efficacy and internal control. Recalling how prior periods of stress were handled successfully may also prompt better outcomes in the rehabilitation setting. Patients in the recovery process spontaneously use many of these strategies, while rehabilitation and mental health professionals can facilitate others.

Variables in Coping

Severity of Injury

The level of impairment itself is not necessarily a determinant of adjustment.[9] In fact, individuals suffering from less severe injuries, such as back pain and concussion, may experience poorer adjustment despite nearly complete physiological healing, secondary to psychological effects such as depression, anxiety, and physical disuse.[3,14,15] Notably, however, there are significant correlations between severity of injury and poor adjustment in individuals with SCIs.[16] Feelings of activity restriction, especially in those activities that are essential to an individual's identity and self-worth (e.g., self- and other-care, work, recreation), have been significantly correlated with adjustment.[9,17] Extent of brain injury and cognitive impairment has also been associated with poorer adjustment. Patients with concomitant spinal cord and brain injuries demonstrated greater family and personal adjustment problems than patients with SCIs alone.[18] Moreover, individuals with severe traumatic brain injuries have been found to be more distressed and rated as more socially and psychologically dysfunctional than patients with SCIs, probably as a result of the former group's cognitive impairments.[16,19]

Age

The relationship between successful long-term adjustment and age at time of injury is unclear. Green et al. found that individuals with injuries occurring before adolescence had poorer self-concepts.[4] Williamson et al.[17] found that adults over the age of 65 had fewer psychological adjustment problems after amputations than younger adults.[9] Notably, Rybarczyk et al.[20] found a correlation between older age and fewer body-related concerns in patients with amputations; however, no associations were noted between age and overall adjustment in this population.[9]

Social Support

The term *social support* has been defined as "the perception that one is cared for, being encouraged to openly express beliefs and feelings, and being given material aid."[2] Cobb[21] hypothesized that social support may have a direct effect on neuroendocrine systems or a more indirect effect via better patient compliance. He found that patients who received social support followed medical recommendations more closely.[2] It is still unclear whether the direct or indirect effects of social support are mediating variables on adjustment, as McNett[22] found that availability of social support was positively correlated with self-concept, but actual use of these supports was not significantly associated with good coping, possibly secondary to the negative feelings associated with dependence on others.[6] Personal variables, such as stable occupational and financial status, when combined with social support, have also been shown to be beneficial for adaptation.[6,23]

Common Acute Adjustment Reactions

Acute onset of disability requires patients to abruptly face severe functional limitations. Decreased ability to ambulate, speak, or perform activities of daily living, including toileting, dressing, and feeding, can be catastrophically immobilizing to patients. They may experience these changes as a profound loss of control and become startlingly aware of their dependence on others. Those with more slowly progressive illnesses such as Parkinson's disease or cancer may confront feelings of demoralization and hopelessness as their abilities continue to decline.

Adaptation to Hospitalization

An inpatient rehabilitation stay can be quite difficult for patients because of unfamiliarity of the institution and separation from loved ones. Feelings of alienation from one's support system frequently result. Many patients also experience anxiety regarding personal finances and medical expenses, the well-being of their families while they are incapacitated, and the status of their vocations. Discharge planning evokes issues of possible further institutionalization and fear of decreased function and poor quality of life at home.

The rehabilitation program prompts a dramatic increase in activity levels, as rigorous physical therapy and occupational therapy regimens are initiated. Patients become part of a larger system that includes rehabilitation professionals as well as peers with injuries and disabilities. Integration with peers either with similar or different difficulties can be jarring. Patients may share rooms and therapy gyms with others who have assistive devices, orthoses, amputations, or ostomies. The lack of privacy can also become a significant issue for some patients, as they are frequently bathed, dressed, and toileted by relative strangers who may also be of the opposite gender. Some individuals have never been touched by anyone except significant others in these ways and may find such interactions distressing. People with traumatic histories of physical or sexual abuse may be exceptionally vigilant about being touched by rehabilitation aides or therapists and may require clinical interventions provided by a psychologist to help optimize their rehabilitation.

Existential Issues

Existential issues, including fear of death and realizations about one's own mortality, may emerge in response to life-threatening injuries. Individuals may begin to question the meaning of their lives, given new limitations. Worries regarding perceived quality of life, loss of goals and dreams, and identity changes secondary to inability to perform previously held family roles and vocations, can prompt significant distress.

Body Image and Sexuality

Major changes in body image and self-esteem may also occur after injuries or chronic illnesses. Some patients experience embarrassment, shame, and disgust in response to their own bodies. As a result, they may be unable or unwilling to look at or touch themselves in affected areas. Moreover, medication effects as well as depression and anxiety may prompt decreased interest in sex or sexual dysfunction, further undermining body image and contributing to negative sexual attitudes. Patients may avoid thinking about or discussing their sexuality and may distance themselves from significant others.

Clinical Consequences of Poor Adaptation

Depression

Some patients have clinically significant difficulty with psychological adaptation in response to the acute and long-term physical, functional, and contextual changes that occur after injury. Rates of depression vary among different rehabilitation populations. It estimated that 20–30% of patients with amputations,[20] SCIs,[11] cerebrovascular accidents,[24] and traumatic brain injuries[25] suffer from clinical depression. Chronic pain patients have been found to have a considerably higher incidence of depression, up to 70%.[26] According to Trexler and Fordyce,[3] prevalence rates of depression among rehabilitation patients exceed those in the general population, indicating that injury and disability can have a significant effect on emotional well-being. Individuals who are clinically depressed, however, represent the minority of rehabilitation patients. Despite the potential difficulties outlined previously, "most patients in rehabilitation settings cope well, even when they have major and disfiguring injuries."[27,28]

Interestingly, many rehabilitation professionals, including mental health professionals, often feel that depression *should* occur in response to injury, impairment, and disability. They may make assumptions regarding patients' emotional functioning that are based largely on their own feelings and experiences. Nonetheless, it is important to outline how depression and poor adjustment can manifest in rehabilitation patients, as well as to review the variables that are associated with poor and successful adjustment.

Patients who experience depressive symptomatology and appear acutely sad or blue are often the easiest to identify. Their distress is evident to those around them because of blunted or flat facial expression and reported feelings of depressed mood. Less commonly recognized symptoms of depression are decreased energy, slowed motor output, sleep or appetite disturbance, poor concentration and decision making, anger or agitation, and decreased interest in social situations or therapy programs. Individuals with these symptoms may be misunderstood and labeled as unmotivated or resistant to treatment. Furthermore, anger and irritability may manifest secondary to depression and feelings of loss of control, which can be difficult for the treatment team to interpret and manage.

Guilt

For patients with chronic medical problems, guilt may arise as a result of maladaptive health behaviors (i.e., smoking, poor regulation of diabetes) that potentially contributed to their illnesses. Individuals who became injured because of alcohol or drug intoxication and risk-taking behaviors may experience guilt, shame, and anger about consequences of their actions. Survivor guilt may also occur in patients who have been involved in multiple-victim traumas.

Anxiety

Anxiety reactions can also manifest in rehabilitation patients, in the form of social avoidance, panic, or excessive worry. Social avoidance can occur as a result of embarrassment regarding functional limitations, assistive devices, personal medical apparatus (e.g., ostomies), perceived disfigurement, and incontinence.[3] Anxiety can also occur secondary to altered sense of body position and fear of falling. Anxious patients may become overwhelmed and disorganized in therapies, seemingly unable to incorporate the information being imparted to them by rehabilitation professionals. Physically, they may appear flushed and diaphoretic, report exaggerated somatic complaints, and try to avoid therapies. In an attempt to lower anxiety levels, consideration should be given to patterns of anxiety reactions and identification of potential precipitants and possibly reinforcing responses.

Patients who have experienced assaults or motor vehicle accidents may be suffering from acute stress disorders. This diagnosis involves an immediate posttraumatic stress reaction that can include increased anxiety, heightened startle responses, re-experiencing of the trauma through intrusive thoughts or flashbacks, and avoidance of things that are reminders of the trauma.[29] These patients may have a steady state of anxiety or have symptoms triggered by specific environmental stimuli, such as being near an automobile or hearing a loud noise.

Denial

The term *denial* is frequently employed in the rehabilitation setting to describe patients who are seemingly unaware of or are emotionally stoic about their illnesses or disabilities. It is generally used as a pejorative label that implies poor coping and adjustment. *Denial* has been defined as "selective, distorted, and restrictive processing of information and a disavowal of painful affects."[30] Mental health professionals often conceptualize denial as a psychological defense that protects individuals from overwhelming levels of anxiety, similar to a shock phenomenon.[31] Patients may use denial as an adaptive coping mechanism until they are able to integrate and manage the reality of their situations. Furthermore, individuals may fluctuate between varying levels of acceptance over time.[31]

Despite these positive interpretations of the denial process, many rehabilitation professionals become distressed when treating patients whom they believe are in denial about their illnesses and limitations. This may be a result of personal expectations and beliefs about what reactions to disability should be. Confrontation of the denial can be tempting, but it is important to note that such interventions can be "counterproductive, as unrealistic expressions of hope can actually reinforce progress through rehabilitation."[3] Direct confrontation can take away people's hope[32] and alliance with rehabilitation professionals. As an alternative, patients should be allowed to face their situations, both cognitively and emotionally, when they are able. More immediate interventions may, however, be indicated if the denial prompts safety risks or psychosocial failures.[3]

Treatment for Adjustment Problems

Overall, many patients benefit from having a mental health professional available to help them to understand and manage the major changes that can occur acutely postinjury or in response to longer term disability issues. They may not have been able to discuss their emotional reactions to their injury or illness in the acute care hospital and may seek an opportunity to do so in the rehabilitation setting. Some individuals feel uncomfortable disclosing sensitive information regarding body image, guilt, or perceived vulnerabilities to close friends and family. Others require participation in psychotherapy to allow them to manage their adjustment problems and help optimize their rehabilitation programs. For a summary of occasions when mental health professionals should be consulted as well as common interventions used to treat adjustment problems, see Table 37-1.

LEARNING

Individuals seek rehabilitation for a wide range of neurologic, vascular, integumentary, cardiopulmonary, and musculoskeletal impairments. A common result of these impairments is a decline in motor functioning. Attempts to maximize self-care, mobility, and vocational skills require a process of motor learning. Other types of learning also occur in the rehabilitation setting, but given the importance of motor learning, the current section focuses primarily on techniques and teaching strategies that can maximize the learning of motor programs. Variables that can have an effect on the teaching of motor skills include type of task to be learned, mode of instruction, use of feedback, context in which tasks are presented, and type and timing of practice.

Goals of Motor Learning

Once goals have been agreed upon and outlined by the treatment team and the patient, the task of teaching new motor skills follows. Information should be imparted to patients in a manner that prompts them to use their intrinsic experiences of their bodies and actions while actively using problem-solving strategies. Self-informed decision making in planning motor sequences and functional skills allows patients to think concretely about how to achieve specific goals one step at a time and

TABLE 37-1
Psychological Interventions for Adjustment Problems

Brief Individual Therapy	Cognitive-Behavioral Therapy	Couple/Family Therapy	Group Therapy	Social Skills Training	Substance Abuse Treatment
Focused on adjustment to injury/disability	Addresses specific negative cognitions/behaviors	Focused on family/systemic issue	Allows for sharing and normalization of experiences	Promotes appropriate social skills	Helps establish and maintain sobriety
Problem-focused on current circumstances and emotional reactions	Reinforces appropriate behaviors and effort in rehabilitation program	Educates families about patient's illness/disability and emotional responses	Developed for specific diagnostic groups	Effective for patients with brain injury and others displaying inappropriate behaviors	Facilitates team monitoring for illicit drug use and drug-seeking/misuse of prescription medications
Used to treat depression, anxiety, body image/sexuality issues, mourning loss of function	Treatment for chronic pain, anger management, anxiety, depression, acute stress disorders	Incorporates sociocultural expectations of family regarding illness, disability, care giving	Facilitates learning from peers regarding diagnosis, course of treatment, recovery	Useful with general rehabilitation patients to familiarize them with societal attitudes regarding disability	May incorporate 12-step programs

facilitates cognitive flexibility in novel situations.[33,34] The ultimate objective is to limit reliance on therapists for sustained guidance and feedback, foster patients' independence, and prompt the generalization of skills to new environments.

Acquisition, Retention, and Transfer of Information

Three components are involved in the learning of new information that are all integral to the attainment of planned goals. *Acquisition* of information refers to the initial learning of a skill or concept. *Retention* occurs when an individual is able to mentally sustain the learned information over time. *Transfer* of information involves the ability to translate the stored information in order to use it to master unfamiliar situations. Various methods of teaching have differential effects on the acquisition, retention, and transfer of information.[33] For example, one approach to teaching a motor sequence, such as employing manual guidance to execute an action, may maximize the initial acquisition of new information, but may limit the amount of information that is actively retained over time. Given these complexities, promoting the mastery of a skill requires agreement between the rehabilitation professional and patient about whether rapid acquisition, retention, or transfer of information is most important to meet the patient's specific goals.

Open and Closed Tasks

Two types of tasks exist in both rehabilitation and real-life settings: open and closed tasks. Closed tasks are predictable because they always remain the same from one trial to another with minimal variation.[33] Many transfers, such as those going from a sit to stand position or from a wheelchair to a mat, are closed tasks. Open tasks, on the other hand, change over time because they occur in diverse environments with varying conditions.[35] An example of an open task is walking on a sidewalk alongside other pedestrians. A person in this situation has to focus on how to ambulate in the chosen direction while simultaneously negotiating individuals passing from behind, approaching, and crossing the intended path. Such a task differs significantly from ambulating in a quiet hallway with specified parameters and instructions readily available.

Successful learning of motor patterns requires that, once mastered, closed tasks should be expanded, thus creating an open task.[36] Such conversion may involve the diversification of the setting in which the task is performed to more natural environments. The patient must use independent problem-solving strategies in areas beyond the therapy gym to anticipate how to negotiate new situations. Moreover, it is desirable, although often difficult practically, to teach a movement or skill in the context in which it typically occurs so that patients are better prepared to manage at home, in the workplace, or while performing daily activities elsewhere.

Augmented Information

Providing extrinsic information via different sensory modalities (i.e., verbally, visually, or manually) is often included in the therapy regimen to complement and direct intrinsic information provided by the patient. Taken together, these modes of teaching and providing feedback are referred to as *augmented information* (AI).[33,37,38] Verbal information can be provided to instruct a patient as to how to perform a task before it is attempted or modeled. Verbal feedback can also be presented during a task, in an attempt to direct the movement in the moment, or after the task is completed, to reflect the degree of success achieved. Similarly, visual information, in the form of modeling the movement *beforehand*, providing visual cues *during* the performance of the task, or mimicking the movement performed by the patient *after* a trial may be employed.[33]

Manual cues and guidance, in the form of passively moving a patient through an action,[34] are also commonly used during instruction of a task, especially when a patient is unable to detect critical information or is lacking an internal reference of the goal of the task.[33] Such inability to intuit the motor skill being taught often occurs in patients who are hemiparetic or experience sensory neglect or inattention. Manual guidance is also used to direct patients with impulsive or erratic behaviors and should then be withdrawn once the task is performed with more forethought and awareness. Individuals with cognitive impairments, language disruption, and dementing illnesses may also benefit from the use of manual guidance if they have difficulty following verbal or visual cues.

Timing of Augmented Information

AI is most effective in hastening the acquisition of skills when it serves as a complement to the intrinsic information and problem-solving strategies generated by the patient.[33] The effects of AI on acquisition, retention, and transfer of information may vary depending on when in the learning process the cues are given.

AI may be beneficial before a task is performed to clarify the goal and help outline a process-oriented strategy for achieving it. Verbal information should revolve around the most important aspects of the movement and should be clear and concise. Visual cues or models may also be introduced before the task is performed, but the patient should first be prompted to think through the problem and consider the sequencing that would be required to perform the movement successfully.[33] The introduction of a picture, written verbal cue, or model may elucidate the qualitative or spatial aspects of a task that can be difficult to explain verbally. According to Majsak,[33] studies on observational learning have shown that modeling done by therapists or experts is less effective for teaching purposes than modeling performed by peers.[39-41] This finding suggests that patients may derive more benefit from receiving instruction in small groups where they may observe the performance of other patients.

AI provided during performance aids the initial acquisition of information; however, declines in retention levels and transfer of skills to new situations may occur.[33] This appears to be a consequence of patients depending on the guidance and feedback of a therapist. Loss of information can occur if continued AI is not present when the task is performed in subsequent trials and is particularly problematic in the context of manual guidance.

AI presented after an action has occurred has the opposite effect. Acquisition may happen more slowly, but the learned information is better retained and transferred for use in varied situations.[33] Allowing an individual to become attuned to an intrinsic experience of the movement or task before offering AI facilitates the use of problem-solving strategies and cognitive flexibility, thus limiting reliance on an external source (e.g., a rehabilitation professional). Swinnen[42] found that patients who were given AI between 3.5 and 8 seconds after performing an action had higher levels of both short-term (minutes to hours) and long-term (4 months) retention of the information they learned than controls who received AI immediately after the action. According to Majsak,[33] allowing patients to evaluate and analyze their own performances while determining how actions could be performed differently before receiving AI optimizes new motor learning.

Role of Augmented Information in Teaching Different Types of Tasks

Feedback or AI is most effective in teaching closed tasks where the development of stereotyped movements is critical.[34] AI may be less useful in the instruction of open tasks because new approaches are required in a varied environment. It is important to note, however, that AI can be tailored for open tasks to prompt the patient's evaluation of the environment where the action is to be performed.[35] Similarly, feedback regarding how the patient developed an appropriate movement strategy and anticipated the environmental features may be useful.

Limitations of Augmented Information and Possible Solutions

Although it can be instrumental in enhancing information acquisition, manual guidance can prevent a patient from sensing an error or inaccurate movement. Manual guidance may also prevent the retention and transfer of information by limiting the patient's independent information processing and problem solving required for the performance of more complicated open tasks.[33] Furthermore, decreased motivation may result if patients perceive that that they are not allowed to make errors.[36] Given these cautions, once a closed task is mastered, the amount of AI should be limited. In order to maximize all three components of learning, namely, acquisition, retention, and transfer of information, the amount or frequency of AI used by rehabilitation professionals should be decreased as soon as possible. Lowering the frequency of AI is commonly referred to as *fading*, which entails slowly tapering the number of trials after which AI is given.[33] According to Winstein et al.,[43] this approach enhances retention better than continued or absent AI.[33] Decreasing the frequency of AI by summarizing the feedback after a certain number of trials may lower initial acquisition rates but promotes greater retention and transfer of information.[44]

Maximizing Performance through the Use of Practice

The idea that practice makes perfect is omnipresent in our culture and has an even stronger importance in the rehabilitation setting. Practice that occurs at one time, or blocked practice, is most contributory toward initial acquisition of information. Randomized distributed practice is less beneficial for learning new information, but more efficacious in promoting retention and transfer of information.[33,45,46] Blocked practice may be carried out relatively automatically, without need for conscious information processing, whereas randomized practice prompts problem solving that is required for the negotiation of tasks in novel situations. Therefore, blocked practice should be employed in the initial acquisition phases of the activity. Once the information has been acquired, randomized practice trials should then occur. This provides greater diversity of action and opportunities to attend to intrinsic information to create problem-solving strategies accordingly.[33,36]

Continued physical practice after therapy sessions is crucial to sustain continuity between treatments. Patients should be given clear instructions regarding their independent practice regimens, with special attention given to desired frequency of practice, number of repetitions recommended, and optimal locations for practice. If possible, it is more beneficial to allow patients to write down the instructions themselves while in the therapy setting than to supply them with printed instruction. For those patients who are unable to write because of their injuries or illnesses, the rehabilitation professional should write the instructions while reviewing them aloud with the patient, thus directly involving the patient in the transfer of information. Simple drawings depicting stick figures conducting motor tasks with cues such as, "Do" or "Don't do," are good complements to narrative instructions, as they are easy for patients to refer to and follow. Between therapy sessions, the availability of videos and photographs of patients themselves performing specific motor or occupational tasks is also useful. These visual cues allow patients to review their performance, learn from their mistakes, and plan for future practice.[34]

Physical practice is undoubtedly instrumental in promoting mastery of motor patterns; however, mental practice should also be employed to bolster the rehabilitation program. Mental practice or visualizing the motor task can be performed easily at any time of the day in any setting. Mental practice has been found to be most beneficial in facilitating the spatial aspects of a movement.[34] Patients should be encouraged to use mental practice to help them sustain engagement in the tasks practiced in therapy sessions, keeping the concepts fresh and accessible, and ultimately, speeding their improvement.

Charting of both physical and mental practice sessions conducted outside of the therapy sessions is helpful, especially when achievement of specific goals is also documented during the time being addressed. This allows patients to review tangibly the work they have done and the investment made, as well as to recognize how their efforts have contributed to their progress.

Learning Problems

The techniques and strategies reviewed in this section have been shown to optimize motor learning in important ways. Employment of these teaching methods, types of feedback, and practice recommendations does not, however, guarantee that learning will occur in all individuals. For patients who have significant difficulty learning motor skills, serious consideration should be given to referral for neuropsychological evaluation. Such evaluations involve the administration of standardized tests that assess different cognitive domains, including, but not limited to, orientation, attention and concentration, short- and long-term memory, language, abstract reasoning, visuospatial skills, judgment and insight, cognitive flexibility, and organizational skills. Specific findings regarding patients' strengths and weaknesses may inform individual rehabilitation programs so that regimens are tailored to meet the particular needs of each patient. This information also allows for compensation of deficits via maximization of preserved abilities and can help to guide rehabilitation professionals regarding how best to treat individual patients, in order to optimize their learning.

Occupational therapists may be helpful in distinguishing organic from behavioral influences on delayed learning. Speech-language pathologists may also make significant contributions to understanding why patients may be having difficulty comprehending and using information provided in physical therapy and occupational therapy. Their expertise with receptive and expressive aphasias can be crucial to patients' success in rehabilitation. Patients who require interventions to improve their speech and cognitive skills often benefit from cognitive remediation therapy in either inpatient or outpatient settings. This is especially true for individuals who may be living without supervision on discharge, as well as for patients who intend to return to work.

There are also patients in the rehabilitation setting who have established or learned different behaviors that interfere in some way with their rehabilitation regimens. Some of the most common behaviors that may have this effect include seeking drugs or abusing pain medication, using the sick role to obtain primary or secondary gain, making demands on the staff, and refusing to attend therapies. Behavioral modification is an intervention employed by psychologists and other mental health professionals to reduce the occurrence of unwanted or inappropriate behaviors. Positive appropriate behaviors are positively reinforced and encouraged, while inappropriate behaviors are negatively reinforced, or given less attention. Consultation with a psychologist may prove effective for treatment of patients with behavioral problems so that such individuals are not unduly punished or isolated. A specific behavioral plan may therefore be generated and shared with other rehabilitation professionals to ensure consistent intervention, thus maximizing the rehabilitation program overall.

MOTIVATION

Definition

Motivation is derived from the Latin root for *moving*[47] and is defined as a stimulus to action, incentive, or drive.[48] *Dorland's Illustrated Medical Dictionary* focuses on the psychological definition as "any of the forces that activate behavior toward satisfying needs or achieving goals."[49] Early motivation theory derived largely from animal research, focused on a biological drive, instinct, or movement toward a basic need such as food or warmth. Maslow theorized that once basic needs are met "man is primarily motivated by his needs to develop and actualize his fullest potentialities and capacities."[50] A more recent and broader understanding of motivation is the "summation of psychological forces manifest as behavior but moderated by the environment."[51]

Only by grasping the full complexities of motivation can rehabilitation professionals abandon the simplistic view of motivation as merely an aspect of an individual's personality. This understanding should reduce the pejorative labeling of certain patients as *unmotivated* and instead focus energy on identifying and mitigating impediments to motivation.

Extrinsic Motivation

Can individuals be truly motivated by the promise of external rewards?[52] Participation in exercise programs by those motivated by intrinsically held goals results in better long-term compliance than those attempting to fulfill an external norm such as weight loss and improved appearance.[25] To be effective the patient must value external rewards to change behavior. Rehabilitation professionals may intervene with techniques of motivational interviewing[53] to help individuals visualize the possibilities of change.

Rehabilitation professionals must educate patients about the possibilities of improvement through participation and the potential negative consequences of not participating. Objective feedback, often in the form of physiological measures such as decreased resting heart rate, improved strength, increased range of motion, or decreased weight provide inspiration that a short-term goal has been achieved because of the patient's effort.

The authority of rehabilitation professionals may be a motivating factor. As authority figures, rehabilitation pro-

fessionals should understand that lack of positive health messages may be misconstrued as tacit acceptance of a negative behavior (e.g., inactivity or smoking). On the other hand, too much authority is perceived as "power over" or paternalistic authority and can be unmotivating.[54] In the same study of elderly women receiving rehabilitation, participants described positive motivation from "power with" or empowerment in which staff work in conjunction with patients regarding the rehabilitation program.[54]

Intrinsic or Self-Motivation

Motivated individuals are found to have a good sense of self-efficacy, the confidence in oneself that one is *able* to perform a task. Confident individuals, in this theory, will more likely attempt something new, resolutely persist, and expect to achieve a goal.[55] Intact executive functioning allows them to appraise their inherent strengths and weaknesses to set appropriate goals and track their progress toward attainment of those goals. They frequently possess optimism and flexibility to allow for reassessment and reframing of their efforts if positive results are not immediately evident. The ability to delay gratification supports the accomplishment of long-term goals that may take years to achieve. Self-motivation can be socially learned, dependent on the capacity for self-reinforcement, and a relatively enduring personality trait.[56,57] The lack of impediments to motivation may allow these individuals to achieve highly in multiple facets of their lives.

Even with this description of self-motivation, recognition of these characteristics on a rehabilitation unit is more difficult than anticipated. King and Barrowclough[58] found no significant agreement between nurses, physicians, and therapists when asked to judge which of their patients were highly motivated.[58] Poor motivation is generally defined as the lack or the slowing of goal achievement, yet poor motivation may be overlooked when it manifests as a patient's anger, decreased initiative, self-doubt, or overly critical comments of the staff.

Goal Setting

Establishment and achievement of appropriate goals are the measures of progress in physical medicine and rehabilitation. Individuals not progressing with expected goals in a rehabilitation program present a challenge to the system. Third-party payers may not continue to pay unless results of the rehabilitation intervention are forthcoming. Moreover, lack of progress is demoralizing to the treatment team as well as the patient. Failure to meet rehabilitation goals may result in health care professionals' blaming the patient for a poor outcome. The pejorative labels *unmotivated* or *noncompliant* may be assigned. This labeling is sometimes used by staff as an excuse for not offering help.[59]

An open dialogue regarding goal setting is integral to the interdisciplinary team approach of rehabilitation and allows for consistency among rehabilitation professionals. Involvement of patients and families in making decisions around goals actively engages them in the rehabilitation process and simultaneously begins their process of education regarding the disability and its rehabilitation. Furthermore, involvement in goal setting can engender a sense of control, sustain motivation, and bolster feelings of self-efficacy. Patients should be consulted regularly about their desires, expectations, and subjective impressions of their progress.

Despite the centrality of mutual goal setting in rehabilitation, some studies indicate that patients often do not participate in the goal-setting process.[60] Furthermore, Wressle[60] found that even when goals are set, patients often focus more on achieving preinjury status rather than short-term functional gains identified by the rehabilitation professionals. In one attempt to measure efficacy as achievement of self-identified goals in cardiac rehabilitation, the results were "unclear and might give misleading results."[61]

To maximize motivation, specific and challenging yet attainable short-term goals must be set. The tasks to be learned should be identified clearly so patients understand what they need to do to achieve those goals. "[V]ague goals such as 'do your best,' or no goals at all, produce lower motivation. Even specific but moderate or easy goals, contrary to what one might expect, are associated with low motivation levels. So, performance effort is inversely related to the likelihood of achieving goals."[62]

TABLE 37-2
Motivation Equation

Perception of **CHANCE** for success	×	Individual **VALUE** of the rehab goal	=	M O T I V A T I O N
Perceived **COST** of achieving goal				

Source: JW Atkinson, JR Bastian, RW Earl, GM Litwin. The achievement of motive, goal setting and probability preferences. J Abnorm Psychol 1960;60:27–36; and RJ Geelen, PH Soons. Rehabilitation: an "everyday" model. Patient Educ Couns 1996;28:69–77.

Although challenging goals may optimize effort, failure to achieve even these short-term objectives can be devastating. Forcing an individual to face reduced abilities prematurely may diminish hope and further hinder progress. If objectives appear too difficult for patients, the objectives must be reformulated to allow for more realistic goal setting.

Motivation Equation

Concentrating on the importance of an individual's assessment of the goals, their perceived cost of participation, and their estimate of possible success helps calculate their motivation equation[63,64] (Table 37-2). Use of this equation may guide rehabilitation professionals in assessing and optimizing motivation.

While rehabilitation professionals may provide objective information regarding the usual course of the illness or outcome from the proposed program, it is the individual's cognitive appraisal and perception of self-efficacy in achieving the goal that are most critical. The *perception of their chance for successful rehabilitation if the necessary effort is made* is the first factor in the motivation equation. Patients who do not believe in their abilities to succeed in the rehabilitation program may do well in a group of individuals with similar pathology and beliefs who nonetheless are progressing by objective measures. The information derived from seeing others achieve may improve an individual's perception of his or her own chance for success.

The second factor is the individual's *value of the rehabilitation goal*. People perform an internal assessment of how worthwhile the proposed goal is. "Will it allow me to better meet my commitments?" "How important is the expected outcome to my values?" "How will achievement of this goal change my life?" Once again, alignment of the goals is critical. For example, an elderly man reluctant to go home with a walker may hold little value in the proposed goal of independent ambulation with this assistive device. However, reframing this goal as independent and safe walking within his home as an interim goal toward ambulation with a cane or no device may be more acceptable.

The denominator in the motivation equation is the *perceived cost of attempting to reach the goal*. The cost may be economic (expense of the therapy or lost work time), risk of failure, pain, fatigue, or loss of time and energy needed to pursue the program (including therapy time and home practice). Significantly, attempting the rehabilitation program may highlight the individual's incapacity because of an inability to achieve goals (i.e., the psychological costs of participating in rehabilitation may seem to grow as the program proceeds). These costs can be addressed through continued encouragement and support from the treatment team.

In general, patients overestimate the costs of rehabilitation in their calculations. The rehabilitation professional should give a frank estimate of the costs rather than ignore the subject. Also, some perceived costs such as exertion or fatigue from the program may be reframed as positive outcomes, gains, or signs of success from the program.

The three factors, the perceived chance of success, the value of the goal, and the cost of participation, each focus on the individual's subjective analysis. This is appropriate because an accurate perceived or believed prognosis on the patient's part is generally the best predictor of success.[65] In contrast, individuals with poor insight reflected by unrealistically high expectations, beyond the capacity expected by the rehabilitation professionals, had the best outcomes in one study.[66] The optimist's expectation of success improved motivation and outcomes.

IMPEDIMENTS TO ADAPTATION, LEARNING, AND MOTIVATION

Although motivation improves adherence to a rehabilitation program, many impediments may impair achievement of goals. Impediments (Table 37-3) may diminish motivation, learning, adaptation, or all three. It is critical to screen the patient in order to diagnose and treat reversible impediments. Comorbid pathologies that are untreatable should at least be enumerated so that expectations of the rehabilitation intervention can be adjusted to reduce patient blaming by rehabilitation staff.

Delirium

Delirium is characterized by a fluctuation in alertness and attention throughout the day. It may be recognized on a rehabilitation unit by discrepant reports from therapists working with the same patient at different times of the day. Delirium, by definition,[29] can be caused by a general medical condition or induced by a medication. Individuals with delirium can develop cognitive impairments in various areas (e.g., memory, language, and disorientation) over a short period of time that are inconsistent with their previous abilities. Furthermore, delirious patients can seem irritable, anxious, psychotic, or combative. Among individuals over 65 years old, 10% of patients admitted to acute care hospitals may suffer from delirium, while an additional 10–15%

TABLE 37-3
Common Impediments to Adaptation, Learning, and Motivation

Delirium
Mood disorders, including depression
Cognitive and neurobehavioral problems
Brain injury: stroke and traumatic brain injury
Frontal lobe pathology
Seizures
Premorbid learning disorders, attention deficit, mental retardation
Dementia
Anxiety
Personality disorders
Substance abuse
Malingering/factitious disorder
Medications
    Psychopharmacologic agents
        Antipsychotics, mood stabilizers, anxiolytics
    Medical pharmacologic agents
        Hypoglycemic agents
        Antihypertensives, β-blockers
        Digitalis
        Sedatives
        Opioids
        Muscle relaxants
Medical illness
    Pain
    Debility
    Sleep deprivation
    Infection
Psychosocial
    Feelings of stigma regarding disability, leading to social withdrawal
    Feelings of social isolation
    Dissatisfaction with family life
    Low self-esteem
Goal setting
    Misalignment of goals
        Secondary gain: financial (e.g., workers' compensation); emotional (attention and release of responsibilities)
        Education: poor recognition of importance of the rehabilitation goal
        Systemic: inappropriate goals
Cultural issues
    Different cultural expectations and beliefs regarding illness and recovery

---

become delirious while hospitalized.[29] As a result of the cognitive and behavioral disturbances, patients with delirium are often unable to focus or learn in therapies and may be mistaken as demented, unmotivated, or actively resistant to treatment.

Brain Injury and Negative Symptoms: Abulia and Indifference

Babinski described sequelae of stroke, including lack of motivation and morbid apathy in 1914.[67] These patients respond poorly to rehabilitation not because of their physical disability but because of the difficulty in motivating them for therapy.[68,69] Some claim that apathy is correlated with lesions of the basal ganglia or posterior limb of the internal capsule.[70,71]

A syndrome of negative symptoms manifested by indifference, apathy, and decreased motivation is found in stroke patients with and without depression.[70] Significantly, presence of negative symptoms was correlated with lengths of stay on an acute rehabilitation unit that were twice as long compared with those patients without significant negative symptoms.[72]

"Of the many behavioral problems that can follow brain injury, passivity and loss of drive (abulia) must rank among the most profoundly debilitating and intractable."[73] Any disruption of the dopaminergic pathways projecting to the nucleus accumbens may impair motivation.[25,73] In addition to brain injury, this syndrome is seen in Parkinson's disease,[74] negative type schizophrenia,[75] and major depression.[76] Certain psychopharmacologic agents can be used to improve initiation. Bromocriptine, a dopamine agonist, improved motivation in brain injury patients.[73] Psychostimulants, such as amphetamine and methylphenidate, acutely release brain dopamine and norepinephrine to improve alertness and attention,[25,77] thereby improving both motivation and learning.

Cognitive and Neurobehavioral

Cognitive and neurobehavioral deficits occur in 25–64% of patients undergoing rehabilitation.[78,79] Moreover, unrecognized cognitive and behavioral problems may be mislabeled as poor motivation.[80] Problems may manifest as a decline in memory, vision, or intellect as well as apraxia, aphasia, agnosia, neglect, distractibility, impulsivity, poor judgment, and diminished safety awareness and orientation difficulties.[28] Therefore, the ability to learn is similarly impaired. Evaluation and intervention by a neuropsychologist is critical to avoid attributing these disorders to poor motivation.

Personality Disorders

To many rehabilitation professionals, a patient's unmotivated behavior or difficulty in adapting to rehabilitation is often attributed to the individual's personality traits and disorders.[29] Personality disorders occur in at least 10% of the general population.[81] Taken as a group these *difficult* patients are described by the staff as splitting, noncompliant, unmotivated, dependent, and needy.[28] These labels may be based on the values and perceptions of the health care providers, not on the behaviors of the patient. Moreover, the same behavior may elicit different responses from different staff members.[82] Therefore, it is important to diagnose personality disorders objectively.[83] Once recognized, the rehabilitation professionals should handle the *difficult* patient through objectivity, limit setting, and compassion.[81,84]

Individuals with personality disorders may remain functional, self-reliant, and motivated at home, but regress under the stress of a disability or the effects of institutionalization. For example, a narcissistic businessman may focus so heavily on his injuries or the insult of requiring care that his involvement in the rehabilitation process is diminished.

Reframing the presentation of goals and expectations may be the best way to treat individuals with personality disorders. Demanding patients may be told that they are indeed entitled to the best care available, but that this still involves their active participation. Involvement of a rehabilitation psychologist or consultation-liaison psychiatrist may be required to best treat such patients and maintain staff cohesion.

Depression

Depression is closely linked to impaired motivation. In fact, lack of interest (i.e., decreased motivation) is a cardinal sign in making the diagnosis of major depressive disorder.[29] Furthermore, lethargy, hypersomnolence, and disturbed concentration may impair learning potential. Pervasive feelings of hopelessness and worthlessness may also diminish normal adaptation and reduce patients' perceptions that they can achieve goals. It is critical to suspect and screen for depression because of its prevalence and its deleterious effect on motivation, learning, and adaptation.

Substance Abuse

Substance abuse, particularly alcohol, is correlated with spinal cord and traumatic brain injuries.[85] Continued use of alcohol and illicit drugs retards learning and delays emotional healing in SCI.[86] Furthermore, staff should be alert to the interaction of pain medications, psychotropic medications, and illicit drugs.

Secondary Gain

A chronically discontented injured worker receiving financial compensation may be poorly motivated to achieve rehabilitation goals of recovery and return to full employment. The individual may, however, be well motivated to continue receiving payment for not working. Rather than being unmotivated the person merely has goals that are not in alignment with those of the therapy staff. A similar dynamic may exist from family and social support of the *sick role*. The rewards of this role may be negated by success in the rehabilitation program. Some patients are wedded to the sick role and supported by oversolicitous family members. Achieving functional independence may therefore not be a valued goal of some individuals.

Cultural Values

Individuals who do not participate fully in their rehabilitation programs may be manifesting cultural values at odds with the values assumed in the rehabilitation setting. These cultural issues are significant in rehabilitation.[87] "Cultures vary in their values and views regarding issues such as dependence/independence, pain, acceptance of body deformities, sexuality, caregiver expectations, and other issues that influence course and outcome."[28]

Malingering

Beyond a misalignment of goals is the more willful and conscious misrepresentation seen in malingering.[29] This must be distinguished from a conversion disorder in which both the motivation and production of symptoms are unconscious. In factitious disorder the motivation is unconscious whereas the production of symptoms is conscious. While the rehabilitation professional may exert considerable effort to ascertain the patient's goals in rehabilitation, malingering can prevent an accurate assessment of the patient's motivating factors. More structured testing by psychologists and neuropsychologists may unmask some malingering patterns.

Medications

Any single medication or combination of drugs that sedates, confuses, or obtunds the patient may prompt slowed or absent learning and impaired motivation.

The list includes, but is not limited to, antihypertensive agents, sedatives, opioids, muscle relaxants, antipsychotic agents, mood stabilizers, and anxiolytics.

CONCLUSION

Adaptation, motor learning, and motivation are interwoven into the rehabilitation process. Facility with the key elements of these issues is essential to rehabilitation professionals. Intrinsic factors, such as self-efficacy, personality, appraisals and attributions, and cognitive abilities, are crucial. At the root of learning, adaptation, and motivation is a patient's internal sense of how one's body should move, how to cope with a disability, and how much effort can be exerted to reach goals. Intrinsic factors, however, are not immutable. Rehabilitation professionals can give support to allow patients as much control as possible to help access to their intrinsic strengths.

Extrinsic factors that significantly influence patients' rehabilitation experiences include techniques in which learning bolsters intrinsic knowledge and adaptation arises from internal reserves. Self-motivation can be enhanced through actively engaging patients in setting goals that they value. Helping individuals to believe that goals are achievable and reducing their perceived costs of participation may further improve motivation and the chance of subsequent achievement.

An individual's access to intrinsic strengths may be hindered by multiple biological, psychological, and social impediments. When impediments to successful adaptation, motor learning, or motivation are suspected, it is incumbent on the rehabilitation professional to identify and mitigate hindrances whenever possible. These efforts will help refocus the rehabilitation team to meet the particular needs of patients and reduce pejorative labeling of individuals as unmotivated or slow learners.

Acknowledgments

The editorial assistance and insight of our colleagues is gratefully recognized. The authors are indebted to Sheila Dugan, MD, PT, Elizabeth Pegg Frates, MD, Lorraine Gomba, MD, Paul Juris, EdD, Ruthanne Lamborghini, PT, Alison Phillips, MD, Debra Knoff Reilly, OT, Miles Tarter, PsyD, Sumer Verma, MD, and Jennifer White, PhD.

REFERENCES

1. Livnek H, Antonak RF. Temporal structure of adaptation to disability. Rehabil Couns Bull 1991;34:298–319.

2. Rohe DE. Psychological Aspects of Rehabilitation. In J De Lisa (ed), Rehabilitation Medicine: Principles and Practice. Philadelphia: JB Lippincott, 1998;189–212.

3. Trexler LE, Fordyce DJ. Psychological

Perspectives on Rehabilitation: Contemporary Assessment and Intervention Strategies. In RL Braddom (ed), Physical Medicine and Rehabilitation. Philadelphia: WB Saunders, 1996;66–81.

4. Green BC, Pratt CC, Grigsby TE. Self-concept among persons with long-term spinal cord injury. Arch Phys Med Rehabil 1984;65:751–754.

5. Swanson B, Cronin-Stubbs D, Sheldon JA. The impact of psychosocial factors on adapting to physical disability: a review of the research literature. Rehabil Nurs 1989;14(2):64–68.

6. Lazarus RS, Folkman S. Stress. Appraisal and Coping. New York: Springer, 1986.

7. Taylor, SE. Psychosocial factors in the course of disease. Paper presented at The Annual Meeting of the Society for Behavioral Medicine. San Francisco, CA, 1997.

8. Rybarczyk B, Nicholas JJ, Nyenhuis DL. Coping with a leg amputation: integrating research and clinical practice. Rehabil Psych 1997;42(3):241–256.

9. Rotter JB. Generalized expectancies for internal versus external control of reinforcement. Psychol Monogr 1966; 80(1):1–28.

10. Buckelew SP, Baumstark KE, Frank RG, Hewet JE. Adjustment following spinal cord injury. Rehabil Psych 1990;35:101–109.

11. Schulz D, Decker S. Long-term adjustment to physical disability: the role of social support, perceived control, and self-blame. J Pers Soc Psychol 1985;48:1162–1172.

12. Pollock SE. Human responses to chronic illness: physiologic and psychosocial adaptation. Nurs Res 1986; 35:90–95.

13. Binder L. Persisting symptoms after mild head injury: a review of the postconcussive syndrome. J Clin Exp Neuropsychol 1986;8:323–346.

14. Fordyce WE. Pain and suffering: a reappraisal. Am Psychol 1988;43:276–283.

15. Evans RL, Hendricks RD, Connis RT, et al. Quality of life after spinal cord injury: a literature critique and meta-analysis. J Am Paraplegia Soc 1994;17:60–66.

16. Fee FA, Fee VC. Psychosocial consequences of concomitant spinal cord injury and traumatic brain injury. Spinal Cord Inj Psychosoc Process 1995;8(3):106–111.

17. Williamson GM, Schulz R, Bridges MW, Behan AM. Social and psychological factors in adjustment to limb amputation. J Soc Behav Pers 1994;9: 249–268.

18. Richards J, Osuna F, Jaworski T, et al. The effectiveness of different methods of defining traumatic brain injury in predicting post-discharge adjustment in a spinal cord injury population. Arch Phys Med Rehabil 1991;72:275–279.

19. Stambrook M, Moore A, Peters L, et al. Head injury and spinal cord injury: differential effects on psychosocial functioning. J Clin Exp Neuropsychol 1991;13(4):521–530.

20. Rybarcayk BD, Nyenhuis DL, Nicholas JJ, et al. Social discomfort and depression in a sample of adults with leg amputations. Arch Phys Med Rehabil 1992;73:1169–1173.

21. Cobb S. Social support as a moderator of life stress. Psychosom Med 1976;38:300–314.

22. McNett SC. Social support, threat, and coping responses and effectiveness in the functionally disabled. Nurs Res 1987;36:98–103.

23. Ben Sira Z. Disability, stress, and readjustment: the function of the professional's latent goals and affective behavior in rehabilitation. Soc Sci Med 1986;23:43–55.

24. Gordon WA, Hibbard MR, Egelko S, et al. Issues in the diagnosis of post-stroke depression. Rehabil Psychol 1991;36:71–88.

25. Kaiser RC. Mental Health. In WR Frontera (ed), Exercise in Rehabilitation Medicine. Champaign, IL: Human Kinetics, 1999;349–372.

26. Roy R, Thomas M, Matas M. Chronic pain and depression: a review. Comp Psychiatry 1984;25:96–105.

27. Bowden ML, Feller I, Tholen D, et al. Self-esteem of severely burned patients. Arch Phys Med Rehabil 1981;61:449–452.

28. Bishop DS, Pet LR. Physical Medicine and Rehabilitation. In JR Rundell, MG Wise (eds), Textbook of Consultation-Liasion Psychiatry. Washington, DC: American Psychiatric Press, 1996;755–780.

29. American Psychiatric Association. Diagnostic and Statistical Manual of Mental Disorders (4th ed). Washington, DC: American Psychiatric Press, 1994.

30. Levine J, Rudy T, Kerns R. A two factor model of denial of illness: a confirmatory factor analysis. J Psychosom Res 1994;38:99–110.

31. Langer, KG. Depression and denial in psychotherapy of persons with disabilities. Am J Psychother 1994; 48(2):181–194.

32. Moore AD, Patterson DR. Psychological intervention with spinal cord injured patients: promoting control out of dependence. Spinal Cord Inj Psychosoc Process 1993;6(1):2–8.

33. Majsak, MJ. Application of motor learning principles to the stroke population. Top Stroke Rehabil 1996;3(2): 27–59.

34. Carr JH, Shepherd RB. A Motor Learning Model for Rehabilitation. In JH Carr, RB Shepherd, J Gordon, et al. (eds), Movement Science—Foundations for Physical Therapy in Rehabilitation. Gaithersburg, MD: Aspen, 1987;31–93.

35. Sullivan, K. Cognitive Rehabilitation. In J Montgomery (ed), Clinics in Physical Therapy: Physical Therapy for Traumatic Brain Injury. New York: Churchill Livingstone, 1995;33–54.

36. Gentile AM. Skill Acquisition: Action, Movement, and Neuromotor Processes. In JH Carr, RB Shepherd, J Gordon, et al. (eds), Movement Science—Foundations for Physical Therapy in Rehabilitation. Gaithersburg, MD: Aspen, 1987;93–155.

37. Newell KM. Skill Learning. In DH Holding (ed), Human Skills. New York: Wiley, 1981.

38. Newell KM. Coordination, Control, and Skill. In D Goodman, RB Wilberg, IM Franks (eds), Differing Perspectives in Motor Learning, Memory, and Control. Amsterdam: North Holland, 1985.

39. McCullagh P. A model status as a determinant of attention in observational learning and performance. J Sports Psych 1987;9:249–260.

40. McCullagh P, Caird JK. Correct and learning models and the use of model knowledge of results in the acquisition and retention of a motor skill. J Hum Mov Stud 1990;18:107–116.

41. Pollack BJ, Lee TD. Effects of the model's skill level on observational motor learning. Res Q Exerc Sport 1992;63:25–29.

42. Swinnen SP. Interpolated activities during the knowledge-of-results delay and post–knowledge-of-results interval: effects on performance and learning. J Exp Psych Learn Mem Cogn 1990;16:692–705.

43. Winstein CJ, Pohl PS, Lewthwaite R. Effects of physical guidance and knowledge of results on motor learning: support for the guidance hypothe-

sis. Res Q for Exerc Sport 1990;16:677–691.

44. Schmidt RA, Swinnen S, Young DE, Shapiro DC. Summary knowledge of results for skill acquisition: support for the guidance hypothesis. J Exp Psych Learn Mem Cogn 1989;15:352–359.

45. Lee TD, Genovese E. Distribution of practice in motor skill acquisition: different effects for discrete and continuous tasks. Res Q Exerc Sport 1988;60:59–65.

46. Magill P, Hall KG. A Review of the Contextual Interference Effect in Motor Skill Acquisition. In RB Wilberg (ed), The Learning, Memory, and Perception of Perceptual-Motor Skills. Amsterdam: North Holland, 1990.

47. Stedman's Medical Dictionary (26th ed). Baltimore: Williams & Wilkins, 1995;1131.

48. Morris W (ed). American Heritage Dictionary of the English Language. Boston: Houghton Mifflin, 1969.

49. Dorland's Illustrated Medical Dictionary (28th ed). Philadelphia: WB Saunders, 1994;1059.

50. Maslow AH. Motivation and Personality. New York: Harper & Bros 1959;105.

51. Petri HL. Motivation: Theory and Research. Belmont, CA: Wadsworth, 1981.

52. Kohn A. Punished By Rewards: The Trouble with Gold Stars, Incentive Plans, A's, Praise and Other Bribes. Boston: Houghton Mifflin, 1993.

53. Miller WR, Rollnick S. Motivational Interviewing. New York: Guilford, 1991.

54. Resnick B. Motivation in geriatric rehabilitation. Image J Nurs Sch 1996; 28:41–45.

55. Bandura A. Self-efficacy: toward a unifying theory of behavioral change. Psychol Rev 1977;84:191–215.

56. Dishman RK, Ickes W. Self-motivation and adherence to therapeutic exercise. J Behav Med 1981;4:421–438.

57. Rhodes R, Morrissey MJ, Ward A. Self-motivation: a driving force for elders in cardiac rehabilitation. Geriatr Nurs 1992;13(2):94–98.

58. King P, Barrowclough C. Rating the motivation of elderly patients on a rehabilitation ward. Clin Rehabil 1989;3:289–291.

59. Wade DT. Stroke rehabilitation and long term care. Lancet 1992;339:791–793.

60. Wressle E, Oberg B, Henriksson C. The rehabilitation process for the geriatric stroke patient: an exploratory study of goal setting and interventions. Disabil Rehabil 1999;2:80–87.

61. Oldridge N, Guyatt G, Crowe J, et al. Goal attainment in a randomized controlled trial of rehabilitation after myocardial infarction. J Cardiopulm Rehabil 1998;19(1):29–34.

62. Locke EA, Latham GP. A Theory of Goal Setting and Task Performance. Englewood Cliffs, NJ: Prentice Hall, 1990.

63. Atkinson JW, Bastian JR, Earl RW, Litwin GM. The achievement of motive, goal setting and probability preferences. J Abnorm Psychol 1960;60:27–36.

64. Geelen RJ, Soons PH. Rehabilitation: an "everyday" model. Patient Educ Couns 1996;28:69–77.

65. Fogel ML, Rosillo RH. Correlation of psychological variables and progress in rehabilitation II: motivation, arthritis and flexibility of goals. Dis Nerv Syst 1969;30:593–601.

66. Herbert CM, Powell GE. Insight and progress in rehabilitation. Clin Rehabil 1989;3:125–130.

67. Babinski MJ. The role of the study of mental disorders in organic cerebral hemiplegia (anosognosia). Rev Neurol 1914;27:845–848.

68. Clark ANG, Mankikar GD. d-Amphetamine in elderly patients refractory to rehabilitation procedures. J Am Geriatric Soc 1979;27:174–177.

69. Dombovy ML, Sandok BA, Basford JR. Rehabilitation for stroke: a review. Stroke 1986;17:363–369.

70. Starkstein SE, Fedoroff JP, Price TR, et al. Apathy following cerebrovascular lesions. Stroke 1993;24:1625–1630.

71. Galynker II, Levinson I, Miner C, Rosenthal RN. Negative symptoms in patients with basal ganglia strokes. Neuropsychiatry Neuropsychol Behav Neurol 1995;8:113–117.

72. Galynker I, Prikhojan A, Phillips E, et al. Negative symptoms in stroke patients and length of stay. J Nerv Ment Dis 1997;185(10):616–620.

73. Powell JH, Al-Adawi S, Morgan J, Greenwood RJ. Motivational deficits after brain injury: effects of bromocriptine in 11 patients. J Neurol Neurosurg Psychiatry 1996;60:416–421.

74. Weddell RA, Weiser R. A double-blind cross-over placebo controlled trial of the effects of bromocriptine on psychomotor function, cognition, and mood in de novo patients with Parkinson's disease. Behav Pharmacol 1995;6:81–91.

75. Liddle PF. The psychomotor disorders: disorders of the supervisory mental processes. Behav Neurol 1993;6:5–14.

76. Brown AS, Gershon S. Dopamine and depression. J Neurol Trauma 1993;91:75–109.

77. Satel SL, Nelson JC. Stimulants in the treatment of depression: a critical review. J Clin Psychiatry 1989;50:241–249.

78. Caplan B. Neuropsychological Assessment in Rehabilitation. In B Caplan (ed), Rehabilitation Psychology Desk Reference. Gaithersburg, MD: Aspen, 1987;247–280.

79. Luxenberg J, Feigenbaum L. Cognitive impairment on a rehabilitation service. Arch Phys Med Rehabil 1986;67:796–798.

80. Goodstein R. Cerebrovascular Accident: A Multidimensional Clinical Problem. In D Krueger (ed), Emotional Rehabilitation of Physical Trauma and Disability. New York: Spectrum, 1984; 111–140.

81. Oldham JM. Personality disorders: current perspectives. JAMA 1994;272: 1770–1776.

82. Crewe N. The Difficult Patient. In D Bishop (ed), Behavioral Problems and the Disabled: Assessment and Management. Baltimore: Williams & Wilkins 1984;98–119.

83. Zimmerman M. Diagnosing personality disorders. Arch Gen Psychiatry 1994;51:225–245.

84. DeLong K, Smith G, Grange J. Does that "difficult" patient have a personality disorder? Emerg Med 1996;Dec:75–96.

85. Heinemann AW. Substance abuse and spinal cord injury. Paraplegia News 1991;45(7):16–17.

86. O'Donnell JJ, Cooper JE, et al. Alcohol, drugs, and spinal cord injury. Alcohol Health Res World 1981;82: 6(2):27–29.

87. Group for the Advancement of Psychiatry, Committee on Handicaps. Report #135: Caring for People With Physical Impairment: The Journey Back. Washington, DC: American Psychiatric Press, 1993.

Index

Note: Page numbers followed by *f* indicate figures; numbers followed by *t* indicate tables.